The GALE ENCYCLOPEDIA of MEDICINE

FOURTH EDITION

The GALE ENCYCLOPEDIA of MEDICINE

FOURTH EDITION

VOLUME
3
F–K

LAURIE J. FUNDUKIAN, EDITOR

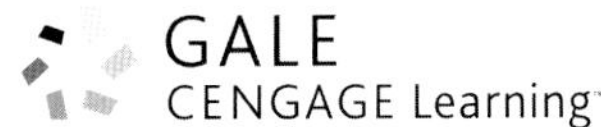

Detroit • New York • S... Maine • London

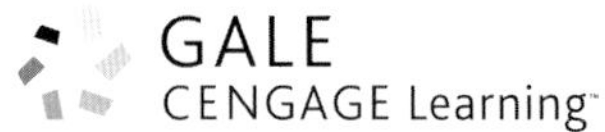

Gale Encyclopedia of Medicine, Fourth Edition

Project Editor: Laurie J. Fundukian

Image Editors: Donna Batten and Kristin Key

Editorial: Donna Batten, Kristin Key, Jacqueline Longe, Kristin Mallegg, Brigham Narins, Jeffrey Wilson, Alejandro Valtierra

Product Manager: Kate Hanley

Editorial Support Services: Andrea Lopeman

Indexing Services: Factiva, a Dow Jones Company

Rights Acquisition and Management: Robyn Young

Composition: Evi Abou-El-Seoud

Manufacturing: Wendy Blurton

Imaging: John Watkins

For product information and technology assistance, contact us at
Gale Customer Support, 1-800-877-4253.
For permission to use material from this text or product,
submit all requests online at **www.cengage.com/permissions.**
Further permissions questions can be emailed to
permissionrequest@cengage.com

Library of Congress Cataloging-in-Publication Data

Gale encyclopedia of medicine—4th ed. Laurie J. Fundukian, editor.
p. ; cm.
Other title: Encyclopedia of medicine
Includes bibliographical references and index.
ISBN 978-1-4144-8646-8 (set : alk. paper) ISBN 978-1-4144-8647-5 (volume 1 : alk. paper)-- ISBN 978-1-4144-8648-2 (volume 2 : alk. paper)--
ISBN 978-1-4144-8649-9 (volume 3 : alk. paper)-- ISBN 978-1-4144-8650-5 (volume 4 : alk. paper)-- ISBN 978-1-4144-8651-2 (volume 5 : alk. paper)--
ISBN 978-1-4144-8633-8 (volume 6 : alk. paper)--
1. Internal medicine--Encyclopedias. I. Fundukian, Laurie J. II. Title: Gale Group III. Title: Encyclopedia of medicine.
[DNLM: 1. Internal Medicine--Encyclopedias--English. 2. Complementary Therapies--Encyclopedias--English. WB 13]

RC41.G35 2011
616.003–dc22 2010053605

Gale
27500 Drake Rd.
Farmington Hills, MI, 48331-3535

ISBN-13: 978-1-4144-8646-8 (set)
ISBN-13: 978-1-4144-8647-5 (vol. 1)
ISBN-13: 978-1-4144-8648-2 (vol. 2)
ISBN-13: 978-1-4144-8649-9 (vol. 3)
ISBN-13: 978-1-4144-8650-5 (vol. 4)
ISBN-13: 978-1-4144-8651-2 (vol. 5)
ISBN-13: 978-1-4144-8633-8 (vol. 6)

ISBN-10: 1-4144-8646-4 (set)
ISBN-10: 1-4144-8647-2 (vol. 1)
ISBN-10: 1-4144-8648-0 (vol. 2)
ISBN-10: 1-4144-8649-9 (vol. 3)
ISBN-10: 1-4144-8650-2 (vol. 4)
ISBN-10: 1-4144-8651-0 (vol. 5)
ISBN-10: 1-4144-8633-2 (vol. 6)

This title is also available as an e-book.
978-1-4144-8691-8
Contact your Gale, a part of Cengage Learning sales representative for ordering information.

Printed in China
1 2 3 4 5 6 7 15 14 13 12 11

CONTENTS

LIST OF ENTRIES

A

B

C

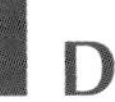

E

F

G

H

M

N

O

P

Q

R

S

T

U

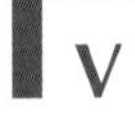

V

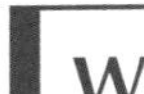

W

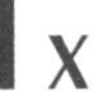

X

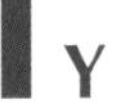

Y

Z

PLEASE READ—IMPORTANT INFORMATION

The *Gale Encyclopedia of Medicine, Fourth Edition* is a health reference product designed to inform and educate readers about a wide variety of health topics such as diseases, disorders and conditions, treatments and diagnostic tests, diets, alternative treatments, and prevention. Gale, Cengage Learning believes the product to be comprehensive, but not necessarily definitive. It is intended to supplement, not replace, consultation with a physician or other healthcare practitioners. While Gale, Cengage Learning has made substantial efforts to provide information that is accurate, comprehensive, and up-to-date, Gale, Cengage Learning makes no representations or warranties of any kind, including without limitation, warranties of merchantability or fitness for a particular purpose, nor does it guarantee the accuracy, comprehensiveness, or timeliness of the information contained in this product. Readers should be aware that the universe of medical knowledge is constantly growing and changing, and that differences of opinion exist among authorities. Readers are also advised to seek professional diagnosis and treatment for any medical condition, and to discuss information obtained from this book with their healthcare provider.

INTRODUCTION

The *Gale Encyclopedia of Medicine 4 (GEM4)* is a one-stop source for medical information on common medical disorders, conditions, tests, treatments, drugs, and other health-related topics, including high-profile diseases such as AIDS, Alzheimer's disease, cancer, and heart disease. This encyclopedia avoids medical jargon and uses language that laypersons can understand, while still providing thorough coverage of each topic. The *Gale Encyclopedia of Medicine 4* fills a gap between basic consumer health resources, such as single-volume family medical guides, and highly technical professional materials.

Scope

More than 1,800 full-length articles are included in the *Gale Encyclopedia of Medicine 4*, including disorders/conditions, tests/procedures, and treatments/therapies. Many common drugs are also covered, with generic drug names appearing first and brand names following in parentheses—e.g., acetaminophen (Tylenol). Prominent individuals in medicine are highlighted as sidebar biographies that accompany the main topical essays. Articles follow a standardized format that provides information at a glance. Rubrics include:

Disorders/Conditions	**Tests/Treatments**
Definition	Definition
Demographics	Purpose
Description	Precautions
Causes and symptoms	Description
Diagnosis	Preparation
Treatment	Aftercare
Prognosis	Risks
Prevention	Normal/abnormal results
Resources	Resources
Key terms	Key terms

In recent years, there has been a resurgence of interest in holistic medicine that emphasizes the connection between mind and body. Aimed at achieving and maintaining good health rather than just eliminating disease, this approach has come to be known as alternative medicine. The *Gale Encyclopedia of Medicine 4* includes a number of essays on alternative therapies, ranging from traditional Chinese medicine to homeopathy and from meditation to aromatherapy. In addition to full essays on alternative therapies, the encyclopedia features specific **Alternative treatment** sections for diseases and conditions that may be helped by complementary therapies. The *Gale Encyclopedia of Medicine 4* also includes entries on diets, nutrition, and general wellness.

Inclusion Criteria

A preliminary list of diseases, disorders, tests, and treatments was compiled from a wide variety of sources, including professional medical guides and textbooks as well as consumer guides and encyclopedias. The general advisory board, made up of public librarians, medical librarians, and consumer health experts, evaluated the topics and made suggestions for inclusion. The list was sorted by category and sent to *GEM4* medical advisors, certified physicians with various medical specialities, for review. Final selection of topics to include was made by the medical advisors in conjunction with the Gale, Cengage Learning editor.

About the Contributors

The essays were compiled by experienced medical writers, including physicians, pharmacists, nurses, and other health care professionals. *GEM4* medical advisors reviewed the completed essays to ensure that they are appropriate, up to date, and medically accurate.

How to Use this Book

The *Gale Encyclopedia of Medicine 4* has been designed with ready reference in mind.

- Straight **alphabetical arrangement** allows users to locate information quickly.
- Bold-faced terms function as **print hyperlinks** that point the reader to related entries in the encyclopedia.
- **Cross-references** placed throughout the encyclopedia direct readers to where information on subjects without entries can be found. Synonyms and acronyms are also cross-referenced.
- Lists of **key terms** are provided where appropriate to define unfamiliar terms or concepts. A **glossary** of key terms is also included at the back of Volume 6.
- Valuable **contact information** for organizations and support groups is included with each entry. The appendix contains an extensive list of organizations arranged in alphabetical order.
- The **resources section** directs users to additional sources of medical information on a topic.
- A comprehensive **general index** allows users to easily target detailed aspects of any topic, including Latin names.

Graphics

The *Gale Encyclopedia of Medicine 4* is enhanced with 765 images, including photos, charts, tables, and detailed illustrations.

ADVISORY BOARD

An advisory board comprised of medical specialists from a variety of backgrounds provided invaluable assistance in the formulation of this encyclopedia. This advisory board performed a myriad of duties, from defining the scope of coverage to reviewing individual entries for accuracy and accessibility. We would therefore like to express our sincere thanks and appreciation for all of their contributions.

Rosalyn S. Carson-Dewitt, MD
Medical Writer and Advisor
Durham, NC

Paul Checchia, MD, FAAP
Director, Pediatric Cardiac Intensive Care Program
St. Louis Children's Hospital
Assistant Professor of Pediatric Critical Care and Cardiology
Washington University School of Medicine
St. Louis, MO

Monique Laberge, PhD
Research Associate
Department of Biochemistry and Biophysics
McGill University
Montreal, Quebec, Canada

Brenda Wilmoth Lerner, RN
Medical Editor and Writer
Montrose, AL

Larry I. Lutwick, MD, FACP
Director, Infectious Diseases
VA Medical Center
Brooklyn, NY

Melinda Granger Oberleitner, RN, DNS
Acting Department Head and Associate Professor
Department of Nursing
University of Louisiana at Lafayette
Lafayette, LA

Sarah Schenker, S.R.D., Ph.D., R.P.H.Nutr.
Nutrition Scientist
British Nutrition Institute
London, England, UK

Chitra Venkatasubramanian, MD
Clinical Assistant Professor, Neurology and Neurological Sciences
Stanford University School of Medicine
Palo Alto, CA

James E. Waun, MD, MA, RPh
Adjunct Assistant Professor of Clinical Pharmacy
Ferris State University
East Lansing, MI

CONTRIBUTORS

Margaret Alic, Ph.D.
Science Writer
Eastsound, WA

Janet Byron Anderson
Linguist/Language Consultant
Rocky River, OH

Lisa Andres, M.S., C.G.C.
Certified Genetic Counselor and Medical Writer
San Jose, CA

Greg Annussek
Medical Writer/Editor
New York, NY

Bill Asenjo, Ph.D.
Science Writer
Iowa City, IA

William Atkins
Medical Writer
Pekin, IL

Sharon A. Aufox, M.S., C.G.C.
Genetic Counselor
Rockford Memorial Hospital
Rockford, IL

Sandra Bain Cushman
Massage Therapist, Alexander Technique Practitioner
Charlottesville, VA

Howard Baker
Medical Writer
North York, Ontario

Laurie Barclay, M.D.
Neurological Consulting Services
Tampa, FL

Jeanine Barone
Nutritionist, Exercise Physiologist
New York, NY

Julia R. Barrett
Science Writer
Madison, WI

Donald G. Barstow, R.N.
Clincal Nurse Specialist
Oklahoma City, OK

Carin Lea Beltz, M.S.
Genetic Counselor and Program Director
The Center for Genetic Counseling
Indianapolis, IN

Linda K. Bennington, C.N.S.
Science Writer
Virginia Beach, VA

Issac R. Berniker
Medical Writer
Vallejo, CA

Kathleen Berrisford, M.S.V.
Science Writer

Bethanne Black
Medical Writer
Atlanta, GA

Jennifer Bowjanowski, M.S., C.G.C.
Genetic Counselor
Children's Hospital Oakland
Oakland, CA

Michelle Q. Bosworth, M.S., C.G.C.
Genetic Counselor
Eugene, OR

Barbara Boughton
Health and Medical Writer
El Cerrito, CA

Cheryl Branche, M.D.
Retired General Practitioner
Jackson, MS

Michelle Lee Brandt
Medical Writer
San Francisco, CA

Maury M. Breecher, Ph.D.
Health Communicator/Journalist
Northport, AL

Ruthan Brodsky
Medical Writer
Bloomfield Hills, MI

Tom Brody, Ph.D.
Science Writer
Berkeley, CA

Leonard C. Bruno, Ph.D.
Medical Writer
Chevy Chase, MD

Diane Calbrese
Medical Sciences and Technology Writer
Silver Spring, MD

Richard H. Camer
Editor
International Medical News Group
Silver Spring, MD

Rosalyn Carson-DeWitt, M.D.
Medical Writer
Durham, NC

Laura Jean Cataldo, RN, Ed.D.
Medical Writer
Myersville, MD

Lata Cherath, Ph.D.
Science Writing Intern
Cancer Research Institute
New York, NY

Linda Chrisman
Massage Therapist and Educator
Oakland, CA

Lisa Christenson, Ph.D.
Science Writer
Hamden, CT

Geoffrey N. Clark, D.V.M.
Editor
Canine Sports Medicine Update
Newmarket, NH

Rhonda Cloos, R.N.
Medical Writer
Austin, TX

Gloria Cooksey, C.N.E
Medical Writer
Sacramento, CA

Amy Cooper, M.A., M.S.I.
Medical Writer
Vermillion, SD

David A. Cramer, M.D.
Medical Writer
Chicago, IL

Esther Csapo Rastega, R.N., B.S.N.
Medical Writer
Holbrook, MA

Arnold Cua, M.D.
Physician
Brooklyn, NY

Tish Davidson, A.M.
Medical Writer
Fremont, CA

Dominic De Bellis, Ph.D.
Medical Writer/Editor
Mahopac, NY

Lori De Milto
Medical Writer
Sicklerville, NJ

Robert S. Dinsmoor
Medical Writer
South Hamilton, MA

Stephanie Dionne, B.S.
Medical Writer
Ann Arbor, MI

Martin W. Dodge, Ph.D.
Technical Writer/Editor
Centinela Hospital and Medical Center
Inglewood, CA

David Doermann
Medical Writer
Salt Lake City, UT

Stefanie B. N. Dugan, M.S.
Genetic Counselor
Milwaukee, WI

Doug Dupler, M.A.
Science Writer
Boulder, CO

Thomas Scott Eagan
Student Researcher
University of Arizona
Tucson, AZ

Altha Roberts Edgren
Medical Writer
Medical Ink
St. Paul, MN

Karen Ericson, R.N.
Medical Writer
Estes Park, CO

L. Fleming Fallon Jr., M.D., Dr.PH
Associate Professor of Public Health
Bowling Green State University
Bowling Green, OH

Karl Finley
Medical Writer
West Bloomfield, MI

Faye Fishman, D.O.
Physician
Randolph, NJ

Janis Flores
Medical Writer
Lexikon Communications
Sebastopol, CA

Risa Flynn
Medical Writer
Culver City, CA

Paula Ford-Martin
Medical Writer
Chaplin, MN

Janie F. Franz
Writer
Grand Forks, ND

Sallie Freeman, Ph.D., B.S.N.
Medical Writer
Atlanta, GA

Rebecca J. Frey, Ph.D.
Research and Administrative Associate
East Rock Institute
New Haven, CT

Cynthia L. Frozena, R.N.
Nurse, Medical Writer
Manitowoc, WI

Jason Fryer
Medical Writer
San Antonio, TX

Ron Gasbarro, Pharm.D.
Medical Writer
New Milford, PA

Julie A. Gelderloos
Biomedical Writer
Playa del Rey, CA

Gary Gilles, M.A.
Medical Writer
Wauconda, IL

Harry W. Golden
Medical Writer
Shoreline Medical Writers
Old Lyme, CT

Debra Gordon
Medical Writer
Nazareth, PA

Megan Gourley
Writer
Germantown, MD

Jill Granger, M.S.
Senior Research Associate
University of Michigan
Ann Arbor, MI

Melinda Granger Oberleitner, RN, DNS
Acting Department Head and Associate Professor
Department of Nursing
University of Louisiana at Lafayette
Lafayette, LA

Alison Grant
Medical Writer
Averill Park, NY

Elliot Greene, M.A.
Former president, American Massage Therapy Association

Massage Therapist
Silver Spring, MD

Peter Gregutt
Writer
Asheville, NC

Laith F. Gulli, M.D.
Consultant Psychotherapist in Private Practice
Lathrup Village, MI

Kapil Gupta, M.D.
Medical Writer
Winston-Salem, NC

Maureen Haggerty
Medical Writer
Ambler, PA

Clare Hanrahan
Medical Writer
Asheville, NC

Ann M. Haren
Science Writer
Madison, CT

Judy C. Hawkins, M.S.
Genetic Counselor
The University of Texas Medical Branch
Galveston, TX

Caroline Helwick
Medical Writer
New Orleans, LA

David Helwig
Medical Writer
London, Ontario

Lisette Hilton
Medical Writer
Boca Raton, FL

Katherine S. Hunt, M.S.
Genetic Counselor
University of New Mexico Health Sciences Center
Albuquerque, NM

Kevin Hwang, M.D.
Medical Writer
Morristown, NJ

Holly Ann Ishmael, M.S., C.G.C.
Genetic Counselor
The Children's Mercy Hospital
Kansas City, MO

Dawn A. Jacob, M.S.
Genetic Counselor
Obstetrix Medical Group of Texas
Fort Worth, TX

Sally J. Jacobs, Ed.D.
Medical Writer
Los Angeles, CA

Michelle L. Johnson, M.S., J.D.
Patent Attorney and Medical Writer
Portland, OR

Paul A. Johnson, Ed.M.
Medical Writer
San Diego, CA

Cindy L. A. Jones, Ph.D.
Biomedical Writer
Sagescript Communications
Lakewood, CO

David Kaminstein, M.D.
Medical Writer
West Chester, PA

Beth A. Kapes
Medical Writer
Bay Village, OH

Janet M. Kearney
Freelance Writer
Orlando, FL

Christine Kuehn Kelly
Medical Writer
Havertown, PA

Bob Kirsch
Medical Writer
Ossining, NY

Joseph Knight, P.A.
Medical Writer
Winton, CA

Melissa Knopper
Medical Writer
Chicago, IL

Karen Krajewski, M.S., C.G.C.
Genetic Counselor
Assistant Professor of Neurology
Wayne State University
Detroit, MI

Jeanne Krob, M.D., F.A.C.S.
Physician, Writer
Pittsburgh, PA

Jennifer Lamb
Medical Writer
Spokane, WA

Richard H. Lampert
Senior Medical Editor
W.B. Saunders Co.
Philadelphia, PA

Jeffrey P. Larson, R.P.T.
Physical Therapist
Sabin, MN

Jill Lasker
Medical Writer
Midlothian, VA

Kristy Layman
Music Therapist
East Lansing, MI

Victor Leipzig, Ph.D.
Biological Consultant
Huntington Beach, CA

Brenda Wilmoth Lerner, RN
Medical Editor and Writer
Montrose, AL

Lorraine Lica, Ph.D.
Medical Writer
San Diego, CA

John T. Lohr, Ph.D.
Assistant Director, Biotechnology Center
Utah State University
Logan, UT

Larry Lutwick, M.D., F.A.C.P.
Director, Infectious Diseases
VA Medical Center
Brooklyn, NY

Suzanne M. Lutwick
Medical Writer
Brooklyn, NY

Nicole Mallory, M.S.
Medical Student
Wayne State University
Detroit, MI

Warren Maltzman, Ph.D.
Consultant, Molecular Pathology
Demarest, NJ

Adrienne Massel, R.N.
Medical Writer
Beloit, WI

Ruth E. Mawyer, R.N.
Medical Writer
Charlottesville, VA

Richard A. McCartney M.D.
Fellow, American College of Surgeons
Diplomat American Board of Surgery
Richland, WA

Bonny McClain, Ph.D.
Medical Writer
Greensboro, NC

Sally C. McFarlane-Parrott
Medical Writer
Ann Arbor, MI

Mercedes McLaughlin
Medical Writer
Phoenixville, CA

Alison McTavish, M. Sc.
Medical Writer and Editor
Montreal, Quebec

Liz Meszaros
Medical Writer
Lakewood, OH

Betty Mishkin
Medical Writer
Skokie, IL

Barbara J. Mitchell
Medical Writer
Hallstead, PA

Mark A. Mitchell, M.D.
Medical Writer
Seattle, WA

Susan J. Montgomery
Medical Writer
Milwaukee, WI

Louann W. Murray, PhD
Medical Writer
Huntington Beach, CA

Bilal Nasser, M. Sc.
Senior Medical Student
Universidad Iberoamericana
Santo Domingo, Domincan Republic

Laura Ninger
Medical Writer
Weehawken, NJ

Nancy J. Nordenson
Medical Writer
Minneapolis, MN

Teresa Odle
Medical Writer
Albuquerque, NM

Lisa Papp, R.N.
Medical Writer
Cherry Hill, NJ

Lee Ann Paradise
Medical Writer
San Antonio, TX

Patience Paradox
Medical Writer
Bainbridge Island, WA

Barbara J. Pettersen
Genetic Counselor
Genetic Counseling of Central Oregon
Bend, OR

Genevieve Pham-Kanter, M.S.
Medical Writer
Chicago, IL

Collette Placek
Medical Writer
Wheaton, IL

J. Ricker Polsdorfer, M.D.
Medical Writer
Phoenix, AZ

Scott Polzin, M.S., C.G.C.
Medical Writer
Buffalo Grove, IL

Elizabeth J. Pulcini, M.S.
Medical Writer
Phoenix, AZ

Nada Quercia, M.S., C.C.G.C.
Genetic Counselor
Division of Clinical and Metabolic Genetics
The Hospital for Sick Children
Toronto, ON, Canada

Ann Quigley
Medical Writer
New York, NY

Robert Ramirez, B.S.
Medical Student
University of Medicine & Dentistry of New Jersey
Stratford, NJ

Kulbir Rangi, D.O.
Medical Doctor and Writer
New York, NY

Esther Csapo Rastegari, Ed.M., R.N./B.S.N.
Registered Nurse, Medical Writer
Holbrook, MA

Toni Rizzo
Medical Writer
Salt Lake City, UT

Martha Robbins
Medical Writer
Evanston, IL

Richard Robinson
Medical Writer
Tucson, AZ

Nancy Ross-Flanigan
Science Writer
Belleville, MI

Anna Rovid Spickler, D.V.M., Ph.D.
Medical Writer
Moorehead, KY

Belinda Rowland, Ph.D.
Medical Writer
Voorheesville, NY

Andrea Ruskin, M.D.
Whittingham Cancer Center
Norwalk, CT

Laura Ruth, Ph.D.
Medical, Science, & Technology Writer
Los Angeles, CA

Karen Sandrick
Medical Writer
Chicago, IL

Kausalya Santhanam, Ph.D.
Technical Writer
Branford, CT

Jason S. Schliesser, D.C.
Chiropractor
Holland Chiropractic, Inc.
Holland, OH

Joan Schonbeck
Medical Writer

Massachusetts Department of Mental Health
Marlborough, MA

Laurie Heron Seaver, M.D.
Clinical Geneticist
Greenwood Genetic Center
Greenwood, SC

Catherine Seeley
Medical Writer

Kristen Mahoney Shannon, M.S., C.G.C.
Genetic Counselor
Center for Cancer Risk Analysis
Massachusetts General Hospital
Boston, MA

Kim A. Sharp, M.Ln.
Writer
Richmond, TX

Judith Sims, M.S.
Medical Writer
Logan, UT

Joyce S. Siok, R.N.
Medical Writer
South Windsor, CT

Jennifer Sisk
Medical Writer
Havertown, PA

Patricia Skinner
Medical Writer
Amman, Jordan

Genevieve Slomski, Ph.D.
Medical Writer
New Britain, CT

Stephanie Slon
Medical Writer
Portland, OR

Linda Wasmer Smith
Medical Writer
Albuquerque, NM

Java O. Solis, M.S.
Medical Writer
Decatur, GA

Elaine Souder, PhD
Medical Writer
Little Rock, AR

Jane E. Spehar
Medical Writer
Canton, OH

Lorraine Steefel, R.N.
Medical Writer
Morganville, NJ

Kurt Sternlof
Science Writer
New Rochelle, NY

Roger E. Stevenson, M.D.
Director
Greenwood Genetic Center
Greenwood, SC

Dorothy Stonely
Medical Writer
Los Gatos, CA

Liz Swain
Medical Writer
San Diego, CA

Deanna M. Swartout-Corbeil, R.N.
Medical Writer
Thompsons Station, TN

Keith Tatarelli, J.D.
Medical Writer

Mary Jane Tenerelli, M.S.
Medical Writer
East Northport, NY

Catherine L. Tesla, M.S., C.G.C.
Senior Associate, Faculty
Dept. of Pediatrics, Division of Medical Genetics
Emory University School of Medicine
Atlanta, GA

Bethany Thivierge
Biotechnical Writer/Editor
Technicality Resources
Rockland, ME

Mai Tran, Pharm.D.
Medical Writer
Troy, MI

Carol Turkington
Medical Writer
Lancaster, PA

Judith Turner, B.S.
Medical Writer
Sandy, UT

Amy B. Tuteur, M.D.
Medical Advisor
Sharon, MA

Samuel Uretsky, Pharm.D.
Medical Writer
Wantagh, NY

Amy Vance, M.S., C.G.C.
Genetic Counselor
GeneSage, Inc.
San Francisco, CA

Michael Sherwin Walston
Student Researcher
University of Arizona
Tucson, AZ

Ronald Watson, Ph.D.
Science Writer
Tucson, AZ

James E. Waun, MD, MA, RPh
Adjunct Assistant Professor of Clinical Pharmacy
Ferris State University
East Lansing, MI

Ellen S. Weber, M.S.N.
Medical Writer
Fort Wayne, IN

Ken R. Wells
Freelance Writer
Laguna Hills, CA

Jennifer F. Wilson, M.S.
Science Writer
Haddonfield, NJ

Kathleen D. Wright, R.N.
Medical Writer
Delmar, DE

Jennifer Wurges
Medical Writer
Rochester Hills, MI

Mary Zoll, Ph.D.
Science Writer
Newton Center, MA

Jon Zonderman
Medical Writer
Orange, CA

Michael V. Zuck, Ph.D.
Medical Writer
Boulder, CO

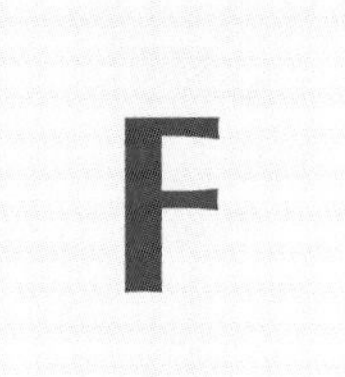

Fabry's disease *see* **Lipidoses**

Facelift

Definition

Facelift surgery is a cosmetic procedure that can involve removing excess skin and fat, tightening muscles, and redraping the remaining skin of the face and neck. This surgery is usually done to counter signs of **aging** produced by sunlight, time, and gravity.

Purpose

The purpose of facelift surgery, also known as facialplasty, rhytidoplasty, or cervicofacial rhytidectomy, is to improve the appearance of the face by removing excess skin and unwanted fat, and tightening some of the underlying muscles. The procedure is designed to counter sagging and looseness in skin and muscle tissue caused by gravity as the patient ages. Facelift surgery will not erase all facial wrinkles, as the term rhytidectomy (which literally means "surgical removal of wrinkles") might imply. Wrinkles around the mouth and eyes, for example, may benefit little from facelift surgery. Other procedures, such as **blepharoplasty**, chemical peel, or dermabrasion, also may be necessary to reduce wrinkling.

Precautions

Patients with other medical conditions should consult with their primary physicians before undergoing facelift surgery. Lung problems, heart disease, and other medical conditions can lead to a higher risk of complications. Patients should tell their surgeon about medications they are taking. Some medications can alter the way their **blood clots**. These include female hormones, **aspirin**, and some non-aspirin **pain** relievers. Surgeons typically instruct patients to stop taking these medications for some time before surgery. This may improve recovery time. In addition, it may lower the risk that a hematoma, or a pocket of blood below the skin, will form. Hematoma formation is the most frequent complication of facelift surgery.

Description

Facelift surgery can usually be performed on an outpatient basis with local anesthetics. Patients typically also receive "twilight anesthesia," an intravenous sedative that helps to lower their awareness of the procedure being performed.

A number of variations of facelift surgery exist. The patient's facial structure, how much correction is needed, and the preferences of the surgeon performing the procedure will help determine which variation is used. In a typical facelift surgery, the surgeon begins by making an incision within the hairline just above the ear. The incision continues down along the front edge of the ear, around the earlobe, and then up and behind the ear extending back into the hairline. The location of this incision is designed to hide any scarring caused by the procedure. The same procedure is repeated on the other side of the face. Using various instruments, the surgeon will then work to separate the skin of the face from its underlying tissue, moving down to the cheek and into the neck area and below the chin. Fat deposits over the cheeks and in the neck may be removed surgically or with **liposuction** at this time. The surgeon will then work to free up and tighten certain bands of muscle and tissue that extend up from the shoulder, below the chin, and up and behind the neck. If these muscles and tissue are not tightened, the looseness and sagging appearance of the skin will return. The surgeon will then trim excess skin from the edges of the original incision, pull the skin back, and staple or suture it into place.

Preparation

Prior to the procedure, a patient meets with his or her surgeon to discuss the surgery, clarify the results

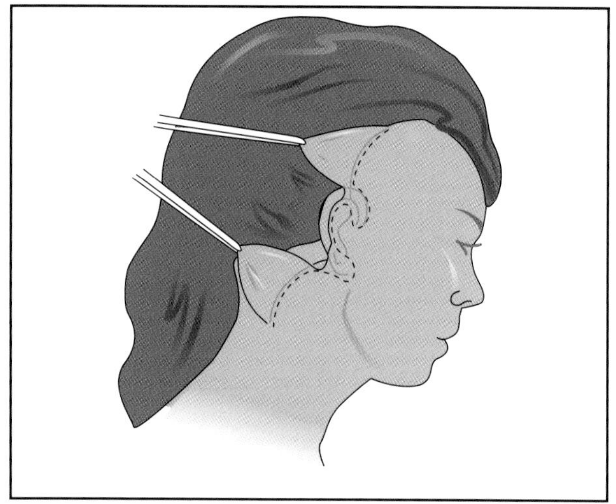

In a typical facelift surgery, the surgeon begins by making an incision within the hairline just above the ear. The incision continues down along the front of the ear, around the earlobe, and then up and behind the ear extending back into the hairline, as shown above. The same procedure is repeated on the other side of the face. The surgeon will then separate the skin from the tissue, remove fat deposits over the cheeks and neck, tighten up muscles and tissues below the chin and upwards behind the neck. The surgeon will then trim excess skin from the original incision, pull the skin back, and suture it into place. *(Illustration by Electronic Illustrators Group. Reproduced by permission of Gale, a part of Cengage Learning.)*

KEY TERMS

Hematoma—A complication of surgery in which a collection of blood forms below the skin.

Rhytidectomy—Another term for facelift surgery, it literally means "wrinkle excision."

Twilight anesthesia—An intravenous mixture of sedatives and other medications that decreases a patient's awareness of the procedure being performed.

that can be achieved, and discuss the potential risks and benefits of the procedure. Having realistic expectations is important in any cosmetic procedure. Patients may be told, for example, that although facelift surgery can improve the contour of the face and neck, other procedures may be necessary to reduce the appearance of wrinkles in some locations. Patients may be instructed to stop taking aspirin, birth control or female hormones, and other medications affecting blood clotting about two weeks before the procedure. Some physicians may instruct the patient to take supplemental vitamins C and K in the belief that this promotes healing. Patients will also be advised to stop **smoking** and to avoid exposure to passive smoke before the procedure and afterward. Some surgeons also recommend **antibiotics** be taken beforehand to limit the risk of infection. Some surgeons also use a steroid injection before or after the procedure, to reduce swelling.

Aftercare

After the surgery, a small tube may be placed under the skin temporarily to reduce the risk of hematoma. The patient may spend a few hours resting in a recovery room to ensure no bleeding has occurred. The patient then returns home. Some surgeons recommend that the patient remain reclining for the next 24 hours, consume a liquid diet, and avoid any movements that lead the neck to flex. Ice packs for the first few days can help to reduce swelling and lower the risk of hematoma. Patients usually continue to take an antibiotic until the first stitches come out about five days after the procedure. The balance are removed seven to ten days later. Most patients return to work and limited activities within two weeks of the procedure.

Risks

The major complication seen following facelift surgery is a hematoma. If a hematoma forms, the patient may have to return to have the stitches reopened to find the source of the bleeding. Most hematomas form within 48 hours of surgery. The typical sign is pain or swelling affecting one side of the face but not the other.

Another risk of facelift surgery is nerve damage. Sometimes it can affect the patient's ability to raise an eyebrow, or distort his or her smile, or leave only limited feeling in the earlobe. Most of these nerve injuries, however, repair themselves within two to six months. Poor healing, infection, and negative reactions to the anesthesia are also risks associated with facelift surgery.

Normal results

Some swelling and bruising is normal following facelift surgery. After these disappear, the patient should see a noticeable improvement in the contour of the face and neck. Most individuals who have facelift surgery find that they are satisfied with the results. Over time, the skin on the neck and face will begin to sag again as normal aging continues. The individual may choose to have additional facelift surgeries in the future to reduce new signs of aging.

Abnormal results

Some individuals may find that their facelift surgeries did not produce the results expected. This is especially likely to be a problem if the individual did not discuss realistic outcomes for the procedure with the surgeon ahead of time. It is generally normal to feel some disappointment with the procedure in the first few weeks afterwards, when bruising and swelling have not yet completely healed. Most people find that they are satisfied with their surgeries a few months later, after the healing process is complete.

Resources

BOOKS

Bailey, Kristen, ed. *Cosmetic Surgery*. Detroit, MI: Greenhaven Press, 2005.

ORGANIZATIONS

American Society for Dermatologic Surgery, 5550 Meadowbrook Dr., Suite 120, Rolling Meadows, IL, 60008, (847) 956-0900, (847) 956-0999, http://www.asds.net/.

American Society of Plastic Surgeons, 444 E. Algonquin Rd., Arlington Heights, IL, 60005, (847) 228-9900, http://www.plasticsurgery.org/.

Richard H. Camer

Factitious disorders

Definition

Factitious disorders are a group of mental disturbances in which patients intentionally act physically or mentally ill without obvious benefits. The name factitious comes from a Latin word that means artificial. These disorders are not **malingering**, which is defined as pretending illness when the "patient" has a clear motive, such as financial gain.

Description

Patients with factitious disorders produce or exaggerate the symptoms of a physical or mental illness by a variety of methods, including contaminating urine samples with blood, taking hallucinogens, injecting themselves with bacteria to produce infections, and other similar behaviors.

No reliable statistics on the frequency of factitious disorders are available, but factitious disorders are more common in men than in women. The following conditions are sometimes classified as factitious disorders:

Munchausen syndrome

Munchausen syndrome refers to patients whose factitious symptoms are dramatized and exaggerated. Many persons with Munchausen go so far as to undergo major surgery repeatedly, and, to avoid detection, at several locations. Many have been employed in hospitals or in healthcare professions. The syndrome's onset is in early adulthood.

Munchausen by proxy

Munchausen by proxy is the name given to factitious disorders in which a parent or other caregiver may but are falsify a child's medical history or tamper with laboratory tests in order to make the child appear sick. Occasionally, the parent may actually injure the child to assure that he or she will be treated.

Ganser's syndrome

Ganser's syndrome is an unusual dissociative reaction to extreme **stress** in which the patient gives absurd or silly answers to simple questions. It has sometimes been labeled as psychiatric malingering, but is more often classified as a factitious disorder.

Causes and symptoms

No single explanation of factitious disorders covers all cases. These disorders are variously attributed to underlying **personality disorders**; **child abuse**; the wish to repeat a satisfying childhood relationship with a doctor; and the desire to deceive or test authority figures. Also, the wish to assume the role of patient and receive care is involved. In many cases, the suffering of a major personal loss has been implicated.

The following are regarded as indications of a factitious disorder:

- dramatic but inconsistent medical history
- extensive knowledge of medicine and/or hospitals
- negative test results followed by further symptom development
- symptoms that occur only when the patient is not being observed
- few visitors
- arguments with hospital staff or similar acting-out behaviors

KEY TERMS

Ganser's syndrome—An unusual factitious disorder characterized by dissociative symptoms and absurd answers to direct questions.

Malingering—Pretending to be sick in order to be relieved of an unwanted duty or obtain some other obvious benefit.

Munchausen by proxy—A factitious disorder in which a parent or other caregiver may falsify a child's medical history or take other action to make a healthy child appear sick.

Munchausen syndrome—A factitious disorder in which the patient's symptoms are dramatized and exaggerated.

- eagerness to undergo operations and other procedures

When patients with factitious disorders are confronted, they usually deny that their symptoms are intentional. They may become angry and leave the hospital. In many cases they enter another hospital, which has led to the nickname "hospital hoboes."

Diagnosis

Diagnosis of factitious disorders is usually based on the exclusion of bona fide medical or psychiatric conditions, together with a combination of the signs listed earlier. In some cases, the diagnosis is made on the basis of records from other hospitals.

Treatment

Treatment of factitious disorders is usually limited to prompt recognition of the condition and the refusal to give unnecessary medications or to perform unneeded procedures. Individuals with factitious disorder do not usually remain in the hospital long enough for effective psychiatric treatment. Some clinicians have tried psychotherapeutic treatment for factitious disorder patients, and anecdotal reports suggest that antidepressant or antipsychotic medications are helpful in certain cases.

Prognosis

Some patients have only one or two episodes of factitious disorders; others develop a chronic form that may be lifelong. Successful treatment of the chronic form appears to be rare.

Resources

BOOKS

McPhee, Stephen, and Maxine Papadakis. *Current Medical Diagnosis and Treatment, 2010*, 49th ed. New York: McGraw-Hill Medical, 2009.

Rebecca J. Frey, PhD

Factor IX deficiency *see* **Hemophilia**

Factor VIII deficiency *see* **Hemophilia**

Failure to thrive

Definition

Failure to thrive (FTT) is used to describe a serious delay in a child's growth or development. This diagnosis usually is applied to infants and children up to two years of age who do not gain or maintain weight as they should. Failure to thrive is not a specific disease, but rather a cluster of symptoms that may come from a variety of sources.

Demographics

Premature infants are at greatest risk for failure to thrive. As many as 10% of hospitalized young children show some signs of failure to thrive. The rate of failure to thrive for non-specific physiological reasons (non-organic failure to thrive) is higher in the United Sates than in other developed countries. Internationally, **malnutrition** is the most common cause of failure to thrive.

Description

Shortly after birth most infants lose some weight. After that expected loss, infants normally gain weight at a steady and predictable rate. When an infant does not gain weight as expected, or continues to lose weight, he or she is not thriving. Failure to thrive may be due to one or more conditions.

Organic failure to thrive (OFTT) implies that the organs involved with digestion and absorption of food are malformed or incomplete so the baby cannot digest its food. Nonorganic failure to thrive (NOFTT) is the most common cause of FTT and implies the baby is not receiving enough food due to economic factors, parental neglect, or psychosocial problems.

KEY TERMS

Esophagus—The muscular tube that leads from the back of the throat to the stomach. Coated with mucus and surrounded by muscles, it pushes food to the stomach by contraction.

Psychosocial—A term referring to the mind's ability, consciously or unconsciously, to adjust and relate the body to its social environment.

Causes and symptoms

Occasionally, underlying physical conditions inhibit an infant's ability to take in, digest, or process food. These defects can occur anywhere in the digestive tract—in the esophagus, stomach, small or large intestine, rectum, or anus. Usually the defect is an incomplete development of the organ, and it must be surgically corrected. Other physical causes of FTT include hormonal abnormalities, chromosomal abnormalities, **cystic fibrosis**, and metabolic disorders. Most physical defects can be detected shortly after birth.

Failure to thrive may also result from lack of available food or the quality of the food offered. This can be due to economic factors in the family, parental beliefs and concepts of **nutrition**, or neglect of the child. In addition, if the infant is breastfed, the quality or quantity of the mother's milk may be the source of the problem.

Psychosocial problems, often stemming from lack of a nurturing parent-child relationship can lead to a failure to thrive. The child may exhibit poor appetite due to depression related to from insufficient attention from parents.

Infants and toddlers whose growth is substantially less than expected, are considered to be suffering from FTT.

Diagnosis

Infants are weighed at birth, and that weight is used as a baseline in future well-baby check-ups. If the infant is not gaining weight at a predictable rate, the doctor will do a more extensive examination. If no apparent physical deformities in the digestive tract exist, the doctor will examine the child's environment. As part of that examination, the doctor will look at the family history of height and weight. In addition, the parents will be asked about feedings, illnesses, and family routines. If the mother is **breastfeeding** the doctor will also evaluate her diet, general health, and well-being as it affects the quantity and quality of her milk.

Treatment

If the baby has an underlying physical reason for failure to thrive, such as a disorder of swallowing mechanism or intestinal problems, correcting that problem should reverse the condition. If the condition is caused by environmental factors, the physician will suggest several ways parents may provide adequate food for the child. Maternal education and parental counseling may also be recommended. In extreme cases, hospitalization or a more nurturing home may be necessary.

Prognosis

The first year of life is important as a foundation for growth and physical and intellectual development in the future. Children with extreme failure to thrive in the first year may never catch up to their peers, even if their physical growth improves. In about one-third of these extreme cases, mental development remains below normal and roughly half will continue to have psychosocial and eating problems throughout life.

When failure to thrive is identified and corrected early, most children catch up to their peers and remain healthy and well-developed.

Prevention

Initial failure to thrive caused by physical defects cannot be prevented but can often be corrected before they become a danger to the child. Maternal education and emotional and economic support systems all help to prevent failure to thrive in those cases where no physical deformity exists.

Resources

OTHER

"Failure to Thrive." MedlinePlus Encyclopedia. August 2, 2009. http://www.nlm.nih.gov/medlineplus/ency/article/000991.htm

"Failure to Thrive." The Merck Manuals Online. January 2007. http://www.merck.com/mmhe/sec23/ch267/ch267j.html

Rabinowitz, Simon S., Madhavi Katturupalli, and Genie Rogers. Failure to Thrive. emedicine.com. May 4, 2010. http://emedicine.medscape.com/article/985007-overview

ORGANIZATIONS

American Academy of Family Physicians, P.O. Box 11210, Shawnee Mission, KS, 66207, (913) 906-6000, (800) 274-2237, (913) 906-6075, http://familydoctor.org.

American Academy of Pediatrics, 141 Northwest Point Blvd., Elk Grove Village, IL, 60007-1098, (847) 434-4000, (847) 434-8000, http://www.aap.org.

American College of Gastroenterology (ACG), P.O. Box 34226, Bethesda, MD, 20827-2260, (301) 263-9000, http://www.acg.gi.org.

American Gastroenterological Association (AGA), 4930 Del Ray Ave., Bethesda, MD, 20814, (310) 654-2055, (301) 654-5920, http://www.gastro.org.

March of Dimes Foundation, 1275 Mamaroneck Ave., White Plains, NY, 10605, (914) 997-4488, askus@marchofdimes.com, http://www.marchofdimes.com.

Dorothy Elinor Stonely
Tish Davidson, A.M.

Fainting

Definition

Fainting, also called syncope, is a transient loss of consciousness and muscle control brought about by an inadequate amount of oxygen reaching the brain.

Demographics

Fainting is a common occurrence. About six people faint for the first time for every 1,000 patient years.

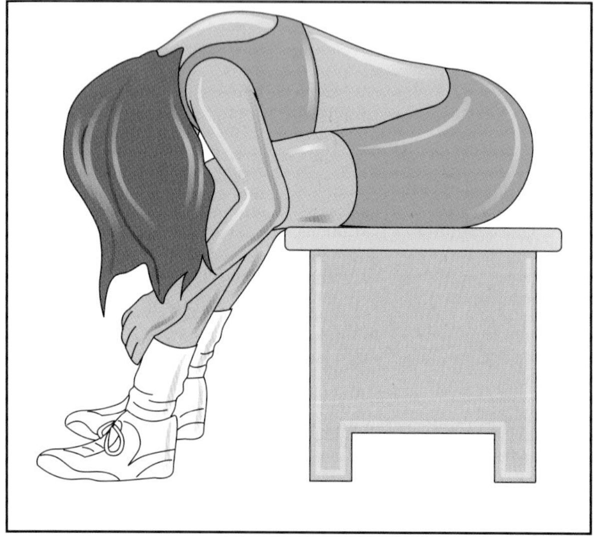

If a person is feeling faint, unconsciousness may be prevented by sitting with the head between the knees, as shown in the illustration above, or by lying flat with the legs raised. *(Illustration by Electronic Illustrators Group. Reproduced by permission of Gale, a part of Cengage Learning.)*

Of these, about 3% will faint again. In people with heart disease, the rate of repeat fainting is about 10%.

The incidence of fainting is about the same worldwide; it appears to be unaffected by gender or ethnicity. However, the elderly are more likely to faint than younger people, and children rarely faint. One reason the elderly are more likely to faint is that fainting often is associated with heart disease, which is much more common in the elderly.

Description

A person who faints temporarily loses consciousness and muscle control. The period of unconsciousness lasts anywhere from a few seconds to a few minutes. Recovery is spontaneous. Fainting normally causes no permanent damage to the brain, although the individual may be injured by falling when losing muscle control.

Physicians distinguish several categories of fainting. Cardiac fainting (cardiac syncope) occurs because heart disease prevents the heart from pumping enough blood to the brain. A person with cardiac syncope tends to faint more than once. Cardiac syncope is a sign of a serious health problem. In a study by the New York Heart Association, 45% of individuals with heart disease and cardiac syncope died within one year compared to 12% of equally ill people who did not faint.

Reflex fainting occurs in response to events such as emotional **stress**, fear, or physical **pain**. Situational fainting occurs reproducibly when the individual assumes a certain posture or performs a specific act. For example, micturation syncope produces a feeling of lightheadedness immediately after urinating. Reflex and situational fainting are not life-threatening and rarely indicate the presence of serious disease.

Orthostatic hypotension occurs when a person rises from lying or sitting to standing. Changing position causes blood pressure to drop suddenly in some people, resulting in a feeling of lightheadedness or a brief faint. Orthostatic **hypotension** can be caused by certain drugs (both prescription and illicit), heavy alcohol consumption, some diseases (e.g., Parkinson's disease, **dementia**) and decreased blood volume (e.g., **dehydration**, severe blood loss).

Risk factors

Risk factors for fainting include heart disease, blood loss, dehydration, emotional distress, heavy use of alcohol, and use of illicit drugs or misuse of prescription drugs. Anemia may contribute to

KEY TERMS

Cardiomyopathy—Disease of the heart muscle.

Patient years—The number of patients multiplied by the number of years that they were followed in a study divided by the number of study events that occurred (in this case, the number of fainting episodes of the group).

Parkinson's disease—A neurological disorder caused by deficiency of dopamine, a neurotransmitter, that assists in transmitting messages between the nerves within the brain. It is characterized by muscle tremor or palsy and rigid movements.

fainting, as may a drop in blood-sugar levels, especially in people with diabetes.

Causes and symptoms

Fainting is caused by inadequate amounts of oxygen reaching the brain. Cardiac syncope can be brought on by **vascular disease**, congestive **heart failure**, irregular heart rhythms (cardiac arrhythmia), heart valve disease, or disease of the heart muscle (**cardiomyopathy**). The causes of less serious types of fainting are based on emotional responses, changes in blood pressure, decreased blood volume, etc. In all cases, the individual feels lightheaded and briefly loses consciousness.

Diagnosis

The goal of diagnosis is to distinguish between fainting and a seizure or **stroke**, and to determine the cause for fainting.

Examination

During an examination, the physician assesses vital signs and takes a medical history, along with a detailed history of the event and circumstances under which fainting occurred. A drug history, including herbal and dietary supplements, is also be taken.

Tests

Depending on initial findings, the age of the individual, and the circumstances surrounding the fainting episode, extensive follow-up cardiac testing may be ordered to look for evidence of heart rhythm irregularities, congestive heart failure, heart valve damage, **heart murmurs**, and blockage of the blood vessels. Neurological tests may be performed.

Treatment

Treatment depends on the underlying cause of the fainting. In cases of reflex and situational fainting, no treatment may be needed. People experiencing orthostatic hypotension are counseled on how to move safely from lying or standing to prevent injury from fainting. People with cardiac fainting continue medical care, most likely supervised by a cardiologist.

Prognosis

People with reflex or situational fainting normally experience no lasting effects from fainting, although they may injure themselves from falling when losing consciousness. Injury is especially likely with the elderly who often break bones when falling.

Individuals who faint because they have heart disease are at increased risk for health problems including stroke and **heart attack**. The outcome of their situation depends on the severity of their heart disease and their response to treatment. Generally, cardiac syncope is a warning sign of serious heart problems that need ongoing medical care.

Prevention

Cardiac syncope is best prevented by following the advice of a cardiologist and taking heart medicine exactly as prescribed. Diabetics can help prevent fainting by monitoring and controlling their blood-sugar levels. Remaining well-hydrated, especially when playing sports or when ill with **diarrhea** and **vomiting**, also can help prevent lightheadedness and fainting.

Resources

OTHER

"Fainting." FamilyDoctor.org. July 2010. http://familydoctor.org/online/famdocen/home/articles/065.html (accessed August 18, 2010).

"Fainting." MedlinePlus. June 26, 2010. http://www.nlm.nih. gov/medlineplus/fainting.html (accessed August 18, 2010).

Morag, Rumm, and Barry E. Brenner. "Syncope." eMedicine. com. May 25, 2010. http://emedicine.medscape.com/article/811669-overview (accessed August 18, 2010).

ORGANIZATIONS

American Academy of Family Physicians, P.O. Box 11210, Shawnee Mission, KS, 66207, (913) 906-6000, (800) 274-2237, (913) 906-6075, http://familydoctor.org.

American Heart Association, 7272 Greenville Ave., Dallas, TX, 75231, (800) 242-8721, http://www.heart.org.

Tish Davidson, AM

Falciparum malaria *see* **Malaria**

Fallopian tube ligation *see* **Tubal ligation**

Fallopian tube removal *see* **Salpingectomy**

Fallopian tube x-rays *see* **Hysterosalpingography**

Famciclovir *see* **Antiviral drugs**

Familial Mediterranean fever

Definition

Familial Mediterranean **fever** (FMF) is an inherited disorder of the inflammatory response characterized by recurring attacks of fever, accompanied by intense **pain** in the abdomen, chest, or joints. Attacks usually last 12–72 hours, and can occasionally involve a skin rash. **Kidney disease** is a serious concern if the disorder is not treated. FMF is most prevalent in people of Armenian, Sephardic-Jewish, Arabic, and Turkish ancestry.

Description

FMF could be described as a disorder of "inappropriate" inflammation. That is, an event that in a normal situation causes a mild or unnoticeable inflammation might cause a severe inflammatory response in someone with FMF. Certain areas of the body are at risk for FMF-related symptoms. A serosa is a serous (fluid-producing) membrane that can be found inside the abdominal cavity (peritoneum), around the lungs (pleura), around the heart (pericardium), and inside the joints (synovium). The symptoms of FMF are due to inflammation of one or more of the serosal membranes (serositis). Thus, FMF is also sometimes called recurrent polyserositis.

During an attack, large numbers of neutrophils, a type of white blood cell, move into the affected areas causing painful inflammation and fever. These episodes may be accompanied by a skin rash or joint pain. In a few cases, chronic arthritis is a problem. **Amyloidosis** is a potentially serious condition in which proteins called amyloids are mistakenly produced and deposited in organs and tissues throughout the body. Left untreated, amyloidosis often leads to kidney failure, which is the major long-term health risk in FMF.

In most cases, the attacks of fever and pain are first noticed in childhood or adolescence. The interval between these episodes may be days or months, and is not predictable. However, during these intervals people with FMF typically lead normal lives. It is not entirely clear what brings on an attack, but people with FMF often report mild physical trauma, physical exertion, or emotional **stress** just prior to the onset of symptoms. Treatment for FMF involves an oral medication called colchicine, which is highly effective for the episodes of fever and pain, as well as for amyloidosis and the kidney disease that can result from it.

FMF is most common in certain ethnic groups from the eastern Mediterranean region, but cases in other ethnic groups in other parts of the world are increasingly being reported. FMF is also known by many other names. They include: recurrent hereditary polyserositis, benign paroxysmal **peritonitis**, familial paroxysmal polyserositis, paroxysmal polyserositis, familial recurrent polyserositis, periodic fever, periodic amyloid syndrome, periodic peritonitis syndrome, Reimann periodic disease, Reimann syndrome, Siegel-Cattan-Mamou syndrome, and Armenian syndrome.

Estimates of the incidence of FMF in specific eastern Mediterranean populations range from one in 2,000 to one in 100, depending on the population studied. Specific mutations in a gene—the MEFV gene—may cause a somewhat different course of the disease. Such mutations are more common in certain ethnic groups. A few mutations in the MEFV gene likely became common in a small population in the eastern Mediterranean several thousand years ago. It is postulated that carrying a single copy of a mutated gene produced a modified (but not abnormal) inflammatory response that may have been protective against some infectious agent at that time. Those who carried a single "beneficial" mutation in the MEFV gene were more likely to survive and reproduce, which may explain the high carrier frequency (up to one in five) in some populations. People of Armenian, Sephardic-Jewish, Arabic, and Turkish ancestry are at greatest risk for FMF. However, a better understanding and recognition of the symptoms of FMF in recent years has resulted in more reports of the condition in other ethnic groups, such as Italians and Armenian-Americans.

Causes and symptoms

FMF is a genetic condition inherited in an autosomal recessive fashion. Mutations in the MEFV gene (short for Mediterranean Fever) on chromosome number 16 are the underlying cause of FMF. Autosomal recessive inheritance implies that a person with FMF has mutations in both copies of the MEFV gene. All genes come in pairs, and one copy of each pair is inherited from each parent. If neither parent of a child with FMF has the condition, it means they carry one mutated copy of the MEFV gene, but also one normal copy, which is enough to protect them from disease. If both parents carry the same autosomal recessive gene, there is a one in four chance in each **pregnancy** that the child will inherit both recessive genes, and thus have the condition.

The MEFV gene carries the instructions for production of a protein called pyrin, named for pyrexia, a medical term for fever. The research group in France that co-discovered the protein named it marenostrin, after ancient Latin words that referred to the Mediterranean Sea. The movement of neutrophils into an area of the body where trauma or infection has occurred is the major cause of inflammation, which is a normal process. Research has shown that pyrin has some function in controlling neutrophils. In a situation where minor trauma or stress occurs, some initial inflammation may follow, but a functional pyrin protein is responsible for shutting down the response of neutrophils once they are no longer needed. An abnormal pyrin protein associated with FMF may be partly functional, but unstable. In some instances, the abnormal pyrin itself seems to be "stressed," and loses its ability to regulate neutrophils and inflammation. Left unregulated, a normal, mild inflammation spirals out of control. Exactly what causes pyrin in FMF to lose its ability to control neutrophils in some situations is not known.

The recurrent acute attacks of FMF typically begin in childhood or adolescence. Episodes of fever and painful inflammation usually last 12–72 hours. About 90% of people with FMF have their first attack by age 20. The group of symptoms that characterizes FMF includes the following:

Fever

An FMF attack is nearly always accompanied by a fever, but it may not be noticed in every case. Fevers are typically 100–104 °F (38–40 °C). Some people experience chills prior to the onset of fever.

Abdominal pain

Nearly all people with FMF experience abdominal pain at one point or another, and for most, it is the most common complaint. The pain can range from mild to severe, and can be diffuse or localized. It can mimic **appendicitis**, and many people with undiagnosed FMF have undergone appendectomies or exploratory surgery of the abdomen, only to have the fever and abdominal pain return.

Chest pain

Pleuritis, also called **pleurisy**, occurs in up to half of the affected individuals in certain ethnic groups. The pain is usually on one side of the chest. **Pericarditis** would also be felt as chest pain.

Joint pain

About 50% of people with FMF experience joint pain during attacks. The pain is usually confined to one joint at a time, and often involves the hip, knee, or ankle. For some people, however, the recurrent joint pain becomes chronic arthritis.

Myalgia

Up to 20% of individuals report muscle pain. These episodes typically last less than two days, and tend to occur in the evening or after physical exertion. Rare cases of muscle pain and fever lasting up to one month have been reported.

Skin rash

A rash, described as erysipelas-like erythema, accompanies attacks in a minority of people, and most often occurs on the front of the lower leg or top of the foot. The rash appears as a red, warm, swollen area about 4–6 in (10–15 cm) in diameter.

Amyloidosis

FMF is associated with high levels in the blood of a protein called serum amyloid A (SAA). Over time, excess SAA tends to be deposited in tissues and organs throughout the body. The presence and deposition of excess SAA is known as amyloidosis. Amyloidosis may affect the gastrointestinal tract, liver, spleen, heart, and testes, but effects on the kidneys are of greatest concern. The frequency of amyloidosis varies among the different ethnic groups, and its overall incidence is difficult to determine because of the use of colchicine to avert the problem. Left untreated, however, those individuals who do develop amyloidosis of the kidneys may require a renal transplant, or may even die of renal failure. The frequency and severity of a person's attacks of fever and serositis seem to have no relation to whether they will develop amyloidosis. In fact, a few people with FMF have been described who have had amyloidosis but apparently no other FMF-related symptoms.

KEY TERMS

Acute phase reactants—Blood proteins whose concentrations increase or decrease in reaction to the inflammation process.

Amyloid—A waxy translucent substance composed mostly of protein, that forms plaques (abnormal deposits) in the brain.

Amyloidosis—Accumulation of amyloid deposits in various organs and tissues in the body such that normal functioning of an organ is compromised.

Colchicine—A compound that blocks the assembly of microtubules–protein fibers necessary for cell division and some kinds of cell movements, including neutrophil migration. Side effects may include diarrhea, abdominal bloating, and gas.

Leukocyte—A white blood cell. The neutrophils are a type of leukocyte.

Leukocytosis—An increase in the number of leukocytes in the blood.

Neutrophil—The primary type of white blood cell involved in inflammation. Neutrophils are a type of granulocyte, also known as a polymorphonuclear leukocyte.

Pericarditis—Inflammation of the pericardium, the membrane surrounding the heart.

Peritonitis—Inflammation of the peritoneum, the membrane surrounding the abdominal contents.

Pleuritis—Inflammation of the pleura, the membrane surrounding the lungs.

Pyrexia—A medical term denoting fevers.

Serositis—Inflammation of a serosal membrane. Polyserositis refers to the inflammation of two or more serosal membranes.

Synovitis—Inflammation of the synovium, a membrane found inside joints.

Other symptoms

A small percentage of boys with FMF develop painful inflammation around the testes. Headaches are a common occurrence during attacks, and certain types of **vasculitis** (inflammation of the blood vessels) seem to be more common in FMF.

Diagnosis

Individually, the symptoms that define FMF are common. Fevers occur for many reasons, and nonspecific pains in the abdomen, chest, and joints are also frequent ailments. Several infections can result in symptoms similar to FMF (Mallaret **meningitis**, for instance), and many people with FMF undergo exploratory abdominal surgery and ineffective treatments before they are finally diagnosed. Membership in a less commonly affected ethnic group may delay or hinder the correct diagnosis.

In general, symptoms involving one or more of the following broad groups should lead to suspicion of FMF: Unexplained recurrent fevers, polyserositis, skin rash, and/or joint pain; abnormal blood studies; and renal or other disease associated with amyloidosis. A family history of FMF or its symptoms would obviously be an important clue, but the recessive nature of FMF means patients usually have no family history. The diagnosis may be confirmed when a person with unexplained fever and pain responds to treatment with colchicine, since colchicine is not known to have a beneficial effect on any other condition similar to FMF. Abnormal results on a blood test typically include **leukocytosis** (elevated number of neutrophils in the blood), an increased **erythrocyte sedimentation rate** (rate at which red blood cells form a sediment in a blood sample), and increased levels of proteins associated with inflammation (called acute phase reactants) such as SAA.

Direct analysis of the MEFV gene for FMF mutations is the only method to be certain of the diagnosis. However, it is not yet possible to detect all MEFV gene mutations that might cause FMF. Thus, if DNA analysis is negative, clinical methods must be relied upon. If both members of a couple were proven to be FMF carriers through **genetic testing**, highly accurate prenatal diagnosis would be available in any subsequent pregnancy.

Similar syndromes of periodic fever and inflammation include familial Hibernian fever and hyperimmunoglobulinemia D syndrome, but both are more rare than FMF.

Treatment

Colchicine is a chemical compound that can be used as a medication, and is frequently prescribed for **gout**. Some years ago, colchicine was discovered to also be effective in reducing the frequency and severity of attacks in FMF. Treatment for FMF at this point consists of taking colchicine daily. Studies have shown that about 75 percent of FMF patients achieve complete remission of their symptoms, and about 95% show marked improvement when taking colchicine. Lower effectiveness has been reported, but there is some question about the number of FMF patients who choose not to take their colchicine between attacks when they are feeling well, and thus lose some of the ability to prevent attacks. Compliance with taking colchicine every day may be hampered by its side effects, which include **diarrhea**, **nausea**, abdominal bloating, and gas. There is a theoretical risk that colchicine use could damage chromosomes in sperms and eggs, or in an embryo during pregnancy, or that it might reduce fertility. However, studies looking at reproduction in men and women who have used colchicine have so far not shown any increased risks. Colchicine is also effective in preventing, delaying, or reversing renal disease associated with amyloidosis.

Other medications may be used as needed to deal with the pain and fever associated with FMF attacks. Dialysis and/or renal transplant might become necessary in someone with advanced kidney disease. Given its genetic nature, there is no cure for FMF, nor is there likely to be in the near future. Any couple that has a child diagnosed with FMF, or anyone with a family history of the condition (especially those in high-risk ethnic groups), should be offered **genetic counseling** to obtain the most up-to-date information on FMF and testing options.

Prognosis

For those individuals who are diagnosed early enough and take colchicine consistently, the prognosis is excellent. Most will have very few, if any, attacks of fever and polyserositis, and will likely not develop serious complications of amyloidosis. The problem of misdiagnosing FMF continues, but education attempts directed at both the public and medical care providers should improve the situation. Future research should provide a better understanding of the inflammation process, focusing on how neutrophils are genetically regulated. That information could then be used to develop treatments for FMF with fewer side effects, and might also assist in developing therapies for other diseases in which abnormal inflammation and immune response are a problem.

ORGANIZATIONS

National Institute of Arthritis and Musculoskeletal and Skin Diseases (NIAMS), 1 AMS Circle, Bethesda, MD, 20892-3675, (301) 495-4484, (301) 718-6366, (877) 226-4267, NIAMSinfo@mail.nih.gov, http://www.niams.nih.gov/.http://niam.com/

National Organization for Rare Disorders, P.O. Box 8923, New Fairfield, CT, 06812-8923, (800) 999-6673, http://www.rarediseases.org.

National Society of Genetic Counselors, 401 N. Michigan Ave., 22nd Floor, Chicago, IL, 60611, (312) 321-6834, nsgc@nsgc.org , http://www.nsgc.org.

Scott J. Polzin, M.S.

Familial polyposis

Definition

Familial polyposis is an inherited condition that primarily affects the large intestine (colon and rectum). Large numbers of projecting masses of swollen and thickened or tumorous membrane (polyps) develop on the inner lining of this part of the bowel. The polyps eventually become malignant.

Demographics

Familial polyposis is a rare disease. Estimates of incidence of the disease vary from one in 7,000 to one in every 31,000 people in the United States. However, it may be very common in affected families. Familial polyposis is inherited in an autosomal dominant pattern. This means that a person with Familial polyposis has a 50% chance of passing the condition down to each of their children. Familial polyposis can also develop in someone with no family history of the disorder due to a new genetic mutation in that individual. It is thought that approximately 1% of all colorectal cancers in the United States can be attributed to Familial polyposis.

Description

Familial polyposis is known by many synonyms, most include some combination of words that reflect what is known about the disease. As the disease is inherited, the word "family" is often included. Because these mushroom-like growths are the most obvious manifestation of the disorder, the word "polyp" is usually in the term as well. Adenoma is frequently included and refers to the particular kind of polyp that is typically discovered. Some of the names found in medical texts and journals include polyposis coli, familial colonic polyposis, multiple familial polyposis, familial adenomatous colon polyposis, adenomatosis of the colon and rectum (ACR), and familial adenomatous polyposis (FAP).

KEY TERMS

Gene—The basic unit of heredity, made of DNA. Each gene occupies a certain location on a chromosome.

Mutation—An alteration in a gene, especially one capable of producing a new trait, or a change in function.

The last term and its abbreviation have been commonly used since the early 1990s.

Familial polyposis or familial adenomatous polyposis is a premalignant disease. This means that a person with FAP, if left untreated, will invariably develop **cancer**. Individuals with this disorder grow hundreds to thousands of polyps throughout their large intestines. The polyps, which may also be called adenomas, commonly develop just after **puberty**. Approximately half of all FAP patients have polyps by age 16. About 90% have detectable polyps by age 25. Usually by age 35–40, one or more of these polyps becomes cancerous. The average age at which patients with FAP tend to develop **colon cancer** is 39 years.

Risk factors

Relatives of individuals with diagnosed FAP are at high risk of having the disease themselves. This condition has no other known risk factors.

Causes and symptoms

FAP is caused by a germline (inherited) mutation in the adenomatous polyposis coli (APC) gene. APC is a tumor suppressor gene, although its exact function is not yet completely understood. Researchers theorize that the normal gene directs the manufacture of a protein that helps control cell growth. The mutated gene section in FAP generates an abnormal protein that does not perform its normal function. Cells grow out of control, causing the development of multiple, sometimes hundreds or thousands of polyps. One or more of these eventually becomes cancerous.

Many individuals develop polyps without displaying any symptoms. Others experience such gastrointestinal problems as **diarrhea**, **constipation**, abdominal cramps, blood in the stool, or weight loss. FAP patients may also develop nonmalignant tumors (desmoid tumors), and/or some bone and dental abnormalities. In addition, they may exhibit a spot on the retina of the eye (congenital hypertrophy of the retinal pigment epithelium, or CHRPE). These eye changes often precede the development of polyposis.

Diagnosis

Tests

The abnormal portion of the gene that causes FAP in most patients can be detected. A blood test can then be performed to identify family members who have the same mutation and who will eventually develop the condition. Children who have a parent with FAP, and siblings of affected patients whose parental history is incomplete, should be evaluated. The polyps characteristic of FAP have been found in children as young as age five. Testing of appropriate individuals should take place as soon as the diagnosis of FAP is established in one member of a family.

Relatives of people with diagnosed FAP should exercise caution regarding where they seek advice and testing. One study of a commercially available blood test found that less than 20% of patients received any **genetic counseling**, and almost one-third of their physicians misinterpreted the test results.

Registries for FAP patients can be found at many sites in the United States. Such a registry specializes in identification, assistance, and education of people with a particular disease, and is usually a separate department in a research hospital. A team of health professionals who have expertise in the disorder staff the registry.

Testing within a research setting and/or at a facility with a registry of patients with FAP is more likely to safeguard against problems, such as the misunderstanding of test results. Patients who participate in a research project sometimes receive counseling, as well as blood tests, at no charge. Insurance coverage varies. Concerns about confidentiality and future insurance and employment discrimination may prompt individuals to pay for the examination out-of- pocket.

Procedures

If the abnormal gene is found in a family member, annual screening for colon polyps is recommended beginning at age 10 to 12 years. Flexible **sigmoidoscopy** is used for this examination. It is usually done in a physician's office, or in a hospital department, most often by a gastroenterologist or a surgeon. Food intake may be restricted for 24 hours prior to the procedure. Before the study, the intestine is cleared of stool by one or more small **enemas**. Some physicians prefer to sedate the patient to help them relax. A flexible, lighted, hollow tube (sigmoidoscope) is inserted into the anus and maneuvered into the large intestine. The physician examines the wall of the colon to look for polyps. If polyps are found, one or more may be removed for biopsy.

Most patients report little discomfort during the examination. The procedure itself takes five to 15 minutes. The patient may be at the facility an hour or more if recovery from **sedation** is needed. If no medication was administered, driving and resumption of normal activities are permitted immediately.

If the diagnosis of FAP is confirmed by sigmoidoscopy or **colonoscopy**, a front- and side-viewing **esophagogastroduodenoscopy** (EGD) procedure is strongly recommended. This procedure helps to determine if adenomas are present in other areas of the gastrointestinal tract such as the stomach and duodenum (small intestine). The second most common site for cancer development other than in the colorectal area in patients with FAP is the duodenum. This test is recommended every one to three years for individuals diagnosed with FAP.

Other screening tests that may be recommended include ultrasounds or CT scans to determine the presence of desmoid tumors in the abdominal area and to check for the development of pancreatic cancer. Ultrasound of the thyroid may be ordered because of the increased risk for **thyroid cancer** in patients with FAP.

In some cases, the portion of the gene responsible for FAP cannot be identified. Family members of these patients cannot have a predictive blood test. The current recommendation for these patients is the same as that for patients with a diagnosed FAP gene: to undergo to an annual examination with flexible sigmoidoscopy. A noninvasive screening **eye examination** to detect CHRPE, associated with FAP, may also be performed.

Treatment

Traditional

The only definitive treatment for FAP is surgical removal of the lower intestine. In very young people, surgical removal of the colon (colectomy) may be delayed until the late teens or early 20s when most patients would be considered psychologically ready for such a procedure. However, surgery may be done at an earlier age if it is determined that the polyps are at an advanced histologic stage.

Several surgical choices are available to treat this condition. Some authorities advocate removal of the colon, leaving the rectum or lowest portion of the intestine in place. The small intestine can be attached to the rectum, allowing normal bowel function. This is often called ileorectal anastomosis. Others argue that this section is also liable to develop polyps, needs to be monitored regularly, and may require eventual removal.

Excision of the entire lower intestine with preservation of normal bowel function is possible. This entails a more complex surgical procedure. The patient may experience more complications and a longer recovery period. However, the risk of polyp development in this area is very low. Periodic examination of the intestine may not be needed once healing is complete.

The more intricate surgery may be referred to as a J-pouch procedure, an ileal pouch-anal anastomosis, a restorative proctocolectomy, or an ileoanal reservoir procedure. It involves creating a "pouch" of tissue from the small intestine, which is attached to the anus. This serves as a reservoir or holding area for stool, much as the rectum does normally. The surgery is often done in several stages. A temporary ileostomy, which creates an opening of the small intestine onto the abdomen, is required. When all procedures are completed, and after a recuperation period, the patient regains normal bowel function through the anus.

Some researchers suggest that as **genetic testing** becomes more developed, the specific portion of the gene involved may dictate the type of surgery chosen. Those at high risk of developing **rectal polyps** may be advised to have the more complex operation. FAP patients considered to be at lower risk for rectal polyps might be counseled to consider the less radical surgery.

Drugs

Medical therapy to treat the adenomatous polyps has been attempted. Some **nonsteroidal anti-inflammatory drugs** have been effective in reducing the number and size of the polyps in colorectal tissue that remains after surgery such as in an ileoanal anastomosis.

Individuals with FAP are at increased risk for cancers of the upper digestive tract including the upper portion of the small bowel (duodenum) and the channels where bile flows (biliary tract). Cancers of the thyroid, pancreas, and adrenal gland are also more commonly found among FAP patients. Periodic examination for the development of malignancy in these areas is considered part of the treatment of FAP. In some cases, such as cancer involving the duodenum, the tests themselves carry a chance of complications. The risk of the study must be weighed against the potential benefits of knowing the results. Desmoid tumors also occur more frequently in patients with FAP. Although they are not malignant, they grow quickly into surrounding tissues, causing many difficulties, even **death** in some cases.

Prognosis

The major cause of death in many patients with FAP remains colorectal cancer. One study suggested that even with improved disease recognition, social and emotional factors, such as fear of surgery, may significantly delay a patient's treatment.

In patients who have undergone colectomy, desmoid tumors and cancers of the upper gastrointestinal tract are the leading causes of death. Medical surveillance is critical for patients with FAP even after surgical removal of the colon.

Prevention

FAP cannot be prevented. Aggressive diagnosis, treatment, and follow-up monitoring are keys to successful management of the disease.

Resources

PERIODICALS

Duncan, R.E., et al. "The Challenge of Developmentally Appropriate Care: Predictive Genetic Testing in Young People for Familial Adenomatous Polyposis." *Familial Cancer* (September 17, 2009).

Galiatsatos, P., and W.D. Foulkes. "Familial Adenomatous Polyposis." *American Journal of Gastroenterology* 101, no. 2 (February 2006): 385–98.

Johnson, M.D., et al. "Outcome Based on Management of Duodenal Adenomas: Sporadic Versus Familial Disease." *Journal of Gastrointestinal Surgery* 67, no. 1 (January 2008): 61–7.

OTHER

Wehbi, M., et al. "Familial Adenomatous Polyposis." *eMedicine*. December 7, 2009. http://emedicine.medscape.com/article/175377-overview (accessed October 4, 2010).

"What are the Risk Factors for Colorectal Cancer?" American Cancer Society. July 9, 2010. http://www.cancer.org/Cancer/ColonandRectumCancer/DetailedGuide/colorectal-cancer-risk-factors (accessed October 4, 2010).

ORGANIZATIONS

Familial Polyposis Registry, Department of Colorectal Surgery, Cleveland Clinic Foundation, 9500 Euclid Ave., Cleveland, OH, 44195-5001, (216) 444-6470.

National Organization for Rare Disorders, 55 Kenosia Ave., P.O. Box 1968, Danbury, CT, 06813-1968, (203) 744-0100, (800) 999-6673, http://www.rarediseases.org.

Ellen S. Weber, MSN
Melinda Granger Oberleitner
RN, DNS, APRN, CNS

Family therapy

Definition

Family therapy is a form of **psychotherapy** that involves all the members of a nuclear or extended family. It may be conducted by a pair or team of therapists. In many cases the team consists of a man and a woman in order to treat gender-related issues or serve as role models for family members. Although some forms of family therapy are based on behavioral or psychodynamic principles, the most widespread form is based on family systems theory. This approach regards the family as a whole, as the unit of treatment, and emphasizes such factors as relationships and communication patterns rather than traits or symptoms in individual members.

Family therapy is a relatively recent development in psychotherapy. It began shortly after World War II, when doctors, who were treating schizophrenic patients, noticed that the patients' families communicated in disturbed ways. The doctors also found that the patients' symptoms rose or fell according to the level of tension between their parents. These observations led to considering a family as an organism or system with its own internal rules, patterns of functioning, and tendency to resist change. The therapists started to treat the families of schizophrenic patients as whole units rather than focusing on the hospitalized member. They found that in many cases the family member with **schizophrenia** improved when the "patient" was the family system. (This should not be misunderstood to mean that schizophrenia is caused by family problems, although family problems may worsen the condition.) This approach of involving the entire family in the treatment plan and therapy was then applied to families with problems other than the presence of schizophrenia.

Family therapy is becoming an increasingly common form of treatment as changes in American society are reflected in family structures. It has led to two further developments: couple's therapy, which treats relationship problems between marriage partners or gay couples; and the extension of family therapy to religious communities or other groups that resemble families.

Purpose

Family therapy is often recommended in the following situations:

- Treatment of a family member with schizophrenia or multiple personality disorder (MPD). Family therapy helps other family members understand their relative's disorder and adjust to the psychological changes that may be occurring in the relative.

- Families with problems across generational boundaries. These would include problems caused by parents sharing housing with grandparents, or children being reared by grandparents.
- Families that deviate from social norms (common-law relationships, gay couples rearing children, etc.). These families may not have internal problems but may be troubled by outsiders' judgmental attitudes.
- Families with members from a mixture of racial, cultural, or religious backgrounds.
- Families who are scapegoating a member or undermining the treatment of a member in individual therapy.
- Families where the identified patient's problems seem inextricably tied to problems with other family members.
- Blended families with adjustment difficulties.

Most family therapists presuppose an average level of intelligence and education on the part of adult members of the family.

Precautions

Some families are not considered suitable candidates for family therapy. They include:

- families in which one, or both, of the parents is psychotic or has been diagnosed with antisocial or paranoid personality disorder
- families whose cultural or religious values are opposed to, or suspicious of, psychotherapy
- families with members who cannot participate in treatment sessions because of physical illness or similar limitations
- families with members who have very rigid personality structures. (Here, members might be at risk for an emotional or psychological crisis)
- families whose members cannot or will not be able to meet regularly for treatment
- families that are unstable or on the verge of breakup

Description

Family therapy tends to be short-term treatment, usually several months in length, with a focus on resolving specific problems such as **eating disorders**, difficulties with school, or adjustments to **bereavement** or geographical relocation. It is not normally used for long-term or intensive restructuring of severely dysfunctional families.

In family-therapy sessions, all members of the family and all therapists (families may have more than one) are present at most sessions. The therapists seek to analyze the process of family interaction and communication as a whole; they do not take sides with specific members. They may make occasional comments or remarks intended to help family members become more conscious of patterns or structures that had been previously taken for granted. Family therapists, who work as a team, also model new behaviors for the family through their interactions with each other during sessions.

Family therapy is based on family-systems theory, which understands the family to be a living organism that is more than the sum of its individual members. Family therapy uses systems theory to evaluate family members in terms of their position or role within the system as a whole. Problems are treated by changing the way the system works rather than trying to "fix" a specific member. Family systems theory is based on several major concepts:

The identified patient

The identified patient (IP) is the family member with the symptom that has brought the family into treatment. The concept of the IP is used by family therapists to keep the family from scapegoating the IP or using him or her as a way of avoiding problems in the rest of the system.

Homeostasis (balance)

The concept of homeostasis means that the family system seeks to maintain its customary organization and functioning over time. It tends to resist change. The family therapist can use the concept of homeostasis to explain why a certain family symptom has surfaced at a given time, why a specific member has become the IP, and what is likely to happen when the family begins to change.

The extended family field

The extended family field refers to the nuclear family, plus the network of grandparents and other members of the extended family. This concept is used to explain the intergenerational transmission of attitudes, problems, behaviors, and other issues.

Differentiation

Differentiation refers to the ability of each family member to maintain his or her own sense of self, while remaining emotionally connected to the family. One mark of a healthy family is its capacity to allow members to differentiate, while family members still feel that they are "members in good standing" of the family.

KEY TERMS

Blended family—A family formed by the remarriage of a divorced or widowed parent. It includes the new husband and wife, plus some or all of their children from previous marriages.

Differentiation—The ability to retain one's identity within a family system while maintaining emotional connections with the other members.

Extended family field—A person's family of origin plus grandparents, in-laws, and other relatives.

Family-systems theory—An approach to treatment that emphasizes the interdependency of family members rather than focusing on individuals in isolation from the family. This theory underlies the most influential forms of contemporary family therapy.

Genogram—A family tree diagram that represents the names, birth order, sex, and relationships of the members of a family. Therapists use genograms to detect recurrent patterns in the family history and to help the members understand their problem(s).

Homeostasis—The tendency of a family system to maintain internal stability and resist change.

Identified patient (IP)—The family member in whom the family's symptom has emerged or is most obvious.

Nuclear family—The basic family unit, consisting of father, mother, and their biological children.

Triangling—A process in which two family members lower the tension level between them by drawing in a third member.

Triangular relationships

Family systems theory maintains that emotional relationships in families are usually triangular. Whenever any two persons in the family system have problems with each other, they will "triangle in" a third member as a way of stabilizing their own relationship. The triangles in a family system usually interlock in a way that maintains family homeostasis. Common family triangles include a child and his or her parents; two children and one parent; a parent, a child, and a grandparent; three siblings; or a husband, wife, and an in-law.

Family therapy can be and is usually provided by clinical social workers or licensed therapists known as marriage and family therapists. Many of these therapists have postgraduate degrees and often become credentialed by the American Association for Marriage and Family Therapy (AAMFT).

Preparation

In some instances, a pediatrician or other primary care provider may have referred the family to a specialist in family therapy. It is estimated that as many as 50 percent of office visits to pediatricians have to do with children's developmental problems that are affecting their families. Some family doctors use symptom checklists or psychological screeners to assess a family's need for therapy.

Family therapists may be either psychiatrists, clinical psychologists, or other professionals certified by a specialty board in marriage and family therapy. They will usually evaluate a family for treatment by scheduling a series of interviews with the members of the immediate family, including young children, and significant or symptomatic members of the extended family. This process allows the therapist(s) to find out how each member of the family sees the problem, as well as to form first impressions of the family's functioning. Family therapists typically look for the level and types of emotions expressed, patterns of dominance and submission, the roles played by family members, communication styles, and the locations of emotional triangles. They will also note whether these patterns are rigid or relatively flexible.

Preparation also usually includes drawing a genogram, which is a diagram that depicts significant persons and events in the family's history. Genograms also include annotations about the medical history and major personality traits of each member. Genograms help in uncovering intergenerational patterns of behavior, marriage choices, family alliances and conflicts, the existence of family secrets, and other information that sheds light on the family's present situation.

Risks

The chief risk in family therapy is the possible unsettling of rigid personality defenses in individuals, or couple relationships that had been fragile before the beginning of therapy. Intensive family therapy may also be difficult for psychotic family members.

Normal results

Normal results vary, but in good circumstances, they include greater insight, increased differentiation of individual family members, improved communication within the family, loosening of previously automatic behavior patterns, and resolution of the problem that led the family to seek treatment.

Resources

BOOKS

Clark, R. Barkley. "Psychosocial Aspects of Pediatrics & Psychiatric Disorders: Psychosocial Assessment of Children & Families." In *Current Pediatric Diagnosis & Treatment*, edited by William W. Hay Jr., et al. Stamford: Appleton & Lange, 1997.

Gurman A.S., et al. Family Therapy and Couple Therapy. In: Sadock B.J., et al. *Kaplan & Sadock's Comprehensive Textbook of Psychiatry*. Philadelphia, PA.: Lippincott Williams & Wilkins, 2005: 2584.

OTHER

Marriage and Family Therapists: The Family-Friendly Mental Health Professionals. American Association for Marriage and Family Therapy (AAMFT). http://www.aamft.org/Press_Room/MFT%20Brochure%207-03.htm. Accessed July 20, 2010.

Rebecca J. Frey, PhD
Karl Finley

Famine fever *see* **Relapsing fever**

Fanconi's syndrome

Definition

Fanconi's syndrome is a set of kidney malfunctions brought about by a variety of seemingly unrelated disorders. Kidney malfunction leads to excessive urine production and excessive thirst, resulting in deficits of water, **calcium**, potassium, magnesium, and other substances in the body. It often leads to bone disease and stunted growth.

Description

Normally, kidneys cleanse the blood and keep its salt, water, and acidity in balance, leaving what the body needs in the blood and putting what the body doesn't need into the urine, which leaves the body. This task is performed in two steps. First, the blood is filtered through a kidney structure with small holes that keep the cells and large molecules in the blood. Second, some of the small molecules in the filtrate, needed by the body, are reabsorbed and returned to the bloodstream.

This reabsorption step is defective in Fanconi's syndrome. As a consequence, substances that are normally reabsorbed, such as glucose, amino acids, small proteins, water, calcium, potassium, magnesium, bicarbonate, and phosphate, are lost and the body becomes overly acidic.

Fanconi's syndrome is also known as Fanconi syndrome, renal Fanconi syndrome, Fanconi renal-tubular syndrome, and Lignac-de Toni-Debré-Fanconi syndrome. Fanconi's anemia, however, is a totally different disease.

Causes and symptoms

Causes

Fanconi's syndrome can be caused by a variety of genetic defects and by certain environmental assaults.

The genetic diseases known to give rise to Fanconi's syndrome are cystinosis (the most common cause in children), **galactosemia**, glycogen storage disease, **hereditary fructose intolerance**, Lowe syndrome, **Wilson disease**, tyrosinemia, medullary cystic disease, vitamin D dependency, and familial idiopathic Fanconi's syndrome.

Environmental assaults that cause Fanconi's syndrome include exposure to heavy metals (like cadmium, lead, mercury, platinum, uranium), certain drugs (like outdated tetracycline and gentamicin), other substances (like Lysol, paraquat, toluene, the amino acid lysine taken as a nutritional supplement), and **kidney transplantation**.

Symptoms

Fanconi's syndrome symptoms related directly to impaired absorption include excessive urine production and urination; excessive thirst; **dehydration**; **constipation**; **anorexia nervosa**; **vomiting**; elevated levels of glucose, phosphate, calcium, uric acid, amino acids, and protein (especially beta$_2$-microglobulin and lysozyme) in the urine; elevated levels of chloride and decreased levels of phosphate and calcium in the blood; and excessively acidic blood.

The most noticeable indirect consequences of impaired reabsorption are two bone diseases: **rickets** and osteomalacia. Rickets affects children and is associated with bone deformities, failure to grow, and difficulty walking. If a person acquires Fanconi's syndrome as an adult, the bone disease is termed osteomalacia and is accompanied by severe bone **pain** and spontaneous

KEY TERMS

Acidosis—Condition where the body is more acidic than normal; associated with headache, nausea, vomiting, and visual disturbances.

Fanconi's anemia—An inherited form of aplastic anemia.

Filtrate—The part of filtered material that flows through the filter.

Idiopathic—Refers to a disease of unknown cause.

Polydipsia—Excessive thirst.

Polyuria—Excessive production of urine.

fractures. Unlike rickets due to **malnutrition**, these diseases cannot be reversed with vitamin D. Muscle weakness and occasional **paralysis** are other indirect consequences of the ineffective reabsorption.

Diagnosis

Diagnosis of Fanconi's syndrome can be made by urine and blood tests. It is also important to find the underlying cause to decide on the best treatment. Other symptoms specific to a particular patient will point to other useful diagnostic tests. For example, high levels of blood galactose in conjunction with symptoms of Fanconi's syndrome indicate the patient is suffering from galactosemia, while high blood levels of cadmium indicate the patient is suffering from cadmium **poisoning**.

Treatment

Fanconi's syndrome is best treated by attacking the underlying cause whenever possible. For example, when cystinosis is treated with the drug cysteamine to lower cystine levels in the body or Wilson disease is treated with penicillamine to lower the levels of copper, accompanying symptoms of Fanconi's syndrome will subside. If the patient has acquired the disease from a heavy metal or another toxic agent, all contact with the toxic agent should stop; the condition will then likely disappear.

Nevertheless, additional treatment will be necessary either when it's not possible to treat the underlying cause or while waiting for the kidneys to resume normal function. This is done by restricting **sodium** chloride (table salt), giving **antacids** to counteract the excessive acidity of the blood, and supplying potassium supplements.

Kidney transplant is the treatment of last resort, used for patients whose kidneys have failed.

Prognosis

Fanconi's syndrome can be reversible. Fanconi's syndrome caused by kidney transplantation usually reverses itself within the first year after **transplant surgery**. When caused by a toxin in the environment, Fanconi's syndrome generally can be reversed by removing the causative agent from the patient's environment. If it is caused by a genetic disease, it can usually be reversed by treating the disease. However, if Fanconi's syndrome is not treated or if treatment is unsuccessful, the kidneys can fail.

Prevention

Fanconi's syndrome caused secondarily by the genetic diseases galactosemia, glycogen-storage disease, hereditary fructose intolerance, and tyrosinemia is prevented by appropriate dietary restrictions to treat the genetic disease, starting in infancy.

Fanconi's syndrome caused by heavy metals and other toxins can be prevented by avoiding these substances.

Resources

OTHER

"Online Mendelian Inheritance in Man." *OMIM Homepage*, http://www.ncbi.nlm.nih.gov/Omim.

ORGANIZATIONS

National Kidney Foundation, Inc. , 30 East 33rd St., New York, NY, 10016, (212) 889-2210, (212) 689-9261, (800) 622-9010, http://www.kidney.org/.

The American Society of Nephrology, 1725 I St., NW, Suite 510, Washington, DC, 20006, (202) 659-0599, (202) 659-0709, http://www.asn-online.org.

Lorraine Lica, PhD

Farsightedness *see* **Hyperopia**

FAS *see* **Fetal alcohol syndrome**

Fasciotomy

Definition

Fasciotomy is a surgical procedure that cuts away the fascia to relieve tension or pressure.

Purpose

The fascia is thin connective tissue covering, or separating, the muscles and internal organs of the body. It varies in thickness, density, elasticity, and composition, and is different from ligaments and tendons.

The fascia can be injured either through constant strain or through trauma. Fasciitis is an inflammation of the fascia. The most common condition for which fasciotomy is performed is plantar fasciitis, an inflammation of the fascia on the bottom of the foot that is sometimes called a heel spur or stone bruise.

Plantar fasciitis is caused by long periods on the feet, being overweight, and wearing shoes that do not support the foot well. Teachers, mail carriers, runners, and others who make heavy use of their feet are especially likely to suffer from plantar fasciitis.

Plantar fasciitis results in moderate to disabling heel **pain**. If nine to 12 months of conservative treatment (reducing time on feet, non-steroidal anti-inflammatory drugs, arch supports) under the supervision of a doctor does not result in pain relief, a fasciotomy may be done. Fasciotomy removes a small portion of the fascia to relieve tension and pain. Connective tissue grows back into the cut space left by the cut, effectively lengthening the fascia.

When a fasciotomy is performed on other parts of the body, it is usually done to relieve pressure from a compression injury to a limb. This type of injury often occurs during contact sports. The blood vessels of the limb are damaged. They swell and leak, causing inflammation. Fluid builds up in the area contained by the fascia. A fasciotomy is done to relieve this pressure and prevent tissue **death**. Similar injury occurs in high voltage electrical **burns** where deep tissue damage occurs.

Precautions

In the case of injury, fasciotomy is done on an emergency basis, and the outcome of the surgery depends largely on the general health of the patient. Plantar fasciotomies are appropriate for most people whose foot problems cannot be resolved in any other way.

Description

Fasciotomy in the limbs is usually done by a surgeon under general or regional anesthesia. An incision is made in the skin, and a small area of fascia is removed where it will best relieve pressure. Then the incision is closed.

Plantar fasciotomy is an endoscopic (performed with the use of an endoscope) procedure. It is done by a foot specialist in a doctor's office or outpatient surgical clinic under **local anesthesia** and takes 20 minutes to one hour. The doctor makes two small incisions on either side of the heel. An endoscope is inserted in one to guide the doctor in identifying the location to make the cut. A tiny knife is inserted in the other. A portion of the fascia is cut from near the heel, after which then the incisions are closed.

KEY TERMS

Endoscope—A tube that contains a tiny camera and light, and that is inserted in the body to allow a doctor to see inside without making a large incision.

Preparation

Little preparation is done before a fasciotomy. When the fasciotomy is related to burn injuries, the fluid and electrolyte status of the patient are constantly monitored.

Aftercare

Aftercare depends on the reason for the fasciotomy. People who have endoscopic plantar fasciotomy can walk without pain almost immediately, return to wearing their regular shoes within three to five days, and return to normal activities within three weeks. Most will need to wear arch supports in their shoes.

Risks

In endoscopic plantar fasciotomy, the greatest risk is that the arch will drop slightly as a result of this surgery, causing other foot problems. Risks involved with other types of fasciotomy are those associated with the administration of anesthesia and the development of **blood clots**.

Normal results

Fasciotomy in the limbs reduces pressure, thus reducing tissue death. Endoscopic plantar fasciotomy has a success rate of 90–95%.

Resources

OTHER

"Plantar fasciitis (heel spur)." http://www.footspecialist.com/sub.php?page = prob_heel_plantar.php.

Tish Davidson, A.M.

Fasting

Definition

Fasting is voluntarily not eating food for varying lengths of time. Fasting is used as a medical therapy for many conditions. It is also a spiritual practice in many religions.

Purpose

Fasting can be used for nearly every chronic condition, including **allergies**, **anxiety**, arthritis, **asthma**, depression, diabetes, headaches, heart disease, high cholesterol, low blood sugar, digestive disorders, mental illness, and **obesity**. Fasting is an effective and safe weight-loss method. It is frequently prescribed as a **detoxification** treatment for those with conditions that may be influenced by environmental factors, such as **cancer** and **multiple chemical sensitivity**. Fasting has been used successfully to help treat people who have been exposed to high levels of toxic materials due to accident or occupation. Fasting is thought to be beneficial as a preventative measure to increase overall health, vitality, and resistance to disease. Fasting is also used as a method of mental and spiritual rejuvenation.

Description

Origins

Used for thousands of years, fasting is one of the oldest therapies in medicine. Many of the great doctors of ancient times and many of the oldest healing systems have recommended it as an integral method of healing and prevention. Hippocrates, the father of Western medicine, believed fasting enabled the body to heal itself. Paracelsus, another great healer in the Western tradition, wrote 500 years ago that "fasting is the greatest remedy, the physician within." **Ayurvedic medicine**, the world's oldest healing system, has long advocated fasting as a major treatment.

Fasting has also been used in nearly every religion in the world, including Christianity, Judaism, Buddhism, and Islam. Many of history's great spiritual leaders fasted for mental and spiritual clarity, including Jesus, Buddha, and Mohammed. In one of the famous political acts of the last century, the Indian leader Mahatma Gandhi fasted for 21 days to promote peace.

Fasting has been used in Europe as a medical treatment for years. Many spas and treatment centers, particularly those in Germany, Sweden, and Russia, use medically supervised fasting. Fasting has gained popularity in American alternative medicine over the past several decades, and many doctors feel it is beneficial. Fasting is a central therapy in detoxification, a healing method founded on the principle that the build-up of toxic substances in the body is responsible for many illnesses and conditions.

The principle of fasting is simple. When the intake of food is temporarily stopped, many systems of the body are given a break from the hard work of digestion. The extra energy gives the body the chance to heal and restore itself, and burning stored calories gets rid of toxic substances stored in the body.

The digestive tract is the part of the body most exposed to environmental threats, including bacteria, viruses, parasites, and toxins. It requires the most immune system support. When food is broken down in the intestines, it travels through the blood to the liver, the largest organ of the body's natural detoxification system. The liver breaks down and removes the toxic by-products produced by digestion, including natural ones and the chemicals now present in the food supply. During fasting, the liver and immune system are essentially freed to detoxify and heal other parts of the body.

Many healers claim that fasting is a particularly useful therapy for Americans and for the modern lifestyle, subjected to heavy **diets**, overeating, and constant exposure to food additives and chemicals. Some alternative practitioners have gone so far as to estimate that the average American is carrying 5-10 pounds of toxic substances in their bodies, for which fasting is the quickest and most effective means of removal.

Physiology of fasting

Through evolution, the body became very efficient at storing energy and handling situations when no food was available. For many centuries, fasting was probably a normal occurrence for most people, and the body adapted to it. It is estimated that even very thin people can survive for 40 days or more without food. The body has a special mechanism that is initiated when no food is eaten. Fasting is not **starvation**, but rather the body's burning of stored energy. Starvation occurs when the body no longer has any stored energy and begins using essential tissues such as organs for an energy source. Therapeutic fasts are stopped long before this happens.

Many physiological changes occur in the body during fasting. During the first day or so, the body uses its glycogen reserves, the sugars that are the basic energy supply. After these are depleted, the body begins using fat. However, the brain, which has high fuel requirements, still needs glucose (sugars converted from glycogen). To obtain glucose for the brain, the body begins to break down muscle tissue during the second day of the fast. Thus, during fasting some muscle loss will occur. To fuel the brain, the body would need to burn over a pound of muscle a day, but the body has developed another way to create energy that saves important muscle mass. This protein-sparing process is called ketosis, which occurs during the third day of a fast for men and the second day for women. In this highly efficient state, the liver begins converting stored fat and other nonessential tissues into ketones, which can be used by the brain, muscles, and heart as energy. It is at this point in the fast that sensations of hunger generally go away, and many people experience normal or even increased energy levels. Hormone levels and certain functions become more stable in this state as well. The goal of most fasts is to allow the body to reach the ketosis state in order to burn excess fat and unneeded or damaged tissue. Thus, fasts longer than three days are generally recommended as therapy.

Weight loss occurs most rapidly during the first few days of a fast, up to 2 pounds per day. In following days, the figure drops to around 0.5 pound per day. An average weight loss of a pound a day for an entire fast can be expected.

Performing a fast

Fasts can be performed for varying lengths of time, depending on the person and his or her health requirements. For chronic conditions, therapists recommend from two to four weeks to get the most benefits. Seven-day fasts are also commonly performed. A popular fasting program for prevention and general health is a three-day fast taken four times per year, at the change of each season. These can be easily performed over long weekends. Preventative fasts of one day per week are used by many people as well.

Juice fasts are also used by many people, although these are not technically fasts. Juice fasts are less intensive than water fasts because the body doesn't reach the ketosis stage. The advantage of juice fasts is that fruit and vegetable drinks can supply extra energy and nutrients. People can fit a few days of juice fasting into their normal schedules without significant drops in energy. Juice fasts are also said to have cleansing and detoxifying effects. The disadvantage of juice fasts is that the body never gets to the ketosis stage, so these fasters are thought to lack the deep detoxification and healing effects of the water fast.

Medical supervision is recommended for any fast over three days. Most alternative medicine practitioners, such as homeopaths, naturopathic doctors, and ayurvedic doctors, can supervise and monitor patients during fasts. Those performing extended fasts and those with health conditions may require blood, urine, and other tests during fasting. There are many alternative health clinics that perform medically supervised fasts as well. Some conventional medical doctors may also supervise patients during fasts. Costs and insurance coverage vary, depending on the doctor, clinic, and requirements of the patient.

Preparations

Fasts must be entered and exited with care. To enter a fast, the diet should be gradually lightened over a few days. First, heavy foods such as meats and dairy products should be eliminated for a day or two. Grains, nuts, and beans should then be reduced for several days. The day before a fast, only easily digested foods like fruits, light salads, and soups should be eaten. During the fast, only pure water and occasional herbal teas should be drunk.

Fasts should be ended as gradually as they are entered, going from lighter to heavier foods progressively. The diet after a fast should emphasize fresh, wholesome foods. Fasters should particularly take care not to overeat when they complete a fast.

Precautions

Fasting isn't appropriate for everyone and, in some cases, could be harmful. Any person undertaking a first fast longer than three days should seek medical supervision. Those with health conditions should always have medical support during fasting. Plenty of water should be taken by fasters since **dehydration** can occur. Saunas and sweating therapies are sometimes recommended to assist detoxification, but should be used sparingly. Those fasting should significantly slow down their lifestyles. Taking time off of work is helpful, or at least reducing the work load. Fasters should also get plenty of rest. **Exercise** should be kept light, such as walking and gentle stretching.

Side effects

Those fasting may experience side effects of **fatigue**, malaise, aches and pains, emotional duress, **acne**, headaches, allergies, swelling, **vomiting**, **bad breath**, and symptoms of colds and flu. These reactions are sometimes called *healing crises*, which are caused by temporarily increased levels of toxins in the body due to elimination and cleansing. Lower energy levels should be expected during a fast.

KEY TERMS

Ayurvedic medicine—A traditional healing system developed in India.

Toxin—A substance that has poisonous effects on the body.

Research and general acceptance

The physiology of fasting has been widely studied and documented by medical science. Beneficial effects such as lowered cholesterol and improved general functioning have been shown. Fasting as a treatment for illness and disease has been studied less, although some studies around the world have shown beneficial results. A 1984 study showed that workers in Taiwan who had severe chemical **poisoning** had dramatic improvement after a 10-day fast. In Russia and Japan, studies have demonstrated fasting to be an effective treatment for mental illness. Fasting has been featured on the cover of medical journals, although mainstream medicine has generally ignored fasting and detoxification treatments as valid medical procedures.

The majority of research that exists on fasting is testimonial, consisting of individual personal accounts of healing without statistics or controlled scientific experiments. In the alternative medical community, fasting is an essential and widely accepted treatment for many illnesses and chronic conditions.

ORGANIZATIONS

Fasting Center International, 32 West Anapurna St., #360, Santa Barbara, CA, 93101, http://www.fasting.com

Douglas Dupler, MA

Fasting blood sugar test *see* **Blood sugar tests**

Fasting plasma glucose test *see* **Blood sugar tests**

Fatigue

Definition

Fatigue is physical and/or mental exhaustion that can be triggered by **stress**, medication, overwork, or mental and physical illness or disease.

Description

Everyone experiences fatigue occasionally. It is the body's way of signaling its need for rest and sleep. But when fatigue becomes a persistent feeling of tiredness or exhaustion that goes beyond normal sleepiness, it is usually a sign that something more serious is amiss.

Physically, fatigue is characterized by a profound lack of energy, feelings of muscle weakness, and slowed movements or central nervous system reactions. Fatigue can also trigger serious mental exhaustion. Persistent fatigue can cause a lack of mental clarity (or feeling of mental "fuzziness"), difficulty concentrating, and in some cases, **memory loss**.

Causes and symptoms

Fatigue may be the result of one or more environmental causes such as inadequate rest, improper diet, work and home stressors, or poor physical conditioning, or one symptom of a chronic medical condition or disease process in the body. Heart disease, low blood pressure, diabetes, end-stage renal disease, iron-deficiency anemia, **narcolepsy**, and **cancer** can cause long-term, ongoing fatigue symptoms. Acute illnesses such as viral and bacterial infections can also trigger temporary feelings of exhaustion. In addition, mental disorders such as depression can also cause fatigue.

A number of medications, including **antihistamines**, **antibiotics**, and blood-pressure medications, may cause drowsiness as a side effect. Individuals already suffering from fatigue who are prescribed one of these medications may wish to check with their healthcare providers about alternative treatments.

Extreme fatigue which persists unabated for at least six months, is not the result of a diagnosed disease or illness, and is characterized by flu-like symptoms such as swollen lymph nodes, **sore throat**, and muscle weakness and/or **pain**, may indicate a diagnosis of **chronic fatigue syndrome**. Chronic fatigue syndrome (sometimes called chronic fatigue immune deficiency syndrome), is a debilitating illness that causes overwhelming exhaustion and a constellation of neurological and immunological symptoms. An estimated 1.5-2 million Americans suffer from the disorder.

Diagnosis

Because fatigue is a symptom of a number of different disorders, diseases, and lifestyle choices, diagnosis may be difficult. A thorough examination and patient history by a qualified healthcare provider is the first step in determining the cause of the fatigue. A physician can rule out physical conditions and diseases that feature fatigue as a symptom, and can also determine if prescription drugs, poor dietary habits, work environment, or other external stressors could be triggering the exhaustion. Several diagnostic tests may also be required to rule out common physical causes of exhaustion. These may include blood tests to check for iron-deficiency anemia.

Diagnosis of chronic fatigue syndrome is significantly more difficult. Because no specific biological marker or conclusive blood test exists to check for the disorder, healthcare providers must rely on the patient's presentation and severity of symptoms to make a diagnosis. In many cases, individuals with chronic fatigue syndrome go through a battery of invasive diagnostic tests and several years of consultation with medical professionals before receiving a correct diagnosis.

Treatment

Conventional medicine recommends the dietary and lifestyle changes as outlined as a first line of defense against fatigue. Individuals who experience occasional fatigue symptoms may benefit from short-term use of caffeine-containing central nervous stimulants, which make people more alert, less drowsy, and improve coordination. However, these should be prescribed with extreme caution, as overuse of the drug can lead to serious **sleep disorders**, like **insomnia**.

Another reason to avoid extended use of **caffeine** is its associated withdrawal symptoms. People who use large amounts of caffeine over long periods build up a tolerance to it. When that happens, they have to use more and more caffeine to get the same effects. Heavy caffeine use can also lead to dependence. If an individual stops using caffeine abruptly, withdrawal symptoms may occur, including **headache**, fatigue, drowsiness, yawning, irritability, restlessness, **vomiting**, or runny nose. These symptoms can go on for as long as a week.

Alternative treatment

The treatment of fatigue depends on its direct cause. Several commonly prescribed treatments for non-specific fatigue include dietary and lifestyle changes, the use of essential oils and herbal therapies, deep-breathing exercises, **traditional Chinese medicine**, and color therapy.

Dietary changes

Inadequate or inappropriate nutritional intake can cause fatigue symptoms. To maintain an adequate energy supply and promote overall physical well-being, individuals should eat a balanced diet and observe the following nutritional guidelines:

- Drink plenty of water. Individuals should try to drink nine to 12 glasses of water a day. Dehydration can reduce blood volume, which leads to feelings of fatigue.
- Eat iron-rich foods (eg., liver, raisins, spinach, apricots). Iron enables the blood to transport oxygen throughout the tissues, organs, and muscles, and diminished oxygenation of the blood can result in fatigue.
- Avoid high-fat meals and snacks. High-fat foods take longer to digest, reducing blood flow to the brain, heart, and the rest of the body while blood flow is increased to the stomach.
- Eat unrefined carbohydrates and proteins together for sustained energy.
- Balance proteins. Limiting protein to 15-20 grams per meal and two snacks of 15 grams is recommended, but not getting enough protein adds to fatigue. Pregnant or breastfeeding women should get more protein.
- Get the recommended daily allowance of B complex vitamins (specifically, pantothenic acid, folic acid, thiamine, and vitamin B_{12}). Deficiencies in these vitamins can trigger fatigue.
- Get the recommended daily allowance of selenium, riboflavin, and niacin. These are all essential nutritional elements in metabolizing food energy.
- Control portions. Individuals should only eat when they're hungry, and stop when they're full. An overstuffed stomach can cause short-term fatigue, and individuals who are overweight are much more likely to regularly experience fatigue symptoms.

Lifestyle changes

Lifestyle factors such as a high-stress job, erratic work hours, lack of social or family support, or erratic sleep patterns can all cause prolonged fatigue. If stress is an issue, a number of relaxation therapies and techniques are available to help alleviate tension, including massage, **yoga**, **aromatherapy**, **hydrotherapy**, progressive relaxation exercises, **meditation**, and **guided imagery**. Some individuals may also benefit from individual or family counseling or **psychotherapy** sessions to work through stress-related fatigue that is a result of family or social issues.

Maintaining healthy sleep patterns is critical to proper rest. Having a set "bedtime" helps to keep sleep on schedule. A calm and restful sleeping environment is also important to healthy sleep. Above all, the bedroom should be quiet and comfortable, away from loud noises and with adequate window treatments to keep sunlight and streetlights out. Removing distractions from the bedroom such as televisions and telephones can also be helpful.

Essential oils

Aromatherapists, hydrotherapists, and other holistic healthcare providers may recommend the use of essential oils of rosemary (*Rosmarinus officinalis*), eucalyptus blue gum (*Eucalyptus globulus*), peppermint, (*Mentha x piperata*), or Scots pine oil (*Pinus sylvestris*) to stimulate the nervous system and reduce fatigue. These oils can be added to bathwater or massage oil as a topical application. Citrus oils such as lemon, orange, grapefruit, and lime have a similar effect, and can be added to a steam bath or vaporizer for inhalation.

Herbal remedies

Herbal remedies that act as circulatory stimulants can offset the symptoms of fatigue in some individuals. An herbalist may recommend an infusion of ginger (*Zingiber officinale*) root or treatment with cayenne (*Capsicum annuum*), balmony (*Chelone glabra*), damiana (*Turnera diffusa*), **ginseng** (*Panax ginseng*), or rosemary (*Rosmarinus officinalis*) to treat ongoing fatigue.

An infusion is prepared by mixing the herb with boiling water, steeping it for several minutes, and then removing the herb from the infusion before drinking. A strainer, tea ball, or infuser can be used to immerse loose herb in the boiling water before steeping and separating it. A second method of infusion is to mix the loose herbal preparation with cold water first, bringing the mixture to a boil in a pan or teapot, and then separating the tea from the infusion with a strainer before drinking.

Caffeine-containing, **central-nervous-system stimulants** such as tea (*Camellia senensis*) and cola (*Cola nitida*) can provide temporary, short-term relief of fatigue symptoms. However, long-term use of caffeine can cause restlessness, irritability, and other unwanted side effects, and in some cases may actually work to increase fatigue after the stimulating effects of the caffeine wear off. To avoid these problems, caffeine intake should be limited to 300 mg or less a day (the equivalent of four to eight cups of brewed, hot tea).

Traditional Chinese medicine

Chinese medicine regards fatigue as a blockage or misalignment of *qi*, or energy flow, inside the human body. The practitioner of Chinese medicine chooses **acupuncture** and/or herbal therapy to rebalance the entire system. The Chinese formula Minot Bupleurum soup (or Xiao Chia Hu Tang) has been used for nearly 2,000 years for the type of chronic fatigue that comes after the flu. In this condition, the person has low-grade **fever**, **nausea**, and fatigue. Additional formulas are helpful in other cases. Acupuncture involves the placement of a series of thin needles into the skin at targeted locations on the body, locations known as acupoints, in order to harmonize the energy flow within the human body.

Deep-breathing exercises

Individuals under stress often experience fast, shallow breathing. This type of breathing, known as chest breathing, can lead to **shortness of breath**, increased muscle tension, inadequate oxygenation of blood, and fatigue. Breathing exercises can both improve respiratory function and relieve stress and fatigue.

Deep-breathing exercises are best performed while laying flat on the back on a hard surface, usually the floor. The knees are bent, and the body (particularly the mouth, nose, and face) is relaxed. One hand should be placed on the chest and one on the abdomen to monitor breathing technique. With proper breathing techniques, the abdomen will rise farther than the chest. The individual takes a series of long, deep breaths through the nose, attempting to raise the abdomen instead of the chest. Air is exhaled through the relaxed mouth. Deep breathing can be continued for up to 20 minutes. After the **exercise** is complete, the individual checks again for body tension and relaxation. Once deep breathing techniques have been mastered, an individual can use deep breathing at any time or place as a quick method of relieving tension and preventing fatigue.

Color therapy

Color therapy, also known as chromatherapy, is based on the premise that certain colors are infused with healing energies. The therapy uses the seven colors of the rainbow to promote balance and healing in the mind and body. Red promotes energy, empowerment, and stimulation. Physically, it is thought to improve circulation and stimulate red blood cell production. Red is associated with the seventh chakra, located at the root; or base of spine. In yoga, the chakras are specific spiritual energy centers of the body.

KEY TERMS

Aromatherapy—The therapeutic use of plant-derived, aromatic essential oils to promote physical and psychological well-being.

Guided imagery—The use of relaxation and mental visualization to improve mood and/or physical well-being.

Hydrotherapy—Hydrotherapy, or water therapy, is use of water (hot, cold, steam, or ice) to relieve discomfort and promote physical well-being.

Therapeutic color can be administered in a number of ways. Practitioners of Ayurvedic, or traditional Indian medicine, wrap their patients in colored cloth chosen for its therapeutic hue. Individuals suffering from fatigue would be wrapped in reds and oranges chosen for their uplifting and energizing properties. Patients may also be bathed in light from a color filtered light source to enhance the healing effects of the treatment.

Individuals may also be treated with color-infused water. This is achieved by placing translucent red colored paper or colored plastic wrap over and around a glass of water and placing the glass in direct sunlight so the water can soak up the healing properties and vibrations of the color. Environmental color sources may also be used to promote feelings of stimulation and energy. Red wall and window treatments, furniture, clothing, and even food may be recommended for their energizing healing properties.

Color therapy can be used in conjunction with both hydrotherapy and aromatherapy to heighten the therapeutic effect. Spas and holistic healthcare providers may recommend red color baths or soaks, which combine the benefits of a warm or hot water soak with energizing essential oils and the fatigue-fighting effects of bright red hues used in color therapy.

Prognosis

Fatigue related to a chronic disease or condition may last indefinitely, but can be alleviated to a degree through some of the treatment options outlined here. Exhaustion that can be linked to environmental stressors is usually easily alleviated when those stressors are dealt with properly.

Chronic fatigue syndrome has no known cure, but steps can be taken to lessen symptoms and improve quality of life for these individuals while researchers continue to seek a cure.

Prevention

Many of the treatments as outlined are also recommended to prevent the onset of fatigue. Getting adequate rest and maintaining a consistent bedtime schedule are the most effective ways to combat fatigue. A balanced diet and moderate exercise program are also important to maintaining a consistent energy level.

Resources

BOOKS

Davis, Martha, Elizabeth Robbins Eshelman, and Matthew McKay.*The Relaxation & Stress Reduction Workbook*. 6th ed. Oakland, CA: New Harbinger Publications, 2008.

Watanabe, Y., et al. *Fatigue Science for Human Health*. Tokyo: Springer Japan, 2008.

Paula Anne Ford-Martin

Fatty liver

Definition

Fatty liver is the collection of excessive amounts of **triglycerides** and other fats inside liver cells.

Demographics

Fatty liver not due to **alcoholism**, is called non-alcoholic fatty **liver disease** (NAFLD) and affects up to 25–35% of the U.S. population. With an increase in **obesity** in the population over the last 30 years, the incidence of NAFLD has also increased, even affecting about 2.5% of the pediatric population. The prevalence of NAFLD among racial and ethnic groups is not well known, although it is thought to affect both sexes equally.

Severe NAFLD (also called steatohepatitis or NASH) affects 2–5% of Americans, is seen in people 40–60 years old, and is more common in women than men. This form of fatty liver is a leading causes of **cirrhosis** (up to 25%) in adults in the United States.

Fatty liver develops in 90–100% of individuals presenting with heavy alcohol use.

Description

Also called steatosis, fatty liver can be a temporary or long-term condition. The condition is not harmful itself, but may indicate some other type of problem. Left untreated, it can contribute to other illnesses. It is usually reversible once the cause of the problem is diagnosed and corrected. Hard return for new para The liver is the organ responsible for changing fats eaten in the diet to types of fat that can be stored and used by the body. Triglycerides are one of the forms of fat stored by the body and used for energy and new cell formation. The breakdown of fats in the liver can be disrupted by alcoholism, **malnutrition**, **pregnancy**, or **poisoning**. In fatty liver, large droplets of fat, containing mostly triglycerides, collect within cells of the liver. The condition is generally not painful and may go unnoticed for a long period of time. In severe cases, the liver can increase to more than three times its normal size, and may be painful and tender.

KEY TERMS

Jaundice—A condition in which where the skin and whites of the eyes take on a yellowish color due to an increase of bilirubin (a compound produced by the liver) in the blood.

Reye's syndrome—A serious, life-threatening illness in children, usually developing after a bout of flu or chickenpox, and often associated with the use of aspirin. Fatal cases show evidence of accumulation of fat in the liver.

Triglycerides—A type of fat consumed in the diet and produced by and stored in the body as an energy source.

Causes and symptoms

The most common cause of fatty liver in the United States is alcoholism. In alcoholic fatty liver, overconsumption of alcohol changes the way that the liver breaks down and stores fats. Often, people with chronic alcoholism also suffer from malnutrition by eating irregularly and not consuming a balanced diet. Conditions that can also cause fatty liver are other forms of malnutrition (especially when there is not enough protein in the diet), obesity, **diabetes mellitus**, and **Reye's syndrome** in children. Pregnancy can cause a rare, but serious form of fatty liver that starts late in pregnancy and may be associated with **jaundice** and liver failure. Some drug overdoses or toxic chemical poisonings, such as carbon tetrachloride, can also cause fatty liver.

Often, fatty liver carries no symptoms. If symptoms occur, they can include **pain** under the rib cage on the right side of the body, swelling of the abdomen, jaundice, and **fever**. Symptoms that occur less often in alcoholic fatty liver, but more often in pregnancy-related fatty liver, are **nausea**, **vomiting**, loss of appetite, and abdominal pain.

Diagnosis

During a **physical examination**, a doctor might notice that the liver is enlarged and tender when the abdomen is palpated (examined with the tips of the fingers while the patient lies flat). Blood tests may be used to determine if the liver is functioning properly. A **liver biopsy**, where a small sample of liver tissue is removed with a long needle or though a very small incision, can be used to confirm fatty liver. In pregnant women, the fatty liver condition is usually associated with another serious complication, pre-eclampsia or **eclampsia**. In this condition, the mother has seriously high blood pressure, swelling, and possibly seizures. Laboratory abnormalities include elevations of the SGOT (serum glutamic-oxaloacetic transaminase) and SGPT (serum glutamic pyruvic transaminase). In many cases alkaline phosphatase will be significantly elevated due to **cholestasis** produced by the fatty infiltration.

Treatment

Treatment involves correcting the condition that caused fatty liver and providing supportive care. In fatty liver caused by alcoholism, the treatment is to give up drinking alcohol and to eat a healthy, well-balanced diet. In fatty liver associated with pregnancy, the recommended treatment is to deliver the baby, if the pregnancy is far enough along. Vitamin and mineral supplements along with nutritional support may be useful.

Prognosis

Fatty liver is usually reversible if recognized and treated. Some long-term tendency toward other types of liver problems may exist, depending on how long and how severe the fatty liver condition was. In pregnant women with the condition, the situation can be life-threatening for both the mother and the infant. Left untreated, it results in a high risk of **death** for both the mother and baby. Severe liver damage that may require a liver transplant can occur in the mother if the condition is not recognized early.

Prevention

Prevention consists of maintaining a well-balanced diet and healthy lifestyle with moderate or no alcohol consumption. Pregnant women require good prenatal care so that symptoms can be recognized and treated as early as possible. To prevent Reye's syndrome, children should not be given **aspirin** to treat symptoms of the flu or other viruses.

Resources

BOOKS

KMS Publishing.com. *Living With Alcoholism: Your Guide To Dealing With Alcohol Abuse And Addiction While Getting The Alcoholism Treatment You Need*. Charleston, SC: CreateSpace, 2010.

Mahl, Thomas, M.D., and John O'Grady. *Liver Disorders*. Oxford, UK: Health Press, 2006.

Qontro Medical Guides. *Reye's Syndrome Medical Guide*. Bel Air, CA: Qontro, 2008.

Younossi, Zobair M.*Practical Management of Liver Diseases*. New York, NY: Cambridge University Press, 2008.

Zein, Nizar., and Kevin M. Edwards. *The Cleveland Clinic Guide to Liver Disorders*. New York, NY: Kaplan Publishing, 2009.

ORGANIZATIONS

American Liver Foundation. 1425 Pompton Ave., Cedar Grove, NJ 07009. (800) 223-0179. http://www.liverfoundation.org.

National Institutes of Health (NIH), 9000 Rockville Pike, Bethesda, MD, 20892, (301) 496-4000, http://www.nih.gov/index.html.

National Organization for Rare Diseases. P.O. Box 8923, Fairfield, CT 06812. (213) 745-6518. http://www.rarediseases.org.

Altha Roberts Edgren
Laura Jean Cataldo, RN, Ed.D.

Febrile agglutination tests *see* **Fever evaluation tests**

Fecal fat test *see* **Stool fat test**

Fecal incontinence

Definition

Fecal incontinence is the inability to control the passage of gas or stools (feces) through the anus. For some people fecal incontinence is a relatively minor problem, as when it is limited to a slight occasional soiling of underwear, but for other people it involves a considerable loss of bowel control and has a devastating effect on quality of life and psychological well-being. Fortunately, professional medical treatment is usually able to restore bowel control or at least substantially reduce the severity of the condition.

Description

Fecal incontinence, also called bowel incontinence, can occur at any age, but is most common among people over the age of 65, who sometimes have to cope with **urinary incontinence** as well. It was reported in 1998 that about 2% of adults experience fecal incontinence at least once a week whereas for healthy independent adults over the age of 65 the figure is about 7%. An extensive American survey, published in 1993, found fecal soiling in 7.1% of the surveyed population, with gross incontinence in 0.7%. For men and women the incidence of soiling was the same, but women were almost twice as likely to suffer from gross incontinence.

The wider public health impact of fecal incontinence is considerable. In the United States, more than $400 million is spent each year on disposable underwear and other incontinence aids. Fecal incontinence is the second most common reason for seeking a nursing home placement. One-third of the institutionalized elderly suffer from this condition. Incontinence sufferers, however, often hesitate to ask their doctors for help because they are embarrassed or ashamed. The 1993 American survey discovered that only one-sixth of those experiencing soiling had sought medical advice, and only one-half of those afflicted with gross incontinence.

Causes and symptoms

Fecal incontinence can result from a wide variety of medical conditions, including childbirth-related anal injuries, other causes of damage to the anus or rectum, and nervous system problems.

Vaginal-delivery **childbirth** is a major cause of fecal incontinence. In many cases, childbirth results in damage to the anal sphincter, which is the ring of muscle that closes the anus and keeps stools within the rectum until a person can find an appropriate opportunity to defecate. Nerve injuries during childbirth may also be a factor in some cases. An ultrasound study of first-time mothers found sphincter injuries in 35%. About one-third of the injured women developed fecal incontinence or an uncontrollable and powerful urge to defecate (urgency) within six weeks of giving birth. Childbirth-related incontinence is usually restricted to gas, but for some women involves the passing of liquid or solid stools.

The removal of **hemorrhoids** by surgery or other techniques (hemorrhoidectomies) can also cause anal damage and fecal incontinence, as can more complex operations affecting the anus and surrounding areas. Anal and rectal infections as well as **Crohn's disease** can lead to incontinence by damaging the muscles that control defecation. For some people, incontinence becomes a problem when the anal muscles begin to weaken in midlife or old age.

Dementia, **mental retardation**, strokes, brain tumors, **multiple sclerosis**, and other conditions that affect the nervous system can cause fecal incontinence by interfering with muscle function or the normal rectal sensations that trigger sphincter contraction and are necessary for bowel control. One study of multiple sclerosis patients discovered that about half were incontinent. Nerve damage caused by long-lasting **diabetes mellitus** (**diabetic neuropathy**) is another condition that can give rise to incontinence.

Diagnosis

Medical assessments in cases of fecal incontinence typically involve three steps: asking questions about the patient's past and current health (the medical history); a **physical examination** of the anal region; and testing for objective information regarding anal and rectal function.

Patient history

The medical history relies on questions that allow the doctor to evaluate the nature and severity of the problem and its effect on the patient's life. The doctor asks, for instance, how long the patient has been suffering from incontinence; how often and under what circumstances incontinence occurs; whether the patient has any control over defecation; and whether the patient has obstacles to defecation in his or her everyday surroundings, such as a toilet that can be reached only by climbing a long flight of stairs. For women who have given birth, a detailed obstetric history is also necessary.

Physical examination

The physical examination begins with a visual inspection of the anus and the area lying between the anus and the genitals (the perineum) for hemorrhoids, infections, and other conditions that might explain the patient's difficulties. During this phase of the examination the doctor asks the patient to bear down. Bearing down enables the doctor to check whether **rectal prolapse** or certain other problems exist. Rectal prolapse means that the patient's rectum has been weakened and drops down through the anus. Next, the doctor uses a pin or probe to **stroke** the perianal skin. Normally this touching, called the anal wink test, causes the anal sphincter to contract and the anus to pucker; if it does not, nerve damage may be present. The final phase of the examination requires the doctor to examine internal structures by carefully inserting a gloved and lubricated finger into the anal canal. This allows the doctor to judge the strength of the anal sphincter and a key muscle (the puborectalis muscle) in maintaining continence; to look for abnormalities such as **scars** and rectal masses; and to learn many other things about the patient's medical situation. At this point the doctor performs the anal wink test again and asks the patient to squeeze and bear down.

Laboratory tests

Information from the medical history and physical examination usually needs to be supplemented by tests that provide objective measurements of anal and rectal function. Anorectal manometry, a common procedure, involves inserting a small tube (catheter) or balloon device into the anal canal or rectum. Among other things, manometry measures pressure levels in the anal canal, rectal sensation, and anal and rectal reflexes. Tests are also available for assessing nerve damage. An anal ultrasound probe can supply accurate images of the anal sphincter and reveal whether injury has occurred. **Magnetic resonance imaging**, which requires the insertion of a coil into the anal canal, is useful at times.

Treatment

Fecal incontinence arising from an underlying condition such as diabetic neuropathy can sometimes be helped by treating the underlying condition. When that does not work, or no underlying condition can be discovered, one approach is to have the patient use a suppository or enema to stimulate defecation at the same time every day or every other day. The goal is to restore regular bowel habits and keep the bowels free of stools. Medications such as loperamide (Imodium) and codeine phosphate are often effective in halting incontinence, but only in less severe cases involving liquid stools or urgency. Dietary changes and exercises done at home to strengthen the anal muscles may also help.

Good results have been reported for **biofeedback** training, although the subject has not been properly researched. In successful cases, patients regain complete control over defecation, or at least improve their control, by learning to contract the external part of the anal sphincter whenever stools enter the rectum. All healthy people have this ability. Biofeedback training begins with the insertion into the rectum of a balloon

KEY TERMS

Anus—The opening at the lower end of the rectum.

Colostomy—A surgical procedure in which an opening is made in the wall of the abdomen to allow a part of the large intestine (the colon) to empty outside the body.

Crohn's disease—A disease marked by inflammation of the intestines.

Defecation—Passage of stools through the anus.

Hemorrhoids—Enlarged veins in the anus or rectum. They are sometimes associated with fecal incontinence.

Rectum—The lower section of the large intestine that holds stools before defecation.

Sphincter—A circular band of muscle that surrounds and encloses an opening to the body or to one of its hollow organs. Damage to the sphincter surrounding the anus can cause fecal incontinence.

Stools—Undigested food and other waste that is eliminated through the anus.

Suppository—A solid medication that slowly dissolves after being inserted into the rectum or other body cavity.

manometry device hooked up to a pressure monitor. The presence of stools in the rectum is simulated by inflating the balloon, which causes pressure changes that are recorded on the monitor. The monitor also records sphincter contraction. By watching the monitor and following instructions from the equipment operator, the patient gradually learns to contract the sphincter automatically in response to fullness in the rectum. Sometimes one training session is enough, but often several are needed. Biofeedback is not an appropriate treatment in all cases, however. It is used only with patients who are highly motivated; who are able, to some extent, to sense the presence of stools in the rectum; and who have not lost all ability to contract the external anal sphincter. One specialist suggests that possibly two-thirds of incontinence sufferers are candidates for biofeedback.

Some people may require surgery. Sphincter damage caused by childbirth is often effectively treated with surgery, however, as are certain other kinds of incontinence-related sphincter injuries. Sometimes surgical treatment requires building an artificial sphincter using a thigh muscle (the gracilis muscle). At one time a **colostomy** was necessary for severe cases of incontinence, but is now rarely performed.

Prognosis

Fecal incontinence is a problem that usually responds well to professional medical treatment, even among elderly and institutionalized patients. If complete bowel control cannot be restored, the impact of incontinence on everyday life can still be lessened considerably in most cases. When incontinence remains a problem despite medical treatment, disposable underwear and other commercial incontinence products are available to make life easier. Doctors and nurses can offer advice on coping with incontinence, and people should never be embarrassed about seeking their assistance. Counseling and information are also available from support groups.

ORGANIZATIONS

International Foundation for Functional Gastrointestinal Disorders, P.O. Box 17864, Milwaukee, WI, 53217-8076, (414) 964-1799, (414) 964-7176, (888) 964-2001, iffd@iffgd.org, http://www.iffgd.org/.

National Association for Continence, P.O. Box 1019, Charleston, SC, 29402-1019, (843) 377-0900, (843) 377-0905, (800) 252-3337, memberservices@nafc.org, http://www.nafc.org.

National Digestive Diseases Information Clearinghouse (NDDIC), 2 Information Way, Bethesda, MD, 20892-3570, (703) 738-4929, (800) 891-5389, http://digestive.niddk.nih.gov.

Howard Baker

Fecal lipids test *see* **Stool fat test**

Fecal occult blood test

Definition

The fecal occult blood test (FOBT) is performed as part of a routine **physical examination** during the examination of the rectum. It is used to detect microscopic blood in the stool and is a screening tool for colorectal **cancer**. The word "occult" in the test's name means that the blood is hidden from view.

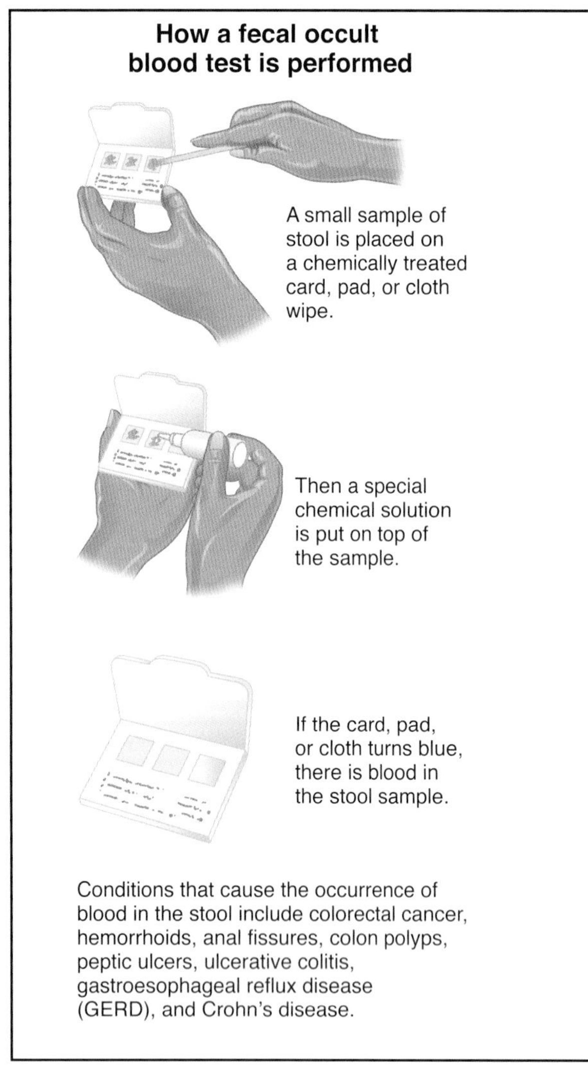

(Illustration by Electronic Illustrators Group. Reproduced by permission of Gale, a part of Cengage Learning.)

Purpose

FOBT uses chemical indicators on stool samples to detect the presence of blood not otherwise visible. Blood originating from or passing through the gastrointestinal tract can signal many conditions requiring further diagnostic procedures and, possibly, medical treatment. These conditions may be benign or malignant; some of them include:

- colon, rectal, and gastric (stomach) cancers
- ulcers
- hemorrhoids
- polyps
- inflammatory bowel disease

KEY TERMS

Endoscopy—The use of a flexible lighted tube inserted into a body opening to evaluate the internal surfaces of an organ.

Globin—The protein component of hemoglobin. Newer fecal occult blood tests screen for the presence of globin in the stool rather than heme.

Guaiac—A compound derived from the wood resin of guaiacum trees. Guaiac reacts with blood in the stool to produce a blue-colored reaction when peroxide is added to the sample.

Heme—The iron-containing pigment found in hemoglobin.

Hemoglobin—The iron-containing protein found in blood that carries oxygen from the lungs to the rest of the body.

Occult—Not visible or easily detected.

- irritations or lesions of the gastrointestinal tract caused by such medications as nonsteroidal anti-inflammatory drugs, also called NSAIDs
- irritations or lesions of the gastrointestinal tract caused by such stomach acid disorders as reflux esophagitis

The FOBT is used routinely (in conjunction with a **rectal examination** performed by a physician) to screen for colorectal cancer, particularly in patients older than 50. The ordering of this test should not be taken as an indication that cancer is suspected. The FOBT must be combined with regular screening **endoscopy** (such as a **sigmoidoscopy**) to detect cancers at an early stage.

Precautions

Certain foods and medicines can influence the test results. Some fruits contain chemicals that prevent the guaiac, the chemical in which the test paper is soaked, from reacting with the blood. **Aspirin** and some NSAIDs irritate the stomach, resulting in bleeding, and should be avoided prior to the examination. Red meat and many vegetables and fruits containing vitamin C also should be avoided for a specified period of time prior to the test. All these factors could produce a false-positive result.

Description

Feces for the stool samples are obtained either by the physician at the rectal examination or by the patient at home, using a small spatula or a collection device. In most cases, the collection of stool samples can easily be done at home, using a kit supplied by the physician. The standard kit contains a specially prepared card on which a small sample of stool will be spread, using a stick provided in the kit. The sample is placed in a special envelope and either mailed or brought in for analysis. When the physician applies hydrogen peroxide to the back of the sample, the paper will turn blue if an abnormal amount of blood is present.

Types of fecal occult blood tests

Hemoccult is the most commonly used fecal occult blood test. It measures the presence of heme, an iron-containing pigment found in hemoglobin. The Hemoccult test takes less than five minutes to perform and may be performed in the physician's office or in the laboratory. The Hemoccult blood test can detect bleeding from the colon as low as 0.5 mg per day.

Newer tests that use anti-hemoglobin antibodies (or immunochemical tests) to detect blood in the stool are also used. These tests screen for globin, the protein component of hemoglobin, rather than heme. Immunochemical tests can detect up to 0.7 mg of hemoglobin in the stool and do not require dietary restrictions. Immunochemical tests:

- are not accurate for screening for stomach cancer
- are more sensitive than Hemoccult tests in detecting colorectal cancer
- are more expensive than Hemoccult tests

HemoQuant, another fecal occult blood test, is used to detect as much as 500 mg/g of blood in the stool. Like the Hemoccult, the HemoQuant test is affected by recent consumption of red meat. It is not affected by chemicals in vegetables.

Fecal blood may also be measured by the amount of chromium in the red blood cells in the feces. The stool is collected for three to 10 days. The test is used in cases where the exact amount of blood loss is required. It is the only test that can exclude blood loss from the gastrointestinal area with accuracy.

A newer fecal occult blood test is based on enzyme immunoassay. This technique does not rely on guaiac, so it is not influenced by diet or medications used prior to the test. The fecal immunoassay test, or FIT, also requires fewer specimen collections. FITs are increasingly replacing the older guaiac-based FOBTs in many settings as of 2010. A 2009 editorial in the *American Journal of Gastroenterology* urged the use of FITs on the grounds that they do not require patients on blood thinners or NSAIDs to stop taking these medications during stool collection and thereby increase their risk of cardiovascular problems.

Two newer tests are based on DNA analysis of stool samples for biological markers of colorectal cancer. The first test of this type, PreGen-Plus, was first used in 2004 but held up for widespread distribution by a warning letter from the U.S. Food and Drug Administration (FDA) in October 2008. ColoSure, a DNA test that measures only one biomarker for colorectal cancer, was made available in the summer of 2008. It retails for about $220. ColoSure is not as accurate as a **colonoscopy** but is less invasive and is intended to be used for patients who resist having a colonoscopy. Widespread use of these new tests remains to be seen. As of 2010, the newer DNA stool tests appear to be cost-effective only in patients who are not compliant with other screening methods for colorectal cancer.

Over-the-counter (OTC) fecal occult blood test kits are now available for purchase at most pharmacies in the United States and Canada. These tests, however, are not as reliable as those performed in doctors' offices or laboratories.

Preparation

For 72 hours prior to collecting samples, patients should avoid red meats, NSAIDs (including aspirin), **antacids**, **steroids**, iron supplements, and vitamin C, including citrus fruits and other foods containing large amounts of vitamin C. Foods like uncooked broccoli, uncooked turnips, cauliflower, uncooked cantaloupe, uncooked radish and horseradish, and parsnips should not be eaten during the 72 hours prior to the examination. Fish, chicken, pork, fruits (other than melons) and many cooked vegetables are permitted in the diet.

People should postpone an FOBT if they are presently having **diarrhea**, **constipation**, a flare-up of **hemorrhoids**, severe **sore throat**, or a menstrual period.

Results

Many factors can result in false-positive and false-negative findings.

Positive results

It is important to note that a true-positive finding signifies only the presence of blood—it is not an indication of cancer. The National Cancer Institute states that, in its experience, less than 10% of all positive results were caused by cancer. The FOBT is positive in 1–5% of the unscreened population and 2–10% of those are found to have cancer. The physician will want to follow up on a positive result with further tests, as indicated by other factors in the patient's history or condition.

Negative results

Alternatively, a negative result (meaning no blood was detected) does not guarantee the absence of **colon cancer**, which may bleed only occasionally or not at all. (Only 50% of colon cancers are FOBT-positive.)

Conclusions

Screening using the FOBT has been demonstrated to reduce the mortality associated with colorectal cancer. However, because only half of colorectal cancers are FOBT-positive, FOBT must be combined with regular screening endoscopy or colonoscopy to increase the accuracy of detection of premalignant colorectal polyps and cancers.

Resources

BOOKS

Kim, Karen E., ed. *Early Detection and Prevention in Colorectal Cancer*. Thorofare, NJ: SLACK, 2009.

Saif, M. Wasif. *Gastrointestinal Malignancies*. New York: Demos Medical Publishing, 2010.

Wilkes, Gail M. *Pocket Guide to Colorectal Cancer*, 2nd ed. Boston: Jones and Bartlett Publishers, 2009.

PERIODICALS

Graser, A., et al. "Comparison of CT Colonography, Colonoscopy, Sigmoidoscopy and Faecal Occult Blood Tests for the Detection of Advanced Adenoma in an Average-risk Population." *Gut* 58 (February 2009): 241–48.

Levin, T.R. "Editorial: It's Time to Make Organized Colorectal Cancer Screening Convenient and Easy for Patients." *American Journal of Gastroenterology* 104 (April 2009): 939–41.

Parekh, M., et al. "As Tests Evolve and Costs of Cancer Care Rise: Reappraising Stool-based Screening for Colorectal Neoplasia." *Alimentary Pharmacology and Therapeutics* 27 (April 2008): 697–712.

Polack, J., and S.H. Itzkowitz. "Practical Advances in Stool Screening for Colorectal Cancer." *Journal of the National Comprehensive Cancer Network* 8 (January 2010): 81–92.

Whitlock, E.P., et al. " Screening for Colorectal Cancer: A Targeted, Updated Systematic Review for the U.S. Preventive Services Task Force." *Annals of Internal Medicine* 149 (November 4, 2008): 638–58.

Young, G.P., and S. Cole. "New Stool Screening Tests for Colorectal Cancer." *Digestion* 76 (January 2007): 26–33.

OTHER

American Cancer Society (ACS). *Colorectal Cancer: Early Detection*. http://www.cancer.org/docroot/CRI/content/CRI_2_6X_Colorectal_Cancer_Early_Detection_10.asp

Cleveland Clinic Foundation. *Fecal Occult Blood Test*. http://my.clevelandclinic.org/services/fecal_occult_blood_test/hic_fecal_occult_blood_test.aspx

Mayo Clinic. *Fecal Occult Blood Test*. http://www.mayoclinic.com/health/fecal-occult-blood-test/MY00620

ORGANIZATIONS

American Cancer Society, 1599 Clifton Rd. NE, Atlanta, GA, 30329, (800) ACS-2345, http://www.cancer.org.

National Cancer Institute (NCI), (800) 4-CANCER (422-6237), http://rex.nci.nih.gov.

Cheryl Branche, M.D.
Rebecca J. Frey, PhD
Brenda W. Lerner

Feldenkrais method

Definition

The Feldenkrais method is an educational system that allows the body to move and function more efficiently and comfortably. Its goal is to re-educate the nervous system and improve motor ability. The system can accomplish much more, relieving pressure on joints and weak points, allowing the body to heal repetitive strain injuries. Continued use of the method can relieve **pain** and lead to higher standards of achievement in sports, the martial arts, dancing, and other physical disciplines.

Pupils are taught to become aware of their movements and to become aware of how they use their bodies, thus discovering possible areas of **stress** and strain. The goal of Feldenkrais is to take the individual from merely functioning, to functioning well, free of pain and restriction of movement. Feldenkrais himself stated that his goal was, "to make the impossible possible, the possible easy, and the easy, elegant."

Purpose

This method of re-educating the nervous system can be beneficial to a wide range of people, including athletes, children, the elderly, martial artists, those who are handicapped, people with special needs, and those with degenerative diseases. It has proved popular with artists, particularly musicians, a number of whom have used Feldenkrais to improve their performance.

The Feldenkrais Guild of North America (FGNA) states that more than half of the those who turn to Feldenkrais practitioners are seeking relief from pain. Many people who have pain from an injury compensate by changing their movements to limit pain. Often these changed movements remain after the pain from the original injury is gone, and new pain may occur. Feldenkrais helps students become aware of the changed movements and allows them to learn new movements that relieve their pain.

Apart from the obvious physical benefits of more efficient movement and freedom from pain and restriction, Feldenkrais practitioners assert that it has other positive benefits for overall physical and mental health, including increased awareness, flexibility, and coordination, and better relaxation. Feldenkrais practitioners have noted other benefits in their students, including improvements in awareness, flexibility, coordination, breathing, digestion, sleep, mood, mental alertness, energy, and range of motion, as well as reduced stress and **hypertension**, and fewer headaches and backaches.

Musicians and athletes can improve their performance in many ways when they learn to use their bodies more efficiently. Feldenkrais can help injured athletes regain lost potential and free them from pain and restriction of movement.

Numerous accounts note remarkable results when Feldenkrais is taught to handicapped children so that they can learn to function despite their limitations. Handicapped people can learn to make full use of whatever potential they have, and to have more confidence in their abilities. Practitioners who specialize in teaching Feldenkrais to those who have handicaps have in many cases allowed the patient to discover ways of performing tasks that were previously thought to be impossible for them.

The elderly, whose movements are often restricted by pain and stiffness, can learn to overcome these obstacles with Feldenkrais instruction. In some instances, even severe cases of arthritis have been conquered. Theoretically, Feldenkrais can make possible renewed levels of energy and freedom from restriction.

MOSHE FELDENKRAIS (1904–1984)

Moshe Feldenkrais was born on the border between Russia and Poland. When he was only a boy of 13, he traveled to Palestine on foot. The journey took a year, and once there, young Feldenkrais worked as a laborer and cartographer, also tutoring others in mathematics. Moving to France in 1933, he graduated in mechanical and electrical engineering from the Ecole des Travaux Publiques de Paris.

Feldendrais became the first person to open a Judo center in Paris after meeting with Jigaro Kano. He was also one of the first Europeans to become a black belt in Judo, in 1936.

Obtaining his Ph.D. at the Sorbonne, he went on to assist Nobel Prize laureate Frédéric Joliot-Curie at the Curie Institute. During World War II in England, he worked on the new sonar anti-submarine research.

Prompted by a recurring leg injury, he applied his knowledge of the martial arts and his training as an engineer to devise a method of re-integrating the body. The concept was that more efficient movement would allow for the treatment of pain or disability, and the better-functioning of the body as a whole. Later on, he would begin to teach what he had learned to others in Tel Aviv.

In addition to many books about judo, including *Higher Judo*, he wrote six books on his method.

Description

Origins

Moshe Feldenkrais (1904–1984) was a Russian-born Israeli physicist and engineer who was also an active soccer player and judo master. He devised his system in response to his own recurring knee injury, which had restricted his movement and caused him great pain over a long period of time. Feldenkrais believed that repeated muscle patterns cause the parts of the brain controlling those muscles to stay in a fixed pattern as well. He thought that the more the muscles are used, the more parts of the brain can be activated. He devised a method of re-educating the neuromuscular system and re-evaluating movement to increase efficiency and reduce stress, using his knowledge of mechanics and engineering, and applying some of his martial arts training.

Feldenkrais is described as being a dual system, with two components: "Awareness Through Movement" and "Functional Integration." The system aims to re-educate the body so that habitual movements that cause strain or pain can be relearned to improve efficiency and eliminate dangerous or painful action.

Feldenkrais helps to translate intention into action. In practice, an individual can learn to achieve his or her highest potential, while at the same time learning to avoid and eliminate stresses, strains, and the possibility of injury.

KEY TERMS

Neuromuscular—The body system of nerves and muscles as they function together.

Repetitive strain injury—Injury resulting from a repeated movement such as typing or throwing a ball.

Functional integration

During this session, the patient wears comfortable clothing, and may sit, stand, walk, or lie on a low padded table. The practitioner helps the pupil by guiding him or her through a number of movements. The practitioner may use touch to communicate with the student, but touch is not used to correct any movements. The purpose of this session is to increase a student's awareness of his or her own movement and become open to different possibilities for movement. The instruction can be focused on a particular activity that the student does every day, or that causes him or her pain. The student can learn to alter habitual movements and re-educate the neuromuscular system. This type of session is particularly useful for those who have limitations originating from misuse, stress, illness, or accident. It can also help athletes and musicians perform to the best of their ability by increasing their possibilities for movement. It offers students the potential for improving their physical and mental performance in addition to heightening the sense of well-being.

Awareness through movement

Feldenkrais's martial arts background can be clearly identified in many of the aspects of Awareness Through Movement (ATM). During group sessions, pupils are taught to become acutely aware of all their movements and to imagine them, so that they can improve the efficiency of their actions in their minds, and put them into practice. Pupils are encouraged to be disciplined about practicing their exercises so they may achieve maximum benefit.

Awareness through movement is described as an exploratory, nonjudgmental process through which pupils are encouraged to observe and learn about themselves and their movements. The range of this therapy is wide, and thousands of different lessons are available to help specific areas.

Preparations

No preparation is necessary for the practice of Feldenkrais, and all are encouraged to seek help from this system. No condition is considered a preclusion to the benefits of Feldenkrais.

Precautions

As with any therapy or treatment, care should be taken to choose a qualified practitioner. Feldenkrais practitioners stress that the body must not be forced to do anything, and if any movement is painful, or even uncomfortable, it should be discontinued immediately and the patient should seek professional help.

Side effects

No known side effects are associated with the practice of Feldenkrais.

Research and general acceptance

Since Feldenkrais began to teach his method, it has gradually gained acceptance as an education system. Published research using the method can be found in United States and foreign publications.

Resources

BOOKS

Davis, Martha. *The Relaxation & Stress Reduction Workbook*. 6th ed. Sydney: ReadHowYouWant, 2009.

Hoffman, Ronald L., and Sidney Stevens. *How to Talk with Your Doctor: The Guide for Patients and Their Physicians Who Want to Reconcile and Use the Best of Conventional and Alternative Medicine*. Laguna Beach, CA: Basic Health, 2010.

Weintraub, Michael I., Ravinder Mamtani, and Marc S. Micozzi, eds. *Complementary and Integrative Medicine in Pain Management*. New York: Springer, 2008.

ORGANIZATIONS

American Pain Society, 4700 W. Lake Ave., Glenview, IL, 60025, (847) 375-4715, http://www.ampainsoc.org.

Benson-Henry Institute for Mind Body Medicine at Massachusetts General Hospital, 151 Merrimac St., 4th Floor, Boston, MA, 02114, (617) 643-6090, http://www.massgeneral.org/bhi.

The Center for Mindfulness in Medicine, Health Care and Society. University of Massachusetts Medical School., 55 Lake Ave., North, Worcester, MA, 01655, (508) 856-2656, (508) 856-1977, mindfulness@umassmed.edu, http://www.umassmed.edu/cfm/.

Feldenkrais Guild of North America, 3611 SW Hood Ave., Suite 100, Portland, OR, 97201, (503) 221-6612, (800) 775-2118, (503) 221-6616, http://www.feldenkrais.com.

Patricia Skinner
Laura Jean Cataldo, RN, EdD

Female circumcision *see* **Female genital mutilation**

Female condom *see* **Condom**

Female genital mutilation

Definition

Female genital mutilation (FGM)—also called female genital cutting (FGC) or female circumcision—is the cutting or partial or total removal of the external female genitalia. It is performed for cultural or other non–medical reasons, most often on girls between the ages of four and ten.

Demographics

The World Health Organization (WHO) estimates that between 100 million and 140 million girls and women have undergone some form of FGM, with as many as three million girls at risk for the procedure each year. FGM is a deeply rooted cultural tradition in some 28 African countries and a few Middle Eastern and Asian nations. Although it is illegal in many countries, including 18 African nations, enforcement is minimal. In the United States it is illegal to perform FGM on anyone under age 18.

Nearly half of all women who have been genitally mutilated live in Egypt or Ethiopia, although the rates of FGM in Egypt and some other countries appear to be on the decline. FGM is practiced to a lesser degree in Indonesia, India, and Pakistan. The countries in which the highest percentages of females are subjected to FGM are as follows (where two percentages are given, the lower percentage refers to girls aged 15–19 and the higher percentage is for women aged 35–39, suggesting that the practice is on the decline):

- Guinea: 99%
- Somalia: 97–99%
- Djibouti: 98%
- Egypt: 81–96%
- Eritrea: 95%
- Mali: 94%
- Sierra Leone: 90%
- Ethiopia: 62–81%
- Gambia: 80%
- Côte d'Ivoire: 28–44%
- Kenya: 15–35%

FGM is practiced by people of all educational levels and social classes and various religions, including Christians, Muslims, and animists. In some countries it is more common in rural areas and in other countries it is more prevalent in cities.

Although FGM is most often performed on girls before they reach **puberty**, it is practiced on women of all ages, from infancy through adulthood. The usual age for FGM varies with the country and region within a country. Sometimes it is performed just before a woman marries or during her first **pregnancy**. In Egypt about 90% of girls are cut between the ages of four and 12. In Yemen more than 75% of girls are cut during the first two weeks of life. In Burkina Faso, Côte d'Ivoire, Egypt, Kenya, and Mali, the age for FGM is decreasing, perhaps because younger children are less able to resist or because in countries where it is illegal, the practice is more easily concealed with younger girls.

Description

FGM includes a wide range of procedures. The simplest form of FGM involves a small cut to the clitoris or labial tissue. A Sunna **circumcision** removes the prepuce—a fold of skin that covers the clitoris—and/or the tip of the clitoris. A clitoridectomy is the removal of the entire clitoris and some or all of the surrounding tissue. Clitoridectomies account for approximately 80% of FGMs. The most extreme form of genital mutilation is excision and infibulation, in which the clitoris and all of the surrounding tissues of the external genitalia are cut away and the remaining skin is sewn together, leaving only a small opening for the passage of urine and menstrual blood. This sewing shut of the vagina is designed to ensure virginity until marriage. Infibulation accounts for approximately 15% of FGM procedures.

FGM is usually performed in the home or some other non–medical setting. Often it is performed by a family member or a local "circumciser," using scissors, knives, razor blades, or other instruments that have not necessarily been sterilized. However in Egypt up to 90% of FGMs are now performed by medical professionals.

With increased immigration to Western countries from regions where female circumcision is common, the practice has come to the attention of health professionals in the United States, Canada, Europe, and Australia. Some families return to their native countries to have their daughters circumcised. In an effort to integrate old customs with modern medical care, some immigrant families have requested that Western physicians perform the procedure. This can place doctors in the difficult position of trying to be sensitive to cultural traditions and choosing between performing female circumcision in a medical facility under anesthesia and sanitary conditions or refusing, knowing that the FGM may be performed without medical supervision. In 2010 the American Academy of Pediatrics, in a controversial change of policy, suggested

KEY TERMS

Circumcision—A procedure, usually with religious or cultural significance, in which the prepuce—the skin covering the tip of the male penis or the female clitoris, is cut away.

Clitoridectomy—A procedure in which the clitoris and possibly some of the surrounding labial tissue at the opening of the vagina is removed.

Clitoris—The small erectile organ at the front of the female vulva that is the site of female sexual pleasure.

Infibulation—A procedure that closes the labia majora to prevent sexual intercourse, leaving only a small opening for the passage of urine and menstrual blood.

Labia majora—The outer fatty folds of the vulva.

Prepuce—The fold of tissue covering the clitoris in females and the tip of the penis in males.

Vulva—The external female genital organs, including the labia majora, labia minora, clitoris, and vestibule of the vagina.

that U.S. doctors be allowed to perform a ceremonial pinprick on girls to prevent them from being sent abroad for FGM.

Causes and symptoms

FGM is practiced for a variety of cultural, social, political, and economic reasons:

- FGM is usually an integral part of community tradition.
- Most parents believe that genital cutting protects—rather than harms—their daughters.
- In some cultures FGM is considered a necessary rite of passage for girls and may even mark their introduction to sexual activity.
- Although FGM represents social and cultural control of female sexuality, some cultures believe that FGM actually empowers women by protecting their family's reputation and ensuring that they will marry.
- Female circumcision is believed to protect a girl's virginity and prevent unwed pregnancy, which could bring shame upon the family.
- In some cultures uncircumcised females are considered to be dirty or unmarriageable and may be treated poorly.
- In some societies FGM is believed to quell female sexual desire.
- Some people believe that their religion requires female circumcision.
- Some people believe in superstitions—that the clitoris will continue to grow if it is not removed or that external genitalia are unclean and can kill an infant during birth.

The effects of FGM depend on the degree of cutting, the cleanliness of the instruments, and the health of the female at the time of the procedure. FGM is usually performed without anesthesia and almost always causes bleeding and **pain**. The pain is usually most severe on the following day when the patient first urinates onto the wound.

The immediate risks of FGM include:

- physical and/or psychological trauma
- hemorrhage (excessive bleeding)
- severe pain
- infection, including abscesses, fever, sepsis (blood infection), shock, tetanus, or gangrene
- death due to excessive blood loss or infection

Long–term complications usually occur with the more severe forms of FGM and include:

- scarring
- poor drainage of urine and menstrual blood, leading to infection
- chronic urinary tract infections
- cysts and abscesses
- incontinence
- pelvic and back pain
- painful menstruation
- very painful sexual intercourse due to scarring of most of the vagina
- lack of sexual pleasure
- inability to undergo normal gynecological exams and procedures
- increased risk for sexually transmitted infections (STIs), including HIV/AIDS, both from contaminated instruments and also because the damaged tissues are more likely to tear during sex, facilitating the transmission of infectious agents

- infertility rates as high as 25–30%, usually related vaginal scarring that makes sexual intercourse difficult
- childbirth complications, including prolonged labor, tearing, heavy bleeding, and infection
- psychological symptoms similar to post–traumatic stress syndrome (PTSD), including anxiety, depression, and sleep abnormalities, although these conditions are rare

Diagnosis

Diagnosis and treatment of FGM requires the care of culturally sensitive gynecologists and women's healthcare specialists who are familiar with the different types of FGM and their complications.

Treatment

Traditional

A girl or young woman who has recently had FGM may require supportive care to control bleeding. Treatment may be necessary for any complications. Women who have undergone FGM may require specialized gynecologic, obstetric, and reproductive care by knowledgeable practitioners.

In the United States female immigrants with FGM often undergo defibulation or **reconstructive surgery** to reverse or repair their genitalia. Some surgical procedures that were originally developed for sex–change operations have been adapted for treating women with FGM. These techniques may involve cutting away scar tissue and skin to expose whatever remains of the clitoris, as well as more extensive reconstruction.

Drugs

Females who have recently undergone FGM may require **antibiotics** to prevent infection.

Prognosis

FGM can adversely affect a woman's quality of life, particularly with regard to sexual enjoyment and **childbirth**. FGM is associated with postpartum hemorrhage, **episiotomy**, extended hospital stays, **stillbirth**, infant resuscitation, and infant and maternal **death**. Circumcised pregnant women sometimes must deliver by Caesarian section.

Prevention

Many national and international medical organizations—including the American Medical Association, Canadian medical associations, and the World Health Organization (WHO)—oppose the practice of female genital mutilation. The United Nations considers FGM to be a violation of human rights and several African and Asian nations have called for an end to the practice. WHO has undertaken a number of projects aimed at decreasing the incidence of FGM. These include:

- a statement addressing the regional status of FGM and encouraging the development of national policies against the practice
- training community workers to oppose FGM
- developing educational materials about FGM for community healthcare workers
- providing alternative job training for circumcisers

Other approaches to halting the practice of FGM include:

- community meetings, discussions, theater productions, and songs
- educational programs conducted by respected local women
- work by Islamic and other religious leaders to change the perception that FGM is required by religion
- substitution of other coming–of–age rituals for girls
- laws prohibiting FGM except as the free choice of an adult woman

Resources

BOOKS

French, Kathy. *Sexual Health*. Ames, IA: Blackwell, 2009.

Levin, Tobe, and Augustine H. Asaah. *Empathy and Rage: Female Genital Mutilation in African Literature*. Boulder, CO: Lynne Rienner Publishers, 2009.

World Health Organization, United Nations Population Fund, Key Centre for Women's Health in Society. *Mental Health Aspects of Women's Reproductive Health: A Global Review of the Literature*. Geneva: World Health Organization, 2009.

Zabus, Chantal J. *Fearful Symmetries: Essays and Testimonies About Excision and Circumcision*. New York: Rodopi, 2008.

PERIODICALS

Adam, Taghreed, et al. "Estimating the Obstetric Costs of Female Genital Mutilation in Six African Countries." *Bulletin of the World Health Organization* 88, no. 4 (April 2010): 281–288.

Auge, Karen. "'I Want to be Like Everyone Else.'" *Denver Post* (March 7, 2010): A1.

Belluck, Pam. "Group Backs Ritual 'Nick' as Female Circumcision Option." *New York Times*. May 7, 2010: A16.

di Giovanni, Janine. "From Torture to Triumph." *Harper's Bazaar* no. 3579 (February 2010): 115.

"Ritual Genital Cutting of Female Minors." *Pediatrics* 125, no. 5 (May 2010): 1088.

OTHER

Feldman–Jacobs, Charlotte, and Donna Clifton. "Female Genital Mutilation/Cutting: Data and Trends Update 2010." Population Reference Bureau. http://www.prb.org/Publications/Datasheets/2010/fgm2010.aspx (accessed September 4, 2010).

"Female Genital Cutting: Frequently Asked Questions." The National Women's Health Information Center. http://womenshealth.gov/faq/female–genital–cutting.cfm (accessed September 4, 2010).

ORGANIZATIONS

African Women's Health Center, Brigham and Women's Hospital, 75 Francis St., Boston, MA, 02115, (617) 732–5500, http://www.brighamandwomens.org/africanwomenscenter.

Center for Reproductive Rights, 120 Wall St., New York, NY, 10005, (917) 637–3600, (917) 637–3666, http://reproductiverights.org.

U.S. Department of Health and Human Services, Office on Women's Health, 200 Independence Ave., SW, Rm. 728E, Washington, DC, 20201, (202) 205–1960, (800) 994–9662, (202) 401–4005, http://www.womenshealth.gov.

World Health Organization, Avenue Appia 20, 1211 Geneva 27, Switzerland, 41 22 791 21 11, 41 22 791 31 11, info@who.int, http://www.who.int/en/.

Altha Roberts Edgren
Margaret Alic, PhD

Female infertility *see* **Infertility**

Female orgasmic disorder

Definition

Female orgasmic disorder (FOD) is the persistent or recurrent inability to achieve orgasm (climax or sexual release) despite adequate sexual arousal and stimulation. FOD is also called orgasmic dysfunction or anorgasmia. It used to be called "inhibited sexual orgasm."

Demographics

The inability to achieve orgasm, discontent with the quality of orgasms, and the ability to achieve orgasm only with a particular type of sexual stimulation are very common sexual complaints among women. It has been suggested that 33–50% of all women are dissatisfied with the frequencies of their orgasms and that fewer than one third of women consistently experience orgasm with sexual activity. However FOD applies to the 10–15% of women have never experienced an orgasm, regardless of the situation or stimulation, and to women who can no longer achieve an orgasm. Women who have never experienced orgasm are more likely to be unmarried, young, and/or sexually inexperienced. FOD has also been associated with **menopause** and **aging**, although many women find that their orgasms increase with age.

Description

When a woman becomes sexually excited, the blood vessels in the pelvic region expand, allowing more blood to flow to the genitals—the same process that occurs when men become sexually excited. This effusion is followed by seepage of fluid into the vagina to provide lubrication before and during intercourse. These events are called the "lubrication–swelling response."

Body tension and blood flow to the pelvic region continue to build as sexual stimulation increases, either by direct pressure on the clitoris or pressure on the walls of the vagina and cervix. An orgasm occurs when the tension is released. It is accompanied by a feeling of intense physical pleasure and involuntary, rhythmic contractions of the pelvic floor muscles and possibly the vagina and uterus. The contractions carry blood away from the genital region. However the exact physiological mechanisms of the female orgasm are not well-understood. Furthermore, women do not necessarily experience orgasms in the same way, and an individual woman may experience orgasms differently at various times and in different situations. Orgasms vary in intensity, length, and the number of contractions, and, unlike men, women can have multiple orgasms in a short period of time. Some 50–80% of women experience orgasm only through direct clitoral stimulation. Mature, more sexually experienced women may find it easier to have orgasms than younger or sexually inexperienced women.

FOD is a type of **sexual dysfunction** that affects the quality of a woman's sexual experience. It often occurs in conjunction with other sexual dysfunctions. Women with FOD experience sexual arousal and lubrication. However as body tension builds, they have extreme difficulty or are completely unable to reach climax and release the tension. This can lead to frustration and less–than–fulfilling sexual experiences for both partners, as well as anger, frustration, and other relationship problems.

According to the American Psychiatric Association's *Diagnostic and Statistical Manual of Mental Disorders,* the *DSM,* a diagnosis of FOD requires that the anorgasmia is not due solely to physiological problems and is not a symptom of another major mental health disorder. However FOD can be caused by a combination of physiological and psychological difficulties. For a diagnosis of FOD the condition also must cause personal distress or relationship problems.

FOD is most often a primary or lifelong condition, in which women never achieve orgasm with any type of stimulation, including self–stimulation (masturbation), direct stimulation of the clitoris by a partner, or vaginal intercourse. Secondary or acquired FOD affects women who have experienced orgasm at least once in the past, but have lost the ability following an illness or emotional trauma or as a side effect of surgery or medication. Acquired FOD is often temporary. Anorgasmia may also be classified as general, which means that orgasm is never achieved under any circumstances or with any partner; or situational, which means that orgasm is only achieved under certain circumstances or with certain types of sexual activity.

Risk factors

Recent studies of twins suggest that genes and heredity play a large role in the development of FOD. A history of sexual or physical **abuse** is also a risk factor for FOD.

Causes and symptoms

FOD is characterized by a woman's inability to achieve orgasm, by extreme difficulty in regularly reaching climax, or having only unsatisfying orgasms. Some women often come close to orgasm but never reach it. FOD can be caused by psychological factors or by a combination of psychological and physiological factors.

Psychological causes of FOD include:

- feelings of isolation, disconnection, or boredom during sex
- shyness or embarrassment
- performance anxiety or sexual activity that is overly goal–oriented, with excessive pressure to achieve orgasm
- past sexual or physical abuse, rape, incest, or other traumatic sexual experiences
- emotional abuse
- fear of pregnancy
- fear of rejection
- fear of loss of control during orgasm
- self–image problems
- relationship problems
- life stresses, such as financial worries, job loss, or divorce
- guilt or negative feelings toward sex or sexual pleasure—attitudes that are usually learned in childhood or adolescence
- religious or cultural beliefs about sex
- other mental health disorders, such as major depression

Various prescription and over–the–counter medications can cause aorgasmia. These include:

- antidepressants called selective serotonin reuptake inhibitors (SSRIs) such as fluoxetine (Prozac), paroxetine (Paxil), and sertraline (Zoloft)
- anti-anxiety drugs such as Xanax
- sedatives such as Halcion
- narcotics
- antihistamines
- blood-pressure medications
- chemotherapy drugs

Other physiological causes of FOD include:

- inadequate sexual stimulation and the inability to discuss or explore more stimulating sexual techniques
- lower estrogen levels during and after menopause, which reduce lubrication and require greater

KEY TERMS

Anorgasmia—A sexual dysfunction characterized by the inability to achieve orgasm.

Clitoris—The small erectile organ at the front of the female vulva that is the site of female sexual pleasure.

Estrogen—Any of several naturally occurring or synthetic steroid hormones that promote the growth and maintenance of the female reproductive system.

Kegel exercises—Repetitive contractions to tone the pubococcygeal muscle for enhancing sexual response during intercourse or controlling incontinence.

Orgasm—The climax of sexual excitement, usually characterized by vaginal contractions by the female and ejaculation of semen by the male.

Testosterone—The primary male sex hormone, which is also produced at low levels in females.

stimulation for relaxing and promoting blood flow to the clitoris and vagina

- other normal aging processes
- smoking, alcohol, or other substance abuse
- hormonal disorders and chronic illnesses that affect general health and sexual interest
- damage to the blood vessels of the pelvic region
- conditions that affect or damage pelvic nerves, including pelvic surgery, multiple sclerosis, diabetes, neurological disease, or spinal cord injury
- pelvic floor prolapse—a loosening of the muscles that support internal pelvic organs
- removal of the clitoris (female genital mutilation), a cultural practice in much of Africa and some regions of the Middle East and Asia

Diagnosis

FOD is often self–diagnosed. However a woman who has never had an orgasm may not realize what is missing in her sexual experience without diagnosis by a physician, women's healthcare specialist, psychiatrist, psychologist, or sex therapist.

Examination

Diagnosis of FOD includes a complete physical exam and medical, psychological, and sexual histories. The clinician or therapist helps determine whether the problem is primary or acquired and general or situational. FOD sometimes occurs in conjunction with sexual aversion disorder and/or **female sexual arousal disorder**, complicating the diagnosis. A diagnosis of FOD requires that:

- Orgasms occur less frequently than would be expected based on the patient's age, sexual experience, and level of sexual stimulation.
- The absence of orgasm results in emotional distress or relationship difficulties.
- The cause is psychological or a combination of psychological and physical factors.
- The absence of orgasm is not a symptom of another psychological disorder, such as depression.

Tests

Blood tests may be performed to measure the levels of estrogen and testosterone.

Treatment

Traditional

Treatment of FOD requires addressing any underlying physiological causes, psychological factors such as depression, and lifestyle factors such as **substance abuse**. Medications may require adjustment. Any associated sexual dysfunctions, such as lack of interest in sex or painful intercourse, must also be addressed. FOD is commonly treated with education, counseling, cognitive behavioral therapy, **psychotherapy**, and/or **sex therapy**.

Psychotherapy or counseling can be effective for treating psychological causes of FOD, especially those causes that are rooted in **sexual abuse**, past sexual or emotional experiences, or cultural taboos. Couples therapy may be used to resolve relationship issues that have either caused or resulted from FOD. These processes require time and a joint commitment by couples.

Sex therapists have specialized training for assisting individuals and couples in overcoming sexual dysfunctions. Sex therapy may include:

- directed exercises for increasing stimulation and decreasing inhibitions
- techniques for relaxation, sexual exploration, and direct clitoral stimulation
- encouragement of masturbation, either by self–-stimulation or with a vibrator
- Kegel exercises for enhancing sexual response
- communication training and relationship enhancement for couples
- desensitization—learning to halt responses that are preventing orgasm, particularly in women with severe sexual anxiety

Drugs

Estrogen or a combination of estrogen and progesterone may be used to treat FOD in menopausal women and others with low hormone levels. FOD is sometimes treated with methyltestosterone, a synthetic form of the male sex hormone testosterone, although this practice is controversial and can have various side effects. Testosterone appears to be most effective for women with low testosterone levels resulting from surgical removal of the ovaries.

Alternative

Zestra is a botanical massage oil that warms the clitoris and may increase sexual arousal and orgasm. L–arginine in various **nutritional supplements** relaxes blood vessels and increases blood flow to the genital area, especially the clitoris.

Home remedies

One of the most important factors in overcoming FOD is open and honest communication between partners about sexuality and sexual techniques. Erotic books or videos may help initiate such conversations. Sometimes focusing on clitoral stimulation is all that is needed to overcome FOD. Experimenting with different sexual positions may improve clitoral stimulation. Using a vibrator during sex can also help trigger orgasms.

Many women have found that Kegel exercises, which involve the repetitive contraction and relaxation of the pelvic floor muscles, can improve both the frequency and intensity of orgasmic experiences. Repeatedly stopping and starting a urine stream identifies the muscles to be exercised, working up to five sets of ten contractions per day. The longer the contractions are held, the more benefit may result.

Prognosis

FOD can often be successfully treated with a combination of psychotherapy and guided sexual exercises. However women should not expect to always achieve orgasm in every situation; nor should they expect to always be satisfied with the strength and quality of their climax. Women whose FOD is not due to an identifiable condition or disorder may be more difficult to treat. Unresolved FOD usually results in a decline in sexual desire and can create resentment and conflict within relationships.

Prevention

Although there is no sure way to prevent FOD, reducing life factors that cause **stress** can be effective. Healthy attitudes toward sex and education about sexual stimulation and responses can help prevent FOD. Seeking counseling or psychotherapy for past trauma or relationship issues can help minimize FOD and other sexual dysfunction problems.

Resources

BOOKS

American Psychiatric Association. *Diagnostic and Statistical Manual of Mental Disorders*, 4th ed., text rev. Arlington, VA: American Psychiatric Association, 2007.

Komisaruk, Barry. R. *The Orgasm Answer Guide*. Baltimore: Johns Hopkins University Press, 2010.

McCabe, Marita P. "Anorgasmia in Women." In: Katherine M. Hertlein, Gerald R. Weeks, and Nancy Gambescia, editors. *Systemic Sex Therapy*. New York: Routledge, 2009.

PERIODICALS

Frank, J. E., et al. "Diagnosis and Treatment of Female Sexual Dysfunction." *American Family Physician* 77 (2008): 635.

Graham, Cynthia A. "The DSM Diagnostic Criteria for Female Orgasmic Disorder." *Archives of Sexual Behavior* 39(2) (April 2010): 256.

OTHER

Berney, Karen. "Female Orgasmic Disorder: 'I'm Not Able to Climax'." Discovery Health. http://health.discovery.com/centers/sex/articles/orgasmic.html (accessed September 26, 2010).

"Female Sexual Dysfunction." MedlinePlus. http://www.nlm.nih.gov/medlineplus/femalesexualdysfunction.html (accessed September 26, 2010).

Mayo Clinic Staff. "Anorgasmia." MayoClinic.com http://www.mayoclinic.com/health/anorgasmia/DS01051/METHOD=print (accessed September 26, 2010).

Mayo Clinic Staff. "Female Sexual Dysfunction." Mayo Clinic.com http://www.mayoclinic.com/print/female–sexual–dysfunction/DS00701/METHOD=print&DSECTION=all (accessed September 26, 2010).

"Orgasmic Dysfunction." MedlinePlus. http://www.nlm.nih.gov/medlineplus/ency/article/001953.htm (accessed September 26, 2010).

ORGANIZATIONS

American Association of Sex Educators, Counselors, and Therapists (AASECT), P.O. Box 1960, Ashland, VA, 23005–1960, (804) 752–0026, (804) 752–0056, aasect@aasect.org, http://www.aasect.org.

American College of Obstetricians and Gynecologists (ACOG), P.O. Box 96920, Washington, DC, 20090–6920, (202) 638–5577, (800) 673–8444, resources@acog.org, http://www.acog.org.

U.S. Department of Health and Human Services, Office on Women's Health, 200 Independence Ave., SW, Rm. 728E, Washington, DC, 20201, (202) 205–1960, (800) 994–9662, (202) 401–4005, http://www.womenshealth.gov.

Tish Davidson, AM
Emily Jane Willingham, PhD
Margaret Alic, PhD

Female sexual arousal disorder

Definition

Female sexual arousal disorder (FSAD) is a woman's persistent or recurrent inability to achieve or maintain an adequate lubrication-swelling response during sexual activity. Sometimes FSAD is defined

ALFRED KINSEY (1894–1956)

Alfred Kinsey became a household name in the 1950s with his groundbreaking research on the sexual mores of American women and men. His two major texts, *Sexual Behavior in the Human Male* (1948) and *Sexual Behavior in the Human Female* (1953), opened the way for research into human sexuality.

Kinsey and his colleagues at the Institute for Sex Research at Indiana University conducted thousands of interviews with men and women about their sexual habits. The 804-page *Sexual Behavior in the Human Male* sold 185,000 copies in its first year and became a *New York Times* bestseller. The work was scientifically based and nonjudgmental, with frank descriptions of biological functions. Although early polls indicated that most Americans were relieved to have an honest and open airing of human sexual practices, there was a tremendous backlash from conservative and religious organizations. *Sexual Behavior in the Human Female* caused an even greater stir. Its more controversial findings included the low incidence of female frigidity, high rates of premarital and extramarital sex, the rapidness of erotic responses, and a detailed discussion of clitoral versus vaginal orgasm. As sales of the book reached 250,000 in the United States alone, Kinsey's methods and motives came under scrutiny. Evangelist Billy Graham stated: "It is impossible to estimate the damage this book will do to the already deteriorating morals of America." Kinsey's research funding was revoked and for the remainder of his life he struggled to find support for his work.

simply as the inability to become sexually aroused or to maintain arousal despite sexual desire. FSAD stems from both physiological and psychological factors. It often results in avoidance of sex, painful intercourse, and sexual tension in relationships.

Demographics

FSAD is common in older women due to decreased hormone production after **menopause** and medical conditions associated with **aging**. However, because FSAD often occurs in combination with other female sexual dysfunctions and can be difficult to distinguish from them, and because women are often reluctant to seek help for FSAD, it is difficult to determine its incidence. There is also disagreement within the medical community concerning the exact demarcations of the various female sexual dysfunctions. One published review of the medical literature found that 22–43% of women experience some form of **sexual dysfunction**. Another study found that about 20% of women have problems with sexual lubrication.

Description

FSAD results from a woman's inability to undergo lubrication and swelling in response to sexual desire and stimulation. This lack of response interferes with sexual desire and satisfying intercourse.

William Masters and Virginia Johnson—the first researchers to extensively examine the physical components of human sexuality—identified four stages of sexual response: excitement, plateau, climax or orgasm, and resolution. More recent models have included emotional aspects of arousal. One model identifies three stages: desire, arousal, and orgasm. FSAD affects the excitement or arousal stage.

The first physiological change in the female body upon becoming aroused or sexually excited is the expansion of the blood vessels in the pelvic region, allowing more blood to flow to the lower abdomen and genitals. Some women experience this as a feeling of fullness in the pelvis, and either consciously or involuntarily contract the muscles in the genital area. The increased blood flow normally results in transudation—the seepage of fluid through the walls of the blood vessels—in this case into the vagina to provide lubrication before and during intercourse. Vaginal lubrication can occur very rapidly, within one minute, and is often very noticeable. The increase in blood flow also expands the upper portion of the vagina, the uterus, and the cervix. The lower third of the vagina, the labia, and the area around the clitoris swell and may tingle. The breasts also swell slightly. Together these physiological changes constitute the lubrication-swelling response, designed to facilitate entry of the penis into the vagina.

With FSAD the lubrication-swelling response is either absent or is not maintained through the completion of sexual activity. The lack of arousal and lubrication can result in painful intercourse (**dyspareunia**), emotional distress, and/or relationship problems. FSAD can be lifelong or acquired and generalized or situation-specific.

Causes and symptoms

The major symptom of FSAD is insufficient transudation, often resulting in painful and unsatisfactory intercourse. In addition to vaginal dryness, there is a

KEY TERMS

Clitoris—The small erectile organ at the front of the female vulva that is the site of female sexual pleasure.

Dyspareunia—Difficult or painful sexual intercourse.

Estrogen—Any of several naturally occurring or synthetic steroid hormones that promote the growth and maintenance of the female reproductive system.

Kegel exercises—Repetitive contractions to tone the pubococcygeal muscle of the pelvic floor for enhancing sexual response during intercourse or controlling incontinence.

Labia—The fatty folds of the vulva.

Testosterone—The primary male sex hormone, which is also produced at low levels in females.

Transudation—The passage of fluid, as through blood vessels into the vagina.

Vulva—The external female genital organs, including the labia majora, labia minora, clitoris, and vestibule of the vagina.

lack of swelling, **tingling**, or throbbing in the genital region. Generalized FSAD occurs with different partners and in many different situations, whereas situation-specific FSAD occurs only with certain partners or under particular circumstances. FSAD can be caused by psychological factors or a combination of psychological and physiological factors. Whereas some women have never had a normal lubrication-swelling response, others develop FSAD from physiological changes, such as illness or emotional trauma, or as a side effect of surgery, **radiation therapy** for **cancer**, or a medication. Physiologically based FSAD can lead to psychological problems that reinforce the disorder.

Arousal disorder that primarily affects the genitals can result from low estrogen or testosterone levels during and after menopause, as well as from vaginal or bladder infections, or changes in the skin around the vulva. Other physiological causes of FSAD include:

- insufficient sexual stimulation
- irritation from contraceptive creams or foams
- smoking, which decreases blood flow throughout the body
- illicit drug use
- lower levels of sex hormones due to breastfeeding
- medical conditions that cause changes in hormone levels, including thyroid disorders, adrenal gland disorders, or removal of the ovaries
- side effects of medications such as antidepressants, antipsychotics, sedatives, high-blood-pressure drugs, or birth control pills or other hormone-containing medications
- reduced blood flow due to damaged blood vessels in the pelvic region, often from medical conditions such as coronary artery disease, high blood pressure, or diabetes
- damage to nerves in the pelvic area, as from diabetes or multiple sclerosis

Psychological causes of FSAD include:

- fear or anxiety around sex
- chronic mild depression (dysthymia)
- emotional stress
- low self-esteem
- past sexual abuse
- emotional abuse
- bereavement
- self-image problems
- relationship problems
- other mental health disorders, including major depression, post-traumatic stress disorder, or obsessive-compulsive disorder

Diagnosis

Since most women occasionally experience difficulties with sexual arousal, a diagnosis of FSAD requires that the deficient lubrication-swelling response is persistent or has occurred intermittently over an extended period and causes emotional distress or relationship difficulties. The *Diagnostic and Statistical Manual of Mental Disorders* (*DSM-IV-TR*) requires that FSAD be caused by psychological factors alone or a combination of psychological and physiological factors. Under these criteria, arousal disorder caused by physiological factors alone, such as injury, illness, or menopause is diagnosed as sexual dysfunction due to a general medical condition. Arousal disorder caused by medication or **substance abuse** alone is diagnosed as substance-induced sexual dysfunction. Arousal difficulties that are symptoms of a major psychological disorder, such as depression, or that result from inadequate sexual stimulation are not considered to be FSAD.

Examination

FSAD is usually diagnosed after a woman reports sexual difficulties to her gynecologist, family doctor, psychotherapist, or sex therapist. The physician will take complete medical, psychological, and sexual histories, including a list of medications and details about sexual symptoms. A **physical examination**, including a gynecological/pelvic exam, will be performed.

Tests

Blood and urine tests may be performed to rule out undiagnosed diabetes or other medical conditions. Hormone levels in the blood may be measured.

Treatment

Traditional

FSAD treatment requires addressing underlying physiological and psychological causes. **Psychotherapy**, either individual or couples therapy, addresses emotions, communication, relationship problems, and problem-solving strategies. **Sex therapy** focuses primarily on the sexual dysfunction. However many couples experiencing sexual dysfunction develop relationship problems and can benefit from traditional psychotherapy even after sexual arousal difficulties are resolved.

The U.S. Food and Drug Administration (FDA) has approved one medical device for treating FSAD. The Eros-Clinical Therapy Device (Eros-CTD) is a small vacuum pump that fits over the clitoral area and exerts a gentle sucking action that stimulates blood flow. In clinical trials the device has proved safe and effective for increasing blood flow, sensation, and vaginal lubrication.

Drugs

Sometimes medications, such as the type or timing of an antidepressant, can be adjusted. Poor lubrication related to decreasing hormone levels associated with menopause can often be successfully treated with **hormone replacement therapy** (HRT), such as estrogen or testosterone. Nonprescription lubricating gels and hormone creams can supplement a woman's natural lubricant. These are especially useful for pre- and postmenopausal women and for those with occasional arousal difficulties.

Research is focusing on new drugs that increase blood flow to the female genitals, thereby improving lubrication. Some of these drugs are aimed at increasing nitric oxide levels, similar to the drug sildenafil (Viagra) for men.

Alternative

A type of **meditation** called mindfulness, which promotes increased awareness and acceptance, has been found to be helpful in treating FSAD, at least when practiced in the context of **group therapy**.

Home remedies

Home remedies for FSAD include:

- Kegel exercises that increase blood flow to the vulvar and vaginal tissues
- relaxation techniques
- aerobic exercise
- changing the circumstances and settings of sexual activity
- sexual activities other than vaginal intercourse
- exploring sexual techniques that increase stimulation
- experimenting with a vibrator, fantasies, or erotic movies
- couples focusing exercises to enhance intimacy, lessen anxiety, and increase arousal

Prognosis

Because of the multiple causes of FSAD individual responses to treatment vary widely. Poor lubrication related to menopause generally has a favorable prognosis. Stress-related causes of FSAD can often be resolved. However couples may need to work through relationship issues that have caused FSAD—or resulted from it—before sexual arousal improves. This process takes time and a joint commitment to problem solving.

Prevention

A healthy, well-balanced diet, adequate rest, regular gynecological exams, and seeking counseling or psychotherapy for problems can minimize the risk for sexual arousal disorder. Aerobic **exercise** and not **smoking** also can help prevent FSAD.

Resources

BOOKS

American Psychiatric Association. *Diagnostic and Statistical Manual of Mental Disorders*, 4th ed., text rev. Arlington, VA: American Psychiatric Association, 2007.

Clinton, Timothy E., and Mark R. Laaser. *The Quick-Reference Guide to Sexuality & Relationship Counseling*. Grand Rapids, MI: Baker Books, 2010.

Rowland, David, and Luca Incrocci. *Handbook of Sexual and Gender Identity Disorders*. Hoboken, NJ: John Wiley & Sons, 2008.

PERIODICALS

Brotto, Lori A., Julia R. Heiman, and Deborah L. Tolman. "Narratives of Desire in Mid-Age Women With and Without Arousal Difficulties." *Journal of Sex Research* 46, no. 5 (September 2009): 387.

Graham, Cynthia A. "The DSM Diagnostic Criteria for Female Sexual Arousal Disorder." *Archives of Sexual Behavior* 39, no. 2 (April 2010): 240.

OTHER

Editorial Staff. "Sexual Dysfunction in Women." *Family-Doctor.org*.http://familydoctor.org/online/famdocen/home/women/reproductive/sex-dys/612.printerview.html

"Female Sexual Dysfunction." *MedlinePlus*.http://www.nlm.nih.gov/medlineplus/femalesexualdysfunction.html

Mayo Clinic Staff. "Female Sexual Dysfunction." *Mayo Clinic.com*. http://www.mayoclinic.com/print/female-sexual-dysfunction/DS00701/METHOD=print&DSECTION=all

Preidt, Robert. "Study Explores Possibility of a Female Viagra." *HealthDay*. http://www.womenshealth.gov/news/english/638088.htm

"Sexual Arousal Disorders." *Merck Manuals Online Medical Library*. http://www.merck.com/mmhe/sec22/ch250/ch250e.html

"Sexual Problems Overview." *MedlinePlus*. http://www.nlm.nih.gov/medlineplus/ency/article/001951.htm

ORGANIZATIONS

American Academy of Family Physicians, 11400 Tomahawk Creek Parkway, Leawood, KS, 66211-2680, (913) 906-6000, (800) 274-6000, (913) 906-6075, http://www.aafp.org/online/en/home.html.

American Association of Sex Educators, Counselors, and Therapists, P.O. Box 1960, Ashland, VA, 23005-1960, (804) 752-0026, (804) 752-0056, aacect@aasect.org, http://www.aasect.org.

American College of Obstetricians and Gynecologists, P.O. Box 96920, Washington, DC, 20090-6920, (202) 638-5577, (800) 673-8444, resources@acog.org, http://www.acog.org.

Tish Davidson, AM
Emily Jane Willingham, PhD
Margaret Alic, PhD

Femoral hernia *see* **Hernia**

Ferritin test *see* **Iron tests**

Fetal alcohol syndrome

Definition

Fetal alcohol syndrome (FAS) is a pattern of **birth defects**, learning, and behavioral problems affecting individuals whose mothers drank alcohol during **pregnancy**.

Demographics

The occurrence FAS/FASD is independent of race, ethnicity, or gender of the individual. Individuals from different genetic backgrounds exposed to similar amounts of alcohol during pregnancy may show different symptoms of FAS. The reported rates of FAS vary widely among different populations studied depending on the degree of alcohol use within the population and the monitoring methods used. Studies by the Centers for Disease Control (CDC) show that, as of 2008, FAS occurs in 0.2 to 1.5 per 1,000 live births in different areas of the United States. FASDs are believed to occur approximately three times as often as FAS.

Description

FAS is the most severe of a range of disorders represented by the term fetal alcohol spectrum disorder (FASD). FAS/FASD is caused by exposure of a developing fetus to alcohol. FASD is used to describe individuals with some, but not all, of the features of FAS. Other terms used to describe specific types of FASD are alcohol-related neurodevelopmental disorder (ARND) and alcohol-related birth defects (ARBD).

FAS is the most common preventable cause of **mental retardation**. This condition was first recognized and reported in the medical literature in 1968 in France and in 1973 in the United States. Alcohol is a teratogen, the term used for any drug, chemical, maternal disease, or other environmental exposure that can cause birth defects or functional impairment in a developing fetus. Some features of FAS that may be present at birth include low birth weight, **prematurity**, and microcephaly. Characteristic facial features may be present at birth or may become more obvious over time. Signs of brain damage include delays in development, behavioral abnormalities, and mental retardation, but affected individuals exhibit a wide range of abilities and disabilities.

FAS is a lifelong condition. It is not curable and has serious long-term consequences. Learning, behavioral, and emotional problems are common in adolescents and adults with FAS/FASD. The costs of FAS to the American economy were estimated in 2006 as $321 million annually.

Risk factors

The only risk factor for a child to develop FAS is the consumption of alcohol by a woman who is

KEY TERMS

Cleft plate—A congenital malformation in which there is an abnormal opening in the roof of the mouth that allows the nasal passages and the mouth to be improperly connected.

IQ—Abbreviation for Intelligence Quotient. Compares an individual's mental age to his/her true or chronological age and multiplies that ratio by 100.

Microcephaly—An abnormally small head.

Miscarriage—Spontaneous pregnancy loss.

Placenta—The organ responsible for oxygen and nutrition exchange between a pregnant mother and her developing baby.

Strabismus—An improper muscle balance of the ocular muscles resulting in crossed or divergent eyes.

Teratogen—Any drug, chemical, maternal disease, or exposure that can cause physical or functional defects in an exposed embryo or fetus.

pregnant. There is no known amount of alcohol use that is safe during pregnancy, nor is there a particular stage of pregnancy during which alcohol use is safe.

Causes and symptoms

The only cause of FAS is maternal use of alcohol during pregnancy. FAS is not a genetic or inherited disorder. Alcohol consumed by the mother freely crosses the placenta and damages the developing fetus. Alcohol use by the father cannot cause FAS. Not all offspring who are exposed to alcohol during pregnancy have signs or symptoms of FAS; individuals of different genetic backgrounds may be more or less susceptible to the damage that alcohol can cause. The amount of alcohol, stage of development of the fetus, and the pattern of alcohol use create the range of symptoms that encompass FASD.

Classic features of FAS include short stature, low birth weight, poor weight gain, microcephaly, and a characteristic pattern of abnormal facial features. These facial features in infants and children may include small eye openings (measured from inner corner to outer corner), epicanthal folds (folds of tissue at the inner corner of the eye), small or short nose, low or flat nasal bridge, smooth or poorly developed philtrum (the area of the upper lip above the colored part of the lip and below the nose), thin upper lip, and small chin. Some of these features are nonspecific, meaning they can occur in other conditions, or be appropriate for age, racial, or family background.

Other major and minor birth defects that have been reported to occur in conjunction with FAS/FASD include **cleft palate**, congenital heart defects, **strabismus**, **hearing loss**, defects of the spine and joints, alteration of the hand creases, small fingernails, and toenails. Since FAS was first described in infants and children, the diagnosis is sometimes more difficult to recognize in older adolescents and adults. Short stature and microcephaly remain common features, but weight may normalize, and the individual may actually become overweight for his/her height. The chin and nose grow proportionately more than the middle part of the face, and dental crowding may become a problem. The small eye openings and the appearance of the upper lip and philtrum may continue to be characteristic. Pubertal changes typically occur at the normal time.

Newborns with FAS may have difficulty nursing due to a poor sucking response, have irregular sleep-wake cycles, decreased or increased muscle tone, seizures or **tremors**. Delays in achieving developmental milestones such as rolling over, crawling, walking, and talking may become apparent in infancy. Behavior and learning difficulties typical in the preschool or early school years include poor attention span, hyperactivity, poor motor skills, and slow language development. Attention deficit-hyperactivity disorder (**ADHD**) is often associated with FASD. Learning disabilities or mental retardation may be diagnosed during this time.

During middle school and high school years the behavioral difficulties and learning difficulties can be significant. Memory problems, poor judgment, difficulties with daily living skills, difficulties with abstract reasoning skills, and poor social skills are often apparent by this time. It is important to note that animal and human studies have shown that neurologic and behavioral abnormalities can be present without characteristic facial features. These individuals may not be identified as having FAS, but may fulfill criteria for alcohol-related neurodevelopmental disorder (ARND).

FASD continues to affect individuals into adulthood. One study looked at FAS adults and found that about 95% had mental health problems, 82% lacked the ability to live independently, 70% had problems staying employed, 60% had been in trouble with the law, and 50% of men and 70% of women were alcohol or drug abusers.

Another long-term study found that the average IQ of the group of adolescents and adults with FAS in the study was 68 (70 is lower limit of the normal range). However, the range of IQ was quite large, ranging from a low of 20 (severely retarded) to a high of 105 (normal). Academic abilities and social skills were also below normal levels. The average achievement levels for reading, spelling, and arithmetic were fourth grade, third grade, and second grade, respectively. The Vineland Adaptive Behavior Scale was used to measure adaptive functioning in these individuals. The composite score for this group showed functioning at the level of a seven-year-old. Daily living skills were at a level of nine years, and social skills were at the level of a six-year-old.

Diagnosis

In 1996, the Institute of Medicine suggested a five-level system to describe the birth defects, learning problems, and behavioral difficulties in offspring of women who drank alcohol during pregnancy. This system contains criteria including confirmation of maternal alcohol exposure, characteristic facial features, growth problems, learning and behavioral problems, and birth defects known to be associated with prenatal alcohol exposure.

FAS is a clinical diagnosis, which means that no blood, x-ray or psychological test can be performed to confirm the suspected diagnosis. The diagnosis is made based on the history of maternal alcohol use, and detailed **physical examination** for the characteristic major and minor birth defects and characteristic facial features. It is often helpful to examine siblings and parents of an individual suspected of having FAS, either in person or by photographs, to determine whether findings on the examination might be familial, of if other siblings may also be affected. Sometimes, genetic tests are performed to rule out other conditions that may present with developmental delay or birth defects. Individuals with developmental delay, birth defects, or other unusual features are often referred to a clinical geneticist, developmental pediatrician, or neurologist for evaluation and diagnosis of FAS. Psychoeducational testing to determine IQ and/or the presence of learning disabilities may also be part of the evaluation process.

Treatment

There is no cure for FAS. The disorder is irreversible. Nothing can change the physical features or brain damage associated with maternal alcohol use during the pregnancy. Children should have psychoeducational evaluation to help plan appropriate educational interventions. Common associated diagnoses such ADHD, depression, or **anxiety** can be recognized and treated. The disabilities that present during childhood persist into adult life. However, some of the behavioral problems mentioned may be avoided or lessened by early and correct diagnosis, better understanding of the life-long complications of FAS, and intervention. The goal of treatment is to help the individual affected by FAS become as independent and successful in school, employment, and social relationships as possible.

Prognosis

The prognosis for FAS/FASD depends on the severity of birth defects and the brain damage present at birth. **Miscarriage**, **stillbirth**, or **death** in the first few weeks of life may be outcomes in very severe cases. Generally individuals with FAS have a long list of mental health problems and associated social difficulties: alcohol and drug problems, inappropriate sexual behavior, problems with employment, trouble with the law, inability to live independently, and often confinement in prison, drug or alcohol treatment centers, or psychiatric institutions.

Some of the factors that have been found to reduce the risk of learning and behavioral disabilities in FAS individuals include diagnosis before the age of six years, stable and nurturing home environments, never having experienced personal violence, and referral and eligibility for disability services. Some physical birth defects associated with FAS are treatable with surgery. The long-term data help in understanding the difficulties that individuals with FAS encounter throughout their lifetime and can help families, caregivers, and professionals provide the care, supervision, education and treatment geared toward their special needs.

Prevention

FAS and FASD are completely preventable by avoiding all use of alcohol while pregnant. Prevention efforts include public education efforts aimed at the entire population, not just women of child bearing age, appropriate treatment for women with high-risk drinking habits, and increased recognition and knowledge about FAS/FASD by professionals, parents, and caregivers.

Resources

BOOKS

Golden, Janet. *Message in a Bottle: The Making of Fetal Alcohol Syndrome*. Cambridge, MA: Harvard University Press, 2006.

Kulp, Jodie. *The Best I Can Be: Living with Fetal Alcohol Syndrome—Effects*. Brooklyn Park, MN: Better Endings New Beginnings, 2006.

Lawryk, Liz. *Finding Perspective: Raising Successful Children Affected by Fetal Alcohol Spectrum Disorders*. Bragg Creek, AB (Canada): OBD Triage Institute, 2005.

Soby, Jeanette M. *Prenatal Exposure to Drugs/Alcohol: Characteristics and Educational Implications of Fetal Alcohol Syndrome and Cocaine/Polydrug Effects*, 2nd ed. Springfield, IL: Charles C Thomas, 2006.

PERIODICALS

Franklin, L., et al. "Children With Fetal Alcohol Spectrum Disorders: Problem Behaviors and Sensory Processing." *American Journal of Occupational Therapy* 62, no. 3 (May–June 2008): 265–273.

Green, J. H. "Fetal Alcohol Spectrum Disorders: Understanding the Effects of Prenatal Alcohol Exposure and Supporting Students." *Journal of School Health* 77, no. 3 (March 2007): 103–108.

OTHER

Chambers, Christine and Keith Vaux. "Fetal Alcohol Syndrome." eMedicine.com, October 20, 2006.[August 29, 2009]. http://emedicine.medscape.com/article/974016-overview

"Fetal Alcohol Syndrome." Medline Plus August 17, 2009 [August 29, 2009]. http://www.nlm.nih.gov/medlineplus/fetalalcoholsyndrome.html

"Fetal Alcohol Spectrum Disorders (FASDs)." United States Centers for Disease Control and Prevention. August 24, 2009 [August 29, 2009]. http://www.cdc.gov/ncbddd/fasd/index.html

ORGANIZATIONS

Fetal Alcohol Spectrum Disorders Center for Excellence, 2101 Gaither Rd., Suite 600, Rockville, MD, 20850, (866) STOP-FAS (786-7327), http://fasdcenter.samhsa.gov.

Fetal Alcohol Syndrome (FAS) World Canada, 250 Scarborough Golf Club Rd., Toronto, ON, Canada, M1J 3G8, (416) 264-8000, (416) 264-8222, info@fasworld.com, http://www.fasworld.com.

March of Dimes Foundation, 1275 Mamaroneck Ave. White Plains, NY, 10605, (914) 997-4488, askus@marchofdimes.com, http://www.marchofdimes.com.

National Institute on Alcohol Abuse and Alcoholism (NIAAA), 5635 Fishers Ln., MSC 9304, Bethesda, MD, 20892-9304, (301) 443-3860, http://www.niaaa.nih.gov.

National Organization on Fetal Alcohol Syndrome (NOFAS), 900 17th St., NW, Suite 910, Washington, DC, 20006, (202) 785-4585, (800) 66-NOFAS , (202) 466-6456, http://www.nofas.org.

Laurie Heron Seaver, M.D.
Tish Davidson, A.M.

Fetal death *see* **Stillbirth**

Fetal hemoglobin test

Definition

Fetal hemoglobin (Hemoglobin F), alkali-resistant hemoglobin, HBF (or Hb F), is the major hemoglobin component in the bloodstream of the fetus. After birth, it decreases rapidly until only traces are found in normal children and adults.wct 2

Purpose

The determination of fetal hemoglobin is an aid in evaluating low concentrations of hemoglobin in the blood (anemia), as well as the hereditary persistence of fetal hemoglobin, and a group of inherited disorders affecting hemoglobin, among which are the thalassemias and sickle cell anemia.

Description

At birth, the newborn's blood is comprised of 60–90% of fetal hemoglobin. The fetal hemoglobin then rapidly decreases to 2% or less after the second to fourth years. By the time of adulthood, only traces (0.5% or less) are found in the bloodstream.

In some diseases associated with abnormal hemoglobin production (see section on Hemoglobinopathy), fetal hemoglobin may persist in larger amounts. When this occurs, the elevation raises the question of possible underlying disease.

For example, HBF can be found in higher levels in hereditary hemolytic **anemias**, in all types of leukemias, in **pregnancy**, diabetes, thyroid disease, and during anticonvulsant drug therapy. It may also reappear in adults when the bone marrow is overactive, as in the disorders of **pernicious anemia**, **multiple myeloma**, and metastatic **cancer** in the marrow. When HBF is increased after age four, it should be investigated for cause.

Hemoglobinopathy

Hemoglobin is the oxygen-carrying pigment found in red blood cells. It is a large molecule made in the bone marrow from two components, heme and globin.

Defects in hemoglobin production may be either genetic or acquired. The genetic defects are further subdivided into errors of heme production (porphyria), and those of globin production (known collectively as the **hemoglobinopathies**).

Hemoglobinopathy is divided into two categories. In the first category, abnormal globin chains give rise

KEY TERMS

Anemia—A disorder characterized by a reduced blood level of hemoglobin, the oxygen-carrying pigment of blood.

Hemolytic anemia—A form of anemia caused by premature destruction of red cells in the blood stream (a process called hemolysis). Hemolytic anemias are classified according to whether the cause of the problem is inside the red blood cell (in which case it is usually an inherited condition), or outside the cell (usually acquired later in life).

to abnormal hemoglobin molecules. In the second category, normal hemoglobin chains are produced but in abnormal amounts. An example of the first category is the disorder of sickle cell anemia, the inherited condition characterized by curved (sickle-shaped) red blood cells and chronic **hemolytic anemia**. Disorders in the second category are called the thalassemias, which are further divided into types according to which amino acid chain is affected (alpha or beta), and whether there is one defective gene (**thalassemia** minor) or two defective genes (thalassemia major).

Preparation

This test requires a blood sample. The patient is not required to be in a **fasting** state (nothing to eat or drink for a period of hours before the test).

Risks

Risks for this test are minimal, but may include slight bleeding from the blood-drawing site, **fainting** or feeling lightheaded after venipuncture, or hematoma (blood accumulating under the puncture site).

Normal results

Reference values vary from laboratory to laboratory but are generally found within the following ranges:

- six months to adult: up to 2% of the total hemoglobin
- newborn to six months: up to 75% of the total hemoglobin

Abnormal results

Greater than 2% of total hemoglobin is abnormal.

Resources

BOOKS

Pagana, Kathleen Deska, and Timothy J. Pagana. *Mosby's Manual of Diagnostic and Laboratory Tests*. 4th ed. St. Louis: Mosby, 2009.

Janis O. Flores

Fetishes *see* **Sexual perversions**

Fever

Definition

A fever is any body temperature elevation over 100 °F (37.8 °C).

Description

A healthy person's body temperature fluctuates between 97 °F (36.1 °C) and 100 °F (37.8 °C), with the average being 98.6 °F (37 °C). The body maintains stability within this range by balancing the heat produced by the metabolism with the heat lost to the environment. The "thermostat" that controls this process is located in the hypothalamus, a small structure located deep within the brain. The nervous system constantly relays information about the body's temperature to the thermostat, which in turn activates different physical responses designed to cool or warm the body, depending on the circumstances. These responses include: decreasing or increasing the flow of blood from the body's core, where it is warmed, to the surface, where it is cooled; slowing down or speeding up the rate at which the body turns food into energy (metabolic rate); inducing shivering, which generates heat through muscle contraction; and inducing sweating, which cools the body through evaporation.

A fever occurs when the thermostat resets at a higher temperature, primarily in response to an infection. To reach the higher temperature, the body moves blood to the warmer interior, increases the metabolic rate, and induces shivering. The "chills" that often accompany a fever are caused by the movement of blood to the body's core, leaving the surface and extremities cold. Once the higher temperature is achieved, the shivering and chills stop. When the infection has been overcome or drugs such as **aspirin** or **acetaminophen** (Tylenol) have been taken, the thermostat resets to normal and the body's cooling

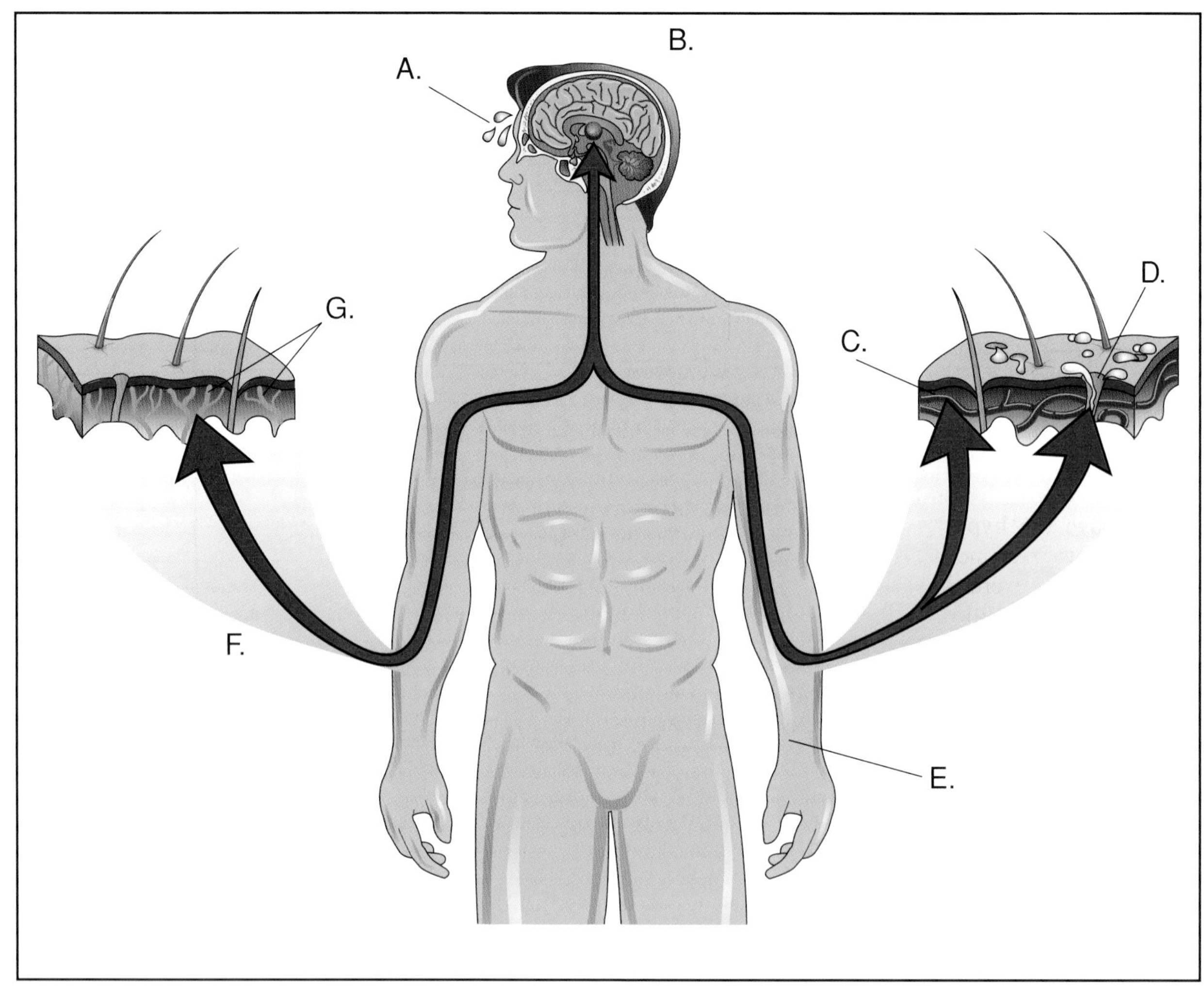

A dramatic rise in body temperature often includes the following symptoms: A. Loss of fluid results in dehydration. B. The hypothalamic set-point is increased, raising metabolism. C. Blood vessels in skin dilate. D. Sweat glands produce excess perspiration. E. Increased pulse rate. F. Increased hypothalmic set-point may introduce chills and shivering to promote heat production from muscles. G. Skin becomes more heat-sensitive. *(Illustration by Electronic Illustrators Group. Reproduced by permission of Gale, a part of Cengage Learning.)*

mechanisms switch on: the blood moves to the surface and sweating occurs.

Fever is an important component of the immune response, though its role is not completely understood. Physicians believe that an elevated body temperature has several effects. The immune system chemicals that react with the fever-inducing agent and trigger the resetting of the thermostat also increase the production of cells that fight off the invading bacteria or viruses. Higher temperatures also inhibit the growth of some bacteria, while at the same time speeding up the chemical reactions that help the body's cells repair themselves. In addition, the increased heart rate that may accompany the changes in blood circulation also speeds the arrival of white blood cells to the sites of infection.

Causes and symptoms

Fevers are primarily caused by viral or bacterial infections, such as **pneumonia** or **influenza**. However, other conditions can induce a fever, including allergic reactions; autoimmune diseases; trauma, such as breaking a bone; **cancer**; excessive exposure to the sun; intense **exercise**; hormonal imbalances; certain drugs; and damage to the hypothalamus. When an infection occurs, fever-inducing agents called pyrogens are released, either by the body's immune system or by the invading cells themselves, that trigger the resetting of the thermostat. In other circumstances, the immune system may overreact (allergic reactions) or become damaged (autoimmune diseases), causing the uncontrolled release of pyrogens. A **stroke** or tumor

KEY TERMS

Antipyretic—A drug that lowers fever, like aspirin or acetaminophen.

Autoimmune disease—Condition in which a person's immune system attacks the body's own cells, causing tissue destruction.

Febrile seizure—Convulsions brought on by fever.

Malignant hyperthermia—A rare, inherited condition in which a person develops a very high fever when given certain anesthetics or muscle relaxants in preparation for surgery.

Meningitis—A potentially fatal inflammation of the thin membrane covering the brain and spinal cord.

Metabolism—The chemical process by which the body turns food into energy, which can be given off as heat.

Pyrogen—A chemical circulating in the blood that causes a rise in body temperature.

Reye's syndrome—A disorder principally affecting the liver and brain, marked by the rapid development of life-threatening neurological symptoms.

can damage the hypothalamus, causing the body's thermostat to malfunction. Excessive exposure to the sun or intensely exercising in hot weather can result in heat stroke, a condition in which the body's cooling mechanisms fail. Malignant hyperthermia is a rare, inherited condition in which a person develops a very high fever when given certain anesthetics or **muscle relaxants** in preparation for surgery.

How long a fever lasts and how high it may go depends on several factors, including its cause, the age of the patient, and his or her overall health. Most fevers caused by infections are acute, appearing suddenly and then dissipating as the immune system defeats the infectious agent. An infectious fever may also rise and fall throughout the day, reaching its peek in the late afternoon or early evening. A low-grade fever that lasts for several weeks is associated with autoimmune diseases such as lupus or with some cancers, particularly leukemia and lymphoma.

Diagnosis

A fever is usually diagnosed using a thermometer. A variety of different thermometers are available, including traditional glass and mercury ones used for oral or rectal temperature readings and more sophisticated electronic ones that can be inserted in the ear to quickly register the body's temperature. For adults and older children, temperature readings are usually taken orally. Younger children who cannot or will not hold a thermometer in their mouths can have their temperature taken by placing an oral thermometer under their armpit. Infants generally have their temperature taken rectally using a rectal thermometer.

As important as registering a patient's temperature is determining the underlying cause of the fever. The presence or absence of accompanying symptoms, a patient's medical history, and information about what he or she may have ingested, any recent trips taken, or possible exposures to illness help the physician make a diagnosis. Blood tests can aid in identifying an infectious agent by detecting the presence of antibodies against it or providing samples for growth of the organism in a culture. Blood tests can also provide the doctor with white blood cell counts. Ultrasound tests, **magnetic resonance imaging** (MRI) tests, or computed tomography (CT) scans may be ordered if the doctor cannot readily determine the cause of a fever.

Treatment

Physicians agree that the most effective treatment for a fever is to address its underlying cause, such as through the administration of **antibiotics**. Also, because a fever helps the immune system fight infection, it usually should be allowed to run its course. Drugs to lower fever (antipyretics) can be given if a patient (particularly a child) is uncomfortable. These include aspirin, acetaminophen (Tylenol), and ibuprofin (Advil). Aspirin, however, should not be given to a child or adolescent with a fever since this drug has been linked to an increased risk of **Reye's syndrome**. Bathing a patient in cool water can also help alleviate a high fever.

A fever requires emergency treatment under the following circumstances:

- newborn (three months or younger) with a fever higher than 100.5 °F (38 °C)
- infant or child with a fever higher than 103 °F (39.4 °C)
- fever accompanied by severe headache, neck stiffness, mental confusion, or severe swelling of the throat

A very high fever in a small child can trigger seizures (febrile seizures) and therefore should be treated immediately. A fever accompanied by the listed symptoms can indicate the presence of a serious infection, such as **meningitis**, and should be brought to the immediate attention of a physician.

Prognosis

Most fevers caused by infection end as soon as the immune system rids the body of the pathogen and do not produce any lasting effects. The prognosis for fevers associated with more chronic conditions, such as autoimmune disease, depends upon the overall outcome of the disorder.

Resources

BOOKS

Fauci, Anthony S., et al., eds. *Harrison's Principles of Internal Medicine*. 17th ed. New York: McGraw-Hill Professional, 2008.

Bridget Travers

Fever blister *see* **Cold sore**

Fever evaluation tests

Definition

Fever evaluation tests, better known as febrile agglutinins tests, are performed to detect the presence of antibodies in the blood that are sensitive to temperature changes. Antibodies are proteins produced by the immune system in response to specific infectious agents, such as viruses or bateria. Febrile agglutinins are antibodies that cause red blood cells to clump, but only when the blood is warmed to temperatures higher than the average body temperature of 98.6 °F (37 °C).

Purpose

The febrile agglutinins test is used to confirm the diagonsis of certain infectious diseases that stimulate the body to produce febrile agglutinins. The disease most commonly diagnosed by this test is **brucellosis**, a infection caused by bacteria belonging to the genus *Brucella* and characterized by intermittent fever, sweating, chills, aches, and mental depression. The test is also used to diagnose certain other infectious diseases: salmonellosis, caused by *Salmonella* bacteria and marked by **nausea** and severe **diarrhea**; rickettsial infections, a group of diseases caused by the bacteria *Rickettsia*; and **tularemia**, also called rabbit fever, a bacterial infection characterized by a high fever and swollen lymph nodes. The febrile agglutinins test can also be used to confirm the presence of two types of **cancer**, leukemia and lymphoma; however, doctors rarely use the test for this purpose, since other diagnostic tests are more reliable.

Description

A febrile agglutinins test can be performed at a doctor's office or a hospital. A nurse or technician will collect a few drops of blood (about 7 mL) in a small tube that has been cooled slightly. The specimen is then taken to a laboratory where it heated and examined for clumping. If the cells clump after warming and unclump as they cool, a febrile agglutinin titer (concentration) of greater than 1:80 is present.

Normal results

The results of febrile agglutinins tests require a doctor's interpretation. In general, however, a normal value is lower than 1:32.

Abnormal results

A value higher than 1:80 suggests a diagnosis for brucellosis or one of the other conditions indicated by this test.

Jill S. Lasker

Fever of unknown origin

Definition

Fever of unknown origin (FUO) refers to the presence of a documented fever for a specified time, for which a cause has not been found after a basic medical evaluation. The classic criteria developed in 1961 included: temperature greater than 101 °F (38.3 °C) for at least three weeks, and inability to find a cause after one week of study. Within the past decade, a revision has been proposed that categorizes FUO into classic, hospital acquired FUO, FUO associated with low white blood counts, and HIV associated FUO (**AIDS** related).

Description

Fever is a natural response of the body that helps in fighting off foreign substances, such as microorganisms, toxins, etc. Body temperature is set by the thermoregulatory center, located in an area in the brain called hypothalamus. Body temperature is not constant all day, but actually is lowest at 6 a.m. and highest around 4–6 p.m. In addition, temperature varies in different regions of the body; for example, rectal and urine temperatures are about one degree Fahrenheit higher than oral temperature and rectal temperature is higher than urine. It is also important to realize that certain normal conditions can effect body temperature, such as **pregnancy**, food ingestion, age, and certain hormonal changes.

Substances that cause fever are known as "pyrogens." Pyrogens come in two types: exogenous and endogenous. Those that originate outside the body, such as bacterial toxins, are called "exogenous" pyrogens. Pyrogens formed by the body's own cells in response to an outside stimulus (such as a bacterial toxin) are called "endogenous" pyrogens.

Researchers have discovered that there are several endogenous pyrogens. These are made up of small groups of amino acids, the building blocks of proteins. These natural pyrogens have other functions in addition to inducing fever; they have been named "cytokines." When cytokines are injected into humans, fever and chills develop within an hour. Interferon, tumor necrosis factor, and various interleukins are the major fever producing cytokines.

The production of fever is a very complex process. Somehow, these cytokines cause the thermoregulatory center in the hypothalamus to reset the normal temperature level. The body's initial response is to conserve heat by vasoconstriction, a process in which blood vessels narrow and prevent heat loss from the skin and elsewhere. This alone will raise temperature by two to three degrees. Certain behavioral activities also occur, such as adding more clothes, seeking a warmer environment, etc. If the hypothalamus requires more heat, then shivering occurs.

Fever is a body defense mechanism. It has been shown that one of the effects of temperature increase is to slow bacterial growth. However, fever also has some downsides: The body's metabolic rate is increased and with it, oxygen consumption. This can have a devastating effect on those with poor circulation. In addition, fever can lead to seizures in the very young.

When temperature elevation occurs for an extended period of time and no cause is found, the term FUO is then used. The far majority of these patients are eventually found to have one of several diseases.

Causes and symptoms

The most frequent cause of FUO is still infection, though the percentage has decreased in recent years. **Tuberculosis** remains an important cause, especially when it occurs outside the lungs. The decrease in infections as a cause of FUO is due in part to improved culture techniques. In addition, technological advances have made it easier to diagnose non-infectious causes. For example, tumors and autoimmune diseases in particular are now easier to diagnose. (An autoimmune disease is one that arises when the body tolerance for its own cell antigenic cell markers disappears.)

Allergies to medications can also cause prolonged fever; sometimes patients will have other symptoms suggesting an allergic reaction, such as a rash.

FUO has many possible causes. Generally though, a diagnosis can be found. About 10% of patients will wind up without a definite cause, and about the same percentage have "factitious fevers" (either self-induced or no fever at all).

Some general symptoms tend to occur along with fever. These are called constitutional symptoms and consist of myalgias (muscle aches), chills, and **headache**.

Diagnosis

Few symptoms in medicine present such a diagnostic challenge as fever. Nonetheless, if a careful, logical, and thorough evaluation is performed, a diagnosis will be found in most cases. The patient's past medical history as well as travel, social, and family history should be carefully searched for important clues.

Usually the first step is to search for an infectious cause. Skin and other screening tests for diseases such as tuberculosis, and examination of blood, urine, and stool, are generally indicated. Antibody levels to a number of infectious agents can be measured; if these are rising, they may point to an active infection.

Various x-ray studies are also of value. In addition to standard examinations, recently developed radiological techniques using ultrasound, computed tomography scan (CT scan) and **magnetic resonance imaging** (MRI) scans are now available. These enable physicians to examine areas that were once accessible only through surgery. Furthermore, new studies using radioactive materials (nuclear medicine), can detect areas of infection and inflammation previously almost impossible to find, even with surgery.

Biopsies of any suspicious areas found on an x-ray exam can be performed by either traditional or newer surgical techniques. Material obtained by biopsy is then

KEY TERMS

AIDS—Acquired immune deficiency syndrome is often represented by these initials. The disease is associated with infection by the human immunodeficiency virus (HIV), and has the main feature of repeated infections, due to failure of certain parts of the immune system. Infection by HIV damages part of the body's natural immunity, and leads to recurrent illnesses.

Antibiotic—A medication that is designed to kill or weaken bacteria.

Computed tomography scan (CT Scan)—A specialized x-ray procedure in which cross-sections of the area in question can be examined in detail. This allows physicians to examine organs such as the pancreas, bile ducts, and others which are often the site of hidden infections.

Magnetic Resonance Imaging (MRI)—This technique is similar to CT Scan, but based on the magnetic properties of various areas of the body to compose images.

NSAID—Nonsteroidal anti-inflammatory drugs are medications such as aspirin and ibuprofen that decrease pain and inflammation. Many can now be obtained without a doctor's prescription.

Ultrasound—A non-invasive procedure based on changes in sound waves of a frequency that cannot be heard, but respond to changes in tissue composition. It is very useful for diagnosing diseases of the gallbladder, liver, and hidden infections, such as abscesses.

examined by a pathologist to look for clues as to the cause of the fever. Evidence of infection, tumor or other diseases can be found in this way. Portions of the biopsy are also sent to the laboratory for culture in an attempt to grow and identify an infectious organism.

Patients with HIV are an especially difficult problem, as they often suffer from many unusual infections. HIV itself is a potential cause of fever.

Treatment

Most patients who undergo evaluation for FUO do not receive treatment until a clear-cut cause is found. **Antibiotics** or medications designed to suppress a fever (such as NSAIDs) will only hide the true cause. Once physicians are satisfied that the fever has no infectious cause, they may use medications such as NSAIDs, or **corticosteroids** to decrease inflammation and diminish constitutional symptoms.

The development of FUO in certain settings, such as that acquired by patients in the hospital or in those with a low white blood count, often needs rapid treatment to avoid serious complications. Therefore, in these instances patients may be placed on antibiotics after a minimal number of diagnostic studies. Once test results are known, treatment can be adjusted as needed.

Prognosis

The outlook for patients with FUO depends on the cause of the fever. If the basic illness is easily treatable and can be found rather quickly, the potential for a cure is quite good. Some patients continue with temperature elevations for six months or more. If no serious disease is found, medications such as NSAIDs are used to decrease the effects of the fever. Careful follow-up and reevaluation is recommended in these cases.

Resources

BOOKS

Fauci, Anthony S., et al., eds.*Harrison's Principles of Internal Medicine*. 17th ed. New York: McGraw–Hill Professional, 2008.

David Kaminstein, MD

Fiber-modified diet *see* **Diets**

Fibrin degradation products *see* **Fibrin split products**

Fibrin split products

Definition

Fibrin split products (FSP) are fragments of protein released from a dissolving clot. The fibrin split products test is one of several tests done to evaluate a person with blood-clotting problems (coagulation), particularly disseminated intravascular coagulation (DIC).

KEY TERMS

Coagulation—The entire process of blood clotting.

Coagulation cascade—A sequence of biochemical activities to stop bleeding by forming a clot.

Disseminated intravascular coagulation (DIC)—A serious medical condition that develops when the normal balance between bleeding and clotting is disturbed. Excessive bleeding and clotting injures body organs, and causes anemia or death.

Fibrin split products (FSP)—Pieces of the protein fibrin released from a dissolving clot.

Fibrinolysis—The clot dissolving portion of the coagulation process.

Titer—A dilution of a substance with an exact known amount of fluid. For example, one part of serum diluted with four parts of saline is a titer of 1:4.

Purpose

High levels of FSP in a person's blood are associated with DIC, a serious medical condition that develops when the normal balance between bleeding and clotting is disturbed. Excessive bleeding and clotting injures body organs, and causes anemia or **death**.

Description

Coagulation begins typically with an injury to some part of the body. The injury sets in motion a cascade of biochemical activities (the coagulation cascade) to stop the bleeding, by forming a clot from a mixture of the blood protein fibrin and platelets.

Once bleeding is stopped, another blood protein dissolves the clot by breaking down the fibrin into fragments. Measurement of these fragments gives information about the clot-dissolving portion of coagulation, called fibrinolysis.

In DIC, the coagulation cascade is triggered in an abnormal way. A blood infection, a **transfusion** reaction, a large amount of tissue damage, such as a burn, a dead fetus, and some cancers can begin the chain of biochemical events leading to **blood clots**. The coagulation cascade becomes overwhelmed with excessive clotting followed by excessive bleeding. As the large number of clots dissolve, fibrin split products accumulate in the blood and encourage even more bleeding.

Laboratory tests for FSP are done on the yellow liquid portion left over after blood clots (serum). A person's serum is mixed with a substance that binds to FSP. This bound complex is measured, and the original amount of FSP is determined. Some test methods give an actual measurement of FSP; some give a titer, or dilution. Methods that provide a titer look for the presence or absence of FSP. If the serum is positive for FSP, the serum is diluted, or titered, and the test is done again. These steps are repeated until the serum is so dilute that it no longer gives a positive result. The last dilution that gives a positive result is the titer reported.

The FSP test is covered by insurance when medically necessary. Results are usually available within one to two hours. Other names for this test are fibrin degradation products, fibrin breakdown products, or FDP.

Preparation

This test requires 0.17 oz (5/14m) of blood. A healthcare worker ties a tourniquet on the patient's upper arm, locates a vein in the inner elbow region, and inserts a needle into that vein. Vacuum action draws the blood through the needle into an attached tube. Collection of the sample takes only a few minutes.

Aftercare

Discomfort or bruising may occur at the puncture site. Pressure applied to the puncture site until the bleeding stops reduces bruising. Warm packs to the puncture site relieve discomfort. The patient may feel dizzy or faint.

Risks

People with coagulation problems may bleed longer than normal. The healthcare provider must make sure bleeding has stopped before leaving the patient unattended.

Normal results

Negative at a less than or equal to 1:4 dilution or less than 10 g/mL.

Abnormal results

High levels of FSP indicate DIC. Results of the test must be interpreted by the physician according to the person's clinical symptoms and medical history. Other conditions that increase blood clotting activity also increase FSP: venous thrombosis, surgery and transplants, blood clots in the lung, certain cancers, and **heart attack** (myocardial infarction).

Resources

BOOKS

McPherson, Richard A., Matthew R Pincus, and John Bernard Henry.*Henry's Clinical Diagnosis and Management by Laboratory Methods*. Philadelphia: Saunders/ Elsevier, 2007.

Nancy J. Nordenson

Fibrinogen test

Definition

Fibrinogen (Factor I) is a protein that originates in the liver. It is converted to fibrin during the blood-clotting process (coagulation).

Purpose

The fibrinogen test aids in the diagnosis of suspected clotting or bleeding disorders caused by fibrinogen abnormalities.

Precautions

This test is not recommended for patients with active bleeding, acute infection or illness, or in those patients who have received blood transfusions within four weeks.

Drugs that may increase fibrinogen levels include estrogens and **oral contraceptives**. Drugs that may cause decreased levels include anabolic **steroids**, androgens, phenobarbital, urokinase, streptokinase, and valproic acid.

Description

Fibrinogen plays two essential roles in the body: It is a protein called an acute-phase reactant that becomes elevated with tissue inflammation or tissue destruction, and it is also a vital part of the "common pathway" of the coagulation process.

In order for blood to clot, fibrinogen must be converted to fibrin by the action of an enzyme called thrombin. Fibrin molecules clump together to form long filaments, which trap blood cells to form a solid clot.

The conversion of fibrinogen to fibrin is the last step of the "coagulation cascade," a series of reactions in the blood triggered by tissue injury and platelet activation. With each step in the cascade, a coagulation factor in the blood is converted from an inactive to an active form. The active form of the factor then activates several molecules of the next factor in the series, and so on, until the final step, when fibrinogen is converted into fibrin.

The factors involved in the coagulation cascade are numbered I, II, and V through XIII. Factor I is fibrinogen, while factor II (fibrinogen's immediate precursor) is called prothrombin. Most of the coagulation factors are made in the liver, which needs an adequate supply of vitamin K to manufacture the different clotting factors.

When fibrinogen acts as an "acute-phase reactant," it rises sharply during tissue inflammation or injury. When this occurs, high fibrinogen levels may be a predictor for an increased risk of heart or circulatory disease. Other conditions in which fibrinogen is elevated are cancers of the stomach, breast, or kidney, and inflammatory disorders like **rheumatoid arthritis**.

Reduced fibrinogen levels can be found in **liver disease**, **prostate cancer**, lung disease, bone marrow lesions, malnourishment, and certain bleeding disorders. The low levels can be used to evaluate disseminated intravascular coagulation (DIS), a serious medical condition that develops when there is a disturbed balance between bleeding and clotting. Other conditions related to decreased fibrinogen levels are those in which fibrinogen is completely absent (congenital afibrinogenemia), conditions in which levels are low (hypofibrinogenemia), and conditions of abnormal fibrinogen (dysfibrinogenemia). Obstetric complications or trauma may also cause low levels. Large-volume blood transfusions cause low levels because banked blood does not contain fibrinogen.

Preparation

This test is performed with a blood sample, which can be drawn at any time of day. The patient does not have to be **fasting** (nothing to eat or drink).

Aftercare

Because a fibrinogen test is often ordered when a bleeding disorder is suspected, the patient should apply pressure or a pressure dressing to the blood-drawn site site for a period of time after blood is drawn, and then reexamine the site for bleeding.

KEY TERMS

Fibrin—The last step in the coagulation process. Fibrin forms strands that add bulk to a forming blood clot to hold it in place and help "plug" an injured blood vessel wall.

Platelet—An irregularly shaped cell-like particle in the blood that is an important part of blood clotting. Platelets are activated when an injury causes a blood vessel to break. They change shape from round to spiny, "sticking" to the broken vessel wall and to each other to begin the clotting process.

Prothrombin—A type of protein called a glycoprotein that is converted to thrombin during the clotting process.

Thrombin—An enzyme that converts fibrinogen into strands of fibrin.

Risks

Risks for this test are minimal, but may include slight bleeding from the blood-drawing site, **fainting** or feeling lightheaded after procedure, or the seeing the accumulation of blood under the puncture site (hematoma).

Normal results

Normal reference ranges are laboratory-specific, but are usually within the following:

- adult: 200 mg/dL–400 mg/dL
- newborn: 125 mg/dL–300 mg/dL

Abnormal results

Spontaneous bleeding can occur with values less than 100 mg/dL.

Resources

BOOKS

Pagana, Kathleen Deska, and Timothy J. Pagana. *Mosby's Manual of Diagnostic and Laboratory Tests*. 4th ed. St. Louis: Mosby, 2009.

Janis O. Flores

Fibroadenoma

Definition

Fibroadenomas are benign breast tumors commonly found in young women. Fibroadenoma means "a tumor composed of glandular (related to gland) and fibrous (containing fibers) tissues."

Description

Breast fibroadenomas, abnormal growths of glandular and fibrous tissues, are most common between the ages of 15 and 30, and are found in 10% of all women (20% of African-American women). They are found rarely in postmenopausal women.

Described as feeling like marbles, these firm, round, movable, and "rubbery" lumps range from 1–5 cm in size. Giant fibroadenomas are larger, lemon-sized lumps. Usually single, from 10–15% of women have more than one.

While some types of breast lumps come and go during the menstrual cycle, fibroadenomas typically do not disappear after a woman's period, and should be checked by a doctor.

Causes and symptoms

The cause of breast fibroadenomas is unknown. They may be dependent upon estrogen, because they are common in premenopausal women, can be found in postmenopausal women taking estrogen, and because they grow larger in pregnant women.

Fibroadenomas usually cause no symptoms and may be discovered during **breast self-examination**, or during a routine check-up.

Diagnosis

When the doctor takes a complete medical history, they will ask when the lump was first noticed, if there were any symptoms or changes in lump size, and if there is any personal or family history of breast disease.

The doctor thoroughly feels the breasts (palpates). Tests are done, usually including **mammography** or ultrasound scans, or surgical removal of cells or tissue for examination under a the microscope (biopsy).

KEY TERMS

Aspiration—To withdraw material with a needle and syringe.

Biopsy—To remove cells or tissue for microscopic examination.

Estrogen—Female sex hormone produced by the ovaries.

Diagnostic tests include:

- mammogram, an x-ray examination of the breast
- ultrasound scan, a technique that uses sound waves to display a two-dimensional image of the breast, showing whether a lump is solid or fluid-filled (cystic)
- fine-needle aspiration biopsy, a minor procedure wherein fluid or cells are drawn out of the lump through a small needle (aspirated)
- core biopsy, a procedure wherein a larger piece of tissue is withdrawn from the lump through a larger needle
- incisional biopsy, a surgical procedure wherein a piece of the lump is removed through an cut (incision)
- excisional biopsy, a surgical procedure wherein the entire lump is removed through an cut (incision)

Most insurance plans cover the costs of diagnosing and treating fibroadenomas.

Treatment

Performed usually in outpatient settings, breast fibroadenomas are removed by **lumpectomy**, or surgical excision under local or **general anesthesia**. Sometimes lumps in younger women are not removed but are monitored by self-examination, yearly doctor check-ups, and mammograms. Surgery is generally recommended for women over 30, and for lumps that are painful or enlarging.

Alternative treatment

Alternative treatments for breast fibroadenomas include a low-fat, high-fiber, vegetarian-type diet; a reduction in **caffeine** intake; supplementation with evening primrose oil (*Oenothera biennis*), flax oil, or fish oil and **vitamins** E and C; and the application of hot compresses to the breast. In addition, a focus on liver cleansing is important to assist the body in conjugation and elimination of excess estrogens. Botanical remedies can be useful in hormone balancing, as can **acupuncture** and homeopathy. Massaging the breasts with castor oil, straight or infused with herbs or essential oils, can help fibroadenomas reduce and dissipate, as well as keep women in touch with changes in their breast tissue.

Prognosis

Breast fibroadenomas are not cancerous. The lumps recur in up to 20% of women. A small number of lumps disappear on their own.

Prevention

Breast fibroadenomas cannot be prevented. They can be discovered early by regular breast self-examination.

ORGANIZATIONS

American College of Obstetricians and Gynecologists (ACOG), P.O. Box 96920, Washington, DC, 20090-6920, (202) 638-5577, http://www.acog.org.

Mercedes McLaughlin

Fibrocystic breast disease *see* **Fibrocystic condition of the breast**

Fibrocystic condition of the breast

Definition

Fibrocystic condition of the breast is a term that may refer to a variety of symptoms: breast lumpiness or tenderness, microscopic breast tissue, and/or the x-ray or ultrasound picture of the breast. It has been called a "wastebasket" diagnosis because a wide range of vaguely defined benign breast conditions may be labeled as fibrocystic condition. It is not a **cancer**, and the majority of types of fibrocystic conditions do not increase the risk of **breast cancer**.

Description

There is no such thing as a normal or typical female breast. Breasts come in all shapes and sizes, with varying textures from smooth to extremely lumpy. The tissues of the female breast change in response to hormone levels, normal **aging**, nursing (**lactation**), weight fluctuations, and injury. To further complicate matters, the breast has several types of tissue; each of these tissue types may respond differently to changes in body chemistry.

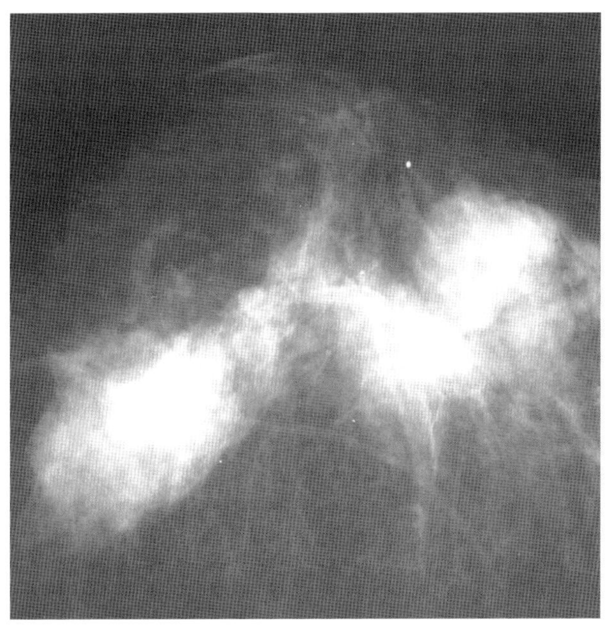

A mammogram of a female breast indicating multiple cysts. *(Custom Medical Stock Photo, Inc. Reproduced by permission.)*

Fibrocystic breast condition may be called fibrocystic disease, although it is clearly not a single, specific disease process. Variations or changes in the way the breast feels or looks on x-ray may cause the condition to be called "fibrocystic change." Other names have been used to refer to this imprecise and ill-defined term: mammary dysplasia, mastopathy, chronic cystic **mastitis**, indurative mastopathy, mastalgia, lumpy breasts, or physiologic nodularity.

Estimates vary, but 40–90% of all women have some evidence of "fibrocystic" condition, change, or disease. It is most common among women between the ages 30 and 50, but may be seen at other ages.

Causes and symptoms

Fibrocystic condition of the breast refers to technical findings on diagnostic testing (signs); however, this discussion focuses on symptoms that may fall under the general category of the fibrocystic condition. First, a brief review of the structure and function of the breast may be useful.

The breast is not supposed to be a soft, smooth organ. It is actually a type of sweat gland. Milk, the breasts' version of sweat, is secreted when the breast receives appropriate hormonal and environmental stimulation.

The normal breast contains milk glands, with their accompanying ducts, or pipelines, for transporting the milk. These complex structures may not only alter in size, but can increase or decrease in number as needed. Fibrous connective tissue, fatty tissue, nerves, blood and lymph vessels, and lymph nodes, with their different shapes and textures, lie among the ever-changing milk glands. It is no wonder that a woman's breasts may not feel uniform in texture and that the "lumpiness" may wax and wane.

The fibrocystic condition refers to the tenderness, enlargement, and/or changing "lumpiness" that many women encounter just before or during their menstrual periods. At this time, female hormones are preparing the breasts for **pregnancy**, by stimulating the milk-producing cells, and storing fluid. Each breast may contain as much as three to six teaspoons of excess fluid. Swelling, with increased sensitivity or **pain**, may result. If pregnancy does not occur, the body reabsorbs the fluid, and the engorgement and discomfort are relieved.

Symptoms of fibrocystic breast condition range from mildly annoying in some women to extremely painful in others. The severity of discomfort may vary from month to month in the same woman. Although sometimes distressing, this experience is the body's normal response to routine hormonal changes.

This cycle of breast sensitivity, pain and/or enlargement, can also result from medications. Some hormone replacement therapies (estrogen and progesterone) used for postmenopausal women can produce these effects. Other medications, primarily, but not exclusively those with hormones may also provoke these symptoms.

Breast pain unrelated to hormone shifts is called "noncyclic" pain. "Trigger-zone breast pain" is a term that may also be used to describe this area-specific pain. This type of pain may be continuous, or it may be felt intermittently. Trauma, such as a blow to the chest area, a prior **breast biopsy**, or sensitivity to certain medications may also underlie this type of pain. Fibrocystic condition of the breast may be cited as the cause of otherwise unexplained breast pain.

Lumps, apart from those clearly associated with hormone cycles, may also be placed under the heading of fibrocystic condition. These lumps stand out from enlarged general breast tissue. Although noncancerous lumps may occur, the obvious concern with such lumps is cancer.

Noncancerous breast lumps include:

- Adenosis. This condition refers to the enlargement of breast lobules, which contain a greater number of glands than usual. If a group of lobules are found near each other, the affected area may be large enough to be felt.

- Cysts. These are fluid-filled sacs in the breast and probably develop as ducts that become clogged with old cells in the process of normal emptying and filling. Cysts usually feel soft and round or oval. However, a cyst deep within the breast may feel hard, as it pushes up against firmer breast tissue. A woman with a cyst may experience pain, especially if it increases in size before her menstrual cycle, as is often the case. Women between the age of 30 and 50 are most likely to develop cysts.
- Epithelial hyperplasia. Also called proliferative breast disease, this condition refers to an overgrowth of cells lining either the ducts or the lobules.
- Fibroadenomas. These are tumors that form in the tissues outside the milk ducts. The cause of fibroadenomas is unknown. They generally feel smooth and firm, with a somewhat rubber-like texture. Typically a fibroadenoma is not attached to surrounding tissue and moves slightly when touched. They are most commonly found in adolescents and women in their early 20s but can occur at any age.
- Fibrosis. Sometimes one area of breast tissue persistently feels thicker or more prominent than the rest of the breast. This feeling may be caused by old hardened scar tissue and/or dead fat tissue as a result of surgery or trauma. Often the cause of this type of breast tissue is unknown.
- Miscellaneous disorders. A number of other benign (noncancerous) breast problems may be placed under the heading of "fibrocystic condition." These problems include disorders that may lead to breast inflammation (mastitis), infection, and/or nipple discharge.

Atypical ductal hyperplasia

Known as atypical ductal hyperplasia (ADH), this is a condition in which the cells lining the milk ducts of the breast are growing abnormally. This condition may appear as spots of **calcium** salts, or calcifications, on the mammogram. A biopsy removed from the breast would confirm the diagnosis. Atypical ductal hyperplasia is not a cancer. In most women, this condition will cause no problems. However, for some women, especially women with family histories of breast cancer, the risk of developing breast cancer is increased. (One study with more than 3,000 female participants indicated that about 20% of the participants who had atypical hyperplasia and a family history of breast cancer, developed breast cancer, as compared to the 8% of participants who developed the disease with atypical hyperplasia and no family history of breast cancer.) For women with ADH and a family history of breast cancer, more frequent mammograms and closer monitoring may be required.

Diagnosis

Breast cancer is the most common concern of women who feel a breast lump or experience an abnormal breast symptom. For peace of mind, and to rule out any possibility of cancer, any newly discovered breast lumps should be brought to the attention of a family physician or an obstetrician-gynecologist. He or she will obtain a history and conduct thorough **physical examination** of the area. Depending on the findings of the physical examination, the patient is usually referred for tests. The most common of these tests include:

- Mammography. A mammogram is an x-ray examination of the breasts. The two major types of abnormalities doctors look for are masses and calcifications; either abnormality may be benign or malignant. The size, shape, and edges of these masses help doctors determine whether or not cancer is present. Sometimes, however, this test may be difficult to interpret, however, due to dense breast tissue.
- Ultrasonography. If a suspicious lump is detected during mammography, an ultrasound (the use of high-frequency sound waves to outline the shape of various organs and tissues in the body) is useful (although not definitive) in distinguishing benign from cancerous growths.
- Ductography. A ductogram (also called a galactogram) is a test that is sometimes useful in evaluating nipple discharge. A very fine tube is threaded into the opening of the duct onto the nipple. A small amount of dye is injected, outlining the shape of the duct on an x-ray, and indicates whether or not there is a mass in the duct.
- Biopsy. If a lump cannot be proven benign by mammography and ultrasound, a breast biopsy may be considered. Usually a tissue sample is removed through a needle (fine-needle aspiration biopsy, or FNAB) to obtain a sample of the lump. The sample is examined under the microscope by a pathologist, and a detailed diagnosis regarding the type of benign lesion or cancer is established. In some cases, however, FNAB may not provide a clear diagnosis, and another type of biopsy (such as a surgical biopsy, core-needle biopsy, or other stereotactic biopsy methods—such as the mammotome or advanced breast biopsy instrument) may be required.

Other breast conditions such as inflammation or infection are usually recognized on the basis of suspicious history, **breastfeeding**, or characteristic

KEY TERMS

Advanced Breast Biopsy Instrument (ABBI)—Uses a rotating circular knife and thin heated electrical wire to remove a large cylinder of abnormal breast tissue.

Lobules—A small lobe or subdivision of a lobe (often on a gland) that may be seen on the surface of the gland by bumps or bulges.

Lymph nodes—Rounded, encapsulated bodies consisting of an accumulation of lymphatic tissue.

Mammotome—A method for removing breast biopsies using suction to draw tissue into an opening in the side of a cylinder inserted into the breast tissue. A rotating knife then cuts tissue samples from the rest of the breast; also known as a vacuum-assisted biopsy.

Stereotactic biopsy—A biopsy taken by precisely locating areas of abnormal growth through the use of delicate instruments.

symptoms such as pain, redness, and swelling. A positive response to appropriate therapies often confirms the diagnosis.

Treatment

Once a specific disorder within the broad category of fibrocystic condition is identified, treatment can be prescribed. There are a number of treatment options for women with a lump that has been diagnosed as benign. If it is not causing a great deal of pain, the growth may be left in the breast. However, some women may choose to have a lump, such as a **fibroadenoma**, surgically removed, especially if it is large. Another option to relieve the discomfort of a painful benign lump is to have the cyst suctioned, or drained. If there is any uncertainty regarding diagnosis, the fluid may be sent to the lab for analysis.

Symptoms of cycle breast sensitivity and engorgement may also be treated with diet, medication, and/or physical modifications. For example,

- Although no scientific data is available to support this claim, many women have reported relief of symptoms when caffeine was reduced or eliminated from their diets. Decreasing salt before and during the period when breasts are most sensitive may also ease swelling and discomfort. Low-fat diets and elimination of dairy products also appear to decrease soreness for some women. However, it may take several months to realize the effects of these various treatments.
- Over-the-counter analgesics such as acetaminophen (Tylenol) or ibuprofen (Advil) may be recommended. In some cases, treatment with prescription drugs such as hormones or hormone blockers may prove successful. Oral contraceptives may also be prescribed.
- Warm soaks or ice packs may provide comfort. A well-fitted support bra can minimize physical movement and do much to relieve breast discomfort. Breast massage may promote removal of excess fluid from tissues and alleviate symptoms. Massaging the breast with castor oil, straight or infused with herbs or essential oils, can help reduce and dissipate fibroadenomas as well as keep women in touch with changes in their breast tissue.
- Infections are often treated with warm compresses and antibiotics. Lactating women are encouraged to continue breastfeeding because it promotes drainage and healing. However, a serious infection may progress to form an abscess that may need surgical drainage.
- Some studies of alternative or complementary treatments, although controversial, have indicated that vitamins A, B complex and E, and mineral supplements may reduce the risk of developing fibrocystic condition of the breast. Evening primrose oil (*Oenothera biennis*), flaxseed oil, and fish oils have been reported to be effective in relieving cyclic breast pain for some women.

Prognosis

Most benign breast conditions carry no increased risk for the development of breast cancer. However, a small percentage of biopsies uncover overgrowth of tissue in a particular pattern in some women; this pattern indicates a 15–20% increased risk of breast cancer over the next 20 years. Strict attention to early detection measures, such as annual mammograms, is especially important for these women.

Prevention

There is no proven method of preventing the various manifestations of fibrocystic condition from occurring. Some alternative health care practitioners believe that eliminating foods high in methyl xanthines (primarily coffee and chocolate) can decrease or reverse fibrocystic breast changes.

Resources

BOOKS

Love, Susan M., with Karen Lindsey. *Dr. Susan Love's Breast Book*. 5th ed. Cambridge, MA: Da Capo Lifelong, 2010.

O'Malley, Frances P., and Sarah E. Pinder. *Breast Pathology*. Edinburgh: Churchill Livingstone/Elsevier, 2006.

OTHER

National Cancer Institute. *Understanding Breast Changes: A Health Guide for All Women*. July 10, 2001. http://www.cancer.gov/cancertopics/screening/understanding-breast-changes.

ORGANIZATIONS

American Cancer Society, 1599 Clifton Rd. NE, Atlanta, GA, 30329, (800) 227-2345, http://www.cancer.org.

American College of Obstetricians and Gynecologists (ACOG), P.O. Box 96920, Washington, DC, 20090-6920, (202) 638-5577, http://www.acog.org.

NCI Office of Communications and Education, 6116 Executive Blvd. Suite 300, Bethesda, MD, 20892-8322, (800) 4-CANCER (422-6237), cancergovstaff@mail.nih.gov, http://www.cancer.gov/aboutnci/cis.

Ellen S. Weber, MSN
Genevieve Slomski, PhD

Fibroids *see* **Uterine fibroids**

Fibromyalgia

Definition

Fibromyalgia is an inflammation of the fibrous or connective tissue (muscles, joints, ligaments, and tendons) of the body. It is characterized by muscle **pain**, **fatigue**, and multiple tender points on the body. Many individuals with fibromyalgia describe the symptoms as similar to the aches and pains of a severe case of the flu. Fibrositis, and fibromyositis are names given to a set of symptoms believed to be caused by the same general problem.

Description

Fibromyalgia is more common than was once thought. According to the American College of Rheumatology, as many as 2–4% of the U.S. population may be affected by the disorder. Fibromyalgia is more prevalent in adults than children, with more women affected than men, particularly women of childbearing age.

KEY TERMS

Connective tissue—Tissue that supports and binds other body tissue and parts.

Lyme disease—An acute recurrent inflammatory disease involving one or a few joints, believed to be transmitted by a tick-borne virus. The condition was originally described in the community of Lyme, Connecticut, but has also been reported in other parts of the United States and other countries. Knees and other large joints are most commonly involved with local inflammation and swelling.

Rheumatology—The study of disorders characterized by inflammation, degeneration of connective tissue, and related structures of the body. These disorders are sometimes collectively referred to as rheumatism.

Causes and symptoms

The exact cause of fibromyalgia is not known. Sometimes it occurs in several members of a family, suggesting that it may be an inherited disorder. Researchers have investigated a number of possible causes, including genetic causes, **sleep disorders**, specific injuries, infections, problems with muscle metabolism, problems with the neurons that transmit information about pain, and nervous system abnormalities. Research is frequently unable to determine if a specific problem, such as sleep disturbances, results from fibromyalgia or are a possible cause of the condition. It is likely that a number of factors must occur in combination to cause fibromyalgia.

Pain is the major symptom with aches, tenderness, and stiffness of multiple muscles, joints, and soft tissues. The pain may move from one part of the body to another. It is most common in the neck, shoulders, chest, arms, legs, hips, and back. Although the pain is present most of the time and may last for years, the severity of the pain may fluctuate.

Symptoms of fatigue may result from the individual's chronic pain coupled with **anxiety** about the problem and how to find relief. The inflammatory process also produces chemicals that are known to cause fatigue. Other common symptoms are tension headaches, difficulty swallowing, recurrent abdominal pain, **diarrhea**, and **numbness** or **tingling** of the extremities. **Stress**, anxiety, depression, or lack of sleep can increase symptoms. Intensity of symptoms is variable, ranging from gradual improvement to episodes of recurrent symptoms.

Diagnosis

Diagnosis is difficult and frequently missed because symptoms of fibromyalgia are vague and generalized. Coexisting nerve and muscle disorders such as **rheumatoid arthritis**, spinal arthritis, or **Lyme disease** may further complicate the diagnostic process. As of 2008, no tests were available to specifically diagnose fibromyalgia. The diagnosis is usually made after ruling out other medical conditions with similar symptoms such as lupus and **hypothyroidism**.

Because of the emotional distress experienced by people with this condition and the influence of stress on the symptoms themselves, fibromyalgia has often been labeled a psychological problem. Although the debate about fibromyalgia continues, research on possible causes of the condition and public awareness campaigns have helped promote fibromyalgia's validity as a physiological problem.

The American College of Rheumatology has developed standards for fibromyalgia that healthcare practitioners can use to diagnose this condition. According to these standards, individuals can be diagnosed with fibromyalgia if they have widespread pain in combination with tenderness in at least 11 of the 18 sites known as trigger points. Trigger point sites include the base of the neck, along the backbone, in front of the hip and elbow, and at the rear of the knee and shoulder.

Treatment

Fibromyalgia has no known cure. Therefore, the goal of treatment is successful symptom management. Treatment usually requires a combination of therapies, including medication, **exercise**, and lifestyle adjustments. On June 21, 2007, the U.S. Food and Drug Administration (FDA) approved the first drug to treat fibromyalgia. Although previously many doctors had prescribed a variety of medications intended to help reduce the symptoms of fibromyalgia, Lyrica (pregabalin) was the first drug approved specifically for the treatment of fibromyalgia. Made by Pfizer, Lyrica was already used to treat pain associated with nerve damage caused by diabetes, pain following **shingles**, and partial seizures. A study of 1,800 patients showed that Lyrica was also effective in treating the pain associated with fibromyalgia in many people. Lyrica was not found to be effective in everyone with fibromyalgia, however, and it can have side effects, including sleepiness, **dizziness**, weight gain, swelling of the feet and hands, blurred vision, and **dry mouth**.

In addition to treatment with medication there are many other ways of managing the symptoms of fibromyalgia. Adequate rest is essential, as is a healthy diet. The diet should include a large variety of fruits and vegetables, which provide the body with trace elements and **minerals** that are necessary for healthy muscles. Avoidance of stimulating foods or drinks (such as coffee) and medications such as **decongestants** prior to bedtime is advised. Individuals should have a clear understanding of their role in the recovery process because it determines the successful management of this condition.

Other treatments found to be helpful include heat and occasionally cold-compress applications. A regular stretching program is often useful. Aerobic activities focusing on increasing the heart rate are the preferred forms of exercise over most other forms of exertion. Exercise programs need to include good warm-up and cool-down sessions, with special attention given to avoiding exercises causing joint pain. **Hydrotherapy** exercises (exercises in a pool or tub) may be useful in providing a low-impact exercise environment while soothing muscle and joint pain.

Massage therapy can be helpful, especially when a family member is instructed on specific massage techniques to manage episodes of increased symptoms. Short sessions are most helpful as repetitious movement can aggravate the condition. Specific attention to mental health, including psychological treatment, may also be important, since depression may precede or accompany fibromyalgia. Relaxation exercises, **yoga**, **aromatherapy**, **guided imagery**, and other relaxation therapies can be useful in easing stress and promoting overall well-being. A Mayo Clinic study released in 2006 found that **acupuncture** can be helpful in relieving the symptoms of fibromyalgia.

Herbalists and aromatherapists may recommend tub soaks or compresses with lavender (*Lavandula angustifolia*), chamomile (*Chamaemelum nobilis*), or juniper (*Juniperus communis*) to soothe muscle and joint pain.

Allopathic treatment

People with fibromyalgia often need a rheumatology consultation (a meeting with a doctor who specializes in disorders of the joints, muscles, and soft tissue) to decide the cause of various rheumatic symptoms, to be educated about fibromyalgia and its treatment, and to exclude other rheumatic diseases. A treatment program must be individualized to meet the patient's needs. The rheumatologist, as the team leader, enlists and coordinates the expertise of other health professionals in the care of the patient.

Prognosis

Fibromyalgia is a chronic health problem. The symptoms sometimes improve and at other times worsen, but they often continue for months to years.

Fibromyalgia can be a stressful and frustrating condition for a majority of patients. Successful treatment often requires a period of trial and error to pinpoint which agents and activities work best for the individual. Support from a health care team and coordination of care through follow-up calls to outside health care providers may be beneficial.

Clinical parameters are **pain management**, improved sleep management, introduction of relaxation techniques (including massage and **biofeedback** if needed), and monitoring alternative treatments and medication. Education is an integral part of the treatment and management of fibromyalgia and its symptoms.

A wide variety of health care providers may be involved in an individual's care, including nurses, physicians, a rheumatologist or other subspecialist, nutritionist, physical therapist, alternative medicine caregiver, or mental health care provider.

Prevention

No known or specific prevention for fibromyalgia exists. However, similar to many other medical conditions, remaining as healthy as possible with a good diet, safe exercise, and adequate rest is the best prevention.

Resources

BOOKS

Bassman, Lynette. *The Feel-Good Guide to Fibromyalgia & Chronic Fatigue Syndrome: A Comprehensive Resource for Recovery*. Oakland, CA: New Harbinger Publications, 2007.

Bested, Alison C., and Alan C. Logan. *Hope and Help for Chronic Fatigue Syndrome and Fibromyalgia*. Nashville, TN: Cumberland House, 2006.

Hu, Fengrui, ed. *Pain Research Progress: Migraine, Fibromyalgia, and Related Pain*. New York: Nova Science, 2007.

Skelly, Mari, and Helen Walker. *Alternative Treatments for Fibromyalgia & Chronic Fatigue Syndrome*, 2nd ed. Alameda, CA: Hunter House, 2007.

Trock, David H. *Living with Fibromyalgia*. Hoboken, NJ: Wiley, 2006.

PERIODICALS

Gallagher, Rollin M. "Fibromyalgia: New Hope for a Medical Dilemma." *Pain Medicine* 8, no. 8 (November/December 2007): 619–620.

Rutledge, Dana R., Kim Jones, and C. Jessie Jones. "Predicting High Physical Function in People with Fibromyalgia." *Journal of Nursing Scholarship* 39, no. 4 (Winter 2007): 319–325.

Sierpina, Victor S. "Is There a Role for Acupuncture in Fibromyalgia?" *Southern Medical Journal* 100, no. 12 (December 2007): 1183–1184.

Smith, Cath, and Leigh Hale. "The Effects of Non-pharmacological Interventions on Fatigue in Four Chronic Illness Conditions: A Critical Review." *Physical Therapy Review* (December 2007): 324–334.

Staud, Roland. "Treatment of Fibromyalgia and Its Symptoms." *Expert Opinion on Pharmacotherapy* (August 2007): 1629–1642.

ORGANIZATIONS

American Pain Society, 4700 W. Lake Ave., Glenview, IL, 60025, (847) 375-4715., http://www.ampainsoc.org.

National Chronic Fatigue Syndrome and Fibromyalgia Association, P.O. Box 18426, Kansas City, MO, 64133, (913) 321-2278, http://www.ncfsfa.org/.

National Fibromyalgia Association, 2121 S. Towne Centre Place, Suite 300, Anaheim, CA, 92806, (714) 921-0150., http://www.fmaware.org.

Paula Ford-Martin
Michele R. Webb
Laura Jean Cataldo, RN, Ed.D.

Fibromyomas *see* **Uterine fibroids**

Fibrous breast lumps *see* **Fibroadenoma**

Fifth disease

Definition

Fifth disease is a mild childhood illness caused by the human parvovirus B19 that causes flu-like symptoms and a rash.

Demographics

Anyone can get the disease, but it occurs more frequently in school-aged children. Outbreaks most often occur in the winter and spring, peaking every four to seven years. About 60% of adults have had the disease by age 20.

Description

Fifth disease got its name because it was fifth on a list of common childhood illnesses that are accompanied by a rash, including **measles**, **rubella** or German measles, **scarlet fever** (or scarlatina), and scarlatinella, a variant of scarlet **fever**. The Latin name for the

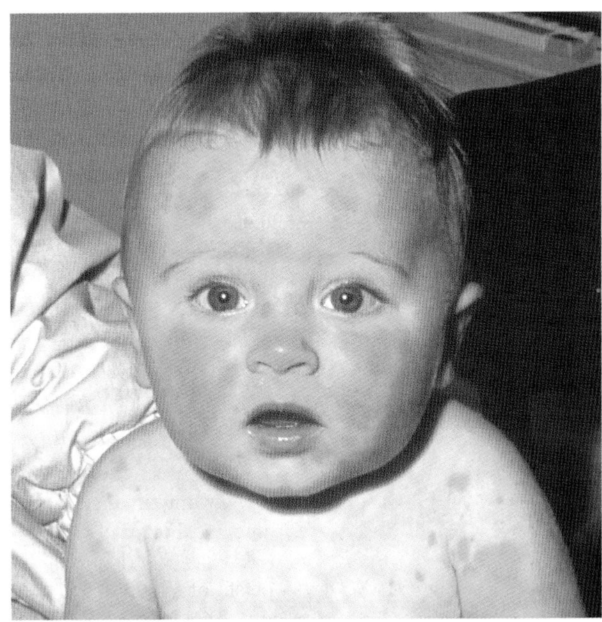

This infant has a rash caused by Fifth disease, or *erythema infectiosum.* *(Custom Medical Stock Photo, Inc. Reproduced by permission.)*

disease is *erythema infectiosum*, meaning infectious redness. It is also called the "slapped cheek disease" because, when the bright red rash first appears on the cheeks, it looks as if the face has been slapped. The disease is usually mild, and both children and adults normally recover quickly without complications. In fact, some individuals exhibit no symptoms and never feel ill.

Causes and symptoms

Fifth disease is caused by the human parvovirus B19, a member of the Parvoviridae family of viruses that lives in the nose and throat of the infected person. The virus is spread through the air by coughing and sneezing. Because the virus needs a rapidly dividing cell in order to multiply, it attacks the red blood cells of the body. Once infected, a person is believed to be immune to re–infection.

Symptoms appear four to 21 days after exposure to the virus. Initial symptoms are flu–like and include **headache**, body ache, **sore throat**, a mild fever of 101 °F (38.3 °C), and chills. It is at this time, before development of the rash, that individuals are contagious. These symptoms last for two to three days. In children, a bright red rash that looks like a slap mark develops suddenly on the cheeks. The rash may be flat or raised and may or may not be itchy. Sometimes, the rash spreads to the arms, legs, and trunk, where it has a lace–like or net–like appearance. The rash can also involve the palms of the hands and soles of the feet. By the time the rash appears, individuals are no longer infectious. On average, the rash lasts for 10–11 days, but may last for as long as five to six weeks. The rash may fade away and then reappear upon exposure to sunlight, hot baths, emotional distress, or vigorous **exercise**.

Adults generally do not develop a rash, but instead may have swollen and painful joints, especially in the hands and feet. In adults, symptoms such as sore throat, headache, muscle and joint **pain**, abdominal pain, **diarrhea**, and **vomiting** occur more frequently than in children and usually are more severe. Joint pain can be arthritis–like and last for several months, especially in women, but the disease does not appear to progress to **rheumatoid arthritis**.

The virus causes the destruction of red blood cells; therefore, a deficiency in the oxygen–carrying capacity of the blood (anemia) can result. In healthy people, the anemia is mild and lasts only a short while. In people with weakened immune systems, either because they have a chronic disease such as HIV infection/AIDS or **cancer** and are immunocompromised; or they are receiving medication to suppress the immune system and are therefore immunosuppressed (e.g., organ transplant recipients), this anemia can be severe and last long after the infection has subsided. Symptoms of anemia include **fatigue**, lack of healthy color, lack of energy, and **shortness of breath**. Some individuals with **sickle cell disease**, iron deficiency, a number of different hereditary blood disorders, and those who have received bone marrow transplantations may be susceptible to developing a potentially life–threatening complication called a transient aplastic crisis, in which the body is temporarily unable to form new red blood cells.

In very rare instances, the virus can cause inflammation of different areas of the body, including the brain (**encephalitis**), the covering of the brain and spinal cord (**meningitis**), the lungs (pneumonitis), the liver (hepatitis), and the heart muscle (**myocarditis**). The virus also can aggravate symptoms for people with an autoimmune disease called **systemic lupus erythematosus** (SLE).

Some concern surrounds fifth disease in pregnant women. Although no association with an increased number of **birth defects** or **mental retardation** has been demonstrated, there is concern that infection during the first three months of **pregnancy** may slightly increase the risk of **miscarriage**. Some concern also exists that infection later in pregnancy may involve a very small risk of premature delivery or **stillbirth**. As a

KEY TERMS

Anemia—A congenital or acquired deficiency in the iron–carrying capacity of the blood.

Antibody—A specific protein produced by the immune system in response to a specific foreign protein or particle called an antigen.

Immunocompromised—A state in which the immune system is weakened or is not functioning properly due to chronic disease.

Immunosuppressed—A state in which the immune system is suppressed by medications during the treatment of other disorders, such as cancer, or following an organ transplantation.

Reye's syndrome—A very serious, rare disease, most common in children, that involves an upper respiratory tract infection followed by brain and liver damage.

Sickle cell disease—A hereditary blood disorder in which red blood cells are misshapen into crescent or sickle shapes resulting in a reduced oxygen–carrying capacity of the lungs.

Systemic lupus erythematosus (SLE)—A chronic, inflammatory, autoimmune disorder in which the individual's immune system attacks, injures, and destroys the body's own organs and tissues. It may affect many organ systems including the skin, joints, lungs, heart, and kidneys.

result, women who get fifth disease while they are pregnant should be monitored closely by a physician.

Diagnosis

Examination

Fifth disease usually is suspected based on a patient's symptoms, including the typical appearance of the bright red rash on the cheeks, patient history, age, and time of year. The physician will exclude other potential causes for the symptoms and rash, including rubella, **infectious mononucleosis**, bacterial infections such as **Lyme disease**, allergic reactions, and SLE.

Tests

In addition, a blood test is available for fifth disease, but it is generally used only for pregnant women and for people who have weakened immune systems or who have blood disorders, such as sickle cell disease. The test involves measuring for a particular antibody or protein that the body produces in response to infection with the human parvovirus B19. The test is 92–97% specific for this disease.

Because fifth disease can pose problems for an unborn fetus exposed to the disease through the mother, testing may also be conducted while a fetus is still in the uterus. This test uses fluid collected from the sac around the fetus (amniotic fluid) instead of blood to detect the viral DNA.

Treatment

In general, no specific treatment for fifth disease is required. The symptoms can be treated using over–the counter medications, such as **acetaminophen** (Tylenol) or ibuprofen (Motrin, Advil). If the rash itches, calamine lotion can be applied. **Aspirin** is not given to children under the age of 18 to prevent the development of a serious illness called **Reye's syndrome**.

Patients who are receiving medications to suppress the immune system in the treatment of some other condition may be allowed to temporarily decrease the medications in order to allow the immune system to combat the infection and recover from the anemia. Those with weakened (not suppressed) immune systems, such as HIV/AIDS patients, may be given immunoglobulin intravenously to help the immune system fight the infection. People with severe anemia or who experience an aplastic crisis may require hospitalization and blood transfusions.

Prognosis

Generally, fifth disease is mild, and patients tend to improve without any complications. In cases where the patient is either immunocompromised or immunosuppressed, a life–threatening aplastic crisis can occur. With prompt treatment, however, the prognosis is good. Mothers who develop the infection while pregnant can pass the infection on to their fetus, and as such, stand a very small increased risk of miscarriage and stillbirth. Tests and treatments, however, can be performed on the fetus while still in the uterus that can reduce the risk of anemia or other complications.

Prevention

Currently, there is no vaccine against fifth disease. Because people with fifth disease are contagious before definitive symptoms appear, it is very difficult to prevent infection. Avoiding contact with persons who exhibit symptoms of a cold and maintaining good personal hygiene by regularly washing hands may minimize the chances of an infection. Pregnant women should avoid exposure to persons infected with the disease and notify their obstetrician immediately if they are exposed so that they can be tested and monitored closely.

Resources

OTHER

"Fifth Disease." MedlinePlus. (May 4, 2010). http://www.nlm.nih.gov/medlineplus/fifthdisease.html (accessed September 17, 2010).

"Parvovirus B19 Infection and Pregnancy." (January 21, 2005). United States Centers for Disease Control and Prevention. http://www.cdc.gov/ncidod/dvrd/revb/respiratory/B19&preg.htm (accessed September 17, 2010).

Zellerman, Glenn. "Erythema Infectiosum (Fifth Disease)" eMedicine.com. (December 8, 2009). http://emedicine.medscape.com/article/1132078-overview (accessed September 17, 2010).

ORGANIZATIONS

National Institute of Allergy and Infectious Diseases, Office of Communications and Government Relations, 6610 Rockledge Dr., MSC 6612, Bethesda, MD, 20892–6612, (301) 496–5717, (866) 284–4107 or TDD: (800)877–8339 (for hearing impaired), (301) 402–3573, http://www3.niaid.nih.gov.

Centers for Disease Control and Prevention (CDC), 1600 Clifton Rd., Atlanta, GA, 30333, (404) 639–3534, (800) CDC–INFO (800–232–4636). TTY: (888) 232–6348, inquiry@cdc.gov, http://www.cdc.gov.

Lata Cherath, PhD
Tish Davidson, AM

Filariasis

Definition

Filiariasis is the name for a group of tropical diseases caused by various thread-like parasitic round worms (nematodes) and their larvae. The larvae transmit the disease to humans through a mosquito bite. Filariasis is characterized by **fever**, chills, **headache**, and **skin lesions** in the early stages and, if untreated, can progress to include gross enlargement of the limbs and genitalia in a condition called **elephantiasis**.

Description

Approximately 170 million people in the tropical and subtropical areas of Southeast Asia, South America, Africa, and the islands of the Pacific are affected by this debilitating parasitic disease. While filariasis is rarely fatal, it is the second leading cause of permanent and long-term disability in the world. The World Health Organization (WHO) has named filariasis one of only six "potentially eradicable" infectious diseases and has embarked upon a 20-year campaign to eradicate the disease.

In all cases, a mosquito first **bites** an infected individual then bites another uninfected individual, transferring some of the worm larvae to the new host. Once within the body, the larvae migrate to a particular part of the body and mature to adult worms. Filariasis is classified into three distinct types according to the part of the body that becomes infected: lymphatic filariasis affects the circulatory system that moves tissue fluid and immune cells (lymphatic system); subcutaneous filariasis infects the areas beneath the skin and whites of the eye; and serous cavity filariasis infects body cavities but does not cause disease. Several different types of worms can be responsible for each type of filariasis, but the most common species include the following: *Wucheria bancrofti, Brugia malayi* (lymphatic filariasis), *Onchocerca volvulus, Loa loa, Mansonella streptocerca, Dracunculus medinensis* (subcutaneous filariasis), *Mansonella pustans*, and *Mansonella ozzardi* (serous cavity filariasis).

The two most common types of the disease are Bancroftian and Malayan filariasis, both forms of lymphatic filariasis. The Bancroftian variety is found throughout Africa, southern and southeastern Asia, the Pacific islands, and the tropical and subtropical regions of South America and the Caribbean. Malayan filariasis occurs only in southern and southeastern Asia. Filariasis is occasionally found in the United States, especially among immigrants from the Caribbean and Pacific islands.

A larvae matures into an adult worm within six months to one year and can live between four and six years. Each female worm can produce millions of larvae, and these larvae only appear in the bloodstream at night, when they may be transmitted, via an insect bite, to another host. A single bite is usually not enough to acquire an infection, therefore, short-term travelers are usually safe. A series of multiple bites over a period of time is required to establish an infection. As a result, those individuals who are regularly active outdoors at night and those who spend more time in remote jungle areas are at an increased risk of contracting the filariasis infection.

KEY TERMS

Abscess—An area of inflamed and injured body tissue that fills with pus.

Antibody—A specific protein produced by the immune system in response to a specific foreign protein or particle called an antigen.

Conjunctiva—The mucous membrane that lines the inside of the eyelid and the exposed surface of the eyeball.

Elephantiasis—A condition characterized by the gross enlargement of limbs and/or the genitalia that is also accompanied by a hardening and stretching of the overlying skin. Often a result of an obstruction in the lymphatic system caused by infection with a filarial worm.

Encephalitis—Inflammation of the brain.

Lymphatic system—The circulatory system that drains and circulates fluid containing nutrients, waste products, and immune cells, from between cells, organs, and other tissue spaces.

Microfilariae—The larvae and infective form of filarial worms.

Nematode—Round worms.

Subcutaneous—The area directly beneath the skin.

Causes and symptoms

In cases of lymphatic filariasis, the most common form of the disease, the disease is caused by the adult worms actually living in the lymphatic vessels near the lymph nodes where they distort the vessels and cause local inflammation. In advanced stages, the worms can actually obstruct the vessels, causing the surrounding tissue to become enlarged. In Bancroftian filariasis, the legs and genitals are most often involved, while the Malayan variety affects the legs below the knees. Repeated episodes of inflammation lead to blockages of the lymphatic system, especially in the genitals and legs. This causes the affected area to become grossly enlarged, with thickened, coarse skin, leading to a condition called elephantiasis.

In conjunctiva filariasis, the worms' larvae migrate to the eye and can sometimes be seen moving beneath the skin or beneath the white part of the eye (conjunctiva). If untreated, this disease can cause a type of blindness known as onchocerciasis.

Symptoms vary, depending on what type of parasitic worm has caused the infection, but all infections usually begin with chills, headache, and fever between three months and one year after the insect bite. Swelling, redness, and **pain** may also occur in the arms, legs, or scrotum. Areas of pus (abscesses) may appear as a result of dying worms or a secondary bacterial infection.

Diagnosis

The disease is diagnosed by taking a patient history, performing a **physical examination**, and by screening blood specimens for specific proteins produced by the immune system in response to this infection (antibodies). Early diagnosis may be difficult because, in the first stages, the disease mimics other bacterial skin infections. To make an accurate diagnosis, the physician looks for a pattern of inflammation and signs of lymphatic obstruction, together with the patient's possible exposure to filariasis in an area where filariasis is common. The larvae (microfilariae) can also be found in the blood, but because mosquitos, which spread the disease, are active at night, the larvae are usually only found in the blood between about 10 p.m. and 2 a.m.

Treatment

Either ivermectin, albendazole, or diethylcarbamazine is used to treat a filariasis infection by eliminating the larvae, impairing the adult worms' ability to reproduce, and by actually killing adult worms. Unfortunately, much of the tissue damage may not be reversible. The medication is started at low doses to prevent reactions caused by large numbers of dying parasites.

While effective, the medications can cause severe side effects in up to 70% of patients as a result either of the drug itself or the massive **death** of parasites in the blood. Diethylcarbamazine, for example, can cause severe allergic reactions and the formation of pus-filled sores (abscesses). These side effects can be controlled using **antihistamines** and anti-inflammatory drugs (**corticosteroids**). Rarely, treatment with diethylcarbamazine in someone with very high levels of parasite infection may lead to a fatal inflammation of the brain (**encephalitis**). In this case, the fever is followed by headache and confusion, then stupor and **coma** caused when massive numbers of larvae and parasites die. Other common drug reactions include **dizziness**, weakness, and **nausea**.

Symptoms caused by the death of the parasites include fever, headache, muscle pain, abdominal pain, **nausea and vomiting**, weakness, dizziness, lethargy, and **asthma**. Reactions usually begin within two days of starting treatment and may last between two and four days.

No treatment can reverse elephantiasis. Surgery may be used to remove surplus tissue and provide a way to drain the fluid around the damaged lymphatic vessels. Surgery may also be used to ease massive enlargement of the scrotum. Elephantiasis of the legs can also be helped by elevating the legs and providing support with elastic **bandages**.

Prognosis

The outlook is good in early or mild cases, especially if the patient can avoid being infected again. The disease is rarely fatal, and with continued WHO medical intervention, even gross elephantiasis is now becoming rare.

Prevention

The best method of preventing filariasis is to avoid repeated bites by the mosquitoes that carry the disease. Some methods of preventing insect bites include the following:

- limit outdoor activities at night, particularly in rural or jungle areas
- wear long sleeves and pants and avoid dark-colored clothing that attracts mosquitoes
- avoid perfumes and colognes
- treat one or two sets of clothing ahead of time with permethrin (Duramon, Permanone).
- wear DEET insect repellent or, especially for children, try citronella or lemon eucalyptus, to repel insects
- if sleeping in an open area or in a room with poor screens, use a bed net to avoid being bitten while asleep
- use air conditioning, the cooler air makes insects less active.

In addition, filariasis can be controlled in highly infested areas by taking ivermectin preventatively before being bitten. Currently, there is no vaccine available, but scientists are working on a preventative vaccine at this time.

Resources

OTHER

Centers for Disease Control.http://www.cdc.gov.

International Society of Travel Medicine. http://www.istm.org.

"Lymphatic Filariasis." *Centers for Disease Control.* http://www.cdc.gov/travel/yellowbk/page117.htm.

ORGANIZATIONS

Centers for Disease Control and Prevention (CDC), 1600 Clifton Rd., Atlanta, GA, 30333, (800) 232-4636, cdcinfo@cdc.gov, http://www.cdc.gov.

Carol A. Turkington

Filgras *see* **Cancer therapy, supportive; Immunologic therapies**

Finasteride

Definition

Finasteride is a drug that belongs to the class of androgen inhibitors, which means that it blocks the production of male sex hormones.

Purpose

Finasteride has two main purposes: the treatment of urinary problems in men caused by benign prostatic hypertrophy (BPH) or enlargement of the prostate gland; and the stimulation of new hair growth in men with male pattern baldness. Finasteride was first approved by the U.S. Food and Drug Administration (FDA) in 1992 under the trade name Proscar as a treatment for BPH. This drug may be used alone or in combination with the drug doxazosin (Cardura) to treat BPH. It received a second FDA approval in December 1997 under the trade name Propecia for the treatment of hair loss in men.

Results of a large clinical trial, the **Prostate Cancer** Prevention Trial, which were released in 2010, revealed that finasteride (Proscar) reduced the risk for prostate **cancer** by as much as 25% in men (ages 55 and older) enrolled in the trial. In the near future, men with an increasing prostate specific antigen (PSA) level and who are considered by their physicians to be at high risk for the development of prostate cancer may be prescribed finasteride to decrease their risk for developing prostate cancer.

Finasteride works to relieve such symptoms of prostate enlargement as urinary urgency, the need to

KEY TERMS

Alopecia—The medical term for baldness.

Androgens—A group of hormones that produce masculine characteristics.

Chemo preventative—Description of a drug given in order to prevent the development of a specific disease.

Dysuria—Painful or difficult urination.

Incontinence—Inability to control urination or defecation.

Nocturia—Excessive need to urinate at night.

Prostate—A gland in males below the bladder that surrounds the urethra. Enlargement of the prostate may cause problems in urination.

Urgency—A sudden and powerful need to urinate.

urinate frequently at night (nocturia), inability to completely empty the bladder, incontinence, or painful urination (dysuria) by blocking the production of DHT. DHT causes the prostate gland to grow and increase pressure on the bladder. As the swollen prostate gradually shrinks, the patient finds it easier to pass urine without discomfort and to empty the bladder completely before going to sleep. Some doctors also prescribe finasteride as pretreatment for prostate surgery, as it lowers the risk of severe bleeding during the operation.

Description

U.S. and Canadian brand names

Finasteride is sold in the United States and Canada under the brand names Proscar (indicated for the treatment of BPH) and Propecia (indicated for the treatment of male pattern baldness). Finasteride inhibits the body's production of an enzyme called 5-alpha-reductase, which is needed to convert testosterone to another androgen called 5-alpha-dihydrotestosterone (DHT). Finasteride is a white powder that can be dissolved in alcohol or chloroform but is very difficult to dissolve in water. Both Proscar and Propecia are manufactured as coated tablets to be taken by mouth.

Recommended dosage

- Proscar: Finasteride for treatment of an enlarged prostate is taken once a day as a 5-mg tablet. The pill may be crushed or broken if the patient finds it hard to swallow.
- Propecia: Finasteride for hair regrowth is taken once a day as a 1-mg tablet. The drug may be taken with or without meals.

Precautions

Finasteride should be stored in a dry place and kept at a temperature between 59°F and 86°F (15–30°C). Heat and moisture may cause the drug to lose its potency.

Tablets, especially crushed or broken tablets, should not be touched by a pregnant woman as the drug can be absorbed through the skin. If the woman is carrying a male fetus, the drug can cause abnormalities in the baby's sex organs. The FDA issued a warning in 2003 that men taking finasteride should not donate blood until one month after the final dose of the drug, on the grounds that their blood could contain high enough levels of the medication to cause **birth defects** in a male baby if given to a pregnant woman.

Patients should be advised that finasteride takes several months to reach its full effect—as long as six months for BPH and three months for hair regrowth. In addition, the drug's effects on the body are not permanent; the prostate will start to enlarge again or the hair growth will be lost if the patient stops taking the drug.

Proscar can affect the results of a prostate-specific antigen (PSA) test for cancer of the prostate.

Finasteride should be used cautiously by men with liver disorders.

Finasteride is not indicated for the treatment of hair loss in women in the United States.

Side effects

Reported side effects from using finasteride include:

- impotence or loss of interest in sex
- lumps or pain in the breast or a discharge from the nipple
- skin rash, itching, or hives
- swelling of the lips or face
- a smaller quantity of ejaculate during intercourse (which does not affect fertility)
- headaches, dizziness, or diarrhea
- pain in the testicles

These side effects are more common with the 5-mg dose, but usually disappear when the drug is discontinued.

Interactions

Finasteride has not been reported to cause significant interactions with other medications.

Resources

BOOKS

Deglin, Judith, April H. Vallerand, and Cynthia A. Sanoski. *Davis's Drug Guide for Nurses*. 12th ed. Philadelphia: F.A. Davis, 2009.

PERIODICALS

Chaudhary, U.B., and J.S. Turner. "Finasteride." *Expert Opinion on Drug Metabolisim and Toxicology* 6, no. 7 (July 6, 2010): 873–81.

Groves-Kirkby, N. "Chemotherapy: Optimizing Finasteride Chemoprevention for Prostate Cancer." *National Review of Clinical Oncology* 7, no. 5 (May 2010): 242.

Smith, A.B., and C.C. Carson. "Finasteride in the Treatment of Patients with Benign Prostatic Hyperplasia: A Review." *Journal of Therapeutics and Clinical Risk Managagement* 5, no. 3 (June 2009): 535–45.

OTHER

"Finasteride." *PubMed Health*. December 1, 2008. http://www.ncbi.nlm.nih.gov/pubmedhealth/PMH0001028 (accessed October 4, 2010).

Rebecca J. Frey, PhD
Melinda Granger Oberleitner, RN, DNS, APRN, CNS

Fingernail removal *see* **Nail removal**

Fingertip injuries

Definition

Fingertip trauma covers cuts, accumulation of blood (hematoma), bone breakage, or **amputation** in the fingertip.

Description

The fingertips are specialized areas of the hand with highly developed sensory and manipulative functions. Large sensory and motor areas located in the brain regulate the precise and delicate functions of fingertips. The fingertip is the site where extensor and flexor tendons insert. Fingertip injuries are extremely common since the hands hold a wide array of objects. In 2001, approximately 10% of all accidents in the United States that were referred for emergency room consults involved the hand. Hand injuries are frequently the result of job injuries and account for 11–14% of on-the-job injuries and 6% of compensation paid injuries. Injury to the nail bed occurs in approximately 15–24% of fingertip injuries.

Fingertip injuries can result in amputation or tissue loss. The injury is assessed whether the bone and underlying tissue are intact and the size of the wound area. The pulp is the area of skin opposite the fingernail and is usually very vulnerable to injury. Pulp injuries commonly occur in persons who use or are in close contact with fast moving mechanical devices. These injuries can crush, cut, and puncture. The fingertips can also be injured by common crushing accidents. This could cause the development of a subungal hematoma (an accumulation of blood under the nail).

At the base of the distal phalanx (the first circular skin fold from the tip) injuries can occur that can fracture the underlying bone in the area. Quite commonly a hammer, closing a door, or sport accidents usually cause these injuries. These **fractures** can be simple, requiring little treatment or more complicated involving the joint. The accident may involve the point of insertion of a tendon. Usually this occurs when the terminal joint is being forced to flex while held straight. This motion typically occurs when tucking in sheets during bed making, a common cause of tendon injury. This injury causes a loss of extension (straightening the finger) ability.

Causes and symptoms

Accidental amputations will usually result in profuse bleeding and tissue loss. Injuries to the pulp can occur as from fast-moving mechanical instruments, such as drills. These injuries may puncture the pulp. Injuries such as a subungal hematoma are caused by a crushing type injury. Fractures typically occur as the result of crushing injuries or tendon avulsion. These crushing injuries are frequently caused during sport injury and can be treated by simple interventions such as **immobilization** or more complex procedures if tendons are affected (the trauma is then treated as a tendon injury). Fractures can cause **pain** and, depending on the extent of swelling, there may be some restriction of movement. Tendon injuries can be caused when the terminal joint is exposed to force flexing motion (moving the finger toward the palm) while held straight.

KEY TERMS

Distal—Movement away from the origin.

Flex—To bend.

Laceration—A cut in the skin

Phalanx—A bone of the fingers or toes.

Tendon—A structure that connects a skeletal muscle to bone.

Diagnosis

The attending clinician should evaluate the injury in a careful and systematic manner. The appearance of the hand can provide valuable information concerning presence of fractures, vascular status, and tendon involvement. Bones and joints should be evaluated for motion and tenderness. Nerves should be examined for sensory (feeling sensations) and motor (movement) functioning. Amputations usually profusely bleed and there is tissue loss. The wound is treated based on loss of tissue, bone, and wound area. Injuries to the pulp can be obvious during inspection. Subungal hematoma usually present a purplish-black discoloration under the nail. This is due to a hematoma underneath the nail. Radiographs may be required to assess the alignment of fractures or detect foreign bodies. Patients usually suffer from pain since injuries to the fingertip bone are usually painful and movement may be partially restricted due to swelling of the affected area. Tendon injuries usually result in the loss of ability to straighten or bend the finger.

Treatment

Amputation in which bone and underlying tissue are intact and the wound area is 1 cm or less, should be cleaned and treated with a dressing. With these types of **wounds**, healthy tissue will usually grow and replace the injured area. Larger wounds may require surgical intervention. Puncture wounds should be cleaned and left open to heal. Patients typically receive **antibiotics** to prevent infection. A procedure called trephining treats subungal hematomas. This procedure is usually done with a straight cutting needle positioned over the nail. The clinician spins the needle with forefinger and thumb until a hole is made through the nail.

Patients who have extensive crush injuries or subungal hematomas involving laceration to skin folds or nail damage should have the nail removed to examine the underlying tissue (called the matrix). Patients who have a closed subungal hematoma with an intact nail and no other damage (no nail disruption or laceration) are treated conservatively. If the fracture is located two-thirds below the fingertip, immobilization using a splint may be needed. Conservative treatment is recommended for crush injuries that fracture the terminal phalanx if a subungal hematoma is not present. Severe fractures near the fist circular skin crease may require surgical correction to prevent irregularity of the joint surface, which can cause difficulty with movement. Injury to a flexor tendon usually requires surgical repair. If this is not possible, the finger and wrist should be placed in a splint with specific positioning to prevent further damage.

Prognosis

Prognosis depends on the extent of traumatic damage to the affected area. Nail lacerations that are not treated may cause nail deformities. When amputation is accompanied with loss of two-thirds of the nail, half of the fingers develop beaking, or a curved nail. Aftercare and follow up are important components of treatment. The patient is advised to keep the hand elevated, check with a clinician two days after treatment, and to splint fractures for two weeks in the extended position. Usually a nail takes about 100 days to fully grow. Healing for an amputation takes about 21-27 days. This markedly decreases in elderly patients, primarily due to a compromised circulation normally part of advancing age.

Resources

BOOKS

Sabiston, David C., et al.*Sabiston Textbook of Surgery: The Biological Basis of Modern Surgical Practice*. Philadelphia: Saunders/Elsevier, 2008.

Laith Farid Gulli, M.D.

First aid

Definition

First aid is the treatment of minor injuries or conditions or immediate care or treatment for a medical emergency that is administered while awaiting professional help.

Purpose

First aid ranges from cleaning and bandaging a minor scrape to saving a life with **cardiopulmonary**

resuscitation (CPR). It is often required to stop bleeding or to stabilize and protect an ill or injured person until they can get to a hospital or emergency help arrives on the scene. First aid may be used to treat:

- cuts, scrapes, and scratches
- nosebleeds
- severe bleeding
- heat exhaustion and heatstroke
- frostnip and frostbite
- burns
- poisoning
- choking
- a foreign object in the eye or nose
- injured or broken bones
- head or spinal injuries
- seizures
- shock
- unconsciousness
- respiratory or heart failure

Demographics

Every year millions of children require first aid for minor injuries, serious accidents, or life-threatening emergencies. For this reason, every home, automobile, daycare, and school should be equipped with a well-stocked first-aid kit and every parent, caregiver, and teacher should be trained in first aid and CPR.

Description

First aid for a minor scrape, cut, or puncture wound may include:

- using sterile gauze, tissue, or a clean, soft cloth to apply gentle, firm pressure to stop bleeding
- cleaning with cool running water or soaking the wound
- using a soft cloth and gentle soap to clean around the injury
- using a soft, damp cloth or tweezers cleaned with rubbing alcohol to remove dirt or debris
- applying antibiotic ointment
- covering with butterfly tape, adhesive strips, or sterile gauze and adhesive tape, if the injury is in an area that could get dirty or rubbed by clothing
- changing bandages daily

For severe bleeding:

- lie down and cover the injured person to prevent loss of body heat
- if possible, elevate the legs to increase blood flow to the brain and prevent fainting or elevate the injured area above the level of the heart to slow bleeding
- apply firm, gentle pressure to the wound for at least 20 minutes
- add more gauze or cloth if needed, without removing the lower layers
- pressure may be applied to a main artery leading to the injured area
- tightly wrap the wound with a bandage or clean cloth and tape
- immobilize the injured part and leave bandages in place once the bleeding has stopped

For a nosebleed:

- sit, leaning slightly forward to drain the blood out of the nose, but with the head above the level of the heart
- squeeze the soft part of the nose, using the thumb and index finger, until the bleeding stops or for at least five minutes
- do not do anything to make the bleeding restart, such as bending over or blowing through the nose

For heat exhaustion or heatstroke:

- rest in a cool, shady spot, with unnecessary clothing removed
- drink plenty of water or other fluids
- be bathed or sprayed with cool water
- be cooled by evaporating water from the skin

For **frostnip** or **frostbite**:

- dress in dry clothing in a warm environment and drink warm fluids
- if emergency help is not immediately available for frostbite, the frozen parts should be immersed in warm water (100°F, 38°C) or treated with warm compresses for 30 minutes
- if warm water is unavailable, gently wrap the affected person in blankets
- thawed areas should be kept still and wrapped to prevent refreezing

For **burns**:

- clothing should be gently removed from around the burn, unless it is stuck to the skin
- first-degree burns should be soaked in cool water for at least five minutes and loosely wrapped with a dry gauze bandage or a clean soft towel or sheet
- second-degree burns should be soaked in cool water for 15 minutes and covered with a dry nonstick dressing that is changed daily

- third-degree burns should be covered with a cool, wet, sterile bandage or clean cloth, without first soaking the burn; if possible, the burned area should be raised above the level of the heart until medical assistance is available
- electrical burns should be covered with gauze without rinsing
- for chemical burns, any contaminated clothing or jewelry should be removed and any dry chemical brushed off the skin; the burn should be gently rinsed with cool, running water for at least 20 minutes; loosely wrapped with a dry, sterile, dressing or gauze or a clean cloth; and rewashed if the pain worsens

If someone begins **choking**, they should be given abdominal thrusts— known as the **Heimlich maneuver**. For an infant under one year:

- place the infant face down over the rescuer's forearm with the head lower than the chest and the neck and head supported with the rescuer's fingers
- apply five quick blows to the infant's back, between the shoulders, with the heel of the free hand
- if no object is ejected, place the infant face-up on a table or floor and give five quick chest thrusts, with two fingers in the middle of the breastbone just below the level of the nipples
- repeat the five back blows and five chest thrusts until the object is dislodged and the infant starts breathing
- if the infant becomes unresponsive or unconscious, CPR must be performed; check the mouth for the object before each rescue breath

To perform the Heimlich maneuver on someone over one year of age (including adults):

- wrap the rescuer's arms around the choking person's waist from behind
- make a fist with one hand and grasp it with the other hand with the thumb just above the person's navel; quickly thrust upward and inward until the object is dislodged or the person begins breathing
- if the person loses consciousness, lower them to the floor for CPR

For a foreign object in the eye:

- sit in a well-lit area.
- pull down the lower lid while the individual looks up and then pull the upper lid while they look down to look for the object
- if the object is floating in the tear film, it can be flushed out with lukewarm water or a saline solution, using an eyecup or small glass

For a foreign object lodged in the nose:

- blow out gently through the nose, but not hard or repeatedly
- if only one nostril is affected, gentle pressure can be used to close the other nostril while blowing out
- if the object is visible, it may be removed with tweezers

For a bone injury:

- remove clothing from the injured limb without moving it
- apply an ice pack wrapped in cloth
- make a simple splint—use anything firm and padded with something soft—to prevent the limb from moving or bending; the splint must extend beyond the joints above and below the injury

A fall from a distance greater than a person's height or a bicycle or automobile accident can result in a head or spinal injury. The injured person should not be moved and the head, neck, and spine should be stabilized until help arrives.

A person having a seizure should:

- be laid on the ground or floor, preferably on the right side, with no nearby objects
- have clothing around the head and neck loosened
- be comforted and remain lying down until fully recovered

A person in **shock** should:

- be laid face-up, unless a head or spinal injury is suspected
- have the legs elevated about 12 in (30 cm), if possible
- have tight clothing loosened
- be covered with a blanket
- be kept warm, still, and comfortable
- may have the lips moistened with water, but should be given nothing by mouth
- be raised to a half-sitting position if vomiting or having trouble breathing, unless there is a head or spinal injury
- should be turned to the side if the child vomits or bleeds from the mouth

An unconscious person should be placed in the recovery position if there is no possibility of a spinal injury. While lying face-up:

- the arm closest to the rescuer is placed by the person's side and tucked under the buttock
- the other arm is placed across the person's chest
- the ankles are crossed with the far leg over the near leg

KEY TERMS

Aloe vera—An extract from the plant *Aloe barbadensis* that is used in skin creams and for treating burns.

Automatic external defibrillator (AED)—An electronic device for restoring regular heart rhythm.

Cardiopulmonary resuscitation (CPR)—A procedure for restoring normal breathing following cardiac arrest. It includes clearing the air passages, mouth-to-mouth artificial respiration, and heart massage by exerting pressure on the chest.

Heimlich maneuver—The application of sudden upward pressure on the upper abdomen to force a foreign object from the trachea of a choking victim; developed by the American surgeon Henry Jay Heimlich.

Shock—Severe depression of vital physiological processes, characterized by paleness, a rapid but weak pulse, rapid and shallow breathing, and low blood pressure; typically caused by injury, severe bleeding, or burns.

Tetanus—An acute infectious disease caused by a toxin produced by the bacterium *Clostridium tetani* and usually introduced into the body through a wound.

- the person is rolled over toward the rescuer by pulling on clothing at the hip, while supporting the head with the other hand
- one arm is bent up and the other down to support the upper and lower body
- the head is tilted back to allow air to move freely in and out of the mouth

If there is **vomiting** or bleeding from the mouth, the person should be rolled to the side in one move, while supporting the neck and back. They should be kept warm and gently restrained if awakened.

CPR should be performed on a someone who is not breathing and is unconscious or unresponsive. The technique used is slightly different for infants, children, and adults.

To perform CPR on an infant:

- place the infant face-up on a hard, flat surface
- tilted back and lift the chin so the mouth opens
- completely cover the mouth and nose of an infant under one year of age and give two rescue breaths
- check to see if the infant's chest rises with each breath; if it does, then begin chest compressions, otherwise repeat breathing
- give the infant 30 chest compressions using two fingers in the middle of the breastbone just below nipple level
- continue the cycle of two breaths and 30 chest compressions until emergency help arrives or the child begins breathing

To perform CPR on a child or an adult:

- place the person face-up on a hard, flat surface
- tilted back and lift the chin so the mouth opens
- completely cover the mouth and give two long rescue breaths
- check to see if the person's chest rises with each breath; if it does, then begin chest compressions, otherwise repeat breathing
- give 30 chest compressions using the heel of the hand on the lower half of the chest for children; for adults, place the heel of one hand on the center of the chest just below the nipples and the other hand on top of the first with the rescuer's body weight over the arms
- continue the cycle of two breaths and 30 chest compressions until emergency help arrives or the child begins breathing

Benefits

First aid can save lives. It can also prevent injuries from worsening or becoming infected and can speed healing.

Precautions

Serious injuries or emergency medical situations require summoning emergency responders, usually by calling 911, or rushing the child to a hospital emergency room or other critical care facility. Precautions for administering first aid depend on the type of injury. The most important precautions include never:

- moving a person if there is any possibility of spinal injury
- applying a tourniquet to stop bleeding
- attempting to remove a deeply imbedded object
- attempting to replace organs
- using direct heat on frostbite or rubbing frostbitten skin

- thawing frostbitten skin if there is a risk of refreezing
- breaking burn blisters or applying ice or any ointment or lotion to burns except under a doctor's direction
- giving anything to someone who may have ingested a toxin and never inducing vomiting, unless directed by the poison control center
- attempting to remove an object embedded in the eyeball or rubbing the eyes
- probing the nose for an object that is not visible and easily grasped
- washing or moving bone injuries
- restraining movement or putting anything in the mouth of a person having a seizure
- attempting to awake an unconscious person by shaking, slapping, or using cold water
- putting a pillow under an unconscious person's head, as this can block an airway

If possible, wear gloves and wash hands before and after administering first aid. It is also a good idea to ensure that a child's **tetanus** shots are current.

Preparation

An individual can prepare for first-aid by taking first-aid classes, learning CPR and renewing CPR certification at least every two years, and by learning to use an automatic external defibrillator (AED).

Basic first aid can be taught to children. It is a good idea for babysitters to also receive training in first aid and CPR.

Every home and automobile should have a well-stocked first-aid kit. Use a container that is clean, strong, and easy to carry and open to store items. First-aid kits are often designed for specific activities, such as hiking, camping, or boating, and should include items geared toward those activities. For example, include ointment for mosquito **bites** in a camping kit. A first-aid manual should also be stored in the kit.

Keep the container out of the reach of young children, but easily accessible to adults and anyone trained in its use. The contents should be checked every three months for missing items and expired medicines. Medicines should be in their original containers and marked with dosage and instructions.

A general purpose first-aid kit should contain:

- emergency and physician phone numbers
- a list of allergies and medications for all family members
- medical consent and medical history forms
- a first-aid manual
- a waterproof flashlight and batteries
- a cell phone and charger
- duct tape
- scissors, tweezers, needles, and safety pins
- a non-mercury, non-glass, oral thermometer
- sterile, disposable gloves
- eye goggles or eye shield
- a breathing barrier or mouthpiece for CPR
- a mylar emergency blanket
- aluminum finger splints
- a tooth-saver kit
- a bulb suction device for flushing out wounds
- instant cold packs
- assorted adhesive bandages, gauze pads, roller gauze, and compress dressings
- adhesive cloth tape
- an elastic (Ace) bandage
- sterile cotton balls and cotton-tipped swabs
- plastic bags for waste
- soap, hand sanitizer, and alcohol wipes
- antiseptic solution or wipes
- sterile eyewash or saline solution
- petroleum jelly or other lubricant
- aloe vera gel
- calamine lotion
- antibiotic ointment or cream
- hydrocortisone ointment or cream
- a medicine cup or spoon and oral medicine syringe
- aspirin, acetaminophen, and ibuprofen
- anti-diarrhea medication
- antihistamines
- decongestant
- cough suppressant
- antacid
- laxatives
- sunscreen
- prescription medications that do not need refrigeration
- any prescribed medical supplies

Aftercare

Most small cuts, scrapes, and abrasions heal without any special care, although it may be necessary to apply an antibiotic ointment. **Bandages** should be changed daily or whenever they become wet or dirty. After a bone injury is treated, the area should be elevated and ice packs or cold compresses should be applied every few hours for 20-minute periods.

Risks

An individual should be cautious about providing first-aid and must assess the situation before getting involved. If the situation is dangerous, such as the scene of an accident, the individual should not intervene and instead contact emergency personnel by dialing 9-1-1.

When coming in contact with blood or other bodily fluids, there may be a risk of infection with HIV or hepatitis virus. Wearing latex gloves can help prevent disease transmission. A mouth-to-mouth barrier device may not protect against contracting an infection when giving rescue breaths.

Resources

BOOKS

American Academy of Pediatrics. *Pediatric First Aid for Parents*. Sudbury, MA: Jones and Bartlett, 2008.

American Red Cross. *First Aid and Safety for Babies and Children*. Yardley, PA: StayWell, 2009.

Borgenicht, David, Justin Heimberg, and Chuck Gonzales. *The Worst-Case Scenario Survival Handbook: Extreme Junior Edition*. San Francisco: Chronicle, 2008.

National Safety Council. *Pediatric First Aid, CPR, and AED*. 2nd ed. Boston: McGraw-Hill Higher Education, 2008.

Porter, Robert S., et al. *The Merck Manual Home Health Handbook*. 3rd ed. Whitehouse Station, NJ: Merck Research Laboratories, 2009.

Subbarao, Italo, Jim Lyznicki, and James J. James. *American Medical Association Handbook of First Aid and Emergency Care*. Rev. and updated ed. New York: Random House Reference, 2009.

PERIODICALS

Onderko, Patty. "How to Save Your Child's Life." *Parenting. Early Years* 24, no. 3 (April 2010): 97–100.

"Qwik Sheet: Teaching Your Kids First Aid." *Pediatrics for Parents* 26, no. 3/4 (March/April 2010): 33–34.

OTHER

American College of Emergency Physicians. "Fast Aid First." Patient Center. http://www.acep.org/patients.aspx (accessed August 18, 2010).

American College of Emergency Physicians. "Home First Aid Kits." Patient Center. http://www3.acep.org/patients.aspx?id=26036 (accessed August 18, 2010).

"Anatomy of a First Aid Kit." American Red Cross. http://www.redcross.org/services/hss/lifeline/fakit.html (accessed August 18, 2010).

"Choking First Aid—Adult or Child Over 1 Year—Series." MedlinePlus. July 8, 2009. http://www.nlm.nih.gov/medlineplus/ency/presentations/100222_1.htm (accessed August 18, 2010).

"First Aid." MedlinePlus. July 9, 2010. http://www.nlm.nih.gov/medlineplus/firstaid.html (accessed August 18, 2010).

"First Aid: Burns." FamilyDoctor.org. November 2009. http://familydoctor.org/online/famdocen/home/healthy/firstaid/after-injury/638.printerview.html (accessed August 18, 2010).

"First Aid: Cuts, Scrapes and Stitches." FamilyDoctor.org. November 2009. http://familydoctor.org/online/famdocen/home/healthy/firstaid/after-injury/041.printerview.html (accessed August 18, 2010).

"First-Aid Kit." KidsHealth. September 2007. http://kidshealth.org/parent/firstaid_safe/home/firstaid_kit.html (accessed August 18, 2010).

"First-Aid Kits: Stock Supplies That Can Save Lives." MayoClinic.com. January 16, 2010. http://www.mayoclinic.com/health/first-aid-kits/FA00067 (accessed August 18, 2010).

ORGANIZATIONS

American Academy of Family Physicians, 11400 Tomahawk Creek Parkway, Leawood, KS, 66211-2680, (913) 906-6000, (800) 274-6000, (913) 906-6075, http://www.aafp.org.

American College of Emergency Physicians, P.O. Box 619911, Dallas, TX, 75261-9911, (972) 550-0911, (800) 798-1822, (972) 580-2816 , membership@acep.org, http://www3.acep.org.

American Red Cross, 2025 E St., NW, Washington, DC, 20006, (202) 303–5000, http://www.redcross.org.

Ready Campaign, Federal Emergency Management Agency, 500 C St., SW, Washington, DC, 20024, (202) 646-3272, ready@dhs.gov, http://www.ready.gov.

Margaret Alic, PhD

Fish and shellfish poisoning

Definition

Fish and shellfish **poisoning** is a common but often unrecognized group of illnesses related to food. Three of these illnesses include ciguatera, scombroid, and paralytic shellfish poisoning.

Ciguatera

Definition

Ciguatera (from the Spanish word for a poisonous snail) is a food-related illness that causes abdominal and neurological symptoms.

Causes and symptoms

Ciguatera is caused by eating fish that have a toxin called ciguatoxin. Scientists believe this toxin is acquired by the fish through the food chain, and is originally produced by small algae microorganisms (dinoflagellates). The fish most likely contaminated with ciguatoxin are those that feed close to tropical reefs, including red snapper, grouper, and barracuda. Larger fish are more likely to contain the toxin. Although not as common in the United States, ciguatera is commonly diagnosed on many of the islands in the Pacific Ocean.

Illness from ciguatera can occur in just a few minutes to about 30 hours after eating. Most cases occur one to six hours after eating the contaminated fish. Initial symptoms are abdominal cramps, **nausea**, **vomiting**, or watery **diarrhea**. The most characteristic symptoms of the illness are those involving the nervous system. These include **numbness and tingling** around the lips, tongue, and mouth; **itching**; **dry mouth**; metallic taste in the mouth; and blurry vision. In more prominent cases, patients may complain of temporary blindness, a slow pulse, and a feeling that their teeth are loose. Patients may also have the strange symptom of reversal of hot and cold sensations on the skin, where cold things feel very hot or painful to the touch. In very severe cases, patients may experience difficulties in breathing or low blood pressure.

Diagnosis

Ciguatera diagnosis is based on the typical combination of symptoms after eating fish. There are no readily available blood or urine tests to detect the poisoning, but some researchers have developed a test for the toxin left on any remaining fish. A person does not have to be in a tropical area to get ciguatera. Fish can be caught from one of these distant areas, and can then be shipped and eaten locally. It is important to report suspected cases to local public health officials because more cases may occur from other contaminated fish.

Treatment

The treatment for this illness is general. Patients are given fluids (by mouth or through a vein) and medications to decrease the itching or to treat **vomiting** and/or diarrhea. The neurological symptoms can cause discomfort and treatment with amitriptyline (a medicine that has been used for depression) may be useful. Other medications may also be given.

Prognosis

Although **death** can occur, almost all patients diagnosed with ciguatera will recover. Recovery, however, can be slow and some symptoms can last for weeks or even months. Symptoms can also be aggravated by other illnesses or alcohol.

Prevention

Knowing the kinds of fish linked to ciguatera can help a person avoid eating high-risk fish. However, more than 400 different kinds of fish have been linked to the disease, even salmon. A particular fish in a given area may be more likely to cause ciguatera than other fish. For example, red snapper is most often the source of ciguatera in the Pacific, while barracuda is more likely to contain the toxin in Florida. This is why it is illegal to sell barracuda in Florida for human consumption. Cooking the fish does not prevent ciguatera.

Scombroid

Definition

Scombroid is a fish-associated illness caused by eating improperly handled fish. Fish linked to this disease are usually in the Scombridae family, which includes yellowfin tuna, skipjack, bonito, and mackerel.

Causes and symptoms

Scombroid occurs after eating fish that has not been properly refrigerated after capture. Unlike ciguatera, the toxins linked with scombroid are not contracted by the fish from its surroundings. Bacteria that are normally found in fish act directly on a chemical (called histidine) in the flesh of fish that are not properly cooled when stored. This interaction produces histamine and other chemicals that cause the illness when the fish is eaten.

Symptoms of scombroid occur quickly after eating the fish, as soon as 10 minutes. Since histamine is released by certain cells in the body during an allergic reaction, scombroid can be confused with a fish allergy. Scombroid causes flushing of the face, sweating, a burning feeling in the mouth or throat, vomiting, diarrhea, and headaches. A rash that looks like a **sunburn** may occur, and a small number of patients have **hives**. Some patients have a metallic or peppery taste in their mouths. In more severe cases, rapid pulse, blurred vision, and difficulty breathing can occur. Symptoms usually last about four hours.

Diagnosis

Like ciguatera, scombroid poisoning is diagnosed based on typical symptoms occurring after eating fish. There are usually no available tests for the patient. Experimentally, however, elevated levels of histamine-related products have been found in the urine. It may be possible for public health officials to test any remaining fish flesh for histamine levels. Improperly refrigerated fish caught in both temperate and tropical waters have been linked to the illness. An outbreak of similar cases may be helpful in correctly diagnosing the problem.

Treatment

The treatment for scombroid is usually general. **Antihistamines** like diphenhydramine (Benadryl) may shorten the duration of the illness, but the illness will go away on its own. Some doctors have found that cimetidine (Tagamet) given through a vein may be helpful as well. In rare, more severe cases, epinephrine (adrenaline) may be used.

Prognosis

Although sometimes dramatic and alarming symptoms can occur, scombroid is usually not serious. The patient should be reassured that scombroid is not a fish allergy.

Prevention

Adequate storage of the target fish will always prevent scombroid. Since the fish does not appear spoiled or smell bad, the consumer cannot detect the risk of the illness before eating the fish. Cooking the fish does not prevent scombroid. Suspected cases should be reported to public health officials.

Paralytic shellfish poisoning

Definition

Paralytic shellfish poisoning (PSP) is a nervous system disease caused by eating cooked or raw shellfish that contain environmental toxins. These toxins are produced by a group of algae (dinoflagellates). It is unclear whether these toxins are related to the "blooming" of the algae, also called red tide because the algae can turn the water reddish brown. PSP occurs mostly in May through November.

Causes and symptoms

PSP develops usually within minutes after eating a contaminated shellfish, most commonly a mussel, clam, or oyster. Symptoms include **headache**, a floating feeling, **dizziness**, lack of coordination, and **tingling** of the mouth, arms, or legs. Muscle weakness causing difficulty swallowing or speaking may occur. Abdominal symptoms such as nausea, vomiting, and diarrhea can also occur. Unlike ciguatera and scombroid, PSP may have a much more serious outcome. PSP may cause difficulty breathing related to weakness or **paralysis** of the breathing muscle. The symptoms may last for six to 12 hours, but a patient may continue to feel weak for a week or more.

Diagnosis

PSP diagnosis is based on symptoms after eating shellfish, even if the shellfish are adequately cooked. No blood or urine test is available to diagnose the illness, but tests in mice to detect the toxin from the eaten fish can be done by public health officials.

Treatment

The treatment of PSP is mostly supportive. If early symptoms are recognized, the doctor will try to flush the toxin from the gastrointestinal tract with medications that create diarrhea. Vomiting may be induced if the patient has no signs of weakness. In cases where the muscles of breathing are weakened, the patient may be placed on a respirator until the weakness goes away. However, this measure is not usually needed. Likewise, the use of a machine to clean the blood (dialysis) has been used in severe cases.

Prognosis

The prognosis for PSP is quite good, especially if the patient has passed the initial 12 hours of illness without needing breathing support. Most deaths occur during this period if breathing help is not available.

Prevention

Measures to control PSP require detecting rising numbers of algae in coastal waters by periodic

KEY TERMS

Algae—Plants that have one cell.

Histamine—A chemical found naturally in the body that produces inflammation and increases blood flow; the uncomfortable symptoms of an allergy attack or an allergic reaction are generally caused by the release of histamine.

Toxin—A poisonous substance usually produced by a living thing.

microscopic examination. By law, shellfish beds are closed when levels of the toxin-producing organisms are above acceptable standards. Cooking the shellfish does not prevent this disease. Suspected cases should be reported to public health officials.

Resources

PERIODICALS

Barton, Erik D., Paula Tanner, Steven G. Turchen, et al. "Ciguatera Fish Poisoning: A Southern California Epidemic." *Western Journal of Medicine* 163, no. 1 (July 1995): 31–35.

Larry I. Lutwick, MD, FACP

Fistula

Definition

A fistula is a permanent abnormal passageway between two organs in the body or between an organ and the exterior of the body.

Description

Fistulas can arise in any part of the body, but they are most common in the digestive tract. They can also develop between blood vessels and in the urinary, reproductive, and lymphatic systems. Fistulas can occur at any age or can be present at birth (congenital). Some are life-threatening, others cause discomfort, while still others are benign and go undetected or cause few symptoms. Diabetics, individuals with compromised immune systems (**AIDS**, **cancer**) and individuals with certain gastrointestinal diseases (**Crohn's disease**, inflammatory bowel disease) are at increased risk of developing fistulas.

Fistulas are categorized by the number of openings they have and whether they connect two internal organs or open through the skin. There are four common types:

- Blind fistulas are open on one end only.
- Complete fistulas have one internal opening and one opening on the skin.
- Horseshoe fistulas are complex fistulas with more than one opening on the exterior of the body.
- Incomplete fistulas are tubes of skin that are open on the outside but closed on the inside and do not connect to any internal structure.

Fistulas of the digestive tract

Anal and rectal fistulas develop in the wall of the anus or rectum. They connect the interior of the body to one or several openings in the skin. Anal and rectal fistulas almost always begin as an inflammation in an anal gland. The inflammation then moves into muscle tissue and develops into an **abscess**. In about half of all cases, the abscess develops into a fistula, degrading the muscle until an opening in the skin is created. About nine people of every 100,000 develop anal fistulas, with men almost twice more likely to develop the condition than women. Although they may develop at any age, the average age for the development of anal fistulas is 38.

Intestinal fistulas can develop in both the large and small intestine. They are commonly associated with diseases such as inflammatory bowel disease (IBD) and Crohn's disease.

Tracheoesophageal fistulas (TEF) are usually **birth defects**. The windpipe, or trachea, is abnormally connected to the esophagus. This allows air to enter the digestive system and makes it possible to breathe food into the lungs (aspiration). In many cases, the esophagus is also incomplete, causing immediate feeding problems. There are several types of TEFs categorized by where the fistula is located and how the esophagus and trachea are connected, but all are life-threatening and require prompt surgery to repair. TEFs occur in about one of every 1,500–3,000 births.

Fistulas of the urinary and reproductive tract

The most common type of fistula involving these systems is a vesicovaginal fistula, in which the woman's vagina is connected to the urinary bladder. This causes leakage of urine from the vagina and results in frequent vaginal and bladder infections. Fistulas may also develop between the vagina and the large intestine (a enterovaginal fistula) so that feces leaks from the vagina. Although both these types of fistulas are uncommon in the developed world, they are common in poor developing countries and result from long, difficult labor and **childbirth**, especially in very young girls. As a result, they are sometimes referred to as obstetric fistulas.

Some experts suggest that in parts of Africa, as many as 3–4 women develop these fistulas for every 1,000 births. Others estimate that as many as 2 million women worldwide are living with unrepaired obstetric fistulas. If left unrepaired, obstetric fistulas cause women to constantly leak urine and feces. As expected, they may suffer severe social issues, extreme hardship and psychological trauma.

Fistulas of the circulatory system

Arteriovenous fistulas (AVF) can develop between an artery and a vein in any part of the body. These fistulas vary in size, length, and frequency. Arteries contain blood carrying oxygen to all parts of the body, while veins carry blood that has given up its oxygen back to the lungs. Connections between arteries and veins cause changes in blood pressure that result in abnormal development of the walls of the arteries and abnormal blood flow. Arteriovenous fistulas that are present at birth are sometimes referred to as **arteriovenous malformations** (AVMs). Many arteriovenous fistulas are present, but not evident at birth, and become obvious only after trauma. AVFs can also be acquired from penetrating trauma.

Causes and symptoms

The causes and symptoms of fistulas vary depending on their location. Anal and rectal fistulas are usually caused by an abscess. Symptoms include constant throbbing **pain** and swelling in the rectal area. Pus is sometimes visible draining from the fistula opening on the skin. Many individuals have a **fever** resulting from the infection causing the abscess.

Vaginal fistulas are caused by infection and trauma to the tissue during childbirth. They are easily detected, because the woman smells unpleasant and leaks urine or feces through her vagina. Rarely these fistulas may develop as a complication of **hysterectomy**.

Tracheoesophageal fistulas are the result of errors in the development of the fetus. They are evident at birth, because the infant is unable to swallow or eat normally and are considered a medical emergency that requires surgery if the infant is to survive.

Arteriovenous fistulas are most often congenital defects. Symptoms vary depending on the size and location of the fistula. Often the skin is bright pink or dark red in the area of the fistula. Individuals may complain of pain. The pain is a result of some tissues not receiving enough oxygen because of abnormal blood flow.

Diagnosis

Tests use to determine the presence of a fistula vary with the location of the fistula. When there is an opening to the outside, the physician may be able to see the fistula and probe it. Various imaging studies such as x-rays, CT scans, barium **enemas**, **endoscopy**, and ultrasonography are used to locate less visible fistulas.

KEY TERMS

Abscess—A collection of pus surrounded by inflamed, infected tissue.

Lymphatic system—The part of the circulatory system that carries lymph, a clear fluid that is involved in immune system response.

Treatment

Anal and rectal fistulas are treated by draining the pus the infected area. The individual also is usually given **antibiotics** to help prevent recurrence of the abscess. If this fails to heal the fistula, surgery may be necessary.

Intestinal fistulas are treated first by reducing the inflammation in the intestine and then, if necessary with surgery. Treatment varies considerably depending on the degree of severity of symptoms the fistula causes. TEFs are always treated with surgery. Obstetric fistulas must also be repaired with surgery. The treatment of arteriovenous fistulas depends on the size and location of the fistula and usually includes surgery.

Alternative treatment

No effective alternative treatments for fistulas are known.

Prognosis

The outcome of fistulas depends on the type and cause of the condition. Surgical repair of obstetric fistulas is almost always successful. Unfortunately, many women in developing countries do not have access to this type of surgery. Treatment of anal and rectal fistulas is almost always successful, although fistulas may recur in up to 18% of individuals. The outcome of surgery on TEFs is highly variable, especially since infants born with this condition often have other developmental abnormalities that may affect the outcome of fistula repair. The degree of successful repair of arteriovenous fistulas depends on their size and location. Uncontrolled bleeding is the most common complication of surgery to repair AVFs.

Prevention

Obstetric fistulas are the only preventable fistulas. These can be prevented with good prenatal and childbirth care and by avoiding **pregnancy** in very young girls. Although anal and rectal fistulas are not preventable, their damage can be minimized by prompt drainage and treatment.

Resources

OTHER

"Fistula." *Medline Plus Medical Encyclopedia*, 29 October 2003 [cited 16 February 2005]. http://www.nlm.nih.gov/medlineplus/ency/article/002365.htm

Legall, Ingrid. *Anal Fistulas and Fissures*, 11 June 2004 [cited 16 February 2005]. http://www.emedicine.com/emerg/topic495.htm.

Morasch, Mark D. and Dipen Maun. *Arteriovenous Fistulas*, 24 October 2003 [cited 16 February 2005]. http://www.emedicine.com/med/topic169.htm.

Zagrodnik, Dennis II. *Fistula-in-Ano*, ii June 2004 [cited 3 March 2005]. http://www.emedicine.com/med/topic2710.htm.

ORGANIZATIONS

American Society of Colon and Rectal Surgeons, 85 W. Algonquin Rd., Suite 550, Arlington Heights, IL, 60005, (847) 290-9184, (847) 290-9203, ascrs@fascrs.org, http://www.fascrs.org/.

Tish Davidson, A.M.

5p-syndrome *see* **Cri du chat syndrome**

Flesh-eating disease

Definition

Flesh-eating disease is more properly called necrotizing fasciitis, a rare condition in which bacteria destroy tissues underlying the skin. This tissue **death**, called necrosis or **gangrene**, spreads rapidly. This disease can be fatal in as little as 12 to 24 hours.

Description

Although the term is technically incorrect, flesh-eating disease is an apt descriptor: The infection appears to devour body tissue. Media reports increased in the middle and late 1990s, but the disease is not new. Hippocrates described it more than three millennia ago and thousands of reports exist from the Civil War. Approximately 500 to 1,500 cases of necrotizing fasciitis occur in the United States each year.

Flesh-eating disease is divided into two types. Type I is caused by anaerobic bacteria, with or without the presence of aerobic bacteria. Type II, also called hemolytic streptococcal gangrene, is caused by group A streptococci; other bacteria may or may not be present. The disease may also be called synergistic gangrene.

Type I fasciitis typically affects the trunk, abdomen, and genital area. For example, Fournier's gangrene is a "flesh-eating" disease in which the infection encompasses the external genitalia. The arms and legs are most often affected in type II fasciitis, but the infection may appear anywhere.

Causes and symptoms

The two most important factors in determining whether a person will develop flesh-eating disease are: the virulence (ability to cause disease) of the bacteria and the susceptibility (ability of a person's immune system to respond to infection) of the person who becomes infected with this bacteria.

In nearly every case of flesh-eating disease, a skin injury precedes the disease. As bacteria grow beneath the skin's surface, they produce toxins. These toxins destroy superficial fascia, subcutaneous fat, and deep fascia. In some cases, the overlying dermis and the underlying muscle are also affected.

Initially, the infected area appears red and swollen and feels hot. The area is extremely painful, which is a prominent feature of the disease. Over the course of hours or days, the skin may become blue-gray, and fluid-filled blisters may form. As nerves are destroyed the area becomes numb. An individual may go into **shock** and develop dangerously low blood pressure. Multiple organ failure may occur, quickly followed by death.

Diagnosis

The appearance of the skin, paired with **pain** and **fever** raises the possibility of flesh-eating disease. An x-ray, **magnetic resonance imaging** (MRI), or **computed tomography scans** (CT scans) of the area reveals a feathery pattern in the tissue, caused by accumulating gas in the dying tissue. Necrosis is evident during exploratory surgery, during which samples are collected for bacterial identification.

KEY TERMS

Aerobic bacteria—Bacteria that require oxygen to live and grow.

Anaerobic bacteria—Bacteria that require the absence of oxygen to live and grow.

CT scan (computed tomography scan)—Cross-sectional x-rays of the body are compiled to create a three-dimensional image of the body's internal structures.

Debridement—Surgical procedure in which dead or dying tissue is removed.

Dermis—The deepest layer of skin.

Fascia, deep—A fibrous layer of tissue that envelopes muscles.

Fascia, superficial—A fibrous layer of tissue that lies between the deepest layer of skin and the subcutaneous fat.

Gangrene—An extensive area of dead tissue.

Hyperbaric oxygen therapy—A treatment in which the patient is placed in a chamber and breathes oxygen at higher-than-atmospheric pressure. This high-pressure oxygen stops bacteria from growing and, at high enough pressure, kills them.

Magnetic resonance imaging (MRI)—An imaging technique that uses a large circular magnet and radio waves to generate signals from atoms in the body. These signals are used to construct images of internal structures.

Necrosis—Abnormal death of cells, potentially caused by disease or infection.

Subcutaneous—Referring to the area beneath the skin.

Treatment

Rapid, aggressive medical treatment, specifically, antibiotic therapy and surgical **debridement**, is imperative. **Antibiotics** may include penicillin, an aminoglycoside or third-generation cephalosporin, and clindamycin or metronidazole. **Analgesics** are employed for pain control. During surgical debridement, dead tissue is stripped away. After surgery, patients are rigorously monitored for continued infection, shock, or other complications. If available, hyperbaric **oxygen therapy** has also be used.

Prognosis

Flesh-eating disease has a fatality rate of about 30%. Diabetes, arteriosclerosis, immunosuppression, **kidney disease**, **malnutrition**, and **obesity** are connected with a poor prognosis. Older individuals and intravenous drug users may also be at higher risk. The infection site also has a role. Survivors may require **plastic surgery** and may have to contend with permanent physical disability and psychological adjustment.

Prevention

Flesh-eating disease, which occurs very rarely, cannot be definitively prevented. The best ways to lower the risk of contracting flesh-eating disease are:

- take care to avoid any injury to the skin that may give the bacteria a place of entry
- when skin injuries do occur, they should be promptly washed and treated with an antibiotic ointment or spray
- people who have any skin injury should rigorously attempt to avoid people who are infected with streptococci bacteria, a bacteria that causes a simple strep throat in one person may cause flesh-eating disease in another
- have any areas of unexplained redness, pain, or swelling examined by a doctor, particularly if the affected area seems to be expanding

Resources

BOOKS

Lewis Tilden, Thomasine E. *Help! What's Eating My Flesh?: Runaway Staph and Strep Infections!* New York: Franklin Watts, 2008.

ORGANIZATIONS

National Necrotizing Fasciitis Foundation, 2731 Porter SW, Grand Rapids, MI, 49509, nnfffeb@aol.com, http://www.nnff.org.

Paul A. Johnson, Ed.M.

Flight medicine *see* **Aviation medicine**

Floppy mitral valve *see* **Mitral valve prolapse**

Flower remedies

Definition

Flower remedies are specially prepared flower essences, containing the healing energy of plants. They are prescribed according to a patient's emotional disposition, as ascertained by the therapist, doctor, or patients themselves.

Purpose

Flower remedies are more homeopathic than herbal in the way they work, effecting energy levels rather than chemical balances. They have been described as "liquid energy." The theory is that they encapsulate the flowers' healing energy, and are said to deal with and overcome negative emotions, and so relieve blockages in the flow of human energy that can cause illness.

Description

Origins

Perhaps the most famous and widely used system is the Bach flower remedies. This system originated in the 1920s when British physician and bacteriologist, Dr. Edward Bach (1886–1936), noticed that patients with physical complaints often seemed to be suffering from **anxiety** or some kind of negative emotion. He concluded that assessing a patient's emotional disposition and prescribing an appropriate flower essence could treat the physical illness. Bach was a qualified medical doctor, but he also practiced homeopathy.

As a result of his own serious illness in 1917, Bach began a search for a new and simple system of medicine that would treat the whole person. In 1930, he gave up his flourishing practice on Harley Street at the Royal London Homeopathic Hospital and moved to the countryside to devote his life to this research. At this point, he ceased to dispense the mixture of homeopathy and allopathic medicine that he had been using. Instead, he began investigating the healing properties of plant essences and discovered that he possessed an "intuition" for judging the properties of each flower. Accordingly, he developed the system of treatment that bears his name, and is also the foundation for all other flower-remedy systems.

The Bach Flower Remedies were ostensibly the only system of significance from the 1920s until in the 1970s, when there was a renewed interest in the subject by doctors working in the field of natural medicine. Perhaps the most notable was Dr. Richard Katz, who was seeking new methods of dealing with modern **stress** and the resulting ailments. He focused on the concept of a psychic, psychological effect and chose to pursue this line of research.

In 1979, Katz founded the Flower Essence Society in California, (FES). This society pledged to further the research and development of Bach's principles. FES hosts a database of more than 100 flower essences from more than 50 countries. FES is now an international organization of health practitioners, researchers, students, and others concerned with flower essence therapy.

The society has connections with an estimated 50,000 active practitioners from around the world, who use flower essence therapy as part of their treatment. FES encourages the study of the plants themselves to determine the characteristics of flower essences. They are compiling an extensive database of case studies and practitioner reports of the use of essences therapeutically, allowing verification and development of the original definitions. They are also engaged in the scientific study of flower essence therapy.

FES says they have developed the theories of Paracelsus and Goethe who researched the "signatures" and "gestures" of botanical specimens, on the premise that the human body and soul are a reflection of the system of nature. FES plant research interprets the therapeutic properties of flower essences according to these insights.

In this regard, they have devised 12 "windows of perception" for monitoring the attributes of plants. Each of these windows reveals an aspect of the plant's qualities, although they maintain that what they are seeking is a "whole which is greater than the sum of its parts." The 12 windows are not considered independent classifications, but more of a blended tapestry of views of the qualities that each plant possesses.

The first window is concerned with the "form" of a plant—its shape classification. The second focuses on its "gesture" or spatial relationship. The third window is a plant's botanical classification: The Flower Essence Society maintains that considering a plant's botanical family is essential to obtaining an overview of its properties as a flower essence. The fourth window concerns the time orientation of a particular specimen regarding the daily and seasonal cycles. Why do some flowers bloom at different times of the day, while others, such as the evening primrose, respond to the moon? The fifth window observes a plant's relationship to its environment. Where a plant chooses to grow, and where it cannot survive, reveals much about its qualities. The sixth window observes a plant's relationship to the Four Elements and the Four Ethers, as FES maintains that plants

EDWARD BACH (1886–1936)

Edward Bach was a graduate of University College Hospital (M.B., B.S., M.R.C.S.) in England. He left his flourishing Harley Street practice in favor of homeopathy, seeking a more natural system of healing than allopathic medicine. He concluded that healing should be as simple and natural as the development of plants, which were nourished and given healing properties by earth, air, water, and sun.

Bach believed that he could sense the individual healing properties of flowers by placing his hands over the petals. His remedies were prepared by floating summer flowers in a bowl of clear stream water exposed to sunlight for three hours.

He developed 38 remedies, one for each of the negative states of mind suffered by human beings, which he classified under seven group headings: fear, uncertainty, insufficient interest in present circumstances, loneliness, over-sensitivity to influences and ideas, despondency or despair, and overcare for the welfare of others. The Bach remedies can be prescribed for plants, animals, and other living creatures as well as human beings.

exist in one of the elemental or etheric forces in addition to their physical life. "Elements" refers to those developed by the Greeks, as opposed to the modern concept of "molecular building blocks." It seems that commonly, two elements predominate in a plant, indicating a polarity of qualities, while two can be said to be recessive. The seventh window relates to a plant's relationship with the other kingdoms of nature: mineral, animal, and human, while the eighth relates to the color and color variations of a plant. Katz explains how the language of color tells us so much about the "soul qualities" of a plant. The ninth window concerns all other sensory perceptions of a plant, such as fragrance, texture, and taste. The 10th window involves assessing the chemical substances and properties; the 11th studies medicinal and herbal uses, as by studying the physical healing properties of plants, we can also understand something of their more subtle effects on the soul. Finally, the 12th window involves the study of the lore, mythology, folk wisdom, and spiritual and ritual qualities associated with a particular plant. Katz relates how in the past, human beings were more in touch with the natural world, and the remnants of this unconscious plant wisdom live on in the form of folklore, mythology, and so on.

Because flower remedies operate on approximately the same principles as homeopathy, practitioners quite often prescribe the two therapies in conjunction with each other. They can also be used concurrently with allopathic medicine.

The system consists of 38 remedies, each for a different disposition. The basic theory is that if the remedy for the correct disposition is chosen, the physical illness resulting from the present emotional state can then be cured. There is a rescue remedy made up of five of the essences—cherry plum, clematis, impatiens, rock star, and star of Bethlehem—that is recommended for the treatment of any kind of physical or emotional shock. Therapists recommended that rescue remedy be kept on hand to help with all emergencies.

The 38 Bach Remedies are:

- agrimony: puts on a cheerful front, hides true feelings, and worries or problems
- aspen: feelings of apprehension, dark foreboding, and premonitions
- beech: critical, intolerant, picky
- centaury: easily comes under the influence of others, weak willed
- cerato: unsure, no confidence in own judgement, intuition, and seeks approval from others
- cherry plum: phobic, fear of being out of control, and tension
- chestnut bud: repeats mistakes, does not learn from experience
- chicory: self-centered, possessive, clingy, demanding, self pity
- clematis: absent minded, dreamy, apathetic, and lack of connection with reality
- crab apple: a "cleanser" for prudishness, self–disgust, feeling unclean
- elm: a sense of being temporarily overwhelmed in people who are usually capable and in control
- gentian: discouraged, doubting, despondent
- gorse: feelings of pessimism, accepting defeat
- heather: need for company, talks about self, and concentrates on own problems
- holly: jealousy, envy, suspicion, anger, and hatred
- honeysuckle: reluctance to enter the present and let the past go
- hornbeam: reluctant to face a new day, weary, can't cope (mental fatigue)
- impatiens: impatience, always in a hurry, and resentful of constraints

- larch: feelings of inadequacy and apprehension, lack of confidence and will to succeed
- mimulus: fearful of specific things, shy, and timid
- mustard: beset by "dark cloud" and gloom for no apparent reason
- oak: courageous, persevering, naturally strong but temporarily overcome by difficulties
- olive: for physical and mental renewal, to overcome exhaustion from problems of long–standing
- pine: for self–reproach, always apologizing, assuming guilt
- red chestnut: constant worry and concern for others
- rock rose: panic, intense alarm, dread, horror
- rock water: rigid–minded, self–denial, restriction
- scleranthus: indecision, uncertainty, fluctuating moods
- star of Bethlehem: consoling, following shock or grief or serious news
- sweet chestnut: desolation, despair, bleak outlook
- vervain: insistent, fanatical, over–enthusiastic
- vine: dominating, overbearing, autocratic, tyrannical
- walnut: protects during a period of adjustment or vulnerability
- water violet: proud, aloof, reserved, enjoys being alone
- white chestnut: preoccupation with worry, unwanted thoughts
- wild oat: drifting, lack of direction in life
- wild rose: apathy, resignation, no point in life
- willow bitter: resentful, dissatisfied, feeling life is unfair

Originally, Bach collected the dew from chosen flowers by hand to provide his patients with the required remedy. This became impractical when his treatment became so popular that production could not keep up with demand. He then set about finding a way to manufacture the remedies, and found that floating the freshly picked petals on the surface of spring water in a glass bowl and leaving them in strong sunlight for three hours produced the desired effect. Therapists explain that the water is "potentized" by the essence of the flowers. The potentized water can then be bottled and sold. For more woody specimens, the procedure is to boil them in a sterilized pan of water for 30 minutes. These two methods produce "mother tinctures" and the same two methods devised by Bach are still used today. Flower essences do not contain any artificial chemical substances, except for alcohol preservative.

Bach remedies cost around $10 each, and there is no set time limit for treatment. It may take days, weeks, or in some cases months. Flower essences cost around $6 each, and there is also no set time for the length of treatment, or the amount of essences that may be taken. These treatments are not generally covered by medical insurance.

Precautions

Bach remedies and flower essences are not difficult to understand, and are considered suitable for self administration. The only difficulty may be in finding the correct suggested remedy, as it can sometimes be tricky to pinpoint an individual's emotional disposition. They are even safe for babies, children, and animals. An important aspect of treatment with flower remedies, is that if you feel instinctively that you need a particular remedy, you are encouraged to act on that instinct. However, it is advisable not to continue a particular remedy once you feel you no longer need it, and to try a different one if you feel that progress is not being made.

The remedies are administered from a stoppered bottle and need to be diluted. Individuals sensitive to alcohol can apply the concentrate directly to temples, wrists, behind the ears, or underarms. They should be kept in a cool dark place; like this they should last indefinitely. However, a diluted remedy should not be kept longer than three weeks. Two drops of each diluted remedy should be taken four times a day, including first thing in the morning and last thing at night. If the rescue remedy is being used, four drops should be used instead. Most therapists recommend that they be taken in spring water, but the remedy can be taken directly from the bottle, if care is taken that the dropper does not touch the tongue, as this would introduce bacteria that would spoil the remedy.

It is not recommended that more than six or seven Bach remedies be used at any one time. Instead, it is preferable to divide a larger amount up into two lots to ensure the optimum effectiveness of the remedies. No combination, or amount of combinations of the remedies can cause any harm, rather they become less effective.

Unlike FES, the Bach Centre does not encourage research to "prove" that the remedies work, preferring that people find out for themselves. They strive to keep the use of the Bach remedies as simple as possible, and to this end they do not keep case records. Bach warned before he died that others would try to change his work and make it more complicated. He was determined to keep it simple so that anyone could use it, and that is why he limited the system to only 38 remedies. The

KEY TERMS

Aura—Emanation of light from living things (plants and animals) that can be recorded by Kirlian photography.

Essence—The constituent of a plant that determines its characteristics.

Potentize—The process of transferring the healing energy of a plant into spring water.

Window—A perspective adopted to assess the property of a given plant.

Centre points out that many who have used Bach's research as a starting point have added other remedies to the list, even some that Bach himself rejected.

Side effects

Flower remedies or essences are generally regarded as being totally safe, and there are no known side effects apart from the rare appearance of a slight rash, which is not a reason to discontinue treatment, says the Bach Centre.

Research and general acceptance

Bach flower remedies and flower essences have not yet officially won the support of allopathic medicine, despite the fact that more and more medical doctors are referring patients for such treatments on the strength of personal conviction. However, it is difficult to discount the scores of testimonials. Some practitioners refer skeptics to the research that has been done regarding the "auras" of living things. Theoretically, the stronger the aura, the more alive an organism is. Flower essences have very strong auras.

Resources

BOOKS

McCabe, Vinton. *The Healing Bouquet: Exploring Bach Flower Remedies*. Laguna Beach, CA: Basic Health, 2007.

ORGANIZATIONS

Flower Essence Society, P.O. Box 459, Nevada City, NV, 95959, (530) 265-9163, (530) 265-0584, (800) 736-9222, info@flowersociety.org, http://www.flowersociety.org/ .

Patricia Skinner

Flu *see* **Influenza**

Flucona *see* **Antifungal drugs, systemic**

Fluke infections

Definition

Fluke infections are diseases of the digestive tract and other organ systems caused by several different species of parasitic flatworms (trematodes) that have complex life cycles involving hosts other than human beings. Trematode comes from a Greek word that means having holes and refers to the external suckers that adult flukes use to draw nourishment from their hosts. Fluke infections are contracted by eating uncooked fish, plants, or animals from fluke-infected waters. Symptoms vary according to the type of fluke infection.

Description

In humans, fluke infections can be classified according to those diseases caused by liver flukes and those caused by lung flukes. Diseases caused by liver flukes include fascioliasis, opisthorchiasis, and clonorchiasis. Cases of liver fluke infection have been reported in Europe and the United States, as well as the Middle East, China, Japan, and Africa. Diseases caused by lung flukes include paragonimiasis. Paragonimiasis is a common infection in the Far East, Southeast Asia, Africa, Central and South America, Indonesia, and the Pacific Islands. It is estimated that

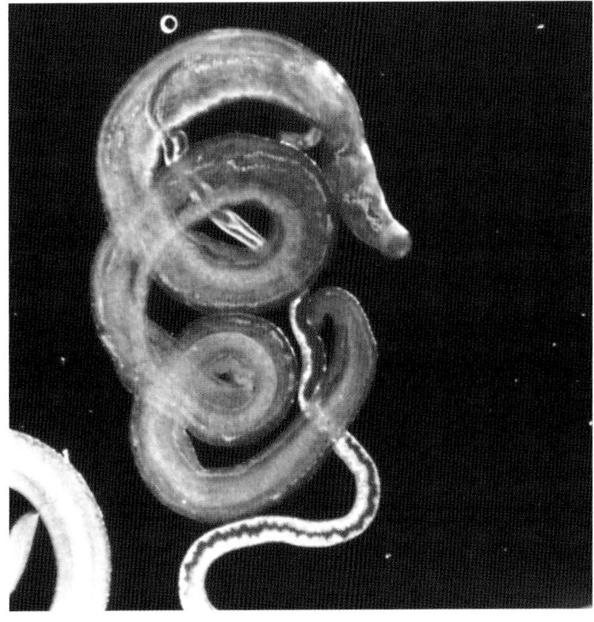

A micrograph of adult intestinal blood flukes, *Schistosoma mansoni*. Humans can become infected while bathing or working in contaminated water. *(Photo Researchers, Inc.)*

between 40 million and 100 million people worldwide suffer from either liver or lung fluke infections.

In their adult stage, liver and lung flukes are symmetrical in shape, ranging between 1/4–1 in in length, and look somewhat like long, plump leaves or blades of grass. They enter through the mouth and can infect any person at any age.

Causes and symptoms

The symptoms of fluke infection differ somewhat according to the type of fluke involved. All forms of liver and lung fluke infection, however, have the following characteristics:

- most persons who get infected do not develop symptoms (asymptomatic)
- the early symptoms of an acute fluke infection are not unique to these diseases alone (nonspecific symptoms)
- infection does not confer immunity against re-infection by the same species or infection by other species of flukes
- infection is usually associated with eating uncooked fish, plants, or animals that live in fresh water

Fascioliasis

Fascioliasis is caused by *Fasciola hepatica*, the sheep liver fluke. The fluke has a three-part life cycle that begins when eggs from a host's feces are deposited in water. The eggs release free-swimming larvae (miracidia) that infect snails. The snails then release free-swimming larvae with tails (cercariae) that form cysts containing larvae in the infective stage (metacercariae) on vegetation growing in fresh water. Humans become infected when they eat watercress, water chestnuts, or other plants covered with the encysted metacercariae.

When a person eats contaminated plants, the cysts are broken open in the digestive system, and the metacercariae leave their cysts, pass through the wall of the intestine, and enter the liver, where they cause inflammation and destroy tissue. After a period of 10–15 weeks in the liver, the adult flukes move to the bile ducts and produce eggs. Acute fascioliasis is marked by abdominal **pain** with **headache**, loss of appetite, anemia, and **vomiting**. Some patients develop **hives**, muscle pains, or a yellow-color to the skin and whites of the eyes (**jaundice**). Chronic forms of the disease may produce complications, including blockage of the bile ducts or the migration of adult flukes to other parts of the body.

Opisthorchiasis and clonorchiasis

These infections are caused by *Clonorchis sinensis*, the Chinese liver fluke, and *Opisthorchis viverrini* or *O. felineus*. The diseases are widespread, affecting more than 20 million people in Japan, China, Southeast Asia, and India. The life cycle of these liver flukes is similar to that of *F. hepatica* except that the etacercariae are encysted in freshwater fish rather than on plants. Dogs, cats, and other mammals that eat raw fish can be infected with opisthorchiasis and clonorchiasis.

The symptoms of opisthorchiasis and clonorchiasis are similar to those of fascioliasis and include both acute and chronic forms. In acute infection, the patient may be tired, have a low-grade **fever**, pains in the joints, a swollen liver, abdominal pain, and a skin rash. The acute syndrome may be difficult to diagnose because the fluke eggs do not appear in the patient's stool for three to four weeks after infection. Patients with the chronic form of the disease experience a loss of appetite, **fatigue**, low-grade fever, **diarrhea**, and an enlarged liver that feels sore when the abdomen is pressed.

Paragonimiasis

Paragonimiasis is caused by a lung fluke, either *Paragonimus westermani* or *P. skrjabini*. These flukes are larger than liver flukes and infect meat- or fish-eating animals as well as humans. Their life cycle is similar to that of liver flukes except that their encysted larvae infect crabs and crayfish rather than plants or fish. Humans can ingest the encysted metacercariae from drinking contaminated water or eating raw or undercooked crabs and crayfish.

In humans, the metacercariae are released from their cysts in the small intestine and migrate to the lungs or the brain in 1% of cases. In the lungs, the flukes lay their eggs and form areas of inflammation covered with a thin layer of fibrous tissue. These areas of infection may eventually rupture, causing the patient to **cough** up fluke eggs, blood, and inflamed tissue. The period between the beginning of the infection and the appearance of the eggs during coughing is about six weeks. Patients with lung infections may have chest pain and fever as well as rust-colored or bloody sputum. Lung infections can lead to **lung abscess**, **pneumonia**, or **bronchitis**. Patients with fluke infections of the brain may experience seizures or a fatal inflammation of brain tissue called **encephalitis**. Some patients also develop diarrhea and abdominal pain or lumps under the skin that contain adult flukes.

KEY TERMS

Aspirator—A medical instrument that uses suction to withdraw fluids from the lungs, digestive tract, or other parts of the body for laboratory testing.

Asymptomatic—Persons who carry a disease and are usually capable of transmitting the disease but, who do not exhibit symptoms of the disease are said to be asymptomatic.

Cercaria (plural, cercariae)—An intermediate-stage of the fluke larva, released into water by infected snails.

Cross-reaction—A reaction that occurs in blood testing when a disease agent reacts to the specific antibody for another disease agent. Cross-reactions are common in blood tests for fluke infections because the different species are closely related.

Encysted—Enclosed in a cyst or capsule. Flukes spend part of their life cycle as encysted larvae.

Fluke—A parasitic flatworm that has external suckers. Flukes are sometimes called trematodes.

Host—The living animal that supplies nutrition to a parasite.

Jaundice—Yellowing of the skin and the whites of the eyes as a result of excess bile in the blood due to an improperly functioning liver.

Metacercaria (plural, metacercariae)—The encysted stage of a fluke larva that produces infection in human beings.

Miracidium (plural, miracidia)—The free-swimming larval form in the life cycle of the liver fluke.

Parasite—An organism that lives on or inside an animal of a different species and feeds on it or draws nutrients from it.

Trematode—Parasitic flatworms or another name for fluke, taken from a Greek word that means having holes.

Diagnosis

Diagnosis of fluke infections is based on a combination of the patient's history, particularly travel or residence in areas known to have flukes, and identification of the fluke's eggs or adult forms. In some patients, the eggs are found in fluid from the lungs, bile duct, or small intestine. Samples of these fluids can be obtained with a suction instrument (aspirator). Because most types of fluke infections are rare in the United States, stool specimens or body fluid samples may need to be sent to a laboratory with experts in unusual diseases or conditions to identify the specific parasite. In some cases, adult flukes may be found in the patient's stools, vomit, sputum, or skin lumps (for lung flukes). In the case of lung flukes, it is important for the doctor to rule out **tuberculosis** as a possible diagnosis. A tuberculosis skin test and **chest x-ray** will usually be sufficient to do this.

Blood tests may be useful in diagnosing fluke infections, but their usefulness is limited because of cross-reactions. A cross-reaction occurs in blood testing when a particular disease agent reacts with antibodies specific to another disease agent. This result means that the doctor may know that the person is infected by flukes but cannot tell from the blood test alone which specific type of fluke is causing the disease. In addition, blood tests for fluke infections cannot distinguish between past and current infections. In some cases, sophisticated imaging techniques, such as **computed tomography scans** (CT scans) or ultrasound scans of the patient's chest or brain (for lung flukes) or abdomen (for liver flukes), are useful in confirming a diagnosis of fluke infection.

Treatment

Liver and lung fluke infections are treated with medications. These include triclabendazole, praziquantel, bithionol, albendazole, and mebendazole. Praziquantel works by paralyzing the flukes' suckers, forcing them to drop away from the walls of the host's blood vessels. In the United States, bithionol is available only from the Centers for Disease Control (CDC). Depending on the species of fluke and the severity of infection, the course of treatment can vary from several days to several weeks. Cure rates vary from 50–95%. Most patients experience mild temporary side effects from these drugs, including diarrhea, **dizziness**, or headache.

Prognosis

The prognosis for recovery from liver fluke infections is good, although patients with serious infections may be more vulnerable to other diseases, particularly if significant liver damage has occurred. Most patients with lung fluke infections also recover, however, severe infections of the brain can cause **death** from the destruction of central nervous system or brain tissue.

Prevention

No vaccines have been developed that are effective against lung or liver fluke infections. Prevention of these infections includes the following measures:

- boiling or purifying drinking water
- avoiding raw or undercooked fish or salads made from fresh aquatic plants; all food eaten in areas with fluke infestations should be cooked thoroughly; pickling or smoking will not kill fluke cysts in fish or shellfish
- control or eradication of the snails that serve as the flukes' intermediate hosts

Resources

BOOKS

McPhee, Stephen, and Maxine Papadakis. *Current Medical Diagnosis and Treatment, 2010*, 49th ed. New York: McGraw–Hill Medical, 2009.

Rebecca J. Frey, PhD

Fluoroquinolones

Definition

Fluoroquinolones are medicines that kill bacteria or prevent their growth.

Purpose

Fluoroquinolones are antimicrobials, medicines used to treat infections caused by microorganisms. Physicians prescribe these drugs for bacterial infections in many parts of the body. For example, they are used to treat bone and joint infections, skin infections, urinary tract infections, inflammation of the prostate, serious ear infections, **bronchitis**, **pneumonia**, **tuberculosis**, some **sexually transmitted diseases** (STDs), and some infections that affect people with **AIDS**.

Description

Fluoroquinolones are available only with a physician's prescription and are sold in tablet and injectable forms. Examples of these medicines are moxifloxacin (Avelox), ciprofloxacin (Cipro), ofloxacin (Floxin), levofloxacin (Levaquin), lomefloxacin (Maxaquin), norfloxacin (Noroxin), enoxacin (Penetrex), gatifloxacin (Tequin), and sparfloxacin (Zagam).

In the wake of the **anthrax** terrorist attacks in the United States in 2001, ciprofloxacin received extensive media attention because it was the only drug labeled as approved by the U.S. Food and Drug Administration (FDA) for both **prophylaxis** and treatment of inhalation anthrax (the most serious form of the disease). However, in late October 2001, the FDA issued a notice clarifying that the antibiotic doxycycline is also approved for anthrax prophylaxis and that doxycycline and amoxicillin are also approved for treatment for all forms of anthrax. The FDA encouraged companies to update labeling of these products with this previously unspecified information.

Recommended dosage

The recommended dosage depends on the type and strength of fluoroquinolone, and the kind of infection for which it is being taken. Check with the physician who prescribed the drug or the pharmacist who filled the prescription for the correct dosage.

To make sure the infection clears up completely, take the medicine for as long as it has been prescribed. Do not stop taking the drug just because symptoms begin to improve. Symptoms may return if the drug is stopped too soon.

Fluoroquinolones work best when they are at constant levels in the blood. To help keep levels constant, take the medicine in doses spaced evenly through the day and night. Do not miss any doses. For best results, take this medicine with a full glass of water and drink several more glasses throughout the day, every day during treatment with the drug. The extra water will help prevent some side effects. Some fluoroquinolones should be taken on an empty stomach; others may be taken with meals. Check package directions or ask the physician or pharmacist for instructions on how to take the medicine.

Precautions

An important precaution for any antibiotic is that unnecessary use or abuse of **antibiotics** can encourage drug-resistant strains of bacteria to develop and proliferate. These drug-resistant strains then become difficult, or even impossible, to treat. Bacteria found in hospitals appear to have become especially resilient, and are causing increasing difficulty for patients and the doctors treating them. Following the U.S. 2001 anthrax attacks, for example, the American Medical Association urged its members not to prescribe ciprofloxacin unnecessarily. One fear is that the overuse of the drug could reduce its effectiveness against infections such as **typhoid fever**, hospital-acquired pneumonia, and others.

Research suggests that fluoroquinolones may cause bone development problems in children and teenagers.

KEY TERMS

Bacteria—Tiny, one-celled forms of life that cause many diseases and infections.

Bronchitis—Inflammation of the air passages of the lungs.

Digestive tract—The stomach, intestines, and other parts of the body through which food passes.

Inflammation—Pain, redness, swelling, and heat that usually develop in response to injury or illness.

Microorganism—An organism that is too small to be seen with the naked eye.

Pneumonia—A disease in which the lungs become inflamed. Pneumonia may be caused by bacteria, viruses, or other organisms, or by physical or chemical irritants.

Prostate—A donut-shaped gland in males below the bladder that contributes to the production of semen.

Sexually transmitted disease (STD)—A disease that is passed from one person to another through sexual intercourse or other intimate sexual contact.

Tendon—A tough band of tissue that connects muscle to bone.

Tuberculosis—An infectious disease that usually affects the lungs, but may also affect other parts of the body. Symptoms include fever, weight loss, and coughing up blood.

Urinary tract—The passage through which urine flows from the kidneys out of the body.

Infants, children, teenagers, pregnant women, and women who are **breastfeeding** should not take this medicine unless directed to do so by a physician.

Although such side effects are rare, some people have had severe and life-threatening reactions to fluoroquinolones. Call a physician immediately if any of these signs of a dangerous reaction occur:

- swelling of the face and throat
- swallowing problems
- shortness of breath
- rapid heartbeat
- tingling of fingers or toes
- itching or hives
- loss of consciousness

Some fluoroquinolones may weaken the tendons in the shoulder, hand, or heel, making the tendons more likely to tear. Anyone who notices **pain** or inflammation in these or other tendon areas should stop taking the medicine immediately and call a physician. Rest and avoid **exercise** until the physician determines whether the tendons are damaged. If the tendons are torn, surgery may be necessary to repair them.

These medicines make some people feel drowsy, dizzy, lightheaded, or less alert. Anyone who takes these drugs should not drive, use machines or do anything else that might be dangerous until they have found out how the drugs affect them.

This medicine may increase sensitivity to sunlight. Even brief exposure to sun can cause a severe **sunburn** or a rash. While being treated with fluoroquinolones, avoid being in direct sunlight, especially between 10 a.m. and 3 p.m.; wear a hat and tightly woven clothing that covers the arms and legs; use a sunscreen with a skin protection factor (SPF) of at least 15; protect the lips with a sun block lipstick; and do not use **tanning** beds, tanning booths, or sunlamps.

Do not take **antacids** that contain aluminum, **calcium**, or magnesium at the same time as fluoroquinolones. The antacids may keep the fluoroquinolones from working as they should. If antacids are needed, take them at least two hours before or two hours after taking norfloxacin or ofloxacin, at least four hours before or two hours after taking ciprofloxacin. Follow the same instructions for taking sucralfate (Carafate), a medicine used to treat stomach ulcers and other irritation in the digestive tract and mouth.

Anyone who has had unusual reactions to fluoroquinolones or related medicines such as cinoxacin (Cinobac) or nalidixic acid (NegGram) in the past should let his or her physician know before taking the drugs again. The physician should also be told about any **allergies** to foods, dyes, preservatives, or other substances.

Before using fluoroquinolones, people with any of these medical problems should make sure their physicians are aware of their conditions:

- kidney disease
- liver disease with kidney disease
- diseases of the brain or spinal cord, including hardening of the arteries in the brain, epilepsy, and other seizure disorders

Taking fluoroquinolones with certain other drugs may affect the way the drugs work or may increase the chance of side effects.

Side effects

The most common side effects are mild **diarrhea**, **nausea**, **vomiting**, stomach or abdominal pain, **dizziness**, drowsiness, lightheadedness, nervousness, sleep problems, and **headache**. These problems usually go away as the body adjusts to the drug and do not require medical treatment unless they are bothersome.

More serious side effects are not common, but may occur. If any of the following side effects occur, check with a physician immediately:

- skin rash or other skin problems such as itching, peeling, hives, or redness
- fever
- agitation or confusion
- hallucinations
- shakiness or tremors
- seizures or convulsions
- tingling of fingers or toes
- pain where the medicine was injected (lasting after the injection)
- pain in the calves, spreading to the heels
- swelling of the calves or lower legs
- swelling of the face or neck
- swallowing problems
- rapid heartbeat
- shortness of breath
- loss of consciousness

Other rare side effects may occur. Anyone who has unusual symptoms after taking fluoroquinolones should get in touch with his or her physician.

Interactions

Fluoroquinolones may interact with other medicines. When this happens, the effects of one or both of the drugs may change or the risk of side effects may be greater. Anyone who takes fluoroquinolones should let the physician know all other medicines he or she is taking. Among the drugs that may interact with fluoroquinolones are:

- antacids that contain aluminum, calcium, or magnesium
- medicines that contain iron or zinc, including multivitamin and mineral supplements
- sucralfate (Carafate)
- caffeine
- blood thinning drugs such as warfarin (Coumadin)
- airway opening drugs (bronchodilators) such as aminophylline, theophylline (Theo-Dur and other brands), and oxtriphylline (choledyl and other brands)
- didanosine (Videx), used to treat HIV infection.

This list does not include every drug that may interact with fluoroquinolones. Be sure to check with a physician or pharmacist before combining fluoroquinolones with any other prescription or nonprescription (over-the-counter) medicine.

Resources

OTHER

"Fluoroquinolones (Systemic)." National Library of medicine. www.nlm.nih.gov/medlineplus/druginfo/fluoroquinolonessystemic202656.html.

Rosalyn Carson-DeWitt, MD

Fluoxetine *see* **Selective serotonin reuptake inhibitors**

Flurbiprofen *see* **Nonsteroidal anti-inflammatory drugs**

Focal glomerulosclе *see* **Nephrotic syndrome**

Folic acid

Definition

Folic acid is a water-soluable vitamin belonging to the B-complex group of **vitamins**. These vitamins help the body break down complex carbohydrates into simple sugars to be used for energy. Excess B vitamins are excreted from the body rather than stored for later use. This is why sufficient daily intake of folic acid is necessary.

Description

Folic acid is also known as folate, or folacin. It is one of the nutrients most often found to be deficient in the Western diet, and there is evidence that deficiency is a problem on a worldwide scale. Folic acid is found in leafy green vegetables, beans, peas and lentils, liver, beets, brussel sprouts, poultry, nutritional yeast, tuna, wheat germ, mushrooms, oranges, asparagus, broccoli, spinach, bananas, strawberries, and cantaloupes. In 1998, the U.S. Food and Drug Administration (FDA) required food manufacturers to add folic acid

KEY TERMS

Homocysteine—An amino acid involved in the breakdown and absorption of protein in the body.

Preeclampsia—A serious disorder of late pregnancy in which the blood pressure rises, there is a large amount of retained fluids, and the kidneys become less effective and excrete proteins directly into the urine.

Raynaud's disease—A symptom of various underlying conditions affecting blood circulation in the fingers and toes and causing them to be sensitive to cold.

Recommended Dietary Allowance (RDA)—Guidelines for the amounts of vitamins and minerals necessary for proper health and nutrition established by the National Academy of Sciences in 1989.

Water-soluble vitamins—Vitamins that are not stored in the body and are easily excreted. They must, therefore, be consumed regularly as foods or supplements to maintain health.

to enriched bread and grain products to boost intake and to help prevent neural tube defects (NTD).

Purpose

Folic acid works together with vitamin B_{12} and vitamin C to metabolize protein in the body. It is important for the formation of red and white blood cells. It is necessary for the proper differentiation and growth of cells and for the development of the fetus. It is also used to form the nucleic acid of DNA and RNA. It increases the appetite and stimulates the production of stomach acid for digestion and it aids in maintaining a healthy liver. A deficiency of folic acid may lead to anemia, in which there is decreased production of red blood cells. This reduces the amounts of oxygen and nutrients that are able to get to the tissues. Symptoms may include **fatigue**, reduced secretion of digestive acids, confusion, and forgetfulness. During **pregnancy**, a folic acid deficiency may lead to **preeclampsia**, premature birth, and increased bleeding after birth.

People who are at high risk of strokes and heart disease may greatly benefit by taking folic acid supplements. An elevated blood level of the amino acid **homocysteine** has been identified as a risk factor for some of these diseases. High levels of homocysteine have also been found to contribute to problems with **osteoporosis**. Folic acid, together with vitamins B_6 and B_{12}, helps break down homocysteine, and may help reverse the problems associated with elevated levels.

Pregnant women have an increased need for folic acid, both for themselves and their child. Folic acid is necessary for the proper growth and development of the fetus. Adequate intake of folic acid is vital for the prevention of several types of **birth defects**, particularly NTDs. The neural tube of the embryo develops into the brain, spinal cord, spinal column, and the skull. If this tube forms incompletely during the first few months of pregnancy a serious, and often fatal, defect results in **spina bifida** or anencephaly. Folic acid, taken from one year to one month before conception through the first four months of pregnancy, can reduce the risk of NTDs by 50–70%. It also helps prevent a **cleft lip and palate**.

Research shows that folic acid can be used to successfully treat cervical dysplasia, a condition diagnosed by a Pap smear, of having abnormal cells in the cervix. This condition is considered to be a possible precursor to **cervical cancer**, and is diagnosed as an abnormal Pap smear. Daily consumption of 1,000 mcg of folic acid for three or more months has resulted in improved cervical cells upon repeat Pap smears.

Studies suggest that long-term use of folic acid supplements may also help prevent lung and **colon cancer**. Researchers have also found that alcoholics who have low folic acid levels face a greatly increased possibility of developing colon cancer.

Preparations

To correct a folic acid deficiency, supplements are taken in addition to food. Since the functioning of the B vitamins is interrelated, it is generally recommended that the appropriate dose of B-complex vitamins be taken in place of single B vitamin supplements. The Recommended Dietary Allowances (RDA) for folate is 400 mcg per day for adults, 600 mcg per day for pregnant women, and 500 mcg for nursing women. Medicinal dosages of up to 1,000-2,000 mcg per day may be prescribed.

Precautions

Folic acid is not stable. It is easily destroyed by exposure to light, air, water, and cooking. Therefore, the supplement should be stored in a dark container in a cold, dry place, such as a refrigerator. Many medications interfere with the body's absorption and use of folic acid. This includes sulfa drugs, sleeping pills, estrogen, anti-convulsants, birth control pills, **antacids**, quinine, and some **antibiotics**. Using large amounts of folic acid (e.g., more than 5,000 mcg per day) can mask a vitamin B_{12} deficiency and thereby risk of irreversible nerve damage.

Side effects

At levels of 5,000 mcg or less, folic acid is generally safe for use. Side effects are uncommon. However, large doses may cause **nausea**, decreased appetite, bloating, gas, decreased ability to concentrate, and **insomnia**. Large doses may also decrease the effects of phenytoin (Dilantin), a seizure medication.

Interactions

As with all B-complex vitamins, it is best to take folic acid with the other B vitamins. Vitamin C is important to the absorption and functioning of folic acid in the body.

Resources

OTHER

"Folic Acid." http://www.cybervitamins.com/folicacid.htm.

"Folic Acid: Coming to A Grocery Store Near You." http://www.mayohealth.org/mayo/9710/htm/folic.htm.

"Folic acid (oral/injectible)." Dr. Koop.com.Inc. 700 N. Mopac, Suite 400, Austin, TX 48731. http://www.drkoop.com/hcr/drugstore/pharmacy/leaflets/english/d00241a1.asp.

Pregnancy and Nutrition Update. http://www.mayohealth.org/mayo/9601/htm/pregvit.htm.

ORGANIZATIONS

Centers for Disease Control and Prevention (CDC), 1600 Clifton Rd., Atlanta, GA, 30333, (800) 232-4636, cdcinfo@cdc.gov, http://www.cdc.gov.

Patience Paradox

Folic acid deficiency anemia

Definition

Folic acid deficiency, an abnormally low level of one of the B **vitamins**, results in anemia characterized by red blood cells that are large in size but few in number.

Description

Folic acid is necessary for growth and cellular repair, since it is a critical component of DNA and RNA as well as essential for the formation and maturation of red blood cells. Folic acid deficiency is one of the most common of all vitamin deficiencies. Although it occurs in both males and females, folic acid deficiency anemia most often affects women over age 30. It becomes increasingly common as age impedes the body's ability to absorb folic acid, a water-soluble vitamin that is manufactured by intestinal bacteria and stored for a short time in the liver. Folic acid deficiency has also been implicated as a cause of neural tube defects in the developing fetus. Recent research has shown that adequate amounts of folic acid can prevent up to one-half of these **birth defects**, if women start taking folic acid supplements shortly before conception. Research from China in 2004 showed that women who were low in B vitamins and folate before conception, though not technically anemic, still had increased risk of lower birth weight babies and adverse **pregnancy** outcome.

A healthy adult needs at least 400 mcg of folic acid every day. Requirements at least double during pregnancy, and increase by 50% when a woman is **breastfeeding**. The average American diet, high in fats, sugar, and white flour, provides about 200 mcg of folic acid, approximately the amount needed to maintain tissue stores of the substance for six to nine months before a deficiency develops. Most of the folic acid in foods (with the exception of the folic acid added to enriched flour and breakfast cereals) occurs as folate. Folate is only about pne-half as available for the body to use as is the folic acid in pills and supplements. Folate also is easily destroyed by sunlight, overcooking, or the storing of foods at room temperature for an extended period of time.

Good dietary sources of folate include:

- leafy green vegetables
- liver
- mushrooms
- oatmeal
- peanut butter
- red beans
- soy
- wheat germ

Causes and symptoms

This condition usually results from a diet lacking in foods with high folic acid content, or from the body's inability to digest foods or absorb foods having high folic acid content. Other factors that increase the risk of developing folic acid deficiency anemia are:

- age
- alcoholism
- birth control pills, anticonvulsant therapy, sulfa antibiotics, and certain other medications
- illness
- smoking
- stress

Fatigue is often the first sign of folic acid deficiency anemia. Other symptoms include:

- anorexia nervosa
- pale skin
- paranoia
- rapid heart beat
- sore, inflamed tongue
- weakness
- weight loss

Diagnosis

Diagnostic procedures include blood tests to measure hemoglobin, an iron-containing compound that carries oxygen to cells throughout the body. Symptoms may be reevaluated after the patient has taken prescription folic acid supplements.

Treatment

Folic acid supplements are usually prescribed, and self-care includes avoiding:

- alcohol
- non-herbal tea, antacids, and phosphates (contained in beer, ice cream, and soft drinks), which restrict iron absorption
- tobacco

A person with folic acid deficiency anemia should rest as often as necessary until restored energy levels make it possible to resume regular activities. A doctor should be seen if **fever**, chills, muscle aches, or new symptoms develop during treatment, or if symptoms do not improve after two weeks of treatment.

Alternative treatment

Alternative therapies for folic acid deficiency anemia may include **reflexology** concentrated on areas that influence the liver and spleen. Increasing consumption of foods high in folate is helpful. Eating a mixture of yogurt (8 oz) and turmeric (1 tsp) also may help resolve symptoms. A physician should be contacted if the tongue becomes slick or smooth or the patient:

- bruises or tires easily
- feels ill for more than five days
- feels weak or out of breath
- looks pale or jaundiced

Prognosis

Although adequate folic acid intake usually cures this condition in about three weeks, folic acid deficiency anemia can make patients infertile or more susceptible to infection. Severe deficiencies can result in congestive **heart failure**.

Prevention

Eating raw or lightly cooked vegetables every day will help maintain normal folic acid levels, as will taking a folic acid supplement containing at least 400 mcg of this vitamin. Because folic acid deficiency can cause birth defects, all women of childbearing age who can become pregnant should consume at least 400 mcg of folic acid daily; a woman who is pregnant should have regular medical checkups, and take a good prenatal vitamin.

Resources

PERIODICALS

Ronnenberg, Alayne G., et al. "Preconception Hemoglobin and Ferritin Concentrations Are Associated With Pregnancy Outcome in a Prospective Cohort of Chinese Women." *The Journal of Nutrition* October 2004: 2586–2592.

Maureen Haggerty
Teresa G. Odle

Follicle-stimulating hormone test

Definition

The follicle-stimulating hormone (FSH) test measures the amount of FSH in the blood. FSH is a hormone that regulates the growth and development of eggs and sperm, and this test is used to diagnose or evaluate disorders involving the pituitary gland and reproductive system.

KEY TERMS

Anovulatory bleeding—Bleeding without release of an egg from an ovary.

Hypopituitarism—Underactivity of the pituitary gland.

Hypothalamus—The part of the brain that controls the endocrine system.

Klinefelter's syndrome—Chromosomal abnormality characterized by small testes and male infertility.

Multiple endocrine neoplasia—Abnormal tissue growth on one or more of the endocrine (hormone-secreting) glands.

Polycystic ovary disease—A condition in which a woman has little or no menstruation, is infertile, has excessive body hair, and is obese. The ovaries may contain several cysts.

Turner syndrome—Chromosomal abnormality characterized by immature reproductive organs in women.

Purpose

FSH testing is performed if a physician suspects the patient may have a disorder involving the reproductive system or pituitary gland. The pituitary gland produces FSH, which stimulates the growth of the sacks (follicles) that surround the eggs in a woman's ovaries. This is important for the process of ovulation, in which the egg is released. In men, FSH stimulates production of sperm. If there are abnormal levels of FSH in the blood it may mean that one of several disorders are present. Normal fluctuations occur as a result of **puberty**, the menstrual cycle, **pregnancy**, and **menopause**.

The FSH test is performed more often on women than on men. In women, it is used to determine if menopause has begun, to diagnose **infertility** and **menstrual disorders** (such as anovulatory bleeding), to measure hormone levels in children who enter puberty at an early age, and to diagnose other disorders. In men, it can be used to determine early puberty, abnormal tissue growth on one or more of the hormone-secreting (endocrine) glands (called multiple endocrine neoplasia), or to diagnose other disorders.

Description

The FSH test is a blood test. Blood will be drawn from the patient and analyzed in a laboratory.

Preparation

In preparation for the test, there are no food or fluid intake restrictions. Patients may be advised to discontinue certain medications for 48 hours before the test. A menstruating woman having hot flashes or irregular periods should be tested on the second or third day of her menstrual cycle. A woman who has missed a period and is having other menopausal symptoms can be tested at any time.

Aftercare

No aftercare is necessary.

Risks

There are no risks associated with this test.

Normal results

Normal FSH test results vary according to age and sexual maturity. The phase of a woman's menstrual cycle or use of birth-control pills also affects test results.

For an adult male, normal results range from about 4–25 units of FSH in every liter of blood (U/L) or about 5–20 micro-international units in every milliliter.

For a premenopausal woman, normal values range from 4–30 U/L or 5–20 micro-international units per milliliter. In a pregnant woman, FSH levels are too low to measure. After menopause, normal values range from 40–250 U/L or 50–100 micro-international units per milliliter.

FSH levels fluctuate during premenopause. If no other symptoms are present, an elevated FSH level should not be interpreted as proof that menopause has begun.

Abnormal results

Anorexia nervosa and disorders of the hypothalamus or pituitary gland can result in abnormally low FSH levels.

Abnormal levels can also indicate:

- infertility
- hypopituitarism
- Klinefelter syndrome (in men)
- turner syndrome
- ovarian failure
- polycystic ovary syndrome

Resources

OTHER

"Follicle-Stimulating Hormone Test." *Health Answers.com* www.healthanswers.com.

Maureen Haggerty

Follicular cysts *see* **Ovarian cysts**

Folliculitis

Definition

Folliculitis is inflammation or infection of one or more hair follicles (openings in the skin that enclose hair).

Description

Folliculitis can affect both women and men at any age. It can develop on any part of the body, but is most likely to occur on the scalp, face, or parts of the arms, armpits, or legs not usually covered by clothing.

Small, yellowish-white blister-like lumps (pustules) surrounded by narrow red rings are usually present with both bacterial folliculitis and fungal folliculitis. Hair can grow through or alongside of the pustules, which sometimes ooze blood-stained pus.

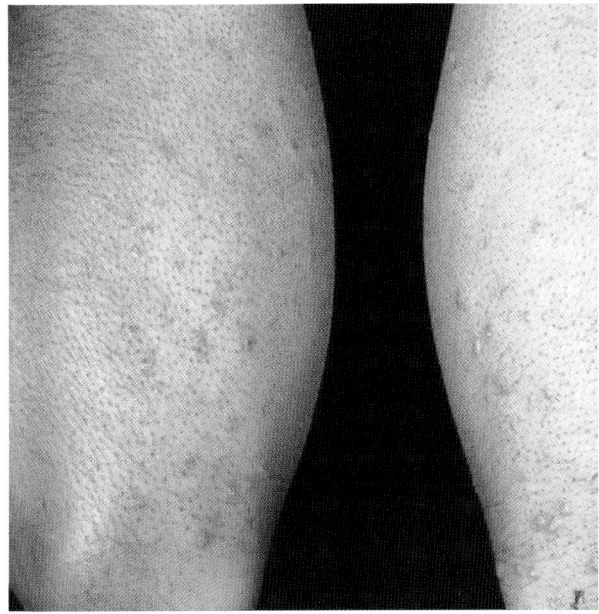

Acne folliculitis. *(Custom Medical Stock Photo, Inc. Reproduced by permission.)*

Folliculitis can cause **boils** and, in rare instances, serious skin infections. Bacteria from folliculitis can enter the blood stream and travel to other parts of the body.

Causes and symptoms

Folliculitis develops when bacteria, such as *Staphylococcus*, or a fungus enters the body through a cut, scrape, surgical incision, or other break in the skin near a hair follicle. Scratching the affected area can trap fungus or bacteria under the fingernails and spread the infection to hair follicles on other parts of the body.

The bacteria that cause folliculitis are contagious. A person who has folliculitis can infect others who live in the same household.

Factors that increase the risk of developing folliculitis include:

- dermatitis
- diabetes
- dirty, crowded living conditions
- eczema
- exposure to hot, humid temperatures
- infection in the nose or other recent illness
- tight clothing

Diagnosis

Diagnosis is based on the patient's medical history and observations. Laboratory analysis of the substance drained from a pustule can be used to distinguish bacterial folliculitis from fungal folliculitis.

Treatment

Bacterial folliculitis may disappear without treatment, but is likely to recur. Non-prescription **topical antibiotics** like Bacitracin, Mycitracin, or Neomycin, gently rubbed on to affected areas three or four times a day, can clear up a small number of bacterial folliculitis pustules. Oral **antibiotics** such as erythromycin (Erythocin) may be prescribed if the infection is widespread. The drug griseofulvin (Fulvicin) and topical antifungal medications are used to treat fungal folliculitis.

A doctor should be notified if:

- pustules spread after treatment has begun or reappear after treatment is completed
- the patient's fever climbs above 100 °F (37.8 °C)
- the patient develops boils or swollen ankles

- redness, swelling, warmth, or pain indicate that the infection has spread
- unexplained new symptoms appear

Alternative treatment

Eating a balanced diet, including protein, complex carbohydrates, healthy fats, fresh fruits and vegetables, and drinking eight to 10 glasses of water a day may stimulate the body's immune system and shorten the course of the infection. Garlic (*Allium sativum*) and goldenseal (*Hydrastis canadensis*), both antiseptic agents against staph infections, may be taken. The daily dosage would vary from person to person and is based on the severity of the infection. **Echinacea** (*Echinacea* spp.) is helpful in modulating immune function. Again, the dosage would vary.

Daily doses of 30–50 mg zinc and 1,000–5,000 mg Vitamin C (taken in equal amounts at several times during the day), and 300–2,000 mg bioflavinoids can also strengthen the body's infection-fighting ability. High doses of **vitamins** and **minerals** should not be used without a doctor's approval.

Prognosis

If properly treated, the symptoms of bacterial folliculitis generally disappear in about two weeks. Fungal folliculitis should clear up within six weeks. But it can worsen if the condition is misdiagnosed and inappropriately treated with steroid creams.

Prevention

Anyone who has a tendency to develop folliculitis should cleanse the skin with antibacterial soap twice a day and before shaving and should not use oily skin lotions. Men should not shave while the beard area is infected. When they begin shaving again, they should use a new blade each time. Women who have had fungal folliculitis should use depilatory creams instead of razors. Daily shampooing can help prevent folliculitis in the scalp. The spread of infection can be prevented by not sharing towels or washcloths.

Resources

OTHER

"Folliculitis." *Thrive Online*. http://thriveonline.oxygen.com.

Maureen Haggerty

Food allergies

Definition

Food **allergies** are the body's abnormal responses to harmless foods; the reactions are caused by the immune system's reaction to some food proteins.

Description

Food allergies are often confused with food intolerance. However, the two conditions have different causes and produce different symptoms. A food allergy is also known as food hypersensitivity. The allergy is caused when a person eats something that the immune system incorrectly identifies as harmful.

Food allergies

About 4% of adults have food allergies according to the National Institute of Allergy and Infectious Diseases (NIAID). The condition affects approximately 6 to 8% of children age 4 and younger.

The immune system works to protect the body and creates food-specific antibodies. The antibodies are proteins that battle antigens, substances that are foreign or initially outside the body. The introduction of an antigen produces the immune response. Antibodies are created to destroy the antigen or counteract its effectiveness.

The food that triggered that reaction is called an allergen. The antibodies are like an alarm system coded to detect the food regarded as harmful. The next time the person eats that food, the immune

Common food allergies

The following food allergens are identified by the Food and Drug Administration (FDA) as the most common and must be clearly labeled on food packaging:

- Milk
- Eggs
- Peanuts
- Tree nuts (such as almonds, cashews, walnuts)
- Fish (such as bass, cod, flounder)
- Shellfish (such as crab, lobster, shrimp)
- Soy
- Wheat

SOURCE: Mayo Clinic, "Food allergies: Watch food labels for these top 8 allergens." Available online at: http://www.mayoclinic.com/health/food-allergies/AA00057 (accessed August 10, 2010).

(Table by PreMediaGlobal. Reproduced by permission of Gale, a part of Cengage Learning.)

system discharges a large amount of histamine and chemicals. This process meant to protect the body against the allergen causes an allergic reaction that can affect the respiratory tract, digestive tract, skin, and cardiovascular system.

Allergic reactions can occur in minutes or in up to two hours after the person ate the food. Symptoms include swelling of the tongue, **diarrhea**, and **hives**. In severe cases, the allergic reaction can be fatal. The most severe reaction is **anaphylaxis**, which could be life-threatening.

Food intolerance

While food allergies involve the immune system, food intolerance is not related to the immune system. For example, a person who is lactose intolerant has a shortage of lactose, the digestive enzyme that breaks down the sugar in milk and dairy products. That person could experience stomach **pain** or bloating several hours after drinking milk.

People who are food-intolerant can sometimes consume that food and not experience intolerance symptoms. Those diagnosed with food allergies must avoid the foods that produce the allergic reactions.

Allergy-producing foods

Although approximately 160 foods produce allergic reactions, about 90% of reactions are caused by some or all items within eight food families. These are milk, eggs, peanuts, tree nuts, fish, shellfish, wheat, and soy. These foods can cause severe reactions. The most adverse reactions are caused by peanuts and tree nuts. According to NIAID, about 0.6% of Americans are impacted by peanut allergies. Approximately 0.4% of Americans have allergic reactions to tree nuts.

Food allergy demographics

Most children have allergies to eggs, milk, peanuts or tree nuts, and soy, according to the American Dietetic Association (ADA). The young generally outgrow their allergies. They are more likely to outgrow milk and soy allergies, according to NIAID. However, children and adults usually allergic to peanuts and tree nuts for life. The most frequent causes of food allergies in adulthood are peanuts, tree nuts, fish, and shellfish.

Allergies are hereditary. There is a tendency for the immune system to create immunoglobulin E (IgE) antibodies in people with family histories of allergies and allergic conditions like hay **fever** and **asthma**, according to NIAID. The likelihood of a child having food allergies increases when both parents are allergic.

Furthermore, people are allergic to the foods that are eaten frequently in their countries. A rice allergy is more common in Japan, and codfish allergies occur more in Scandinavian countries, according to NIAID.

Causes and symptoms

Food allergies are caused by the immune system's reaction to a food item that it believes is harmful. When the food is digested, the immune system responds by creating immunoglobulin E (IgE) antibodies as a defense. The antibodies are proteins found in the bloodstream. Formed to protect the body against harmful substances, the antibodies are created after the person's first exposure to the allergen.

The majority of food allergies are caused by foods in eight families. In some families, every food causes an allergic reaction. In other families like shellfish, a person may be allergic to one species, but able to eat others. The allergy-inducing foods include:

- Milk. The dairy family includes milk, ice cream, yogurt, butter, and some margarines. Nondairy foods that contain casein must be avoided. Prepared foods that contain milk range from breads and doughnuts to sausage and soup, according to the ADA.
- Eggs. Although a person may be allergic to either the egg white or yolk, the entire egg must be avoided because there is a risk of cross-contamination. Eggs are an ingredient in mayonnaise. Moreover, products such as baked goods, breads, pasta, yogurt, and batter on fried foods may contain eggs. In addition, some egg-substitute products contain egg whites.
- Peanuts. Peanuts grow in the ground and are legumes like lentils and chickpeas. A person with a peanut allergy may not be allergic to other legumes or tree nuts. Products to be avoided include peanuts, peanut butter, peanut oil, and some desserts and candy. In addition, some Asian dishes are prepared with a peanut sauce. Tree nuts include almonds, cashews, pecans, walnuts, Brazil nuts, chestnuts, hazelnuts, macadamia nuts, pine nuts, pistachios, and hickory nuts. Products containing tree nuts include nut oil, nut oil, desserts, candy, crackers, and barbecue sauce. A person may be allergic to one type of nut but able to eat other nuts. That should be determined after consulting with a doctor.
- Fish. Fish allergy is generally diagnosed as an allergy to all fish species because the allergen is similar among the different species.
- Shellfish. Shellfish species include lobster, crab, shrimp, clams, oysters, scallops, mollusks, and crawfish. An allergy to one type of shellfish may indicate an allergy to others.

- Wheat. Wheat is a grain found in numerous foods including breads, cereals, pastas, lunch meats, desserts, and bulgar. It is also found in products such as enriched flour and farina.
- Soy. The soybean is a legume, and people who have this allergy are rarely allergic to peanuts or other legumes. Soy is an ingredient in many processed foods including crackers and baked goods, sauces, and soups. There is also soy in canned tuna, according to the ADA.

The chemical reaction

During the initial exposure, many IgE antibodies are created. These attach to mast cells. These cells are located in tissue throughout the body, especially in areas such as the nose, throat, lungs, skin, and gastrointestinal tract. These are also the areas where allergic reactions occur.

The antibodies are in place, and a reaction is triggered the next time the person eats the food regarded as harmful. As the allergen reacts with the IgE, the body releases histamine and other chemicals. Histamine is a chemical located in the body's cells. When released during an allergic reaction, histamine and other chemicals cause symptoms like inflammation.

The type of allergic reaction depends on where the antibodies are released, according to NIAID. Chemicals released in the ears, nose, and throat could cause the mouth to itch. The person may also have difficulty breathing or swallowing. If the allergen triggers a reaction in the gastrointestinal tract, the person could experience stomach pain or diarrhea. An allergic reaction that affects skin cells could produce hives. This condition also known as urticaria is an allergic reaction characterized by **itching**, swelling, and the presence of patchy red areas called wheals.

Severe allergic reaction

Anaphylaxis is a severe allergic reaction that is potentially life-threatening. Also known as an anaphylactic reaction, this condition requires immediate medical attention. The reaction occurs within seconds or up to several hours after the person ate the allergy-inducing food.

Symptoms can include difficulty breathing, a **tingling** feeling in the mouth, and a swelling in the tongue and throat. The person may experience hives, **vomiting**, abdominal cramps, and diarrhea. There is also a sudden drop in blood pressure. Anaphylaxis may be fatal if not treated promptly.

Each year, some 150 Americans die from food-induced anaphylaxism, according to NIAID. The casualties are generally adolescents and young adults. The risk increases for people who have allergies and asthma. Also at increased risk are people who experienced previous episodes of a naphylaxis.

The peanut is one of the primary foods that trigger an anaphylactic reaction. Tree nuts also cause the reaction. The nuts generally linked to anaphylaxis are almonds, Brazil nuts, cashews, chestnuts, hazelnuts, macadamia nuts, pecans, pine nuts, pistachios and walnuts. Fish, shellfish, and eggs can also set off the reaction, according to the ADA.

Cross-reactivity

Cross-reactivity is the tendency of a person with one allergy to reaction to another allergen. A person allergic to crab might also be allergic to shrimp. In addition, someone with ragweed sensitivity could experience sensations when trying to eat melons during ragweed pollinating season, according to NIAID. The person's mouth would start itching, and the person wouldn't be able to eat the melon. The cross-reaction happens frequently with cantaloupes. The condition is known as oral allergy syndrome.

Diagnosis

Food allergies are diagnosed by first determining whether a person has an allergy or if symptoms are related to a condition like food intolerance. The medical professional may be a board-certified allergist, a doctor with education and experience in treating allergies. However, some health plans may require that the patient first see a family practice doctor.

If food allergies are suspected, the doctor will take a detailed case history. The doctor asks the patient if there is a family history of allergies. Other questions are related to the patient's adverse reactions.

The doctor's questions include how the food was prepared, the amount eaten and what time the reaction happened. The patient describes the symptoms and actions taken to relieve them. The doctor also asks if the patient had other similar experiences when eating that food.

The patient receives a physical exam. In addition, the doctor may ask the patient to keep a food diary, a log of what the person eats for one to two weeks. The medical history and the food diary are used in conjunction with testing to diagnose the patient.

Allergy tests

Doctors generally start the testing process with a skin test or a blood test. The prick skin test, which is also known as the scratch test, examines the patient's reaction to a solution containing a protein that triggers allergies.

The doctor places a drop of the substance on the patient's arm or back. The doctor then uses a needle to prick or scratch the skin. This allows the potential allergen to enter the patient's skin. If more than one food allergy is suspected, the test is repeated with other proteins applied to the skin. After about 15 minutes, the doctor can read the reactions on the patient's skin.

If there is no reaction, the patient is probably not allergic to that food. The possibility of an allergy is indicated by the presence of a wheal, a bump that resembles a mosquito bite. The wheal signifies a positive reaction to the test. However, the test may show a false positive, which is a reaction to a food that does not cause allergies.

The skin test is not appropriate for people who are severely allergic or have skin conditions like **eczema**. Those people are given the RAST (radioallergosorbent test). This test measures the presence of food-specific IgE in the blood. After a sample of the patient's blood is taken, it is sent to a laboratory. The sample is tested with different foods. Levels of antibodies are measured, and the reactions to different proteins are ranked. While measurement systems may vary, a high ranking indicates a high number of antibodies. Lab results are generally completed within a week.

Results to this test may not be conclusive. A negative test may not have identified antibodies in the patient's blood. Positive results make it probable but not definite that the patient has allergies.

Costs for blood and skin tests will vary, with fees typically ranging from $10 to more than $300. Insurance may cover some of the cost. While both tests are reliable, they aren't 100% accurate. If questions remain, the diagnosis takes into account the patient's medical history and the food diary. If necessary, the patient is put on a special diet.

Elimination diet

If the skin or blood test shows strong positive results, the doctor may put the patient on an elimination diet. This is done when needed to narrow the list of suspected allergens. The person stops eating the foods suspected of causing the allergic reaction. That food is eliminated from the diet for from two to four weeks. If allergy symptoms improve, the food is probably an allergen.

If more confirmation is needed, the doctor may ask the patient to start eating the food again. The elimination diet procedure is generally not utilized if the patient initially had a severe reaction.

Food challenges

Other tests called food challenges may be performed. The challenges are done in a medical setting, with a doctor present. The patient is given capsules that each contain a different food. Some capsules contain allergy-producing foods. Other capsules may be placebos that won't produce a reaction.

The patient swallows the capsule, and the doctor watches for an allergic reaction. In an open food challenge, doctor and patient are aware of the capsule contents. In a single-blind food challenge, only the doctor knows. In a double-blind challenge, neither doctor nor patient knows the contents.

Challenges are rarely authorized by health care providers. Testing is time-consuming and many allergens are difficult to evaluate with the challenges, according to NIAID.

Treatment

The treatment for food allergies is to avoid eating the food that causes the allergy. This preventive treatment includes reading food labels. Manufacturers are required by the U.S. Food and Drug Administration to list a product's ingredients on the label. However, if there is a question about an ingredient, the person should contact the manufacturer before eating the food. When dining out, people should ask if food contains the allergen or ingredients contain the allergy-inducing foods.

When reading food labels, people with food allergies should know that:

- Words indicating the presence of milk include lactose, ghee, and whey.
- Words signifying eggs in a product include albumin, globulin, and ovomucin.
- While it is apparent that peanuts are an ingredient in a product like peanut butter, there could be peanuts in hydrolyzed plant protein and hydrolyzed vegetable protein.
- People with tree nut allergies should carefully read the labels of products such as cereals and barbecue sauce.
- The American Dietetic Association cautions that surimi, an ingredient in imitation seafood, is made from fish muscle. Furthermore, fish in the form of

anchovies is sometimes an ingredient in Worcestshire sauce.

- Words on labels that signal the presence of wheat include gluten, sietan, and vital gluten.

Allergies and children

Parents of children with food allergies need to monitor their children's food choices. They also must know how to care for the child if there is an allergic reaction. Parents need to notify the child's school about the condition. Caregivers should be informed, too. Both the school and caregivers should know how to handle an allergic reaction. Care must be taken because a highly allergic person could react to a piece of food as small as 1/44,000 of a peanut kernel, according to NIAID.

Living with severe allergies

Despite precautions, people may accidentally eat something that causes an allergic reaction. People with severe allergies must be prepared to treat the condition and prevent an anaphylactic reaction. A medical alert bracelet should be worn. This informs people that the person has a food allergy and could have severe reactions.

To reduce the risks from an anaphylactic reaction, the person carries a syringe filled with epinephrine, which is adrenaline. This is a prescription medication sold commercially as the EpiPen auto injector. While prices vary, one syringe costs about $50.

The person with allergies must know how to inject the epinephrine. It is helpful for other family members to know how to do this, and parents of an allergic child must be trained in the procedure.

The person is injected at the first sign of a severe reaction. Medical attention is required, and the person should be taken to an emergency room. The person will be treated and monitored because there could be a second severe reaction about four hours after the initial one.

Allergy treatment research

There was no cure for food allergies as of the spring of 2005. That could change, with some relief available for people diagnosed with peanut allergies. According to a study reported on in 2003 in the *New England Journal of Medicine*, 84 people who took the drug TNX-901 had a decrease in their IgE antibody levels.

Organizations including the Food Allergy & Anaphylaxis Network (FAAN) lauded the results of the study that was conducted from July of 1999 through March of 2002. Work on that study was stopped in 2004 when biotechnology companies Genentech, Novartis, and Tanox concentrated efforts instead on use of an asthma medication for treating peanut allergies. Research started in June of 2004 on omalizumab, a medication sold commercially as Xolair. The study of Xolair's effectiveness was expected to take from two to three years.

Alternative treatment

The only treatment for food allergies is for a person to stop eating the food that causes the allergies. Some alternative treatments may be helpful in easing the symptoms caused by allergies. However, people should check with their health care providers before embarking on an alternative treatment.

Prognosis

Food allergies cannot be cured, but they can be managed. The allergen-inducing foods should be avoided. These foods should be replaced with others that provide the **vitamins** and nutrients needed for a healthy diet. Organizations including the American Dietetic Association recommend the following dietetic changes:

- Milk is a source of calcium and vitamins A and D. For people with milk allergies, alternate choices of calcium include calcium-fortified orange juice and cereal.
- Since eggs are an ingredient in products like bread, egg-free sources of grains are an alternate source of vitamin B.
- Peanuts are a source of vitamin E, niacin, and magnesium. Other sources of these nutrients include other legumes, meat, and grains.
- Fish is a source of protein and nutrients like B vitamins and niacin. Alternate sources of these nutrients should be sought.
- Wheat is a source of many nutrients including niacin and riboflavin. The person allergic to wheat should substitute products made from grains such as oat, corn, rice and barley.
- Although soybeans are rich in nutrients, very little soy is used in commercial products. As a result, a person with this food allergy would not need to find a safe substitute in order to get needed nutrients.

Prevention

People prevent the return of food allergies by following treatment guidelines. These include avoiding the foods that cause allergic reactions, reading food labels, and taking measures to prevent an anaphylactic reaction.

Anaphylaxis is a major concern after a diagnosis of severe food allergies. To reduce the risks associated this reaction, people with food allergies should wear medical alert bracelets and never go anywhere without epinephrine. If possible, family members or friends of adults with allergies should learn how to administer this medication.

The American Dietetic Association advises people to develop an emergency plan. ADA recommendations include preparing a list of the foods the person is allergic to, three emergency contacts, the doctor's name, and a description of how to treat the reaction. This list is kept with the epinephrine syringe.

Resources

BOOKS

Brostoff, Jonathan, and Linda Gamlin.*The Complete Guide to Food Allergy and Intolerance*. Kingsbridge: Quality Health, 2008.

Wood, Robert A., and Joe Kraynak.*Food Allergies for Dummies*. Hoboken, NJ: Wiley, 2007.

OTHER

Food Allergy An Overview. National Institute of Allergy and Infectious Diseases. July 2004. [cited March 30, 2005]. http://www.niaid.nih.gov/publications/pdf/foodallergy.pdf.

Peanut Anti-IgE Study Update. The Food Allergy & Anaphylaxis Network. September 2, 2004 [cited April 5]. http://www.foodallergy.org/Research/antiigetherapy.html.

ORGANIZATIONS

American Academy of Allergy, Asthma & Immunology, 555 East Wells Street, Suite 1100, Milwaukee, WI, 53202-3823, (414) 272-6071, http://www.aaaai.org.

American Dietetic Association, 120 S. Riverside Plaza, Suite 2000, Chicago, IL, 60606-6995, (312) 899-0040, (800) 877-1600, http://www.eatright.org/.

National Institute of Allergies and Infectious Diseases, 6610 Rockledge Drive, MSC 6612, Bethesda, MD, 20892-6612, (301) 496-5717, (301) 402-3573, (866) 284-4107, ocpostoffice@niaid.nih.gov, http://www.niaid.nih.gov.

The Food Allergy & Anaphylaxis Network, 11781 Lee Jackson Hwy., Suite 160, Fairfax, VA, 22033-3309, (703) 691-2713, (800) 929-4040, http://www.foodallergy.org.

Liz Swain,

Food poisoning

Definition

Food poisoning is a general term for health problems arising from eating contaminated food. Food may be contaminated by bacteria, viruses, environmental toxins, or toxins present within the food itself, such as the poisons in some mushrooms or certain seafood. Symptoms of food poisoning usually involve **nausea**, **vomiting** and/or **diarrhea**. Some food-borne toxins can affect the nervous system.

Description

Every year millions of people suffer from bouts of **vomiting** and diarrhea each year that they blame on "something I ate." These people are generally correct. Each year in the United States, one to two bouts of diarrheal illness occur in every adult. The Centers for Disease Control and Prevention (CDC) estimates that six to 33 million cases of food poisoning occur in the United States annually. Many cases are mild and pass so rapidly that they are never diagnosed. Occasionally a severe outbreak creates a newsworthy public health hazard.

Classical food poisoning, sometimes incorrectly called ptomaine poisoning, is caused by a variety of different bacteria. The most common are *Salmonella*, *Staphylococcus aureus*, ***Escherichia coli*** O157:H7 or other *E. coli strains*, *Shigella*, and *Clostridium botulinum*. Each has a slightly different incubation period

Common pathogens causing food poisoning

Pathogen	Common host(s)
Campylobacter	Poultry
Clostridium botulinum	Home and improperly canned foods
Escherichia coli 0157:H7 (*E. coli*)	Undercooked, contaminated ground beef
Listeria monocytogenes	Found in a variety of raw foods, such as uncooked meats and vegetables, and in processed foods that become contaminated after processing
Salmonella	Poultry, eggs, meat, and milk
Shigella	This bacteria is transmitted through direct contact with an infected person or from food or water that have become contaminated
Vibrio vulnificus	Contaminated seafood

(Table by PreMediaGlobal. Reproduced by permission of Gale, a part of Cengage Learning.)

ALICE CATHERINE EVANS (1881–1975)

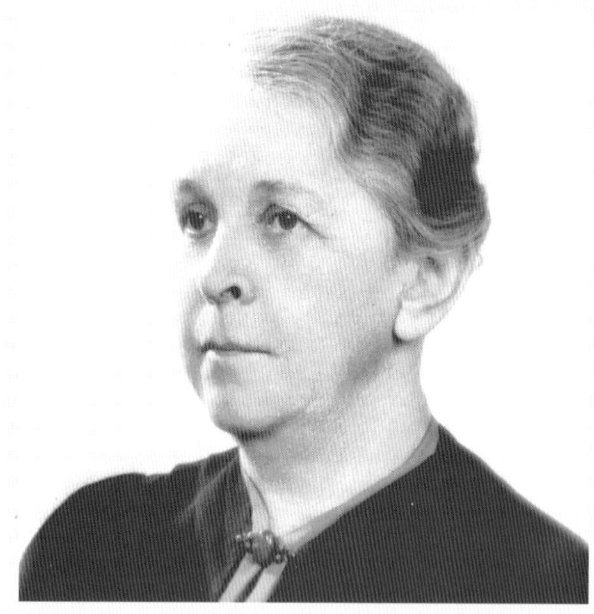

(© Corbis.)

Alice Catherine Evans was born on January 29, 1881, in Neath, Pennsylvania. Evans was the second of two children born to Anne Evans and William Howell. Evans taught grade school for four years because she could not afford to pay college tuition. Following her time as a teacher, Evans enrolled at the Cornell University College of Agriculture, earning her B.S. degree. Evans' professor recommended her for a scholarship, which she received, and she began her master's degree program at the University of Wisconsin where she earned her degree in 1910.

In 1911, Evans took a position with the University of Wisconsin's Dairy Division as a researcher studying cheese-making instead of continuing her education. In 1913, she moved to Washington, D.C., with the division and worked with a team on identifying the cause of contamination in raw cow's milk. By 1917, Evans' research had shown that the bacteria responsible for undulant (Malta) fever was very similar to one found when a cow experienced a spontaneous abortion. When administered to guinea pigs, the two bacteria produced similar results. Her findings were met with much skepticism but, as time went on, Evans' research began to gain support. She continued to document cases of the disease and to argue for the pasteurization process. Finally, after 1930, officials responsible for public health and safety realized the need for this process, which ultimately became a standard procedure. Evans retired from her position with the National Institute of Health in 1945 and died on September 5, 1975.

and duration, but all except *C. botulinum* cause inflammation of the intestines and diarrhea. Sometimes food poisoning is called bacterial **gastroenteritis** or infectious diarrhea. Food and water can also be contaminated by viruses (such as the Norwalk agent that causes diarrhea and the viruses of **hepatitis A** and E), environmental toxins (heavy metals), and poisons produced within the food itself (**mushroom poisoning** or **fish and shellfish poisoning**).

Careless food handling during the trip from farm to table creates conditions for the growth of bacteria that make people sick. Vegetables that are eaten raw, such as lettuce, may be contaminated by bacteria in soil, water, and dust during washing and packing. Home canned and commercially canned food may be improperly processed at too low a temperature or for too short a time to kill the bacteria.

Raw meats carry many food-borne bacterial diseases. The United States Food and Drug Administration (FDA) estimates that 60% or more of raw poultry sold at retail carry some disease-causing bacteria. Other raw meat products and eggs are contaminated to a lesser degree. Thorough cooking kills the bacteria and makes the food harmless. However, properly cooked food can become re-contaminated if it comes in contact with plates, cutting boards, countertops, or utensils that were used with raw meat and not cleaned and sanitized.

Cooked foods can also be contaminated after cooking by bacteria carried by food handlers or from bacteria in the environment. It is estimated that 50% of healthy people have the bacteria *Staphylococcus aureus* in their nasal passages and throat, and on their skin and hair. Rubbing a runny nose, then touching food can introduce the bacteria into cooked food. Bacteria flourish at room temperature, and will rapidly grow into quantities capable of making people sick. To prevent this growth, food must be kept hot or cold, but never just warm.

Although the food supply in the United States is probably the safest in the world, anyone can get food poisoning. Serious outbreaks are rare. When they occur, the very young, the very old, and those with immune system weaknesses have the most severe and life-threatening cases. For example, this group is 20 times more likely to become infected with the *Salmonella* bacteria than the general population.

Travel outside the United States to countries where less attention is paid to sanitation, water purification, and good food handling practices increases the chances that a person will get food poisoning. People living in institutions such as nursing homes are also more likely to get food poisoning.

Causes and symptoms

The symptoms of food poisoning occur because food-borne bacteria release toxins or poisons as a byproduct of their growth in the body. These toxins (except those from *C. botulinum*) cause inflammation and swelling of the stomach, small intestine and/or large intestine. The result is abdominal muscle cramping, vomiting, diarrhea, **fever**, and the chance of **dehydration**. The severity of symptoms depends on the type of bacteria, the amount consumed, and the individual's general health and sensitivity to the bacterial toxin.

Salmonella

According to a 2001 report from the CDC, *Salmonella* caused almost 50,000 culture-confirmed cases of food poisoning in the United States annually. However, between two and four million probably occur each year. *Salmonella* is found in egg yolks from infected chickens, in raw and undercooked poultry and in other meats, dairy products, fish, shrimp, and many more foods. The CDC estimates that one out of every 50 consumers is exposed to a contaminated egg yolk each year. However, thorough cooking kills the bacteria and makes the food harmless. *Salmonella* is also found in the feces of pet reptiles such as turtles, lizards, and snakes.

About one out of every 1,000 people get food poisoning from *Salmonella*. Of these, two-thirds are under age 20, with the majority under age nine. Most cases occur in the warm months between July and October.

Symptoms of food poisoning begin eight to 72 hours after eating food contaminated with *Salmonella*. These include traditional food poisoning symptoms of abdominal **pain**, diarrhea, vomiting, and fever. The symptoms generally last one to five days. Dehydration can be a complication in severe cases. People generally recover without antibiotic treatment, although they may feel tired for a week after the active symptoms subside.

Staphylococcus aureus

Staphylococcus aureus is found on humans and in the environment in dust, air, and sewage. The bacteria is spread primarily by food handlers using poor sanitary practices. Almost any food can be contaminated, but salad dressings, milk products, cream pastries, and any food kept at room temperature, rather than hot or cold are likely candidates.

It is difficult to estimate the number of cases of food poisoning from *Staphylococcus aureus* that occur each year, because its symptoms are so similar to those caused by other foodborne bacteria. Many cases are mild and the victim never sees a doctor.

Symptoms appear rapidly, usually one to six hours after the contaminated food is eaten. The acute symptoms of vomiting and severe abdominal cramps without fever usually last only three to six hours and rarely more than 24 hours. Most people recover without medical assistance. Deaths are rare.

Escherichia coli (E. coli)

There are many strains of *E. coli*, and not all of them are harmful. The strain that causes most severe food poisoning is *E. coli O157:H7*. Food poisoning by *E. coli* occurs in three out of every 10,000 people. Food-borne *E. coli* is found and transmitted mainly in food derived from cows such as raw milk, raw or rare ground beef and fruit or vegetables that are contaminated.

Symptoms of food poisoning from *E. coli* are slower to appear than those caused by some of the other food-borne bacteria. *E. coli* produces toxins in the large intestine rather than higher up in the digestive system. This accounts for the delay in symptoms and the fact that vomiting rarely occurs in *E. coli* food poisoning.

One to three days after eating contaminated food, the victim with *E. coli O157:H7* begins to have severe abdominal cramps and watery diarrhea that usually becomes bloody within 24 hours. There is little or no fever, and rarely does the victim vomit. The bloody, watery diarrhea lasts from one to eight days in uncomplicated cases.

Campylobacter jejuni (C. jejuni)

According to the FDA, *C. jejuni* is the leading cause of bacterial diarrhea in the United States. It is responsible for more cases of bacterial diarrhea than *Shigella* and *Salmonella* combined. Anyone can get food poisoning from *C. jejuni*, but children under five and young adults between the ages of 15 and 29 are more frequently infected.

C. jejuni is carried by healthy cattle, chickens, birds, and flies. It is not carried by healthy people in the United States or Europe. The bacteria is also found ponds and stream water. The ingestion of only a few hundred *C. jejuni* bacteria can make a person sick.

Symptoms of food poisoning begin two to five days after eating food contaminated with *C. jejuni*. These symptoms include fever, abdominal pain, nausea, **headache**, muscle pain, and diarrhea. The diarrhea can be watery or sticky and may contain blood. Symptoms last from seven to 10 days, and relapses occur in about one quarter of people who are infected. Dehydration is a common complication. Other complications such as arthritis-like joint pain and **hemolytic-uremic syndrome** (HUS) are rare.

Shigella

Shigella is a common cause of diarrhea in travelers to developing countries. It is associated with contaminated food and water, crowded living conditions, and poor sanitation. The bacterial toxins affect the small intestine.

Symptoms of food poisoning by *Shigella* appear 36–72 hours after eating contaminated food. These symptoms are slightly different from those associated with most foodborne bacteria. In addition to the familiar watery diarrhea, nausea, vomiting, abdominal cramps, chills and fever occur. The diarrhea may be quite severe with cramps progressing to classical **dysentery**. Up to 40% of children with severe infections show neurological symptoms. These include seizures caused by fever, confusion, headache, lethargy, and a stiff neck that resembles **meningitis**.

The disease runs its course usually in two to three days but may last longer. Dehydration is a common complication. Most people recover on their own, although they may feel exhausted, but children who are malnourished or have weakened immune systems may die.

Clostridium botulinum (C. botulinum)

C. botulinum, which causes both adult **botulism** and infant botulism, is unlike any of the other foodborne bacteria. First, *C. botulinum* is an anaerobic bacterium in that it can only live in the absence of oxygen. Second, the toxins from *C. botulinum* are neurotoxins. They poison the nervous system, causing **paralysis** without the vomiting and diarrhea associated with other foodborne illnesses. Third, toxins that cause adult botulism are released when the bacteria grows in an airless environment outside the body. They can be broken down and made harmless by heat. Finally, botulism is much more likely to be fatal even in tiny quantities.

Adult botulism outbreaks are usually associated with home canned food, although occasionally commercially canned or vacuum packed foods are responsible for the disease. *C. botulinum* grows well in non-acidic, oxygen-free environments. If food is canned at too low heat or for too brief a time, the bacteria is not killed. It reproduces inside the can or jar, releasing its deadly neurotoxin. The toxin can be made harmless by heating the contaminated food to boiling for ten minutes. However, even a very small amount of the *C. botulinum* toxin can cause serious illness or **death**.

Symptoms of adult botulism appear about 18–36 hours after the contaminated food is eaten, although there are documented times of onset ranging from four hours to eight days. Initially a person suffering from botulism feels weakness and **dizziness** followed by double vision. Symptoms progress to difficulty speaking and swallowing. Paralysis moves down the body, and when the respiratory muscles are paralyzed, death results from asphyxiation. People who show any signs of botulism poisoning must receive immediate emergency medical care to increase their chance of survival.

Infant botulism is a form of botulism first recognized in 1976. It differs from food-borne botulism in its causes and symptoms. Infant botulism occurs when a child under the age of one year ingests the spores of *C. botulinum*. These spores are found in soil, but a more common source of spores is honey.

The *C. botulinum* spores lodge in the baby's intestinal tract and begin to grow, producing their neurotoxin. Onset of symptoms is gradual. Initially the baby is constipated. This is followed by poor feeding, lethargy, weakness, drooling, and a distinctive wailing cry. Eventually, the baby loses the ability to control its head muscles. From there the paralysis progresses to the rest of the body.

Diagnosis

One important aspect of diagnosing food poisoning is for doctors to determine if a number of people have eaten the same food and show the same symptoms of illness. When this happens, food poisoning is strongly suspected. The diagnosis is confirmed when the suspected bacteria is found in a **stool culture** or a fecal smear from the person. Other laboratory tests are used to isolate bacteria from a sample of the contaminated food. Botulism is usually diagnosed from its distinctive neurological symptoms, since rapid treatment is essential. Many cases of food poisoning go undiagnosed, since a definite diagnosis is not necessary to effectively treat the symptoms. Because it takes time for symptoms to develop, it is not necessarily the most recent food one has eaten that is the cause of the symptoms.

KEY TERMS

Diuretic—Medication that increases the urine output of the body.

Electrolytes—Salts and minerals that produce electrically charged particles (ions) in body fluids. Common human electrolytes are sodium chloride, potassium, calcium, and sodium bicarbonate. Electrolytes control the fluid balance of the body and are important in muscle contraction, energy generation, and almost all major biochemical reactions in the body.

Lactobacillus acidophilus—This bacteria is found in yogurt and changes the balance of the bacteria in the intestine in a beneficial way.

Platelets—Blood cells that help the blood to clot.

Treatment

Treatment of food poisoning, except that caused by *C. botulinum*, focuses on preventing dehydration by replacing fluids and electrolytes lost through vomiting and diarrhea. Electrolytes are salts and **minerals** that form electrically charges particles (ions) in body fluids. Electrolytes are important because they control body fluid balance and are important for all major body reactions. Pharmacists can recommend effective, pleasant-tasting, electrolytically balanced replacement fluids that are available without a prescription. When more fluids are being lost than can be consumed, dehydration may occur. Dehydration more likely to happen in the very young, the elderly, and people who are taking **diuretics**. To prevent dehydration, a doctor may give fluids intravenously.

In very serious cases of food poisoning, medications may be given to stop abdominal cramping and vomiting. Anti-diarrheal medications are not usually given. Stopping the diarrhea keeps the toxins in the body longer and may prolong the infection.

People with food poisoning should modify their diet. During period of active vomiting and diarrhea they should not try to eat and should drink only clear liquids frequently but in small quantities. Once active symptoms stop, they should eat bland, soft, easy to digest foods for two to three days. One example is the BRAT diet of bananas, rice, applesauce, and toast, all of which are easy to digest. Milk products, spicy food, alcohol and fresh fruit should be avoided for a few days, although babies should continue to breastfeed. These modifications are often all the treatment that is necessary.

Severe bacterial food poisonings are sometimes treated with **antibiotics**. Trimethoprim and sulfamethoxazole (Septra, Bactrim), ampicillin (Amcill, Polycill) or ciprofloxacin (Ciloxan, Cipro) are most frequently used.

Botulism is treated in a different way from other bacterial food poisonings. Botulism antitoxin is given to adults, but not infants, if it can be administered within 72 hours after symptoms are first observed. If given later, it provides no benefit.

Both infants and adults require hospitalization, often in the intensive care unit. If the ability to breathe is impaired, patients are put on a mechanical ventilator to assist their breathing and are fed intravenously until the paralysis passes.

Alternative treatment

Alternative practitioners offer the same advice as traditional practitioners concerning diet modification. In addition they recommend taking charcoal tablets, *Lactobacillus acidophilus*, *Lactobacillus bulgaricus*, and citrus seed extract. An electrolyte replacement fluid can be made at home by adding one teaspoon of salt and four teaspoons of sugar to one quart of water. For food poisoning other than botulism, two homeopathic remedies, either *Arsenicum album* or *Nux vomica*, are strongly recommended.

Prognosis

Most cases of food poisoning (except botulism) clear up on their own within one week without medical assistance. The ill person may continue feel tired for a few days after active symptoms stop. So long as the ill person does not become dehydrated, there are few complications. Deaths are rare and usually occur in the very young, the very old and people whose immune systems are already weakened.

Complications of *Salmonella* food poisoning include arthritis-like symptoms that occur three to four weeks after infection. Although deaths from *Salmonella* are rare, they do occur. Most deaths caused by *Salmonella* food poisoning have occurred in elderly people in nursing homes.

Adults usually recover without medical intervention, but many children need to be hospitalized as the result of *E. coli* food poisoning. *E. coli* toxins may be absorbed into the blood stream where they destroy red blood cells and platelets. Platelets are important in blood clotting. About 5% of victims develop hemolytic-uremic syndrome which results in sudden kidney failure and makes dialysis necessary. (Dialysis is a medical procedure used to filter the body's waste product when the kidneys have failed).

Botulism is the deadliest of the bacterial foodborne illnesses. With prompt medical care, the death rate is less than 10%.

Prevention

Food poisoning is almost entirely preventable by practicing good sanitation and good food handling techniques. These include:

- Keep hot foods hot and cold foods cold.
- Cook meat to the recommended internal temperature, use a meat thermometer to check and cook eggs until they are no longer runny.
- Refrigerate leftovers promptly, do not let food stand at room temperature.
- Avoid contaminating surfaces and other foods with the juices of uncooked meats.
- Wash fruits and vegetables before using.
- Purchase pasteurized dairy products and fruit juices.
- Throw away bulging or leaking cans or any food that smells spoiled.
- Wash hands well before and during food preparation and after using the bathroom.
- Sanitize food preparation surfaces regularly.

Resources

OTHER

U. S. Food and Drug Administration. Center for Food Safety and Applied Nutrition. *Bad Bug Book*. http://vm.cfsan.fda.gov.

Suzanne M. Lutwick, MPH

Foot acupressure *see* **Reflexology**

Foot care

Definition

Foot care involves all aspects of preventative and corrective care of the foot and ankle. Doctors specializing in foot care are called podiatrists.

Purpose

During an average lifetime, each person walks about 115,000 miles and three-quarters of people have foot problems at some point in their lives.

Foot problems can arise from wearing ill-fitting shoes, from general wear and tear, as a result of injury, or as a complication of disease. People with **diabetes mellitus** or circulatory diseases are 20 times more likely to have foot problems than the general public.

Podiatrists are doctors who specialize in treating the foot and ankle. Other doctors who have experience with foot problems are family physicians, orthopedists, sports medicine specialists, and those who care for diabetics. Problems with the feet include foot **pain**, joint inflammation, plantar **warts**, fungal infections (like **athlete's foot**), nerve disorders, torn ligaments, broken bones, bacterial infections, and tissue injuries (like **frostbite**).

Precautions

People with diabetes or circulatory disorders should be alert to even small foot problems. In these people, a break in the skin can lead to infection, **gangrene**, and **amputation**.

Description

Daily foot care for people likely to develop foot problems includes washing the feet in tepid water with mild soap and oiling the feet with vegetable oil or a lanolin-based lotion. Toenails should be cut straight across above the level of the skin after soaking the feet in tepid water. **Corns and calluses** should not be cut. If they need removal, it should be done under the care of a doctor. Athletes foot and plantar warts should also be treated by a doctor if they develop in high risk patients.

Many people with diabetes or circulatory disorders have problems with cold feet. These problems can be reduced by avoiding **smoking** tobacco (smoking constricts the blood vessels), wearing warm socks, not crossing the legs while sitting or not sitting in one position too long, or avoiding constricting stockings.

People with circulatory problems should not use heating pads or hot water bottles on their feet, as even moderate heat can damage the skin if circulation is impaired.

Preparation

No special preparation other than an understanding of the nature of foot problems is necessary to begin routine foot care.

Aftercare

Foot care is preventative and should be ongoing throughout a person's life.

Risks

There are no risks associated with foot care. The risks are in ignoring the feet and allowing problems to develop.

Normal results

With regular care, foot disorders such as infections, skin ulcers, and gangrene can be prevented.

ORGANIZATIONS

American Diabetes Association, 1701 North Beauregard St., Alexandria, VA, 22311, (800) 342-2383, AskADA@diabetes.org, http://www.diabetes.org/.

American Podiatric Medical Association, 9312 Old Georgetown Rd., Bethesda, MD, 20814-1621, (301) 581-9200, http://www.apma.org.

Tish Davidson, A.M.

Foreign bodies *see* **Foreign objects**

Foreign objects

Definition

Foreign means "originating elsewhere" or simply "outside the body." Foreign objects, also known as foreign bodies, typically become lodged in the eyes, ears, nose, airways, and rectum of human beings.

Demographics

Swallowing foreign bodies is a fairly common pediatric emergency; about 80,000 cases involving persons 19 years old or younger are reported each year to the 67 poison control centers in the United States. In a recent survey of the parents of 1,500 children, 4% reported that their children had swallowed a foreign object of some kind. The highest incidence of swallowed foreign bodies is in children between the ages of six months and four years.

The type of object most frequently swallowed varies somewhat across different historical periods and cultures. A recent study comparing the Jackson collection of foreign bodies removed from children between 1920 and 1932 with data collected from North American children's hospitals between 1988 and 2000 found that coins have replaced safety pins as the objects most commonly swallowed by American children. In Asia, fish bones are a frequent offender because fish is a dietary staple in most countries of the Far East.

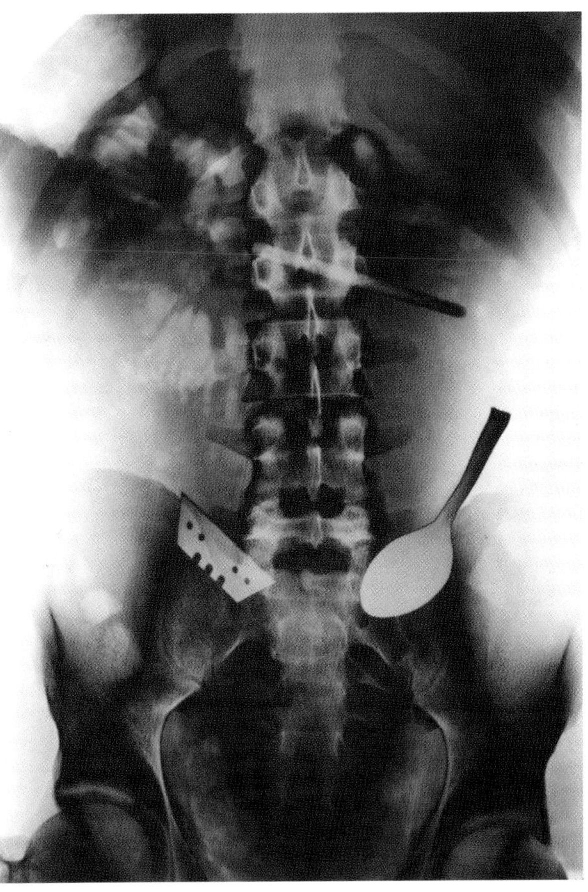

X-ray of swallowed spoon and blade in the intestine. *(Photo Researchers, Inc.)*

In younger children, boys are at slightly greater risk than girls (53–47%) of swallowing foreign objects. Among teenagers, males are at a much higher risk than females of swallowing foreign bodies or inserting them into the rectum.

Younger children usually swallow or insert foreign objects into their bodies accidentally, usually as a result of play or exploring their environment. Adolescents are more likely to swallow or insert foreign bodies intentionally as a risk-taking behavior, a bid for attention, or while under the influence of drugs or alcohol. A small minority of teenagers who harm themselves by swallowing or inserting foreign bodies have **schizophrenia** or another psychotic disorder.

Description

Both children and adults experience problems caused by foreign objects getting stuck in their bodies.

Young children are naturally curious and may intentionally put shiny objects, such as coins or button batteries, into their mouths. They also like to stick things in their ears and up their noses. Adults may accidentally swallow a non-food object or inhale a foreign body that gets stuck in the throat. Even if an object like a toothpick successfully passes through the esophagus and into the stomach, it can get stuck inside the rectum. Airborne particles can lodge in the eyes of people at any age.

Foreign bodies can be in hollow organs (like swallowed batteries) or in tissues (like bullets). They can be inert or irritating. If they irritate, they will cause inflammation and scarring. They can bring infection with them or acquire it and protect it from the body's immune defenses. They can obstruct passageways either by their size or by the scarring they cause. Some can be toxic.

Causes and symptoms

Eyes

Dust, dirt, sand, or other airborne material can lodge in the eyes, causing minor irritation and redness. More serious damage can be caused by hard or sharp objects that penetrate the surface and become embedded in the cornea or conjunctiva (the mucous membranes around the inner surface of the eyelids). Swelling, redness, bleeding from the surface blood vessels, sensitivity to light, and sudden vision problems are all symptoms of foreign matter in the eyes.

Ears and nose

Children will sometimes put things into their noses, ears, and other openings. Beans, popcorn kernels, raisins, and beads are just a few of the many items that have been found in these bodily cavities. On occasion, insects may fly into the ears and nose. **Pain**, **hearing loss**, and a sense of something stuck in the ear are symptoms of foreign bodies in the ears. A smelly, bloody discharge from one nostril is a symptom of foreign bodies in the nose.

Airways and stomach

At a certain age children will eat anything. A very partial list of items recovered from young stomachs includes: coins, chicken bones, fish bones, beads, rocks, plastic toys, pins, keys, round stones, marbles, nails, rings, batteries, ball bearings, screws, staples, washers, a heart pendant, a clothespin spring, and a toy soldier. Some of these items pass right on through and come out the other end. The progress of metal objects has been successfully followed with a metal detector. Others, like sharp bones, can get stuck and cause trouble. Batteries are corrosive and must be removed immediately.

Some objects can be inhaled unintentionally. The most commonly inhaled item is probably a peanut. A crayon and a cockroach have been found in a child's windpipes. These items always cause symptoms (difficulty swallowing and spitting up saliva, for instance) and may elude detection for some time while the child is being treated for **asthma** or recurring **pneumonia**.

Adults are not exempt from unusual inedibles. Dental devices are commonly swallowed. Adults with mental illness or subversive motives may swallow inappropriate objects, such as toothbrushes.

Rectum

Sometimes a foreign object will successfully pass through the throat and stomach only to get stuck at the juncture between the rectum and the anal canal. Items may also be self-introduced to enhance sexual stimulation and then get stuck. Sudden sharp pain during elimination may signify that an object is lodged in the rectum. Other symptoms vary depending upon the size of the object, its location, how long it has been in place, and whether or not infection has set in.

Diagnosis

The symptoms are as diverse as the objects and their locations. The most common manifestation of a foreign object anywhere in the body is infection. Even if the object started out sterile, germs may still be introduced. Blockage of passageways—breathing, digestive or excretory—is another result. Pain is common.

Treatment

Eyes

Small particles like sand may be removable without medical help, but if the object is not visible or cannot be retrieved, prompt emergency treatment is necessary. Trauma to the eyes can lead to loss of vision. Before attempting any treatment, the person should move to a well-lit area where the object can be better viewed. Hands should be washed and only clean, preferably sterile, materials should make contact with the eyes. If the particle is small, it may be dislodged by blinking or pulling the upper lid over the lower lid and flushing out the speck. A clean cloth can also be used to remove the particle. Once the object is

KEY TERMS

Bronchoscope—An illuminated instrument that is inserted into the airway to inspect and retrieve objects from the bronchial tubes.

Conjunctiva—Mucous membranes around the inner surface of the eyelid.

Cornea—The rounded, transparent portion of the eye that covers the pupil and iris and lets light into the interior

Endoscopy—The surgical use of long, thin instruments that have both viewing and operating capabilities.

Heimlich maneuver—An emergency procedure for removing a foreign object lodged in the airway that is preventing the person from breathing.

removed, the eye should be rinsed with clean, lukewarm water or an opthalmic wash.

If the foreign object cannot be removed at home, the eye should be lightly covered with sterile gauze to discourage rubbing. A physician will use a strong light and possibly special eye drops to locate the object. Surgical tweezers can effectively remove many objects. An antibiotic sterile ointment and a patch may be prescribed. If the foreign body has penetrated the deeper layers of the eye, an ophthalmic surgeon will be consulted for emergency treatment.

Ears and nose

A number of ingenious extraction methods have been devised for removing foreign objects from the nose and ears. A bead in a nostril, for example, can be popped out by blowing into the mouth while holding the other nostril closed. Insects can be floated out of the ear by pouring warm (not hot) mineral oil, olive oil, or baby oil into the ear canal. Items that are lodged deep in the ear canal are more difficult to remove because of the possibility of damaging the ear drum. These require emergency treatment from a qualified physician.

Airways and stomach

Mechanical obstruction of the airways, which commonly occurs when food gets lodged in the throat, can be treated by applying the **Heimlich maneuver**. If the object is lodged lower in the airway, a bronchoscope (a special instrument to view the airway and remove obstructions) can be inserted. If the object is blocking the entrance to the stomach, a fiberoptic endoscope (an illuminated instrument that views the interior of a body cavity) may be used. The physician typically administers a sedative and anesthetizes the throat. The foreign object will then either be pulled out or pushed into the stomach, depending on whether or not the physician thinks it will pass through the digestive tract on its own. Objects in the digestive tract that are not irritating, sharp, or large may be followed as they continue on through. Sterile objects that are not causing symptoms may be left in place. Surgical removal of the offending object is necessary if it is causing symptoms.

Rectum

A rectal retractor can remove objects that a physician can feel during **physical examination**. Surgery may be required for objects deeply lodged within the recturm.

Prevention

Using common sense and following safety precautions are the best ways to prevent foreign objects from entering the body. Parents and other child care providers should toddler-proof their homes. Batteries should be stored in a locked cabinet and properly disposed of after use. To minimize the chance of youngsters inhaling food, parents should not allow children to eat while walking or playing. Adults should chew food thoroughly and not talk while chewing. Many eye injuries can be prevented by wearing safety glasses while using tools

Resources

PERIODICALS

Al-Sebeih, Khalid, Khairy-Alhag Abu-Shara, and Amro Sobeih. "Extraluminal Perforation Complicating Foreign Bodies in the Upper Aerodigestive Tract." *The Annals of Otology, Rhinology & Laryngology* 119, no. 5 (May 1, 2010): 284-8.

Gilchrist, B. F., et al. "Pearls and Perils in the Management of Prolonged, Peculiar, Penetrating Esophageal Foreign Bodies in Children." *Journal of Pediatric Surgery* 32, no. 10 (October 1997): 1429-31.

Shivakumar, A., et al. "Foreign Bodies in Upper Digestive Tract." *Indian Journal of Otolaryngology and Head and Neck Surgery* 58, no. 1 (January-March 2006): 63-68.

J. Ricker Polsdorfer, MD
Karl Finley

47, XXY syndrome *see* **Klinefelter syndrome**

Fourn *see* **Flesh-eating disease**

Fracture repair

Definition

Fracture repair is the process of rejoining and realigning the ends of broken bones. This procedure is usually performed by an orthopedist, general surgeon, or family doctor. In cases of an emergency, **first aid** measures should be evoked for temporary realignment and **immobilization** until proper medical help is available.

Purpose

Fracture repair is required when there is a need for restoration of the normal position and function of the broken bone. Throughout the stages of fracture healing, the bones must be held firmly in the correct position. In the event the fracture is not properly repaired, malalignment of the bone may occur, resulting in possible physical dysfunction of the bone or joint of that region of the body.

Precautions

Precautions for fracture repair are anything found to be significant with patients' medical diagnosis and history. This would include an individual's tolerance to anesthesia and the presence of bleeding disorders that may be present to complicate surgery.

Description

Fracture repair is applied by means of **traction**, surgery, and/or by immobilization of the bones. The bone fragments are aligned as close as possible to the normal position without injuring the skin. Metal wires or screws may be needed to align smaller bone fragments. Once the broken ends of the bone are set, the affected area is immobilized for several weeks and kept rigid with a sling, plaster cast, brace or splint. With the use of traction, muscle pull on the fracture site is overcome by weights attached to a series of ropes running over pulleys. Strategically implanted electrical stimulation devices have proven beneficial in healing a fracture site, especially when the fracture is healing poorly and repair by other means is difficult.

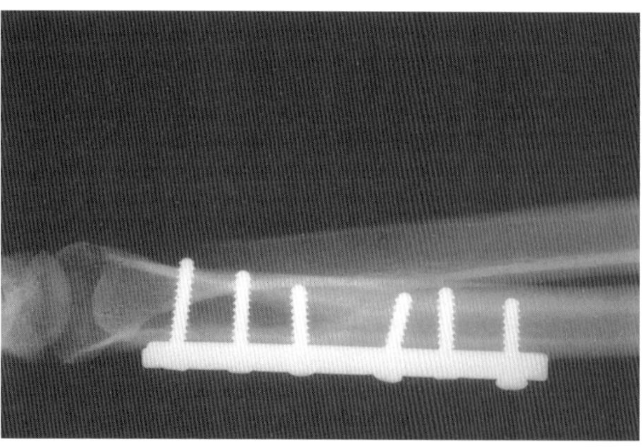

An x-ray image of a healing fracture. *(Custom Medical Stock Photo, Inc. Reproduced by permission.)*

Preparation

Emergency splinting may be required to immobilize the body part or parts involved. When fracture repair is necessary, the procedure is often performed in a hospital but can also be successfully done in an outpatient surgical facility, doctor's office or emergency room. Before any surgery for fracture repair, blood and urine studies may be taken from the patient. X-rays may follow this if not previously acquired. It has been noted however, that not all **fractures** are immediately apparent on an initial x-ray examination. In this case, where a fracture is definitely suspected the extent of the fracture can be properly diagnosed by repeating the x-rays 10–14 days later. Depending upon the situation, local or **general anesthesia** may be used for fracture repair.

Aftercare

After surgery, x-rays may be again taken through the cast or splint to evaluate if rejoined pieces remain in good position for healing. This is usually performed either before the application of the splint or at least before the patient is awakened from the general anesthesia. The patient needs to be cautious not to place excess pressure on any part of the cast until it is completely dry. The patient also should avoid excess pressure on the operative site until complete healing has taken place and the injury has been re-examined by the physician. If the cast becomes exposed to moisture it may soften and require repair. The patient should also be instructed to keep the injured region propped up whenever possible to reduce the possibility of swelling.

Risks

Surgical risks of fracture repair are greater in patients over 60 years of age because the bones often taking longer to heal properly. **Obesity** may place extra stress on the healing site, affecting healing and possibly risking reinjury. **Smoking** may slow the healing process after fracture repair, as well as poor **nutrition**, **alcoholism**, and chronic illness. Some medications may affect

KEY TERMS

Compound fracture—A fracture in which the broken end or ends of the bone have torn through the skin. Compound fractures are also known as open fractures

Staphylococcal infection—An infection caused by any of several pathogenic species of Staphylococcus, commonly characterized by the formation of abscesses of the skin or other organs.

Streptococcal infection—An infection caused by a pathogenic bacteria of one of several species of the genus Streptococcus or their toxins. Almost any organ in the body may be involved.

the fracture site, causing poor union. Such medications include anti-hypertensives and cortisone.

Possible complications following fracture repair include excessive bleeding, improper fit of joined bone ends, pressure on nearby nerves, delayed healing, and a permanent incomplete healing of the fracture. If there is a poor blood supply to the fractured site with one of the portions of broken bone not properly supplied by the blood, the bony portion will die and healing of the fracture will not take place. This is called aseptic necrosis. Poor immobilization of the fracture from improper casting which permits motion between the bone parts may prevent healing and repair of the bone with possible deformity. Infection can interfere with bone repair. This risk is greater in the case of a compound fracture (a bone fracture causing an open wound) where ideal conditions are present for severe streptococcal and **staphylococcal infections**. Occasionally, fractured bones in the elderly may possibly never heal properly. The risk is increased when nutrition is poor.

Normal results

Once the procedure for fracture repair is completed, the body begins to produce new tissue to bridge the broken pieces. At first, this tissue (called a callus) is soft and easily injured. Later, the body deposits bone **minerals** until the callus becomes a solid piece of bone. The fracture site is thus strengthened further with extra bone. It usually takes about six weeks for a broken bone to heal together. The exact time required for healing depends on the type of fracture and the extent of damage. Before the use of x-rays, fracture repair was not always accurate, resulting in crippling deformities. With modern x-ray technology, the physician can view the extent of the fracture, check the setting following the repair, and be certain after the procedure that the bones have not moved from their intended alignment. Children's bones usually heal relatively rapidly.

Abnormal results

Abnormal results of fracture repair include damage to nearby nerves or primary blood vessels. Improper alignment causing deformity is also an abnormal outcome, however, with today's medical technology it is relatively rare.

Resources

OTHER

Griffith, H. Winter. "Fracture Repair." *ThriveOnline*. 1998. http://thriveonline.oxygen.com.

Jeffrey P. Larson, RPT

Fractures

Definition

A fracture is a complete or incomplete break in a bone resulting from the application of excessive force.

Description

A fracture usually results from traumatic injury to bones causing the continuity of bone tissues or bony cartilage to be disrupted or broken. Fracture classifications include simple, compound, incomplete and complete. Simple fractures (more recently called "closed") are not obvious as the skin has not been ruptured and remains intact. Compound fractures (now commonly called "open") break the skin, exposing bone and causing additional soft tissue injury and possible infection. A single fracture means that one fracture only has occurred and multiple fractures refer to more than one fracture occurring in the same bone. Fractures are termed complete if the break is completely through the bone and described as incomplete or "greenstick" if the fracture occurs partly across a bone shaft. This latter type of fracture is often the result of bending or crushing forces applied to a bone.

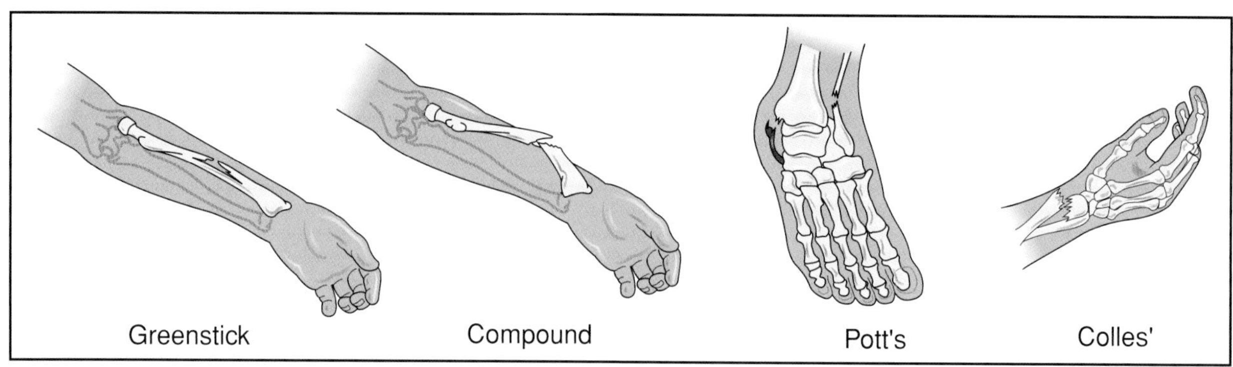

Fractures usually result from a traumatic injury to a bone where the continuity of bone tissues or bony cartilage is disrupted or broken. The illustrations above feature common sites where fractures occur. *(Illustration by Electronic Illustrators Group. Reproduced by permission of Gale, a part of Cengage Learning.)*

Fractures are also named according to the specific part of the bone involved and the nature of the break. Identification of a fracture line can further classify fractures. Types include linear, oblique, transverse, longitudinal, and spiral fractures. Fractures can be further subdivided by the positions of bony fragments and are described as comminuted, non-displaced, impacted, overriding, angulated, displaced, avulsed, and segmental. Additionally, an injury may be classified as a fracture-dislocation when a fracture involves the bony structures of any joint with associated dislocation of the same joint.

Fractures line identification

Linear fractures have a break that runs parallel to the bone's main axis or in the direction of the bone's shaft. For example, a linear fracture of the arm bone could extend the entire length of the bone. Oblique and transverse fractures differ in that an oblique fracture crosses a bone at approximately a 45° angle to the bone's axis. In contrast, a transverse fracture crosses a bone's axis at a 90° angle. A longitudinal fracture is similar to a linear fracture. Its fracture line extends along the shaft but is more irregular in shape and does not run parallel to the bone's axis. Spiral fractures are described as crossing a bone at an oblique angle, creating a spiral pattern. This break usually occurs in the long bones of the body such as the upper arm bone (humerus) or the thigh bone (femur).

Bony fragment position identification

Comminuted fractures have two or more fragments broken into small pieces, in addition to the upper and lower halves of a fractured bone. Fragments of bone that maintain their normal alignment following a fracture are described as being non-displaced. An impacted fracture is characterized as a bone fragment forced into or onto another fragment resulting from a compressive force. Overriding is a term used to describe bony fragments that overlap and shorten the total length of a bone. Angulated fragments result in pieces of bone being at angles to each other. A displaced bony fragment occurs from disruption of normal bone alignment with deformity of these segments separate from one another. An avulsed fragment occurs when bone fragments are pulled from their normal position by forceful muscle contractions or resistance from ligaments. Segmental fragmented positioning occurs if fractures in two adjacent areas occur, leaving an isolated central segment. An example of segmental alignment is when the arm bone fractures in two separate places, with displacement of the middle section of bone.

Causes and symptoms

Individuals with high activity levels appear to be at greater risk for fractures. This group includes children and athletes participating in contact sports. Because of an increase in bone brittleness with **aging**, elderly persons are also included in this high-risk population. Up to the age of 50, more men suffer from fractures than women due to occupational hazards. However, after the age of 50, women are more prone to fractures than men. Specific diseases causing an increased risk for fractures include Paget's disease, **rickets**, **osteogenesis imperfecta**, **osteoporosis**, bone **cancer** and tumors, and prolonged disuse of a non-functional body part such as after a **stroke**.

Symptoms of fractures usually begin with **pain** that increases with attempted movement or use of the area and swelling at the involved site. The skin in the area may be pale and an obvious deformity may be present. In more severe cases, there may be a loss of pulse below the fracture site, such as in the extremities, accompanied by **numbness**, **tingling**, or **paralysis** below the fracture. An open or compound fracture is often accompanied by bleeding or bruising. If the lower limbs or pelvis are fractured, pain and resistance to movement usually accompany the injury causing difficulty with weight bearing.

Diagnosis

Diagnosis begins immediately with an individual's own observation of symptoms. A thorough medical history and physical exam by a physician often reveals the presence of a fracture. An x-ray of the injured area is the most common test used to determine the presence of a bone fracture. Any x-ray series performed involves at least two views of the area to confirm the presence of the fracture because not all fractures are apparent on a single x-ray. Some fractures are often difficult to see and may require several views at different angles to see clear fracture lines. In some cases, CT, MRI or other imaging tests are required to demonstrate fracture. Sometimes, especially with children, the initial x-ray may not show any fractures but repeat seven to 14 days later may show changes in the bone(s) of the affected area. If a fracture is open and occurs in conjunction with soft tissue injury, further laboratory studies are often conducted to determine if blood loss has occurred.

In the event of exercise-related stress fractures (micro-fractures due to excessive stress), a tuning fork can provide a simple, inexpensive test. The tuning fork is a metal instrument with a stem and two prongs that vibrate when struck. If an individual has increased pain when the tuning fork is placed on a bone, such as the tibia or shinbone, the likelihood of a stress fracture is high. Bone scans also are helpful in detecting stress fractures. In this diagnostic procedure, a radioactive tracer is injected into the bloodstream and images are taken of specific areas or the entire skeleton by CT or MRI.

Treatment

Treatment depends on the type of fracture, its severity, the individual's age and general health. The first priority in treating any fracture is to address the entire medical status of the patient. Medical personnel are trained not allow a painful, deformed limb to distract them from potentially life-threatening injury elsewhere or **shock**. If an open fracture is accompanied by serious soft tissue injury, it may be necessary to control bleeding and the shock that can accompany loss of blood.

First aid is the appropriate initial treatment in emergency situations. It includes proper splinting, control of blood loss, and monitoring vital signs such as breathing and circulation.

Immobilization

Immobilization of a fracture site can be done internally or externally. The primary goal of immobilization is to maintain the realignment of a bone long enough for healing to start and progress. Immobilization by external fixation uses splints, casts, or braces. This may be the primary and only procedure for fracture treatment. Splinting to immobilize a fracture can be done with or without **traction**. In emergency situations if the injured individual must be moved by someone other than a trained medical person, splinting is a useful form of fracture management. It should be done without causing additional pain and without moving the bone segments. In a clinical environment, plaster of Paris casts are used for immobilization. Braces are useful as they often allow movement above and below a fracture site. Treatments for stress fractures include rest and decreasing or stopping any activity that causes or increases pain.

Fracture reduction

Fracture reduction is the procedure by which a fractured bone is realigned in normal position. It can be either closed or open. Closed reduction refers to realigning bones without breaking the skin. It is performed with manual manipulation and/or traction and is commonly done with some kind of anesthetic. Open reduction primarily refers to surgery that is performed to realign bones or fragments. Fractures with little or no displacement may not require any form of reduction.

Traction is used to help reposition a broken bone. It works by applying pressure to restore proper alignment. The traction device immobilizes the area and maintains realignment as the bone heals. A fractured bone is immobilized by applying opposing force at both ends of the injured area, using an equal amount of traction and countertraction. Weights provide the traction pull needed or the pull is achieved by positioning the individual's body weight appropriately. Traction is a form of closed reduction and is sometimes used as an alternative to surgery. Since it restricts movement of the affected limb or body part, it may confine a person to bed rest for an extended period of time.

A person may need open reduction if there is an open, severe, or comminuted fracture. This procedure allows a physician to examine and surgically correct associated soft tissue damage while reducing the

KEY TERMS

Avulsion fracture—A fracture caused by the tearing away of a fragment of bone where a strong ligament or tendon attachment forcibly pulls the fragment away from the bone tissue.

Axis—A line that passes through the center of the body or body part.

Comminuted fracture—A fracture where there are several breaks in a bone creating numerous fragments.

Compartment syndrome—Compartment syndrome is a condition in which a muscle swells but is constricted by the connective tissue around it, which cuts off blood supply to the muscle.

Contrast hydrotherapy—A series of hot and cold water applications. A hot compress (as hot as an individual can tolerate) is applied for three minutes followed by an ice cold compress for 30 seconds. These applications are repeated three times each and ending with the cold compress.

Osteogenesis imperfecta—A genetic disorder involving defective development of connective tissues, characterized by brittle and fragile bones that are easily fractured by the slightest trauma.

Osteoporosis—Literally meaning "porous bones," this condition occurs when bones lose an excessive amount of their protein and mineral content, particularly calcium. Over time, bone mass and strength are reduced leading to increased risk of fractures.

Paget's disease—Chromic disorder of unknown cause, usually affecting middle aged and elderly people, characterized by enlarged and deformed bones. Excessive breakdown and formation of bone tissue occurs with Paget's disease and can cause bone to weaken, resulting in bone pain, arthritis, deformities, and fractures.

Reduction—The restoration of a body part to its original position after displacement, such as the reduction of a fractured bone by bringing ends or fragments back into original alignment. The useof local or general anesthesia usually accompanies a fracture reduction. If performed by outside manipulation only, the reduction is described as closed; if surgery is necessary, it is described as open.

Rickets—A condition caused by the dietary deficiency of vitamin D, calcium, and usually phosphorus, seen primarily in infancy and childhood, and characterized by abnormal bone formation.

Traction—The process of placing a bone, limb, or group of muscles under tension by applying weights and pulleys. The goal is to realign or immobilize the part or to relieve pressure on that particular area to promote healing and restore function.

fracture and, if necessary, applying internal or external devices. Internal fixation involves the use of metallic devices inserted into or through bone to hold the fracture in a set position and alignment while it heals. Devices include plates, nails, screws, and rods. When healing is complete, the surgeon may or may not remove these devices. Virtually any hip fracture requires open reduction and internal fixation so that the bone will be able to support the patient's weight.

Alternative treatment

In addition to the importance of **calcium** for strong bones, many alternative treatment approaches recommend use of mineral supplements to help build and maintain a healthy, resilient skeleton. Some physical therapists use electro-stimulation over a fractured site to promote and expedite healing. Chinese traditional medicine may be helpful by working to reconnect chi through the meridian lines along the line of a fracture. Homeopathy can enhance the body's healing process. Two particularly useful homeopathic remedies are *Arnica* (*Arnica montana*) and *Symphytum* (*Symphytum officinalis*). If possible, applying contrast **hydrotherapy** to an extremity (e.g., a hand or foot) of a fractured area can assist healing by enhancing circulation.

Prognosis

Fractures involving joint surfaces almost always lead to some degree of arthritis of the joint. Fractures can normally be cured with proper first aid and appropriate aftercare. If determined necessary by a physician, the fractured site should be manipulated, realigned, and immobilized as soon as possible. Realignment has been shown to be much more difficult after six hours. Healing time varies from person to person with the elderly generally needing more time to heal completely. A non-union fracture may result when a fracture does not heal, such as in the case of an elderly person or an individual with medical complications. Recovery is complete when there is no bone motion at the fracture site, and x rays indicate complete healing. Open fractures may lead to bone infections, which delay the healing process. Another possible complication is compartment syndrome, a painful condition resulting from the expansion of enclosed tissue and that may occur when a body part is immobilized in a cast.

Prevention

Adequate calcium intake is necessary for strong bones and can help decrease the risk of fractures. People who do not get enough calcium in their **diets** can take a calcium supplement. **Exercise** can help strengthen bones by increasing bone density, thereby decreasing the risk of fractures from falls. A University of Southern California study reported that older people who exercised one or more hours per day had approximately half the incidence of hip fractures as those who exercised fewer than 30 minutes per day or not at all.

Fractures can be prevented if safety measures are taken seriously. These measures include using seat belts in cars and encouraging children to wear protective sports gear. Estrogen replacement for women past the age of 50 has been shown to help prevent osteoporosis and the fractures that may result from this condition. In one study, elderly women on estrogen replacement therapy demonstrated the lowest occurrence of hip fractures when compared to similar women not on estrogen replacement therapy.

Resources

BOOKS

Johnson, Donald, and Robert A. Pedowitz. *Practical Orthopaedic Sports Medicine and Arthroscopy*. Philadelphia : Lippincott Williams & Wilkins, 2007.

Morrey, Bernard F. *Master Techniques in Orthopaedic Surgery*. 3rd ed. Philadelphia: Wolters Kluwer Health / Lippincott Williams & Wilkins, 2007.

Starkey, Chad, and Glen Johnson. *Athletic Training and Sports Medicine*. 4th ed. Sudbury, MA: Jones and Bartlett, 2006.

Wiss, Donald A. *Fractures*. Philadelphia: Lippincott Williams & Wilkins, 2006.

OTHER

"About the Human." http://orthopedics.about.com/health/orthopedics/blhipfracture.htm.

Family Practice Notebook.com. http://www.fpnotebook.com.

National Library of Medicine. http://medlineplus.adam.com/ency/article/000001.htm.

University of Iowa. http://www.vh.org/Providers/ClinRef/FPHandbook/Chapter06/18-6.html.

ORGANIZATIONS

American Academy of Orthopaedic Surgeons, 6300 North River Rd., Rosemont, IL, 60018-4262, (847) 823-7186, (847) 823-8125, pemr@aaos.org, http://www.aaos.org.

American College of Sports Medicine (ACSM), 401 West Michigan St., P.O. Box 1440, Indianapolis, IN, 46202-3233, (317) 637-9200, (317) 634-7817, http://www.acsm.org.

Children's Orthopedics of Atlanta, 5445 Meridian Mark Rd., Suite 250, Atlanta, GA, 30342, (404) 255-1933, (404) 256-7924, http://www.childrensortho.com.

Nemours Foundation, 10140 Centurion Parkway, Jacksonville, FL, 32256, (904) 697-4100, (904) 697-4220, http://www.nemours.org.

L. Fleming Fallon, Jr., MD, DrPH

Fragile X syndrome

Definition

Fragile X syndrome is the most common form of inherited **mental retardation**. Individuals with this condition have developmental delay, variable levels of mental retardation, and behavioral and emotional difficulties. They may also have characteristic physical traits. Generally, males are affected with moderate mental retardation and females with mild mental retardation.

Description

Fragile X syndrome is also known as Martin-Bell syndrome, Marker X syndrome, and FRAXA syndrome. It is the most common form of inherited mental retardation. Fragile X syndrome is caused by a mutation in the FMR-1 gene, located on the X chromosome. The role of the gene is unclear, but it is probably important in early development.

In order to understand fragile X syndrome it is important to understand how human genes and chromosomes influence this condition. Normally, each cell in the body contains 46 chromosomes (23 pairs). These chromosomes consist of genetic material (DNA) needed for the production of proteins, which lead to growth, development, and physical/intellectual characteristics. The first 22 pairs of chromosomes are the same in males and females. The remaining two chromosomes are called the sex chromosomes (X and Y). The sex chromosomes determine whether a person is male or female. Males have only one X chromosome, which is inherited from the mother at conception, and they receive a Y chromosome from the father. Females inherit two X chromosomes, one from each parent. Fragile X syndrome is caused by a mutation in a gene called FMR-1. This gene is located on the X chromosome. The FMR-1 gene is thought to play an important role in the development of the brain, but the exact way that the gene acts in the body is not fully understood.

Fragile X syndrome affects males and females of all ethnic groups. It is estimated that about one in 4,000-6,250 males are affected with fragile X syndrome. There are approximately one-half as many females with fragile X syndrome as there are males. The carrier frequency in unaffected females is one in 100-600, with one study finding a carrier frequency of one in 250.

Causes and symptoms

For reasons not fully understood, the CGG sequence in the FMR-1 gene can expand to contain between 54 and 230 repeats. This stage of expansion is called a premutation. People who carry a premutation do not usually have symptoms of fragile X syndrome, although there have been reports of individuals with a premutation and subtle intellectual or behavioral symptoms. Individuals who carry a fragile X premutation are at risk to have children or grandchildren with the condition. Female premutation carriers may also be at increased risk for earlier onset of **menopause**; however, premutation carriers may exist through several generations of a family and no symptoms of fragile X syndrome will appear.

The size of the premutation can expand over succeeding generations. Once the size of the premutation exceeds 230 repeats, it becomes a full mutation and the FMR-1 gene is disabled. Individuals who carry the full mutation may have fragile X syndrome. Since the FMR-1 gene is located on the X chromosome, males are more likely to develop symptoms than females. This is because males have only one copy of the X chromosome. Males who inherit the full mutation are expected to have mental impairment. A female's normal X chromosome may compensate for her chromosome with the fragile X gene mutation. Females who inherit the full mutation have an approximately 50% risk of mental impairment. The phenomenon of an expanding trinucleotide repeat in successive generations is called anticipation. Another unique aspect of fragile X syndrome is that mosaicism is present in 15–20% those affected by the condition. Mosaicism is when there is the presence of cells of two different genetic materials in the same individual.

The mutation involves a short sequence of DNA in the FMR-1 gene. This sequence is designated CGG. Normally, the CGG sequence is repeated between six to 54 times. People who have repeats in this range do not have fragile X syndrome and are not at increased risk to have children with fragile X syndrome. Those affected by fragile X syndrome have expanded CGG repeats (more than 200) in the first exon of the FMR1 gene (the full mutation)

Fragile X syndrome is inherited in an X-linked dominant manner (characters are transmitted by genes on the X chromosome). When a man carries a premutation on his X chromosome, it tends to be stable and usually will not expand if he passes it on to his daughters (he passes his Y chromosome to his sons). Thus, all of his daughters will be premutation carriers like he is. When a woman carries a premutation, it is unstable and can expand as she passes it on to her children, therefore a man's grandchildren are at greater risk of developing the syndrome. There is a 50% risk for a premutation carrier female to transmit an abnormal mutation with each **pregnancy**. The likelihood for the premutation to expand is related to the number of repeats present; the higher the number of repeats, the greater the chance that the premutation will expand to a full mutation in the next generation. All mothers of a child with a full mutation are carriers of an FMR-1 gene expansion. Ninety-nine% of patients with fragile X syndrome have a CGG expansion, and less than 1% have a point mutation or deletion on the FMR1 gene.

Individuals with fragile X syndrome appear normal at birth but their development is delayed. Most boys with fragile X syndrome have mental impairment. The severity of mental impairment ranges from learning disabilities to severe mental retardation. Behavioral problems include attention deficit and hyperactivity at a young age. Some may show aggressive behavior in adulthood. Short attention span, poor eye contact, delayed and disordered speech and language, emotional instability, and unusual hand mannerisms (hand flapping or hand biting) are also seen frequently. Characteristic physical traits appear later in childhood. These traits include a long and narrow face, prominent jaw, large ears, and enlarged testes. In females who carry a full mutation, the physical and behavioral features and mental retardation tend to be less severe. About 50% of females who have a full mutation are mentally retarded. Other behavioral characteristics include whirling, spinning, and occasionally **autism**.

Children with fragile X syndrome often have frequent ear and sinus infections. Nearsightedness and

KEY TERMS

Amniocentesis—A procedure performed at 16–18 weeks of pregnancy in which a needle is inserted through a woman's abdomen into her uterus to draw out a small sample of the amniotic fluid from around the baby. Either the fluid itself or cells from the fluid can be used for a variety of tests to obtain information about genetic disorders and other medical conditions in the fetus.

CGG or CGG sequence—Shorthand for the DNA sequence: cytosine-guanine-guanine. Cytosine and guanine are two of the four molecules, otherwise called nucleic acids, that make up DNA.

Chorionic villus sampling (CVS)—A procedure used for prenatal diagnosis at 10-12 weeks gestation. Under ultrasound guidance a needle is inserted either through the mother's vagina or abdominal wall and a sample of cells is collected from around the early embryo. These cells are then tested for chromosome abnormalities or other genetic diseases.

Chromosome—A microscopic thread-like structure found within each cell of the body that consists of a complex of proteins and DNA. Humans have 46 chromosomes arranged into 23 pairs. Changes in either the total number of chromosomes or their shape and size (structure) may lead to physical or mental abnormalities.

FMR-1 gene—A gene found on the X chromosome. Its exact purpose is unknown, but it is suspected that the gene plays a role in brain development.

Mitral valve prolapse—A heart defect in which one of the valves of the heart (which normally controls blood flow) becomes floppy. Mitral valve prolapse may be detected as a heart murmur but there are usually no symptoms.

Premutation—A change in a gene that precedes a mutation; this change does not alter the function of the gene.

X chromosome—One of the two sex chromosomes (the other is Y) containing genetic material that, among other things, determine a person's gender.

lazy eye are also common. Many babies with fragile X syndrome may have trouble with sucking and some experience digestive disorders that cause frequent gagging and **vomiting**. A small percentage of children with fragile X syndrome may experience seizures. Children with fragile X syndrome also tend to have loose joints which may result in joint **dislocations**. Some children develop a curvature in the spine, flat feet, and a heart condition known as **mitral valve prolapse**.

Diagnosis

Any child with signs of developmental delay of speech, language, or motor development with no known cause should be considered for fragile X testing, especially if there is a family history of the condition. Behavioral and developmental problems may indicate fragile X syndrome, particularly if there is a family history of mental retardation. Definitive identification of the fragile X syndrome is made by means of a genetic test to assess the number of CGG sequence repeats in the FMR-1 gene. Individuals with the premutation or full mutation may be identified through **genetic testing**. Genetic testing for the fragile X mutation can be done on the developing baby before birth through **amniocentesis** or **chorionic villus sampling** (CVS), and is 99% effective in detecting the condition due to trinucleotide repeat expansion. Prenatal testing should only be undertaken after the fragile X carrier status of the parents has been confirmed and the couple has been counseled regarding the risks of recurrence. While prenatal testing is possible to do with CVS, the results can be difficult to interpret and additional testing may be required.

Treatment

Presently there is no cure for fragile X syndrome. Management includes such approaches as **speech therapy**, **occupational therapy**, and **physical therapy**. The expertise of psychologists, special education teachers, and genetic counselors may also be beneficial. Drugs may be used to treat hyperactivity, seizures, and other problems. Establishing a regular routine, avoiding overstimulation, and using calming techniques may also help in the management of behavioral problems. Children with a troubled heart valve may need to see a heart specialist and take medications before surgery or dental procedures. Children with frequent ear and sinus infections may need to take medications or have special tubes placed in their ears to drain excess fluid. Mainstreaming of children with fragile X syndrome into regular classrooms is encouraged because they do well imitating behavior. Peer tutoring and positive reinforcement are also encouraged.

Prognosis

Early diagnosis and intensive intervention offer the best prognosis for individuals with fragile X syndrome. Adults with fragile X syndrome may benefit from vocational training and may need to live in a supervised setting. Life span is typically normal.

A 2004 study found that men who are carriers of the fragile X gene but have not have the mutation severe enough to have fragile X syndrome may begin to show signs of tremor disorder, gait instability and memory impairment as they age. The higher prevalence of these symptoms among grandfathers of children with fragile x syndrome was noted so a study was done to investigate their symptoms compared to men of the same age without the mutation. About 17% of the grandfathers in their 50s had the condition, 37% of those in their 60s, 47% of men in their 70s and 75% of men in their 80s. Often, these men have been diagnosed with other diseases such as Parkinson's or Alzheimer's rather than with fragile X-associated tremor/ataxia syndrome, the name which has been given to these late symptoms from the fragile x mutation.

Resources

PERIODICALS

Kirn, Timothy F. "New Fragile X Often Misdiagnosed as Parkinson's." *Clinical Psychiatry News* March 2004: 84.

OTHER

"Fragile X Site Mental Retardation 1; FMR1." *Online Mendelian Inheritance in Man.* March 6, 2001. http://www.ncbi.nlm.nih.gov/omim/300624.

Tarleton, Jack, and Robert A. Saul. "Fragile X Syndrome." *GeneClinics* March 6, 2001. http://www.geneclinics.org.

ORGANIZATIONS

FRAXA Research Foundation, 45 Pleasant St., Newburyport, MA, 01950, (978) 462-1866, kclapp@fraxa.org, http://www.fraxa.org.

The Arc, 1660 L St., NW, Suite 301, Washington, DC, 20036, (202) 534-3700, (202) 534-3731, (800) 433-5255, info@thearc.org, http://thearc.org.

The National Fragile X Foundation, (925) 938-9300, (925) 938-9315, (800) 688-8765, http://www.fragilex.org.

Nada Quercia, MS, CCGC
Teresa G. Odle

Frambesia *see* **Yaws**

Francisella tularensis infection *see* **Tularemia**

Fresh cell therapy *see* **Cell therapy**

Friedreich's ataxia

Definition

Friedreich's ataxia (FA) is an inherited, progressive nervous system disorder causing loss of balance and coordination.

Description

Ataxia is a condition marked by impaired coordination. Friedreich's ataxia is the most common inherited ataxia, affecting between 3,000–5,000 people in the United States. FA is an autosomal recessive disease, which means that two defective gene copies must be inherited to develop symptoms, one from each parent. A person with only one defective gene copy will not show signs of FA, but may pass along the gene to offspring. Couples with one child affected by FA have a 25% chance in each **pregnancy** of conceiving another affected child.

Causes and symptoms

Causes

The gene for FA codes for a protein called frataxin. Normal frataxin is found in the cellular energy structures known as mitochondria, where it is thought to be involved in regulating the transport of iron. In FA, the frataxin gene on chromosome 9 is expanded with nonsense information known as a "triple repeat." This extra DNA interferes with normal production of frataxin, thereby impairing iron transport. Normally, there are 10-21 repeats of the frataxin gene. In FA, this sequence may be repeated between 200-900 times. The types of symptoms and severity of FA seems to be associated with the number of repetitions. Patients with more copies have more severe symptomatology. Researchers are still wrestling with how frataxin and the repeats on chromosome 9 are involved in causing FA. One theory suggests that FA develops in part because defects in iron transport prevent efficient use of cellular energy supplies.

The nerve cells most affected by FA are those in the spinal cord involved in relaying information between muscles and the brain. Tight control of movement requires complex feedback between the muscles promoting a movement, those restraining it, and the brain. Without this control, movements become uncoordinated, jerky, and inappropriate to the desired action.

Symptoms

Symptoms of FA usually first appear between the ages of 8 and 15, although onset as early as 18 months or as late as age 25 is possible. The first symptom is usually gait incoordination. A child with FA may graze doorways when passing through, for instance, or trip over low obstacles. Unsteadiness when standing still and deterioration of position sense is common. Foot deformities and walking up off the heels often results from uneven muscle weakness in the legs. **Muscle spasms and cramps** may occur, especially at night.

Ataxia in the arms follows, usually within several years, leading to decreased hand-eye coordination. Arm weakness does not usually occur until much later. Speech and swallowing difficulties are common. **Diabetes mellitus** may also occur. **Nystagmus**, or eye tremor, is common, along with some loss of visual acuity. **Hearing loss** may also occur. A side-to-side curvature of the spine (**scoliosis**) occurs in many cases, and may become severe.

Heartbeat abnormalities occur in about two thirds of FA patients, leading to **shortness of breath** after exertion, swelling in the lower limbs, and frequent complaints of cold feet.

Diagnosis

Diagnosis of FA involves a careful medical history and thorough **neurological exam**. Lab tests include **electromyography**, an electrical test of muscle, and a nerve conduction velocity test. An electrocardiogram may be performed to diagnose heart arrhythmia.

Direct DNA testing is available, allowing FA to be more easily distinguished from other types of ataxia. The same test may be used to determine the presence of the genetic defect in unaffected individuals, such as siblings.

Treatment

There is no cure for FA, nor any treatment that can slow its progress. Amantadine may provide some limited improvement in ataxic symptoms, but is not recommended in patients with cardiac abnormalities. Physical and **occupational therapy** are used to maintain range of motion in weakened muscles, and to design adaptive techniques and devices to compensate for loss of coordination and strength. Some patients find that using weights on the arms can help dampen the worst of the uncoordinated arm movements.

Heart **arrhythmias** and diabetes are treated with drugs specific to those conditions.

Prognosis

The rate of progression of FA is highly variable. Most patients lose the ability to walk within 15 years of symptom onset, and 95% require a wheelchair for mobility by age 45. Reduction in lifespan from FA complications is also quite variable. Average age at **death** is in the mid-thirties, but may be as late as the mid-sixties. As of mid-1998, the particular length of the triple repeat has not been correlated strongly enough with disease progression to allow prediction of the course of the disease on this basis.

KEY TERMS

Ataxia—A condition marked by impaired coordination.

Scoliosis—An abnormal, side-to-side curvature of the spine.

Prevention

There is no way to prevent development of FA in a person carrying two defective gene copies.

Resources

BOOKS

Cecil, Russell L., Lee Goldman, and D. A. Audiello.*Cecil Medicine*. 23rd ed, Philadelphia: Saunders Elsevier, 2008.

Fauci, Anthony S., et al., eds. *Harrison's Principles of Internal Medicine*. 17th ed. New York: McGraw–Hill Professional, 2008.

ORGANIZATIONS

Muscular Dystrophy Association, 3300 East Sunrise Dr., Tucson, AZ, 85718, (800) 572-1717, http://www.mdausa.org.

Rosalyn Carson-DeWitt, MD

Frostbite and frostnip

Definition

Frostbite is the term for damage to the skin and other tissues caused by freezing. Frostnip is a milder form of cold injury; it is sometimes described as the first stage of frostbite.

Demographics

Frostbite is most likely to occur among military personnel, people who work outdoors in cold weather, mountain climbers, skiers and other winter sports

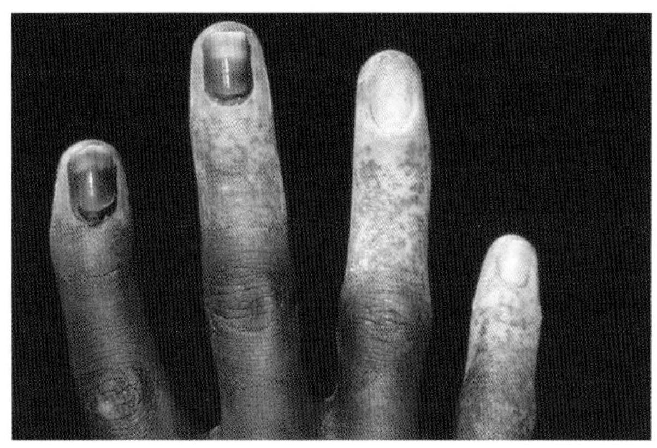

A human hand with frostbite. *(SIU/Photo Researchers, Inc.)*

participants, homeless people, travelers stranded outside in cold weather, and people who live close to the polar regions. In a few cases frostbite is caused by industrial accidents, when workers who must handle liquid nitrogen or other liquefied gases fail to protect their hands or use proper safety equipment. It is estimated that frostbite in North America and northern Europe causes 2.5 hospital admissions per 100,000 people annually. The true rate is unknown because there is no standardized reporting system for this disorder.

Most frostbite victims are male, but this ratio is thought to reflect occupational choices and interest in high-risk outdoor sports rather than a genetic factor.

According to U.S. military statistics, African American male soldiers are 4 times as likely and African American female soldiers 2.2 times as likely to suffer frostbite as their Caucasian or Native American counterparts. Pacific Islanders and other ethnic and racial groups from warmer climates are also thought to be more likely to suffer frostbite. British Army findings are similar. In addition to race, certain diseases, including diabetes, thyroid disorders, arthritis, and some infections increase a person's risk of developing frostbite during exposure to cold.

Most frostbite victims are middle-aged adults between the ages of 35 and 50; one study found the average age of patients treated for frostbite is 41.

Description

Frostbite is most likely to affect the face, hands, and feet; however, the shins, knees, and the outer portions of the eyes may also be affected. Freezing of exposed tissues results in the formation of ice crystals inside the cell wall. There is a variation of frostbite known as mountain frostbite, which affects mountain climbers and others exposed to extremely cold temperatures at high altitude. It combines tissue freezing with oxygen deprivation and general body **dehydration**.

Risk factors

Risk factors for frostbite and frostnip include:

- military service or employment that requires being outdoors for long periods of time in cold weather or cold climates
- participation in mountain climbing, alpine skiing, or other winter sports
- homelessness
- alcohol or substance abuse
- mental illness
- previous exposure to frostbite or cold injury
- (Nicotine causes blood vessels to constrict, thus lowering the body's ability to circulate blood to the hands, feet, and face.)
- malnutrition
- underlying infection
- medical conditions that affect a person's ability to feel or respond to cold, including dehydration, exhaustion, diabetes, or circulatory disorders

Causes and symptoms

Causes

Frostbite is caused by exposure of skin and underlying tissues to extreme cold, usually environmental. When the skin is exposed to temperatures at or below 32°F (0°C), the blood vessels in the skin start to constrict. This closing down of the blood flow in the extremities is the body's protective strategy for preserving normal body temperature in the body core (the heart and other internal organs).

Skin exposed to temperatures a little below the freezing mark can take hours to freeze, but very cold skin can freeze in minutes or seconds. Air temperature, wind speed, and moisture all affect how cold the skin becomes. A strong wind can lower skin temperature considerably by dispersing the thin protective layer of warm air that surrounds our bodies. Wet clothing readily draws heat away from the skin because water is a potent conductor of heat. The evaporation of moisture on the skin also produces cooling. For these reasons, wet skin or clothing on a windy day can lead to frostbite even if the air temperature is above the freezing mark.

Three nearly simultaneous physiological processes underlie frostbite injury: tissue freezing, tissue hypoxia, and the release of inflammatory mediators. Tissue

KEY TERMS

Amputation—Surgical removal of a limb.

Debridement—The medical term for the surgical removal of dead or damaged soft tissue.

Dermis—The layer of skin just below the epidermis.

Epidermis—The outermost layer of the skin.

Gangrene—Decay and death of soft tissue due to loss of blood supply.

Hypoxia—The medical term for deprivation of an adequate oxygen supply, either to specific tissues or to the entire organism.

freezing causes ice crystal formation and other changes that damage and eventually kill cells. Much of this harm occurs because the ice produces pressure changes that cause water (crucial for cell survival) to flow out of the cells. Tissue hypoxia (oxygen deficiency) occurs when the blood vessels in the hands, feet, and other extremities narrow in response to cold. Among its many tasks, blood transfers body heat to the skin, which then dissipates the heat into the environment. Blood vessel narrowing is the body's way of protecting vital internal organs at the expense of the extremities by reducing heat flow away from the core. However, blood also carries life-sustaining oxygen to the skin and other tissues, and narrowed vessels result in oxygen starvation. Narrowing also causes acidosis (an increase in tissue acidity) and increases blood viscosity (thickness). Ultimately, blood stops flowing through the capillaries (the tiny blood vessels that connect the arteries and veins) and **blood clots** form in the arterioles and venules (the smallest arteries and veins). Damage also occurs to the endothelial cells that line the blood vessels. Hypoxia, blood clots, and endothelial damage lead, in turn, to the release of inflammatory mediators (substances that act as links in the inflammatory process), which promote further endothelial damage, hypoxia, and cell destruction.

Symptoms

The early stage of frostbite is sometimes called frostnip. Short-term symptoms include loss of feeling or aching **pain** in the affected part, followed by redness of the skin and tissue swelling. Unfortunately, a victim is often unaware of frostbite until someone else points it out because the frozen tissues are numb. Long-term symptoms include intense pain in the affected part, **tingling** sensations, cracks in the skin, dry skin, loss of fingernails, joint stiffness, loss of bone or muscle tissue, and increased sensitivity to cold. If left untreated, frostbitten skin gradually darkens and blisters after a few hours. Skin destroyed by frostbite is completely black, looks burnt, and may hang loosely from the underlying tissues.

Diagnosis

Diagnosis of frostbite is usually made in the field on the basis of the appearance of the frostbitten parts of the body. Some doctors use a four-degree classification of injuries:

- First-degree: The epidermis (outermost layer of the skin) is reddened, swollen, and may look waxy. There is also a loss of sensation in the affected skin.
- Second-degree: The skin is reddened, swollen, and has formed blisters filled with a clear or milky fluid.
- Third-degree: The blisters are filled with blood and the skin begins to turn black.
- Fourth-degree: The epidermis, dermis, and underlying muscles, tendons, and bones are damaged.

Examination

Examination of the patient usually has to be done at the scene rather than in a doctor's office, although it can also be conducted in an ambulance, helicopter, or other emergency medical transport. The doctor will examine the condition of the affected parts, including skin color, the presence of blisters, and other features. If the patient has also been injured in an accident, the doctor will also evaluate the patient for sprains, broken bones, and internal injuries.

Tests

A technique that can be used to diagnose the extent of soft-tissue injury after frostbite is technetium scintigraphy. This is a technique in which radioactive technetium is administered intravenously. The radioactive element is taken up differently by healthy and damaged tissue, and the pattern of "hot spots" and "cold spots" as traced by a scanner allows the doctor to tell whether and where deep tissues have been damaged by frostbite. Scintigraphy can also be used to monitor the recovery of the injured tissues following emergency treatment.

X-rays and other imaging studies will not help in diagnosing frostbite but may be used to evaluate the injured person for broken or fractured bones.

Treatment

Traditional

FROSTBITE. Emergency medical help should always be summoned whenever frostbite is suspected. While waiting for help to arrive, one should, if possible, remove wet or tight clothing and put on dry, loose clothing or wraps. A splint and padding are used to protect the injured area. The patient should not be allowed to walk on frostbitten toes or feet, as the weight of the body will cause further damage to tissue—unless walking is the only way the patient can get to shelter.

Rubbing the area with snow or anything else is dangerous. The key to prehospital treatment is to avoid partial thawing and refreezing, which releases more inflammatory mediators and makes the injury substantially worse. For this reason, the affected part must be kept away from such heat sources as campfires and car heaters. In addition, the injured person should not be given alcohol or tranquilizers, as these will increase loss of body heat. Experts advise rewarming in the field only when emergency help will take more than two hours to arrive and refreezing can be prevented.

Because the outcome of a frostbite injury cannot be predicted at first, all hospital treatment follows the same route. Treatment begins by rewarming the affected part for 15–30 minutes in water at a temperature of 104–108 °F (40–42.2 °C). This rapid rewarming halts ice crystal formation and dilates narrowed blood vessels. Aloe vera (which acts against inflammatory mediators) is applied to the affected part, which is then splinted, elevated, and wrapped in a dressing. Depending on the extent of injury, blisters may be debrided (cleaned by removing foreign material) or simply covered with aloe vera. Except when injury is minimal, treatment generally requires a hospital stay of several days, during which **hydrotherapy** and **physical therapy** are used to restore the affected part to health. Experts recommend a cautious approach to tissue removal, and advise that 22–45 days must pass before a decision on **amputation** can safely be made.

If frostbitten skin is not treated and its blood vessels are affected, **gangrene** may set in. Gangrene is the **death** of soft tissue due to loss of blood supply. It may be treated by surgical removal of the affected tissue if caught early; otherwise, the surgeon may have to amputate the affected digit or limb to prevent bacterial infections from spreading from the dead tissue to the rest of the body.

FROSTNIP. Frostnipped fingers are helped by blowing warm air on them or holding them under one's armpits. Other frostnipped areas can be covered with warm hands. The injured areas should never be rubbed.

Drugs

The goals of medical therapy for frostbite are pain control and prevention of such complications as further tissue damage or infection. Patients being treated in the hospital for severe frostbite may be given morphine for **pain management** as **narcotics** are needed in most cases to reduce the excruciating pain that occurs as sensation returns during rewarming. A **tetanus** shot and penicillin G are used to prevent infection, and the patient is given ibuprofen or another NSAID to combat inflammation.

Alternative

Alternative practitioners suggest several kinds of treatment to speed recovery from frostbite after leaving the hospital. Bathing the affected part in warm water or using contrast hydrotherapy can help enhance circulation. Contrast hydrotherapy involves a series of hot and cold water applications. A hot compress (as hot as the patient can stand) is applied to the affected area for three minutes followed by an ice cold compress for 30 seconds. These applications are repeated three times each, ending with the cold compress. Nutritional therapy to promote tissue growth in damaged areas may also be helpful.

Homeopathic and botanical therapies may also assist recovery from frostbite. Homeopathic *Hypericum* (*Hypericum perforatum*) is recommended when nerve ending are affected (especially in the fingers and toes) and *Arnica* (*Arnica montana*) is prescribed for **shock**. Cayenne pepper (*Capsicum frutescens*) can enhance circulation and relieve pain. Drinking hot ginger (*Zingiber officinale*) tea also aids circulation. Other possible approaches include **acupuncture** to avoid permanent nerve damage and **oxygen therapy**.

Prognosis

Patients with early recovery of sensation in the affected part, blisters filled with clear fluid, and healthy-appearing skin color have a better prognosis for full recovery than those whose skin has turned bluish, has blood-filled blisters, and looks frozen.

People who have recovered from frostbite have an increased risk of another episode during future exposures to cold. They should take extra precautions to dress properly for extreme cold or avoid it altogether. They may also notice that the frostbitten parts of their body are more sensitive to ordinary cold weather, and ache or tingle whenever they are outdoors.

The extreme throbbing pain that many frostbite sufferers endure for days or weeks after rewarming is not the only prolonged symptom of frostbite. Other possible consequences of frostbite include skin—color changes, nail deformation or loss, joint stiffness and pain, **hyperhidrosis** (excessive sweating), and heightened sensitivity to cold. For everyone, a degree of sensory loss lasting at least four years—and sometimes a lifetime—is inevitable. About 65% of people with severe frostbite will eventually develop arthritis in the affected hand, foot, or leg.

Prevention

With the appropriate knowledge and precautions, frostbite can be prevented even in the coldest and most challenging environments. Appropriate clothing and footwear are essential. To prevent heat loss and keep the blood circulating properly, clothing should be worn loosely and in layers. Covering the hands, feet, and head is also crucial for preventing heat loss; mittens are better than gloves for keeping hands warm. Outerwear should be wind- and water-resistant; and wet clothing and footwear must be replaced as quickly as possible. People should also be aware of the early warning signs of frostbite, which include redness of the skin, prickling sensations, and **numbness**.

Alcohol and drugs should be avoided because of their harmful effects on judgment and reasoning. Experts also warn against alcohol use and **smoking** in the cold because of the circulatory changes they produce. Paying close attention to the weather report before venturing outdoors and avoiding such unnecessary risks as driving in isolated areas during a blizzard are also important precautionary measures. In addition, when traveling in cold weather, people should carry emergency supplies and warm clothing in case they become stranded. Last, people who are hiking or skiing in cold temperatures should use a buddy system in case one person is injured and must be evacuated quickly.

Resources

BOOKS

Auerbach, Paul S., Howard J. Donner, and Eric A. Weiss. *Field Guide to Wilderness Medicine*, 3rd ed. Philadelphia: Mosby/Elsevier, 2008.

Forgey, William W., ed. *Wilderness Medical Society Practice Guidelines for Wilderness Emergency Care*, 5th ed. Guilford, CT: Falcon Guide, 2006.

Giesbrecht, Gordon G. *Hypothermia, Frostbite, and Other Cold Injuries: Prevention, Survival, Rescue and Treatment*, 2nd ed. Seattle, WA: Mountaineers Books, 2006.

PERIODICALS

Bruen, K.G., and W.F. Gowski. "Treatment of Digital Frostbite: Current Concepts." *Journal of Hand Surgery* 34 (March 2009): 553—54.

Burgess, J.E., and F, Macfarlane. "Retrospective Analysis of the Ethnic Origins of Male British Army Soldiers with Peripheral Cold Weather Injury." *Journal of the Royal Army Medical Corps* 155 (March 2009): 11–15.

Imray, C., et al. "Cold Damage to the Extremities: Frostbite and Non-freezing Cold Injuries." *Postgraduate Medical Journal* 85 (September 2009): 481–88.

Mohr, W.J., et al. "Cold Injury." *Hand Clinics* 25 (November 2009): 481–96.

Rehman, H., and A. Seguin. "Images in Clinical Medicine: Frostbite." *New England Journal of Medicine* 361 (December 17, 2009): 2461.

Schlagenhauf, P., et al. "Sex and Gender Differences in Travel-associated Disease." *Clinical Infectious Diseases* 50 (March 15, 2010): 826–32.

Sheridan, R.L., et al. "Case Records of the Massachusetts General Hospital: Case 41-2009. A 16-year-old Boy with Hypothermia and Frostbite." *New England Journal of Medicine* 362 (December 31, 2009): 2654–2662.

OTHER

Centers for Disease Control and Prevention (CDC). *Winter Weather: Frostbite*. http://emergency.cdc.gov/disasters/winter/staysafe/frostbite.asp

Mayo Clinic. *Frostbite*. http://www.mayoclinic.com/health/frostbite/DS01164

Mechem, C. Crawford. "Frostbite." *eMedicine*, February 5, 2010. http://emedicine.medscape.com/article/770296-overview

MedlinePlus Medical Encyclopedia. *Frostbite*. http://www.nlm.nih.gov/medlineplus/ency/article/000057.htm

ORGANIZATIONS

American College of Emergency Physicians (ACEP), 1125 Executive Circle, Irving, TX, 75038-2522, (972) 550-0911, (800) 798-1822, 972-580-2816, http://www.acep.org/.

Centers for Disease Control and Prevention (CDC), 1600 Clifton Rd., Atlanta, GA, 30333, (800) 232-4636, cdcinfo @cdc.gov, http://www.cdc.gov.

Wilderness Medical Society (WMS), 2150 S 1300 E, Suite 500, Salt Lake City, UT, 84106, (801) 990-2988, (801) 990-2987, wms@wms.org, http://www.wms.org/.

International Society of Travel Medicine (ISTM), 315 W. Ponce de Leon Ave., Suite 245, Decatur, GA, United States, 30030, (404) 373-8282, (404) 373-8283, istm@istm.org, https://www.istm.org/.

Howard Baker
Rebecca J. Frey, PhD

Frostnip *see* **Frostbite and frostnip**

FSH test *see* **Follicle-stimulating hormone test**

Fugu poisoning

Definition

Fugu poisoning occurs when a person eats the flesh of a fugu, also known as a puffer fish, which contains lethal toxins.

Description

Fugu, also known as puffer fish, blowfish, or globefish, has long been a food delicacy in Japan, but has only been introduced in the United States in the last 30-40 years. The fugu and related species may contain a tetrodotoxin, an extremely potent neurotoxin and one of the most toxic substances known, which produces critical illness and often **death**. Between January 1 and April 1, 2002, at least 10 cases of fugu poisoning were reported in the United States, according to the Centers for Disease Control and Prevention (CDC) in Atlanta. All persons recovered from the poisonings. All of the fish came from the Atlantic Ocean off the coast of Titusville, Florida. Fugu caught in southern U.S. waters, such as the Gulf of Mexico, may also be toxic. Tetrodotoxin has been detected in pufferfish throughout the Pacific Ocean and the Baja California coastal region. Cases of fugu poisoning are sporadically diagnosed, but many more are not recognized or reported. The earliest cases reported to the CDC involved poisonings in Florida during the mid-1970s. Since 1950, only three known fatalities have occurred in the United States, all in Florida.

The dangers of puffer fish consumption have long been recognized. Artifacts recovered from an Egyptian tomb indicate that puffer fish poisoning has been known since approximately 2400-2700 B.C. In journals covering expeditions from 1772-1775, Pacific explorer Captain James Cook provided a vivid description of what some believe to be puffer fish poisoning. Fugu are found in waters throughout the world. Scientists have found that toxic fugu have unique exocrine glands for the secretion of tetrodotoxin. The fish appear to actively produce the toxin, rather than passively acquire it from the environment. For these fish, tetrodotoxin may serve as a natural defense mechanism to repel predators. The flesh of the fugu is generally eaten raw in paper-thin slices, known as sashimi. Part of the reported delight in eating fugu is the **tingling** oral sensation induced by minute amounts of tetrodotoxin in the flesh. For this reason, eating fugu is considered an "experience," rather than just a meal in Japan. The experience is expensive, however, since a plate of this delicacy can cost as much as $500.

Causes and symptoms

The most common symptoms of fugu poisioning are tingling and burning of the mouth and tongue, **numbness**, drowsiness, and incoherent speech. These symptoms usually occur 30 minutes to two hours after ingestion of the fish, depending on the amount of toxin ingested. In severe cases, ataxia (the inability to coordinate the movements of muscles), muscle weakness, **hypotension** (low blood pressure) and cardiac **arrhythmias** (irregular heartbeat) may develop, followed by muscle twitching and respiratory **paralysis**, and death can occur. In several cases, people died within 17 minutes after eating pufferfish.

Diagnosis

The initial diagnosis is usually made by observation of early symptoms, including an abnormal or unexplained tingling, pricking, or burning sensation on the skin around the mouth and throat. Definitive diagnosis can only be made in a medical laboratory by examination of the ingested fish and identification of the specific toxins. Ill persons should be advised to proceed to a hospital emergency department and contact their local poison control center.

Treatment

There is no antidote for fugu poisoning, therefore treatment is limited to supportive measures and the removal of the unabsorbed toxin. If spontaneous **vomiting** does not occur, it should be induced. Gastric lavage (stomach washing) with an alkaline solution has been suggested, as well as **endoscopy** to remove the poison from the proximal small bowel. Following lavage, **activated charcoal** is reported to effectively bind the toxin. Other steps include administration of oxygen, assisted breathing, intravenous atropine for bradycardia (slow heartbeat) and intravenous fluids, along with dopamine, to manage hypotension. Since tetrodotoxins and opiates are similar, use of an opiate antagonist may be useful, according to the American Academy of Family Physicians.

Alternative treatment

There is no alternative medicine treatment for fugu poisoning.

KEY TERMS

Ataxia—A lack of muscle control.

Arrhythmia—An irregularity in the normal rhythm or force of the heartbeat.

Atropine—A poisonous alkaloid obtained from belladonna or related plants, used medically to dilate the pupils of the eyes and to stop spasms.

Endoscopy—The use of a medical instrument consisting of a long tube inserted into the body, usually through a small incision, for diagnostic examination and surgical procedures.

Exocrine—Relating to external secretion glands, such as sweat glands or salivary glands that release a secretion through a duct to the surface of an organ.

Hypotension—Low blood pressure.

Lavage—The washing out of a hollow body organ, for example, the stomach, using a flow of water.

Neurotoxin—A substance that damages, destroys, or impairs the functioning of nerve tissue.

Prognosis

The mortality rate may be as high as 60%. Epidemiologic evidence suggests that recovery can be expected if an affected person survives beyond 24 hours. After 24 hours, a person with fugu poisoning usually makes a full recovery.

Prevention

The only prevention is not to eat any of the species of fugu that contain toxins.

Resources

BOOKS

Olson, Kent R. *Poisoning & Drug Overdose*. 5th ed. New York: McGraw–Hill Medical, 2006.

PERIODICALS

Currie, Bart J. "Marine Antivenoms." *Journal of Toxicology: Clinical Toxicology* (April 2003): 301–308.

"Fugu Fish Sequenced." *Applied Genetics News* (August 2002).

Scully, Mary-Louise. "Tingling Away in Titusville, Florida." *Infectious Disease Alert* (August 1, 2002): 165–167.

ORGANIZATIONS

American Association of Poison Control Centers, 515 King St., Suite 510, Alexandria, VA, 22314, (703) 894-1858, (703) 683-2812, (800) 222-1222, info@aapcc.org, http://www.aapcc.org.

Ken R. Wells

Fugue *see* **Dissociative disorders**

FUO *see* **Fever of unknown origin**

Furosemide *see* **Diuretics**

Furunculosis *see* **Boils**

Fusobacterium infection *see* **Anaerobic infections**

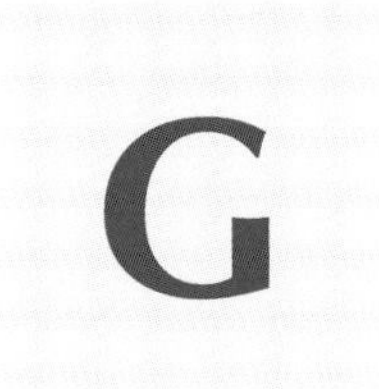

G6PD deficiency *see* **Glucose-6-phosphate dehydrogenase deficiency**

Galactorrhea

Definition

Galactorrhea is the secretion of breast milk in men, or in women who are not **breastfeeding** an infant.

Description

Lactation, or the production of breast milk, is a normal condition occurring in women after delivery of a baby. Many women who have had children may even be able to express a small amount of breast milk from the nipple up to two years after **childbirth**. Galactorrhea, or hyperlactation, however, is a rare condition that can occur in both men and women, where a white or grayish fluid is secreted by the nipples of both breasts. While this condition is not serious in itself, galactorrhea can indicate more serious conditions, including hormone imbalances or the presence of tumors.

Causes and symptoms

Causes

Galactorrhea is associated with a number of conditions. The normal production of breast milk is controlled by a hormone called prolactin, which is secreted by the pituitary gland in the brain. Any condition that upsets the balance of hormones in the blood or the production of hormones by the pituitary gland or sexual organs can stimulate the production of prolactin.

Often, a patient with galactorrhea will have a high level of prolactin in the blood. A tumor in the pituitary gland can cause this overproduction of prolactin. At least 30% of women with galactorrhea, menstrual abnormalities, and high prolactin levels have a pituitary gland tumor. Other types of brain tumors, head injuries, or **encephalitis** (an infection of the brain) can also cause galactorrhea.

Tumors or growths in the ovaries or other reproductive organs in women, or in the testicles or related sexual organs of men, can also stimulate the production of prolactin. Any discharge of fluid from the breast after a woman has passed **menopause** may indicate **breast cancer**. However, most often the discharge associated with breast **cancer** will be from one breast only. In galactorrhea both breasts are usually involved. The presence of blood in the fluid discharged from the breast could indicate a benign growth in the breast tissue itself. In approximately 10–15% of patients with blood in the fluid, carcinoma of the breast tissue is present.

A number of medications and drugs can also cause galactorrhea as a side-effect. Hormonal therapies (like **oral contraceptives**), drugs for treatment of depression or other psychiatric conditions, tranquilizers, morphine, heroin, and some medications for high blood pressure can cause galactorrhea.

Several normal physiologic situations can cause production of breast milk. Nipple stimulation in men or women during sexual intercourse may induce lactation, for women particularly during or just after **pregnancy**.

Even after extensive testing, no specific cause can be determined for some patients with galactorrhea.

Symptoms

The primary symptom of galactorrhea is the discharge of milky fluid from both breasts. In women, galactorrhea may be associated with **infertility**, menstrual cycle irregularities, hot flushes, or amenorrhea–a condition where menstruation stops completely. Men may experience loss of sexual interest and **impotence**. Headaches and visual disturbances have also been associated with some cases of galactorrhea.

KEY TERMS

Amenorrhea—Abnormal cessation of menstruation.

Bromocriptine—Also known as Parlodel, the main drug used to treat galactorrhea by reducing levels of the hormone prolactin.

Hyperlactation—Another term for galactorrhea.

Lactation—The production of breast milk.

Diagnosis

Galactorrhea is generally considered a symptom that may indicate a more serious problem. Collection of a thorough medical history, including pregnancies, surgeries, and consumption of drugs and medications is a first step in diagnosing the cause of galactorrhea. A **physical examination**, along with a breast examination, will usually be conducted. Blood and urine samples may be taken to determine levels of various hormones in the body, including prolactin and compounds related to thyroid function.

A mammogram (an x ray of the breast) or an ultrasound scan (using high frequency sound waves) might be used to determine if there are any tumors or cysts present in the breasts themselves. If a tumor of the pituitary gland is suspected, a series of computer assisted x rays called a computed tomography scan (CT scan) may be done. Another procedure that may be useful is a **magnetic resonance imaging** (MRI) scan to locate tumors or abnormalities in tissues.

Treatment

Treatment for galactorrhea will depend on the cause of the condition and the symptoms. The drug bromocriptine is often prescribed first to reduce the secretion of prolactin and to decrease the size of **pituitary tumors**. This drug will control galactorrhea symptoms and in many cases may be the only therapy necessary. Oral estrogen and progestins (hormone pills, like birth control pills) may control symptoms of galactorrhea for some women. Surgery to remove a tumor may be required for patients who have more serious symptoms of **headache** and vision loss, or if the tumor shows signs of enlargement despite drug treatment. **Radiation therapy** has also been used to reduce tumor size when surgery is not possible or not totally successful. A combination of drug, surgery, and radiation treatment can also be used.

Galactorrhea is more of a nuisance than a real threat to health. While it is important to find the cause of the condition, even if a tumor is discovered in the pituitary gland, it may not require treatment. With very small, slow-growing tumors, some physicians may suggest a "wait and see" approach.

Prognosis

Treatment with bromocriptine is usually effective in stopping milk secretion, however, symptoms may recur if drug therapy is discontinued. Surgical removal or radiation treatment may correct the problem permanently if it is related to a tumor. Frequent monitoring of hormone status and tumor size may be recommended.

Prevention

There is no way to prevent galactorrhea. If the condition is caused by the use of a particular drug, a patient may be able to switch to a different drug that does not have the side-effect of galactorrhea.

Resources

BOOKS

McPhee, Stephen, and Maxine Papadakis.*Current Medical Diagnosis and Treatment, 2010*, 49th ed. New York: McGraw–Hill Medical, 2009.

Altha Roberts Edgren

Galactosemia

Definition

Galactosemia is an inherited disease in which the transformation of galactose to glucose is blocked, allowing galactose to increase to toxic levels in the body. If galactosemia is untreated, high levels of galactose cause **vomiting**, **diarrhea**, lethargy, low blood sugar, brain damage, **jaundice**, liver enlargement, **cataracts**, susceptibility to infection, and **death**.

Description

Galactosemia is a rare but potentially life-threatening disease that results from the inability to metabolize galactose. Serious consequences from galactosemia can be prevented by screening newborns at birth with a simple blood test.

Galactosemia is an inborn error of metabolism. "Metabolism" refers to all chemical reactions that take place in living organisms. A metabolic pathway is a series of reactions where the product of each step in the series is the starting material for the next step. Enzymes are the chemicals that help the reactions occur. Their ability to function depends on their structure, and their structure is determined by the deoxyribonucleic acid (DNA) sequence of the genes that encode them. Inborn errors of metabolism are caused by mutations in these genes which do not allow the enzymes to function properly.

Sugars are sometimes called "the energy molecules," and galactose and glucose are both sugars. For galactose to be utilized for energy, it must be transformed into something that can enter the metabolic pathway that converts glucose into energy (plus water and carbon dioxide). This is important for infants because they typically get most of their nutrient energy from milk, which contains a high level of galactose. Each molecule of lactose, the major sugar constituent of milk, is made up of a molecule of galactose and a molecule of glucose, and so galactose makes up 20% of the energy source of a typical infant's diet.

Three enzymes are required to convert galactose into glucose-1-phosphate (a phosphorylated glucose that can enter the metabolic pathway that turns glucose into energy). Each of these three enzymes is encoded by a separate gene. If any of these enzymes fail to function, galactose build-up and galactosemia result. Thus, there are three types of galactosemia with a different gene responsible for each.

Every cell in a person's body has two copies of each gene. Each of the forms of galactosemia is inherited as a recessive trait, which means that galactosemia is only present in individuals with two mutated copies of one of the three genes. This also means that carriers, with only one copy of a gene mutation, will not be aware that they are carrying a mutation (unless they have had a genetic test), as it is masked by the normal gene they also carry and they have no symptoms of the disease. For each step in the conversion of galactose to glucose, if only one of the two copies of the gene controlling that step is normal (i.e. for carriers), enough functional enzyme is made so that the pathway is not blocked at that step. If a person has galactosemia, both copies of the gene coding for one of the enzymes required to convert glucose to galactose are defective and the pathway becomes blocked. If two carriers of the same defective gene have children, the chance of any of their children getting galactosemia (the chance of a child getting two copies of the defective gene) is 25% (one in four) for each **pregnancy**.

Classic galactosemia occurs in the United States about one in every 50,000–70,000 live births.

Causes and symptoms

Galactosemia I

Galactosemia I (also called classic galactosemia), the first form to be discovered, is caused by defects in both copies of the gene that codes for an enzyme called galactose-1-phosphate uridyl transferase (GALT). There are 30 known different mutations in this gene that cause GALT to malfunction.

Newborns with galactosemia I appear normal at birth, but begin to develop symptoms after they are given milk for the first time. Symptoms include **vomiting**, diarrhea, lethargy (sluggishness or **fatigue**), low blood glucose, jaundice (a yellowing of the skin and eyes), enlarged liver, protein and amino acids in the urine, and susceptibility to infection, especially from gram negative bacteria. Cataracts (a grayish white film on the eye lens) can appear within a few days after birth. People with galactosemia frequently have symptoms as they grow older even though they have been given a galactose-free diet. These symptoms include **speech disorders**, cataracts, ovarian atrophy, and **infertility** in females, learning disabilities, and behavioral problems.

Galactosemia II

Galactosemia II is caused by defects in both copies of the gene that codes for an enzyme called galactokinase (GALK). The frequency of occurrence of galactosemia II is about one in 100,000–155,000 births.

Galactosemia II is less harmful than galactosemia I. Babies born with galactosemia II will develop cataracts at an early age unless they are given a galactose-free diet. They do not generally suffer from liver damage or neurologic disturbances.

Galactosemia III

Galactosemia III is caused by defects in the gene that codes for an enzyme called uridyl diphosphogalactose-4-epimerase (GALE). This form of galactosemia is very rare.

There are two forms of galactosemia III, a severe form, which is exceedingly rare, and a benign form. The benign form has no symptoms and requires no special diet. However, newborns with galactosemia III, including the benign form, have high levels of galactose-1-phosphate that show up on the initial screenings for elevated galactose and galactose-1-phosphate. This situation illustrates one aspect of the importance of follow-up enzyme function tests. Tests showing normal levels of GALT and GALK allow people affected by the benign form of galactosemia III to enjoy a normal diet.

KEY TERMS

Casein hydrolysate—A preparation made from the milk protein casein, which is hydrolyzed to break it down into its constituent amino acids. Amino acids are the building blocks of proteins.

Catalyst—A substance that changes the rate of a chemical reaction, but is not physically changed by the process.

Enzyme—A protein that catalyzes a biochemical reaction or change without changing its own structure or function.

Galactose—One of the two simple sugars, together with glucose, that makes up the protein, lactose, found in milk. Galactose can be toxic in high levels.

Glucose—One of the two simple sugars, together with galactose, that makes up the protein, lactose, found in milk. Glucose is the form of sugar that is usable by the body to generate energy.

Lactose—A sugar made up of of glucose and galactose. It is the primary sugar in milk.

Metabolic pathway—A sequence of chemical reactions that lead from some precursor to a product, where the product of each step in the series is the starting material for the next step.

Metabolism—The total combination of all of the chemical processes that occur within cells and tissues of a living body.

Recessive trait—An inherited trait or characteristic that is outwardly obvious only when two copies of the gene for that trait are present.

The severe form has symptoms similar to those of galactosemia I, but with more severe neurological problems, including seizures. Only two cases of this rare form has been reported .

Diagnosis

The newborn screening test for classic galactosemia is quick and straightforward; all but three states require testing on all newborns. Blood from a baby who is two to three days old is usually first screened for high levels of galactose and galactose-1-phosphate. If either of these compounds is elevated, further tests are performed to find out which enzymes (GALT, GALK, or GALE) are present or missing. DNA testing may also be performed to confirm the diagnosis.

If there is a strong suspicion that a baby has galactosemia, galactose is removed from the diet right away. In this case, an initial screen for galactose or galactose-1-phosphate will be meaningless. In the absence of galactose in the diet, this test will be negative whether the baby has galactosemia or not. In this case, tests to measure enzyme levels must be given to find out if the suspected baby is indeed galactosemic.

In addition, galactosemic babies who are refusing milk or vomiting will not have elevated levels of galactose or galactose phosphate, and their condition will not be detected by the initial screen. Any baby with symptoms of galactosemia (for example, vomiting) should be given enzyme tests.

Treatment

Galactosemia I and II are treated by removing galactose from the diet. Since galactose is a breakdown product of lactose, the primary sugar constituent of milk, this means all milk and foods containing milk products must be totally eliminated. Other foods like legumes, organ meats, and processed meats also contain considerable galactose and must be avoided. Pills that use lactose as a filler must also be avoided. Soy-based and casein hydrolysate-based formulas are recommended for infants with galactosemia.

Treatment of the severe form of galactosemia III with a galactose-restricted diet has been tried, but this disorder is so rare that the long-term effects of this treatment are unknown.

Prognosis

Early detection in the newborn period is the key to controlling symptoms. Long-term effects in untreated babies include severe **mental retardation**, **cirrhosis** of the liver, and death. About 75% of the untreated babies die within the first two weeks of life. On the other hand, with treatment, a significant proportion of people with galactosemia I can lead nearly normal lives, although speech defects, learning disabilities, and behavioral problems are common. A 2004 study revealed that children and adolescents with classic galactosemia often have lower quality of life than peers without the disease, exhibiting problems with cognition (thinking and intellectual skills) and social function. In addition, cataracts due to galactosemia II can be completely prevented by a galactose-free diet.

Prevention

Since galactosemia is a recessive genetic disease, the disease is usually detected on a newborn screening test, since most people are unaware that they are carriers of a gene mutation causing the disease. For couples with a previous child with galactosemia, prenatal diagnosis is available to determine whether a pregnancy is similarly affected. Families in which a child has been diagnosed with galactosemia can have DNA testing which can enable other more distant relatives to determine their carrier status. Prospective parents can then use that information to conduct family planning or to prepare for a child with special circumstances. Children born with galactosemia should be put on a special diet right away, to reduce the symptoms and complications of the disease.

Resources

PERIODICALS

Bosch, Annet M., et al. "Living With Classical Galactosmeia: Health-related Quality of Life Consequences." *Pediatrics* May 2004: 1385–1387.

OTHER

"GeneCards: Human Genes, Proteins and Diseases." http://bioinfo.weizmann.ac.il/cards.

"Vermont Newborn Screening Program." http://healthvermont.gov/regs/newborn_screening_reg.aspx.

ORGANIZATIONS

Association for Neuro-Metabolic Disorders, 5223 Brookfield Lane, Sylvania, OH, 43560-1809, (419) 885-1809.

National Endocrine and Metabolic Diseases Information Service, 6 Information Way, Bethesda, MD, 20892–3569, (703) 738–4929, (888) 828–0904, endoandmeta@info.niddk.nih.gov, http://endocrine.niddk.nih.gov.

Parents of Galactosemic Children, PO Box 2401, Mandeville, LA, 70470-2401, (866) 9007421, http://www.galactosemia.org.

Amy Vance, MS, CGC
Teresa G. Odle

Gallbladder cancer

Definition

Cancer of the gallbladder is cancer of the pear-shaped organ that lies on the undersurface of the liver.

Description

Bile from the liver is funneled into the gallbladder by way of the cystic duct. Between meals, the gallbladder stores a large amount of bile. To do this, it must absorb much of the water and electrolytes from the bile. In fact, the inner surface of the gallbladder is the most absorptive surface in the body. After a meal, the gallbladder's muscular walls contract to deliver the bile back through the cystic duct and eventually into the small intestine, where the bile can help digest food.

Demographics

About 5,000 people are diagnosed with gallbladder cancer each year in the United States, making it the fifth most common gastrointestinal cancer. It is more common in females than males and most patients are elderly. Southwest American Indians have a particularly high incidence— six times that of the general population.

Causes and symptoms

Gallstones are the most significant risk factor for the development of gallbladder cancer. Roughly 75 to 90 percent of patients with gallbladder cancer also have gallstones. Larger gallstones are associated with a higher chance of developing gallbladder cancer. Chronic inflammation of the gallbladder from infection also increases the risk for gallbladder cancer.

Unfortunately, sometimes cancer of the gallbladder does not produce symptoms until late in the disease. When symptoms are evident, the most common is **pain** in the upper right portion of the abdomen, underneath the right ribcage. Patients with gallbladder cancer may also report symptoms such as **nausea**, **vomiting**, weakness, **jaundice**, skin **itching**, **fever**, chills, poor appetite, and weight loss.

Diagnosis

Gallbladder cancer is often misdiagnosed because it mimics other more common conditions, such as gallstones, **cholecystitis**, and **pancreatitis**. But the imaging tests that are utilized to evaluate these other conditions can also detect gallbladder cancer. For example, ultrasound is a quick, noninvasive imaging test that reliably diagnoses gallstones and cholecystitis. It can also detect the presence of gallbladder cancer as well as show how far the cancer has spread. If cancer is suspected, a computed tomography scan is useful in confirming the presence of an abnormal mass and further demonstrating the size and extent of the tumor. Cholangiography, usually performed to evaluate a patient with jaundice, can also detect gallbladder cancer.

KEY TERMS

Cholangiography—Radiographic examination of the bile ducts after injection with a special dye

Cholecystitis—Inflammation of the gallbladder, usually due to infection

Computed tomography—A radiology test by which images of cross-sectional planes of the body are obtained

Jaundice—Yellowish staining of the skin and eyes due to excess bilirubin in the bloodstream

Metastasis—The spread of tumor cells from one part of the body to another through blood vessels or lymphatic vessels

Pancreatitis—Inflammation of the pancreas

Stent—Slender hollow catheter or rod placed within a vessel or duct to provide support or maintain patency

Ultrasound—A radiology test utilizing high frequency sound waves

There are no specific laboratory tests for gallbladder cancer. Tumors can obstruct the normal flow of bile from the liver to the small intestine. Bilirubin, a component of bile, builds up within the liver and is absorbed into the bloodstream in excess amounts. This can be detected in a blood test, but it can also manifest clinically as jaundice. Elevated bilirubin levels and clinical jaundice can also occur with other conditions, such as gallstones.

On occasion, gallbladder cancer is diagnosed incidentally. About one percent of all patients who have their gallbladder removed for symptomatic gallstones are found to have gallbladder cancer. The cancer is found either by the surgeon or by the pathologist who inspects the gallbladder with a microscope.

Treatment

Staging of gallbladder cancer is determined by the how far the cancer has spread. The effectiveness of treatment declines as the stage progresses. Stage I cancer is confined to the wall of the gallbladder. Approximately 25% of cancers are at this stage at the time of diagnosis. Stage II cancer has penetrated the full thickness of the wall, but has not spread to nearby lymph nodes or invaded adjacent organs. Stage III cancer has spread to nearby lymph nodes or has invaded the liver, stomach, colon, small intestine, or large intestine. Stage IV disease has invaded very deeply into two or more adjacent organs or has spread to distant lymph nodes or organs by way of metastasis.

Early Stage I cancers involving only the innermost layer of the gallbladder wall can be cured by simple removal of the gallbladder. Cancers at this stage are sometimes found incidentally when the gallbladder is removed in the treatment of gallstones or cholecystitis. The majority of patients have good survival rates. Late Stage I cancers, which involve the outer muscular layers of the gallbladder wall, are generally treated in the same way as Stage II or III cancers. Removal of the gallbladder is not sufficient for these stages. The surgeon also removes nearby lymph nodes as well as a portion of the adjacent liver (radical surgery). Survival rates for these patients are considerably worse than for those with early Stage I disease. Patients with early Stage IV disease may benefit from radical surgery, but the issue is controversial. Late Stage IV cancer has spread too extensively to allow complete excision. Surgery is not an option for these patients.

Other therapies

When long-term survival is not likely, the focus of therapy shifts to improving quality of life. Jaundice and blockage of the stomach are two problems faced by patients with advanced cancer of the gallbladder. These can be treated with surgery, or alternatively, by special interventional techniques employed by the gastroenterologist or radiologist. A stent can be placed across the bile ducts in order to re-establish the flow of bile and relieve jaundice. A small feeding tube can be placed in the small intestine to allow feeding when the stomach is blocked. Pain may be treated with conventional pain medicines or a celiac **ganglion** nerve block.

Current **chemotherapy** or **radiation therapy** cannot cure gallbladder cancer, but they may offer some benefit in certain patients. For cancer that is too advanced for surgical cure, treatment with chemotherapeutic agents such as 5-fluorouracil may lengthen survival for a few months. The limited benefit of chemotherapy must be weighed carefully against its side effects. Radiation therapy is sometimes used after attempted surgical resection of the cancer to extend survival for a few months or relieve jaundice.

Resources

BOOKS

Abeloff, Martin D., et al. *Clinical Oncology*. 4th ed. New York: Churchill Livingstone/Elsevier, 2008.

Sabiston, David C., et al. *Sabiston Textbook of Surgery: The Biological Basis of Modern Surgical Practice*. Philadelphia: Saunders/Elsevier, 2008.

OTHER

National Cancer Institute Cancer Trials web site. http://www.cancertrials.gov.

Kevin O. Hwang, MD

Gallbladder disease *see* **Cholecystitis**

Gallbladder nuclear medicine scan

Definition

A nuclear medicine scan of the gallbladder is used to produce a set of images that look like x rays. The procedure uses a small amount of radioactive dye which is injected into the body. The dye accumulates in the organ, in this case, the gallbladder. A special camera called a scintillation or gamma camera produces images based on how the dye travels through the system and how the radiation is absorbed by the tissues. The procedure is also called cholescintigraphy or a hepatobiliary scan.

Purpose

A nuclear medicine scan can be used to diagnose disease and to find abnormalities in a body organ. A gallbladder scan can detect **gallstones**, tumors, or defects of the gallbladder. It can also be used to diagnose blockages of the bile duct that leads from the gallbladder to the small intestine. Unlike ultrasound, a gallbladder nuclear medicine scan can assess gallbladder function.

Precautions

Women who are pregnant or **breastfeeding** should tell their doctors before a scan is performed. Some medications or even eating a high fat meal before the procedure can interfere with the results of the scan.

Description

The gallbladder is a small pear-shaped sac located under the liver. The liver produces bile, a yellowish-green mixture of salts, acids, and other chemicals, that are stored in the gallbladder. Bile is secreted into the small intestine to help the body digest fats from foods.

Gallbladder disease, gallstones, **cancer**, or other abnormalities can cause **pain** and other symptoms. A gallbladder condition might be suspected if a patient has chronic or occasional pain in the upper right side of the abdomen. The pain may be stabbing and intense with sudden onset or it may be more of a dull, occasional ache. Loss of appetite, **nausea and vomiting** can also occur. **Fever** may indicate the presence of infection. **Jaundice**, a yellowing of the skin and whites of the eyes, may also indicate that the gallbladder is involved.

A gallbladder nuclear medicine scan may be used to diagnose gallstones, blockage of the bile duct or other abnormalities, and to assess gallbladder functioning and inflammation (**cholecystitis**). The scan is usually performed in a hospital or clinical radiology department. The patient lies on an examination table while a small amount of radioactive dye is injected into a vein in the arm. This dye circulates through the blood and collects in the gallbladder. As the dye moves through the gallbladder, a series of pictures is taken using a special camera called a *scintillation* or *gamma camera*. This procedure produces images that look like x rays. The test usually takes one to two hours to complete, but can last up to four hours.

The results of the scan are read by a radiologist, a doctor specializing in x rays and other types of scanning techniques. A report is sent, usually within 24 hours, to the doctor who will discuss the results with the patient.

Preparation

The patient may be required to withhold food and liquids for up to eight hours before the scan.

KEY TERMS

Cholecystitis—Inflammation of the gallbladder.

Cholescintigraphy—Another term for a gallbladder nuclear medicine scan.

Hepatobiliary scan—Another term for a gallbladder nuclear medicine scan.

Scintillation or gamma camera—A camera, somewhat like an x-ray machine, used to photograph internal organs after the patient has been injected with a radioactive material.

Aftercare

No special care is required after the procedure. Once the scan is complete, the patient can return to normal activities.

Risks

Nuclear medicine scans use a very small amount of radioactive material, and the risk of radiation is minimal. Very rarely, a patient may have a reaction to the dye material used.

Normal results

A normal scan shows a gallbladder without gallstones. There will be no evidence of growths or tumors, and no signs of infection or swelling. The normal gallbladder fills with bile and secretes it through the bile duct without blockages.

Abnormal results

An abnormal scan may show abnormal gallbladder emptying (suggesting gallbladder dysfunction or inflammation), or gallstones in the gallbladder or in the bile duct. The presence of tumors, growths or other types of blockages of the duct or the gallbladder itself could also appear on an abnormal scan.

Resources

OTHER

"Nuclear Medicine." Washington Radiology Associates Page. http://www.wrapc.com.

Altha Roberts Edgren

Gallbladder surgery *see* **Cholecystectomy**

Gallbladder x rays

Definition

This is an x-ray exam of the gallbladder (GB), a sac-like organ that stores bile that is located under the liver. The study involves taking tablets containing dye (contrast) which outline any abnormalities when x rays are taken the following day. The test was once the standard for diagnosing diseases of the GB such as **gallstones**, but is used less frequently now. This is due to advances in diagnostic ultrasound, which is quick, accurate and doesn't involve exposure to ionizing radiation. When functional parameters of the gallbladder need to be demonstrated, scintigraphy is now the study of choice. OCG, however, can be useful when a gallbladder is contracted down due to the presence of many, many gallstones. It can also help determine whether the cystic duct is clear, prior to surgical procedures such as **lithotripsy**. OCG may also be used to evaluate gallbladder disease that doesn't involve gallstones, such as adenomyomatosis of the gallbladder or cholesterolosis of the gallbladder.

Purpose

This test, also known as an oral cholecystogram or OCG, is usually ordered to help physicians diagnose disorders of the gallbladder, such as gallstones and tumors, which show up as solid dark structures. It is performed to help in the investigation of patients with upper abdominal **pain**. The test also measures gallbladder function, as the failure of the organ to visualize can signify a non-functioning or diseased gallbladder. The gallbladder may also not visualize if the bilirubin level is over 4 and the study should not be performed under these circumstances.

Precautions

Your physician must be notified if you are pregnant or allergic to iodine. Patients with a history of severe kidney damage, have an increased risk of injury or side effects from the procedure. In those cases, ultrasound is commonly used instead of the x-ray examination. Some people experience side effects from the contrast material (dye tablets), especially **diarrhea**. During preparation for the test, patients should not use any **laxatives**. Diabetics should discuss the need for any adjustment in medication with their physician.

Description

The exam is performed in the radiology department. The night before the test, patients swallow six tablets (one at a time) that contain the contrast (x-ray dye). The following day at the hospital, the radiologist examines the gallbladder with a fluoroscope (a special x ray that projects the image onto a video monitor). Sometimes, patients are then asked to drink a highfat formula that will cause the gallbladder to contract and release bile. X rays will then be taken at various intervals. There is no discomfort from the test. If the gallbladder is not seen, the patient may be asked to return the following day for x rays.

Preparation

The day before the test patients are instructed to eat a high fat lunch (eggs, butter, milk, salad oils,

KEY TERMS

Bile—A yellow-green liquid produced by the liver, which is released through the bile ducts into the small intestines to help digest fat.

Bilirubin—A reddish-yellow pigment formed from the destruction of red blood cells, and metabolized by the liver. Levels of bilirubin in the blood increase in patients with liver disease or blockage of the bile ducts.

Ultrasound—A non-invasive procedure based on changes in sound waves of a frequency that cannot be heard, but respond to changes in tissue composition. It requires no preparation and no radiation occurs; it has become the "gold standard" for diagnosis of stones in the gallbladder, but is less accurate in diagnosing stones in the bile ducts. Gallstones as small as 2 mm can be identified.

or fatty meats), and a fat-free meal (fruits, vegetables, bread, tea or coffee, and only lean meat) in the evening. Two hours after the evening meal, six tablets containing the contrast medium, are taken, one a time. After that, no food or fluid is permitted until after the test.

Aftercare

No special care is required after the study.

Risks

There is a small chance of an allergic reaction to the contrast material. In addition, there is low radiation exposure. X rays are monitored and regulated to provide the minimum amount of radiation exposure needed to produce the image. Most experts feel that the risk is low compared with the benefits. Pregnant women and children are more sensitive to the risks of x rays, and the risk versus benefits should be discussed with the treating physician.

Normal results

The x ray will show normal structures for the age of the patient. The gallbladder should visualize, and be free of any solid structures, such as stones, polyps, etc.

Abnormal results

Abnormal results may show gallstones, tumors, or cholesterol polyps (a tumor growing from the lining that is usually noncancerous). Typically stones will "float" or move around as the patient changes position, whereas tumors will stay in the same place.

Resources

OTHER

"Gall Bladder Exam." Harvard Medical School. http://www.bih.harvard.edu/radiology/Modalities/Xray/xraysSubdivsf/gallbl.html.

"Gallstones." National Institutes of Health. http://www.niddk.nih.gov/health/digest/pubs/gallstns/gallstns.htm.

Rosalyn Carson-DeWitt, MD

Gallium scan of the body

Definition

A gallium scan of the body is a nuclear medicine test that is conducted using a camera that detects gallium, a form of radionuclide, or radioactive chemical substance.

Purpose

Most gallium scans are ordered to detect cancerous tumors, infections, or areas of inflammation in the body. Gallium is known to accumulate in inflamed,

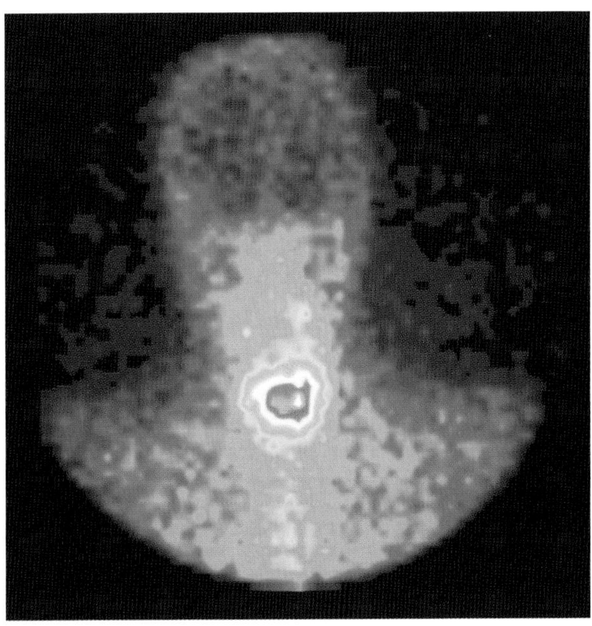

Gallium scan highlighting the thyroid gland. *(Photo Researchers, Inc.)*

infected, or cancerous tissues. The scans are used to determine whether a patient with an unexplained **fever** has an infection and the site of the infection, if present. Gallium scans also may be used to evaluate **cancer** following **chemotherapy** or **radiation therapy**.

Precautions

Children and women who are pregnant or **breast-feeding** are only given gallium scans if the potential diagnostic benefits will outweigh the risks.

Description

The patient will usually be asked to come to the testing facility 24–48 hours before the procedure to receive the injection of gallium. Sometimes, the injection will be given only four to six hours before the study or as long as 72 hours before the procedure. The timeframe is based on the area or organs of the body being studied.

For the study itself the patient lies very still for approximately 30–60 minutes. A camera is moved across the patient's body to detect and capture images of concentrations of the gallium. The camera picks up signals from any accumulated areas of the radionuclide. In most cases, the patient is lying down throughout the procedure. Back (posterior) and front (anterior) views will usually be taken, and sometimes a side (lateral) view is used. The camera may occasionally touch the patient's skin, but will not cause any discomfort. A clicking noise may be heard throughout the procedure; this is only the sound of the scanner registering radiation.

Preparation

The intravenous injection of gallium is done in a separate appointment prior to the procedure. Generally, no special dietary requirements are necessary. Sometimes the physician will ask that the patient have light or clear meals within a day or less of the procedure. Many patients will be given **laxatives** or an enema prior to the scan to eliminate any residual gallium from the bowels.

Aftercare

There is generally no aftercare required following a gallium scan. However, women who are breastfeeding who have a scan will be cautioned against breast-feeding for four weeks following the exam.

Risks

There is a minimal risk of exposure to radiation from the gallium injection, but the exposure from one gallium scan is generally less than exposure from x rays.

KEY TERMS

Benign—Not cancerous. Benign tumors are not considered immediate threats, but may still require some form of treatment.

Gallium—A form of radionuclide that is used to help locate tumors and inflammation (specifically referred to as GA67 citrate).

Malignant—This term, usually used to describe a tumor, means cancerous, becoming worse and possibly growing.

Nuclear medicine—A subspecialty of radiology used to show the function and anatomy of body organs. Very small amounts of radioactive substances, or tracers, are detected with a special camera as they accumulate in certain organs and tissues.

Radionuclide—A chemical substance, called an isotope, that exhibits radioactivity. A gamma camera, used in nuclear medicine procedures, will pick up the radioactive signals as the substance gathers in an organ or tissue. They are sometimes referred to as tracers.

Normal results

A radiologist trained in nuclear medicine or a nuclear medicine specialist will interpret the exam results and compare them to other diagnostic tests. It is normal for gallium to accumulate in the liver, spleen, bones, breast tissue, and large bowel.

Abnormal results

An abnormal concentration of gallium in areas other than those where it normally concentrates may indicate the presence of disease. Concentrations may be due to inflammation, infection, or the presence of tumor tissue. Often, additional tests are required to determine if the tumors are malignant (cancerous) or benign.

Even though gallium normally concentrates in organs such as the liver or spleen, abnormally high concentrations will suggest certain diseases and conditions. For example, Hodgkin's or non-Hodgkin's lymphoma may be diagnosed or staged if there is abnormal gallium activity in the lymph nodes. After a patient receives cancer treatment, such as radiation therapy or chemotherapy, a gallium scan may help to find new or recurring tumors or to record regression of a treated tumor. Physicians can narrow causes of liver problems by noting abnormal gallium activity in the liver.

Gallium scans also may be used to diagnose lung diseases or a disease called **sarcoidosis**, in the chest.

Resources

OTHER

"A Patient's Guide to Nuclear Medicine." *University of Iowa Virtual Hospital*. July 2, 2001. http://www.vh.org/Patients/IHB/Rad/NucMed/PatGuideNucMed/PatGuideNucMed.html.

ORGANIZATIONS

American Cancer Society, 1599 Clifton Rd. NE, Atlanta, GA, 30329, (800) 227-2345, http://www.cancer.org.

American College of Nuclear Medicine, 1850 Samuel Morse Drive, Reston, VA, 20190-5316, (703) 326-1190, (703) 708-9015.

American Liver Foundation, 75 Maiden Lane, Suite 603, New York, NY, 10038, (212) 668-1000, (212) 483-8179, http://www.liverfoundation.org.

Society of Nuclear Medicine (SNM), 1850 Samuel Morse Dr., Reston, VA, 20190, (703) 708-9000, (703) 708-9015, http://www.snm.org.

Teresa Odle

Gallstone removal

Definition

Also known as cholelithotomy, gallstone removal is the medical procedure that rids the gallbladder of calculus buildup.

Purpose

The gallbladder is not a vital organ. Its function is to store bile, concentrate it, and release it during digestion. Bile is supposed to retain all of its chemicals in solution, but commonly one of them crystallizes and forms sand, gravel, and finally stones.

The chemistry of **gallstones** is complex and interesting. Like too much sugar in solution, chemicals in bile will form crystals as the gallbladder draws water out of the bile. The solubility of these chemicals is based on the concentration of three chemicals, not just one–bile acids, phospholipids, and cholesterol. If the chemicals are out of balance, one or the other will not remain in solution. Certain people, in particular the Pima tribe of Native Americans in Arizona, have a genetic predisposition to forming gallstones. Scandinavians also have a higher than average incidence of this disease. Dietary fat and cholesterol are also implicated in their formation. Overweight women in their middle years constitute the vast majority of patients with gallstones in every group.

As the bile crystals aggregate to form stones, they move about, eventually occluding the outlet and preventing the gallbladder from emptying. This creates symptoms. It also results in irritation, inflammation, and sometimes infection of the gallbladder. The pattern is usually one of intermittent obstruction due to stones moving in and out of the way. All the while the gallbladder is becoming more scarred. Sometimes infection fills it with pus–a serious complication.

On occasion a stone will travel down the cystic duct into the common bile duct and get stuck there. This will back bile up into the liver as well as the gallbladder. If the stone sticks at the Ampulla of Vater, the pancreas will also be plugged and will develop **pancreatitis**. These stones can cause a lot of trouble.

Bile is composed of several waste products of metabolism, all of which are supposed to remain in liquid form. The complex chemistry of the liver depends on many chemical processes, which depend in turn upon the chemicals in the diet and the genes that direct those processes. There are greater variations in the output of chemical waste products than there is allowance for their cohabitation in the bile. Incompatible mixes result in the formation of solids.

Gallstones will cause the sudden onset of **pain** in the upper abdomen. Pain will last for 30 minutes to several hours. Pain may move to the right shoulder blade. **Nausea** with or without **vomiting** may accompany the pain.

Precautions

Individuals suffering from sickle cell anemia, children, and patients with large stones may seek other treatments.

Description

Laparoscopic cholecystectomy

Surgery to remove the entire gallbladder with all its stones is usually the best treatment, provided the patient is able to tolerate the procedure. Over the past decade, a new technique of removing the gallbladder using a laparoscope has resulted in quicker recovery and much smaller surgical incisions than the six-inch gash under the right ribs that used to be standard. Not everyone is a candidate for this approach.

If a stone is lodged in the bile ducts, additional surgery must be done to remove it. After surgery, the surgeon will ordinarily leave in a drain to collect bile until

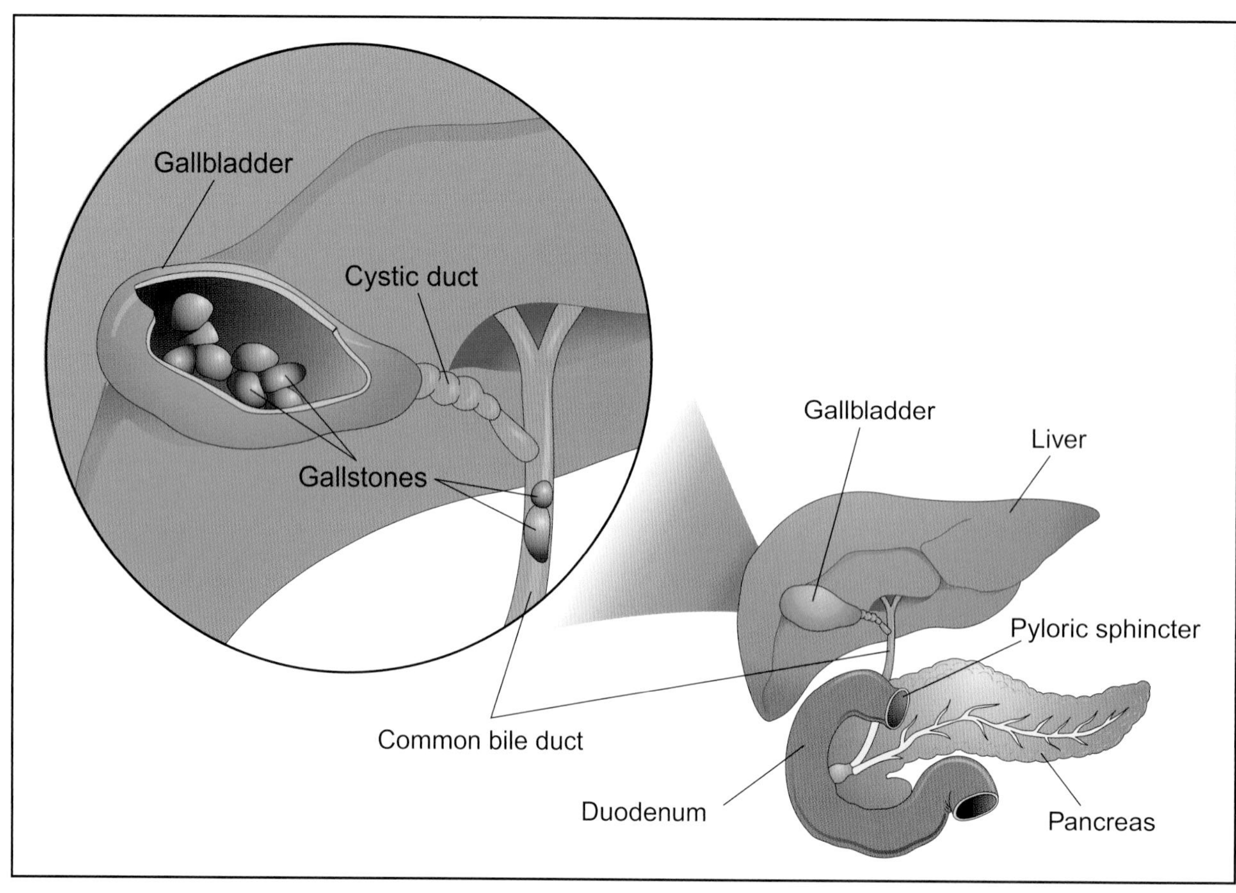

Gallstone removal, also known as cholelithotomy, usually involves the surgical removal of the entire gallbladder, but in recent years the procedure done by laparoscopy has resulted in smaller surgical incisions and faster recovery time. *(Illustration by Electronic Illustrators Group. Reproduced by permission of Gale, a part of Cengage Learning.)*

the system is healed. The drain can also be used to inject contrast material and take x rays during or after surgery.

Endoscopic retrograde cholangiopancreatoscopy (ERCP)

A procedure called endoscopic retrograde cholangiopancreatoscopy (ERCP) allows the removal of some bile duct stones through the mouth, throat, esophagus, stomach, duodenum, and biliary system without the need for surgical incisions. ERCP can also be used to inject contrast agents into the biliary system, providing superbly detailed pictures.

Cholelithotomy

Rare circumstances require different techniques. Patients too ill for a complete **cholecystectomy** (removal of the gallbladder), sometimes only the stones are removed, a procedure called cholelithotomy. But that does not cure the problem. The liver will go on making faulty bile, and stones will reform, unless the composition of the bile is altered.

Ursodeoxycholic acid

For patients who cannot receive the laparoscopic procedure, there is also a nonsurgical treatment in which ursodeoxycholic acid is used to dissolve the gallstones. Extracorporeal shock-wave **lithotripsy** has also been successfully used to break up gallstones. During the procedure, high-amplitude sound waves target the stones, slowly breaking them up.

Preparation

There are a number of imaging studies that identify gallbladder disease, but most gallstones will not show up on conventional x rays. That requires contrast agents given by mouth that are excreted into the bile. Ultrasound is very useful and can be enhanced by doing it through an endoscope in the stomach. CT (**computed tomography scans**) and MRI (**magnetic resonance**

KEY TERMS

Cholecystectomy—Surgical removal of the gallbladder.

Cholelithotomy—Surgical incision into the gallbladder to remove stones.

Contrast agent—A substance that causes shadows on x rays (or other images of the body).

Endoscope—One of several instruments designed to enter body cavities. They combine viewing and operating capabilities.

Jaundice—A yellow color of the skin and eyes due to excess bile that is not removed by the liver.

Laparoscopy—Surgery through pencil-sized viewing instruments and tools so that incisions need be less than half an inch long.

imaging) scanning are not used routinely but are helpful in detecting common duct stones and complications.

Aftercare

Without a gallbladder, stones rarely reform. Patients who have continued symptoms after their gallbladder is removed may need an ERCP to detect residual stones or damage to the bile ducts caused by the stones before they were removed. Once in a while the Ampulla of Vater is too tight for bile to flow through and causes symptoms until it is opened up.

Resources

BOOKS

Sleisenger, Marvin H., et al.*Sleisenger & Fordtran's Gastrointestinal and Liver Disease: Pathophysiology, Diagnosis, Management*. St. Louis, Mo.: MD Consult, 2009.

J. Ricker Polsdorfer, MD

Gallstones

Definition

A gallstone is a solid crystal deposit that forms in the gallbladder, which is a pear–shaped organ that stores bile salts until they are needed to help digest fatty foods. Gallstones can migrate to other parts of the digestive tract and cause severe **pain** with life–threatening complications.

Demographics

Gallstones are the most common of all gallbladder problems. They are responsible for 90% of gallbladder and bile duct disease, and are the fifth most common reason for hospitalization of adults in the United States. Over half a million people per year in the United States develop symptoms of or complications from gallstones that require removal of the gallbladder.

Gallstones usually develop in adults between the ages of 20 and 50; about 20% of patients with gallstones are over 40. The risk of developing gallstones increases with age. At least 20% of people over 60 have a single large stone or as many as several thousand smaller ones. The gender ratio of gallstone patients changes with age. Young women are between two and six times as likely to develop gallstones as are men in the same age group. In patients over 50, the condition affects men and women with equal frequency. The lifetime risk for developing gallstones is 50% in women and about 30% in men. Mexican Americans and Native Americans develop gallstones more often than any other segment of the population.

Description

Gallstones vary in size and chemical structure. A gallstone may be as tiny as a grain of sand or as large as a golf ball. Eighty percent of gallstones are composed of cholesterol. They are formed when the liver produces more cholesterol than digestive juices can liquefy. The remaining 20% of gallstones are composed of **calcium** and an orange–yellow waste product called bilirubin. Bilirubin gives urine its characteristic color and sometimes causes **jaundice**.

Risk factors

Some risk factors associated with the development of cholesterol gall stones include:

- female gender
- increasing age
- Mexican or Native American ancestry
- history of multiple pregnancies
- conditions which result in gallbladder stasis (decreased movement or flow of bile in the gallbladder) such as rapid weight loss and high spinal cord injuries

Women who take oral birth control pills containing estrogen, women using other estrogen–dispensing birth control devices, and some men who are prescribed estrogen and/or estrogen–like drugs for the treatment of **prostate cancer** are also at high risk. Up to 25% of

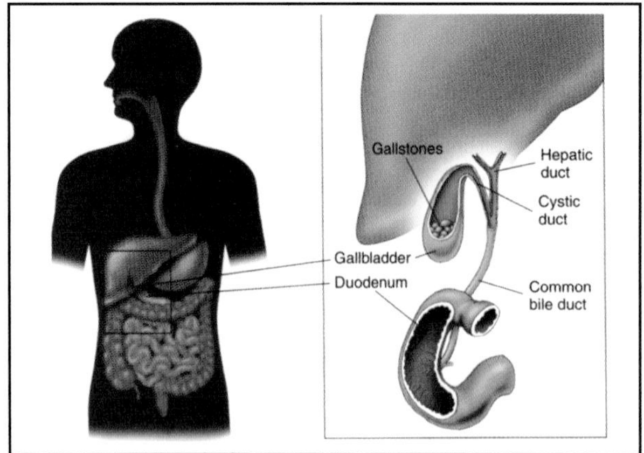

Gallstones form in the gallbladder but can migrate to other parts of the body via the bile duct. *(Illustration by Frank Forney. Reproduced by permission of Gale, a part of Cengage Learning.)*

people who develop gallstones develop the stones as a result of hereditary predisposition.

Definitions

Gallstones can cause several different disorders. Cholelithiasis is defined as the presence of gallstones within the gallbladder itself. Choledocholithiasis is the presence of gallstones within the common bile duct that leads into the first portion of the small intestine (the duodenum). The stones in the duct may have been formed inside it or carried there from the gallbladder. These gallstones prevent bile from flowing into the duodenum. Ten percent of patients with gallstones have choledocholithiasis, which is sometimes called common–duct stones. Patients who do not develop infection usually recover completely from this disorder.

Cholecystitis is a disorder marked by inflammation of the gallbladder. It is usually caused by the passage of a stone from the gallbladder into the cystic duct, which is a tube that connects the gallbladder to the common bile duct. In five to 10 percent of cases, however, cholecystitis develops in the absence of gallstones. This form of the disorder is called acalculous cholecystitis. Cholecystitis causes painful enlargement of the gallbladder and is responsible for 10–25% of all gallbladder surgery. Chronic cholecystitis is most common in the elderly. The acute form is most likely to occur in middle–aged adults.

Cholesterolosis or cholesterol polyps is characterized by deposits of cholesterol crystals in the lining of the gallbladder. This condition may be caused by high levels of cholesterol or inadequate quantities of bile salts, and is usually treated by surgery.

Gallstone **ileus**, which results from a gallstone's blocking the entrance to the large intestine, is most common in elderly people. Surgery usually cures this condition.

Narrowing (stricture) of the common bile duct develops in as many as five percent of patients whose gallbladders have been surgically removed. This condition is characterized by inability to digest fatty foods and by abdominal pain, which sometimes occurs in spasms. Patients with stricture of the common bile duct are likely to recover after appropriate surgical treatment.

Causes and symptoms

Gallstones are caused by an alteration in the chemical composition of bile. Bile is a digestive fluid that helps the body absorb fat. Gallstones tend to run in families. In addition, high levels of estrogen, insulin, or cholesterol can increase a person's risk of developing them.

Pregnancy or the use of birth control pills can slow down gallbladder activity and increase the risk of gallstones. So can diabetes, **pancreatitis**, and **celiac disease**. Other factors influencing gallstone formation are:

- infection
- obesity
- intestinal disorders
- coronary artery disease or other recent illness
- multiple pregnancies
- a high–fat, low–fiber diet
- smoking
- heavy drinking
- rapid weight loss

Gallbladder attacks usually follow a meal of rich, high–fat foods. The attacks often occur in the middle of the night, sometimes waking the patient with intense pain that ends in a visit to the emergency room. The pain of a gallbladder attack begins in the abdomen and may radiate to the chest, back, or the area between the shoulders. Other symptoms of gallstones include:

- inability to digest fatty foods
- low-grade fever
- chills and sweating
- nausea and vomiting
- indigestion
- gas
- belching
- clay-colored bowel movements

KEY TERMS

Acalculous cholecystitis—Inflammation of the gallbladder that occurs without the presence of gallstones.

Bilirubin—A reddish–yellow waste product produced by the liver that colors urine and is involved in the formation of some gallstones.

Celiac disease—Inability to digest wheat protein (gluten), which causes weight loss, lack of energy, and pale, foul–smelling stools.

Cholecystectomy—Surgical removal of the gallbladder.

Cholecystitis—Inflammation of the gallbladder.

Choledocholithiasis—The presence of gallstones within the common bile duct.

Cholelithiasis—The presence of gallstones within the gallbladder.

Cholesterolosis—Cholesterol crystals or deposits in the lining of the gallbladder.

Common bile duct—The passage through which bile travels from the cystic duct to the small intestine.

Gallstone ileus—Obstruction of the large intestine caused by a gallstone that has blocked the intestinal opening.

Lithotripsy—A nonsurgical technique for removing gallstones by breaking them apart with high–frequency sound waves.

Diagnosis

Examination

Gallstones may be diagnosed by a family doctor, a specialist in digestive problems (a gastroenterologist), or a specialist in internal medicine. The doctor will first examine the patient's skin for signs of jaundice and feel (palpate) the abdomen for soreness or swelling.

Tests

After the basic **physical examination**, the doctor will order blood counts or blood chemistry tests to detect evidence of bile duct obstruction and to rule out other illnesses that cause **fever** and pain, including stomach ulcers, **appendicitis**, and heart attacks.

Procedures

More sophisticated procedures used to diagnose gallstones include:

- Ultrasound imaging. Ultrasound is noninvasive, has an accuracy (sensitivity) rate of 96% in detecting gallstones, and is the least expensive imaging technique.
- Cholecystography (cholecystogram, gallbladder series, gallbladder x ray). This type of study shows how the gallbladder contracts after the patient has eaten a high–fat meal.
- Fluoroscopy. This imaging technique allows the doctor to distinguish between jaundice caused by pancreatic cancer and jaundice caused by gallbladder or bile duct disorders.
- Endoscopy (ERCP). ERCP uses a special dye to outline the pancreatic and common bile ducts and locate the position of the gallstones.
- Radioisotopic scan. This technique reveals blockage of the cystic duct.

Treatment

Watchful waiting

One–third of all patients with gallstones never experience a second attack. For this reason many doctors advise watchful waiting after the first episode. Reducing the amount of fat in the diet or following a sensible plan of gradual weight loss may be the only treatments required for occasional mild attacks. A patient diagnosed with gallstones may be able to manage more troublesome episodes by:

- applying heat to the affected area
- resting and taking occasional sips of water
- using non–prescription forms of acetaminophen (Tylenol or Anacin–3)

A doctor should be notified if pain intensifies or lasts for more than three hours; if the patient's fever rises above 101°F (38.3°C); or if the skin or whites of the eyes turn yellow.

Surgery

Surgical removal of the gallbladder (**cholecystectomy**) is the most common conventional treatment for recurrent attacks. Laparoscopic surgery, the technique most widely used, is a safe, effective procedure that involves less pain and a shorter recovery period than traditional open surgery. In this technique, the doctor makes a small cut (incision) in the patient's abdomen and removes the gallbladder through a long tube called a laparoscope.

Nonsurgical approaches

Patients who are too ill for surgery may benefit from gradual medical dissolution therapy with ursodeoxycholic acid (ursodiol). This technique typically requires months of therapy before stones are dissolved.

Alternative treatment

Alternative therapies, like non–surgical treatments, may provide temporary relief of gallstone symptoms. Alternative approaches to the symptoms of gallbladder disorders include homeopathy, Chinese traditional herbal medicine, and **acupuncture**. Dietary changes may also help relieve the symptoms of gallstones. Since gallstones seem to develop more often in people who are obese, eating a balanced diet, exercising, and losing weight may help keep gallstones from forming.

Prognosis

Forty percent of all patients with gallstones have "silent gallstones" that produce no symptoms. Silent stones, discovered only when their presence is indicated by tests performed to diagnose other symptoms, do not require treatment.

Gallstone problems that require treatment can be surgically corrected. Although most patients recover, some develop infections that must be treated with **antibiotics**.

In rare instances, severe inflammation can cause the gallbladder to burst. The resulting infection can be fatal.

Prevention

The best way to prevent gallstones is to minimize risk factors. Obese adults who lose large amounts of weight very quickly including those who undergo **bariatric surgery** are at high risk for the development of gallstones. Prophylactic treatment with ursodeoxycholic acid may be prescribed in these situations.

Participation in regular **exercise** may decrease the probability of gallstone formation in some people.

Resources

PERIODICALS

Halldestam, I., E. Kullman, and K. Borch. "Incidence of and Potential Risk Factors for Gallstone Disease in a General Population Sample." *British Journal of Surgery*. 92(11) (November 2009): 1315–22.

OTHER

Heuman, D.M., A.A. Mihas, and J. Allen. "Cholelithiasis." eMedicine. March 17, 2010. http://www.emedicine.medscape.com (accessed September 10, 2010).

ORGANIZATIONS

National Institute of Diabetes and Digestive and Kidney Diseases (NIDDK), Building 31, Room 9A06, 31 Center Drive, MSC 2560, Bethesda, MD, 20892–2560, (301) 496–3583, http://www.niddk.nih.gov.

Maureen Haggerty
Melinda Granger Oberleitner, RN, DNS, APRN, CNS

Gamete intrafallopian transfer *see* **Infertility therapies**

Gamma-glutamyl transferase test *see* **Liver function tests**

Gamma globulin

Definition

Gamma globulin is a type of protein found in the blood. When Gamma globulins are extracted from the blood of many people and combined, they can be used to prevent or treat infections.

Purpose

This medicine is used to treat or prevent diseases that occur when the body's own immune system is not effective against the disease. When disease-causing agents enter the body, they normally trigger the production of antibodies, proteins that circulate in the blood and help fight the disease. Gamma globulin contains some of these antibodies. When Gamma globulins are taken from the blood of people who have recovered from diseases such as **chickenpox** or hepatitis, they can be given to other people to make them temporarily immune to those diseases. With hepatitis, for example, this is done when someone who has not been vaccinated against hepatitis is exposed to the disease.

Some diseases or disorders that may require treatment with Gamma globulin include:

- skin diseases such as lupus erythematosus and scleroderma
- hematologic disorders such as idiopathic thrombocytopenia purpura (ITP)

KEY TERMS

Hepatitis—Inflammation of the liver caused by a virus, chemical or drugs. There are several different types of hepatitis, including the most common forms: hepatitis A, hepatitis B, and hepatitis C.

Immune system—The body's natural defenses against disease and infection.

Inflammation—Pain, redness, swelling, and heat that usually develop in response to injury or illness.

- Kawasaki disease
- graft versus host disease associated with bone marrow, stem cell, and other transplant procedures

Description

Gamma globulin, also known as immunoglobulin, immune serum globulin or serum therapy, is injected either into a vein (the most common method) or into a muscle. When injected into a vein, it produces results more quickly than when injected into a muscle.

U.S. brand names

Some of the brand names of products that contain Gamma globulin and that are sold in the United States include:

- Gammagard S/D
- Gammar-IV
- Gamimmune-N
- Iveegam
- Polygam S/D
- Sandoglobulin
- Venoglobulin-I or Venoglobulin-S
- Carimune/Panglobulin
- Gamunex

Recommended dosage

Doses are different for different people and depend on the person's body weight and the condition for which he or she is being treated.

Precautions

Anyone who has had unusual reactions to Gamma globulin in the past should let his or her physician know before taking the drugs again. The physician should also be told about any **allergies** to foods, dyes, preservatives, or other substances.

Individuals who have a history of reactions to blood products or who have experienced a blood product **transfusion** reaction in the past should inform their health care providers prior to receiving Gamma globulin products.

People who have certain medical conditions may have problems if they take Gamma globulins. For example:

- Gamma globulins may worsen heart problems or deficiencies of immunoglobin A (IgA, a type of antibody.)
- Certain patients with low levels of Gamma globulins in the blood (conditions called aGamma globulinemia and hypoGamma globulinemia) may be more likely to have side effects when they take Gamma globulin.
- Patients receiving Gamma globulin who have a history of liver and/or kidney problems should be monitored closely while receiving this product.

Side effects

Minor side effects such as **headache**, backache, joint or muscle **pain**, and a general feeling of illness usually go away as the body adjusts to this medicine. These problems do not need medical attention unless they continue.

Other side effects, such as breathing problems or a fast or pounding heartbeat, should be brought to a physician's attention immediately.

Anyone who shows the following signs of overdose should check with a physician immediately:

- unusual tiredness or weakness
- dizziness
- nausea
- vomiting
- fever
- chills
- tightness in the chest
- red face
- sweating

Interactions

Anyone who takes Gamma globulin should let the physician know all other medicines he or she is taking and should ask whether interactions with Gamma globulin could interfere with treatment.

Resources

OTHER

Scheinfeld, Noah S., and John E. Godwin. "Intravenous Immunoglobulin." *eMedicine*. September 22, 2010. http://emedicine.medscape.com/article/210367-overview (accessed October 6, 2010).

Nancy Ross-Flanigan
Melinda Granger Oberleitner, RN, DNS, APRN, CNS

Gamma knife surgery

Definition

Gamma knife surgery, also referred to as stereotactic radiosurgery, utilizes intersecting radiation beams targeted to a specific location in the brain to treat brain tumors and other abnormalities within the brain. Despite the name, no surgical incisions are required with this type of procedure.

Purpose

Gamma Knife radiosurgery is used to treat benign and malignant brain tumors which are considered to be inoperable because of their location in the brain which makes them inaccessible to conventional surgical approaches. This type of radiosurgery is also effective in treating **cancer** which has spread or metastasized to the brain.

Gamma Knife surgery can also be used to treat many conditions including the following:

- tumors of the pituitary gland which are located deep in brain tissue
- benign tumors such as schwannomas or acoustic neuromas which affect the acoustic nerve and can lead to problems with balance and hearing if left untreated
- trigeminal neuralgia, a condition which causes severe facial pain
- arteriovenous malformations (AVMs), a condition in which abnormal veins and arteries connect directly to each other rather than through the normal anatomic network of smaller blood vessels known as capillaries

Gamma Knife surgery is also increasingly used to treat patients with tumors in areas other than the brain. Recent studies report the effectiveness of this technology on the treatment of inoperable lung tumors and in the treatment of cancers of the head and neck.

Demographics

According to the manufacturer, the number of patients treated with Gamma Knife surgery has increased by more than 300% over the past five years and more than 500,000 people have received treatment utilizing this technology to date. There are over 125 Gamma Knife treatment centers in the United States.

Description

Gamma Knife technology was developed in the 1950s by Dr. Lars Leksell, a Swedish professor of **neurosurgery**, and radiation biologist, Borje Larsson, who pioneered the use of radiation beams in combination with stereotactic or precise guiding devices that could focus the beams with surgical precision. Thus, the term stereotactic (guided) radio(radiation) surgery was coined. In 1967, the first Gamma Knife device, which used cobalt–60 as the radiation source, was constructed. Gamma Knife technology became available in the United States in 1987.

Current Gamma Knife technology utilizes cobalt–60 photon radiation to deliver the radiation dose to targeted areas within the brain with pinpoint accuracy while sparing adjacent normal tissue from the deleterious effects of radiation. The radiation dose is calculated specifically for each patient taking into account tumor type, tumor shape, and tumor location including tumor depth. The precise dose to be delivered is determined based on the results of highly sophisticated imaging tests such as angiograms, **magnetic resonance imaging** (MRI), and/or computed tomography (CT) scans. Currently, most neurosurgeons use one MRI scan to determine the area to be treated. The results of these imaging tests are then placed into dose planning software which can model the affected area in 3 dimensions. The specific dose, individualized for each patient, is based on the results obtained from the treatment planning software, and is calculated by a radiation oncologist and a medical physicist.

Despite being called surgery, no actual surgery and no blade or knife is involved in the treatment process. There is no incision made in Gamma Knife surgery and no brain tissue is removed from the body. Radiation, delivered by a machine, is targeted into the affected brain tissue while sparing adjacent normal tissue.

Each Gamma Knife treatment unit can store 200 sources of cobalt–60 radiation. Thousands of radiation beams can then be generated from these sources and targeted to the area of the brain to be treated.

KEY TERMS

Benign—Not cancerous.

Malignant—Cancerous.

Radiosurgery—Precise delivery of a large dose of radiation to a targeted area within the brain.

Stereotactic—Precise guidance or positioning.

Each individual beam does not contain enough energy to harm normal tissue as it passes through brain tissue to reach the target. However, when all of the beams intersect and converge on the target, the combined effect of the energy in all of the radiation beams is powerful enough to treat the tissue in the area. According to the manufacturer, by keeping the patient immobilized during the actual treatment in combination with using three–dimensional treatment planning that is computer–aided, the radiation dose can be targeted with such precision that the level of accuracy is about one–tenth of one millimeter, which is about the thickness of an individual strand of human hair. The end result is that the calculated radiation dose reaches the targeted tissue, adjacent normal tissue is spared and the entire process is accomplished in a single treatment session.

Preparation

Unlike other **radiation therapy** procedures which may require multiple daily treatment visits, treatment using Gamma Knife technology is typically completed in one visit to the treatment center and is done on an outpatient basis. The patient will be asked not to consume food or water past midnight the night before the procedure is scheduled. Patients should ask their physicians if they may consume a small amount of water with their medications, however. Patients should inform the physician if they are taking oral medications or insulin to control diabetes.

Patients will also be asked if they are allergic to shellfish or iodine in anticipation of radiologic imaging techniques they will undergo as part of the treatment planning process. Patients should inform the staff if they have any implanted medical devices such as **pacemakers**, cardiac stents, artificial heart valves and other similar devices.

The staff at most treatment facilities will instruct the patient not to wear jewelry or makeup, including nail polish, on the day of the procedure. Once the treatment planning process begins the patient will be asked to remove eyeglasses, **contact lenses**, dentures, and wigs.

Preparation for treatment involves application of a stereotactic head frame. The frame, which is comprised of lightweight aluminum material, is attached to the head using four screws after **local anesthesia** is applied to the sites where the screws will be inserted. The primary purpose of the head frame is to allow for the precise targeting of the area within the brain which is to be treated. Hair will not be cut or shaved to position the head frame. The frame is designed to limit movement during radiologic imaging procedures such as magnetic resonance imaging (MRI) and/or computed tomography (CT) scanning and during the actual treatment process. An angiogram may also be required depending on the particular condition being treated. During the imaging process, a device called a coordinate box is affixed to the head frame. The coordinate box provides reference points on the images to facilitate development of a treatment plan. The time needed to secure the head frame and to complete the imaging tests, which are part of the treatment planning process, typically takes several hours. Results of the imaging tests are directed to a computerized planning system. The patient is allowed to rest while the treatment plan is being individualized and customized for that specific patient, however the head frame must remain attached during this time.

Once treatment planning is complete, the actual treatment begins. The patient remains awake during treatment and may be able to listen to music during the procedure. The actual treatment may take a few minutes or more than an hour depending on the size, location, and configuration of the area in the brain being targeted for treatment. The patient can communicate with the staff during the treatment if necessary and will be monitored at all times with audio and video monitoring.

While wearing the head frame which is then attached to a helmet located inside the treatment machine, the patient is positioned on a movable treatment table. The treatment table moves into a section of the treatment machine that is shaped like a dome. The patient may not know unless told that the treatment has started because the treatment itself is silent and does not cause **pain** nor is the patient able to feel any radiation.

Aftercare

Once the treatment is completed, the head frame is removed and the patient may be allowed to go home. Patients who have undergone **angiography** may have to lie still and remain at the treatment center for several hours to ensure that bleeding from the angiogram catheter entry and exit site does not occur and that swelling at the site is minimized. Rarely, some patients may have to be monitored overnight.

Some individuals may experience minor **headache** and pain at the site on the scalp where the head frame was affixed. Some patients may also experience minor swelling at the site. The effects from the actual radiation treatment are not immediate and may not be felt for weeks, months, or longer after the treatment. Most individuals can return to their regular routine in one to two days after treatment.

After the procedure, some patients may experience swelling in brain tissue adjacent to the area being treated. The swelling can usually be controlled with oral **steroids**.

Follow–up care usually involves additional images of the area which can be obtained by angiography, MRI, and/or CT scans. The results of these imaging studies are compared to the studies done before the procedure to determine whether the stereotactic radiosurgery procedure was effective.

Risks

Due to the noninvasive nature of this procedure, there are minimal risks involved with Gamma Knife surgery. Some patients, especially pediatric patients, may require **sedation** and/or anesthesia to complete the treatment planning process and the actual treatment. Rarely, a small number of these patients may experience side–effects and risks associated with sedation and/or anesthesia.

Resources

PERIODICALS

Patil, C.G., Pricola, K., Garg, S.K., Bryant, A., & Black, K.L. "Whole Brain Radiation Therapy (WBRT) Alone Versus WBRT and Radiosurgery for Treatment of Brain Metastasis."*Cochrane Database Syst Rev*.(June 2010); 16; 6.

Serizawa, T., Yamamoto, M., Nagano, O., et al. "Gamma Knife Surgery for Metastatic Brain Tumors."*J Neurosurg*. (Dec 2008); 109, Supp.118–21.

Short, S., & Tobias, J. "Radiosurgery for Brain Tumors." *BMJ*.(June 2010); 340.

OTHER

"Gamma–knife Radiosurgery." The Mayo Clinic. October 10, 2008 (accessed September 6, 2010). http://www.mayoclinic.com

"Gamma Knife Surgery: Information for Patients." Elekta Instruments (accessed September 6, 2010). http://www.gammaknife.org

ORGANIZATIONS

International Radiosurgery Association, 2002 N. 2nd Street, Harrisburg, PA, 17110, (717) 260-9809, http://www.irsa.org.

Melinda Granger Oberleitner, RN, DNS, APRN, CNS

Ganglion

Definition

A ganglion is a small, usually hard bump above a tendon or in the capsule that encloses a joint. A ganglion is also called a synovial **hernia** or synovial cyst.

Description

A ganglion is a non-cancerous cyst filled with a thick, jelly-like fluid. Ganglions can develop on or beneath the surface of the skin and usually occur between the ages of 20 and 40.

Most ganglions develop on the hand or wrist. This condition is common in people who bowl or who play handball, raquetball, squash, or tennis. Runners and

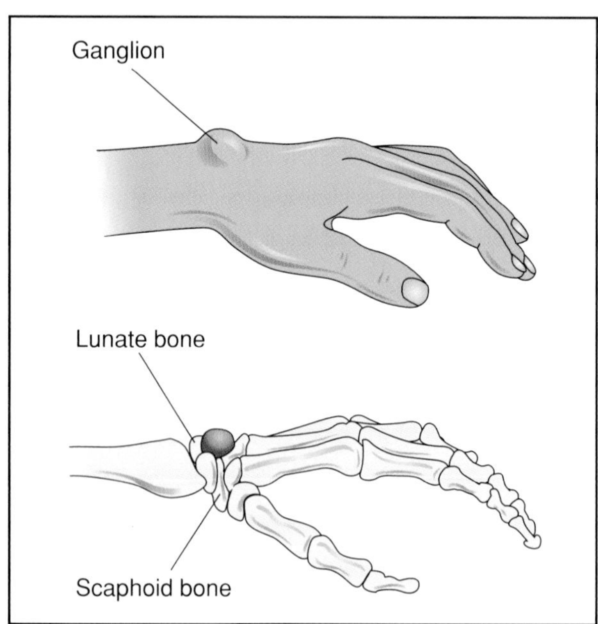

A ganglion is a non-cancerous cyst filled with a thick, jelly-like fluid. Ganglions can develop on or beneath the surface of the skin, most likely on the hand or wrist, although runners and skiers often develop them on the foot. *(Illustration by Electronic Illustrators Group. Reproduced by permission of Gale, a part of Cengage Learning.)*

athletes who jump, ski, or play contact sports often develop foot ganglions.

Causes and symptoms

Mild sprains or other repeated injuries can irritate and tear the thin membrane covering a tendon, causing fluid to leak into a sac that swells and forms a ganglion.

Ganglions are usually painless, but range of motion may be impaired. Flexing or bending the affected area can cause discomfort, as can continuing to perform the activity that caused the condition.

Cysts on the surface of the skin usually develop slowly but may result from injury or severe strain. An internal ganglion can cause soreness or a dull, aching sensation, but the mass cannot always be felt. Symptoms sometimes become evident only when the cyst causes pressure on a nerve or outgrows the membrane surrounding it.

Diagnosis

Diagnosis is usually made through **physical examination** as well as such imaging studies as x ray, ultrasound, and **magnetic resonance imaging** (MRI). Fluid may be withdrawn from the cyst and evaluated.

Treatment

Some ganglions disappear without treatment, and some reappear despite treatment.

Acetaminophen (Tylenol) or other over-the-counter **analgesics** can be used to control mild **pain**. **Steroids** or local anesthetics may be injected into cysts that cause severe pain or other troublesome symptoms. Surgery performed in a hospital operating room or an outpatient facility, is the only treatment guaranteed to remove a ganglion. The condition can recur if the entire cyst is not removed.

A doctor should be notified if the surgical site drains, bleeds, or becomes

- inflamed
- painful
- swollen or if the patient feels ill or develops:
- head or muscle aches
- dizziness
- fever following surgery

The patient may bathe or shower as usual, but should keep the surgical site dry and covered with a bandage for two or three days after the operation. Patients may resume normal activities as soon as they feel comfortable doing so.

Prognosis

Possible complications include excessive post-operative bleeding and infection of the surgical site. Calcification, or hardening, of the ganglion is rare.

Prevention

Exercises that increase muscle strength and flexibility can prevent ganglions. Warming and cooling down before and after workouts may also decrease the rate of developing ganglions.

Resources

OTHER

"Ganglion Cysts." American Society for Surgery of the Hand. (Accessed November 21, 2010). http://www.assh.org/Public/HandConditions/Pages/GanglionCysts.aspx.

Maureen Haggerty

Gangrene

Definition

Gangrene is the term used to describe the decay or **death** of an organ or tissue caused by a lack of blood supply. It is a complication resulting from infectious or inflammatory processes, injury, or degenerative changes associated with chronic diseases, such as **diabetes mellitus**.

Description

Gangrene may be caused by a variety of chronic diseases and post–traumatic, post–surgical, and

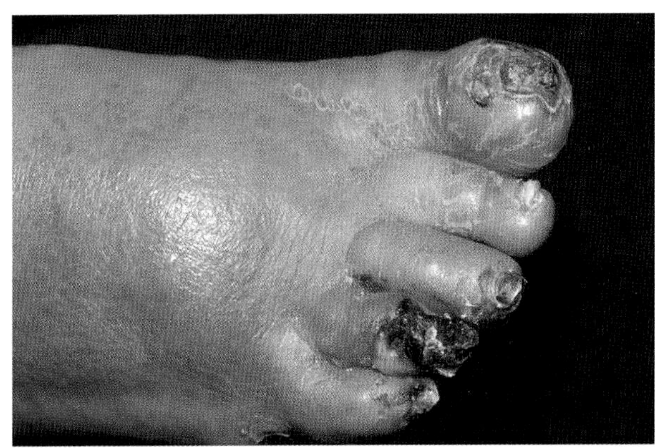

A close-up of gangrene in the toes of a diabetic patient. *(Photo Researchers, Inc.)*

spontaneous causes. There are three major types of gangrene: dry, moist, and gas (a type of moist gangrene).

Dry gangrene is a condition that results when one or more arteries become obstructed. In this type of gangrene, the tissue slowly dies, due to receiving little or no blood supply, but does not become infected. The affected area becomes cold and black, begins to dry out and wither, and eventually drops off over a period of weeks or months. Dry gangrene is most common in persons with advanced blockages of the arteries (arteriosclerosis) resulting from diabetes.

Moist gangrene may occur in the toes, feet, or legs after a crushing injury or as a result of some other factor that causes blood flow to the area to stop suddenly. When blood flow ceases, bacteria begin to invade the muscle and thrive, multiplying quickly without interference from the body's immune system.

Gas gangrene, also called myonecrosis, is a type of moist gangrene that is commonly caused by bacterial infection by *Clostridium welchii, Cl. perfringes, Cl. septicum, Cl. novyi, Cl. histolyticum, Cl. sporogenes*, or other species that are capable of thriving under conditions where there is little oxygen (anaerobic conditions). Once present in tissue, these bacteria produce gasses and toxins as they grow. Normally inhabiting the gastrointestinal, respiratory, and female genital tract, they often infect thigh **amputation wounds**, especially in those individuals who have lost control of their bowel functions (incontinence). Gangrene, incontinence, and debility often occur together in patients with diabetes, and it is in the amputation stump of diabetic patients that gas gangrene is often found to occur.

Other causative organisms for moist gangrene include various bacterial strains, including those of the *Streptococcus* and *Staphylococcus* genera. A serious, but rare form of infection with Group A *Streptococcus* can impede blood flow and, if untreated, can progress to synergistic gangrene, more commonly called necrotizing fasciitis, or infection of the skin and tissues directly beneath the skin.

Chronic diseases, such as diabetes mellitus, arteriosclerosis, or diseases affecting the blood vessels, such as **Buerger's disease** or Raynaud's disease, can cause gangrene. Post–traumatic causes of gangrene include compound fractures, **burns**, and injections given under the skin or in a muscle. Gangrene may occur following surgery, particularly in individuals with diabetes mellitus or other long–term (chronic) disease. In addition, gas gangrene can be also be a complication of dry gangrene or occur spontaneously in association with an underlying **cancer**.

In the United States, approximately 50% of moist gangrene cases are the result of a severe traumatic injury, and 40% occur following surgery. Car and industrial accidents, crush injuries, and gunshot wounds are the most common traumatic causes. Because of prompt surgical management of wounds with the removal of dead tissue, the incidence of gangrene from trauma has significantly diminished. Surgeries involving the bile ducts or intestine are the most frequent procedures causing gangrene. Approximately two–thirds of cases affect the extremities, and the remaining one–third involve the abdominal wall.

Symptoms

Areas of either dry or moist gangrene are initially characterized by a red line on the skin that marks the border of the affected tissues. As tissues begin to die, dry gangrene may cause some **pain** in the early stages or may go unnoticed, especially in the elderly or in those individuals with diminished sensation to the affected area. Initially, the area becomes cold, numb, and pale before later changing in color to brown, then black. This dead tissue will gradually separate from the healthy tissue and fall off.

Moist gangrene and gas gangrene are distinctly different. Gas gangrene usually involves muscle, rather than skin. In moist or gas gangrene, there is a sensation of heaviness in the affected region that is followed by severe pain. The pain is caused by swelling resulting from fluid or gas accumulation in the tissues. This pain peaks, on average, between one to four days following the injury, with a range of eight hours to several weeks. The swollen skin may initially be blistered, red, and warm to the touch before progressing to a bronze, brown, or black color. In approximately 80% of cases, the affected and surrounding tissues may produce crackling sounds (crepitus), as a result of gas bubbles accumulating under the skin. The gas may be felt beneath the skin (palpable). In wet gangrene, the pus is foul–smelling, while in gas gangrene, there is no true pus, just an almost "sweet" smelling watery discharge.

Fever, rapid heart rate, rapid breathing, altered mental state, loss of appetite, **diarrhea**, **vomiting**, and vascular collapse may also occur if bacterial toxins are allowed to spread in the bloodstream. Gas gangrene can be a life–threatening condition and should receive prompt medical attention

KEY TERMS

Aerobic—Organism that grows and thrives only in environments containing oxygen.

Anaerobic—Organism that grows and thrives in an oxygen–free environment.

Arteriosclerosis—Build–up of fatty plaques in arteries that can lead to the obstruction of blood flow.

Aseptic—Without contamination by bacteria or other microorganisms.

Crepitus—A crackling sound.

Gram stain—A staining procedure used to visualize and classify bacteria. The Gram stain procedure allows the identification of purple (Gram positive) organisms and red (Gram negative) organisms.

Hyperbaric oxygen—Medical treatment in which oxygen is administered in specially designed chambers, under pressures greater than that of the atmosphere, in order to treat specific medical conditions.

Incontinence—A condition characterized by the inability to control urination or bowel functions.

Myonecrosis—The destruction or death of muscle tissue.

Sepsis—The spreading of an infection in the bloodstream.

Thrombosis—The formation of a blood clot in a vein or artery that may obstruct local blood flow or may dislodge, travel downstream, and obstruct blood flow at a remote location.

Diagnosis

A diagnosis of gangrene will be based on a combination of patient history, a **physical examination**, and results of blood and other laboratory tests. A physician will look for a history of recent trauma, surgery, cancer, or chronic disease. Blood tests will be used to determine whether infection is present and determine the extent to which an infection has spread.

A sample of drainage from a wound, or obtained through surgical exploration, may be cultured with oxygen (aerobic) and without oxygen (anaerobic) to identify the microorganism causing the infection and to aid in determining which antibiotic will be most effective. The sample obtained from a person with gangrene will contain few, if any, white blood cells and, when stained (with Gram stain) and examined under the microscope, will show the presence of purple (Gram positive), rod–shaped bacteria.

X–ray studies and more sophisticated imaging techniques, such as computed tomography scans (CT) or **magnetic resonance imaging** (MRI), may be helpful in making a diagnosis since gas accumulation and muscle death (myonecrosis) may be visible. These techniques, however, are not sufficient alone to provide an accurate diagnosis of gangrene.

Precise diagnosis of gas gangrene often requires surgical exploration of the wound. During such a procedure, exposed muscle may appear pale, beefy–red, or in the most advanced stages, black. If infected, the muscle will fail to contract with stimulation, and the cut surface will not bleed.

Treatment

Gas gangrene is a medical emergency because of the threat that infection will spread rapidly via the bloodstream and infect vital organs. It requires immediate surgery and administration of **antibiotics**.

Areas of dry gangrene that remain free from infection (aseptic) in the extremities are most often left to wither and fall off. Treatments applied to the wound externally (topically) are generally not effective without adequate blood supply to support wound healing. Assessment by a vascular surgeon, along with x rays to determine blood supply and circulation to the affected area, can help determine whether surgical intervention would be beneficial.

Once the causative organism has been identified, moist gangrene requires the prompt initiation of intravenous, intramuscular, and/or topical broad–spectrum antibiotic therapy. In addition, the infected tissue must be removed surgically (**debridement**), and amputation of the affected extremity may be necessary. Pain medications (**analgesics**) are prescribed to control discomfort. Intravenous fluids and, occasionally, blood transfusions are indicated to counteract **shock** and replenish red blood cells and electrolytes. Adequate hydration and **nutrition** are vital to wound healing.

Although still controversial, some cases of gangrene are treated by administering oxygen under pressure greater than that of the atmosphere (hyperbaric) to the patient in a specially designed chamber. The theory behind using hyperbaric oxygen is that more oxygen will dissolve in the patient's bloodstream, and therefore, more oxygen will be delivered to the gangrenous areas. By providing optimal oxygenation, the body's ability to fight off bacterial infection are believed to be improved, and there is a direct toxic effect on bacteria that thrive in an oxygen–free environment. Some studies have shown that the use of hyperbaric oxygen produces marked pain relief, reduces the number of amputations required, and reduces the extent of surgical debridement required. Patients receiving hyperbaric oxygen treatments must be monitored closely for evidence of oxygen toxicity. Symptoms of this toxicity include slow heart rate, profuse sweating, ringing in the ears, shortness of breath, **nausea and vomiting**, twitching of the lips/cheeks/eyelids/nose, and convulsions.

The emotional needs of the patient must also be met. The individual with gangrene should be offered moral support, along with an opportunity to share questions and concerns about changes in body image. In addition, particularly in cases where amputation was required, physical, vocational, and rehabilitation therapy will also be required.

Prognosis

Except in cases where the infection has been allowed to spread through the blood stream, prognosis is generally favorable. Anaerobic wound infection can progress quickly from initial injury to gas gangrene within one to two days, and the spread of the infection in the blood stream is associated with a 20–25% mortality rate. If recognized and treated early, however, approximately 80% of those with gas gangrene survive, and only 15–20% require any form of amputation. Unfortunately, the individual with dry gangrene often has multiple other health problems that complicate recovery, and it is usually those other system failures that can prove fatal.

Prevention

Patients with diabetes or severe arteriosclerosis should take particular care of their hands and feet because of the risk of infection associated with even a minor injury. Education about proper **foot care** is vital. Diminished blood flow as a result of narrowed vessels will not lessen the body's defenses against invading bacteria. Measures taken towards the reestablishment of circulation are recommended whenever possible. Any abrasion, break in the skin, or infected tissue should be cared for immediately. Any dying or infected skin must be removed promptly to prevent the spread of bacteria.

Penetrating abdominal wounds should be surgically explored and drained, any tears in the intestinal walls closed, and antibiotic treatment begun early. Patients undergoing elective intestinal surgery should receive preventive antibiotic therapy. Use of antibiotics prior to and directly following surgery has been shown to significantly reduce the rate of infection from 20–30% to four to eight percent.

Resources

BOOKS

Holt, Tim, and Sudhesh Kumar. *ABC of Diabetes (ABC Series)*, 6th ed. Hoboken, NJ: BMJ Books, 2010.

Murray, Craig, editor. *Amputation, Prosthesis Use, and Phantom Limb Pain: An Interdisciplinary Perspective.* New York, NY: Springer, 2009.

Pierce, Dino Paul. *The Diabetes Handbook: Create Awareness and a New You.* Charleston, SC: CreateSpace, 2009.

Vaughn, Richard, A. *Beating The Odds: 64 Years of Diabetes Health.* Charleston, SC: CreateSpace, 2010.

ORGANIZATIONS

American Diabetes Association, 1701 North Beauregard St., Alexandria, VA, 22311, (800) DIABETES (800–342–2383), http://www.diabetes.org.

Centers for Disease Control and Prevention (CDC), 1600 Clifton Rd., Atlanta, GA, 30333, (404) 498–1515, (800) 311–3435, http://www.cdc.gov.

Center for Disability Information and Referral, Indiana Institute on Disability and Community, 2853 East Tenth St., Bloomington, IN, 47408–2696, (812) 855–9396, http://www.iidc.indiana.edu/cedir.

Kathleen D. Wright, RN
Laura Jean Cataldo, RN, Ed.D.

Gas embolism

Definition

Gas **embolism**, also called air embolism, is the presence of gas bubbles in the bloodstream that obstruct circulation.

Description

Gas embolism may occur with decompression from increased pressure; it typically occurs in ascending divers who have been breathing compressed air. If a diver does not fully exhale upon ascent, the air in the lungs expands as the pressure decreases, overinflating the lungs and forcing bubbles of gas (emboli) into the bloodstream. When gas emboli reach the arteries to the brain, the blood blockage causes unconsciousness.

KEY TERMS

Compressed air—Air that is held under pressure in a tank to be breathed underwater by divers. A tank of compressed air is part of a diver's scuba (self-contained underwater breathing apparatus) gear.

Compression—An increase in pressure from the surrounding water that occurs with increasing diving depth.

Decompression—A decrease in pressure from the surrounding water that occurs with decreasing diving depth.

Emboli—Plural of embolus. An embolus is something that blocks the blood flow in a blood vessel. It may be a gas bubble, a blood clot, a fat globule, a mass of bacteria, or other foreign body. It usually forms somewhere else and travels through the circulatory system until it gets stuck.

Hyperbaric chamber—A sealed compartment in which patients are exposed to controlled pressures up to three times normal atmospheric pressure. Hyperbaric treatment may be used to regulate blood gases, reduce gas emboli, and provide higher levels of oxygen more quickly in cases of severe gas poisoning.

Recompression—Restoring the elevated pressure of the diving environment to treat gas embolism by decreasing bubble size.

Gas embolism is second only to drowning as a cause of **death** among divers.

Gas embolism may also result from trauma or medical procedures such as catheterization and open heart surgery that allow air into the circulatory system.

Causes and symptoms

Gas embolism occurs independent of diving depth; it may occur in as little as 6 ft of water. It is frequently caused by a diver holding his breath during ascent. It may also result from an airway obstruction or other condition that prevents a diver from fully exhaling.

The primary sign of gas embolism is immediate loss of consciousness; it may or may not be accompanied by convulsions.

Diagnosis

Any unconscious diver should be assumed to be the victim of gas embolism, regardless of whether consciousness was lost during or promptly after ascent. A doctor may also find pockets of air in the chest around the lungs and sometimes a collapsed lung from overinflation and rupture. Coughing up blood or a bloody froth around the mouth are visible signs of lung injury.

Treatment

Prompt **recompression treatment** in a hyperbaric (high-pressure) chamber is necessary to deflate the gas bubbles in the bloodstream, dissolve the gases into the blood, and restore adequate oxygenated blood flow to the brain and other organs. Recompression by returning the diver to deeper water will not work, and should not be attempted. The patient should be kept lying down and given oxygen while being transported for recompression treatment.

Before the diver receives recompression treatment, other lifesaving efforts may be necessary. If the diver isn't breathing, artificial respiration (also called mouth-to-mouth resuscitation or rescue breathing) should be administered. In the absence of a pulse, **cardiopulmonary resuscitation** (CPR) must be performed.

Prognosis

The prognosis is dependent upon the promptness of recompression treatment and the extent of the damage caused by oxygen deprivation.

Prevention

All divers should receive adequate training in the use of compressed air and a complete evaluation of fitness for diving. People with a medical history of lung cysts or spontaneous collapsed lung (**pneumothorax**), and those with active **asthma** or other lung disease must not dive, for they would be at extreme risk for gas embolism. Patients with conditions such as **alcoholism** and drug abuse are also discouraged from diving. Individuals with certain other medical conditions such as diabetes may be able to dive safely with careful training and supervision.

ORGANIZATIONS

American College of Hyperbaric Medicine, 9875 South Franklin Drive, Suite 300, Franklin, Wisconsin, 53132, (414) 385-2943, (414) 385-8721, http://www.achm.org.

Divers Alert Network, 6 West Colony Place, Durham, NC, 27705, (919) 684-2948, (919) 490-6630, (800) 446-2671, http://www.diversalertnetwork.org.

Undersea and Hyperbaric Medical Society, 21 West Colony Place, Suite 280, Durham, NC, 27705, (919) 490-5140, (919) 490-5149, (877) 533-UHMS (8467), uhms@uhms@org, http://www.uhms.org.

Bethany Thivierge

Gas gangrene *see* **Gangrene**

Gastrectomy

Definition

Gastrectomy is the surgical removal of all or part of the stomach.

Purpose

Gastrectomy is performed for several reasons, most commonly to remove a malignant tumor or to cure a perforated or bleeding stomach ulcer.

Description

Gastrectomy for cancer

Removal of the tumor, often with removal of surrounding lymph nodes, is the only curative treatment for various forms of gastric (stomach) **cancer**. For many patients, this entails removing not just the tumor but part of the stomach as well. The extent to which lymph nodes should also be removed is a subject of some debate, but some studies show additional survival benefit associated with removal of a greater number of lymph nodes.

Gastrectomy, either total or subtotal (also called partial), is the treatment of choice for gastric adenocarcinomas, primary gastric lymphomas (originating in the stomach), and the rare leiomyosarcomas (also called gastric **sarcomas**). Adenocarcinomas are by far the most common form of **stomach cancer** and are less curable than the relatively uncommon lymphomas, for which gastrectomy offers good odds for survival.

After gastrectomy, the surgeon may "reconstruct" the altered portions of the digestive tract so that it continues to function. Several different surgical techniques are used, but, generally speaking, the surgeon attaches any remaining portion of the stomach to the small intestine.

Gastrectomy for gastric cancer is almost always done by the traditional "open" surgery technique, which requires a wide incision to open the abdomen. However, some surgeons use a laparoscopic technique that requires only a small incision. The laparoscope is connected to a tiny video camera that projects a picture of the abdominal contents onto a monitor for the surgeon's viewing. The stomach is operated on through this incision.

The potential benefits of laparoscopic surgery include less postoperative **pain**, decreased hospitalization, and earlier return to normal activities. The use of laparoscopic gastrectomy is limited, however. Only patients with early stage gastric cancers or those whose surgery is only intended for palliation—pain and symptomatic relief rather than cure—should be considered for this minimally invasive technique. It can only be performed by surgeons experienced in this type of surgery.

Gastrectomy for ulcers

Gastrectomy is also occasionally used in the treatment of severe peptic ulcer disease or its complications. While the vast majority of peptic ulcers (gastric ulcers in the stomach or duodenal ulcers in the duodenum) are managed with medication, partial gastrectomy is sometimes required for peptic ulcer patients who have complications. These include patients who do not respond satisfactorily to medical therapy, those who develop a bleeding or perforated ulcer, and those who develop pyloric obstruction, a blockage to the exit from the stomach.

The surgical procedure for severe ulcer disease is also called an antrectomy, a limited form of gastrectomy in which the antrum, a portion of the stomach, is removed. For duodenal ulcers, antrectomy may be combined with other surgical procedures that are aimed at reducing the secretion of gastric acid, which is associated with ulcer formation. This additional surgery is commonly a **vagotomy**, surgery on the vagus nerve that disables the acid-producing portion of the stomach.

Preparation

Before undergoing gastrectomy, patients may need a variety of tests, such as x rays, **computed tomography**

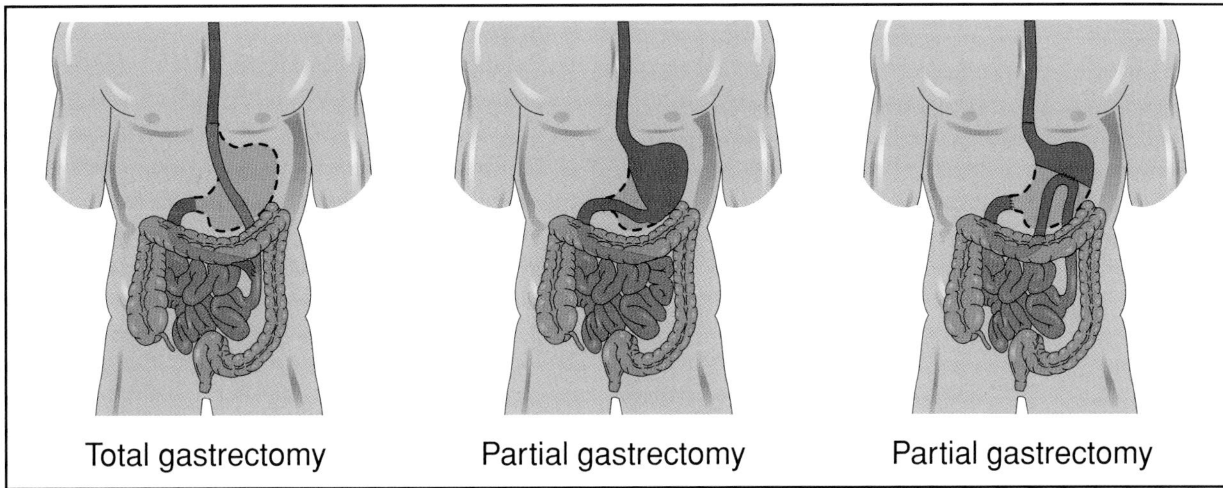

Gastrectomy, the surgical removal of all or part of the stomach, is performed primarily to remove a malignant tumor or to cure a bleeding stomach ulcer. Following the gastrectomy, the surgeon may reconstruct the altered portions of the digestive tract so that it continues to function. *(Illustration by Electronic Illustrators Group. Reproduced by permission of Gale, a part of Cengage Learning.)*

scans (CT scans), ultrasonography, or endoscopic biopsies (microscopic examination of tissue), to assure the diagnosis and localize the tumor or ulcer. **Laparoscopy** may be done to diagnose a malignancy or to determine the extent of a tumor that is already diagnosed. When a tumor is strongly suspected, laparoscopy is often performed immediately before the surgery to remove the tumor; this avoids the need to anesthetize the patient twice and sometimes avoids the need for surgery altogether if the tumor found on laparoscopy is deemed inoperable.

Aftercare

It is important to follow any instructions that have been given for postoperative care. Major surgery usually requires a recuperation time of several weeks.

Risks

Surgery for peptic ulcer is effective, but it may result in a variety of postoperative complications. After gastrectomy, as many as 30% of patients have significant symptoms. An operation called highly selective vagotomy is now preferred for ulcer management, and is safer than gastrectomy.

After a gastrectomy, several abnormalities may develop that produce symptoms related to food intake. This happens largely because the stomach, which serves as a food reservoir, has been reduced in its capacity by the surgery. Other surgical procedures that often accompany gastrectomy for ulcer disease can also contribute to later symptoms: vagotomy, which lessens acid production and slows stomach emptying, and **pyloroplasty**, which enlarges the opening between the stomach and small intestine to facilitate emptying of the stomach.

Some patients experience light-headedness, heart **palpitations** or racing heart, sweating, and **nausea and vomiting** after a meal. These may be symptoms of "dumping syndrome," as food is rapidly "dumped" into the small intestine from the stomach. This is treated by adjusting the diet and pattern of eating, for example, eating smaller, more frequent meals, and limiting liquids.

Patients who have abdominal bloating and pain after eating, frequently followed by **nausea and vomiting**, may have what is called the afferent loop syndrome. This is treated by surgical correction. Patients who have early satiety (feeling of fullness after eating), abdominal discomfort, and **vomiting** may have bile reflux **gastritis** (also called bilious vomiting), which is also surgically correctable. Many patients also experience weight loss.

Reactive **hypoglycemia** is a condition that results when blood sugar becomes too high after a meal, stimulating the release of insulin, about two hours after eating. A high-protein diet and smaller meals are advised.

Ulcers recur in a small percentage of patients after surgery for peptic ulcer, usually in the first few years. Further surgery is usually necessary.

Vitamin and mineral supplementation is necessary after gastrectomy to correct certain deficiencies, especially vitamin B_{12}, iron, and folate. Vitamin D and **calcium** are also needed to prevent and treat the bone problems that often occur. These include softening

KEY TERMS

Antrectomy—A surgical procedure for ulcer disease in which the antrum, a portion of the stomach, is removed.

Laparoscopy—The examination of the inside of the abdomen through a lighted tube, sometimes accompanied by surgery.

and bending of the bones, which can produce pain, and **osteoporosis**, a loss of bone mass. According to one study, the risk for spinal **fractures** may be as high as 50% after gastrectomy.

Depending on the extent of surgery, the risk for post-operative **death** after gastrectomy for gastric cancer has been reported as 1–3% and the risk of nonfatal complications as 9–18%.

Normal results

Overall survival after gastrectomy for gastric cancer varies greatly by the stage of disease at the time of surgery. For early gastric cancer, the five-year survival rate is up to 80–90%; for late-stage disease, the prognosis is bad. For gastric adenocarcinomas that are amenable to gastrectomy, the five-year survival rate is 10–30%, depending on the location of the tumor. The prognosis for patients with gastric lymphoma is better, with five-year survival rates reported at 40–60%.

Most studies have shown that patients can have an acceptable quality of life after gastrectomy for a potentially curable gastric cancer. Many patients will maintain a healthy appetite and eat a normal diet. Others may lose weight and not enjoy meals as much. Some studies show that patients who have total gastrectomies have more disease-related or treatment-related symptoms after surgery and poorer physical function than patients who have subtotal gastrectomies. There does not appear to be much difference, however, in emotional status or social activity level between patients who have undergone total versus subtotal gastrectomies.

Resources

BOOKS

Sleisenger, Marvin H., et al. *Sleisenger & Fordtran's Gastrointestinal and Liver Disease: Pathophysiology, Diagnosis, Management*. St. Louis, Mo.: MD Consult, 2009.

Caroline A. Helwick

Gastric acid determination

Definition

Gastric acid determination, also known as stomach acid determination, gastric analysis, or basal gastric secretion, is a procedure to evaluate gastric (stomach) function. The test specifically determines the presence of gastric acid, as well as the amount of gastric acid secreted. It is often done in conjunction with the gastric acid stimulation test, a procedure that measures gastric acid output after injection of a drug to stimulate gastric acid secretion.

Purpose

The purpose of the gastric acid determination is to evaluate gastric function by measuring the amount of acid as suctioned directly from the stomach. The complete gastric acid determination includes the basal gastric secretion test, which measures acid secretion while the patient is in a **fasting** state (nothing to eat or drink), followed by the gastric acid stimulation test, which measures the secretion of gastric acid for one hour after injection of pentagastrin or a similar drug that stimulates gastric acid output. The Gastric acid stimulation test is done when the basal secretion test suggests abnormalities in gastric secretion. It is normally performed immediately afterward.

The basal gastric secretion test is indicated for patients with obscure gastric **pain**, loss of appetite, and weight loss. It is also utilized for suspected peptic (related to the stomach) ulcer, severe stomach inflammation (**gastritis**), and Zollinger-Ellison (Z-E) syndrome (a condition in which a pancreatic tumor, called a **gastrinoma**, stimulates the stomach to secrete excessive amounts of acid, resulting in peptic ulcers). Because external factors like the sight or odor of food, as well as psychological **stress**, can stimulate gastric secretion, accurate testing requires that the patient be relaxed and isolated from all sources of sensory stimulation. Abnormal basal secretion can suggest various gastric and duodenal disorders, so further evaluation requires the gastric acid stimulation test.

The gastric acid stimulation test is indicated when abnormalities are found during the basal secretion test. These abnormalities can be caused by a number of disorders, including duodenal ulcer, **pernicious anemia**, and gastric **cancer**. The test will detect abnormalities, but x rays and other studies are necessary for a definitive diagnosis.

KEY TERMS

Achlorhydria—An abnormal condition in which hydrochloric acid is absent from the secretions of the gastric glands in the stomach.

Pernicious anemia—One of the main types of anemia, caused by inadequate absorption of vitamin B_{12}. Symptoms include tingling in the hands, legs, and feet, spastic movements, weight loss, confusion, depression, and decreased intellectual function.

Zollinger-Ellison syndrome—A rare condition characterized by severe and recurrent peptic ulcers in the stomach, duodenum, and upper small intestine, caused by a tumor, or tumors, usually found in the pancreas. The tumor secretes the hormone gastrin, which stimulates the stomach and duodenum to produce large quantities of acid, leading to ulceration. Most often cancerous, the tumor must be removed surgically; otherwise total surgical removal of the stomach is necessary.

Precautions

Because both the basal gastric secretion test and the gastric acid stimulation test require insertion of a gastric tube (intubation) through the mouth or nasal passage, neither test is recommended for patients with esophageal problems, **aortic aneurysm**, severe gastric hemorrhage, or congestive **heart failure**. The gastric acid stimulation test is also not recommended in patients who are sensitive to pentagastrin (the drug used to stimulate gastric acid output).

Description

This test, whether performed for basal gastric acid secretion, gastric acid stimulation, or both, requires the passage of a lubricated rubber tube, either by mouth or through the nasal passage, while the patient is in a sitting or reclining position on the left side. The tube is situated in the stomach, with proper positioning confirmed by fluoroscopy or x ray.

Basal gastric acid secretion

After a wait of approximately 10–15 minutes for the patient to adjust to the presence of the tube, and with the patient in a sitting position, specimens are obtained every 15 minutes for a period of 90 minutes. The first two specimens are discarded to eliminate gastric contents that might be affected by the stress of the intubation process. The patient is allowed no liquids during the test, and saliva must be ejected to avoid diluting the stomach contents.

The four specimens collected during the test constitute the *basal acid output*. If analysis suggests abnormally low gastric secretion, the gastric acid stimulation test is performed immediately afterward.

Gastric acid stimulation test

After the basal samples have been collected, the tube remains in place for the gastric acid stimulation test. Pentagastrin, or a similar drug that stimulates gastric acid output, is injected under the skin (subcutaneously). After 15 minutes, a specimen is collected every 15 minutes for one hour. These specimens are called the *poststimulation specimens*. As is the case with the basal gastric secretion test, the patient can have no liquids during this test, and must eject saliva to avoid diluting the stomach contents.

Preparation

The patient should be fasting (nothing to eat or drink after the evening meal) on the day prior to the test, but may have water up to one hour before the test. **Antacids**, anticholinergics, cholinergics, alcohol, H_2-receptor antagonists (Tagamet, Pepcid, Axid, Zantac), reserpine, adrenergic blockers, and adrenocorticosteroids should be withheld for one to three days before the test, as the physician requests. If pentagastrin is to be administered for the gastric acid secretion test, medical supervision should be maintained, as possible side effects may occur.

Aftercare

Complications such as **nausea**, **vomiting**, and abdominal distention or pain are possible following removal of the gastric tube. If the patient has a **sore throat**, soothing lozenges may be given. The patient may also resume the usual diet and any medications that were withheld for the test(s).

Risks

There is a slight risk that the gastric tube may be inserted improperly, entering the windpipe (trachea) and not the esophagus. If this happens, the patient may have a difficult time breathing or may experience a coughing spell until the tube is removed and reinserted properly. Also, because the tube can be difficult to swallow, if a patient has an overactive gag reflex, there may be a transient rise in blood pressure due to **anxiety**.

Normal results

Reference values for the *basal gastric secretion test* vary by laboratory, but are usually within the following ranges:

- men: 1–5 mEq/h
- women: 0.2–3.8 mEq/h

Reference values for the *gastric acid stimulation test* vary by laboratory, but are usually within the following ranges:

- men: 18–28 mEq/h
- women: 11–21 mEq/h

Abnormal results

Abnormal findings in the *basal gastric secretion test* are considered nonspecific and must be evaluated in conjunction with the results of a gastric acid stimulation test. Elevated secretion may suggest different types of ulcers; when markedly elevated, Zollinger-Ellison syndrome is suspected. Depressed secretion can indicate gastric cancer, while complete absence of secretion (achlorhydria) may suggest pernicious anemia.

Elevated gastric secretion levels in the gastric acid stimulation test may be indicative of duodenal ulcer; high levels of secretion again suggest Zollinger-Ellison syndrome.

Resources

BOOKS

Pagana, Kathleen Deska, and Timothy J. Pagana. *Mosby's Manual of Diagnostic and Laboratory Tests*. 4th ed. St. Louis: Mosby, 2009.

Janis O. Flores

Gastric bypass

Definition

A gastric bypass is one type of elective bariatric (weight-loss) surgery done on the digestive system to help morbidly obese people lose weight. Gastric bypass surgery is also called malabsorptive surgery because it creates an alternate route for food traveling through the digestive system that bypasses a section of the small intestine where many nutrients are absorbed.

Purpose

Gastric bypass surgery is intended to treat severe (morbid) **obesity** in people who have tried unsuccessfully to lose weight and whose excess weight threatens their health and well being. Obesity is defined by the body mass index (BMI). The BMI calculation compares weight to height. Adults age 20 and older are evaluated as follows:

- BMI below 18.5: underweight
- BMI 18.5–24.9: normal weight
- BMI 25.0–29.9: overweight
- BMI 30 and above: obese
- BMI 40 and above: morbidly or severely obese

Obesity is linked to an increased likelihood of developing more than 20 different diseases and disorders, including high blood pressure (**hypertension**), type 2 diabetes, heart disease, **stroke**, deep vein **blood clots**, fatty **liver disease**, **sleep apnea**, **heartburn**, **gastroesophageal reflux disease** (GERD), gallstone disease, arthritis, **colon cancer**, breathing problems, and depression. Gastric bypass surgery reduces the amount of nutrients that are absorbed from food. It is performed in conjunction with bariatric restriction surgery in which the size of the stomach is reduced through surgical application of a band or stomach staples that close off a portion of the stomach. People who have had restriction surgery can eat only small amounts at a time before feeling full. Reduced food intake along with reduced nutrient absorption can lead to dramatic weight loss.

Demographics

Obesity is the second leading cause (after tobacco use) of preventable **death** in the United States. The number of overweight and obese Americans has steadily increased since 1960. According to the National Institutes of Health, in 2006, 34% of Americans were overweight and 27% were obese. Of these, 15 million were morbidly obese, however, less than 1% chose to undergo a surgical weight-loss procedure.

The number of all surgical weight-loss procedures has increased rapidly. In 1995, only 20,000 weight-loss surgeries were performed in the United States. By 2006, 170,000 of these surgeries were done. In 2006, the United States government agreed to pay for certain bariatric surgeries for individuals who qualified

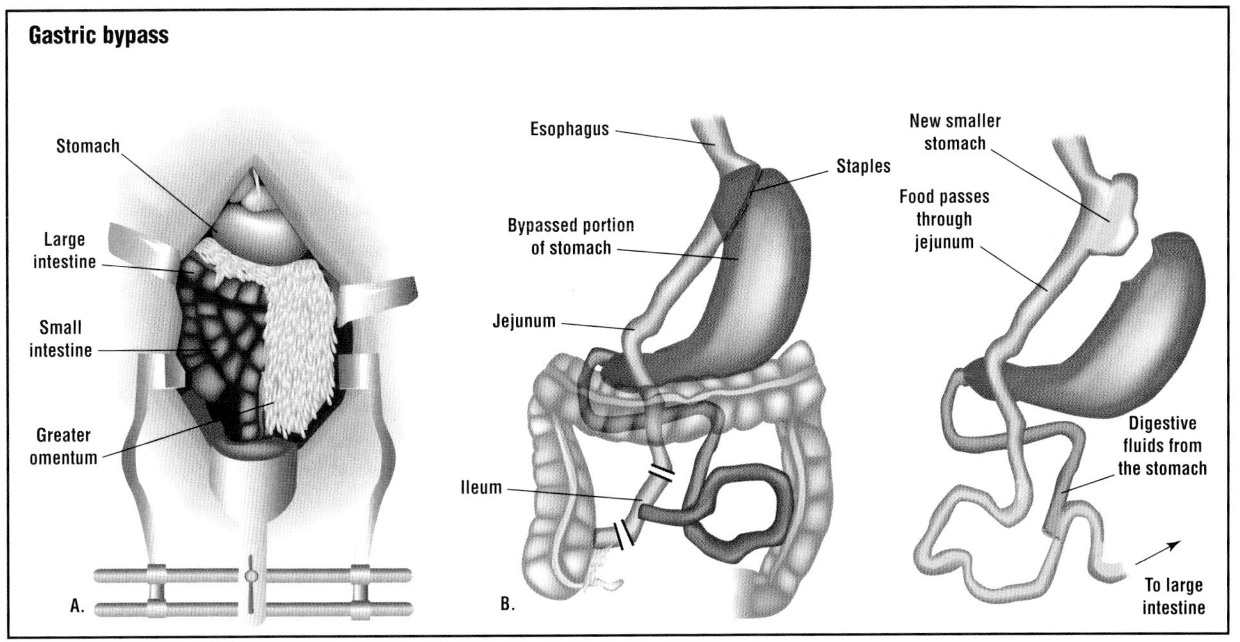

In this Roux-en-Y gastric bypass, a large incision is made down the middle of the abdomen (A). The stomach is separated into two sections. Most of the stomach will be bypassed, so food will no longer go to it. A section of jejunum (small intestine) is then brought up to empty food from the new smaller stomach (B). Finally, the surgeon connects the duodenum to the jejunum, allowing digestive secretions to mix with food further down the jejunum. *(Illustration by PreMediaGlobal. Reproduced by permission of Gale, a part of Cengage Learning.)*

for Medicare. At that time, about 395,000 Americans ages 65–69 were medically eligible for **obesity surgery**. With Medicare coverage, it is likely that more older people will have weight-loss surgery. In 2006, the average patient having **bariatric surgery** was a woman in her late 30s who weighed about 300 pounds (135 kg).

Description

There are several different variations on gastric bypass, all of which are malabsorptive surgeries designed to lower caloric intake by reducing the amount of nutrients absorbed by the digestive system. These include:

- gastric bypass with long gastrojejunostomy
- Roux-en-Y (RNY) gastric bypass
- transected (Miller) RNY bypass
- laparoscopic RNY bypass
- vertical (Fobi) gastric bypass
- distal RNY bypass
- biliopancreatic (BPD) diversion

All bariatric procedures create an alternate route for food through the digestive system so that the food bypasses part of the intestine. These procedures are accompanied by a procedure to reduce the size of the stomach so that less food can be comfortably consumed. Choice of procedure relies on the patient's overall health status and on the surgeon's judgment and experience.

In the operating room, the patient is put under **general anesthesia** by the anesthesiologist. Once the patient is asleep, an endotracheal tube is placed through the mouth into the trachea (windpipe) to connect the patient to a respirator during surgery. A urinary catheter is also placed in the bladder to drain urine during surgery and for the first two days after surgery. This also allows the surgeon to monitor the patient's hydration. A nasogastric (NG) tube is also placed through the nose to drain secretions and is typically removed the morning after surgery.

The most common gastric bypass operation is the Roux-en-Y (RNY) gastric bypass. In this surgery, a small stomach pouch is created by stapling and banding the stomach. The pouch is about the size of an egg and initially can hold 1–2 oz (30–60 mL), as compared to the 40–50 oz (1.2–1.5 L) held by a normal stomach. It is created along the more muscular side of the stomach, which makes it less likely to stretch over time.

Next, a Y-shaped piece of intestine is attached to the pouch on one end, and the jejunum, or middle part

KEY TERMS

Gastrojejunostomy—A surgical procedure in which the stomach is surgically connected to the jejunum (middle portion of the small intestine).

Gastroesophageal reflux disease (GERD)—A condition in which gastric juice from the stomach backs up into the bottom of the esophagus and causes irritation, inflammation, or erosion of the cells lining the esophagus.

Heartburn—A pain in the center of the chest behind the breastbone caused by the contents of the stomach flowing backwards (refluxing) into the lower end of the esophagus and causing irritation.

Hernia—The protrusion of a loop or section of an organ or tissue through an abnormal opening.

Laparoscopy—The examination of the inside of the abdomen through a lighted tube (endoscope), sometimes accompanied by surgery done through a small incision.

Malabsorption—Poor absorption of materials in the digestive system.

Morbidly obese—Definition of a person who is 100 lb (45 kg) or more than 50% overweight and has a body mass index above 40.

Osteoporosis—A condition found in older individuals in which bones decrease in density and become fragile and more likely to break. It can be caused by lack of vitamin D and/or calcium in the diet.

Sleep apnea—A temporary interruption in breathing during sleep.

Small intestine—Consists of three sections: duodenum (nearest the stomach), jejunum, and ileum (nearest the colon or large intestine). Different nutrients are absorbed in different sections of the small intestine.

Type 2 diabetes—Sometimes called adult-onset diabetes, this disease prevents the body from properly using glucose (sugar), but can often be controlled with diet and exercise.

of the small intestine, on the other. This allows food to bypass the duodenum, or first part of the small intestine, where nutrients are absorbed. The food then continues normally through the rest of the small intestine and the large intestine.

The RNY gastric bypass can also be performed laparoscopically. The result is the same as an open surgery RNY, except that instead of opening the patient with a long incision on the stomach, surgeons make a small incision and insert a pencil-thin optical instrument called a laparoscope, to project a picture to a TV monitor. The laparoscopic RNY results in smaller **scars**, as usually only three to four small incisions are made. The average time required to complete the laparoscopic RNY gastric bypass is approximately two hours.

The great advantage of Roux-en-Y gastric bypass is that individuals lose, on average, 60–70% of their excess weight and are able to maintain the weight loss for 10 years or more. As a result, most obesity-related health problems are substantially reduced or cured when weight is lost and that weight loss is maintained. Medicare usually pays for this surgery.

However, Roux-en-Y surgery also has some serious disadvantages, including:

- This surgery is more difficult for the surgeon than restrictive surgeries, and involves permanently altering the digestive system.
- Many vitamins and minerals are absorbed in the part of the small intestine bypassed by this surgery. The individual must commit to a lifetime of taking nutritional supplements to prevent serious vitamin and mineral deficiencies.
- Tearing, bleeding, and infection at the sites where the incisions and reconnections are potentially fatal complications.
- Dumping syndrome may occur in response to meals high in sugar. Dumping occurs when food moves too fast through the intestine and causes symptoms of nausea, bloating, weakness, sweating, fainting, and diarrhea.

Biliopancreatic diversion (BPD), another type of malabsorptive surgery, bypasses an even longer section of the small intestine. In BPD, about two-thirds of the stomach is surgically withdrawn, leaving a pouch that can hold about 3 cups of food. A bypass is then created to the ileum, or final portion of the small intestine. In all, about 9 ft (3 m) of intestine are bypassed. As a result, many fewer calories and nutrients are absorbed. The main advantage of BPD is the large amount of excess weight—between 75% and 80%—that is lost over the first two years and the health benefits that this loss brings. Medicare would usually pay for this surgery. Disadvantages are the same as for Roux-en Y surgery, but nutrient deficiencies are greater. Because fat is poorly digested as a result of this surgery, bowel movements are frequent and stools are especially foul smelling.

Diagnosis/Preparation

A diagnosis of obesity relies on a body weight assessment based on the body mass index (BMI) and waist circumference measurements. Waist circumference exceeding 40 in (101 cm) in men and 35 in (89 cm) in women increases disease risk. Gastric bypass as a weight-loss treatment is considered only for morbidly obese patients whose health is impaired by their obesity. To be candidates for gastric bypass surgery, individuals need to have failed at serious attempts to lose weight in the past, be in good mental health, demonstrate an understanding of the risks associated with this surgery, and be willing to make a lifetime commitment to changing eating habits.

Before the surgery, the patient will undergo a physical and psychological examination and receive nutritional counseling. To prepare for the surgery itself, an intravenous (IV) line is placed, and the patient may be given a sedative to help relax before going to the operating room.

Aftercare

Patients experience postoperative **pain** and the other common discomforts of major surgery, such as the NG tube and a dry mouth. Pain is managed with medication. A large dressing covers the surgical incision on the abdomen of the patient and is usually removed by the second day in the hospital. Short showers 48 hours after surgery are usually allowed. Patients are also fitted with special socks to improve blood flow in their legs and prevent blood clot formation. At the surgeon's discretion, some patients may have a **gastrostomy** tube (g-tube) inserted during surgery to drain secretions from the larger bypassed portion of the stomach. After a few days, it will be clamped and will remain closed. When inserted, the g-tube usually remains for another four to six weeks. It is kept in place in the unlikely event that the patient may need direct feeding into the stomach.

By the evening after surgery or the next day at the latest, patients are usually able to sit up or walk around. Gradually, physical activity may be increased, with normal activity resuming three to four weeks after surgery. Patients are also taught breathing exercises and are asked to cough frequently to clear their lungs of mucus. Postoperative pain medication is prescribed to ease discomfort and initially administered by an epidural. At the time patients are discharged from the hospital, they will be given oral medications for pain. Most patients will typically have a three-day hospital stay if their surgery is uncomplicated.

After gastric bypass or BPD, the individual does not eat anything for one or two days, giving the bowel time to rest. During this time, all **nutrition** is given intravenously. Once the person begins eating, the diet will include:

- liquids such as juice, broth, milk, or diluted cooked cereal for two or three days
- pureed foods that have the texture of baby food for two or three weeks while the stomach heals; these foods must be smooth and contain no large pieces
- soft foods such as ground meat and soft-cooked fruits and vegetables for about eight weeks
- regular food can be eaten in very small amounts

Most people begin by eating six tiny meals a day. These meals should be high in protein. Food must be chewed thoroughly. Liquids are drunk between meals, not with them. Vitamin and mineral supplements are essential.

Risks

Gastric bypass surgery has many of the same risks associated with other major abdominal operations. Life-threatening complications or death are rare, occurring in less than 1% of patients. Significant side effects, such as wound healing problems, difficulty in swallowing food, infections, and extreme **nausea**, can occur in 10–20% of patients. Blood clots after major surgery are rare, but extremely dangerous; if they occur, they may require re-hospitalization and anticoagulants (blood-thinning medications).

Some risks are specific to gastric bypass surgery, including:

- Dumping syndrome. Usually occurs when sweet foods are eaten or when food is eaten too quickly. When the food enters the small intestine, it causes cramping, sweating, and nausea.
- Abdominal hernias. These are the most common complications, requiring follow-up surgery. Incisional hernias occur in 10–20% of patients and require follow-up surgery.
- Narrowing of the stoma. The stoma, or opening between the stomach and intestines, can sometimes become too narrow, causing vomiting. The stoma can be repaired by an outpatient procedure that uses a small endoscopic balloon to stretch it.
- Gallstones. They develop in more than a third of obese patients undergoing gastric surgery. Gallstones are clumps of cholesterol and other matter that accumulate in the gallbladder. Rapid or major weight loss increases a person's risk of developing gallstones.
- Leakage of stomach and intestinal contents. Leakage of stomach and intestinal contents from the staple

and suture lines into the abdomen can occur. This is a rare occurrence and sometimes seals itself. If not, another operation is required.

- Nutritional deficiencies. People who have gastric bypass surgery or BPD need extensive nutritional counseling and must take vitamin and mineral supplements for the rest of their lives. Most iron and **calcium** is absorbed in the duodenum, the first part of the intestine that is bypassed by these operations. Calcium deficiency can lead to **osteoporosis**, and iron deficiency can cause anemia.

In BPD, only 25% of the fat in food is absorbed because so much of the small intestine is bypassed. The fat-soluble **vitamins** A, D, E, and K are absorbed along with fat. When the body absorbs too little fat, inadequate amounts of these fat-soluble vitamins are absorbed, so dietary supplements containing these vitamins must be taken. Other vitamins that may not be absorbed in adequate amounts are vitamin B_{12}, **folic acid**, and vitamin B_1 (thiamine). Research published in the journal *Neurology* in March 2007 found that a very small number of people developed a brain disorder called Wernicke encephalopathy 4–12 weeks after bariatric surgery. This disorder is caused by a deficiency of vitamin B_1. Most of the people who developed the disorder had failed to take their vitamin supplements as prescribed after surgery.

Normal results

Most people who have surgery for obesity lose anywhere from 50–80% of their excess weight. However, quite a few put pounds back on beginning several years after surgery. The main reason for weight gain is noncompliance with their nutrition and **exercise** plan. Also, over time the size of the stomach pouch in restrictive surgeries tends to stretch, allowing people to eat more and still feel comfortable. On the positive side, people who lose weight through surgery almost always see great improvement in any obesity-related diseases they have.

According to the *American Journal of Medicine*, gastric bypass surgery resolves Type 2 Diabetes in over 80 percent of morbidly obese people. They also are asking for more research to determine the benefits for non-obese diabetics as well.

Alternatives

Surgical alternatives

Lap-band and adjustable gastric band restrictive surgery used alone represent alternatives to gastric bypass surgery. Lap-Band surgery achieves restriction by placing a saline (salt water) filled bag around the stomach, pinching off a portion of it leaving only a small pouch at the top. The exit to the pouch is narrowed so that the rate at which the pouch empties is slowed. Because the pouch is so small, the individual can only eat about half a cup of food at a time without feeling nauseated. Since there is no cutting, stapling, or stomach rerouting involved, the procedure is the least invasive of all weight-loss surgeries. Patients generally experience less pain and scarring, and their hospital stay is shorter than with malabsorptive surgeries. In addition, a port allows access to the saline bag, so that the size of the stomach pouch can be adjusted without additional surgery. This surgery is reversible; the band or saline bag can be removed and the digestive system will function normally. Weight loss averages 50–65% of the excess body weight during the first two years. The procedure is often covered by Medicare.

Gastric band surgery uses a different technique to reduce the size of the stomach. The United States Food and Drug Administration (FDA) approved this surgery in 2001. Its long-term effects have not been studied.

Vertical banded gastroplasty (VBG) is also known as stomach stapling. This surgery is performed less often than lap-band surgery. With VBG, part of the stomach is stapled shut, making it smaller so that individuals feel full sooner. The advantage of VBG is that the procedure is quick and has few complications. Disadvantages are that average weight loss is less than with other weight-loss surgeries, and staples can pull out allowing small leaks between the stomach and the abdomen to develop. Infection is possible, but rare (less than 1%).

Nonsurgical alternatives

Diet and nutrition counseling is the main nonsurgical method of weight loss. Diet therapy involves instruction on how to adjust a diet to reduce the number of calories eaten. Reducing calories moderately is essential in achieving gradual and steady weight and in maintaining the loss. Strategies of diet and nutrition therapy include teaching individuals about the calorie content of different foods, food composition (fats, carbohydrates, and proteins), reading nutrition labels, types of foods to buy, and how to prepare foods. To be healthful, a diet must provide balanced nutrition along with calorie reduction.

Physical activity, especially when combined with a healthy low-calorie diet is another nonsurgical way to lose weight. Moderate physical activity, progressing to 30 minutes or more five or more days a week, is recommended for weight loss. Physical activity has also been reported to be a key part of maintaining weight loss. Abdominal fat and, in some cases, waist circumference can be modestly reduced through physical activity. Strategies of successful weight loss through long-term physical activity involve selecting enjoyable activities that can be scheduled into a regular daily routine.

Behavior therapy aims to improve diet and physical activity patterns and develop habits and new behaviors that promote weight loss. Behavioral therapy strategies for weight loss and maintenance include keeping a food and exercise diary, identifying high-risk situations such as having high-calorie foods in the house and learning to avoiding these situations, using non-food rewards for specific actions such as exercising regularly, developing realistic goals and modifying false beliefs about weight loss and body image, developing a social support network (family, friends, or colleagues), and joining a support group that will encourage weight loss in a positive and motivating manner.

Drug therapy is another nonsurgical alternative option for treating obesity. The United States Food and Drug Administration (FDA) has approved three prescription drugs for treating obesity: orlistat (Xenical), phentermine (an appetite suppressant available under more than a dozen trade names), and sibutramine (Meridia in the United States, Reductil in Europe). In 2007, orlistat became available in the United States as an over-the-counter (nonprescription) drug under the name Alli. These drugs alone are not magic bullets for weight loss and should be used in addition to calorie reduction and regular exercise.

Resources

BOOKS

Apple, Robin F. James Lock, and Rebecka Peebles. *Is Weight Loss Surgery Right for You?* New York: Oxford University Press, 2006.

Furtado, Margaret M. and Lynette Schultz. *Recipes for Life after Weight-Loss Surgery: Delicious Dishes for Nourishing the New You.* Gloucester, MA: Fair Winds Press, 2007.

Kurian, Marina S., Barbara Thompson, and Brian K. Davidson. *Weight Loss Surgery for Dummies* Hoboken, NJ: Wiley, 2005.

Leach, Susan M. *Before & After, Revised Edition: Living and Eating Well After Weight-Loss Surgery*. New York: Morrow Cookbooks, 2007.

OTHER

"Calculate Your Body Mass Index." *United States Department of Health and Human Services*, March 26, 2007 [cited January 5, 2008]. http://www.nhlbisupport.com/bmi (accessed March 30, 2008).

" Gastric Bypass Surgery: What Can You Expect?" *Mayo Clinic*, October 5, 2007 [cited January 5, 2008]. http://www.mayoclinic.com/health/gastric-bypass/HQ01465 (accessed March 30, 2008).

"Gastrointestinal Surgery for Severe Obesity." *Weight-control Information Network (WIN)*, December 2004 [cited January 5, 2008]. http://win.niddk.nih.gov/publications/gastric.htm (accessed March 30, 2008).

ORGANIZATIONS

American Obesity Association, 1250 24th Street, NW, Suite 300, Washington, DC, 20037, (202) 776-7711, http://www.obesity.org.

American Society for Bariatric Surgery, 7328 West University Avenue, Suite F, Gainesville, FL, 32607, (352) 331-4900, http://www.asbs.org.

Monique Laberge, PhD
Karl Finley
Brenda Lerner

Gastric carcinoma *see* **Stomach cancer**

Gastric emptying scan

Definition

A gastric emptying scan (GES) is an x-ray exam using special radioactive material that allows physicians to identify abnormalities related to emptying of the stomach. Diseases that involve changes in the way the stomach contracts (motility disorders) are best diagnosed by this test.

Purpose

The study is used most frequently to evaluate patients who have symptoms suggestive of decreased, delayed, or rapid gastric emptying, and no visible abnormality to explain their symptoms.

Symptoms pointing to a delay in gastric emptying are non-specific, and may be due to a number of causes, such as ulcers, diabetes, tumors, and others. These symptoms include **nausea**, upper abdominal bloating, and at times **vomiting**. Another significant symptom is called "early satiety," which means feeling full after eating only a small amount of food. In some patients, weight loss is also present. In addition to symptoms, the finding of a large amount of material in the stomach after an overnight fast suggests abnormal emptying, but does not distinguish between an actual blockage or an irregularity

KEY TERMS

Endoscopy—The examination of the inside of an organ with an instrument that has a light at the end of it and an optical system for examination of the organ.

Motility—Motility is spontaneous movement. One example is the automatic stomach contractions that move the food content along from the stomach into the intestines. A motility disease is one that involves changes in the way the stomach contracts.

in gastric contractions. It is therefore essential to find out what is causing material to remain in the stomach.

Since many diseases can produce the above symptoms, structural lesions (such as tumors or regions of narrowing or scar tissue) need to be ruled out first. This is usually done by upper gastrointestinal series test or by **endoscopy** (examination of the inside of an organ, in this instance the stomach, with an instrument that has a light at the end of it and an optical system for examination of the organ). Once it is clear that a mechanical or physical lesion is not the cause of symptoms, attempts to document an abnormality in the nervous or muscular function of the stomach is then begun. GES is usually the first step in that evaluation.

Precautions

The exam should not be performed on pregnant women, but is otherwise quite safe. Since eggs are usually used to hold the radioactive material, patients should notify their physician if they are allergic to eggs. However, other materials can be used in place of an egg.

Description

Gastric emptying scans have undergone several changes since the initial studies in the late 1970s. During the study, patients are asked to ingest an egg sandwich containing a radioactive substance (for example, technetium) that can be followed by a special camera. The emptying of the material from the stomach is then followed and displayed both in the form of an image, as well as the percentage emptied over several hours (generally two and four hours). Studies are in progress using substances that are not radioactive, but this procedure is not available to the patient as of yet.

Preparation

The only preparation involved is for the patient to fast overnight before the test.

Risks

The radiation exposure during the study is quite small and safe, unless the patient is pregnant.

Normal results

There are several different measurements considered normal, depending on the radioactive material and solid meal used. The value is expressed as a percentage of emptying over a period of time. For a technetium-filled egg sandwich, normal emptying is 78 minutes for half the material to leave the stomach, with a variation of 11 minutes either way.

Abnormal results

GES scan studies that show emptying of the stomach in a longer than accepted period is abnormal. Severity of test results and symptoms do not always match; therefore, the physician must carefully interpret these findings. Diabetic injury to the nerves that supply the stomach (called diabetic gastroparesis) is one of the most common causes of abnormal gastric motility. However, up to 30% of patients have no obvious cause to explain the abnormal results and symptoms. These cases are called idiopathic (of unknown cause). GES is often used to follow the effect of medications used for treatment of motility disorders.

ORGANIZATIONS

American Pseudo-Obstruction & Hirschsprung's Society, 158 Pleasant St., North Andover, MA, 01845-2797, (978) 685-4477, (978) 685-4488, aphs@tiac.net.

David Kaminstein, MD

Gastric lavage *see* **Stomach flushing**
Gastric stapling *see* **Obesity surgery**
Gastric ulcers *see* **Ulcers (digestive)**

Gastrinoma

Definition

Gastrinomas are tumors associated with a rare gastroenterological disorder known as Zollinger-Ellison syndrome (ZES). They occur primarily in the pancreas and duodenum (beginning of the small intestine) and secrete large quantities of the hormone gastrin, triggering gastric acid production that produces ulcers. They may be malignant (cancerous) or benign.

Description

Gastrinomas are an integral part of the Zollinger-Ellison syndrome (ZES). In fact, ZES is also known as gastrinoma. This syndrome consists of ulcer disease in the upper gastrointestinal tract, marked increases in the secretion of gastric acid in the stomach, and tumors of the islet cells in the pancreas. The tumors produce large amounts of gastrin that are responsible for the characteristics of Zollinger-Ellison syndrome, namely severe ulcer disease. Although usually located within the pancreas, they may occur in other organs.

Gastrinomas may occur randomly and sporadically, or they may be inherited as part of a genetic condition called multiple endocrine neoplasia type 1 (MEN-1) syndrome. About half of persons with MEN-1 have gastrinomas, which tend to be more numerous and smaller than tumors in sporadic cases.

About half of ZES patients have multiple gastrinomas, which can vary in size from 1–20 mm. Gastrinomas found in the pancreas are usually much larger than duodenal gastrinomas. About two thirds of gastrinomas are malignant (cancerous). These usually grow slowly, but some may invade surrounding sites rapidly and metastasize (spread) widely. Sometimes, gastrinomas are found only in the lymph nodes, and it is uncertain whether these malignancies have originated in the lymph nodes or have metastasized from a tumor not visible in the pancreas or duodenum.

There is some evidence that the more malignant form of gastrinomas is more frequent in larger pancreatic tumors, especially in females and in persons with a shorter disease symptom duration and higher serum gastrin levels.

Causes and symptoms

Most persons with gastrinomas secrete profound amounts of gastric acid, and almost all develop ulcers, mostly in the duodenum or stomach. Early in the course of the disease, symptoms are typical of peptic ulcers, however once the disease is established, the ulcers become more persistent and symptomatic, and may respond poorly to standard anti-ulcer therapy. Abdominal pain is the predominant symptom of ulcer disease. About 40% of patients have **diarrhea** as well. In some patients, diarrhea is the primary symptom of gastrinoma.

Diagnosis

Persons with gastrinomas have many of the same symptoms as persons with ulcers. Their levels of gastric acid, however, are usually far greater than those in common ulcer disease. Gastrinomas are usually diagnosed by a blood test that measures the level of gastrin in the blood. Patients with gastrinomas often have gastrin levels more than 200 pg/mL, which is 4–10 times higher than normal. Serum gastrin levels as high as 450,000 pg/mL have occurred.

When the serum gastrin test does not show these extremely high levels of gastrin, patients may be given certain foods or injections in an attempt to provoke a response that will help diagnose the condition. The most useful of these provocative tests is the secretin injection test (or secretin stimulation or provocative test), which will almost always produce a positive response in persons with gastrinomas but seldom in persons without them.

Surgically, gastrinomas are often difficult to locate, even with careful inspection. They may be missed in at least 10–20% of patients with ZES. Gastrinomas are sometimes found only because they have metastasized and produced symptoms related to the spread of malignancy. Such metastasis may be the most reliable indication of whether the gastrinoma is malignant or benign.

Diagnostic imaging techniques help locate the gastrinomas. The most sophisticated is an x-ray test called radionuclide octreotide scanning (also known as somatostatin receptor scintigraphy or 111In pentetreotide SPECT). A study by the National Institutes of Health (NIH) found this test to be superior to other imaging methods, such as computed tomography scan (CT) or **magnetic resonance imaging** (MRI), in pinpointing the location of tumors and guiding physicians in treatment.

Approximately half of all gastrinomas do not show up on imaging studies. Therefore, exploratory surgery is often recommended to try to locate and remove the tumors.

Treatment

Therapy for gastrinomas should be individualized, since patients tend to have varying degrees of disease and symptoms. Treatment is aimed at eliminating the overproduction of gastric acid and removing the gastrin-producing tumors.

Drugs

Gastrinomas may not be easily treated by the standard anti-ulcer approaches. The medical treatment

KEY TERMS

Gastrin—A hormone secreted in the stomach that is involved in the production of gastric acid. Overproduction of gastric acid contributes to peptic ulcer formation.

Multiple endocrine neoplasia type 1 (MEN-1)—An inherited condition marked by multiple malignancies of the pituitary gland, parathyroid gland, and islet cells of the pancreas. About half of MEN-1 patients with pancreatic islet cell tumors will have gastrinomas, gastrin-producing tumors that lead to ulcer disease.

Peptic ulcer—An eroded area in the stomach lining or in the first part of the duodenum (beginning of the small intestine).

Serum gastrin test—A laboratory test that is performed on a blood sample to determine that level of the hormone gastrin. High levels of gastrin indicate the presence a duodenal ulcer or a gastrinoma.

Sporadic—Occurring at random or by chance, and not as a result of a genetically determined, or inherited, trait.

of choice is with drugs called **proton pump inhibitors**, such as omeprazole or lansoprazole, daily. These drugs are potent inhibitors of gastric acid. High doses of H-2 receptor antagonists may also reduce gastric acid secretion, improve symptoms, and induce ulcer healing. These drugs must be continued indefinitely, since even a brief discontinuation will cause ulcer recurrence. **Antacids** may provide some relief, but it is usually not longlasting or healing.

Surgery

Because of the likelihood that gastrinomas may be malignant, in both sporadic tumors and those associated with the inherited MEN-1 syndrome, surgery to locate and remove gastrinomas is frequently advised. It is now known that complete surgical removal of gastrinomas can cure the overproduction of gastrin, even in patients who have metastases to the lymph nodes. Surgery in patients with MEN-1 and ZES, however, remains controversial since the benefit is less clear.

Freedom from disease after surgery is judged by improved symptoms, reduced gastric acid production, reduced need for drug therapy, normalization of serum gastrin levels, and normalization of results from the secretin stimulation test and imaging studies.

Prognosis

Medical therapy often controls symptoms, and surgery may or may not cure gastrinoma. About 50% of ZES patients in whom gastrinomas are not removed will die from malignant spread of the tumor. In patients with gastrinomas as part of MEN-1 syndrome, the cure rate is extremely low.

A NIH study of patients who had surgical removal of gastrinomas found that 42% were disease-free one year after surgery and 35% were disease-free at five years. Disease recurrences can often be detected with a serum gastrin test or secretin stimulation test.

When gastrinomas are malignant, they often grow slowly. The principal sites of metastasis are the regional lymph nodes and liver, but they may also spread to other structures. About one quarter of patients with gastrinomas have liver metastases at the time of diagnosis. This appears to be more frequent with pancreatic gastrinomas than duodenal gastrinomas.

Metastases of malignant gastrinomas to the liver is very serious. Survival five years after diagnosis is 20–30%, however patients with gastrinomas found only in the lymph nodes have been known to live as long as 25 years after diagnosis, without evidence of further tumor spread. In fact, the life expectancy of patients with gastrinomas that have spread to the lymph nodes is no different from that of patients with gastrinomas that cannot even be found at surgery for about 90%, five years after diagnosis.

ORGANIZATIONS

National Digestive Diseases Information Clearinghouse (NDDIC), 2 Information Way, Bethesda, MD, 20892-3570, (703) 738-4929, (800) 891-5389, http://digestive.niddk.nih.gov.

Caroline A. Helwick

Gastritis

Definition

Gastritis commonly refers to inflammation of the lining of the stomach, but the term is often used to cover a variety of symptoms resulting from stomach lining inflammation and symptoms of burning or discomfort. True gastritis comes in several forms and is diagnosed using a combination of tests. In the 1990s, scientists discovered that the main cause of true gastritis is infection from a bacterium called *Helicobacter pylori* (*H. pylori*).

Description

Gastritis should not be confused with common symptoms of upper abdominal discomfort. It has been associated with resulting ulcers, particularly peptic ulcers. And in some cases, chronic gastritis can lead to more serious complications.

Nonerosive H. pylori gastritis

The main cause of true gastritis is *H. pylori* infection. *H. pylori* is indicated in an average of 90% of patients with chronic gastritis. This form of nonerosive gastritis is the result of infection with *Helicobacter pylori* bacterium, a microorganism whose outer layer is resistant to the normal effects of stomach acid in breaking down bacteria.

The resistance of *H. pylori* means that the bacterium may rest in the stomach for long periods of times, even years, and eventually cause symptoms of gastritis or ulcers when other factors are introduced, such as the presence of specific genes or ingestion of **nonsteroidal anti-inflammatory drugs** (NSAIDS). Study of the role of *H. pylori* in development of gastritis and peptic ulcers has disproved the former belief that **stress** lead to most stomach and duodenal ulcers and has resulted in improved treatment and reduction of stomach ulcers. *H. pylori* is most likely transmitted between humans, although the specific routes of transmission are continuously under study.

Erosive and hemorrhagic gastritis

After *H. pylori*, the second most common cause of chronic gastritis is use of nonsteroidal anti-inflammatory drugs. These commonly used **pain** killers, including **aspirin**, fenoprofen, ibuprofen and naproxen, among others, can lead to gastritis and peptic ulcers. Other forms of erosive gastritis are those due to alcohol and corrosive agents or due to trauma such as ingestion of foreign bodies.

Other forms of gastritis

Clinicians differ on the classification of the less common and specific forms of gastritis, particularly since there is so much overlap with *H. pylori* in development of chronic gastritis and complications of gastritis. Other types of gastritis that may be diagnosed include:

- Acute stress gastritis–the most serious form of gastritis which usually occurs in critically ill patients, such as those in intensive care. Stress erosions may develop suddenly as a result of severe trauma or stress to the stomach lining.
- Atrophic gastritis is the result of chronic gastritis which is leading to atrophy, or decrease in size and wasting away, of the gastric lining. Gastric atrophy is the final stage of chronic gastritis and may be a precursor to gastric cancer.
- Superficial gastritis is a term often used to describe the initial stages of chronic gastritis.
- Uncommon specific forms of gastritis include granulomatous, eosiniphilic and lymphocytic gastritis.

Causes and symptoms

Nonerosive H. pylori gastritis

H. pylori gastritis is caused by infection from the *H. pylori* bacterium. The route of its transmission is under study as clinicians believe there are numerous routes for the bacterium. Its prevalence and distribution differs in nations around the world. The presence of *H. pylori* has been detected in 86–99% of patients with chronic superficial gastritis. However, physicians are still learning about the link of *H. pylori* to chronic gastritis and peptic ulcers, since many patients with *H. pylori* infection do not develop symptoms or peptic ulcers. *H. pylori* is also seen in 90–100% of patients with duodenal ulcers.

Symptoms of *H. pylori* gastritis include abdominal pain and reduced acid secretion in the stomach. However, the majority of patients with *H. pylori* infection suffer no symptoms, even though the infection may lead to ulcers and resulting symptoms. Ulcer symptoms include dull, gnawing pain, often two to three hours after meals and pain in the middle of the night when the stomach is empty.

Erosive and hemorrhagic gastritis

The most common cause of this form of gastritis is use of NSAIDS. Other causes may be **alcoholism** or stress from surgery or critical illness. The role of NSAIDS in development of gastritis and peptic ulcers depends on the dose level. Although even low doses of aspirin or other nonsteroidal anti-inflammatory drugs may cause some gastric upset, low doses generally will not lead to gastritis. However, as many as 10–30% of patients on higher and more frequent doses of NSAIDS, such as those with chronic arthritis, may develop gastric ulcers. Studies were underway to understand the role of *H. pylori* in gastritis and ulcers among patients using NSAIDS.

Patients with erosive gastritis may also show no symptoms. When symptoms do occur, they may include **anorexia nervosa**, gastric pain, **nausea and vomiting**.

Other Forms of Gastritis

Less common forms of gastritis may result from a number of generalized diseases or from complications of chronic gastritis. Any number of mechanisms may cause various less common forms of gastritis and they may differ slightly in their symptoms and clinical signs. However, they all have in common inflammation of the gastric mucosa.

Diagnosis

Nonerosive H. pylori gastritis

H. pylori gastritis is easily diagnosed through the use of the urea breath test. This test detects active presence of *H. pylori* infection. Other serological tests, which may be readily available in a physician's office, may be used to detect *H. pylori* infection. Newly developed versions offer rapid diagnosis. The choice of test will depend on cost, availability and the physician's experience, since nearly all of the available tests have an accuracy rate of 90% or better. **Endoscopy**, or the examination of the stomach area using a hollow tube inserted through the mouth, may be ordered to confirm diagnosis. A biopsy of the gastric lining may also be ordered.

Erosive or hemorrhagic gastritis

Clinical history of the patient may be particularly important in the diagnosis of this type of gastritis, since its cause is most often the result of chronic use of NSAIDS, alcoholism, or other substances.

Other forms of gastritis

Gastritis that has developed to the stage of duodenal or gastric ulcers usually requires endoscopy for diagnosis. It allows the physician to perform a biopsy for possible malignancy and for *H. pylori*. Sometimes, an upper gastrointestinal x-ray study with barium is ordered. Some diseases such as Zollinger-Ellison syndrome, an ulcer disease of the upper gastrointestinal tract, may show large mucosal folds in the stomach and duodenum on radiographs or in endoscopy. Other tests check for changes in gastric function.

Treatment

H. pylori gastritis

The discovery of *H. pylori's* role in development of gastritis and ulcers has led to improved treatment of chronic gastritis. In particular, relapse rates for duodenal and gastric ulcers has been reduced with successful treatment of *H. pylori* infection. Since the infection can be treated with **antibiotics**, the bacterium can be completely eliminated up to 90% of the time.

Although *H. pylori* can be successfully treated, the treatment may be uncomfortable for patients and relies heavily on patient compliance. Clinicians are attempting to identify the best treatment method based on simplicity, patient cooperation and results. As of 2010, no single antibiotic had been found which would eliminate *H. pylori* on its own, so a combination of antibiotics has been prescribed to treat the infection.

DUAL THERAPY. Dual therapy involves the use of an antibiotic and a proton pump inhibitor. **Proton pump inhibitors** help reduce stomach acid by halting the mechanism that pumps acid into the stomach. This also helps promote healing of ulcers or inflammation. Dual therapy has not been proven to be as effective as triple therapy, but may be ordered for some patients who can more comfortably handle the use of less drugs and will therefore more likely follow the two-week course of therapy.

TRIPLE THERAPY. As of early 1998, triple therapy was the preferred treatment for patients with *H. pylori* gastritis. It is estimated that triple therapy successfully eliminates 80–95% of *H. pylori* cases. This treatment regimen usually involves a two-week course of three drugs. An antibiotic such as amoxicillin or tetracycline, and another antibiotic such as clarithomycin or metronidazole are used in combination with bismuth subsalicylate, a substance found in the over-the-counter medication, Pepto-Bismol, which helps protect the lining of the stomach from acid. Physicians were experimenting with various combinations of drugs and time of treatment to balance side effects with effectiveness. Side effects of triple therapy are not serious, but may cause enough discomfort that patients are not inclined to follow the treatment.

OTHER TREATMENT THERAPIES. Scientists have experimented with quadruple therapy, which adds an antisecretory drug, or one which suppresses gastric secretion, to the standard triple therapy. One study showed this therapy to be effective with only a week's

KEY TERMS

Duodenal—Refers to the duodenum, or the first part of the small intestine.

Gastric—Relating to the stomach.

Mucosa—The mucous membrane, or the thin layer which lines body cavities and passages.

Ulcer—A break in the skin or mucous membrane. It can fester and pus like a sore.

course of treatment in more than 90% of patients. Short course therapy was attempted with triple therapy involving antibiotics and a proton pump inhibitor and seemed effective in eliminating *H. pylori* in one week for more than 90% of patients. The goal is to develop the most effective therapy combination that can work in one week of treatment or less.

MEASURING H. PYLORI TREATMENT EFFECTIVENESS. In order to ensure that *H. pylori* has been eradicated, physicians will test patients following treatment. The breath test is the preferred method to check for remaining signs of *H. pylori*.

Treatment of erosive gastritis

Since few patients with this form of gastritis show symptoms, treatment may depend on severity of symptoms. When symptoms do occur, patients may be treated with therapy similar to that for *H. pylori*, especially since some studies have demonstrated a link between *H. pylori* and NSAIDS in causing ulcers. Avoidance of NSAIDS will most likely be prescribed.

Other forms of gastritis

Specific treatment will depend on the cause and type of gastritis. These may include prednisone or antibiotics. Critically ill patients at high risk for bleeding may be treated with preventive drugs to reduce risk of acute stress gastritis. If stress gastritis does occur, the patient is treated with constant infusion of a drug to stop bleeding. Sometimes surgery is recommended, but is weighed with the possibility of surgical complications or **death**. Once torrential bleeding occurs in acute stress gastritis, mortality is as high as greater than 60%.

Alternative treatment

Alternative forms of treatment for gastritis and ulcers should be used cautiously and in conjunction with conventional medical care, particularly now that scientists have confirmed the role of *H. pylori* in gastritis and ulcers. Alternative treatments can help address gastritis symptoms with diet and **nutritional supplements**, herbal medicine and **ayurvedic medicine**. It is believed that zinc, vitamin A and beta-carotene aid in the stomach lining's ability to repair and regenerate itself. Herbs thought to stimulate the immune system and reduce inflammation include **echinacea** (*Echinacea* spp.) and goldenseal (*Hydrastis canadensis*). Ayurvedic medicine involves **meditation**. There are also certain herbs and nutritional supplements aimed at helping to treat ulcers.

Prognosis

The discovery of *H. pylori* has improved the prognosis for patients with gastritis and ulcers. Since treatment exists to eradicate the infection, recurrence is much less common. The only patients requiring treatment for *H. pylori* are those at high risk because of factors such as NSAIDS use or for those with ulcers and other complicating factors or symptoms. Research will continue into the most effective treatment of *H. pylori*, especially in light of the bacterium's resistance to certain antibiotics. Regular treatment of patients with gastric and duodenal ulcers has been recommended, since H. pylori plays such a consistently high role in development of ulcers. It is believed that *H. pylori* also plays a role in the eventual development of serious gastritis complications and cancer. Detection and treatment of *H. pylori* infection may help reduce occurrence of these diseases. The prognosis for patients with acute stress gastritis is much poorer, with a 60 percent or higher mortality rate among those bleeding heavily.

Prevention

The widespread detection and treatment of *H. pylori* as a preventive measure in gastritis has been discussed but not resolved. Until more is known about the routes through which *H. pylori* is spread, specific prevention recommendations are not available. Erosive gastritis from NSAIDS can be prevented with cessation of use of these drugs. An education campaign was launched in 1998 to educate patients, particularly an **aging** population of arthritis sufferers, about risk for ulcers from NSAIDS and alternative drugs.

Resources

PERIODICALS

Podolski, J. L. "Recent Advances in Peptic Ulcer Disease: H. pylori Infection and Its Treatement." *Gastroenterology Nursing* 19, no. 4: 128–136.

OTHER

American College of Gastroenterology Page. http://www.acg.org.

ORGANIZATIONS

National Digestive Diseases Information Clearinghouse (NDDIC), 2 Information Way, Bethesda, MD, 20892-3570, (703) 738-4929, (800) 891-5389, http://digestive.niddk.nih.gov.

Teresa Odle,

Gastroduodenostomy (Billroth I) *see* **Ulcer surgery**

Gastroenteritis

Definition

Gastroenteritis is a catchall term for infection or irritation of the digestive tract, particularly the stomach and intestine. It is frequently referred to as the stomach or intestinal flu, although the **influenza** virus is not associated with this illness. Major symptoms include **nausea and vomiting**, **diarrhea**, and abdominal cramps. These symptoms are sometimes also accompanied by **fever** and overall weakness. Gastroenteritis typically lasts about three days. Adults usually recover without problem, but children, the elderly, and anyone with an underlying disease are more vulnerable to complications such as **dehydration**.

Demographics

Gastroenteritis is an uncomfortable and inconvenient ailment, but it is rarely life-threatening in the United States and other developed nations. However, an estimated 220,000 children younger than age five are hospitalized with gastroenteritis symptoms in the United States annually. Of these children, 300 die as a result of severe diarrhea and dehydration. In developing nations, diarrheal illnesses are a major source of mortality. Worldwide, inadequate treatment of gastroenteritis kills 5 to 8 million people per year, and is a leading cause of **death** among infants and children under the age of 5. Annually, worldwide, rotaviruses are estimated to cause 800,000 deaths in children below age five.

Description

Typically, children are more vulnerable to rotaviruses, the most significant cause of acute watery diarrhea. For this reason, much research has gone into developing a vaccine to protect children from this virus. Adults can be infected with rotaviruses, but these infections typically have minimal or no symptoms. Children are also susceptible to adenoviruses and astroviruses, which are minor causes of childhood gastroenteritis. Adults experience illness from astroviruses as well, but the major causes of adult viral gastroenteritis are the caliciviruses and SRSVs. These viruses also cause illness in children. The SRSVs are a type of calicivirus and include the Norwalk, Southhampton, and Lonsdale viruses. These viruses are the most likely to produce **vomiting** as a major symptom.

Bacterial gastroenteritis is frequently a result of poor sanitation, the lack of safe drinking water, or contaminated food–conditions common in developing nations. Natural or man-made disasters can make underlying problems in sanitation and food safety worse. In developed nations, the modern food production system potentially exposes millions of people to disease-causing bacteria through its intensive production and distribution methods. Common types of bacterial gastroenteritis can be linked to *Salmonella* and *Campylobacter* bacteria; however, ***Escherichia coli*** 0157 and *Listeria monocytogenes* are creating increased concern in developed nations. **Cholera** and Shigella remain two diseases of great concern in developing countries, and research to develop long-term vaccines against them is underway.

Causes and symptoms

Gastroenteritis arises from ingestion of viruses, certain bacteria, or parasites. Food that has spoiled may also cause illness. Certain medications and excessive alcohol can irritate the digestive tract to the point of inducing gastroenteritis. Regardless of the cause, the symptoms of gastroenteritis include diarrhea, **nausea** and **vomiting**, and abdominal pain and cramps. Sufferers may also experience bloating, low fever, and overall tiredness. Typically, the symptoms last only two to three days, but some viruses may last up to a week.

A usual bout of gastroenteritis shouldn't require a visit to the doctor. However, medical treatment is essential if symptoms worsen or if there are complications. Infants, young children, the elderly, and persons with underlying disease require special attention in this regard.

The greatest danger presented by gastroenteritis is dehydration. The loss of fluids through diarrhea and vomiting can upset the body's electrolyte balance, leading to potentially life-threatening problems such as heart beat abnormalities (arrhythmia). The risk of dehydration increases as symptoms are prolonged. Dehydration should be suspected if a dry mouth, increased or excessive thirst, or scanty urination is experienced.

If symptoms do not resolve within a week, an infection or disorder more serious than gastroenteritis may be involved. Symptoms of great concern include a high fever (102° F [38.9°C] or above), blood or mucus

KEY TERMS

Dehydration—A condition in which the body lacks the normal level of fluids, potentially impairing normal body functions.

Electrolyte—An ion, or weakly charged element, that conducts reactions and signals in the body. Examples of electrolytes are sodium and potassium ions.

Glucose—A sugar that serves as the body's primary source of fuel.

Influenza—A virus that affects the respiratory system, causing fever, congestion, muscle aches, and headaches.

Intravenous (IV) therapy—Administration of intravenous fluids.

Microflora—The bacterial population in the intestine.

Pathogenic bacteria—Bacteria that produce illness.

Probiotics—Bacteria that are beneficial to a person's health, either through protecting the body against pathogenic bacteria or assisting in recovery from an illness.

in the diarrhea, blood in the vomit, and severe abdominal pain or swelling. These symptoms require prompt medical attention.

Diagnosis

The symptoms of gastroenteritis are usually enough to identify the illness. Unless there is an outbreak affecting several people or complications are encountered in a particular case, identifying the specific cause of the illness is not a priority. However, if identification of the infectious agent is required, a stool sample will be collected and analyzed for the presence of viruses, disease-causing (pathogenic) bacteria, or parasites.

Treatment

Gastroenteritis is a self-limiting illness which will resolve by itself. However, for comfort and convenience, a person may use over-the-counter medications such as Pepto Bismol to relieve the symptoms. These medications work by altering the ability of the intestine to move or secrete spontaneously, absorbing toxins and water, or altering intestinal microflora. Some over-the-counter medicines use more than one element to treat symptoms.

If over-the-counter medications are ineffective and medical treatment is sought, a doctor may prescribe a more powerful anti-diarrheal drug, such as motofen or lomotil. Should pathogenic bacteria or parasites be identified in the patient's stool sample, medications such as **antibiotics** will be prescribed.

It is important to stay hydrated and nourished during a bout of gastroenteritis. If dehydration is absent, the drinking of generous amounts of nonalcoholic fluids, such as water or juice, is adequate. **Caffeine**, since it increases urine output, should be avoided. The traditional BRAT diet–bananas, rice, applesauce, and toast–is tolerated by the tender gastrointestinal system, but it is not particularly nutritious. Many, but not all, medical researchers recommend a diet that includes complex carbohydrates (e.g., rice, wheat, potatoes, bread, and cereal), lean meats, yogurt, fruit, and vegetables. Milk and other dairy products shouldn't create problems if they are part of the normal diet. Fatty foods or foods with a lot of sugar should be avoided. These recommendations are based on clinical experience and controlled trials, but are not universally accepted.

Minimal to moderate dehydration is treated with oral rehydrating solutions that contain glucose and electrolytes. These solutions are commercially available under names such as Naturalyte, Pedialyte, Infalyte, and Rehydralyte. Oral rehydrating solutions are formulated based on physiological properties. Fluids that are not based on these properties–such as cola, apple juice, broth, and sports beverages–are not recommended to treat dehydration. If vomiting interferes with oral rehydration, small frequent fluid intake may be better tolerated. Should oral rehydration fail or severe dehydration occur, medical treatment in the form of intravenous (IV) therapy is required. IV therapy can be followed with oral rehydration as the patient's condition improves. Once normal hydration is achieved, the patient can return to a regular diet.

Alternative treatment

Symptoms of uncomplicated gastroenteritis can be relieved with adjustments in diet, herbal remedies, and homeopathy. An infusion of meadowsweet (*Filipendula ulmaria*) may be effective in reducing nausea and stomach acidity. Once the worst symptoms are relieved, slippery elm (*Ulmus fulva*) can help calm the digestive tract. Of the homeopathic remedies available, *Arsenicum album*, **ipecac**, or *Nux vomica* are three said to relieve the symptoms of gastroenteritis.

Probiotics, bacteria that are beneficial to a person's health, are recommended during the recovery phase of gastroenteritis. Specifically, live cultures of *Lactobacillus acidophilus* are said to be effective in soothing the digestive tract and returning the intestinal flora to normal. *L. acidophilus* is found in live-culture yogurt, as well as in capsule or powder form at health food stores. The use of probiotics is found in folk remedies and has some support in the medical literature. Castor oil packs to the abdomen can reduce inflammation and also reduce spasms or discomfort.

Prognosis

Gastroenteritis is usually resolved within two to three days and there are no long-term effects. If dehydration occurs, recovery is extended by a few days.

Prevention

There are few steps that can be taken to avoid gastroenteritis. Ensuring that food is well-cooked and unspoiled can prevent bacterial gastroenteritis, but may not be effective against viral gastroenteritis.

Resources

BOOKS

Craig SA, Zich DK. Gastroenteritis. In: Marx JA, ed. *Rosen's Emergency Medicine: Concepts and Clinical Practice, 7th ed.* Philadelphia, Pa: Mosby Elsevier; 2009: chap 92.

Sodha SV, Griffin PM, Hughes JM. Foodborne disease. In: Mandell GL, Bennett JE, Dolin R, eds. *Principles and Practice of Infectious Diseases, 7th ed.* Philadelphia, Pa: Elsevier Churchill Livingstone; 2009: chap 99.

Julia Barrett
Karl Finley

Gastroesophageal reflux disease

Definition

Gastroesophageal reflux disease (GERD) is a condition in which stomach acids and other stomach contents backflow into the esophagus, the tube leading from the mouth to the stomach, causing a burning sensation in the middle of the chest known as **heartburn**.

Gastroesophageal reflux disease (GERD) relief

Diet and lifestyle modifications:

- Eat smaller but more frequent meals
- Avoid common triggers (including tomato sauces, fried or spicy foods, alcohol, and caffeinated beverages)
- Lose excess weight
- Sleep with the head elevated
- Avoid eating before bed

Over-the-counter medications:

- Antacids (Tums*, Rolaids)
- OTC acid blockers (Pepcid AC, Prilosec OTC)

Prescription medications:

- Proton pump inhibitors (Nexium, Prevacid)
- Pro-motility drugs (Propulsid)
- Prescription-strength antacids (Carafate)
- Prescription-strength H2 blockers (Zantac, Tagamet)

*Drug names are provided as examples but are not meant to be recommendations or wholly representative of the treatments available.

SOURCE: The American College of Gastroenterology, "Heartburn or Gastroesophageal Reflux Disease (GERD)." Available online at: http://www.acg.gi.org/patients/women/whatisgerd.asp (accessed August 19, 2010).

(Table by PreMediaGlobal. Reproduced by permission of Gale, a part of Cengage Learning.)

Demographics

Estimates of the number of people in the United States with GERD may be significantly underreported because some people who experience heartburn self-treat through over-the-counter medications and are never officially diagnosed with GERD unless a more serious condition occurs. The American College of Gastroenterology estimates that about 60 million Americans experience heartburn at least once a month; of these, 15 million experience the condition daily. Other estimates suggest that 7% of the population has heartburn daily, and of these individuals, 20–40% have GERD, while heartburn in the remaining individuals arises from other causes. GERD occurs in all races and at all ages but is most common in people over age 40 years. Men and women are equally affected, although white men are ten times more likely to develop Barrett's esophagus (a precursor of **esophageal cancer**) than women.

Description

The mechanism behind GERD is a weakness in the lower esophageal sphincter (LES), causing stomach acids to back into the esophagus. The LES is a muscle located at the bottom of the esophagus that acts as a doorkeeper to the stomach. Normally, when food is

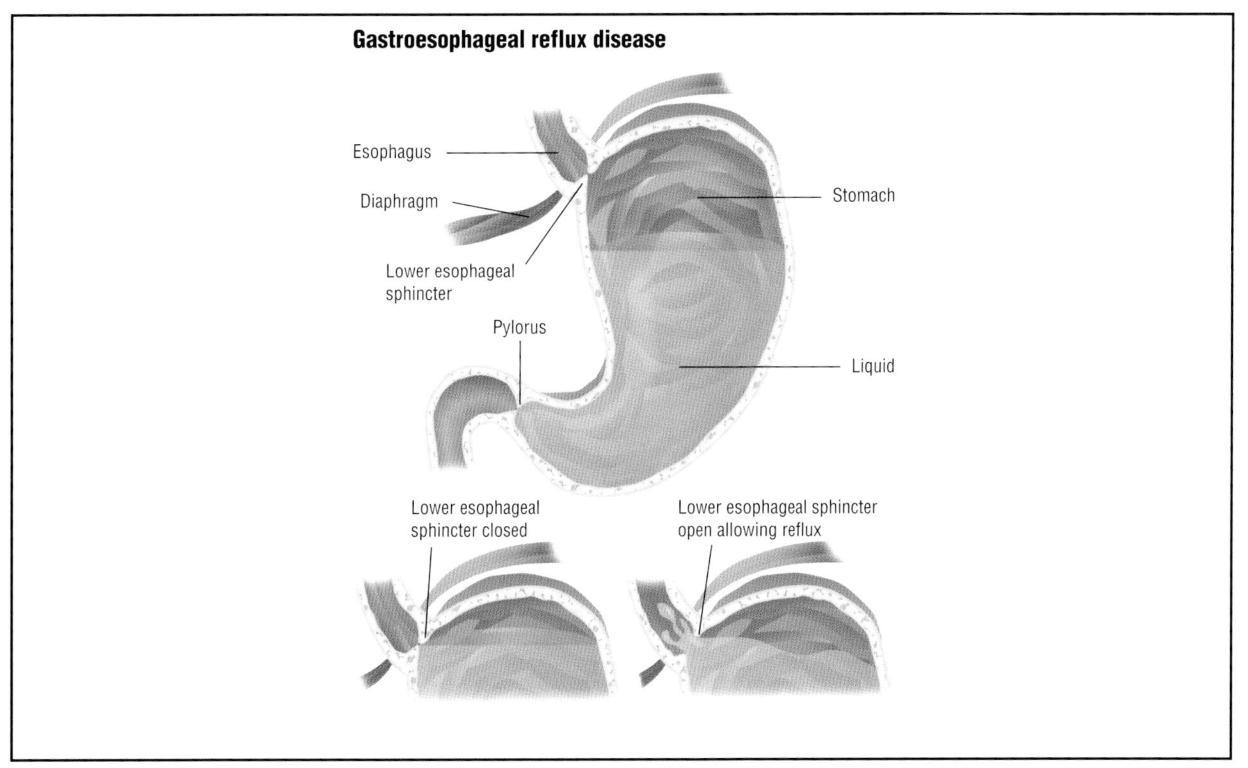

Normally, the lower esophageal sphincter keeps the stomach contents contained with the stomach (top). However, with gastroesophageal reflux disease, the sphincter opens, allowing the acidic contents to flow up the esophagus. *(Illustration by PreMediaGlobal. Reproduced by permission of Gale, a part of Cengage Learning.)*

eaten, it passes through the esophagus into the stomach, and the LES closes to keep the highly acidic stomach contents from washing back into the esophagus. Although a malfunctioning LES can be present from birth and can cause infants and children to complain of stomachaches and have frequent bouts of **vomiting**, GERD is most often seen in adults.

The esophagus risks being damaged every time stomach acids wash into it. Constant irritation by stomach acids can cause esophagitis, a condition in which the esophagus becomes red and irritated. Because the lining of the esophagus is thinner and less acid-resistant than the stomach or the intestines, untreated GERD over many years can cause ulcers to develop in the esophagus. These can bleed and can, in turn, result in anemia. Scar tissue can also build up.

The body may try to protect the esophagus by developing a thick lining made up of cells like those in the stomach and intestine. This is known as Barrett's esophagus and is a pre-cancerous condition that can lead to **cancer** of the esophagus.

Some people have trouble eating because there is a feeling that something is in their throats or that their food keeps getting stuck when they eat. This may be a serious condition called dysphagia, which develops from long-term GERD. It is a narrowing of the esophagus, caused by a thickening of the lining in response to acids from the stomach. When swallowing hurts, the condition is called odynophagia. This type of GERD often is referred to as silent reflux because no other symptoms are reported.

Everyone experiences heartburn occasionally, especially after overeating or eating fatty foods. Continued heartburn, though, can disrupt sleep. Moreover, if stomach acids keep bathing the esophagus, chronic inflammation of the lower esophagus can occur. In addition, if stomach material from the esophagus finds its way into the windpipe (trachea), it can enter the lungs, leading to **asthma** and **pneumonia**. For elderly individuals who are bedridden, aspiration of stomach contents can cause **choking**, infection, and even suffocation and **death**.

Causes and symptoms

Causes

Often, a structural abnormality called a **hiatal hernia** is the cause of constant reflux and GERD. In a hiatal hernia, a part of the stomach protrudes through a whole in the diaphragm (a sheet of muscle that separates the abdominal cavity from the chest cavity). This condition is more common in older individuals. Impaired motility in the stomach also can be a factor in GERD. In this case, the stomach nerves or muscles do not allow the stomach and the esophagus to contract normally, thereby allowing acid to build up in the esophagus. **Scleroderma**, a disease that causes muscular tissue to thicken, can affect digestive muscles and keep the LES open.

Lifestyle factors affect the development of GERD. Being overweight or pregnant increases abdominal pressure, and can cause the LES to remain open, thus allowing the stomach contents to squeeze into the esophagus. Wearing tight clothing around the abdomen, eating large meals, and lying down after eating can keep the LES open. Some foods may act as triggers for GERD, including chocolate, peppermint, high fat foods, citrus foods, tomato products, and onions. Smoking can stimulate acid production in the stomach and also can relax the LES. Consuming alcoholic, caffeinated, and carbonated drinks also can contribute to GERD.

Some medications have been linked to the development of GERD. They include high blood pressure medications such as **calcium channel blockers**, nitrate heart medications, asthma drugs such as theophylline, antidepressants, sedatives such as diazepam (Valium), and corticosteroid drugs. Nitrates in foods also may trigger GERD. Non-steroidal anti-inflammatory drugs (NSAIDs) such as **aspirin**, ibuprofen, and naproxen can irritate the stomach and lead to GERD.

Symptoms

Although heartburn is the characteristic symptom of GERD, people with this condition also may experience other symptoms. Regurgitation of stomach acid into the mouth (sometimes called water brash) is often present. Some individuals report abdominal pain, difficulty in swallowing, **nausea**, morning hoarseness, **sore throat**, coughing, **wheezing**, or a need to repeatedly clear the throat. Others experience **vomiting** or frequent burping or **hiccups**. A few note weight loss or **snoring**.

Some people do not experience noticeable symptoms. This is or milder forms of common GERD symptoms, but they experienced more instances of difficulty swallowing, vomiting, anemia, and weight loss. The study also found that abdominal pain and heartburn seemed to decrease with age and that GERD in the elderly most often was related to nonsteroidal anti-inflammatory drug (NSAID) use.

Having heartburn several times a week or waking up with heartburn at night is a good indicators that an appointment should be made for evaluation by a physician. If symptoms disturb sleep or interfere with work or leisure activities, a doctor should be consulted. Losing weight, breathing difficulties, vomiting blood, or has producing black, tarry stool, indicate that a doctor should be seen immediately. In addition, if an individual has been treated by a family physician for GERD for more than two years, a consultation with a gastroenterologist (a doctor specializing in diseases of the digestive system) usually is recommended.

Diagnosis

Examination

Because GERD is common, it often will be diagnosed after the doctor takes a thorough medical history, listens carefully for GERD symptoms, and does a **physical examination**. If the patient responds positively to treatment, no further tests are ordered. However, if the patient has serious symptoms such as intense pain, vomiting blood, or rapid weight loss, the doctor will investigate these through a series of tests. In addition, if the patient has been complaining of heartburn for a long time or has been treated for GERD for more than two years, other tests will likely be ordered to gauge the extent of damage done to the esophagus.

Procedures

The most common procedures are the upper gastrointestinal (GI) series and the upper GI **endoscopy**. The upper GI series examines the esophagus, stomach, and the duodenum (the first section of the small intestine). The patient drinks a cup of barium (barium swallow), a metallic, chalky liquid that coats the digestive track and makes it show up on x rays. X rays or images are then taken as the barium flows down the esophagus, into the stomach, and into the duodenum. The patient may be asked to turn to the side so that the technician can gently massage the stomach to move the barium into the duodenum. Images are sent to a video monitor where the doctors and technicians observe the behavior of the upper digestive tract and snap still images from the monitor.

The upper GI series can reveal anatomical changes in the esophagus, such as a hiatal hernia or esophageal narrowing. It also can assess damage to the esophagus, detect stomach ulcers or ulcers in the duodenum, and determine whether an intestinal blockage is present.

The upper GI endoscopy, also called the **esophagogastroduodenoscopy** (EGD), offers a more complete picture of what is happening in the upper digestive tract. It is the test of choice for many gastroenterologists.

Before the endoscopy, the patient receives a mild sedative, and then the doctor inserts a small, flexible tube down the patient's throat. At the end of the tube is a light, a tiny camera, and a small instrument used to take tissue samples (biopsies). The camera broadcasts live images from the esophagus and stomach to a video monitor. Using these tools, the doctor can capture still images for further diagnosis and can examine suspicious areas more closely with the camera or by taking tissue samples. The EGD allows the doctor to determine the extent of damage to the esophagus and to rule out serious complications such as Barrett's esophagus. Mild GERD may show no damage to the esophagus at all.

Another test, esophageal manometry, measures pressure within the esophagus and how well the LES functions. A thin tube is inserted through the nose and down the throat. Coupled with the 24-hour pH probe study, esophageal manometry becomes the best determinant of GERD because it monitors how often the patient has reflux into the esophagus during a full day. One episode of acid reflux is considered having a pH of less than 4.0 for at least 15–30 seconds. This test can determine if there is a correlation between episodes of acid reflux and other symptoms, such as chronic **cough**, wheezing, or **sleep apnea**.

To do a pH probe study, a small computer is attached to the outside end of the thin tube in the patient's nose, and the computer is worn around the waist or over the shoulder. The patient goes home, carries on a normal routine, then comes back to have the probe removed and the results analyzed.

A more comfortable form of the 24-hour pH probe study is the Bravo pH probe that is placed in the esophagus during endoscopy. This tiny probe transmits data to a miniature recorder the size of a paper clip that is worn around the waist. Eventually, the probe makes its way through the digestive system and is passed in the patient's stool in a week to ten days.

Sometimes, chest x rays are ordered to check for pneumonia or lung damage due to aspiration of stomach contents.

Treatment

The preferred treatments for GERD are lifestyle changes and drugs.

Lifestyle changes

Either prescribed alone or in combination with drug therapy, lifestyle changes can ease many GERD symptoms. Food choices, the timing of meals, and the size of meals are key lifestyle factors. Individuals should avoid foods that trigger GERD and eat smaller, more frequent meals. Doing so helps to control the amount of acid in the stomach. Individuals also should stop eating three hours before lying down. Lying down after eating can cause stomach contents to backflow into the esophagus. In addition, elevating the head of the bed about six inches may help keep acid within the stomach. Losing weight and avoiding slumping will reduce pressure on the stomach.

Drugs

Drugs often are prescribed along with lifestyle changes, even in the early stages of the disease. Commonly, the first medications prescribed are over-the-counter **antacids** and/or histamine-2 receptor blockers (H2 blockers). Antacids, such as Gaviscon, Tums, Maalox, and Mylanta, help neutralize acid already in the stomach or esophagus but do nothing to heal inflammation. Some have a foaming agent that helps prevent acid from backflowing into the esophagus. Unless otherwise instructed by a doctor, antacids can be used every day for three weeks. If taken longer, they can produce **diarrhea**, interfere with **calcium** absorption in the body, and increase levels of magnesium, which can damage the kidneys. Antacids are not recommended for individuals taking drugs to correct **hypothyroidism**.

Common H2 blockers are nizatidine (Axid), ranitidine (Zantac), famotidine (Pecid), and cimetidine (Tagamet). At half the strength of their prescription counterparts, these over-the-counter medications block acid production, but they have no effect on acid already present in the stomach. These drugs should be taken thirty minutes to one hour before meals. H2 blockers do not work as quickly as antacids, but they produce longer relief and are effective in reducing acid reflux at night. These drugs can heal mild esophageal damage but are not strong enough to heal serious injury. Standard dosage for 6–12 weeks has been found to relieve symptoms in half of GERD patients using H2 blockers.

If symptoms do not improve, proton-pump inhibitors (PPIs) may be given. PPIs can be bought without a prescription and, like H2 blockers, are also available in stronger strengths with a prescription. PPIs include esomeprazole (Nexium), omeprazole (Prilosec), lansoprazole (Prevacid), and rabeprazole (Aciphex). These drugs block the production of an enzyme that aids in acid formation. PPIs can reduce stomach acid by more than 95%. They are used to treat GERD and can heal some gastric and duodenal ulcers and prevent upper GI tract bleeding. PPIs are contraindicated for people with **liver disease** and may make the intestinal tract more susceptible to bacterial infections.

KEY TERMS

Calcium channel blocker—A drug that lowers blood pressure by regulating calcium-related electrical activity in the heart.

Dysphagia—Difficulty in swallowing, as if something is stuck in the throat.

Esophagogastroduodenoscopy (EGD)—A test that involves visually examining the lining of the esophagus, stomach, and upper duodenum with a flexible fiber-optic endoscope.

Esophagus—The muscular tube that leads from the back of the throat to the stomach. Coated with mucus and surrounded by muscles, it pushes food to the stomach by contraction.

Fundoplication—A surgical procedure that tightens the lower esophageal sphincter by stretching and wrapping the upper part of the stomach around the sphincter.

Gastroenterologist—A physician who specializes in diseases of the digestive system.

H2 Blockers—Medications used to treat some GERD symptoms, for example, Tagamet, Pepcid, Axid.

Heartburn—A burning sensation in the chest that can sometimes also be felt in the neck, throat, and face. It is the primary symptom of GERD.

Hiatal hernia—A condition in which part of the stomach protrudes above the diaphragm next to the esophagus.

Laparoscopic surgery—A minimally invasive surgery in which a camera and surgical instruments are inserted through a small incision.

Lower esophageal sphincter (LES)—A muscular ring at the base of the esophagus that keeps stomach contents from entering back into the esophagus.

Odynophagia—Pain felt when swallowing.

pH—A measure of the acidity of a fluid. On a scale of 1–14, a pH of 7 is neutral. Higher pH readings are alkaline and lower pH readings are acidic.

Silent reflux—An acid reflux problem that does not have marked symptoms but can cause chronic, recurrent respiratory symptoms much like asthma.

Sleep apnea—A sleep disorder in which breathing stop briefly then resumes on its own. These pauses can occur many times each night, resulting in poor quality sleep.

Water brash—The flow of saliva and stomach acid back up the esophagus and into the throat or lungs.

In addition to PPIs, the doctor may prescribe coating agents, such as sucralfate (Carfate), to cover the sores and mucous membranes of the esophagus and stomach. This acts as a protective barrier.

Some doctors also a prokinetic agent to tighten the LES and promote faster emptying of the stomach. Metaclopramide (Reglan) is the only prokinetic drug approved for use in the United States. Many doctors are reluctant to use prokinetic drugs because they have serious side effects.

Surgery

If all other treatments fail, surgery is a final option. A surgical procedure called fundoplication creates a one-way valve into the stomach. During surgery, the doctor wraps a part of the stomach around the esophagus and sews it down. This procedure can be done laparoscopically, a less invasive surgical method in which the doctor makes small cuts into the abdomen to insert a camera and the surgical instruments. Laparoscopic surgery produces very little scarring and has a faster recovery rate than traditional open surgery. However, the benefits of fundoplication have been challenged in some studies.

Certain endoscopy treatments can be used to repair the upper digestive tract instead of using surgery. Plication allows the doctor to stitch tears in the esophagus or narrow the LES. The Stretta procedure uses radiofrequency energy to cause the LES sphincter to tighten. The Enteryx procedure lets the doctor inject a bulking material into the LES to narrow it. As of 2010, these procedures were not widely available but were being used at some larger medical centers.

Alternative treatments

Alternative remedies include eating bananas or drinking chamomile or ginger tea. Chamomile should be avoided by people who have ragweed **allergies**. Some people eat licorice to balance the acid output in the stomach and to increase the mucous coating of the esophagus, but this is contraindicated for people with high blood pressure. Teas made from marsh mallow root, papaya, fennel, and catnip are also suggested treatments for heartburn, as well as eating papayas.

Homeopathic remedies most recommended are Nux vomica, Carbo vegetabilis, and Srsenicum album. **Acupuncture** and **acupressure** have also been used to treat heartburn.

Home Remedies

In addition to the lifestyle changes listed above, a common home remedy offering temporary relief is drinking water with sodium bicarbonate (baking soda) in it. However, this remedy can also add uncomfortable gas to the stomach, more sodium to the diet, which can increase blood pressure, and the excessive bicarbonate can produce rebound hyperacidity with worsening symptoms.

Prognosis

In most cases, GERD is easily managed. Between 80% and 90% of individuals improve with drug therapy. However, the length of treatment varies. Some patients may not see improvement for several weeks or months. Some patients can experience relief after two to three months of treatment and are able to modify their lifestyle to minimize symptoms so that medications are reduced or discontinued. Many patients with serious, persistent GERD may need to take medications for the rest of their lives.

Even with successful treatment, some patients experience acid breakthrough. This response occurs when symptoms appear even though the patient has faithfully taken medications. Some patients on PPIs may be symptom free during the day but wake up at night with heartburn. Sometimes, an H2 blocker is given to the patient at night in addition to PPI medications. Some patients on H2 blockers may benefit from a combination pill that contains an antacid and an H2 blocker.

Untreated GERD can lead to the development of Barrett's esophagus. Barrett's is a pre-cancerous condition. Many times it can be reversed with proper treatment of GERD.

Prevention

Symptoms of GERD can be prevented by taking drugs as prescribed, avoiding alcohol, not **smoking**, eating smaller meals, limiting fatty foods, and eliminating trigger foods. Individuals should avoid belts and tight clothing around the waist and try to lose excess weight. Individuals may chew gum or suck on hard candies to increase saliva production, which can sooth the esophagus and wash the acid back to the stomach. People with heartburn should wait two hours after eating before exercising and plan not to eat anything at least three hours before lying down. Finally, elevating the head of the bed at least six inches and sleeping on the left side may reduce nighttime heartburn.

Resources

BOOKS

Burns, David L. and Neeral L. Shah. *100 Questions & Answers About Gastroesophageal Reflux Disease (GERD)*. Sudbury, MA: Jones and Bartlett Publishers, 2007

Wendland, Barbara E., and Lisa Marie Ruffolo. *Chronic Heartburn: Managing Acid Reflux and GERD Through Understanding, Diet, and Lifestyle*. Toronto, Ontario, Canada: Robert Rose, 2006.

PERIODICALS

Wellbery, Caroline. "GERD Symptoms Differ with Patient Age." *American Family Physician* (March 15, 2007): 906.

OTHER

Gastroesophageal Reflux in Children and Adolescents. National Digestive Diseases Information Clearinghouse. August 2006. http://digestive.niddk.nih.gov/ddiseases/pubs/gerinchildren

GERD. MedlinePlus February 4, 2010. http://www.nlm.nih.gov/medlineplus/gerd.html

The Word on GERD. American College of Gastroenterology. Undated [accessed February 7, 2010]. http://www.acg.gi.org/patients/gerd/word.asp

ORGANIZATIONS

American College of Gastrolenterology (ACG), P.O. Box 34226, Bethesda, MD, 20827-2260, (301) 263-9000, http://www.acg.gi.org.

American Gastroenterological Association (AGA), 4930 Del Ray Avenue, Bethesda, MD, 20814, (310) 654-2055, (301) 654-5920, www.gastro.org.

International Foundation for Functional Gastrointestinal Disorders, P. O. Box 170864, MilwaukeeWI, USA, 53217-8076, (414) 964-1799, (USA only) (888) 964-2001, (414) 964-7176, iffgdiffgd.org, http://www.iffgd.org.

National Digestive Diseases Information Clearinghouse (NDDIC)., 2 Information Way, Bethesda, MD, 20892-3570, (800) 891-5389; TTY (866) 569-1162 , (703) 738-4929, info@niddk.nih.gov, http://digestive.niddk.nih.gov.

Janie F. Franz
Tish Davidson, AM

Gastrointestinal bleeding studies *see* **GI bleeding studies**

Gastrointestinal study *see* **Liver nuclear medicine scan**

Gastrojejunostomy *see* **Ulcer surgery**

Gastroschisis *see* **Abdominal wall defects**

Gastrostomy

Definition

Gastrostomy is a surgical procedure for inserting a tube through the abdomen wall and into the stomach. The tube is used for feeding or drainage.

Purpose

Gastrostomy is performed because a patient temporarily or permanently needs to be fed directly through a tube in the stomach. Reasons for feeding by gastrostomy include **birth defects** of the mouth, esophagus, or stomach, and problems sucking or swallowing.

Gastrostomy is also performed to provide drainage for the stomach when it is necessary to bypass a long-standing obstruction of the stomach outlet into the small intestine. Obstructions may be caused by peptic ulcer scarring or a tumor.

Precautions

Gastrostomy is a relatively simple procedure. As with any surgery, patients are more likely to experience complications if they are smokers, obese, use alcohol heavily, or use illicit drugs. In addition, some prescription medications may increase risks associated with anesthesia.

Description

Gastrostomy, also called gastrostomy tube insertion, is surgery performed by a general surgeon to give an external opening into the stomach. Surgery is performed either when the patient is under general anesthesia–where the patient feels as if he is in a deep sleep and has no awareness of what is happening–or under **local anesthesia**. With local anesthesia, the patient is awake, but the part of the body cut during the operation is numbed.

A small incision is made on the left side of the abdomen; then, an incision is made through the stomach. A small, flexible, hollow tube, usually made of polyvinylchloride or rubber, is inserted into the stomach. The stomach is stitched closed around the tube, and the incision is closed. The procedure is performed at a hospital or free-standing surgery center.

The length of time the patient needs to remain in the hospital depends on the age of the patient and the patient's general health. In some cases, the hospital stay can be as short as one day, but often is longer. Normally, the stomach and abdomen heal in five to seven days.

The cost of the surgery varies, depending on the age and health of the patient. Younger, sicker patients require more intensive, thus more expensive, care.

Preparation

Prior to the operation, the doctor will perform **endoscopy** and take x rays of the gastrointestinal tract. Blood and urine tests will also be performed, and the patient may meet with the anesthesiologist to evaluate any special conditions that might affect the administration of anesthesia.

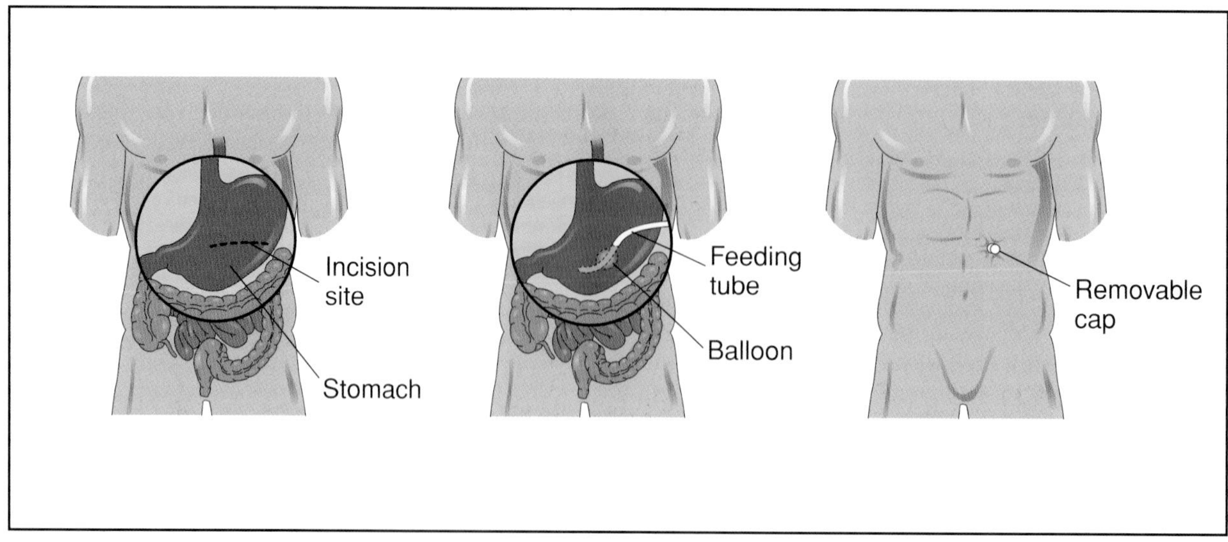

Gastrostomy is a procedure in which the surgeon makes an opening into the stomach and inserts a feeding tube for feeding or for drainage. *(Illustration by Electronic Illustrators Group. Reproduced by permission of Gale, a part of Cengage Learning.)*

KEY TERMS

Endoscopy—A procedure in which an instrument containing a camera is inserted into the gastrointestinal tract so that the doctor can visually inspect the gastrointestinal system.

Aftercare

Immediately after the operation, the patient is fed intravenously for at least 24 hours. Once bowel sounds are heard, indicating that the gastrointestinal system is working, the patient can begin clear liquid feedings through the tube. Gradually feedings are increased.

Patient education concerning use and care of the gastrostomy tube is very important. Patients and their families are taught how to recognize and prevent infection around the tube, how to feed through the tube, how to handle tube blockage, what to do if the tube pulls out, and what normal activities can be continued.

Risks

There are few risks associated with this surgery. The main complications are infection, bleeding, dislodgment of the tube, stomach bloating, **nausea**, and **diarrhea**.

Normal results

The patient is able to eat through the gastrostomy tube, or the stomach can be drained through the tube.

Resources

OTHER

"Stomach Tube Insertion." HealthAnswers.com. www.healthanswers.com.

Tish Davidson, A.M.

Gaucher disease

Definition

Gaucher disease is a rare genetic disorder that results in accumulation of fatty molecules called cerebrosides. It can have serious effects on numerous body organs including the liver, spleen, bones and central nervous system. Treatments based on molecular biology are becoming available, but are very expensive.

Description

Gaucher disease was first described by the French physician Philippe Gaucher in 1882. It is the most common of a class of diseases called lysosomal storage diseases, each of which is characterized by the accumulation of a specific chemical substance (a different substance depending on the exact disease). Gaucher disease is characterized by a wide array of different symptoms and the severity of the disease ranges from undetectable to lethal.

Three forms of the disease are recognized: Types I, II and III. Type I is by far the most common and shows the mildest symptoms. It is non-neuronopathic, meaning that the nervous system is not attacked. The onset of Type I can occur at any age in childhood or adult life with the average age of onset at about 21 years. Some affected individuals are have no symptoms throughout adult life. Type II, the infantile form, accounts for less than 1% of patients with Gaucher disease. It is neuronopathic (attacks the nervous system); nervous system effects are severe, and victims often die within the first year of life. Type III most often has its onset during childhood and has some of the features of both the adult and infantile forms. This affects less than 5% of persons with Gaucher disease.

Gaucher disease is caused by the absence, or near absence, of activity of an enzyme called glucocerebrosidase (GC). The normal action of GC is to break down a common molecule called glucocerebroside. If not broken down, glucocerebroside accumulates in certain cells to levels that can cause damage, especially in the spleen, liver, and bone. The common link among these organs is that they house a cell type called a macrophage. A macrophage is a large cell that surrounds and consumes a foreign substance (such as bacteria) in the body. The cellular structures in which glucocerebroside accumulates are called lysosomes.

The three forms of Gaucher disease also differ in their population genetics. Type I is most common in persons of eastern European (Ashkenazi) Jewish descent. Among this population, the disease occurs at a rate of one in 450 live births and about one in 10 to 15 persons are carriers, making it the most common genetic disease affecting Jewish people. The other two types are equally frequent in all ethnic groups. Type II occurs at a rate of one in 100,000 live births, while Type III is estimated to occur in one in 50,000 live births.

Causes and symptoms

Lack of the GC enzyme is caused by a mutation in the glucocerebrosidase gene. The gene is located on chromosome 1. There have been more than 100 mutations described in this gene that causes Gaucher disease. Gaucher disease is inherited in an autosomal recessive pattern. This means that two defective gene copies must be inherited, one from each parent, for the disease to manifest itself. Persons with only one gene mutation are carriers for the disorder. A person who is a carrier for Gaucher disease does not have any symptoms and does not know he or she is a carrier unless he or she has had specific testing. When both parents are carriers for Gaucher disease, there is a one in four chance (25%) in each **pregnancy** for a child to have Gaucher disease. There is a two in three chance that a healthy sibling of an affected child is a carrier.

The results of Gaucher disease are widespread in the body and include excessive growth of the liver and spleen (hepatosplenomegaly), weakening of bones, and, in acute cases, severe nervous system damage. Many patients experience "bone crises," which are episodes of extreme **pain** in their bones.

There is a wide array of other problems that occur with Gaucher disease, such as anemia (fewer than normal red blood cells). Just how these other symptoms are caused is not known. Nor is it known why some patients have very mild disease and others have much more significant problems. Even identical twins with the disease can have differing symptoms.

Diagnosis

Diagnosis of Gaucher disease, based initially on the symptoms described above, can be confirmed by microscopic, enzymatic, and molecular tests. Biopsy (surgical removal of tissue from a problem area) of tissue is helpful for microscopic diagnosis. When biopsy tissue is examined under the microscope, cells will appear swollen and will show characteristic features of the cytoplasm (part of the cell body along with the nucleus) and nucleus. Enzyme tests will show deficiency (<30% of normal levels) of the enzyme GC. Molecular analysis of DNA samples looking at four of the more common mutations will show defects in the gene for GC in 95% of Ashkenazi Jewish individuals and in 75% of non-Jewish people. Diagnosis can be performed prenatally (before birth) if the parents' mutations are known using **amniocentesis** or **chorionic villus sampling**.

Diagnosis as to which of the three types of Gaucher disease an individual has is based on the symptoms, rather than on test results.

Treatment

Until the 1990s, only supportive therapy could be offered. **Analgesics** are used to control pain. Orthopedic treatment is used for bone **fractures**. In some cases, surgical removal of the spleen may be necessary. Several treatments for anemia have been used, including vitamin and iron supplements, blood transfusions, and bone marrow transplants.

The newest form of treatment for Gaucher disease is enzyme replacement therapy, in which GC can be administered intravenously. The enzyme can be prepared either by purification from placentas (alglucerase) or by recombinant DNA manufacturing techniques (imiglucerase). Either way, the cost of treatment ranges from $100,000 to $400,000 per year, which can prevent many from obtaining treatment.

Enzyme replacement is effective at reducing most Gaucher symptoms. The notable exception is neurologic damage in Type II disease, which remains unimproved by this treatment. This treatment is not recommended for individuals who are asymptomatic. The efficacy for the treatment of Type III Gaucher disease is not known. Many questions remain about enzyme replacement therapy in regard to dosage, and method and frequency of administration. The treatment program should be individualized for each patient.

Prognosis

A patient's expected lifespan varies greatly with the type of Gaucher disease. Infants with Type II disease have a life span of one to four years. Patients with Types I and III of the disease have highly variable outcomes with some patients dying in childhood and others living full lives. Little is known about the reasons for this variability.

Prevention

Genetic counseling is advised for individuals with Gaucher disease and for their relatives to accurately assess risk and discuss testing options. For couples who previously had a child with Gaucher or in situations

KEY TERMS

Cerebrosides—Fatty carbohydrates that occur in the brain and nervous system.

Enzymatic replacement therapy—A treatment method used to replace missing enzymes. It is possible to synthesize enzymes and then inject them intravenously into patients.

Glucocerebroside—A cerebroside that contains glucose in the molecule.

where both parents are carriers for known Gaucher mutations, prenatal diagnosis is available to determine whether a pregnancy is affected. Families in which a person has been diagnosed with Gaucher disease can have DNA testing, which enables other relatives to determine their carrier status. Prospective parents can then use that information to conduct family planning or to prepare for a child who may have special circumstances.

Families in which both parents are known to be a carrier of a mutation for Gaucher disease could consider preimplantation genetic diagnosis. This relatively new procedure can select an embryo without both Gaucher disease mutations prior to implantation of the embryo into the uterus. This technique is only available at selected genetics centers.

As of the early 2000s, population screening for Gaucher disease is not standard of care.

Resources

OTHER

"Cerezyme." Genzyme Therapeutics. http://www.cerezyme.com.

"Gaucher Disease: Current Issues in Diagnosis and Treatment." http://text.nlm.nih.gov/nih/ta/www/16.html.

National Foundation for Jewish Genetic Diseases (NFJGD). http://www.nfjgd.org.

ORGANIZATIONS

Children's Gaucher Research Fund, 8110 Warren Court, Granite Bay, CA, 95746, (916) 797-3700, (916) 797-3707, research@childrensgaucher.org, http://www.childrensgaucher.org.

Genetic Alliance, Inc., 4301 Connecticut Ave., NW, Suite 404, Washington, DC, 20008-2369, (202) 966-5557, (202) 966-8553, info@geneticalliance.org, http://www.geneticalliance.org.

National Gaucher Foundation, 2227 Idlewood Road, Suite 6, Tucker, GA, 30084, (770) 934-2911, (800) 504-3189, ngf@gaucherdisease.org, http://www.gaucherdisease.org.

National Organization for Rare Disorders, P.O. Box 8923, New Fairfield, CT, 06812-8923, (800) 999-6673, http://www.rarediseases.org.

Amy Vance, MS, CGC

Gay and lesbian health

Definition

Lesbian, gay, bisexual, and transgender (LGBT) individuals are as diverse as the general population in terms of race, ethnicity, age, religion, education, income, and family history. A number of health concerns are unique to or shared by the LGBT community, however, including an increased risk of certain cancers, infectious and **sexually transmitted diseases** (STDs), and mental health disorders, issues relating to **nutrition** and weight, tobacco use, and **substance abuse**, and discrimination by health care and insurance providers.

Description

The definitions of different sexual identities have shifted over the years, as have the perceptions and stereotypes of the general population. Because of the wide range of behaviors and identities that exist in the LGBT community, it is difficult to develop an inclusive definition. It is generally accepted, however, that gay men and lesbians are sexually attracted to or participate in sexual behaviors with individuals of the same gender, while bisexual men and women are sexually attracted to or participate in sexual behaviors with individuals of both genders. Transgender individuals live part or full-time in a gender role opposite to their genetic sex.

Estimates suggest that approximately 2.8% of men and 1.4% of women identify as being gay, lesbian, or bisexual while 9.1% of men and 4.3% of women have participated in sexual behavior with someone of the same gender at least once. The true extent of the transgender community has not been well researched in the United States. Note that estimates of the LGBT community are based on self-reported information and actual rates may be higher.

Certain issues arise when trying to define sexual orientation. Many gay men and lesbians have participated in or continue to participate in sexual activities with members of the opposite sex but choose not to identify as heterosexuals or bisexuals. Others have never participated in sexual activities at all yet still identify as gay, lesbian, or bisexual. Some men and women identifying as bisexuals are in long-term, monogamous relationships with individuals of the same or opposite sex. Male-to-female (MTF) or female-to-male (FTM) transgender individuals may or may not identify themselves as gay or lesbian.

The implications of these identity issues are far-reaching. Misdiagnoses or improper medical recommendations might be made by health care providers who have mistakenly assumed sexual behaviors or risks from the patient's stated identity. For example, a provider might incorrectly assume that a lesbian patient has never had sexual intercourse with a male and therefore would not have contracted STDs. It has been difficult to closely estimate the numbers of LGBT individuals in the United States because of varying definitions. Likewise, the statistics in medical or social studies and surveys on LGBT issues might vary widely depending on what definitions were provided for the respondents. Because of this, many researchers have opted for the more inclusive terms of "men who have sex with men" (MSM) and "women who have sex with women" (WSW) to categorize gay, lesbian, and bisexual respondents.

Important health care issues

Many LGBT individuals have difficulty revealing their sexual identity ("coming out") to their health care providers. They may fear discrimination from providers or believe that their confidentiality might be breached. In some cases health care workers have been poorly trained to address the needs of LGBT individuals, have difficulty communicating with their LGBT patient, or feel uncomfortable providing care for LGBT patients. In addition, many questions posed in questionnaires or examinations are heterosexually biased (e.g., asking a lesbian which birth control methods she uses).

Other reasons why LGBT individuals are often hesitant to share their sexual identity are more logistical. Many insurance companies deny benefits to long-term partners on the basis that they are not married. LGBT patients may have inadequate access to health care, either because they live in a remote rural area or in the crowded inner city. Some same-sex partners encounter discrimination in hospitals and clinics when they are denied the rights usually given to spouses of a patient such as visiting, making medical decisions, and participating in consultations with physicians.

Some of the health concerns and risk factors that are relevant to LGBT individuals may be shared by the general population, while others are more specific to the LGBT community, and still others are specific to different subgroups of LGBT individuals. These health concerns may be grouped into the following areas of concern:

- Sexual behavior issues: STDs such as human immunodeficiency virus (HIV) and acquired immune deficiency syndrome (AIDS), hepatitis A virus (HAV), hepatitis B virus (HBV), bacterial vaginosis, gonorrhea, chlamydia, and genital warts (human papillomavirus or HPV); anal, ovarian, and cervical cancer.
- Cultural issues: body image, nutrition, weight, and eating disorders; drug and alcohol abuse; tobacco use; parenting and family planning.
- Discrimination issues: inadequate medical care; harassment at work, school, or home; difficulty in obtaining housing, insurance coverage, or child custody; violence.
- Sexual identity issues: conflicts with family, friends, and work mates; psychological issues such as anxiety, depression, and suicide; economic hardship.

CANCER. Cancer is the second leading cause of **death** (after heart disease) in the United States. In 2008, it was estimated that about 1.4 million individuals were diagnosed with cancer and about 565,600 lost their lives as a result. LGBT individuals are at an increased risk for certain types of cancers.

Several studies indicated that lesbians appear to have a higher risk for developing uterine, breast, cervical, endometrial, and ovarian cancers This is partially related to higher rates of risk factors such as **obesity**, alcohol use, tobacco use, and nulliparity (not bearing children). Lesbians are less likely than heterosexual women to visit a doctor for routine Pap screening that can detect **cervical cancer**. Lesbians also have additional risk of developing **ovarian cancer**, due to inadequate access to health care, nulliparity, and not using **oral contraceptives** (use of oral contraceptives has been shown to decrease the risk of getting ovarian cancer).

Gay and bisexual men (or more generally, men who have sex with men [MSM]) are at higher risk of developing non-Hodgkin's lymphoma, Hodgkin's disease, and **anal cancer**. **Kaposi's sarcoma**, an AIDS-associated cancer, are also found in the gay community at rates higher than the general population. Anal cancer is associated with transmission of human papillomavirus (HPV), and the risk factors associated with MSM are also associated with increased rates of anal cancer (i.e. **smoking**, having many sexual partners, and receiving anal intercourse).

AIDS. The United States Centers for Disease Control and Prevention (CDC) estimated that in 2006, 944,000 people in the United States had been diagnosed with **AIDS** since the disease was identified in 1981. In 2006, an additional 1–1.2 million Americans were diagnosed as infected with HIV but not yet showing symptoms (HIV positive). However, in early 2009, the CDC issued a statement that they now thought that earlier the HIV-positive estimates were too low, as many more people than were originally estimated are living with unreported or undiagnosed HIV infection. More than 70% of HIV infections are transmitted through sexual contact. Traditionally in the United States, the majority of cases were found in homosexual

KEY TERM

Nulliparity—The condition of being nulliparous, or not bearing offspring.

or bisexual men. In 2007, about half of new HIV cases were acquired by men having sex with other men.

PSYCHIATRIC DISORDERS. In 1973, the American Psychiatric Association removed homosexuality from their list of mental disorders. Nevertheless, American society has been slow to fully accept of members of the LGBT community. As a result, members of this community often find themselves rejected by their families, socially stigmatized for their sexual orientation, treated unequally by laws and the justice system, and subject to physical and emotional **abuse** for their lifestyles. These pressures, plus the continuing **stress** caused by the need some LGBT individuals feel to conceal their sexual orientation from family, LGBT employers, and larger society lead to an increased occurrence of depressive illness, **anxiety disorders**, and drug and alcohol abuse.

NUTRITION AND BODY IMAGE. Diet and nutritional factors are associated with a number of diseases including cancer, **stroke**, diabetes, heart disease, and **osteoporosis**. It has been shown that lesbians are more likely than heterosexual women to be obese, have a higher body mass index (BMI), have a nutritionally poorer diet, and have higher rates of smoking and alcohol use, but they are also more likely to have a healthier body image than heterosexual women. Gay men and adolescents, on the other hand, have been shown to have increased rates of eating disorder behaviors than heterosexual men (e.g. **anorexia nervosa**, bulimia, and **binge eating**) and a poorer body image.

DRUG, ALCOHOL, AND TOBACCO USE. Marijuana and **cocaine** use has been shown to be higher among lesbians than heterosexual women. The incidence of the use of some drugs is higher in gay men than heterosexual men; these include marijuana, psychedelic drugs, ecstasy, **barbiturates**, and stimulants such as amyl or butyl nitrate ("poppers"). Although alcohol use has declined in the LGBT community since the 1990s, the rate is still higher among young LGBT individuals.

Cigarette smoking is responsible for 430,000 deaths a year in the United States, with an estimated 3,000 nonsmokers dying as a result of exposure to secondhand smoke. In 2004 the rate of smoking among all adults was 28%. In contrast, 50% of gay men, lesbians and bisexuals were noted to be smokers. Lesbians are more than two times as likely to become heavy smokers than heterosexual women.

Prevention

There are numerous ways that health care providers can improve the access to and experience of health care services for LGBT individuals. These include:

- rewording questionnaires and examinations to be inclusive of LGBT patients
- providing referrals to social service agencies and counseling services that are LGBT-friendly
- taking educational courses that are sensitive to the needs of LGBT patients
- treating the families of LGBT patients as one would the families of heterosexual patients
- maintaining the strictest code of confidentiality
- developing and maintaining health care centers or clinics that address LGBT-specific needs
- asking non-threatening questions to determine if a person is at risk of an STD
- educating patients of risk factors associated with STDs, possible vaccines, and treatments available
- providing services to individuals in the process of disclosing their sexual identity and, if applicable, their families

Resources

BOOKS

Makadon, Harvey J., et al. eds. *The Fenway Guide to Lesbian, Gay, Bisexual, and Transgender Health*. Philadelphia: American College of Physicians, 2008.

Spinelli, Frank. *The Advocate Guide to Gay Men's Health and Wellness*. New York: Alyson Books, 2008.

OTHER

"Gay, Lesbian and Transgender Health." *MedlinePlus*. January 12, 2009 [cited February 25, 2009]. http://www.nlm.nih.gov/medlineplus/gaylesbianandtransgenderhealth.html

"Lesbian Health." *WomensHealth.gov*. January 1, 2005 [cited February 25, 2009]. http://womenshealth.gov/faq/lesbian-health.cfm

"Sexual Orientation." *American Psychiatric Association*. [cited October 18, 2010]. http://healthyminds.org/More-Info-For/GayLesbianBisexuals.aspx

ORGANIZATIONS

Gay and Lesbian Medical Association, 459 Fulton Street, Suite 107, San Francisco, CA, (415) 255-4547, (415) 255-4784, info@glma.org, http://www.glma.org.

Parents, Familes and Friends of Lesbians and Gays (PFLAG), 1726 M Street NW, Suite 400, Washington, DC, 20036, (202) 467-8180, (202) 467-8194, info@pflag.org, http://community.pflag.org.

Stéphanie Dionne
Teresa G. Odle
Tish Davidson, A. M.

Gender identity disorder

Definition

The psychological diagnosis gender identity disorder (GID) is used to describe a male or female that feels a strong identification with the opposite sex and experiences considerable distress because of their actual sex.

Description

Gender identity disorder can affect children, adolescents, and adults. Individuals with gender identity disorder have strong cross-gender identification. They believe that they are, or should be, the opposite sex. They are uncomfortable with their sexual role and organs and may express a desire to alter their bodies. While not all persons with GID are labeled as transsexuals, there are those who are determined to undergo sex change procedures or have done so, and, therefore, are classified as transsexual. They often attempt to pass socially as the opposite sex. Transsexuals alter their physical appearance cosmetically and hormonally, and may eventually undergo a sex-change operation.

Children with gender identity disorder refuse to dress and act in sex-stereotypical ways. It is important to remember that many emotionally healthy children experience fantasies about being a member of the opposite sex. The distinction between these children and gender identity disordered children is that the latter experience significant interference in functioning because of their cross-gender identification. They may become severely depressed, anxious, or socially withdrawn.

Causes and symptoms

The cause of gender identity disorder is not known. It has been theorized that a prenatal hormonal imbalance may predispose individuals to the disorder. Problems in the individual's family interactions or family dynamics have also been postulated as having some causal impact.

KEY TERMS

Cross-dressing—Dressing in clothing that is stereotypical of the opposite sex.

Gender identity disorder (GID)—A strong and lasting cross-gender identification and persistent discomfort with one's biological gender (sex) role. This discomfort must cause a significant amount of distress or impairment in the functioning of the individual.

Transsexual—A person with gender identity disorder who has an overwhelming desire to change anatomic sex; one who seeks hormonal or surgical treatment to change sex.

The *Diagnostic and Statistical Manual of Mental Disorders*, Fourth Edition (*DSM-IV*), the diagnostic reference standard for United States mental health professionals, describes the criteria for gender identity disorder as an individual's strong and lasting cross-gender identification and their persistent discomfort with their biological gender role. This discomfort must cause a significant amount of distress or impairment in the functioning of the individual.

DSM-IV specifies that children must display at least four of the following symptoms of cross-gender identification for a diagnosis of gender identity disorder:

- a repeatedly stated desire to be, or insistence that he or she is, the opposite sex
- a preference for cross-dressing
- a strong and lasting preference to play make-believe and role-playing games as a member of the opposite sex or persistent fantasies that he or she is the opposite sex
- a strong desire to participate in the stereotypical games of the opposite sex
- a strong preference for friends and playmates of the opposite sex

Diagnosis

Gender identity disorder is typically diagnosed by a psychiatrist or psychologist, who conducts an interview with the patient and takes a detailed social history. Family members may also be interviewed during the assessment process. This evaluation usually takes place in an outpatient setting.

Treatment

Treatment for children with gender identity disorder focuses on treating secondary problems such as depression and **anxiety**, and improving self-esteem. Treatment may also work on instilling positive identifications with the child's biological gender. Children typically undergo psychosocial therapy sessions; their parents may also be referred for family or individual therapy.

Transsexual adults often request hormone and surgical treatments to suppress their biological sex characteristics and acquire those of the opposite sex. A team of health professionals, including the treating psychologist or psychiatrist, medical doctors, and several surgical specialists, oversee this transitioning process. Because of the irreversible nature of the surgery, candidates for sex-change surgery are evaluated extensively and are often required to spend a period of time integrating themselves into the cross-gender role before the procedure begins. Counseling and peer support are also invaluable to transsexual individuals.

Prognosis

Long-term follow up studies have shown positive results for many transsexuals who have undergone sex-change surgery. However, significant social, personal, and occupational issues may result from surgical sex changes, and the patient may require **psychotherapy** or counseling.

Resources

OTHER

The National Transgender Guide. http://www.tgguide.com.

ORGANIZATIONS

American Academy of Child and Adolescent Psychiatry (AACAP), 3615 Wisconsin Ave. NW, Washington, DC, 20013-3007, (202) 966-7300, (202) 966-2891, communications@aacap.org, http://www.aacap.org.

Paula Anne Ford-Martin

Gender reassignment surgery *see* **Sex reassignment surgery**

Gene therapy

Gene therapy is a rapidly growing field of medicine in which genes are introduced into the body to treat diseases. Genes control heredity and provide the basic biological code for determining a cell's specific functions. Gene therapy seeks to provide genes that correct or supplant the disease-controlling functions of cells that are not, in essence, doing their job. Somatic gene therapy introduces therapeutic genes at the tissue or cellular level to treat a specific individual. Germ-line gene therapy inserts genes into reproductive cells or possibly into embryos to correct genetic defects that could be passed on to future generations. Initially conceived as an approach for treating inherited diseases, like **cystic fibrosis** and Huntington's disease, the scope of potential gene therapies has grown to include treatments for cancers, arthritis, and infectious diseases. Although gene therapy testing in humans has advanced rapidly, many questions surround its use. For example, some scientists are concerned that the therapeutic genes themselves may cause disease. Others fear that germ-line gene therapy may be used to control human development in ways not connected with disease, like intelligence or appearance.

The biological basis of gene therapy

Gene therapy has grown out of the science of genetics or how heredity works. Scientists know that life begins in a cell, the basic building block of all multicellular organisms. Humans, for instance, are made up of trillions of cells, each performing a specific function. Within the cell's nucleus (the center part of a cell that regulates its chemical functions) are pairs of chromosomes. These threadlike structures are made up of a single molecule of DNA (deoxyribonucleic acid), which carries the blueprint of life in the form of codes, or genes, that determine inherited characteristics.

A DNA molecule looks like two ladders with one of the sides taken off both and then twisted around each other. The rungs of these ladders meet (resulting in a spiral staircase-like structure) and are called base pairs. Base pairs are made up of nitrogen molecules and arranged in specific sequences. Millions of these base pairs, or sequences, can make up a single gene, specifically defined as a segment of the chromosome and DNA that contains certain hereditary information. The gene, or combination of genes formed by these base pairs ultimately direct an organism's growth and characteristics through the production of certain chemicals, primarily proteins, which carry out most of the body's chemical functions and biological reactions.

Scientists have long known that alterations in genes present within cells can cause inherited diseases like cystic fibrosis, sickle-cell anemia, and **hemophilia**. Similarly, errors in the total number of chromosomes can cause conditions such as **Down syndrome** or **Turner syndrome**. As the study of genetics advanced, however, scientists learned that an altered genetic sequence can

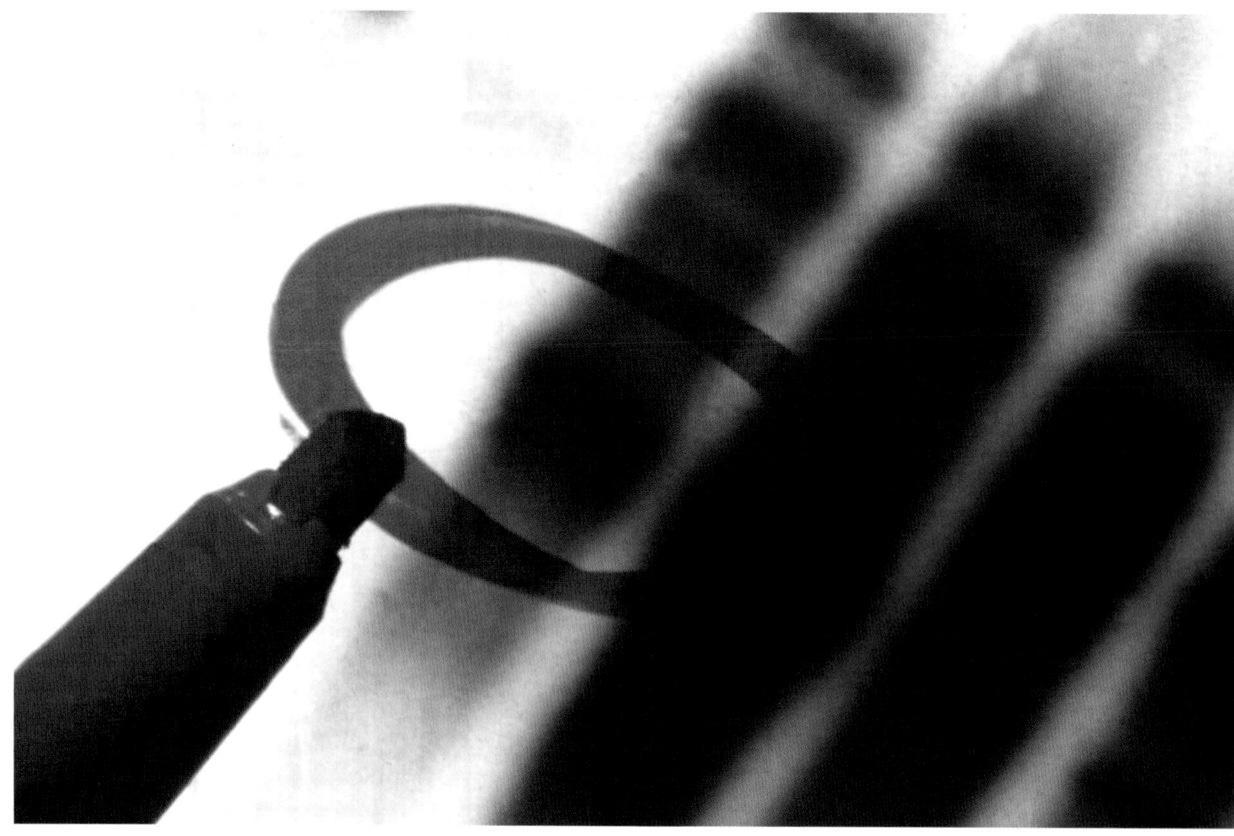

Early detection of cancer. The researcher's pen marks a band on a DNA sequencing autogradiogram confirming a bladder cancer. *(Custom Medical Stock Photo, Inc. Reproduced by permission.)*

also make people more susceptible to diseases, like **atherosclerosis**, **cancer**, and even **schizophrenia**. These diseases have a genetic component, but are also influenced by environmental factors (such as diet and lifestyle). The objective of gene therapy is to treat diseases by introducing functional genes into the body to alter the cells involved in the disease process by either replacing missing genes or providing copies of functioning genes to replace nonfunctioning ones. The inserted genes can be naturally occurring genes that produce the desired effect or may be genetically engineered (or altered) genes.

Scientists have known how to manipulate a gene's structure in the laboratory since the early 1970s through a process called gene splicing. The process involves removing a fragment of DNA containing the specific genetic sequence desired then inserting it into the DNA of another gene. The resultant product is called recombinant DNA and the process is genetic engineering.

There are basically two types of gene therapy. Germ-line gene therapy introduces genes into reproductive cells (sperm and eggs) or someday possibly into embryos in hopes of correcting genetic abnormalities that could be passed on to future generations. Most of the current work in applying gene therapy, however, has been in the realm of somatic gene therapy. In this type of gene therapy, therapeutic genes are inserted into tissue or cells to produce a naturally occurring protein or substance that is lacking or not functioning correctly in an individual patient.

Viral vectors

In both types of therapy, scientists need something to transport either the entire gene or a recombinant DNA to the cell's nucleus, where the chromosomes and DNA reside. In essence, vectors are molecular delivery trucks. One of the first and most popular vectors developed were viruses because they invade cells as part of the natural infection process. Viruses have the potential to be excellent vectors because they have a specific relationship with the host in that they colonize certain cell types and tissues in specific organs. As a result, vectors are chosen according to their attraction to certain cells and areas of the body.

One of the first vectors used was the retrovirus. Because these viruses are easily cloned (artificially reproduced) in the laboratory, scientists have studied them extensively and learned a great deal about their biological action. They have also learned how to remove the genetic information which governs viral replication, thus reducing the chances of infection.

Retroviruses work best in actively dividing cells, but cells in the body are relatively stable and do not divide often. As a result, these cells are used primarily for *ex vivo* (outside the body) manipulation. First, the cells are removed from the patient's body, and the virus, or vector, carrying the gene is inserted into them. Next, the cells are placed into a nutrient culture where they grow and replicate. Once enough cells are gathered, they are returned to the body, usually by injection into the blood stream. Theoretically, as long as these cells survive, they will provide the desired therapy.

Another class of viruses, called the adenoviruses, may also prove to be good gene vectors. These viruses can effectively infect nondividing cells in the body, where the desired gene product is then expressed naturally. In addition to being a more efficient approach to gene transportation, these viruses, which cause respiratory infections, are more easily purified and made stable than retroviruses, resulting in less chance of an unwanted viral infection. However, these viruses live for several days in the body, and some concern surrounds the possibility of infecting others with the viruses through sneezing or coughing. Other viral vectors include **influenza** viruses, Sindbis virus, and a herpes virus that infects nerve cells.

Scientists have also delved into nonviral vectors. These vectors rely on the natural biological process in which cells uptake (or gather) macromolecules. One approach is to use liposomes, globules of fat produced by the body and taken up by cells. Scientists are also investigating the introduction of raw recombinant DNA by injecting it into the bloodstream or placing it on microscopic beads of gold shot into the skin with a "gene-gun." Another possible vector under development is based on dendrimer molecules. A class of polymers (naturally occurring or artificial substances that have a high molecular weight and formed by smaller molecules of the same or similar substances), is "constructed" in the laboratory by combining these smaller molecules. They have been used in manufacturing Styrofoam, polyethylene cartons, and Plexiglass. In the laboratory, dendrimers have shown the ability to transport genetic material into human cells. They can also be designed to form an affinity for particular cell membranes by attaching to certain sugars and protein groups.

History of gene therapy

In the early 1970s, scientists proposed "gene surgery" for treating inherited diseases caused by faulty genes. The idea was to take out the disease-causing gene and surgically implant a gene that functioned properly. Although sound in theory, scientists, then and now, lack the biological knowledge or technical expertise needed to perform such a precise surgery in the human body.

However, in 1983, a group of scientists from Baylor College of Medicine in Houston, Texas, proposed that gene therapy could one day be a viable approach for treating Lesch-Nyhan disease, a rare neurological disorder. The scientists conducted experiments in which an enzyme-producing gene (a specific type of protein) for correcting the disease was injected into a group of cells for replication. The scientists theorized the cells could then be injected into people with Lesch-Nyhan disease, thus correcting the genetic defect that caused the disease.

As the science of genetics advanced throughout the 1980s, gene therapy gained an established foothold in the minds of medical scientists as a promising approach to treatments for specific diseases. One of the major reasons for the growth of gene therapy was scientists' increasing ability to identify the specific genetic malfunctions that caused inherited diseases. Interest grew as further studies of DNA and chromosomes (where genes reside) showed that specific genetic abnormalities in one or more genes occurred in successive generations of certain family members who suffered from diseases like intestinal cancer, manic-depression, **Alzheimer's disease**, heart disease, diabetes, and many more. Although the genes may not be the only cause of the disease in all cases, they may make certain individuals more susceptible to developing the disease because of environmental influences, like **smoking**, pollution, and **stress**. In fact, some scientists theorize that all diseases may have a genetic component.

On September 14, 1990, a four-year-old girl with a genetic disorder that prevented her body from producing a crucial enzyme became the first person to undergo gene therapy in the United States. Because her body could not produce adenosine deaminase (ADA), she had a weakened immune system, making her extremely susceptible to severe, life-threatening infections. W. French Anderson and colleagues at the National Institutes of Health's Clinical Center in Bethesda, Maryland, took white blood cells (which are crucial to proper immune system functioning) from the girl, inserted ADA producing genes into them, and then transfused the cells back into the patient. Although the young girl continued to show an increased ability to produce ADA, debate arose as to whether the improvement resulted from the gene therapy or from an additional drug treatment she received.

Nevertheless, a new era of gene therapy began as more and more scientists sought to conduct clinical trial (testing in humans) research in this area. In that same year, gene therapy was tested on patients with melanoma (skin cancer). The goal was to help them produce antibodies (disease fighting substances in the immune system) to battle the cancer.

These experiments have spawned an ever-growing number of attempts at gene therapies designed to perform a variety of functions in the body. For example, a gene therapy for cystic fibrosis aims to supply a gene that alters cells, enabling them to produce a specific protein to battle the disease. Another approach was used for brain cancer patients, in which the inserted gene was designed to make the cancer cells more likely to respond to drug treatment. Gene therapy for patients who have artery blockage, which can lead to strokes, induces the growth of new blood vessels near clogged arteries, thus ensuring normal blood circulation.

Currently, there are a host of new gene therapy agents in clinical trials. In the United States, both nucleic acid-based (*in vivo*) treatments and cell-based (*ex vivo*) treatments are being investigated. Nucleic acid-based gene therapy uses vectors (like viruses) to deliver modified genes to target cells. Cell-based gene therapy techniques remove cells from the patient in order to genetically alter them then reintroduce them to the patient's body. Presently, gene therapies for the following diseases are being developed: cystic fibrosis (using adenoviral vector), HIV infection (cell-based), **malignant melanoma** (cell-based), Duchenne **muscular dystrophy** (cell-based), hemophilia B (cell-based), **kidney cancer** (cell-based), **Gaucher disease** (retroviral vector), **breast cancer** (retroviral vector), and lung cancer (retroviral vector). When a cell or individual is treated using gene therapy and successful incorporation of engineered genes has occurred, the cell or individual is said to be *transgenic*.

The medical establishment's contribution to transgenic research has been supported by increased government funding. In 1991, the U.S. government provided $58 million for gene therapy research, with increases in funding of $15–40 million dollars a year over the following four years. With fierce competition over the promise of societal benefit in addition to huge profits, large pharmaceutical corporations have moved to the forefront of transgenic research. In an effort to be first in developing new therapies, and armed with billions of dollars of research funds, such corporations are making impressive strides toward making gene therapy a viable reality in the treatment of once elusive diseases.

Diseases targeted for treatment by gene therapy

The potential scope of gene therapy is enormous. More than 5,000 diseases have been identified as resulting directly from abnormal genes, and countless others that may be partially influenced by a person's genetic makeup. Initial research has concentrated on developing gene therapies for diseases whose genetic origins have been established and for other diseases that can be cured or ameliorated by substances genes produce.

The following are examples of potential gene therapies. People suffering from cystic fibrosis lack a gene needed to produce a salt-regulating protein. This protein regulates the flow of chloride into epithelial cells, (the cells that line the inner and outer skin layers) which cover the air passages of the nose and lungs. Without this regulation, patients with cystic fibrosis build up a thick mucus that makes them prone to lung infections. A gene therapy technique to correct this abnormality might employ an adenovirus to transfer a normal copy of what scientists call the cystic fibrosis transmembrane conductance regulator, or CTRF, gene. The gene is introduced into the patient by spraying it into the nose or lungs.

Familial **hypercholesterolemia** (FH) is also an inherited disease, resulting in the inability to process cholesterol properly, which leads to high levels of artery-clogging fat in the blood stream. Patients with FH often suffer heart attacks and strokes because of blocked arteries. A gene therapy approach used to battle FH is much more intricate than most gene therapies because it involves partial surgical removal of patients' livers (*ex vivo* transgene therapy). Corrected copies of a gene that serve to reduce cholesterol build-up are inserted into the liver sections, which are then transplanted back into the patients.

Gene therapy has also been tested on patients with **AIDS**. AIDS is caused by the human **immunodeficiency** virus (HIV), which weakens the body's immune system to the point that sufferers are unable to fight off diseases like pneumonias and cancer. In one approach, genes that produce specific HIV proteins have been altered to stimulate immune system functioning without causing the negative effects that a complete HIV molecule has on the immune system. These genes are then injected in the patient's blood stream. Another approach to treating AIDS is to insert, via white blood cells, genes that have been genetically engineered to produce a receptor that would attract HIV and reduce its chances of replicating.

Several cancers also have the potential to be treated with gene therapy. A therapy tested for melanoma, or skin cancer, involves introducing a gene with an anti-cancer protein called tumor necrosis factor (TNF) into test tube samples of the patient's own cancer cells, which are then reintroduced into the patient. In brain cancer, the approach is to insert a specific gene that increases the cancer cells' susceptibility to a common drug used in fighting the disease.

Gaucher disease is an inherited disease caused by a mutant gene that inhibits the production of an enzyme called glucocerebrosidase. Patients with Gaucher disease have enlarged livers and spleens and eventually their bones deteriorate. Clinical gene therapy trials focus on inserting the gene for producing this enzyme.

Gene therapy is also being considered as an approach to solving a problem associated with a surgical procedure known as balloon **angioplasty**. In this procedure, a stent (in this case, a type of tubular scaffolding) is used to open the clogged artery. However, in response to the trauma of the stent insertion, the body initiates a natural healing process that produces too many cells in the artery and results in restenosis, or reclosing of the artery. The gene therapy approach to preventing this unwanted side effect is to cover the outside of the stents with a soluble gel. This gel contains vectors for genes that reduce this overactive healing response.

The Human Genome Project

Although great strides have been made in gene therapy in a relatively short time, its potential usefulness has been limited by lack of scientific data concerning the multitude of functions that genes control in the human body. For instance, it is now known that the vast majority of genetic material does not store information for the creation of proteins, rather, it is involved in the control and regulation of gene expression, and is therefore much more difficult to interpret. Even so, each individual cell in the body carries thousands of genes coding for proteins, with some estimates as high as 150,000 genes. For gene therapy to advance to its full potential, scientists must discover the biological role of each of these individual genes and where the base pairs that make them up are located on DNA.

To address this issue, the National Institutes of Health initiated the Human Genome Project in 1990. Led initially by James D. Watson, one of the co-discoverers of the chemical makeup of DNA, the project's 15-year goal was to map the entire human genome (a combination of the words gene and chromosomes). Watson was replaced in 1993 by Dr. Francis Collins, and the name of the project's center was officially changed to the National Human Genome Research Institute (NHGRI) in 1997. A genome map would clearly identify the location of all genes as well as the more than three billion base pairs that make them up. With a precise knowledge of gene locations and functions, scientists may one day be able to conquer or control diseases that have plagued humanity for centuries.

Scientists working at NHGRI have identified an average of one new gene a day, but many expect this rate of discovery to increase. Their goal was to determine the exact location of all the genes on human DNA and the exact sequence of the base pairs that make them up by 2005. A "rough draft" of the genome was finished in 2000, with the complete genome essentially sequenced by April 2003, two years earlier than planned. A number of regions of the genome, however, remain incompletely sequenced as of 2010. These include the central regions of the chromosomes, known as centromeres, and the end regions of the chromosomes, the telomeres. Both these regions are highly repetitive DNA sequences millions of base pairs in length that are difficult to sequence given the limits of current technology. The best current estimate is that about 93% of the genome has been completely sequenced as of early 2010.

Some of the genes already identified through the Human Genome Project include a gene that predisposes people to **obesity**, one associated with programmed cell death (apoptosis), a gene that guides HIV viral reproduction, and the genes of inherited disorders like **Huntington disease**, Lou Gehrig's disease, and some colon and breast cancers. As the human genome is completed, there will be more information available for gene therapy research and implementation.

Future of gene therapy

Gene therapy seems elegantly simple in its concept: supply the human body with a gene that can correct a biological malfunction that causes a disease. However, there are many obstacles and some distinct questions concerning the viability of gene therapy. For example, viral vectors must be carefully controlled lest they infect the patient with a viral disease. Some vectors, like retroviruses, can also enter cells functioning properly and interfere with the natural biological processes, possibly leading to other diseases. Other viral vectors, like the adenoviruses, are often recognized and destroyed by the immune system so their therapeutic effects are short-lived. Maintaining gene expression so that the gene will perform its role properly after vector delivery is difficult. As a result, some therapies need to be repeated often to provide long-lasting benefits.

One of the most pressing issues, however, is gene regulation. Genes work in concert to regulate their functioning. In other words, several genes may play a part in turning other genes on and off. For example, certain genes work together to stimulate cell division and growth, but if these are not regulated, the inserted genes could cause tumor formation and cancer. Another difficulty is learning how to make the gene go into action only when needed. For the best and safest therapeutic effort, a specific gene should turn on, for example, when certain levels of a protein or enzyme are low and must be replaced. But the gene should also remain dormant when not needed to ensure it does not oversupply a substance and disturb the body's delicate chemical makeup.

One approach to gene regulation is to attach other genes that detect certain biological activities and then react as a type of automatic off-and-on switch that regulates the activity of the other genes according to biological cues. Although still in the rudimentary stages, researchers are making headway in inhibiting some gene functioning by using a synthetic DNA to block gene transcriptions (the copying of genetic information). This approach may have implications for gene therapy.

Ethics of gene therapy

While gene therapy holds promise as a revolutionary approach to treating disease, ethical concerns over its use and ramifications have been expressed by scientists and lay people alike. For example, since much needs to be learned about how these genes actually work and their long-term effect, is it ethical to test these therapies on humans, where they could have a disastrous result? As with most clinical trials concerning new therapies, including many drugs, the patients participating in these studies have usually not responded to more established therapies and are often so ill the novel therapy is their only hope for long-term survival.

Another questionable outgrowth of gene therapy is that scientists could possibly manipulate genes to genetically control traits in human offspring that are not health-related. For example, perhaps a gene could be inserted to ensure that a child would not be bald, a seemingly harmless goal. However, what if genetic manipulation was used to alter skin color, prevent homosexuality, or ensure good looks? If a gene is found that can enhance intelligence of children who are not yet born, will everyone in society, the rich and the poor, have access to the technology or will it be so expensive only the elite can afford it?

The Human Genome Project, which plays such an integral role for the future of gene therapy, also has social repercussions. If individual genetic codes can be determined, will such information be used against people? For example, will someone more susceptible to a disease have to pay higher insurance premiums or be denied health insurance altogether? Will employers discriminate between two potential employees, one with a "healthy" genome and the other with genetic abnormalities?

Some of these concerns can be traced back to the eugenics movement popular in the first half of the twentieth century. This genetic "philosophy" was a societal movement that encouraged people with "positive" traits to reproduce while those with less desirable traits were sanctioned from having children. Eugenics was used to pass strict immigration laws in the United States, barring less suitable people from entering the country lest they reduce the quality of the country's collective gene pool. Probably the most notorious example of eugenics in action was the rise of Nazism in Germany, which resulted in the Eugenic Sterilization Law of 1933. The law required sterilization for those suffering from certain disabilities and even for some who were simply deemed "ugly." To ensure that this novel science is not abused, many governments have established organizations specifically for overseeing the development of gene therapy. In the United States, the Food and Drug Administration (FDA) and the National Institutes of Health (NIH) require scientists to take a precise series of steps and meet stringent requirements before approving clinical trials.

In fact, gene therapy has been immersed in more controversy and surrounded by more scrutiny in both the health and ethical arena than most other technologies (except, perhaps, for cloning) that promise to substantially change society. Despite the health and ethical questions surrounding gene therapy, the field will continue to grow and is likely to change medicine faster than any previous medical advancement.

Resources

BOOKS

Jorde, Lynn B., John C. Carey, and Michael J. Bamshad. *Medical Genetics*, 4th ed. Philadelphia: Mosby/Elsevier, 2010.

Marcovitz, Hal. *Gene Therapy Research*. San Diego, CA: ReferencePoint Press, 2009.

Walther, Wolfgang, and Ulrike Stein, eds. *Gene Therapy of Cancer: Methods and Protocols*, 2nd ed. New York: Humana Press, 2009.

PERIODICALS

Agarwalla, P.K., et al. "Virally Mediated Immunotherapy for Brain Tumors." *Neurosurgery Clinics of North America* 21 (January 2010): 167–79.

Costerton, W.J., et al. "Prospecting Gene Therapy of Implant Infections." *International Journal of Artificial Organs* 32 (September 2009): 689–95.

Germani, A., et al. "Regenerative Therapy in Peripheral Artery Disease." *Cardiovascular Therapeutics* 27 (Winter 2009): 289–304.

Reilly, M.M., and M.E. Shy. "Diagnosis and New Treatments in Genetic Neuropathies." *Journal of Neurology, Neurosurgery, and Psychiatry* 80 (December 2009): 1304–14.

Rew, L., et al. "A Systematic Review of Literature about the Genetic Testing of Adolescents." *Journal for Specialists in Pediatric Nursing* 14 (October 2009): 284–94.

Via, M., et al. "Recent Advances of Genetic Ancestry Testing in Biomedical Research and Direct-to-Consumer Testing." *Clinical Genetics* 76 (September 2009): 225–35.

OTHER

Human Genome Project Information. *Gene Therapy*. http://www.ornl.gov/sci/techresources/Human_Genome/medicine/genetherapy.shtml

National Cancer Institute (NCI). *Gene Therapy for Cancer: Questions and Answers*. http://www.cancer.gov/cancertopics/factsheet/Therapy/gene

Katherine Hunt, MS
Rebecca J. Frey, PhD
Brenda W. Lerner

General adaptation syndrome

Definition

General adaptation syndrome, or GAS, is a term used to describe the body's short-term and long-term reactions to **stress**.

Stressors in humans include such physical stressors as **starvation**, being hit by a car, or suffering through severe weather. Additionally, humans can suffer such emotional or mental stressors as the loss of a loved one, the inability to solve a problem, or even having a difficult day at work.

Description

Originally described by Hans Selye (1907–1982), an Austrian-born physician who emigrated to Canada in 1939, the general adaptation syndrome represents a three-stage reaction to stress. Selye explained his choice of terminology as follows: "I call this syndrome *general* because it is produced only by agents which have a general effect upon large portions of the body. I call it *adaptive* because it stimulates defense...I call it a *syndrome* because its individual manifestations are coordinated and even partly dependent upon each other."

Selye thought that the general adaptation syndrome involved two major systems of the body, the nervous system and the endocrine (or hormonal) system. He then went on to outline what he considered as three distinctive stages in the syndrome's evolution. He called these stages the alarm reaction (AR), the stage of resistance (SR), and the stage of exhaustion (SE).

Stage 1: Alarm reaction (AR)

The first stage of the general adaptation stage, the alarm reaction, is the immediate reaction to a stressor. In the initial phase of stress, humans exhibit a "fight or flight" response, which prepares the body for physical activity. However, this initial response can also decrease the effectiveness of the immune system, making persons more susceptible to illness during this phase.

Stage 2: Stage of resistance (SR)

Stage 2 might also be named the stage of adaptation, instead of the stage of resistance. During this phase, if the stress continues, the body adapts to the stressors it is exposed to. Changes at many levels take place in order to reduce the effect of the stressor. For example, if the stressor is starvation (possibly due to anorexia), the person might experienced a reduced desire for physical activity to conserve energy, and the absorption of nutrients from food might be maximized.

Stage 3: Stage of exhaustion (SE)

At this stage, the stress has continued for some time. The body's resistance to the stress may gradually be reduced, or may collapse quickly. Generally, this means the immune system, and the body's ability to resist disease, may be almost totally eliminated. Patients who experience long-term stress may succumb to heart attacks or severe infection due to their reduced immunity. For example, a person with a stressful job may experience long-term stress that might lead to high blood pressure and an eventual **heart attack**.

KEY TERMS

Adjustment disorder—A disorder defined by the development of significant emotional or behavioral symptoms in response to a stressful event or series of events within the normal range of human experience.

Cortisol—A steroid hormone released by the cortex (outer portion) of the adrenal gland when a person is under stress.

Eustress—A term that is sometimes used to refer to positive stress.

Stress management—A set of techniques and programs intended to help people deal more effectively with stress in their lives by analyzing the specific stressors and taking positive actions to minimize their effects. Most stress management programs deal with job stress and workplace issues.

Stressor—A stimulus or event that provokes a stress response in an organism. Stressors can be categorized as acute or chronic, and as external or internal to the organism.

Stress, a useful reaction?

The reader should note that Dr. Selye did not regard stress as a purely negative phenomenon; in fact, he frequently pointed out that stress is not only an inevitable part of life but results from intense joy or pleasure as well as fear or **anxiety**. "Stress is not even necessarily bad for you; it is also the spice of life, for any emotion, any activity, causes stress." Some later researchers have coined the term "eustress" or pleasant stress, to reflect the fact that such positive experiences as a job promotion, completing a degree or training program, marriage, travel, and many others are also stressful.

Selye also pointed out that human perception of and response to stress is highly individualized; a job or sport that one person finds anxiety-provoking or exhausting might be quite appealing and enjoyable to someone else. Looking at one's responses to specific stressors can contribute to better understanding of one's particular physical, emotional, and mental resources and limits.

Causes and symptoms

Stress is one cause of general adaptation syndrome. The results of unrelieved stress can manifest as **fatigue**, irritability, difficulty concentrating, and difficulty sleeping. Persons may also experience other symptoms that are signs of stress. Persons experiencing unusual symptoms, such as hair loss, without another medical explanation might consider stress as the cause.

The general adaptation syndrome is also influenced by such universal human variables as overall health and nutritional status, sex, age, ethnic or racial background, level of education, socioeconomic status (SES), genetic makeup, etc. Some of these variables are biologically based and difficult or impossible to change. For example, recent research indicates that men and women respond somewhat differently to stress, with women being more likely to use what is called the "tend and befriend" response rather than the classical "fight or flight" pattern. These researchers note that most of the early studies of the effects of stress on the body were conducted with only male subjects.

Selye's observation that people vary in their perceptions of stressors was reflected in his belief that the stressors themselves are less dangerous to health than people's maladaptive responses to them. He categorized certain diseases, ranging from cardiovascular disorders to inflammatory diseases and mental disorders as "diseases of adaptation," regarding them as "largely due to errors in our adaptaive response to stress" rather than the direct result of such outside factors as germs, toxic substances, etc.

Diagnosis

GAS by itself is not an official diagnostic category but rather a descriptive term. A person who consults a doctor for a stress-related physical illness may be scheduled for blood or urine tests to measure the level of cortisol or other stress-related hormones in their body, or imaging studies to evaluate possible abnormalities in their endocrine glands if the doctor thinks that these tests may help to establish or confirm a diagnosis.

The American Psychiatric Association (APA) recognizes stress as a factor in **anxiety disorders**, particularly **post-traumatic stress disorder** (PTSD) and **acute stress disorder** (ASD). These two disorders are defined as symptomatic reactions to extreme traumatic stressors (war, natural or transportation disasters, criminal assault, **abuse**, hostage situations, etc.) and differ chiefly in the time frame in which the symptoms develop. The APA also has a diagnostic category of **adjustment disorders**, which are characterized either by excessive reactions to stressors within the normal range of experience (e.g., academic examinations, relationship breakups, being fired from a job) or by significant impairment in the person's occupational or social functioning.

Treatment

Treatment of stress-related illnesses typically involves one or more **stress reduction** strategies. Stress reduction strategies generally fall into one of three categories: avoiding stressors; changing one's reaction to the stressor(s); or relieving stress after the reaction to the stressor(s). Many mainstream as well as complementary or alternative (CAM) strategies for stress reduction, such as exercising, listening to music, **aromatherapy**, and massage relieve stress after it occurs.

Many psychotherapeutic approaches attempt to modify the patient's reactions to stressors. These approaches often include an analysis of the patient's individual patterns of response to stress; for example, one commonly used set of categories describes people as "speed freaks," "worry warts," "cliff walkers," "loners," "basket cases," and "drifters." Each pattern has a recommended set of skills that the patient is encouraged to work on; for example, worry warts are advised to reframe their anxieties and then identify their core values and goals in order to take concrete action about their worries. In general, persons wishing to improve their management of stress should begin by consulting a medical professional with whom they feel comfortable to discuss which option, or combination of options, they can use.

Selye himself recommended an approach to stress that he described as "living wisely in accordance with natural laws." In his now-classic book *The Stress of Life* (1956), he discussed the following as important dimensions of living wisely:

- Adopting an attitude of gratitude toward life rather than seeking revenge for injuries or slights.
- Acting toward others from altruistic rather than self-centered motives.
- Retaining a capacity for wonder and delight in the genuinely good and beautiful things in life.
- Finding a purpose for one's life and expressing one's individuality in fulfilling that purpose.
- Keeping a healthy sense of modesty about one's goals or achievements.

Resources

BOOKS

Beers, Mark H., Robert S. Porter, and Thomas V. Jones, eds. *The Merck Manual of Diagnosis and Therapy*. 18th ed. Whitehouse Station, NJ: Merck Research Laboratories, 2006.

PERIODICALS

Cosen-Binker, L. I., M. G. Binker, G. Negri, and O. Tiscornia. "Influence of Stress in Acute Pancreatitis and Correlation with Stress-Induced Gastric Ulcer." *Pancreatology* 4 (July 2004): 470–484.

Motzer, S. A., and V. Hertig. "Stress, Stress Response, and Health." *Nursing Clinics of North America* 39 (March 2004): 1–17.

OTHER

"Stress management, General adaptation syndrome, GAS." http://www.holisticonline.com/stress/stress_GAS.htm.

ORGANIZATIONS

American Psychiatric Association (APA), 1000 Wilson Boulevard, Suite 1825, Arlington, VA, 22209, (888) 357-7924, apa@psych.org, http://www.psych.org.

Canadian Institute of Stress, Hans Selye Foundation, Medcan Clinic Office, Suite 1500, 150 York Street, Toronto, ON, Canada, M5H 3S5, (416) 236-4218, info@stresscanada.org, http://www.stresscanada.org.

National Institute of Mental Health (NIMH), 6001 Executive Boulevard, Bethesda, MD, 20892, (301) 443-4513, (301) 443-4279, (866) 615-6464, nimhinfo@nih.gov, http://www.nimh.nih.gov.

The American Institute of Stress, 124 Park Avenue, Yonkers, NY, 10703, (914) 963-1200, (914) 965-6267, Stress125@optonline.net, http://www.stress.org.

Michael V. Zuck, PhD
Rebecca J. Frey, PhD

General anesthetic *see* **Anesthesia, general**

General surgery

Definition

General surgery is the treatment of injury, deformity, and disease using operative procedures.

Purpose

General surgery is frequently performed to alleviate suffering when a cure is unlikely through medication alone. It can be used for routine procedures performed in a physician's office, such as **vasectomy**, or for more complicated operations requiring a medical team in a hospital setting, such as laparoscopic **cholecystectomy** (removal of the gallbladder). Areas of the body treated by general surgery include the stomach, liver, intestines, appendix, breasts, thyroid gland, salivary glands, some arteries and veins, and the skin. The brain, heart, eyes, and feet, to name only a few, are areas that require specialized surgical repair.

New methods and techniques are less invasive than previous practices, permitting procedures that were considered impossible in the past. For example, microsurgery has been used in reattaching severed body parts by successfully reconnecting small blood vessels and nerves.

Precautions

Patients who are obese, smoke, have bleeding tendencies, or are over 60, need to follow special precautions, as do patients who have recently experienced an illness such as **pneumonia** or a **heart attack**. Patients on medications such as heart and blood pressure medicine, blood thinners, **muscle relaxants**, tranquilizers, insulin, or sedatives, may require special lab tests prior to surgery and special monitoring during surgery. Special precautions may be necessary for patients using mind-altering drugs such as **narcotics**, psychedelics, hallucinogens, **marijuana**, sedatives, or **cocaine** since these drugs may interact with the anesthetic agents used during surgery.

Description

In earlier times, surgery was a dangerous and dirty practice. Until the middle of the 19th century, as many patients died of surgery as were cured. With the discovery and development of **general anesthesia** in the mid-1800s, surgery became more humane. And as knowledge about infections grew, surgery became more successful as sterile practices were introduced into the operating room. The last 50 years of the 20th century have seen continued advancements.

Types of general surgery

General surgery experienced major advances with the introduction of the endoscope. This is an instrument for visualizing the interior of a body canal or a hollow organ. Endoscopic surgery relies on this pencil-thin instrument, capable of its own lighting system and small video camera. The endoscope is inserted through tiny incisions called portals. While viewing the procedure on a video screen, the surgeon then operates with various other small, precise instruments inserted through one or more of the portals. The specific area of the body treated determines the type of endoscopic surgery performed. For example, **colonoscopy** uses an endoscope, which can be equipped with a device for obtaining tissue samples for visual examination of the colon. Gastroscopy uses an endoscope inserted through the mouth to examine the interior of the stomach. **Arthroscopy** refers to joint surgery, and abdominal procedures are called laparoscopies.

Endoscopy is used in both treatment and diagnosis especially involving the digestive and female reproductive systems. Endoscopy has advantages over many other surgical procedures, resulting in a quicker recovery and shorter hospital stay. This non-invasive technique is being used for appendectomies, gallbladder surgery, hysterectomies and the repair of shoulder and knee ligaments. However, endoscopy does not come without limitations such as complications and high operating expense. Also, endoscopy doesn't offer advantages over conventional surgery in all procedures. Some literature states that as general surgeons become more experienced in their prospective fields, additional non-invasive surgery will be a more common option to patients.

ONE-DAY SURGERY. One-day surgery is also termed same-day, or outpatient surgery. Surgical procedures usually take two hours or less and involve minimal blood loss and a short recovery time. In the majority of surgical cases, oral medications control postoperative **pain**. Cataract removal, **laparoscopy**, **tonsillectomy**, repair of broken bones, **hernia repair**, and a wide range of cosmetic procedures are common same-day surgical procedures. Many individuals prefer the convenience and atmosphere of one-day surgery centers, as there is less competition for attention with more serious surgical cases. These centers are accredited by the Joint Commission on Accreditation of Healthcare Organizations or the Accreditation Association for Ambulatory Health Care.

Preparation

The preparation of patients has advanced significantly with improved diagnostic techniques and procedures. Before surgery the patient may be asked to undergo a series of tests including blood and urine studies, x rays and specific heart studies if the patient's past medical history and/or physical exam warrants this testing. Before any general surgery the physician will explain the nature of the surgery needed, the reason for the procedure, and the anticipated outcome. The risks involved will be discussed along with the types of anesthesia utilized. The expected length of recovery and limitations imposed during the recovery period are also explained in detail before any general surgical procedure.

KEY TERMS

Appendectomy—Removal of the appendix.

Endoscope—Instrument for examining visually the inside of a body canal or a hollow organ such as the stomach, colon, or bladder.

Hysterectomy—Surgical removal of part or all of the uterus.

Laparoscopic cholecystectomy—Removal of the gallbladder using a laparoscope, a fiberoptical instrument inserted through the abdomen.

Microsurgery—Surgery on small body structures or cells performed with the aid of a microscope and other specialized instruments.

Portal—An entrance or a means of entrance.

Surgical procedures most often require some type of anesthetic. Some procedures require only **local anesthesia**, produced by injecting the anesthetic agent into the skin near the site of the operation. The patient remains awake with this form of medication. Injecting anesthetic agents into a primary nerve located near the surgical site produces block anesthesia (also known as regional anesthesia), which is a more extensive local anesthesia. The patient remains conscious, but is usually sedated. General anesthesia involves injecting anesthetic agents into the blood stream and/or inhaling medicines through a mask placed over the patient's face. During general anesthesia, the patient is asleep and an airway tube is usually placed into the windpipe to help keep the airway open.

As part of the preoperative preparation, the patient will receive printed educational material and may be asked to review audio or videotapes. The patient will be instructed to shower or bathe the evening before or morning of surgery and may be asked to scrub the operative site with a special antibacterial soap. Instructions will also be given to the patient to ingest nothing by mouth for a determined period of time prior to the surgical procedure.

Aftercare

After surgery, blood studies and a laboratory examination of removed fluid or tissue are often performed especially in the case of **cancer** surgery. After the operation, the patient is brought to a recovery room and vital signs, fluid status, **dressings** and surgical drains are monitored. Pain medications are offered and used as necessary. Breathing exercises are encouraged to maximize respiratory function and leg exercises are encouraged to promote adequate circulation and prevent pooling of blood in the lower extremities. Patients must have a responsible adult accompany them home if leaving the same day as the surgery was performed.

Risks

One of the risks involved with general surgery is the potential for postoperative complications. These complications include—but are not limited to—pneumonia, internal bleeding, and wound infection as well as adverse reactions to anesthesia.

Normal results

Advances in diagnostic and surgical techniques have increased the success rate of general surgery by many times compared to the past. Today's less invasive surgical procedures have reduced the length of hospital stays, shortened recovery time, decreased postoperative pain and decreased the size of surgical incision. On the average, a conventional abdominal surgery requires a three to six-day hospital stay and three to six-week recovery time.

Abnormal results

Abnormal results from general surgery include persistent pain, swelling, redness, drainage or bleeding in the surgical area and surgical wound infection resulting in slow healing.

ORGANIZATIONS

American Medical Association, 515 N. State St., Chicago, IL, 60654, (800) 621-8335, http://www.ama-assn.org.

Jeffrey P. Larson, RPT

Generalized anxiety disorder

Definition

Generalized **anxiety** disorder is a condition characterized by "free floating" anxiety or apprehension not linked to a specific cause or situation.

Description

Some degree of fear and anxiety is perfectly normal. In the face of real danger, fear makes people more alert and prepares the body to fight or flee (the "fight or flight" response). When people are afraid, their hearts beat faster and they breathe faster in anticipation of the physical activity that will be required of them. Sometimes people can become anxious even when there is no identifiable cause, and this anxiety can become overwhelming and very unpleasant, interfering with their daily lives. People with debilitating anxiety are said to be suffering from **anxiety disorders**, such as **phobias**, panic disorders, and generalized anxiety disorder. The person with generalized anxiety disorder generally has chronic (officially, having more days with anxiety than not for at least six months), recurrent episodes of anxiety that can last days, weeks, or even months.

Causes and symptoms

Generalized anxiety disorder afflicts between 2–3% of the general population, and is slightly more common in women than in men. It accounts for almost one-third of cases referred to psychiatrists by general practitioners.

Generalized anxiety disorder may result from a combination of causes. Some people are genetically predisposed to developing it. Psychological traumas that occur during childhood, such as prolonged separation from parents, may make people more vulnerable as well. Stressful life events, such as a move, a major job change, the loss of a loved one, or a divorce, can trigger or contribute to the anxiety.

Psychologically, the person with generalized anxiety disorder may develop a sense of dread for no apparent reason—the irrational feeling that some nameless catastrophe is about to happen. Physical symptoms similar to those found with **panic disorder** may be present, although not as severe. They may include trembling, sweating, heart **palpitations** (the feeling of the heart pounding in the chest), **nausea**, and "butterflies in the stomach."

According to the *Diagnostic and Statistical Manual of Mental Disorders*, 4th edition, a person must have at least three of the following symptoms, with some being present more days than not for at least six months, in order to be diagnosed with generalized anxiety disorder:

- restlessness or feeling on edge
- easily fatigued
- difficulty concentrating
- irritability

KEY TERMS

Cognitive behavioral therapy—A psychotherapeutic approach that aims at altering cognitions—including thoughts, beliefs, and images—as a way of altering behavior.

Panic attack—A time-limited period of intense fear accompanied by physical and cognitive symptoms. Panic attacks may be unexpected or triggered by specific internal or external cues.

- muscle tension
- sleep disturbance

While generalized anxiety disorder is not completely debilitating, it can compromise a person's effectiveness and quality of life.

Diagnosis

Anyone with chronic anxiety for no apparent reason should see a physician. The physician may diagnose the condition based on the patient's description of the physical and emotional symptoms. The doctor will also try to rule out other medical conditions that may be causing the symptoms, such as excessive **caffeine** use, thyroid disease, **hypoglycemia**, cardiac problems, or drug or alcohol withdrawal. Psychological conditions, such as depressive disorder with anxiety, will also need to be ruled out.

In June 2004, the Anxiety Disorders Association of America released follow-up guidelines to help primary care physicians better diagnose and manage patients with generalized anxiety disorder. They include considering the disorder when medical causes for general, vague physical complaints cannot be ruled out. Since generalized anxiety disorder often co-occurs with **mood disorders** and **substance abuse**, the clinician may have to treat these conditions as well, and, therefore, must consider them in making the diagnosis.

Treatment

Drugs

Over the short term, a group of tranquilizers called **benzodiazepines**, such as clonazepam (Klonipin), may help ease the symptoms of generalized anxiety disorder. Sometimes **antidepressant drugs**, such as amitryptiline (Elavil), or **selective serotonin reuptake inhibitors** (SSRIs), such as paroxetine (Paxil), escitalopram (Lexapro), and venlafaxine (Effexor), which also has norepinephrine, may be preferred. Other SSRIs are fluoxetine (Prozac) and sertraline (Zoloft).

Alternative

Psychotherapy can be effective in treating generalized anxiety disorder. The therapy may take many forms. In some cases, psychodynamically-oriented psychotherapy can help patients work through this anxiety and solve problems in their lives. Cognitive behavioral therapy aims to reshape the way people perceive and react to potential stressors in their lives. Relaxation techniques have also been used in treatment, as well as in prevention efforts.

Prognosis

When properly treated, most patients with generalized anxiety disorder experience improvement in their symptoms.

Prevention

While preventive measures have not been established, a number of techniques may help manage anxiety, such as relaxation techniques, breathing exercises, and distraction—putting the anxiety out of one's mind by focusing thoughts on something else.

Resources

BOOKS

Kase, Larina, and Deborah Roth Ledley. *Anxiety Disorders*. Hoboken, NJ: John Wiley and Sons, 2007.

Otto, Michal, and Stefan Hofmann, eds. *Avoiding Treatment Failures in the Anxiety Disorders (Series in Anxiety and Related Disorders)*. New York: Springer, 2009.

Pelletier, Kenneth R. "CAM Therapies for Specific Conditions: Anxiety." In *The Best Alternative Medicine*, Part II. New York: Simon & Schuster, 2007.

Texas, Nami, and Deborah Rose. *Diagnosis—Anxiety Disorders: Visions for Tomorrow—The Basics (Volume 1)*. Charleston, SC: CreateSpace, 2009.

PERIODICALS

"Guidelines to Assist Primary Care Physicians in Diagnosing GAD." *Psychiatric Times* (July 1, 2004): 16.

Sherman, Carl. "GAD Patients Often Require Combined Therapy." *Clinical Psychiatry News* (August 2004): 12–14.

ORGANIZATIONS

American Psychiatric Association, 1000 Wilson Boulevard, Suite 1825, Arlington, VA, 22209, (703) 907-7300, http://www.psych.org.

Anxiety Disorders Association of America, 8730 Georgia Ave., Suite 600, Silver Spring, MD, 20910, (240) 485-1001, http://www.adaa.org.

National Institute of Mental Health (NIMH, Mental Health Public Inquiries, 6001 Executive Boulevard Room 8184, MSC 9663, Bethesda, MD, 20892-9663, (668) 227-6464, http://www.nimh.nih.gov.

National Alliance on Mental Illness (NAMI), 3803 N. Fairfax Dr., Ste. 100, Arlington, VA, 22201, (703) 524-7600, (800) 950-NAMI (6264), (703) 524-9094, http://www.nami.org.

National Mental Health Association (NMHA), 2000 N. Beauregard Street, 6th Floor, Alexandria, VA, 22311, (703) 684-7722, (800) 969-NMHA, (703) 684-5968, http://www1.nmha.org.

Robert Scott Dinsmoor
Teresa G. Odle
Laura Jean Cataldo, RN, EdD

Genetic counseling

Definition

Genetic counseling is a communication process by which personal genetic risk information is translated into practical information for families. Genetic counselors are commonly health care professionals with specialized training and experience in the areas of medical genetics and counseling. They work as members of a healthcare team, providing individuals and families with information on the nature, inheritance, and implications of genetic disorders to help them make informed medical and personal decisions.

Purpose

Specifically, the process of genetic counseling assists families by:

- Helping families understand information about birth defects or genetic disorders. This includes explaining patterns of inheritance, recurrence risks, natural history of diseases, and genetic testing options.
- Providing nondirective supportive counseling regarding emotional issues related to a diagnosis or testing options.
- Helping individuals or families make decisions that they are comfortable with based on their personal ethical and religious standards.
- Connecting families with appropriate resources, such as support groups or specific types of medical clinics, locally and nationally.

As of 2008, 25 universities were offering genetic counseling study programs in the United States and Canada meeting the rigorous accreditation criteria established by the American Board of Genetic

Counseling (ABGC). Most genetic counseling programs are two-year programs that include course work, clinical rotations and an independent research project. Most applicants enter the field from variety of disciplines, including biology, genetics, psychology, and nursing.

Description

Genetic counselors work with people concerned about the risk of an inherited disease. These patients represent several different patient populations. Prenatal genetic counseling is provided to couples that have an increased risk for **birth defects** or inherited conditions and are expecting a child or planning a **pregnancy**. Pediatric genetic counseling is provided to families with children suspected of having a genetic disorder or with children previously diagnosed with a genetic disorder. Adult genetic counseling is provided to adults with clinical features of an inherited disease or a family history of an inherited disease. **Cancer** genetic counseling is provided to those with a strong family history of certain types of cancer.

Prenatal genetic counseling

There are several different reasons a person or couple may seek prenatal genetic counseling. If a woman is age 35 or older and pregnant, there is an increased chance that the fetus may have a change in the number of chromosomes present. Changes in chromosome number may lead to **mental retardation** and birth defects. **Down syndrome** is the most common change in chromosome number that occurs more often in the fetuses of older women. Couples may seek prenatal genetic counseling because of abnormal results of screening tests performed during pregnancy. A blood test called the alpha fetal protein (AFP) test is offered to all pregnant women. This blood test screens for Down syndrome, open spine defects (**spina bifida**) and another type of mental retardation caused by a change in chromosome number called Trisomy 18. When this test is abnormal, further tests are offered to get more information about the chance of these conditions in the fetus. Another reason that people seek prenatal genetic counseling is a family history of birth defects or inherited diseases. In some cases, blood tests on the parents may be available to indicate if their children would be at risk of being affected. Genetic counselors assess risk in each case, help patients understand their risks and explore how patients feel about or cope with these risks.

Prenatal tests that are offered during genetic counseling include level II ultrasounds, maternal serum AFP screening, **chorionic villus sampling** (CVS), and **amniocentesis**. Level II ultrasound is a detailed ultrasound surveying fetal anatomy for birth defects. Ultrasound is limited to detection of structural changes in anatomy and cannot detect changes in chromosome number. The maternal serum AFP screening is used to indicate if a pregnant woman has a higher or lower chance of certain birth defects. This test can only change the chances for a birth defect. The screening cannot diagnose a birth defect. CVS is a way of learning how many chromosomes is present in a fetus. A small piece of placental tissue is obtained for these studies during the tenth to twelfth weeks of pregnancy. Amniocentesis is also a way of learning how many chromosomes are present in a fetus. Amniotic fluid is obtained for these studies, usually between 16 and 18 weeks of pregnancy. There is a small risk for **miscarriage** with both of these tests. Genetic counseling regarding these procedures involves the careful explanation of benefits and limitations of each testing option. The counselor also tries to explore how patients feel about prenatal testing and the impact of such testing on the pregnancy. Genetic counselors are supportive of any decision a patient makes about whether or not to have prenatal tests performed.

Pediatric genetic counseling

Families or pediatricians seek genetic counseling when a child has features of an inherited condition. Any child who is born with more than one birth defect, mental retardation, or dysmorphic features has an increased chance of having a genetic syndrome. A common type of mental retardation in males for which **genetic testing** is available is **fragile X syndrome**. Genetic testing is also available for many other childhood illnesses such as **hemophilia** and **muscular dystrophy**. Genetic counselors work with medical geneticists to determine if a genetic syndrome is present. This process includes a careful examination of family history, medical history of the child, review of pertinent medical records in the family, a **physical examination** of the child, and sometimes blood work or other diagnostic tests. If a diagnosis is made, then the medical geneticist and genetic counselor review what is known about the inheritance of the condition, the natural history of the condition, treatment options, further examinations that may be needed for health problems common in the diagnosed syndrome and resources for helping the family. The genetic counselor also helps the family adjust to the diagnosis by emotional support and counseling. Many families are devastated by receiving a diagnosis, learning of the likely outcome for the child, and by the loss of the hoped–for healthy child. There would also be a discussion about recurrence risks in the family and who else in the family may be at risk.

Adult genetic counseling

Adults seek genetic counseling when a person in the family decides to be tested for a known genetic condition in the family, when an adult begins exhibiting symptoms of an inherited condition or when there is a new diagnosis of someone with an adult onset disorder in the family. In addition, sometimes the birth of a child with obvious features of a genetic disease leads to diagnosis of a parent who is affected more mildly. Genetic counseling for adults may lead to the consideration of presymptomatic genetic testing. Testing a person to determine if they will be symptomatic for a condition before the symptoms occur is an area of controversy. **Huntington disease** is an example of a genetic disease for which presymptomatic testing is available. Huntington disease is a neurological disease resulting in **dementia**. Onset of the condition is between 30 to 50 years of age. Huntington disease is inherited in an autosomal dominant pattern. If a person has a parent with the disease, their risk of being affected is 50%. Would presymptomatic testing relieve or create **anxiety**? Would a person benefit from removal of doubt about being affected? Would knowing help a person with life planning? Genetic counselors help patients sort through their feelings about such testing and whether or not the results would be helpful to them.

Cancer genetic counseling

A family history of early onset breast, ovarian, or **colon cancer** in multiple generations of a family is a common reason a person would seek a genetic counselor that works with cancer patients. While most cancer is not inherited, there are some families in which a dominant gene is present and causing the disease. The genetic counselor is able to discuss with a patient the chance that the cancer in the family is related to a dominantly inherited gene. The counselor can also discuss the option of testing for the breast and **ovarian cancer** genes, BRCA1 and BRCA2. In some cases the person seeking testing has already had cancer, and in others they have not. Therefore, presymptomatic testing is also an issue in cancer genetics. Emotional support is important for these patients as they have often lost close relatives from cancer and are fearful of their own risks. For families in which a dominant form of cancer is detected through genetic testing, a plan for increased surveillance for the disease can be made.

KEY TERMS

Carrier—An individual who possesses a genetic mutation associated with a recessive disorder, but who usually does not display symptoms of that disease. Carriers are able to pass the mutation on to their offspring.

Consangunity—Related from a common ancestor; blood relative.

Dominant inheritance—A pattern of inheritance in which a trait or disease is conferred by one gene or allele. A parent with a disorder caused by a dominant allele has a 50% chance of passing the trait for disease to their offspring.

Recessive inheritance—A pattern of inheritance where both parents carry the gene responsible for a trait or disease (although they seldom show symptoms). Their offspring will have a 25% chance of having the trait or disease. Recessive inheritance is also responsible for disorders such as hemophilia, where the mother carries the affected gene on the X chromosome and passes it to her son.

Pedigree

In all types of genetic counseling, an important aspect of the genetic counseling session is information gathering about family and medical history. Information gathering is performed by drawing a chart called a pedigree. A pedigree is made of symbols and lines that represent the family history. To accurately assess the risk of inherited diseases, information about three generations of the family, including health status and/or cause of **death**, is usually needed. If the family history is complicated, information from more distant relatives may be helpful, and medical records may be requested for any family members who have had a genetic disorder. Through an examination of the family history a counselor may be able to discuss the probability of future occurrence of genetic disorders.

ETHNICITY. In taking a family history, a genetic counselor asks for the patient's ethnicity or ancestral origin. There are some ethnic groups that have a higher chance of being carriers of specific genetic diseases. For instance, the chance that an African American is a carrier of a gene for **sickle cell disease** is 1 in 10 individuals. People of Jewish ancestry are more likely to be carriers of several conditions including **Tay–Sachs disease**, Canavan disease and **cystic fibrosis**. People of Mediterranean ancestry are more likely to be carriers of a type of anemia called **thalassemia**. Genetic counselors discuss inheritance patterns of these diseases, carrier risks, and genetic screening or testing options.

CONSANGUNITY. Another question a genetic counselor asks in taking a family history is if the couple is related to one another by blood. The practice of marrying or having children with relatives is infrequent in the United States, but is more common in some countries. When two people are related by blood, there is an increased chance for their children to be affected with conditions inherited in a recessive pattern. In recessive inheritance, each parent of a child affected with a disease carries a single gene for the disease. The child gets two copies, one from each parent, and is affected. People who have a common ancestor are more likely than unrelated people to be carriers of genes for the same recessively inherited genes. Depending on family history and ethnic background, blood tests can be offered to couples to get more information about the chance for these conditions to occur.

EXPOSURES DURING PREGNANCY. During prenatal genetic counseling, the counselor will ask about pregnancy history. If the patient has taken a medication or has had a harmful exposure (like radiation), the genetic counselor can discuss the possibility of harmful effects. Ultrasound is often a useful tool to look for some affects of exposures.

Ethical issues in genetic counseling

Prenatal diagnosis of anomalies or chromosomal abnormalities leads to a decision about whether or not a couple wishes to continue a pregnancy. Some couples chose to continue a pregnancy. Prenatal gives them additional time to emotionally prepare for the birth of the child and to gather resources. Others choose not to continue a pregnancy in which problems have been diagnosed. These couples have unique emotional needs. Often the child is very much a desired addition to the family and parents are devastated that the child is not healthy. Presymptomatic testing for adult onset disorders and cancer raise difficult issues regarding the need to know and the reality of dealing with abnormal results before symptoms. The National Society of Genetic Counselors (NSGC) has established a Code of Ethics to guide genetic counselors in caring for patients. The NSGC Code of Ethics, last updated in 2006, is based on four ethical principles:

- Beneficience is the promotion of personal well being in others. The genetic counselor is an advocate for the patient.
- Nonmaleficience is the idea of doing no harm to a patient.
- Autonomy is recognizing the value of the individual, the person's abilities and their point of view. Important aspects of autonomy are truthfulness with patients, respecting confidentiality, and practicing informed consent.
- Justice is providing equal care for all, freedom of choice, and providing a high quality of care.

Perhaps the main ethical principle of genetic counseling is the attempt to provide nondirective counseling. This requires a patient–centered approach by providing care focused on the thoughts and feelings of the patient. Five percent of the Human Genome Project budget is assigned to research involving the best way to deal with ethical issues that arise as new genetic tests become available. Genetic counselors can help patients navigate through the unfamiliar territory of genetic testing.

Resources

BOOKS

Evans, Christine. *Genetic Counselling: A Psychological Approach.* Cambridge, UK: Cambridge University Press, 2006.

Harper, Peter S. *Practical Genetic Counselling*, 6th edition, London, UK: Hodder Arnold Publication, 2004.

Veach, Patricia McCarthy. *Facilitating the Genetic Counseling Process: A Practice Manual.* New York, NY: Springer, 2003.

PERIODICALS

Aalfs, C. M., et al. "A Comparison of Counselee and Counselor Satisfaction in Reproductive Genetic Counseling."*Clinical Genetics* 72, no. 2 (August 2007): 74–82.

Micheil Innes, A. "Molecular Genetic Testing and Genetic Counseling."*Handbook of Clinical Neurology* 87 (2007): 517–531.

Mikkelsen, E. M., et al. "Psychosocial Consequences of Genetic Counseling: A Population–Based Follow–Up Study."*Breast Journal* 15, no. 1 (January–February 2009): 61–68.

Mittman, I. S., and K. Downs. "Diversity in Genetic Counseling: Past, Present and Future."*Journal of Genetic Counseling* 17, no. 4 (August 2008): 301–313.

Moskowitz, S. M., et al. "Clinical Practice and Genetic Counseling for Cystic Fibrosis and CFTR–Related Disorders."*Genetics in Medicine* 10, no. 12 (December 2008): 851–868.

Norton, M. E. "Genetic Screening and Counseling."*Current Opinion in Obstetrics & Gynecology* 20, no. 2 (April 2008): 157–1634.

Sekizawa, A., et al. "Recent Advances in Non–Invasive Prenatal DNA Diagnosis Through Analysis of Maternal Blood."*Journal of Obstetrics and Gynaecology* 33, no. 6 (December 2007): 747–764.

Simon, M. S., and N. Petrucelli. "Hereditary Breast and Ovarian Cancer Syndrome : the Impact of Race on

Uptake of Genetic Counseling and Testing." *Methods in Molecular Biology* 471 (2009): 487–500.

Smets, E., et al. "Comparing Genetic Counseling with Non-Genetic Health Care Interactions: Two of a Kind?"- *Patient Education and Counseling* 68, no. 3 (November 2007): 225–234.

Veach, P. M., et al. "Coming Full Circle: A Reciprocal-Engagement Model of Genetic Counseling Practice." *Journal of Genetic Counseling* 16, no. 6 (December 2007): 713–728.

OTHER

"FAQs about Genetic Counselors." Information Page. NSGC.http://www.nsgc.org/consumer/faq_consumers.cfm (accessed February 4, 2010).

"Genetic Counselling." Information Page. Mount Sinai Hospital. http://www.mtsinai.on.ca/pdmg/Tests/gencounsel.htm (accessed February 4, 2010).

"Genetic Counselling." Information Page. Sick Kids. http://www.sickkids.ca/CGenetics/section.asp?s = Genetic + Counselling&sID = 12834 (accessed February 4, 2010).

"Genetic Counselling." Information Page. AboutKidshealth. http://www.aboutkidshealth.ca/pregnancy/Genetic-Counselling.aspx?articleID = 7550&categoryID = PG-nh2-04h (accessed February 4, 2010).

"What is a Genetic Counsellor?" Information Page. CAGC. http://www.cagc-accg.ca/content/view/12/26/ (accessed February 4, 2010).

ORGANIZATIONS

March of Dimes Foundation, 1275 Mamaroneck Avenue, White Plains, NY, 10605, (914) 428–7100, (888) MODIMES (663–4637), (914) 428–8203, askus@marchofdimes.com, http://www.marchofdimes.com.

National Office of Public Health Genomics, 4770 Buford Highway Mailstop K–89, White Plains, Atlanta, GA, (770) 488–8510, (888) MODIMES (663–4637), (770) 488–8355, genetics@cdc.gov, http://www.cdc.gov/genomics.

National Society of Genetic Counselors, 401 N. Michigan Ave., Chicago, IL, 60611, (312) 321–6834, (312) 673–6972, nsgc@nsgc.org, http://www.nsgc.org.

Sonja Rene Eubanks, MS, CGC
Brenda W. Lerner

Genetic studies *see* **Genetic testing**

Genetic testing

Definition

A genetic test seeks to identify changes in a person's chromosomes, genes, or proteins, that are associated with inherited disorders. Genetic testing is performed to determine if a person has or will develop a certain disease or could pass a disease to his or her offspring. Genetic tests also determine whether or not couples are at a higher risk than the general population for having a child affected with a genetic disorder.

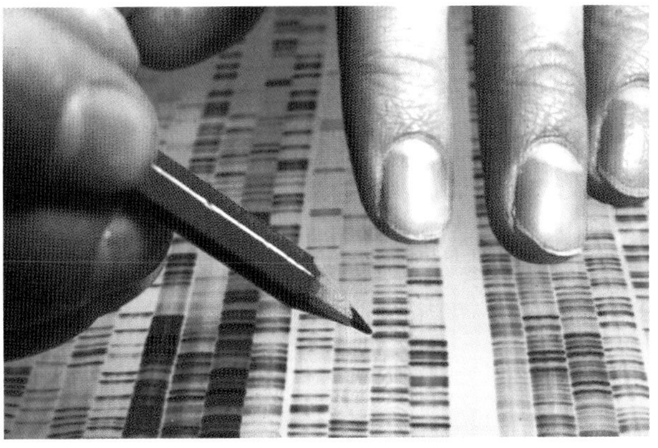

A scientist examines a DNA sequencing autogradiogram on a light box. *(Photo Researchers, Inc.)*

Purpose

Some families or ethnic groups have a higher incidence of a certain disease than does the population as a whole. For example, individuals from Eastern European, Ashkenazi Jewish descent are at higher risk for carrying genes for rare conditions that occur much less frequently in populations from other parts of the world. Before having a child, a couple from such a family or ethnic group may want to know if their child would be at risk of having that disease. Genetic testing for this type of purpose is called genetic screening.

During **pregnancy**, the baby's cells can be studied for certain genetic disorders or chromosomal problems such as **Down syndrome**. Chromosome testing is most commonly offered when the mother is 35 years or older at the time of delivery. When there is a family medical history of a genetic disease or there are individuals in a family affected with developmental and physical delays, genetic testing may also be offered during pregnancy. Genetic testing during pregnancy is called prenatal diagnosis.

Prior to becoming pregnant, couples who are having difficulty conceiving a child or who have suffered multiple miscarriages may be tested to see if a genetic cause can be identified.

A genetic disease may be diagnosed at birth by doing a physical evaluation of the baby and observing characteristics of the disorder. Genetic testing can help to confirm the diagnosis made by the physical evaluation. In addition, genetic testing is used routinely on all newborns to screen for certain genetic diseases which can affect a newborn baby's health shortly after birth.

There are several genetic diseases and conditions in which the symptoms do not occur until adulthood. One such example is Huntington's disease. This is a serious disorder affecting the way in which individuals walk, talk and function on a daily basis. Genetic testing may be able to determine if someone at risk for the disease will in fact develop the disease.

Some genetic defects may make a person more susceptible to certain types of **cancer**. Testing for these defects can help predict a person's risk. Other types of genetic tests help diagnose and predict and monitor the course of certain kinds of cancer, particularly leukemia and lymphoma.

Description

Gene tests

Gene tests look for signs of a disease by examining DNA taken from a person's blood, body fluids or tissues. The tests can look for large changes, such as a gene that has a section missing or added, or small changes, such as a missing, added, or altered chemical base within the DNA strand. Other important changes can be genes with too many copies, genes that are too active, genes that are turned off, or those that are lost entirely.

Various techniques are used for gene tests. Direct DNA sequencing examines the direct base pair sequence of a gene for specific gene mutations. Some genes contain more than 100,000 bases; a mutation of any one base can make the gene nonfunctional and cause disease. The more mutations possible, the less likely it is for a test to detect all of them. This test is usually done on white blood cells from a person's blood, but can also be performed on other tissues. There are different ways in which to perform direct DNA mutation analysis. When the specific genetic mutation is known, it is possible to perform a complete analysis of the genetic code, also called direct sequencing. There are several different lab techniques used to test for a direct mutation. One common approach begins by using chemicals to separate DNA from the rest of the cell. Next, the two strands of DNA are separated by heating. Special enzymes (called restriction enzymes) are added to the single strands of DNA; they then act like scissors and cut the strands in specific places. The DNA fragments are then sorted by size through a process called electrophoresis. A special piece of DNA, called a probe, is added to the fragments. The probe is designed to bind to specific mutated portions of the gene. When bound to the probe, the mutated portions appear on x–ray film with a distinct banding pattern.

Another gene test technique is indirect DNA testing. Family linkage studies are done to study a disease when the exact type and location of the genetic alteration is not known, but the general location on the chromosome has been identified. These studies are possible when a chromosome marker has been found associated with a disease. Chromosomes contain certain regions that vary in appearance between individuals. These regions are called polymorphisms and do not cause a genetic disease to occur. If a polymorphism is always present in family members with the same genetic disease, and absent in family members without the disease, it is likely that the gene responsible for the disease is near that polymorphism. The gene mutation can be indirectly detected in family members by looking for the polymorphism.

To look for the polymorphism, DNA is isolated from cells in the same way it is for direct DNA mutation analysis. A probe is added that will detect the large polymorphism on the chromosome. When bound to the probe, this region will appear on x–ray film with a distinct banding pattern. The pattern of banding of a person being tested for the disease is compared to the pattern from a family member affected by the disease.

Linkage studies have disadvantages not found in direct DNA mutation analysis. These studies require multiple family members to participate in the testing. If key family members choose not to participate, the incomplete family history may make testing other members useless. The indirect method of detecting a mutated gene also causes more opportunity for error.

Chromosome tests

Various genetic syndromes are caused by structural chromosome abnormalities. To analyze a person's chromosomes, his or her cells are allowed to grow and multiply in the laboratory until they reach a certain stage of growth. The length of growing time varies with the type of cells. Cells from blood and bone marrow take one to two days; fetal cells from amniotic fluid take 7–10 days.

When the cells are ready, they are placed on a microscope slide using a technique to make them burst open, spreading their chromosomes. The slides are stained: the stain creates a banding pattern unique to each chromosome. Under a microscope, the chromosomes are counted, identified, and analyzed based on their size, shape, and stained appearance.

Types of chromosome tests include the karyotype test and the FISH (fluorescent in situ hybridization) test. In a karyotype test, the chromosomes are counted, and a photograph is taken of the chromosomes from one or more cells as seen through the microscope. Then the chromosomes are cut out and arranged side-by-side with their partner in ascending numerical order, from largest to smallest. The karyotype is done either manually or using a computer attached to the microscope. The FISH test identifies specific regions on chromosomes using fluorescent DNA probes. FISH analysis can find small pieces of chromosomes that are missing or have extra copies and that can be missed by the karyotype test.

Biochemical tests

Genes contain instructions for making proteins and abnormal protein levels can be indicative of a genetic disorder. Biochemical tests look at the level of key proteins. This level can identify genes that are not working normally. These types of tests are typically used for newborn screening. For example, this screening can detect infants who have metabolic conditions such as **phenylketonuria** (PKU).

Applications of genetic testing

Newborn screening

In the United States, genetic testing is used most often for newborn screening, a major public health program which can find disorders in newborns that have long-term health effects. Newborn screening tests infant blood samples for abnormal or missing gene products. Every year, millions of newborn babies have their blood samples tested for potentially serious genetic diseases. As of 2009, newborn screening programs were testing for disorders that can cause **infectious disease**, premature **death**, hearing disorders, and heart problems. A new technology called tandem mass spectrometry allows screening of up to 30 other metabolic disorders.

Carrier testing

An individual who has a gene associated with a disease but never exhibits any symptoms of the disease is called a carrier. A carrier is a person who is not affected by the mutated gene he or she possesses, but can pass the gene to an offspring. Genetic tests have been developed that tell prospective parents whether or not they are carriers of certain diseases. If one or both parents are a carrier, the risk of passing the disease to a child can be predicted.

To predict the risk, it is necessary to know if the gene in question is autosomal or sex–linked. If the gene is carried on any one of chromosomes 1–22, the resulting disease is called an autosomal disease. If the gene is carried on the X or Y chromosome, it is called a sex–linked disease.

Sex–linked diseases, such as the bleeding condition **hemophilia**, are usually carried on the X chromosome. A woman who carries a disease–associated gene on one of her X chromosomes has a 50% chance of passing that gene to her son. A son who inherits that gene will develop the disease because he does not have another normal copy of the gene on a second X chromosome to compensate for the abnormal copy. A daughter who inherits the disease–associated gene from her mother will be at risk for having a son affected with the disease.

The risk of passing an autosomal disease to a child depends on whether the gene is dominant or recessive. A prospective parent carrying a dominant gene has a 50% chance of passing the gene to a child. A child needs to receive only one copy of the mutated gene to be affected by the disease.

If the gene is recessive, a child needs to receive two copies of the mutated gene, one from each parent, to be affected by the disease. When both parents are carriers, their child has a 25% chance of inheriting two copies of the mutated gene and being affected by the disease; a 50% chance of inheriting one copy of the mutated gene, and being a carrier of the disease but not affected; and a 25% chance of inheriting two normal genes. When only one parent is a carrier, a child has a 50% chance of inheriting one mutated gene and being an unaffected carrier of the disease, and a 50% chance of inheriting two normal genes.

Cystic fibrosis is a disease that affects the lungs and pancreas and is discovered in early childhood. It is the most common autosomal recessive genetic disease found in the Caucasian population: one in 25 people of Northern European ancestry are carriers of a mutated cystic fibrosis gene. The gene, located on chromosome 7, was identified in 1989.

The gene mutation for cystic fibrosis is detected by a direct DNA test. Over 600 mutations of the cystic fibrosis gene have been found; each of these mutations cause the same disease. Tests are available for the most common mutations. Tests that check for the 86 of the most common mutations in the Caucasian population will detect 90% of carriers for cystic fibrosis. (The percentage of mutations detected varies according to the individual's ethnic background). If a person tests negative, it is likely, but not guaranteed that he or she does not have the gene. Both parents must be carriers of the gene to have a child with cystic fibrosis.

Tay–Sachs disease, also autosomal recessive, affects children primarily of Ashkenazi Jewish descent. Children with this disease usually die between the ages of two and five. This disease was previously detected by looking for a missing enzyme. The mutated gene has now been identified and can be detected using direct DNA mutation analysis.

Presymptomatic testing

Not all genetic diseases show their effect immediately at birth or early in childhood. Although the gene mutation is present at birth, some diseases do not appear until adulthood. If a specific mutated gene responsible for a late–onset disease has been identified, a person from an affected family can be tested before symptoms appear.

Huntington disease is one example of a late–onset autosomal dominant disease. Its symptoms of mental confusion and abnormal body movements do not appear until middle to late adulthood. The chromosome location of the gene responsible for Huntington chorea was located in 1983 after studying the DNA from a large Venezuelan family affected by the disease. Ten years later the gene was identified. A test is now available to detect the presence of the expanded base pair sequence responsible for causing the disease. The presence of this expanded sequence means the person will develop the disease.

Another late onset disease, Alzheimer's, does not have as well a understood genetic cause as Huntington disease. The specific genetic cause of Alzheimer disease is not as clear. Although many cases appear to be inherited in an autosomal dominant pattern, many cases exist as single incidents in a family. Like Huntington, symptoms of mental deterioration first appear in adulthood. Genetic research has found an association between this disease and genes on four different chromosomes. The validity of looking for these genes in a person without symptoms or without family history of the disease is still being studied.

CANCER SUSCEPTIBILITY TESTING. Cancer can result from an inherited (germline) mutated gene or a gene that mutated sometime during a person's lifetime (acquired mutation). Some genes, called tumor suppressor genes, produce proteins that protect the body from cancer. If one of these genes develops a mutation, it is unable to produce the protective protein. If the second copy of the gene is normal, its action may be sufficient to continue production, but if that gene later also develops a mutation, the person is vulnerable to cancer. Other genes, called oncogenes, are involved in the normal growth of cells. A mutation in an oncogene can cause too much growth, which is the beginning of cancer.

Direct DNA tests are currently available to look for gene mutations identified and linked to several kinds of cancer. People with a family history of these cancers are those most likely to be tested. If one of these mutated genes is found, the person is more susceptible to developing the cancer. The likelihood that the person will develop the cancer, even with the mutated gene, is not always known because other genetic and environmental factors are also involved in the development of cancer.

Cancer susceptibility tests are most useful when a positive test result can be followed with clear treatment options. In families with **familial polyposis** of the colon, testing a child for a mutated APC gene can reveal whether or not the child needs frequent monitoring for the disease. In families with potentially fatal familial medullary **thyroid cancer** or multiple endocrine neoplasia type 2, finding a mutated RET gene in a child provides the opportunity for that child to have preventive removal of the thyroid gland. In the same way, MSH1 and MSH2 mutations can reveal which members in an affected family are vulnerable to familiar colorectal cancer and would benefit from aggressive monitoring.

In 1994, a mutation linked to early–onset familial breast and **ovarian cancer** was identified. BRCA1 is located on chromosome 17. Women with a mutated form of this gene have an increased risk of developing breast and ovarian cancer. A second related gene, BRCA2, was later discovered. Located on chromosome 13, it also carries increased risk of breast and ovarian cancer. Although both genes are rare in the general population, they are slightly more common in women of Ashkenazi Jewish descent.

When a woman is found to have a mutation in one of these genes, the likelihood that she will get breast or ovarian cancer increases, but not to 100%. Other genetic and environmental factors influence the outcome.

Testing for these genes is most valuable in families where a mutation has already been found. BRCA1 and BRCA2 are large genes; BRCA1 includes 100,000 bases. More than 120 mutations to this gene have been discovered, but a mutation could occur in any one of the bases. Studies show tests for these genes may miss 30% of existing mutations. The rate of missed mutations, the unknown disease likelihood in spite of a positive result and the lack of a clear preventive response to a positive result, make the value of this test for the general population uncertain.

Prenatal and postnatal chromosome analysis

Chromosome analysis is performed on fetal cells primarily when the mother is age 35 or older at the time of delivery, has experienced multiple miscarriages, or reports a family history of a genetic abnormality. Prenatal testing is done on the fetal cells from a **chorionic villus sampling** (from the baby's developing placenta) at 10–12 weeks or from the amniotic fluid (the fluid surrounding the baby) at 16–18 weeks of pregnancy. Cells from amniotic fluid grow for 7–10 days before they are ready to be analyzed. Chorionic villi cells have the potential to grow faster and can be analyzed sooner.

Chromosome analysis using blood cells is done on a child who is born with or later develops signs of **mental retardation** or physical malformation. In the older child, chromosome analysis may be done to investigate developmental delays.

Extra or missing chromosomes cause mental and physical abnormalities. A child born with an extra chromosome 21 (trisomy 21) has Down syndrome. An extra chromosome 13 or 18 also produce well known syndromes. A missing X chromosome causes **Turner syndrome** and an extra X in a male causes **Klinefelter syndrome**. Other abnormalities are caused by extra or missing pieces of chromosomes. **Fragile X syndrome** is a sex–linked disease that causes mental retardation in males.

Chromosome material may also be rearranged, such as the end of chromosome 1 moving to the end of chromosome 3. This is called a chromosomal translocation. If no material is added or deleted in the exchange, the person may not be affected. Such an exchange, however, can cause **infertility** or abnormalities if passed to children.

Evaluation of a man and woman's infertility or repeated miscarriages will include blood studies of both to check for a chromosome translocation. Many chromosome abnormalities are incompatible with life; babies with these abnormalities often miscarrry during the first trimester. Cells from a baby that died before birth can be studied to look for chromosome abnormalities that may have caused the death.

Diagnostic testing

This type of genetic testing is used to confirm a diagnosis when a person has signs or symptoms of a genetic disease. The genetic test used depends on the disease for which a person is tested. For example, if a patient has physical features indicative of Down syndrome, a chromosomal test is used. To test for Duchenne **muscular dystrophy**, a gene test is done to look for missing sections in the dystrophin gene.

Chromosome tests are also used to diagnose certain cancers, particularly leukemia and lymphoma, which are associated with changes in chromosomes: extra or missing complete chromosomes, extra or missing portions of chromosomes, or exchanges of material (translocations) between chromosomes. Studies show that the locations of the chromosome breaks are at locations of tumor suppressor genes or oncogenes.

Chromosome analysis on cells from blood, bone marrow, or solid tumor helps diagnose certain kinds of leukemia and lymphoma and often helps predict how well the person will respond to treatment. After treatment has begun, periodic monitoring of these chromosome changes in the blood and bone marrow gives the physician information as to the effectiveness of the treatment.

A well-known chromosome rearrangement is found in chronic myelogenous leukemia. This leukemia is associated with an exchange of material between chromosomes 9 and 22. The resulting smaller chromosome 22 is called the Philadelphia chromosome.

Pharmacogenetic testing

Among the latest types of genetic testing is pharmacogenetic testing. This test examines a person's genes to gain information on how drugs would be broken down by the body. Pharmacogenetic testing aims to design drug treatments that are specific to each person. For example, a test used in patients who have chronic myelogenous leukemia can show which patients would benefit from a medicine called Gleevac. Another test looks at a liver enzyme called cytochrome P450, which breaks down certain types of drugs. Gene mutations can affect the ability of the body to break down certain drugs and people with a less active form of P450 might be taking excessive levels of a drug. Pharmacogenetic testing seeks to help patients obtain the right amount of a medication.

Precautions

Because genetic testing is not always accurate and because there are privacy concerns for the individual receiving a genetic test, **genetic counseling** should always be performed prior to genetic testing. A genetic counselor is an individual with a master's degree in genetic counseling. A medical geneticist is a physician specializing and board certified in genetics.

KEY TERMS

Autosomal disease—A disease caused by a gene mutation located on a chromosome other than a sex chromosome.

Karyotype—A photomicrograph (picture taken through a microscope) of a person's 46 chromosomes, lined up in 23 pairs, that is used to identify some types of genetic disorders.

Oncogene—A gene that causes normal cell growth, but if mutated or expressed at high levels, encourages normal cells to change into cancerous cells.

Sex-linked genetic disorder—A disease or disorder caused by a gene mutation located on the X (female) or Y (male) chromosome.

Translocation—The rearrangement or exchange of segments of chromosomes that does not alter the total number of chromosomes, but sometimes results in a genetic disorder or disease.

A genetic counselor reviews the person's family history and medical records and the reason for the test. The counselor explains the likelihood that the test will detect all possible causes of the disease in question (known as the sensitivity of the test), and the likelihood that the disease will develop if the test is positive (known as the positive predictive value of the test).

Learning about the disease in question, the benefits and risks of both a positive and a negative result, and what treatment choices are available if the result is positive, will help prepare the person undergoing testing. During the genetic counseling session, the individual interested in genetic testing will be asked to consider how the test results will affect his or her life, family, and future decisions.

After this discussion, the person should have the opportunity to indicate in writing that he or she gave informed consent to have the test performed, verifying that the counselor provided complete and understandable information.

A variety of genetic tests are now increasingly being offered directly to consumers, usually over the Internet. Such genetic testing usually involves scraping a few cells from inside the cheek and mailing the sample to a test laboratory, where the test is performed. People considering such genetic tests, should discuss the issue with their health-care provider or a genetic counselor.

Preparation

Most tests for genetic diseases of children and adults are done on blood. To collect the 5–10 mL of blood needed, a healthcare worker draws blood from a vein in the inner elbow region. Collection of the sample takes only a few minutes.

Prenatal testing is done either on amniotic fluid or a chorionic villus sampling. To collect amniotic fluid, a physician performs a procedure called **amniocentesis**. An ultrasound is done to find the baby's position and an area filled with amniotic fluid. The physician inserts a needle through the woman's skin and the wall of her uterus and withdraws 5–10 mL of amniotic fluid. Placental tissue for a chorionic villus sampling is taken through the cervix. Each procedure takes approximately 30 minutes.

Bone marrow is used for chromosome analysis in a person with leukemia or lymphoma. The person is given **local anesthesia**. Then the physician inserts a needle through the skin and into the bone (usually the sternum or hip bone). One–half to 2 mL of bone marrow is withdrawn. This procedure takes approximately 30 minutes.

Aftercare

After blood collection the person can feel discomfort or bruising at the puncture site or may become dizzy or faint. Pressure to the puncture site until the bleeding stops reduces bruising. Warm packs to the puncture site relieve discomfort.

The chorionic villus sampling, amniocentesis and bone marrow procedures are all done under a physician's supervision. The person is asked to rest after the procedure and is watched for weakness and signs of bleeding.

Risks

Collection of amniotic fluid and chorionic villus sampling have the risk of **miscarriage**, infection, and bleeding; the risks are higher for the chorionic villus sampling. Because of the potential risks for miscarriage, 0.5% following the amniocentesis and 1% following the chorionic villus sampling procedure, both of these prenatal tests are offered to couples, but not required. A woman should tell her physician immediately if she has cramping, bleeding, fluid loss, an increased temperature, or a change in the baby's movement following either of these procedures.

After bone marrow collection, the puncture site may become tender and the person's temperature may rise. These are signs of a possible infection.

Genetic testing involves other nonphysical risks. Many people fear the possible loss of privacy about personal health information. Other family members may be affected by the results of a person's genetic test. Privacy of the person tested and the family members affected is a consideration when deciding to have a test and to share the results.

A positive result carries a psychological burden, especially if the test indicates the person will develop a disease later in life, such as Huntington's chorea. The news that a person may be susceptible to a specific kind of cancer, while it may encourage positive preventive measures, may also negatively shadow many decisions and activities.

A genetic test result may also be inconclusive meaning no definitive result can be given to the individual or family. This may cause the individual to feel more anxious and frustrated and experience psychological difficulties.

Prior to undergoing genetic testing, individuals need to learn from the genetic counselor the likelihood that the test could miss a mutation or abnormality.

Results

A normal result for chromosome analysis is 46, XX or 46, XY. This means there are 46 chromosomes (including two X chromosomes for a female or one X and one Y for a male) with no structural abnormalities. A normal result for a direct DNA mutation analysis or linkage study includes no gene mutations found.

There can be some benefits from genetic testing when the individual tested is not found to carry a genetic mutation. Those who learn with great certainty they are no longer at risk for a genetic disease may choose not to undergo prophylactic therapies and may feel less anxious and relieved.

An abnormal chromosome analysis report will include the total number of chromosomes and will identify the abnormality found. Tests for gene mutations will report the mutations found.

There are many ethical issues to consider with an abnormal prenatal test result. Many of the diseases tested for during a pregnancy, cannot be treated or cured. In addition, some diseases tested for during pregnancy, may have a late-onset of symptoms or have minimal effects on the affected individual.

Before making decisions based on an abnormal test result, the person should meet again with a genetic counselor to fully understand the meaning of the results, learn what options are available based on the test result, and what are the risks and benefits of each of those options.

Resources

BOOKS

Betta, Michella, ed. *The Moral, Social, and Commercial Imperatives of Genetic Testing and Screening: The Australian Case.* New York, NY: Springer, 2006.

Hart, Anne. *How to Safely Tailor Your Food, Medicines & Cosmetics to Your Genes: A Consumer's Guide to Genetic Testing Kits from Ancestry to Nourishment.* Lincoln, NE: iUniverse, 2003.

Institute of Medicine of the National Academies. *Cancer–Related Genetic Testing and Counseling: Workshop Proceedings.* Washington, DC: National Academies Press, 2007.

Lemmens, Trudo, et al. *Reading the Future? : Legal and Ethical Challenges of Predictive Genetic Testing.* Montreal, QC, Canada: Editions Themis, 2007.

Sharpe, Neil F., and Ronald F. Carter. *Genetic Testing: Care, Consent and Liability.*New York, NY: Wiley–Liss, 2006.

Zallen Teichler, Doris. *To Test or Not To Test: A Guide to Genetic Screening and Risk.* Piscataway, NJ: Rutgers University Press, 2008.

PERIODICALS

Bandelt, H. J. "The Brave New Era of Human Genetic Testing."*Bioessays* 30, no. 11–12 (November 2008): 1246–1251.

Borry, P., et al. "Predictive Genetic Testing in Minors for Adult-Onset Genetic Diseases."*Mount Sinai Journal of Medicine* 75, no. 3 (May–June 2008): 287–296.

Clarke, A. J., and C. Gaff. "Challenges in the Genetic Testing of Children for Familial Cancers."*Archives of Disease in Childhood* 93, no. 11 (November 2008): 911–9141.

Goodeve, A. "Molecular Genetic Testing of Hemophilia A."*Seminars in Thrombosis and Hemostasis* 34, no. 6 (September 2008): 4911–501.

Kuehn, B. M. "Risks and Benefits of Direct-to-Consumer Genetic Testing Remain Unclear."*Journal of the American Medical Association* 300, no. 13 (October 2008): 1503–1505.

Micheil Innes, A. "Molecular Genetic Testing and Genetic Counseling."*Handbook of Clinical Neurology* 87 (2007): 517–531.

Rich, T. A., and M. Salazar. "Genetic Risk Assessment, Counseling and Testing."*Surgical Oncology Clinics of North America* 18, no. 1 (January 2009): 19–38.

Tutt, A., and A. Ashworth. "Can Genetic Testing Guide Treatment in Breast Cancer?"; *European Journal of Cancer* 44, no. 18 (December 2008): 2774–2780.

Valente, E. M., et al. "Genetic Testing for Pediatric Neurological Disorders." *Lancet Neurology* 7, no. 12 (December 2008): 1113–1126.

OTHER

Human Genome Project Information. "Pharmacogenitics." http://www.ornl.gov/sci/techresources/Human_Genome/medicine/pharma.shtml (accessed February 3, 2010).

March of Dimes. "Your First Tests." http://www.marchofdimes.com/pnhec/159_519.asp (accessed February 3, 2010).

National Human Genome Research Institute. "Frequently Asked Questions About Genetic Testing." http://www.genome.gov/19516567 (accessed February 3, 2010.).

National Human Genome Research Institute. "Genetic Testing." http://www.genome.gov/10002335 (accessed February 3, 2010).

National Institutes of Health. "Genetic Testing." http://www.nlm.nih.gov/medlineplus/genetictesting.html (accessed February 3, 2010).

ORGANIZATIONS

EuroGentest, Gasthuisberg O&N, Herestraat 49, Box 602, Leuven, Belgium, 3000, (+32)16 345860, (+32) 16 34599, http://www.eurogentest.org.

March of Dimes Foundation, 1275 Mamaroneck Avenue, White Plains, NY, 10605, (914) 428–7100, (888) MODIMES (663–4637), (914) 428–8203, askus@marchofdimes.com, http://www.marchofdimes.com.

National Office of Public Health Genomics, 4770 Buford Highway Mailstop K–89, White Plains, Atlanta, GA, (770) 488–8510, (888) MODIMES (663–4637), (770) 488–8355, genetics@cdc.gov, http://www.cdc.gov/genomics.

National Society of Genetic Counselors, 401 N. Michigan Ave., Chicago, IL, 60611, (312) 321–6834, (312) 673–6972, nsgc@nsgc.org, http://www.nsgc.org.

Katherine S. Hunt, MS
Brenda W. Lerner

Genital herpes

Definition

Genital herpes is a sexually transmitted disease caused by a herpes virus. The disease is characterized by the formation of fluid–filled, painful blisters in the genital area. However, many people who are infected with the virus may not have symptoms and may be unaware they are infected.

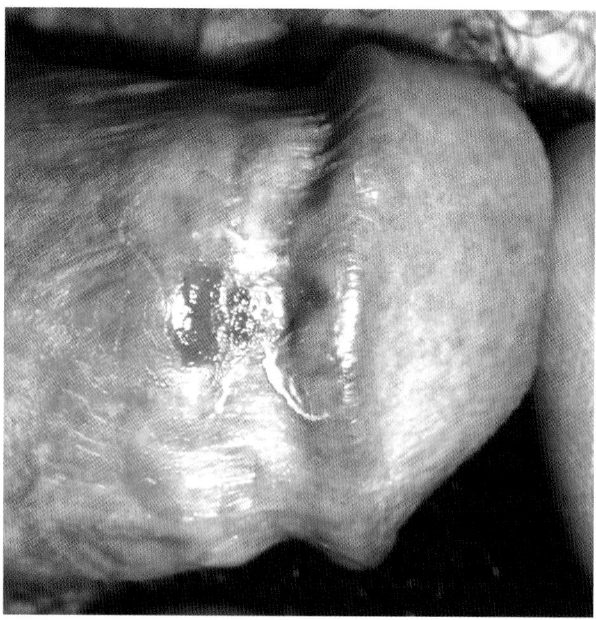

A close-up view of a man's penis with a blister (center of image) caused by the herpes simplex virus. *(Custom Medical Stock Photo, Inc. Reproduced by permission.)*

Demographics

It is estimated that almost 536 million people world–wide between the ages of 15–49 years are living with the herpes simplex type 2 virus (HSV–2). The lowest prevalence of the infection is in Western Europe. Approximately 30 million people in North America are infected with genital herpes. About 17% of the adult population in the United States have antibodies to HSV–2 while almost 60% have antibodies to HSV–1. Newly diagnosed cases of primary genital herpes are increasingly caused by the herpes simplex virus type 1 (HSV–1).

More women (one out of four) than men (one out of eight) have antibodies to the herpes simplex virus. The racial differences for herpes type 2 antibodies are whites, 17.6%; blacks, 45.9%; and Mexican Americans, 22.3%. The occurrence of antibodies to herpes type 1 is higher in blacks.

Interestingly, only 2.6% of adults report that they have had genital herpes.

Description

Genital herpes (herpes genitalis, herpes progenitalis) is characterized by the formation of fluid–filled blisters on the genital organs of men and women. The word "herpes" comes from the Greek adjective *herpestes,* meaning *creeping,* which refers to the serpent–like pattern

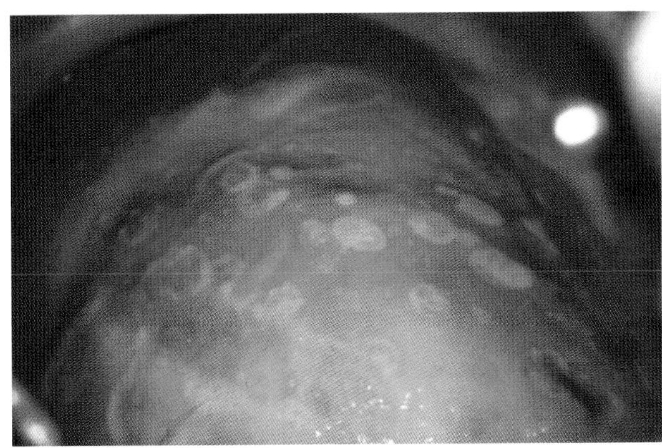

Female cervix covered with herpes lesions.
(Photo Researchers, Inc.)

that the blisters may form. Genital herpes is considered to be a sexually transmitted disease which means that it can be spread from person–to–person by sexual contact. Herpes may be spread by vaginal, anal, or oral sexual activity. In addition, genital herpes may be spread by an infected mother to a baby when the baby passes through the birth canal during the delivery process. It is not spread by objects (such as a toilet seat or doorknob), swimming pools, hot tubs, or through the air.

Genital herpes is a disease resulting from an infection by a herpes simplex virus. There are eight different kinds of human herpes viruses. Only two of these, herpes simplex types 1 and 2, can cause genital herpes. It has been commonly believed that herpes simplex virus type 1 infects above the waist (causing **cold sores**) and herpes simplex virus type 2 infects below the waist (causing genital sores). This generalization is not completely true. Both herpes virus type 1 and type 2 can cause herpes lesions on the lips or genitals, but recurrent cold sores are almost always type 1. The two viruses seem to have evolved to more likely infect at one site or the other, especially with regard to recurrent disease.

Viruses are different from bacteria. While bacteria are independent and can reproduce on their own, viruses cannot reproduce without the help of a cell. Viruses enter human cells and modify them in such as way as to make more virus. A human cell infected with herpes virus releases thousands of new viruses before it is killed by the virus. The cell death and resulting tissue damage causes the actual sores. The highest risk for spreading the virus is the time period beginning with the appearance of blisters and ending with scab formation.

Herpes virus can also infect a cell and instead of making the cell produce new viruses, it hides inside the cell and waits. Herpes virus hides in cells of the nervous system called "neurons." This period is called "latency." A latent virus can remain inside neurons for days, months, or even years. At some future time, the virus "awakens" and causes the cell to produce thousands of new viruses, which causes an active infection. Sometimes an active infection occurs without visible sores. Therefore, an infected person can spread herpes virus to other people even in the absence of sores.

This process of latency and active infection is best understood by considering the genital sore cycle. An active infection is obvious because sores are present. The first infection is called the "primary" infection. This active infection is then controlled by the body's immune system and the sores heal. In between active infections, the virus is latent. At some point in the future, latent viruses become activated and once again cause sores. These episodes are called "recurrent infections" or "outbreaks." Genital sores caused by herpes type 1 recur much less frequently than sores caused by herpes type 2.

Although the factors that trigger latent viruses to activate are not known, several conditions seem to bring on infections. These factors include illness, tiredness, exposure to ultraviolet light (sunlight, **tanning** beds), menstruation, **stress**, immunosuppression, sexual intercourse, and genital trauma.

In the United States, approximately 22% of pregnant women are infected with HSV–2. Newborn babies who are infected with herpes virus experience a very severe, and possibly fatal disease. This disease is called "neonatal herpes infection."

The risk to the neonate varies depending on the time the mother was infected. If the mother was infected prior to the **pregnancy** or during early pregnancy, the risk for infection to the neonate is about one percent. If a woman becomes infected in the last trimester, the risk of neonatal infection is as high as 30 to 50%. The higher risk for infection in late pregnancy is attributed to an inadequate time to develop the antibodies needed to suppress replication of the virus before labor begins.

In the United States, one in 3,000–5,000 babies born will be infected with the herpes virus. Babies can become infected during passage through the birth canal, but can also become infected during the pregnancy if the mother's membranes rupture early. Doctors will perform a **Cesarean section** on women who go into labor with active genital herpes.

Causes and symptoms

While anyone can be infected by herpes virus, not everyone will show symptoms. Risk factors for genital herpes include: early age at first sexual activity, multiple sexual partners, history of unprotected sexual intercourse, and a medical history of other sexually–transmitted diseases.

Most patients with genital herpes experience a prodrome (symptoms of oncoming disease) of **pain**, burning, **itching**, or **tingling** at the site where blisters will form. This prodrome stage may last anywhere from a few hours, to one to two days. The herpes infection prodrome can occur for both the primary infection and recurrent infections. The prodrome for recurrent infections may be severe and cause a severe burning or stabbing pain in the genital area, legs, or buttocks.

Primary genital herpes

The first symptoms of herpes usually occur within three to seven days after contact with an infected person, but may take up to two weeks. Symptoms of the primary infection are usually more severe than those of recurrent infections. For up to 70% of patients, the primary infection causes symptoms which affect the whole body (called "constitutional symptoms") including tiredness, **headache**, **fever**, chills, muscle aches, loss of appetite, as well as painful, swollen lymph nodes in the groin. These symptoms are greatest during the first three to four days of the infection and disappear within one week. The primary infection is more severe in women than in men.

Following the prodrome herpes pimples which turn into blisters, which are similar on men and women, begin to appear. First, small red bumps appear. These bumps quickly become fluid–filled blisters. In dry areas, the blisters become filled with pus and take on a white to gray appearance, become covered with a scab, and heal within two to three weeks. In moist areas, the fluid–filled blisters burst and form painful ulcers which drain before healing. New blisters may appear over a period of one week or longer and may join together to form very large ulcers. The pain is relieved within two weeks and the blisters and ulcers heal without scarring by two to six weeks.

Women can experience a very severe and painful primary infection. Herpes blisters first appear on the labia majora (outer lips), labia minora (inner lips), and entrance to the vagina. Blisters often appear on the clitoris, at the urinary opening, around the anal opening, and on the buttocks and thighs. In addition, women may get herpes blisters on the lips, breasts, fingers, and eyes. The vagina and cervix are almost always involved, which causes a watery discharge. Other symptoms that occur in women are: painful or difficult urination (83%), swelling of the urinary tube (85%), **meningitis** (36%), and throat infection (13%).

KEY TERMS

Groin—The region of the body that lies between the abdomen and the thighs.

Latent virus—An inactive virus which is in a dormant state within a cell. Herpes virus is latent in cells of the nervous system.

Prodrome—Symptoms which warn of the beginning of disease. The herpes prodrome consists of pain, burning, tingling, or itching at a site before blisters are visible.

Recurrence—The return of an active herpes infection following a period of latency.

Ulcer—A painful, pus–draining, depression in the skin caused by an infection.

Most women develop painful, swollen lymph nodes (lymphadenopathy) in the groin and pelvis. About one in ten women get a vaginal yeast infection as a complication of the primary herpes infection.

In men, the herpes blisters usually form on the penis but can also appear on the scrotum, thighs, and buttocks. Fewer than half of the men with primary herpes experience constitutional symptoms. Thirty to forty percent of men have a discharge from the urinary tube. Some men develop painful swollen lymph nodes (lymphadenopathy) in the groin and pelvis. Although less frequently than women, men too may experience painful or difficult urination (44%), swelling of the urinary tube (27%), meningitis (13%), and throat infection (7%).

Recurrent genital herpes

Several (five to eight) outbreaks of genital herpes per year occur in 60–90% of those infected with the herpes virus. About 40% of the persons infected with herpes simplex virus type 2 will experience six or more outbreaks each year. Genital herpes recurrences are less severe than the primary infection; however, women still experience more severe symptoms and pain than men. Constitutional symptoms are not usually present. Blisters will appear at the same sites during each outbreak. Usually there are fewer blisters, less pain, and the time period from the beginning of symptoms to healing is shorter than the primary infection. One out of every four women experience painful or difficult urination during recurrent infection. Both men and women may develop lymphadenopathy.

Diagnosis

Because genital herpes is so common, it is diagnosed primarily by symptoms. It can be diagnosed and treated by the family doctor or nurse practitioner, dermatologists (doctors who specialize in skin diseases), urologists (doctors who specialize in the urinary tract diseases of men and women and the genital organs of men), gynecologists (doctors who specialize in the diseases of women's genital organs) and **infectious disease** specialists. The diagnosis and treatment of this infectious disease should be covered by most insurance providers.

Examination

The health care practitioner will examine the patient for typical signs of genital herpes such as shallow, painful ulcers, and swelling in areas where herpes lesions are present. The lymph nodes in the groin will be palpated during the **physical examination**. These lymph nodes are often tender and painful to the touch.

Because newborns who are infected with herpes virus may be born to mothers who have no symptoms of infection it is important to check all newborn babies for symptoms. Any skin sore should be sampled to determine if it is caused by herpes simplex. Babies should be checked for sores in their mouth and for signs of herpes infection in their eyes.

Tests

Laboratory tests may be performed to look for the virus. Because healing sores do not shed much virus, a sample from an open sore would be taken for viral culture. A sterile cotton swab is wiped over open sores and the sample used to infect human cells in culture. Cells which are killed by herpes virus have a certain appearance under microscopic examination. The results of this test are available within two to ten days. Other areas which may be sampled, depending upon the disease symptoms in a particular patient, include the urinary tract, vagina, cervix, throat, eye tissues, and cerebrospinal fluid.

Direct staining and microscopic examination of the lesion sample may also be used. A blood test may be performed to see if the patient has antibodies to herpes virus. The results of blood testing are available within one day. The disadvantage of this blood test is that it usually does not distinguish between herpes type 1 and 2, and only determines that the patient has had a herpes infection at some point in his or her life. Therefore, the viral culture test must be performed to be absolutely certain that the sores are caused by herpes virus.

Because genital sores can be symptoms of many other diseases, the doctor must determine the exact cause of the sores. The above mentioned tests are performed to determine that herpes virus is causing the genital sores. Other diseases which may cause genital sores are **syphilis**, **chancroid**, **lymphogranuloma venereum**, **granuloma inguinale**, herpes zoster, erythema multiform, Behçet's syndrome, inflammatory bowel disease, **contact dermatitis**, **candidiasis**, and **impetigo**.

Treatment

Traditional

There is no cure for herpes virus infections. There are **antiviral drugs** available which have some effect in lessening the symptoms and decreasing the length of herpes outbreaks. There is evidence that some may also prevent future outbreaks. These antiviral drugs work by interfering with the replication of the virus and are most effective when taken as early in the infection process as possible. For the best results, drug treatment should begin during the prodrome stage before blisters are visible. Depending on the length of the outbreak, drug treatment can continue for up to 10 days.

Drugs

Antiviral agents such as acyclovir (Zovirax), famciclovir (Famvir), and valacyclovir (Valtrex) appear to be equally effective as treatment agents for primary genital HSV infection although treatment with acyclovir is typically less expensive. The drugs, which are most frequently given orally to treat uncomplicated cases of genital herpes, should be started within 72 hours of the appearance of lesions to be most effective. Beginning treatment within this time frame appears to decrease the duration of the outbreak and often lessens the severity of the infection.

Currently, recommended doses and treatment schedules for these drugs are:

- acyclovir, 400 mg by mouth three times per day
- famciclovir, 250 mg by mouth three times per day
- valacyclovir, 1000 mg by mouth two times per day

Duration of treatment is usually seven to ten days.

Treatment of recurrent episodes

Treatment strategies for recurrent episodes of genital herpes depend on the frequency of the episodes and the severity of the outbreaks among other considerations. These strategies include:

- No treatment may be recommended for individuals who experience infrequent outbreaks and/or minimal symptoms with outbreaks.
- Chronic suppressive therapy is recommended for people with very frequent recurrences and for individuals who are HSV–seropositive with uninfected sexual partners. This strategy involves daily antiviral therapy.
- Episodic therapy may be used by individuals to treat outbreaks of the infection as they occur. Patients should be counseled to begin treatment with antivirals when prodromal symptoms (tingling, itching, burning, pain) begin and before herpes pimples and blisters occur.

Treatment for complicated genital herpes infection

Complicated genital herpes includes those cases in which there is involvement of the central nervous system such as in cases of aseptic meningitis, **encephalitis**, or tranverse myelitis associated with the herpes infection. Other complications can include hepatitis, pneumonitis, and HSV infection which is wide–spread. The Centers for Disease Control (CDC) recommends treatment with intravenous acyclovir at a dose of five to 10 mg/kg every eight hours for two to seven days or longer as the treatment for complicated cases of genital herpes. Treatment is continued until clinical improvement is noted. Following conclusion of intravenous antiviral therapy, the patient is started on oral antiviral therapy for at least an additional 10 days. Some patients may require longer duration of treatment.

Neonatal herpes

Newborn babies with herpes virus infections are treated with intravenous acyclovir. The duration of treatment, which may last 21 days or longer, depends on the extent of the infection and on the baby's response to therapy. Treatment with antivirals and other supportive measures has greatly reduced deaths and increased the number of babies who appear normal at one year of age. However, because neonatal herpes infection is so serious, even with treatment babies may not survive, or may suffer nervous system damage.

Alternative

An imbalance in the amino acids lysine and arginine is thought to be one contributing factor in herpes virus outbreaks. A ratio of lysine to arginine that is in balance (that is more lysine than arginine is present) seems to help the immune system work optimally. Thus, a diet that is rich in lysine may help prevent recurrences of genital herpes. Foods that contain high levels of lysine include most vegetables, legumes, fish, turkey, beef, lamb, cheese, and chicken. Patients may take 500 mg of lysine daily and increase to 1,000 mg three times a day during an outbreak. Intake of the amino acid arginine should be reduced. Foods rich in arginine that should be avoided are chocolate, peanuts, almonds, and other nuts and seeds.

Clinical experience indicates a connection between high stress and herpes outbreaks. Some patients respond well to **stress reduction** and relaxation techniques. **Acupressure** and massage may relieve tiredness and stress. **Meditation**, **yoga**, **tai chi**, and **hypnotherapy** can also help relieve stress and promote relaxation.

Some herbs, including **echinacea** (*Echinacea* spp.) and garlic (*Allium sativum*), are believed to strengthen the body's defenses against viral infections. Red marine algae (family Dumontiaceae), both taken internally and applied topically, is thought to be effective in treating herpes type I and type II infections. Other topical treatments may be helpful in inhibiting the growth of the herpes virus, in minimizing the damage it causes, or in helping the sores heal. Zinc sulphate ointment seems to help sores heal and to fight recurrence. Lithium succinate ointment may interfere with viral replication. An ointment made with glycyrrhizinic acid, a component of licorice (*Glycyrrhiza glabra*), seems to inactivate the virus. Topical applications of vitamin E or tea tree oil (*Melaleuca* spp.) help dry up herpes sores. Results of one study indicated that using an ointment containing propolis, a waxy substance made by bees, helped in healing herpes lesions. Individuals using the ointment four times a day for 10 days reported improvement in the lesions. Other research seems to indicate that the herb Prunella vulgaris and an edible mushroom, Rozites caperata (also known as gypsy mushroom) contain chemicals that may be helpful in fighting the effects of HSV–1 and HSV–2. Specific combinations of homeopathic remedies may also be helpful treatments for genital herpes.

Home remedies

There are several things that a patient may do to lessen the pain of genital sores. Over–the–counter pain relievers such as **aspirin**, **acetaminophen**, or ibuprofen may help to reduce the pain associated with a herpes outbreak. Wearing loose fitting clothing and cotton underwear is helpful. Removing clothing or wearing loose pajamas while at home may reduce pain. Soaking in a tub of warm water and using a blow dryer on the "cool" setting to dry the infected area is helpful however, most clinicians recommend keeping infected areas dry most of the time. Putting an ice pack on the affected area for 10 minutes, followed by five minutes off and then repeating this procedure may relieve pain. Application of a baking soda compress to sores may be soothing.

Prognosis

Although physically and emotionally painful, genital herpes is usually not a serious disease. The primary infection can be severe and may require hospitalization for treatment. Complications of the primary infection may involve the cervix, urinary system, anal opening, and the nervous system. Persons who have a decreased ability to produce an immune response to infection (called "immunocompromised") due to disease or medication are at risk for a very severe, and possibly fatal, herpes infection. Even with antiviral treatment, neonatal herpes infections can be fatal or cause permanent nervous system damage.

Prevention

The only way to prevent genital herpes is to avoid contact with infected persons. This is not an easy solution because many people are not aware that they are infected and can easily spread the virus to others. Avoid all sexual contact with an infected person during a herpes outbreak. Because herpes virus can be spread at any time, condom use is recommended to prevent the spread of virus to uninfected partners. At this time, there is no vaccine available to prevent genital herpes.

Resources

BOOKS

Levine, G.I. "Herpes, Genital." In Dominino, F.J., ed. *The Five Minute Clinical Consult 2009*, 17th ed. Philadelphia: Wolters, Kluwer Health/Lippincott Williams, and Wilkins, 2009

PERIODICALS

Gupta,R., T. Warren, and A. Wald. "Genital Herpes." *Lancet*. 370 (2007): 2127–2137.

Phillip, S.S., et al. "Evaluation of a New Point–of–Care Serologic Assay for Herpes Simplex Virus Type 2 Infection." *Clinical Infectious Diseases*. 47 (2008): e79–e82.

Sen, P. and S.E. Barton. "Genital Herpes and Its Management." *BMJ* 334 (2007): 1048–1052.

Xu, F., et al. "Trends in Herpes Simplex Virus Type 1 and type 2 Seroprevalence in the United States." *JAMA*. 296 (2006): 964–973.

OTHER

Genital Herpes – CDC Fact Sheet. Centers for Disease Control and Prevention. http://www.cdc.gov/st d/Herpes/STDFact-Herpes.htm (accessed on August 31, 2010).

ORGANIZATIONS

Centers for Disease Control and Prevention (CDC), 1600 Clifton Road, Atlanta, GA, 30333, (800) 232–4636, cdcinfo@cdc.gov, http://www.cdc.gov.

Belinda Rowland, PhD
Melinda Granger Oberleitner, RN,DNS,APRN,CNS

Genital warts

Definition

Genital **warts**, which are also called condylomata acuminata or venereal warts, are growths in the genital area caused by a sexually transmitted papillomavirus. A papillomavirus is a virus that produces papillomas, or benign growths on the skin and mucous membranes.

Description

Genital warts are the most common sexually transmitted disease (STD) in the general population. It is estimated that 1% of sexually active people between the ages of 18 and 45 have genital warts; however, polymerase chain reaction (PCR) testing indicates that as many as 40% of sexually active adults carry the human papillomavirus (HPV) that causes genital warts.

Genital warts vary somewhat in appearance. They may be either flat or resemble raspberries or cauliflower in appearance. The warts begin as small red or pink

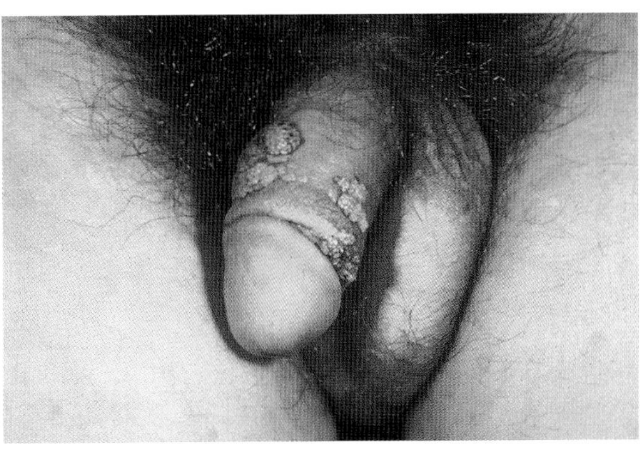

Man with genital warts. *(Custom Medical Stock Photo, Inc. Reproduced by permission.)*

growths and grow as large as four inches across, interfering with intercourse and **childbirth**. The warts grow in the moist tissues of the genital areas. In women, they occur on the external genitals and on the walls of the vagina and cervix; in men, they develop in the urethra and on the shaft of the penis. The warts then spread to the area behind the genitals surrounding the anus.

Risk factors for genital warts include:

- multiple sexual partners
- infection with another STD
- pregnancy
- anal intercourse
- poor personal hygiene
- heavy perspiration

Causes and symptoms

There are about 80 types of human papillomavirus. Genital warts are caused by HPV types 1, 2, 6, 11, 16, and 18. HPV is transmitted by sexual contact. The incubation period varies from one to six months.

The symptoms include bleeding, **pain**, and odor as well as the visible warts.

Diagnosis

The diagnosis is usually made by examining scrapings from the warts under a darkfield microscope. If the warts are caused by HPV, they will turn white when a 5% solution of white vinegar is added. If the warts reappear, the doctor may order a biopsy to rule out **cancer**.

Treatment

No treatment for genital warts is completely effective because therapy depends on destroying skin infected by the virus. There are no drugs that will kill the virus directly.

Medications

Genital warts were treated until recently with applications of podophyllum resin, a corrosive substance that cannot be given to pregnant patients. A milder form of podophyllum, podofilox (Condylox), has been introduced. Women are also treated with 5-fluorouracil cream, bichloroacetic acid, or trichloroacetic acid. All of these substances irritate the skin and require weeks of treatment.

Genital warts can also be treated with injections of interferon. Interferon works best in combination with podofilox applications.

KEY TERMS

Condylomata acuminata—Another name for genital warts.

Papilloma—A benign growth on the skin or mucous membrane. Viruses that cause these growths are called human papillomaviruses (HPVs).

Podophyllum resin—A medication derived from the May apple or mandrake and used to treat genital warts.

Surgery

Surgery may be necessary to remove warts blocking the patient's vagina, urethra, or anus. Surgical techniques include the use of liquid nitrogen, electrosurgery, and **laser surgery**.

Prognosis

Genital warts are benign growths and are not cancerous by themselves. Repeated HPV infection in women, however, appears to increase the risk of later **cervical cancer**. Women infected with HPV types 16 and 18 should have yearly cervical smears. Recurrence is common with all present methods of treatment—including surgery—because HPV can remain latent in apparently normal surrounding skin.

Prevention

The only reliable method of prevention is sexual abstinence. The use of **condoms** minimizes but does not eliminate the risk of HPV transmission. The patient's sexual contacts should be notified and examined.

Resources

BOOKS

Larsen, Laura. *Sexually Transmitted Diseases Sourcebook*. 4th ed. Detroit, MI: Omnigraphics, 2009.

McPhee, Stephen, and Maxine Papadakis.*Current Medical Diagnosis and Treatment, 2010*, 49th ed. New York: McGraw–Hill Medical, 2009.

Rebecca J. Frey, PhD

Gentamicin *see* **Aminoglycosides**

Germ cell tumors

Definition

Germ cell tumors (GCTs) are solid tumors which are diagnosed in children, adolescents, and less frequently, in adults. The term germ cell tumor alludes to the term "germinate" rather than to the term "germ" as it relates to bacterial or other related organisms that are capable of causing disease. These tumors arise from germ cells that develop into reproductive tissue such as testicular and ovarian cells. GCTs can be benign tumors or malignant (cancerous) tumors.

Demographics

The incidence of GCTs appears to be increasing. Malignant germ cell tumors account for about 3% of all cases of **cancer** occurring in children and adolescents prior to age 20 years. Malignant GCTs are more commonly diagnosed in adolescents between the ages of 15 and 19 years and account for about 14% of all cancers which occur in this age group.

Description

GCTs appear to arise from primitive germs cells. During embryo development, these germ cells migrate from the yolk sac down the midline of the body to the pelvis and eventually to the gonads, or reproductive organs. During fetal development, some of the cells may migrate to abnormal sites other than the gonads, however. Therefore, GCTs are classified as gonadal GCTs or extragonadal GCTs, meaning they occur in tissues that are not reproductive tissue. About 90% of GCTs are gonadal in origin.

Malignant GCTs can be further histologically classified according to the origin of the tumor. In young children, GCTs are classified as yolk sac tumors, which can arise from extragonadal, ovarian, or testicular tissue, or dysgerminoma, which arises from ovarian tissue and is rarely diagnosed in young children. In adolescents and in young adults, malignant GCTs can be classified as follows:

- seminoma – germinomas which arise from testicular tissue
- dysgerminoma – germinomas which arise from ovarian tissue
- germinoma –extagonadal origin
- yolk sac tumor –extragonadal, ovarian and testicular origin; also termed endodermal sinus tumors
- choriocarcinoma –extragonadal, ovarian, and testicular origin; a rare tumor type
- embryonal carcinoma –arises from testicular tissue
- mixed germ cell tumors – arises from extragonadal and ovarian tissue

Testicular and mediastinal seminomas are most likely to be diagnosed in adolescent and young adult males while ovarian dysgerminomas are more likely to be diagnosed in adolescent and young adult females. Most children who are diagnosed with a malignant GCT are most likely to have a yolk sac component to their tumors.

Some of the malignant GSTs secrete abnormal proteins such as alpha–fetaprotein (AFP) and beta–human chorionic gonadotropin (b–HCG) which are considered to be **tumor markers**. For example, yolk sac tumors secrete AFP while germinomas (such as seminoma and dysgerminoma) and choriocarcinomas produce b–HCG. Serum levels of these tumor markers can be monitored during treatment to determine the response of the tumor to the treatment.

Risk factors

Specific risk factors related to the development of GCTs have not been identified. However, patients diagnosed with certain genetic or hereditary syndromes or disorders appear to be at higher risk for the development of some types of GCTs. For example, individuals with **Klinefelter syndrome** appear to be at increased risk for the development of extragonadal GCT and patients with Swyer syndrome may be at increased risk for the development of germinomas.

KEY TERMS

Embryo—The human organism in the earliest stages of development.

Extragonadal—Occurring outside of the gonads or outside of the reproductive organs.

Gonads—The reproductive organs; testes in males and ovaries in females.

Histology—The study of the structure, composition, and function of tissues of organs.

Tumor marker—A biochemical substance produced and released or secreted by a tumor.

Yolk sac—A sac made of membranous tissue that is attached to the embryo and provides nutrition to the embryo.

Causes and symptoms

The specific cause of most cases of GCTs is unknown at this time. Some individuals with certain genetic or hereditary syndromes and disorders appear to be at higher risk for the development of some types of GCTs. In addition, several chromosomal abnormalities are being studied to determine their exact role in causing GCTs.

Symptoms of GCTs are linked to the size and location of the tumor. Symptoms may include:

- a swelling or mass of tissue that can be palpated
- abnormal shape or size of the testicle
- excessive hair growth
- early puberty
- hormonal abnormalities such as diabetes
- headache
- weakness in the lower extremities
- constipation

Diagnosis

Examination

A complete history and **physical examination** will be conducted. The suspected tumor mass will be examined and palpated. A focused assessment and examination will be conducted based on the location of the suspected tumor.

Tests

Levels of tumor markers such as AFP and b–HCG should be assessed prior to surgical intervention. Lactate dehydrogenase levels will also be determined. Tests which should be conducted prior to **chemotherapy** administration include a **complete blood count** (CBC) with differential and **platelet count**, tests to determine baseline kidney function such as the glomerular filtration rate and creatinine clearance rate, uric acid levels, **liver function tests**, and electrolyte levels as well as the levels of **calcium** and magnesium in the body.

Radiologic procedures which may be utilized include chest xray and magnetic imaging scanning (MRI) to evaluate for metastasis to the lungs, computed tomography (CT) and/or MRI scanning of the abdomen and/or pelvis if tumor is suspected in those locations, and bone scans to further determine extent of metastasis. Other tests which may be done, depending on the location of the tumor, include CT or MRI scans of the brain, ultrasounds of the abdomen and pelvis, testicular ultrasounds, and **positron emission tomography (PET)** scans to detect relapse of tumor. In addition, **pulmonary function tests** may be done to establish baseline pulmonary function prior to the start of chemotherapy administration.

Treatment

Treatment for these relatively rare types of cancer should be conducted at pediatric cancer centers experienced in treating GCTs. Factors which play a role in determining optimum treatment for GCTs include the histology of the tumor, tumor stage, the location of the primary tumor and the patient's age. Clinicians treating these children and adolescents will attempt to maximize the potential for survival while attempting to minimize the risk for adverse long–term side effects such as the development of second cancers, and other serious physical and cognitive impairments.

Currently, multimodality therapy is utilized including surgery and administration of chemotherapy. Based on the factors described above, treatment options may include:

- surgical removal of the tumor followed by strict surveillance for tumor relapse
- biopsy of the tumor to obtain a definitive diagnosis, followed by preoperative chemotherapy administration which includes a platinum–based chemotherapy drug, followed by surgical removal of all remaining tumor
- surgical removal of the tumor followed by platinum–based chemotherapy administration.

Currently, the standard chemotherapy regimen for children and adults diagnosed with malignant nonseminomatous GCTs includes the drugs cisplatin, etoposide and bleomycin. However, children are given fewer doses of bleomycin than adults.

There are different treatment options for malignant testicular GCTs in boys than for adolescents and young adult males which vary by stage of disease at the time of diagnosis and age of the patient. Treatment options for childhood ovarian GCT includes a multimodality approach which may utilize surgery, observation, and chemotherapy. Current standard treatment options for childhood malignant extragonadal GCTs varies by patient age, tumor location, tumor histology, and stage at time of diagnosis and may include surgery and chemotherapy administration.

Prognosis

The 5–year survival rate for gonadal GCTs increased from 89% to 98% in children younger than age 15 years between 1975 and 2002 according to the National Cancer Institute. The 5–year survival rate for adolescents diagnosed with gonadal GCTs between the ages of 15 and 19 years increased from 70% to 95% during that same time period.

The 5–year survival rate for extragonadal GCTs increased from 42% to 83% in children younger than age 15 years between 1979 and 2002. The 5–year survival rate for adolescents between the ages of 15 and 19 years increased from 80% to 95% during that same time period.

Prevention

As the cause of most cases of childhood GCTs is not currently known, there are no ways to prevent development of GCTs. Children diagnosed with specific congenital or hereditary syndromes or disorders which increase their risk of developing GCTs should be screened for GCTs.

Resources

PERIODICAL

Horton, Z., Schlatter, M., & Schultz, S. "Pediatric Germ Cell Tumors."*Surg Oncol.* (2007); 16(3): 205–13.

McIntyre, A., Gilbert, D., Goddard, N. et al. "Genes, Chromosomes, and the Development of Testicular Germ Cell Tumors of Adolescents and Adults."*Genes Chromosomes and Cancer*. (2008); 47(7): 547–57.

McKenney, J.K., Heerema-McKenney, A., & Rouse, R.V. "Extragonadal Germ Cell Tumors: A Review with Emphasis on Pathologic Features, Clinical Prognostic Variables, and Differential Diagnostic Considerations." *Adv Anat Pathol.* (2007); 14(2): 69–92.

Palenzuela, G., Martin, E., Meunier, A., et al. "Comprehensive Staging Allows for Excellent Outcome in Patients with Localized Malignant Germ Cell Tumor of the Ovary."*Ann Surg.* (2008); 248(5): 836–41.

OTHER

Adkins, E.S. "Teratomas and Other Germ Cell Tumors." eMedicine. May 29, 2008 [cited September 5, 2010]. http://www.emedicine.medscape.com

"Childhood Extracranial Germ Cell Tumors Treatment (PDQ)." National Cancer Institute. June 24, 2010 [cited September 5, 2010]. http://www.cancer.gov

ORGANIZATIONS

Candlelighters Childhood Cancer Family Alliance. , 8323 Southwest Freeway, Suite 435, Houston, Texas, 77074, (713) 270-4700, (713) 270-9802, http//www.candle.org.

CureSearch for Children's Cancer, National Childhood Cancer Foundation, 4600 East West Highway, Suite 600, Bethesda, Maryland, 20814-3457, (800) 458–6223 (U.S. and Canada), info@curesearch.org, http://www.curesearch.org.

Genetic and Rare Disease Information Center (GARD), P.O. Box 8126, Gaithersburg, Maryland, 20898-8126, (888) 205-2311, (301) 251-4911, http://www.rarediseases.info.nih.gov/GARD.

St. Jude's Children's Research Hospital, 262 Danny Thomas Place, Memphis, Tennessee, 38105, (901) 595-3300, http://www.stjude.org.

Melinda Granger Oberleitner, RN, DNS, APRN, CNS

German measles *see* **Rubella**

Gestalt therapy

Definition

Gestalt therapy is a humanistic therapy technique that focuses on gaining an awareness of emotions and behaviors in the present rather than in the past. The therapist does not interpret experiences for the patient. Instead, the therapist and patient work together to help the patient understand him/herself. This type of therapy focuses on experiencing the present situation rather than talking about what occurred in the past. Patients are encouraged to become aware of immediate needs, meet them, and let them recede into the background. The well-adjusted person is seen as someone who has a constant flow of needs and is able to satisfy those needs.

Purpose

In Gestalt therapy (from the German word meaning *form*), the major goal is self-awareness. Patients work on uncovering and resolving interpersonal issues during therapy. Unresolved issues are unable to fade into the background of consciousness because the needs they represent are never met. In Gestalt therapy, the goal is to discover people connected with a patient's unresolved issues and try to engage those people (or images of those people) in interactions that can lead to a resolution. Gestalt therapy is most useful for patients open to working on self-awareness.

Precautions

The choice of a therapist is crucial. Some people who call themselves "therapists" have limited training in Gestalt therapy. It is important that the therapist be a licensed mental health professional. Additionally, some individuals may not be able to tolerate the intensity of this type of therapy.

Description

Gestalt therapy has developed into a form of therapy that emphasizes medium to large groups, although many Gestalt techniques can be used in one-on-one therapy. Gestalt therapy probably has a greater range of formats than any other therapy technique. It is practiced in individual, couples, and family therapies, as well as in therapy with children.

Ideally, the patient identifies current sensations and emotions, particularly ones that are painful or disruptive. Patients are confronted with their unconscious feelings and needs, and are assisted to accept and assert those repressed parts of themselves.

The most powerful techniques involve role-playing. For example, the patient talks to an empty chair as they imagine that a person associated with an unresolved issue is sitting in the chair. As the patient talks to the "person" in the chair, the patient imagines that the person responds to the expressed feelings. Although this technique may sound artificial and might make some people feel self-conscious, it can be a powerful way to approach buried feelings and gain new insight into them.

Sometimes patients use battacca bats, padded sticks that can be used to hit chairs or sofas. Using a battacca bat can help a patient safely express anger. A patient may also experience a Gestalt therapy marathon, where the participants and one or more facilitators have non-stop **group therapy** over a weekend. The effects of the intense emotion and the lack of sleep can eliminate many psychological defenses and allow significant progress to be made in a short time. This is true only if the patient has adequate psychological strength for a marathon and is carefully monitored by the therapist.

Preparation

Gestalt therapy begins with the first contact. There is no separate diagnostic or assessment period. Instead, assessment and screening are done as part of the ongoing relationship between patient and therapist. This assessment includes determining the patient's willingness and support for work using Gestalt methods, as well as determining the compatibility between the patient and the therapist. Unfortunately, some "encounter groups" led by poorly trained individuals do not provide adequate pre-therapy screening and assessment.

Aftercare

Sessions are usually held once a week. Frequency of sessions held is based on how long the patient can go between sessions without losing the momentum from the previous session. Patients and therapists discuss when to start sessions, when to stop sessions, and what kind of activities to use during a session. However, the patient is encouraged and required to make choices.

Risks

Disturbed people with severe mental illness may not be suitable candidates for Gestalt therapy. Facilities that provide Gestalt therapy and train Gestalt therapists vary. Since there are no national standards for these Gestalt facilities, there are no set national standards for Gestalt therapy or Gestalt therapists.

Normal results

Scientific documentation on the effectiveness of Gestalt therapy is limited. Evidence suggests that this type of therapy may not be reliably effective.

Abnormal results

This approach can be anti-intellectual and can discount thoughts, thought patterns, and beliefs. In the hands of an ineffective therapist, Gestalt procedures can become a series of mechanical exercises, allowing the therapist as a person to stay hidden. Moreover, there is a potential for the therapist to manipulate the patient with powerful techniques, especially in therapy marathons where **fatigue** may make a patient vulnerable.

ORGANIZATIONS

Association for the Advancement of Gestalt Therapy, 400 East 58th St, New York, NY, 10022, (212) 486-1581, http://www.aagt.org.

David James Doermann

Gestational diabetes

Definition

Gestational diabetes is an abnormal increase blood sugar (glucose) levels that occurs during **pregnancy** in some women. Unlike other types of diabetes, gestational diabetes first appears during pregnancy and then disappears after the woman gives birth.

Demographics

Studies have found that in the United States between 3% and 10% of women experience diabetes

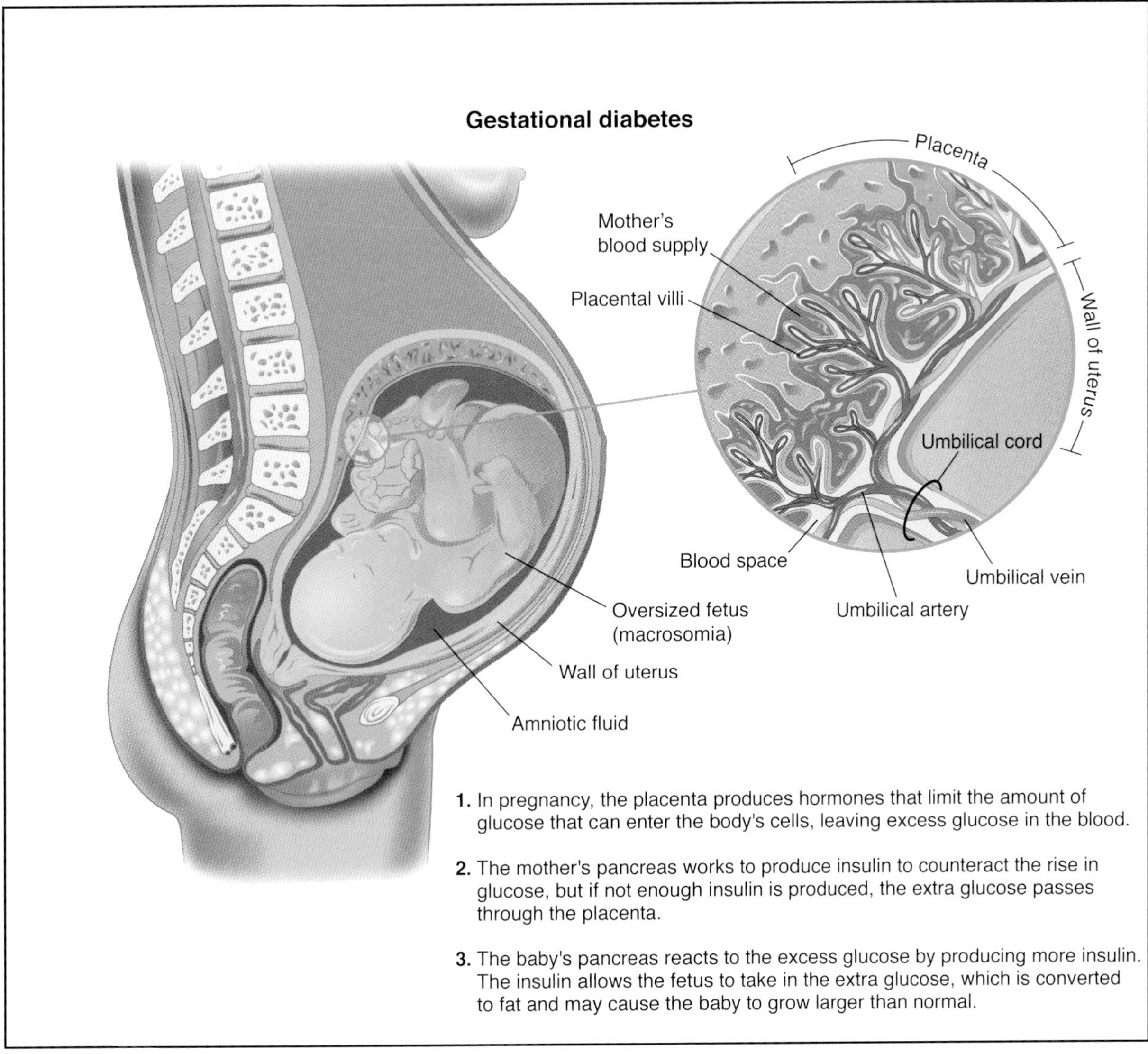

(Illustration by Electronic Illustrators Group. Reproduced by permission of Gale, a part of Cengage Learning.)

during pregnancy. Ninety percent of these women develop gestational diabetes, about 8% have pre-existing type 2 (insulin resistant) diabetes, while about 1% have pre-existing type 1 (insulin deficiency) diabetes.

Race and ethnicity strongly affect the rate of development of gestational diabetes. Only about 1.4–2% of Caucasian women develop gestational diabetes, while as many as 15% of Native American women from tribes in the Southwest United States develop the disorder. Between 5% and 8% of Hispanic Americans, African Americans, and Asian Americans develop gestational diabetes. If a woman experiences gestational diabetes, the chance of her developing it again in future pregnancies is as high as 68%.

Description

Carbohydrates (sugars and starches) found in foods such as sweets, potatoes, pasta, and breads, are broken down during digestion into glucose, a simple sugar that circulates in the blood and is used by cells for energy. The level of glucose changes depending on what food and how much of it a person eats. The level usually is highest about two hours after a meal. However, in order for the body to remain healthy, blood glucose levels must stay stable with certain narrow limits. In healthy people, the hormone insulin regulates the blood glucose level by controlling how much glucose enters cells. Once in cells, glucose either is used to meet the immediate energy needs of the cell or stored in liver, muscle, or fat cells for later release when blood glucose levels are low. In people with diabetes, this regulatory mechanism does not function correctly, and glucose builds up in the blood, a condition called hyperglycemia.

There are three types of diabetes. In type 1 diabetes, the pancreas, a digestive system organ, does not make any insulin or does not make enough insulin to properly regulate blood glucose levels. People with type 1 diabetes must control their blood glucose through diet, **exercise**, and most importantly, through the regular injection of synthetic or animal insulin.

In type 2 diabetes, the pancreas makes enough insulin, but cells become unresponsive to it, a condition called **insulin resistance**. As a result, adequate amounts of glucose cannot enter these cells, and glucose builds up in the blood. Many people with type 2 diabetes can control their blood glucose level through diet and exercise. Others must take supplemental insulin either by mouth (orally) or by injection.

In gestational diabetes, the pancreas makes insulin, but the placenta, which allows the fetus to obtain nourishment, produces hormones (e.g., estrogens, progesterone, and chorionic somatomammotropin) that increase the insulin resistance of cells. These hormones are at their highest levels during the third trimester of pregnancy. Their presence reduces the amount of glucose that can enter cells, so that more remains in the blood and hyperglycemia occurs. Most pregnant women do not develop gestational diabetes because the pancreas produces additional quantities of insulin (as much as 50% more than normal in the third trimester) in order to compensate for insulin resistance caused by pregnancy hormones. However, when a woman's pancreas cannot produce enough extra insulin, blood levels of glucose stay abnormally high, and the woman develops gestational diabetes.

Risk factors

Women at risk for gestational diabetes include those who:

- are overweight
- have a family history of diabetes
- have previously given birth to a very large, heavy baby
- have previously had a baby who was stillborn, or born with a birth defect
- have an unusually large amount of amniotic fluid (the cushioning fluid within the uterus that surrounds the developing fetus)
- are over 30 years of age
- belong to an ethnic group known to experience higher rates of gestational diabetes
- have a history of gestational diabetes during a pregnancy

Causes and symptoms

Since increasing levels of pregnancy hormones cause gestational diabetes, it develops in late in pregnancy when pregnancy hormones are at their highest levels. Often women with gestational diabetes have few symptoms. However, leaving gestational diabetes undiagnosed and untreated is risky to the developing fetus. Left untreated, the mother's blood glucose levels will remain consistently high, and these same high levels will occur in the blood of the fetus. The fetal pancreas responds to the high level glucose by secreting large amounts of insulin. This insulin allows the fetal cells to take in excess glucose that is converted into fat and stored. This conversion process uses oxygen that may be needed for other fetal processes. Low oxygen levels can lead to an increased risk of heart, breathing, and vision problems. Increased fat storage causes many babies born to women with gestational diabetes to be unusually large, often large enough to cause more difficult deliveries that may require the use of forceps, suction, or **cesarean section**.

Furthermore, when the baby is born, it will have an abnormally high level of insulin in the blood. After birth, when the mother and baby are no longer attached to each other via the placenta and umbilical cord, the baby will no longer be receiving the mother's high level of blood glucose. The infant's high level of insulin, however, will quickly use up the glucose circulating in the infant's bloodstream. The baby is then at risk for having a dangerously low level of blood glucose, a condition called **hypoglycemia**. When this occurs, it is easily resolved by giving the baby glucose from an external source.

Diagnosis

Since gestational diabetes often exists with no symptoms detectable by the mother, and since its existence puts the developing baby at risk for developmental abnormalities, screening for the disorder is a routine part of pregnancy care. This screening usually is done between the 26th and 28th week of pregnancy. At this point in the pregnancy, the placental hormones have reached a sufficient level to cause insulin

KEY TERMS

Glucose—A simple sugar that is the final product of the breakdown of carbohydrates.

Glycemic index—A ranking from 1–100 of how much carbohydrate-containing foods raise blood sugar levels within two hours after being eaten. Foods with a glycemic index of 50 or lower are considered "good."

Hormone—A chemical messenger that is produced by one type of cell and travels through the bloodstream to change the metabolism of a different type of cell.

Insulin—A hormone produced by the pancreas that is central to the processing of sugars and carbohydrates in the diet.

Placenta—An organ that is attached to the inside wall of the mother's uterus and to the fetus via the umbilical cord. The placenta allows oxygen and nutrients from the mother's bloodstream to pass into the unborn baby.

Type 1 diabetes—A chronic immune system disorder in which the pancreas does not produce sufficient amounts of insulin, a hormone that enables cells to use glucose for energy. Also called juvenile diabetes, it must be treated with insulin injections.

Type 2 diabetes—Formerly called adult-onset diabetes. In this form of diabetes, the pancreas either does not make enough insulin or cells become insulin resistant and do not use insulin efficiently.

resistance. Screening for gestational diabetes involves the pregnant woman drinking a special solution that contains exactly 50 grams of glucose. An hour later, the woman's blood is drawn and tested for its glucose level. A level less than 140 mg/dL is considered normal.

When the screening glucose level is over 140 mg/dL, a special three-hour glucose tolerance test is performed. This involves following a special diet for three days before the test. This diet is set up to contain at least 150 grams of carbohydrates each day. Just before the test, the woman is instructed to eat and drink nothing except water for 10–14 hours. A blood sample is then tested to determine the fasting glucose level. The woman then drinks a special solution containing exactly 100 grams of glucose, and her blood is tested every hour for the next three hours. If two or more of these levels are elevated over normal, then the woman is considered to have gestational diabetes.

Treatment

Treatment for gestational diabetes depends on the severity of the diabetes. Mild forms can be treated with changes in diet. Women may be put on strict, detailed **diets**, and instructed to stay within a certain range of calorie intake. Exercise sometimes is used to help reduce blood glucose levels. Women often are asked to regularly measure their blood glucose level. This is done by poking a finger with a needle called a lancet, putting a drop of blood on a special type of paper, and feeding the paper into a meter that analyzes and reports the blood glucose level. Self-monitoring of blood glucose helps to manage gestational diabetes and prevent complications. When diet and exercise do not keep blood glucose levels within an acceptable range, a woman may need to take regular shots of insulin.

Prognosis

Prognosis for women with gestational diabetes and their infants is generally good. Almost all such women have blood glucose levels that return to normal after the birth of their baby. However, research has shown that nearly half of these women who have gestational diabetes will develop type 2 diabetes within 15 years.

Pregnant women who have type 1 or type 2 diabetes that is poorly controlled have 4–8 times the chance of having a baby born with a birth defect than women who do not have diabetes. The risk is much lower for babies born to women who develop gestational diabetes because their fetus is exposed to high glucose levels for a much shorter time and only near the end of pregnancy after most organs are already formed. However, the child of a mother with gestational diabetes has a greater-than-normal chance of developing diabetes sometime in adulthood. A woman who has had gestational diabetes during one pregnancy has about a 68% chance of having it again during any subsequent pregnancies. Women who had gestational diabetes usually have their blood glucose levels tested at the post-partum checkup or after stopping **breastfeeding**.

Prevention

There is no known way to prevent gestational diabetes since it is caused by the effects of normal hormones of pregnancy. However, the effects of insulin resistance can be best handled through careful attention to diet, avoiding becoming overweight throughout life, and participating in reasonable exercise and avoiding **smoking**.

Resources

BOOKS

American College of Obstetricians and Gynecologists, Women's, Health Care Physicians. *Your Pregnancy and Childbirth: Month to Month*, 5th ed. Washington, DC: American College of Obstetricians and Gynecologists, 2010.

BOOKS

Harms, Roger W. *Mayo Clinic Guide to a Healthy Pregnancy*. Rochester, MN: Mayo Clinic, 2004.

Roizen, Michael F., and Mehmet C. Oz. *You Having a Baby: The Owner's Manual to a Happy and Healthy Pregnancy*. New York: Free Press, 2009.

OTHER

Diabetes and Pregnancy. Medline Plus. January 6, 2010. http://www.nlm.nih.gov/medlineplus/diabetesandpregnancy.html

Diabetes and Pregnancy Frequently Asked Questions. United States Centers for Disease Control and Prevention. October 5, 2005. http://www.cdc.gov/ncbddd/bd/diabetespregnancyfaqs.htm

Prenatal Care. National Women's Health Information Center March 6, 2009. http://www.womenshealth.gov/faq/prenatal-care.cfm

Routine Tests in Pregnancy. American College of Obstetri cians and Gynecologists January 2009. http://www. acog.org/publications/patient_education/bp133.cfm

ORGANIZATIONS

American College of Obstetricians and Gynecologists, P.O. Box 96920, Washington, DC, 20090-6920, (202) 638-5577, http://www.acog.org.

American Diabetes Association, 1701 North Beauregard Street, Alexandria, VA, 22311, (800) DIABETES (342-2383), askADA@diabetes.org, http://www.diabetes.org.

American Pregnancy Association, 431 Greenway Drive, Suite 800, Irving, TX, 75038, (972) 550-0140, (972) 550-0800, Questions@AmericanPregnancy.org, http://www.americanpregnancy.org.

National Diabetes Education Program, One Diabetes Way, Bethesda, MD, 20814-9692, (301) 496-3583, http://www.ndep.nih.gov.

Rosalyn Carson-DeWitt, MD
Tish Davidson, AM

GI bleeding studies

Definition

GI bleeding studies uses radioactive materials in the investigation of bleeding from the gastrointestinal (GI) tract. These studies go under various names such as "GI bleeding scans" or "Tagged red blood cell scans." They are performed and interpreted by radiologists (physicians who specialize in diagnosis and treatment of diseases by means of x rays or related substances).

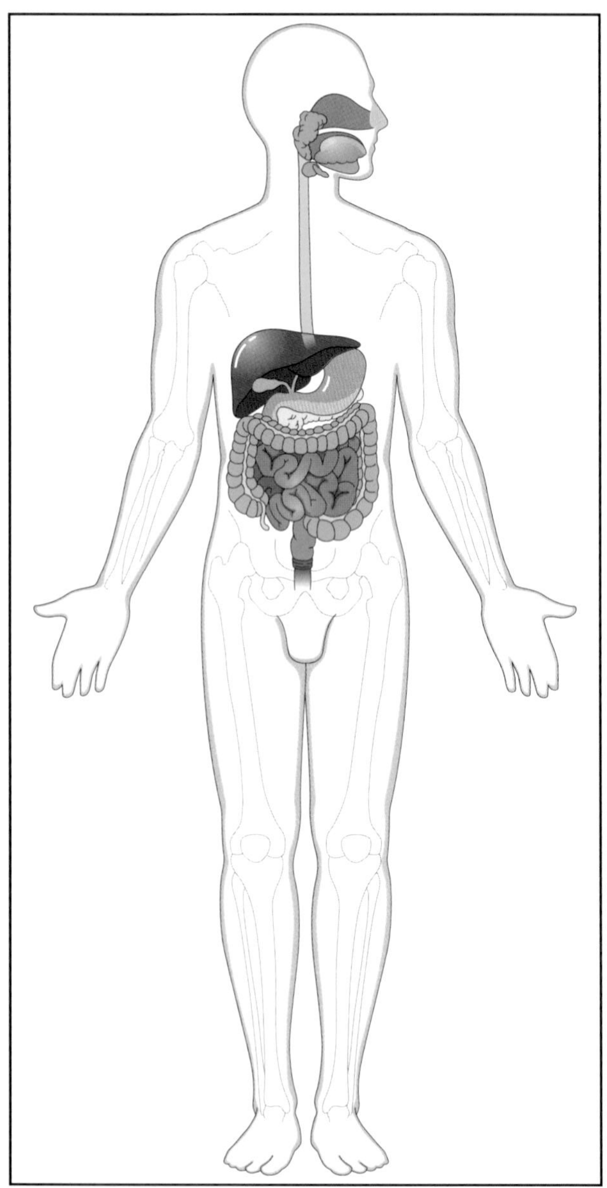

Diagram of the human digestive system. *(Illustration by Argosy, Inc. Reproduced by permission of Gale, a part of Cengage Learning.)*

KEY TERMS

Endoscope, Endoscopy—An endoscope as used in the field of gastroenterology is a thin flexible tube which uses a lens or miniature camera to view various areas of the gastrointestinal tract. The performance of an exam using an endoscope is referred by the general term endoscopy. Diagnosis through biopsies or other means and therapeutic procedures can be done with these instruments.

Purpose

These studies are designed to find the source of blood loss from the GI tract; that is the stomach, small bowel, or colon. They work best when bleeding is either too slow, intermittent, or too rapid to be identified by other means, such as **endoscopy**, upper GI series, or **barium enema**.

They are particularly useful when other methods have not been able to determine the site or cause of bleeding.

Precautions

Because of the use of radioactive materials, these studies are best avoided in pregnant patients. Another important relates to the interpretation of these tests, whether normal or abnormal. Since these studies are far from perfect, they can only be used as "guides" as to the cause or site of bleeding. In most instances, further studies must be performed to confirm their findings.

Description

Bleeding scans are based on the accumulation of radioactive material as it exits from the vessels during a bleeding episode. Blood is first withdrawn from the patient. Then, the blood, along with a radioactive substance is injected into a vein and over several hours scans measuring radioactivity are performed. The studies were initially reported to be very sensitive and accurate; however, critical evaluation of these tests have shown them to be less accurate than originally believed.

Preparation

No preparation is needed for these tests. They are often done on an "emergency" basis.

Aftercare

No special care is needed after the exam.

Risks

Bleeding scans are free of any risks or side-effects, aside from the fact that they should best be avoided in **pregnancy**.

Normal results

A normal exam would fail to show any evidence of accumulation of radioactive material on the scan. However, scans may be normal in as many as 70% of patients who later turn out to have significant causes of bleeding. This is known as a false-negative result. A patient must be bleeding at the same time the scan is performed for it to be seen. Therefore, not finding evidence of a bleeding source during the study, can be misleading.

Abnormal results

The accumulation of radioactive material indicating a "leakage" of blood from the vessels is abnormal. The scan gives a rough, though not exact, guide as to the location of the bleeding. It can tell where the bleeding may be, but usually not the cause. Thus, extreme caution and skill is needed in interpreting these scans, and decisions involving surgery or other treatment should await more definitive tests.

Resources

BOOKS

Sleisenger, Marvin H., et al.*Sleisenger & Fordtran's Gastrointestinal and Liver Disease: Pathophysiology, Diagnosis, Management*. St. Louis, Mo.: MD Consult, 2009.

David Kaminstein, MD

Giant-cell arteritis *see* **Temporal arteritis**

Giardia lamblia infection *see* **Giardiasis**

Giardiasis

Definition

Giardiasis is a common intestinal infection spread by eating contaminated food, drinking contaminated water, or through direct contact with the organism that causes the disease, *Giardia lamblia*. Giardiasis is found throughout the world and is a common cause

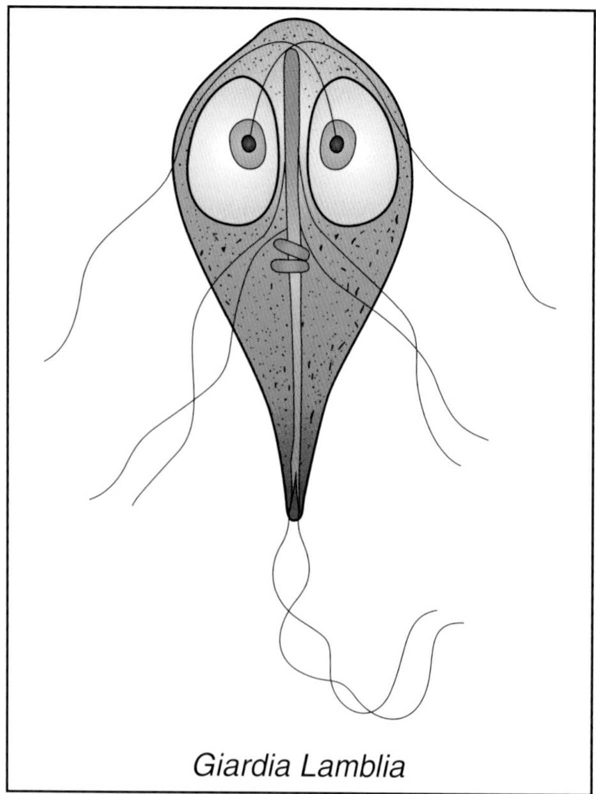

Infection with the protozoon *Giardia lamblia*, shown above, causes diarrhea in humans. *(Illustration by Electronic Illustrators Group. Reproduced by permission of Gale, a part of Cengage Learning.)*

of traveller's **diarrhea**. In the United States it is a growing problem, especially among children in child-care centers.

Giardiasis case reports in the United States[1] (including Guam and Puerto Rico), 2006–2008

Year	Number of cases	Number of outbreak cases[2]
2006	19,239	393
2007	19,794	346
2008	19,140	189

[1]*Giardia* is not a reputable condition in five states (IN, KY, MS, NC, TX).
[2]Number of cases linked to a known outbreak.

SOURCE: Centers for Disease Control and Prevention, "Giardiasis Surveillance—United States, 2006–2008," *MMWR Surveillance Summaries* 59, no. SS—6 (June 11, 2010):15–25. Available online at: http://www.cdc.gov/mmwr/preview/mmwrhtml/ss5906a2.htm (accessed September 20, 2010).

(Table by PreMediaGlobal. Reproduced by permission of Gale, a part of Cengage Learning.)

Description

Giardia is one of the most common intestinal parasites in the world, infecting as much as 20% of the entire population of the earth. It is common in overcrowded developing countries with poor sanitation and a lack of clean water. Recent tests have found *Giardia* in 7% of all stool samples tested nationwide, indicating that this disease is much more widespread than was originally believed. It has been found not only in humans, but also in wild and domestic animals.

Giardiasis is becoming a growing problem in the United States, where it affects three times more children than adults. In recent years, giardiasis outbreaks have been common among people in schools or daycare centers and at catered affairs and large public picnic areas. Children can easily pass on the infection by touching contaminated toys, changing tables, utensils, or their own feces, and then touching other people. For this reason, infection spreads quickly through a daycare center or institution for the developmentally disabled.

Unfiltered streams or lakes that may be contaminated by human or animal wastes are a common source of infection. Outbreaks can occur among campers and hikers who drink untreated water from mountain streams. While 20 million Americans drink unfiltered city water from streams or rivers, giardiasis outbreaks from tainted city water have been rare. Most of these problems have occurred not due to the absence of filters, but because of malfunctions in city water treatment plants, such as a temporary drop in chlorine levels. It is possible to become infected in a public swimming pool, however, since *Giardia* can survive in chlorinated water for about 15 minutes. During that time, it is possible for an individual to swallow contaminated pool water and become infected.

Causes and symptoms

Giardiasis is spread by food or water contaminated by the *Giardia lamblia* protozoan organism found in the human intestinal tract and feces. When the cysts are ingested, the stomach acid degrades the cysts and releases the active parasite into the body. Once within the body, the parasites cling to the lining of the small intestine, reproduce, and are swept into the fecal stream. As the liquid content of the bowel dries up, the parasites form cysts, which are then passed in the feces. Once excreted, the cysts can survive in water for more than three months. The parasite is spread further by direct fecal-oral contamination, such as can occur if food is prepared without adequate hand-washing, or by ingesting the cysts in water or food.

Giardiasis is not fatal, and about two-thirds of infected people exhibit no symptoms. Symptoms will not occur until between one and two weeks after infection. When present, symptoms include explosive, watery diarrhea that can last for a week or more and, in chronic cases, may persist for months. Because the infection interferes with the body's ability to absorb fats from the intestinal tract, the stool is filled with fat. Other symptoms include foul-smelling and greasy feces, stomach pains, gas and bloating, loss of appetite, **nausea and vomiting**. In cases in which the infection becomeschronic, lasting for months or years, symptoms might include poor digestion, problems digesting milk, intermittent diarrhea, **fatigue**, weakness, and significant weight loss.

Diagnosis

Diagnosis can be difficult because it can be easy to overlook the presence of the giardia cysts during a routine inspection of a stool specimen. In the past, the condition has been diagnosed by examining three stool samples for the presence of the parasites. However, because the organism is shed in some stool samples and not others, the infection may not be discovered using this method.

A newer, more accurate method of diagnosing the condition is the enzyme-linked immunosorbent assay (ELISA) that detects cysts and antigen in stool, and is approximately 90% accurate. While slightly more expensive, it only needs to be done once and is therefore less expensive overall than the earlier test.

Treatment

Acute giardiasis can usually be allowed to run its natural course and tends to clear up on its own. **Antibiotics** are helpful, however, in easing symptoms and preventing the spread of infection. Medications include metronidazole, furazolidone and paromomycin. Healthy carriers with no symptoms do not need antibiotic treatment. If treatment should fail, the patient should wait two weeks and repeat the drug course. Anyone with an impaired immune system (immunocompromised), such as a person with **AIDS**, may need to be treated with a combination of medications.

Prognosis

Giardiasis is rarely fatal, and when treated promptly, antibiotics usually cure the infection. While most people respond quickly to treatment, some have lingering symptoms and suffer with diarrhea and cramps for long periods, losing weight and not growing well. Those most at-risk for a course like this are the elderly, people with a weakened immune system, malnourished children, and anyone with low stomach acid.

KEY TERMS

Antibody—A specific protein produced by the immune system in response to a specific foreign protein or particle called an antigen.

Antigen—A substance (usually a protein) identified as foreign by the body's immune system, triggering the release of antibodies as part of the body's defense mechanism.

Enzyme-linked immunosorbent assay (ELISA)—A laboratory technique used to detect specific antigens or antibodies. It can be used to diagnose giardiasis.

Giardia lamblia—A type of protozoa with a whip-like tail that infects the human intestinal tract, causing giardiasis. The protozoa will not spread to other parts of the body.

Immunocompromised—A state in which the immune system is suppressed or not functioning properly.

Prevention

The best way to avoid giardiasis is to avoid drinking untreated surface water, especially from mountain streams. The condition also can be minimized by practicing the following preventive measures:

- thoroughly washing hands before handling food
- maintaining good personal cleanliness
- boiling any untreated water for at least three minutes
- properly disposing of fecal material

Children with severe diarrhea (and others who are unable to control their bowel habits) should be kept at home until the stool returns to normal. If an outbreak occurs in a daycare center, the director should notify the local health department. Some local health departments require a follow-up stool testing to confirm that the person is no longer contagious. People not in high-risk settings can return to their routine activities after recovery.

Resources

OTHER

Centers for Disease Control. http://www.cdc.gov/ncidod/EID/eidtext.htm.

International Society of Travel Medicine. http://www.istm.org.

ORGANIZATIONS

Centers for Disease Control and Prevention (CDC), 1600 Clifton Road, Atlanta, GA, 30333, (800) 232-4636, cdcinfo@cdc.gov, http://www.cdc.gov.

Carol A. Turkington

Gigantism *see* **Acromegaly and gigantism**

Gilchrist's disease *see* **Blastomycosis**

Gilles de la Tourette's syndrome *see* **Tourette syndrome**

Gingivitis *see* **Periodontal disease**

Ginkgo biloba

Definition

Ginkgo biloba, known as the kew tree, ginkyo, or duck-foot tree, is one of the oldest trees on Earth. Known for its heartiness and resilience, Ginkos survived the Atom Bomb attack on Hiroshima, Japan in 1945.

The Ginkgo is indigenous to China, Japan, and Korea and, when planted, thrives in North America and Europe.

Description

Ginkgo trees may grow to 122 ft (37.2 m) tall and measure 4 ft (1.2 m) in girth. They are grown on plantations in the United States, France, South Korea, and Japan.

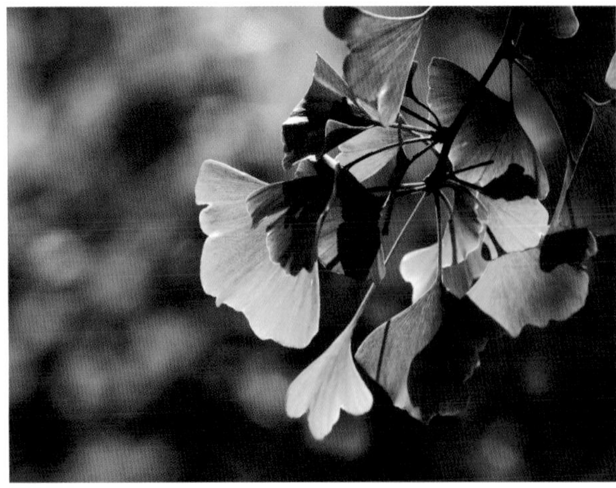

Ginkgo biloba leaves. *(© iStockPhoto/Ma Sai.)*

Purpose

In Chinese medicine, leaf extracts have been traditionally used to treat **asthma**, **allergies**, **premenstrual syndrome**, ringing in the ears, age-related **memory loss** and **dementia**. Standardized leaf extracts are currently used to treat memory loss and early Alzheimer's and circulation problems in the hands and legs.

Preparations

There are more than 40 chemical compounds extractable from Ginkgo leaves. The compounds have complex interactions, making precise cause and effect relationships between them difficult to asses.

Ginkgo acts to dilate blood vessels and increase blood flow in the brain, hands and legs and can relax smooth muscles in the lungs. It also acts as a blood thinner by interfering with platelet aggregation.

Precautions

Though used as medicines, herbal products like Ginko are regulated like dietary supplements in the United States. Thus, manufacturers are responsible only for their production processes. Imported herbals may not have met our manufacturing standards. Approval of herbals is based on traditional use, not demonstrated safety and effectiveness. Before an herbal can be withdrawn from the market, the FDA must prove that it is unsafe.

In therapeutic doses of 120-240mg per day, Ginkgo is generally safe and non-toxic. Approximately 2% of people taking Ginko may experience **headache**, restlessness, mild abdominal discomfort and **diarrhea**.

Ginko interferes with platelets, crucial components in blood clotting, and should not be taken for at least two days prior to having surgery or dental work.

Ginko may increase the blood-thinning effects of warfarin.

Drug-herbal and herbal-herbal interactions are not well understood and have not been thoroughly tested. Patients must be careful observers of themselves as they take new drugs or herbs, or as they take these products regularly over many months.

Side effects

Plum-like fruits of female Ginko trees may cause **contact dermatitis**. Taken internally, seeds may cause headache, **nausea**, diarrhea, and even seizures when taken in large amounts.

Resources

OTHER

"Gingko (Gingko biloba L)." National Standard. Mayo Clinic online. http://www.mayoclinic/health/gingko-biloba/NS_patient-ginkgo.

James Waun, MD, RPh

Ginseng

Definition

Ginseng is an herb derived from the roots of different plants in the Araliacea family that is native to Asia and North America. It is also called Asian ginseng, Asiatic ginseng, Chinese ginseng, and Korean ginseng. Russian ginseng is not a true member of the ginseng family.

Description

Highest quality ginseng root is harvested in the fall from three to six-year-old plants.

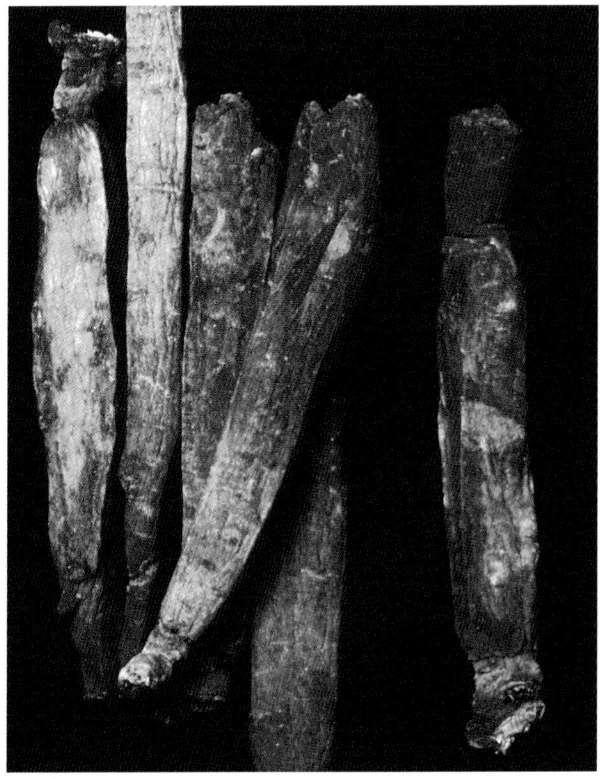

Dried Korean ginseng. *(Custom Medical Stock Photo, Inc. Reproduced by permission.)*

Purpose

Evidence suggests that ginseng boosts immune systems and increases the effectiveness of **antibiotics** during treatment for respiratory infections.

Ginseng has some antioxidant effects that may protect the heart and lower low density lipoproteins, bad cholesterol.

Ginseng may lower blood sugar. Long term effects of the herb on type II diabetes are unknown and safe, effective doses for use in this condition have not been established.

Ginseng is used to improve the overall sense of well being during recovery from illness and to boost stamina and mental and physical performance.

It is sometimes used to treat **erectile dysfunction** and relieve symptoms of **menopause**.

preparations

Carefully cleansed, dried and ground ginseng root is available as teas and in tablets, capsules, liquid extracts and as topical creams.

Precautions

Though used as medicines, herbal products are regulated like dietary supplements in the United States. Manufacturers are responsible only for their production processes. Manufacturing standards, and combinations of herbs within herbal products, may vary.

The potency of many herbal products sold in stores varies from what is stated on their labels.

There is no reliable evidence on the long-term side effects of taking ginseng; some advocates for the herb recommend limiting its use to three months.

Side effects

Some people are allergic to ginseng.

Side effects include **headache**, intestinal and sleep disturbances

Long-term use of ginseng may result in skin **rashes**, **itching**, loss of appetite, **diarrhea**, **anxiety**, excitability, depression and **insomnia**.

Occasionally, headaches, **dizziness**, rapid heart rate or **palpitations** (pounding sensation in the chest) occur.

Some people taking ginseng experience an estrogen-like effect with swelling and tenderness in the breasts, or post-menopausal bleeding.

Because of the possible estrogen effect, ginseng should not be used by people with hormone-related conditions like breast or uterine **cancer** or **endometriosis**.

Ginseng effects the liver enzyme that decomposes many drugs, and can alter their effects. For instance, it may reduce the effects of the blood thinner warfarin and increase the effects of drugs taken to reduce blood pressure.

Interactions

Ginseng may reduce the effectiveness of the blood-thinner warfarin and increase the likelihood **blood clots**.

Ginseng may increase the potential for bleeding for people taking blood thinners like **aspirin**, Plavix, and nonsteroidal anti inflammatory drugs like ibuprofen.

People who take ginseng and monoamine oxidase inhibitor antidepressants (MAOI) are more likely to experience headaches and insomnia.

Ginseng may either increase or decrease the effects drugs taken for heart disease and high blood pressure.

Resources

OTHER

"Asian ginseng." National Center for Complementary and Alternative Medicine. http://nccam.nih.gov/health/asianginseng.

James Waun, MD, RPh

Glaucoma

Definition

Glaucoma is a condition in which the optic nerve is subject to damage—usually, but not always, because of excessively high intraocular pressure (pressure within the eye, also called IOP). If untreated, the optic nerve damage results in progressive, permanent vision loss, starting with unnoticeable blind spots in the field of vision, progressing to tunnel vision, and then to blindness. Glaucoma can result in irreversible damage to the optic nerve. It is one of the leading causes of irreversible blindness in the United States and world-wide, and is the leading cause of blindness among African Americans and older adults in the United States. Because there are usually no symptoms early on in the disease, about half of the people with glaucoma do not even know they have the condition.

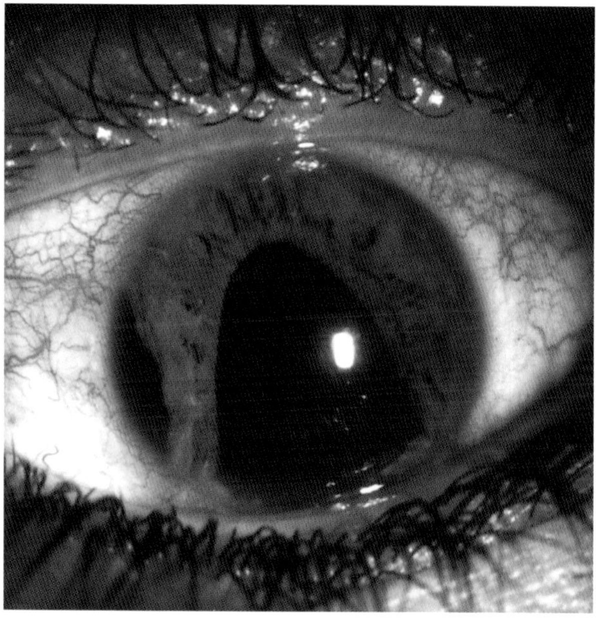

A close-up view of an inflamed eye with acute glaucoma and an irregularly enlarged pupil. *(Custom Medical Stock Photo, Inc. Reproduced by permission.)*

Description

More than two million people in the United States have glaucoma, and 80,000 of those are legally blind as a result of the disease. Glaucoma can strike any age group, even newborn infants. Susceptibility to the disease, however, increases with age. African Americans are at a three times higher risk of glaucoma than the rest of the population.

Glaucoma is a class of diseases. There are at least 20 different forms that can be divided into two categories: open-angle glaucoma and narrow-angle glaucoma. To understand what glaucoma is and what these terms mean, it is useful to understand eye structure.

Eyes are sphere-shaped. A tough, non-leaky protective sheath (the sclera) covers the entire eye, except for the clear cornea at the front and the optic nerve at the back. Light comes into the eye through the cornea, then passes through the lens, which focuses it onto the retina (the innermost surface at the back of the eye). The rods and cones of the retina transform the light energy into electrical messages, which are transmitted to the brain by the bundle of nerves known as the optic nerve.

The iris, the colored part of the eye shaped like a round picture frame, is between the dome-shaped cornea and the lens. It controls the amount of light that enters the eye by opening and closing its central hole (pupil) like the diaphragm in a camera. The iris, cornea, and lens are bathed in a liquid called the aqueous humor, which is somewhat similar to plasma. This liquid is continually produced by nearby ciliary tissues and moved out of the eye into the bloodstream by a system of drainage canals (called the trabecular meshwork). The drainage area is located in front of the iris, in the angle formed between the iris and the point at which the iris appears to meet the inside of the cornea.

Glaucoma occurs if the aqueous humor is not removed rapidly enough or if it is made too rapidly, causing pressure to build-up. The high pressure distorts the shape of the optic nerve and destroys the nerve. Destroyed nerve cells result in blind spots in places where the image from the retina is not being transmitted to the brain.

Open-angle glaucoma accounts for over 90% of all cases. It is called "open-angle" because the angle between the iris and the cornea is open, allowing drainage of the aqueous humor. It is usually chronic and progresses slowly. In narrow-angle glaucoma, the angle where aqueous fluid drainage occurs is narrow, and therefore may drain slowly or may be at risk of becoming closed. A closed-angle glaucoma attack is usually acute, occurring when the drainage area is blocked. This can occur, for example, if the iris and lens suddenly adhere to each other and the iris is pushed forward. In patients with very narrow angles, this can occur when the eyes dilate (e.g., when entering a dark room, or if taking certain medications).

Congenital glaucoma occurs in babies and is the result of incomplete development of the eye's drainage canals during embryonic development. An infant with congenital glaucoma may have enlarged, hazy corneas; show signs of being extremely sensitive to light; and have very teary eyes. The eye may also seem enlarged or bulging. The best way to detect childhood glaucoma is for children to have a regular and complete **eye examination**. Microsurgery can often correct the defects or they can be treated with a combination of medicine and surgery.

One rare form of open-angle glaucoma, normal tension glaucoma, is different. People with normal-tension glaucoma have optic nerve damage in the presence of normal IOP. The mechanism of this disease is a mystery but is generally detected after an examination of the optic nerve. Those at higher risk for this form of glaucoma are people with a familial history of normal tension glaucoma, people of Japanese ancestry, and people with a history of systemic heart disease such as irregular heart rhythm.

Glaucoma is also a secondary condition of over 60 widely diverse diseases and can also result from injury, inflammation, tumor, or in advanced cases of cataract or diabetes.

Causes

Glaucoma is the result of disruptions of normal processes to maintain pressure within the eye tissue. The iris, cornea, and lens of the eye are bathed in a nutritive liquid called the aqueous humor, which is made by cells within the eye. Excess fluid is continually removed by a spongy meshwork of drainage canals. Glaucoma occurs if there is a build up of the aqueous humor due to poor drainage or overproduction. As the fluid builds up there is increased pressure on the retina at the back of the eye. This increased pressure reduces the blood supply to the nerves of the retina and causes the nerves to die, which may distort and destroy the optic nerve. As nerve cells are destroyed, blind spots develop, and there is a progressive loss of vision. A change in the production and strength of collagen may also contribute to the onset of the disease. Collagen is a protein that helps maintain the structure and function of eye tissue. **Stress** and **allergies** may aggravate glaucoma symptoms.

It is probable that most cases of glaucoma are partially due to a genetic predisposition. At least 10 defective genes have been identified that may cause glaucoma. Although in the late 2000s there were still many unknown factors that trigger the disease, a number of processes have been implicated. They include age-related changes, congenital abnormalities, injuries to the eye tissue, and problems related to other eye diseases. Vision loss in all forms of glaucoma is caused by damage to the optic nerve, the retina, and the collagen protein that makes up eye tissue. Use of certain medications, including antihypertensives, **antihistamines**, anticholinergics, and antidepressants may also contribute to the development of glaucoma. Corticosteroid eye drops, which are often used for other eye disorders, may destroy the integrity of eye tissue. Other types of eye drops may cause the pupils to dilate, increasing intraocular eye pressure (IOP), which may also lead to glaucoma in those who have a tendency to the disease.

Symptoms

Chronic open-angle glaucoma at first develops without noticeable symptoms. The pressure buildup is gradual, and it does not bring on discomfort. Moreover, the vision loss is too gradual to be noticed at first, and the brain compensates for blind spots. Over an extended period of time, though, the elevated pressure pushes against and damages the optic nerve and the retina. If glaucoma is left untreated, vision loss becomes evident, and the condition becomes painful.

Acute closed-angle glaucoma is obvious from the beginning. The symptoms are blurred vision, severe eye **pain**, sensitivity to light, **nausea and vomiting**, dilated pupils, reddened eyes, and halos visualized around lights. The corneas may become hazy in appearance. Acute closed-angle glaucoma is an emergency situation. It needs to be treated immediately. Congenital glaucoma is evident at birth. Symptoms are bulging eyes, cloudy corneas, enlarged corneas, excessive teariness, and sensitivity to light.

Risk factors that increase the probability of developing glaucoma include:

- ocular hypertension, a slightly increased IOP
- age over 40
- diabetic conditions
- high blood pressure
- migraine headaches
- nearsightedness, farsightedness, and other visual disturbances
- a family history of glaucoma
- being of African American or Hispanic ethnicity

Diagnosis

Sometimes glaucoma can be diagnosed with a routine eye exam by an ophthalmologist, who can make a definitive diagnosis of glaucoma. IOP, defects in the field of vision, and the appearance of the optic nerve, are all considered in the diagnosis of glaucoma. Visual field tests (perimetry) can detect blind spots in a patient's field of vision before the patient is aware of them. An instrument, known as a tonometer, is used to measure eye pressure. Since IOP can vary throughout the day, a person may have to return for several visits to measure eye pressure at different times of the day. An ophthalmoscope is used to examine the inner aspects and the back of the eyes, including the optic nerve, for changes and damage. A slit lamp may be used to allow the doctor further examination of the eye. Another test, gonioscopy, can distinguish between narrow-angle and open-angle glaucoma. A gonioscope allows visualization of the angle between the iris and the cornea. A subsequent technology is optical coherence tomography (OCT) that produces high-resolution images of the anterior segment of the eye and is a noninvasive procedure. As of 2007, it was primarily used in conjunction with gonioscopy in diagnosing and assessing glaucoma.

Intraocular pressure can vary throughout the day. For that reason, the doctor may have a patient return for several visits to measure the IOP at different times of the day.

Treatment

The first line of glaucoma treatment is the use of prescription eyedrops. Several classes of medications are effective at lowering IOP and thus preventing optic nerve damage in chronic and neonatal glaucoma. **Beta blockers** (e.g., timolol), carbonic anhydrase inhibitors (e.g., acetazolamide), and alpha-2 agonists (e.g., brimonidine tartrate) inhibit aqueous humor production. Miotics (e.g., pilocarpine) and prostaglandin analogues (e.g., latanoprost) increase the outflow of aqueous humor.

It is important for patients to inform their doctors of any health conditions they have or any medications they take, including over-the counter drugs. Certain drugs used to treat glaucoma are not prescribed for patients with pre-existing conditions. The drugs prescribed to treat glaucoma all have side effects, so patients taking them should be monitored closely, especially for cardiovascular, pulmonary, and behavioral symptoms. Each medication lowers IOP by a different amount, and a combination of medications may be necessary. To ensure that IOP is lowered sufficiently, it is important that patients take their medications and be monitored regularly. IOP should be measured three to four times per year.

Normal-tension glaucoma is treated by reducing IOP to less-than-normal levels, on the theory that overly susceptible optic nerves are less likely to be damaged at lower pressures. Research underway may point to better treatments for this form of glaucoma.

Attacks of acute closed-angle glaucoma are medical emergencies. IOP is rapidly lowered by successive deployment of acetazolamide, hyperosmotic agents, a topical beta-blocker, and pilocarpine. Epinephrine should not be used because it exacerbates angle closure.

Trabeculectomy, to open the drainage canals or make an opening in the iris, can be effective in increasing the outflow of aqueous humor. This surgery is usually successful, but the effects often last less than one year. Nevertheless, this is an effective treatment for patients whose IOP is not sufficiently lowered by drugs and for those who can't tolerate the drugs.

Laser peripheral iridotomy is a procedure used almost exclusively to treat narrow angle glaucoma. It involves creating a small opening in the peripherial iris that allows aqueous fluid to drain from behind the iris

KEY TERMS

Agonist—A drug that mimics one of the body's own molecules.

Alpha-2 agonist—A class of drugs that bind to and stimulate alpha-2 adrenergic receptors, causing responses similar to those of adrenaline and noradrenaline, by inhibiting aqueous humor production.

Aqueous humor—A transparent liquid, contained within the eye, that is composed of water, sugars, vitamins, proteins, and other nutrients.

Beta-blocker—A class of drugs that bind beta-adrenergic receptors and thereby decrease the ability of the body's own natural epinephrine to bind to those receptors, leading to the reduction of aqueous humor secretion.

Carbonic anhydrase inhibitor—A class of diuretic drugs that inhibit the enzyme carbonic anhydrase, an enzyme involved in producing bicarbonate, which is required for aqueous humor production by the ciliary tissues in the eye. Thus, inhibitors of this enzyme inhibit aqueous humor production. Some side effects are urinary frequency, kidney stones, loss of the sense of taste, depression, and anemia.

Cornea—The clear, bowl-shaped structure at the front of the eye located in front of the colored part of the eye. The cornea lets light into the eye and partially focuses it.

Gonioscope—An instrument that consists of a magnifier and a lens equipped with mirrors and sits on the patient's cornea.

Hyperosmotic drugs—Refers to a class of drugs for glaucoma that increase the osmotic pressure in the blood, which then pulls water from the eye into the blood.

Iris—The colored part of the eye just behind the cornea and in front of the lens that controls the amount of light sent to the retina.

Laser cyclophotocoagulation—A procedure used for severe glaucoma in patients who have not responded well to previous treatments. The laser partially destroys the tissues that make the fluid of the eye.

Laser peripheral iridotomy—This procedure makes a drainage hole in the iris allowing the fluid to drain from the eye.

Laser trabeculoplasty—In this procedure the laser attempts to open the normal drainage channels of the eye so fluid can drain more effectively.

Lens (the crystalline lens)—A transparent structure in the eye that focuses light onto the retina.

Miotic—A drug that causes pupils to contract.

Ophthalmoscope—An instrument, with special lighting, designed to view structures in the eye.

Optic nerve—The nerve that carries visual messages from the retina to the brain.

Prostaglandin—A group of molecules that exert local effects on a variety of processes including fluid balance, blood flow, and gastrointestinal function.

Prostaglandin analogue—A class of drugs that are similar in structure and function to prostaglandin.

Retina—The light-sensitive layer of the eye.

Sclera—The tough, fibrous, white outer protective covering that surrounds the eye.

Tonometry—The measurement of pressure.

Trabecular meshwork—A sponge-like tissue located near the cornea and iris that functions to drain the aqueous humor from the eye into the blood.

directly to the anterior chamber. This procedure typically result in "opening up" the narrow angle between the iris and the cornea, in essence converting a narrow angle into an open angle.

Argon laser trabeculoplasty is usually recommended when medications have not been able to sufficiently control IOP, although it is increasingly advocated as primary therapy for patients who are not good candidates for the use of glaucoma medications or who cannot use eyedrops. In this procedure, the beam of an argon laser is directed at the trabecular meshwork. Typically about 180° of the trabecular meshwork is treated with laser spots. As a result of this procedure, the drainage of aqueous fluid out of the eye increases, thus lowering IOP.

Gene therapy may also be part of future treatments. A mutation in the gene myocilin is believed to cause most cases of juvenile glaucoma, and 3–4% of adult glaucoma. Researchers are investigating drugs that inhibit myocilin production. The drug therapy would not just treat IOP, but also could be used before glaucoma's onset.

Vitamin C, vitamin B_1 (thiamine), chromium, zinc, and rutin may reduce IOP.

Patients using alternative methods to attempt to prevent optic nerve damage should be advised they also need the care of a traditionally trained ophthalmologist or optometrist who is licensed to treat glaucoma, so that IOP and optic nerve damage can be monitored.

Since the early 1970s, a number of scientific studies reported that the active agents in **marijuana** *Cannabis sativa* are effective in lowering intraocular pressure (IOP) in people with glaucoma. One study reported that people with glaucoma who smoked marijuana had a 25% to 30% drop in IOP that lasted three to four hours. Under federal law, the use, possession, or sale of marijuana is illegal in the United States. However, as of 2007, twelve states had legalized the medical use of marijuana. In 2005, the U.S. Supreme Court ruled that federal laws against medical marijuana take precedence over state laws, allowing for continued federal prosecution against people who use marijuana for medical purposes. Despite the ruling, medical marijuana programs continue in several states, including California. The active agents in marijuana are cannabinol, cannabidiol, and delta-9-tetrahydrocannabinol (THC). A synthetic version of THC, dronabinol (Marinol), is available in the United States and can be legally prescribed for a number of conditions, including glaucoma.

Expected results

If glaucoma is left untreated, optic nerve damage will result in a progressive loss of vision. Once blindness develops due to glaucoma, it cannot be reversed. With early treatment and monitoring, however, serious vision loss can usually be prevented.

Prevention

While glaucoma is not preventable, early detection and treatment can help to prevent serious damage to vision. Those with risk factors should have regular eye exams and avoid medicines that tend to be implicated in the development of glaucoma, including some over-the-counter cold and allergy medications. All medications should be checked for their ingredients. Alternatives for drugs that aggravate glaucoma should be discussed with a healthcare provider.

Patients with narrow angles should avoid certain medications (even over-the-counter medications, such as some cold or allergy medications).Any person who is glaucoma-susceptible (i.e. narrow angles and borderline IOPs) should read the warning labels on over-the-counter medicines and inform their physicians of products they are considering taking. **Steroids** may also raise IOP, so patients may need to be monitored more frequently if it is necessary to use steroids for another medical condition.

Health care team roles

Nursing and allied health professionals play an important part in the diagnosis and treatment of glaucoma. Skilled ophthalmic technicians and assistants record the patient history and perform many of the preliminary tests. Depending on skill level, these ophthalmic assistants may perform measurement of visual acuity under both low and high illumination, assessment of ocular motility and binocularity, visual fields, measurement of IOPs with tonometers, evaluation of pupillary responses, and refraction.

Before surgical procedures, nurses and assistants also prepare the operating room (OR). Many ophthalmologists now have their own ambulatory surgery centers where skilled technicians and ophthalmic nurses play a critical role in preparing the OR and patients for the surgery. Ophthalmic nurses also assist the ophthalmologists during surgery and discuss outcomes with patients post-operatively.

Nurses and assistants assist patients by explaining the sometimes difficult regimen of glaucoma medication. In some cases, patients require several doses of a combination of medications. Ophthalmic nurses and assistants show patients the correct technique for inserting eyedrops, and reinforce the physician's instructions for medication compliance.

Patient education

Ophthalmic assistants and nurses help to ensure that patients return to the physician's office in a timely manner so that IOPs can be monitored. Nurses and assistants also emphasize the importance of adhering to the eyedrop schedule to keep IOPs at a lower level, and answer any questions concerning proper eyedrop instillation.

Resources

BOOKS

Bello, Joan. *The Benefits of Marijuana: Physical, Psychological, & Spiritual.* Boca Raton, FL: Lifeservices Press, 2007.

Choplin, Neil T., and Diane C. Lundy, eds. *Atlas of Glaucoma*, 2nd ed. New York: Informa Healthcare, 2007.

Wauters, Ambika. *The Homeopathy Bible: The Definitive Guide to Remedies.* New York: Sterling, 2007.

PERIODICALS

Fanelli, James L. "Do We Monitor or Medicate? When New Patients May Be At Risk for Glaucoma Development, Should You Initially Monitor Them or Immediately Begin Treatment?" *Review of Optometry* (January 15, 2008): 81(2).

Guttman, Cheryl. "Glaucoma 2007: The Year in Review: Specialists Turn Their Focus to Diagnostics, New

Surgical Modalities." *Ophthalmology Times* (December 15, 2007): 18(8).

Kabat, Alan G., and Joseph W. Sowka. "Just Say No: Ganja for Glaucoma? A Simple Answer Still Works Best for This Difficult Question." *Review of Optometry* (February 15, 2007): 138(2).

Parham, Marti. "What Blacks Must Know About Glaucoma." *Jet* (January 21, 2008): 40.

Pirisi, Angela. "Your 20/20 Diet for Eye Health: Focus in on Foods and Supplements that May Keep Your Eyes and Vision at Their Peak." *Better Nutrition* (October 2007): 54(3).

Schwartz, Gail F. "Patience Adherence and Persistence with Glaucoma Therapy." *Ophthalmology Times* (December 15, 2007): S3(3).

Sowka, Joseph W, Alan G. Kabat. "Treating Kids Who Have Glaucoma: What do you do Medically When Children Have Glaucoma?" *Review of Optometry* (July 15, 2006):95-96.

Takma, Julia. "Imaging Enhancements Offer Surgeons Greater Precision: Cataract, Refractive, Glaucoma Specialists Enabled to Better Plan for Pre-op, Evaluate Post-op." *Ophthalmology Times* (November 1, 2007): 59(3).

ORGANIZATIONS

American Academy of Ophthalmology., PO Box 7424, San Francisco, CA, 94120-7424, (415) 561-8500, http://www.aao.org.

Glaucoma Foundation., 80 Maiden Lane, Suite 1206, New York, NY, 10038, (212) 285-0080, http://www.glaucomafoundation.org.

National Eye Institute., 31 Center Dr., MSC 2510, Bethesda, MD, 20892-2510, (301) 496-5248, http://www. nei.nih.gov.

Optometric Glaucoma Society., 5553 Taft Ave., Oakland, CA, 94618, (925) 557-4181, http://www.optometricglaucomasociety.org.

Mary Bekker
Bonny McClain
Patience Paradox
Laura Jean Cataldo, RN, Ed.D.

Glaucoma surgery *see* **Trabeculectomy**

Glioma *see* **Brain tumor**

Glipizide *see* **Antidiabetic drugs**

Glomerulonephritis

Definition

Acute glomerulonephritis is an inflammatory disease of both kidneys predominantly affecting children from ages two to 12. Chronic glomerulonephritis can develop over a period of 10–20 years and is most often

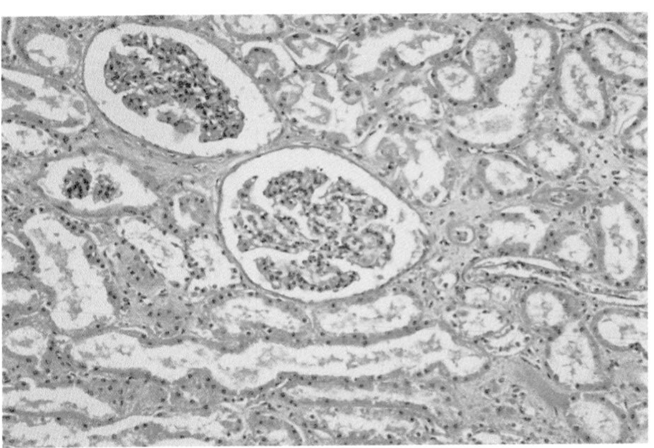

A close-up view of glomerulonephritis affecting the kidney. *(Custom Medical Stock Photo, Inc. Reproduced by permission.)*

associated with other systemic disease, including diabetes, **malaria**, hepatitis, or **systemic lupus erythematosus**.

Description

Acute glomerulonephritis is an inflammation of the glomeruli, bundles of tiny vessels inside the kidneys. The damaged glomeruli cannot effectively filter waste products and excess water from the bloodstream to make urine. The kidneys appear enlarged, fatty, and congested.

Causes and symptoms

Acute glomerulonephritis most often follows a streptococcal infection of the throat or skin. In children, it is most often associated with an upper respiratory infection, **tonsillitis**, or **scarlet fever**. Kidney symptoms usually begin two to three weeks after the initial infection. Exposure to certain paints, glue or other organic solvents may also be the causative agent. It is thought that the kidney is damaged with exposure to the toxins that are excreted into the urine.

Mild glomerulonephritis may produce no symptoms, and diagnosis is made with laboratory studies of the urine and blood. Individuals with more severe cases of the disease may exhibit:

- fatigue
- nausea and vomiting
- shortness of breath
- disturbed vision
- high blood pressure
- swelling, especially noted in the face, hands, feet, and ankles
- blood and protein in the urine, resulting in a smoky or slightly red appearance

KEY TERMS

Dialysis—A process of filtering and removing waste products from the bloodstream. Two main types are hemodialysis and peritoneal dialysis. In hemodialysis, the blood flows out of the body into a machine that filters out the waste products and routes the cleansed blood back into the body. In peritoneal dialysis, the cleansing occurs inside the body. Dialysis fluid is injected into the peritoneal cavity and wastes are filtered through the peritoneum, the thin membrane that surrounds the abdominal organs.

Glomeruli—Groups of tiny blood vessels with very thin walls that function as filters in the kidney. Glomeruli become inflamed and are destroyed in the disease process of glomerulonephritis.

Renal—Relating to the kidneys, from the Latin word *renes.*

The individual with chronic glomerulonephritis may discover their condition with a routine physical exam revealing high blood pressure, or an eye exam showing vascular or hemorrhagic changes. The kidneys may be reduced to as little as one-fifth their normal size, consisting largely of fibrous tissues.

Diagnosis

Diagnosis of glomerulonephritis is established based on medical history, combined with laboratory studies. A "dipstick" test of urine will reveal increased protein levels. A 24 hour urine collection allows measurement of the excretion of proteins and creatinine. Creatinine clearance from the bloodstream by the kidneys is considered an index of the glomerular filtration rate. Blood studies may reveal a low blood count, and may also be checked for the presence of a streptococcal antibody titer(a sophisticated blood test indicating presence of streptococcal infection). A **kidney biopsy** may also be performed, using ultrasound to guide the needle for obtaining the specimen.

Treatment

The main objectives in the treatment of acute glomerulonephritis are to:

- decrease the damage to the glomeruli
- decrease the metabolic demands on the kidneys
- improve kidney function

Bedrest helps in maintaining adequate blood flow to the kidney. If residual infection is suspected, antibiotic therapy may be needed. In the presence of fluid overload, **diuretics** may be used to increase output with urination. Iron and vitamin supplements may be ordered if anemia develops, and antihypertensives, if high blood pressure accompanies the illness. In order to rest the kidney during the acute phase, decreased **sodium** and protein intake may be recommended. The amount of protein allowed is dependent upon the amount lost in the urine, and the requirements of the individual patient. Sodium limitations depend on the amount of **edema** present. Fluid restrictions are adjusted according to the patient's urinary output and body weight.

An accurate daily record of the patient's weight, fluid intake and urinary output assist in estimating kidney function. The patient must be watched for signs of complications and recurrent infection. As edema is reduced and the urine becomes free of protein and red blood cells, the patient is allowed to increase activity. A woman who has had glomerulonephritis requires special medical attention during **pregnancy**.

Prognosis

In acute glomerulonephritis, symptoms usually subside in two weeks to several months, with 90% of children recovering without complications and adults recovering more slowly. Chronic glomerulonephritis is a disease that tends to progress slowly, so that there are no symptoms until the kidneys can no longer function. The resultant renal failure may require dialysis or kidney transplant.

Prevention

Prevention of glomerulonephritis is best accomplished by avoiding upper respiratory infections, as well as other acute and chronic infections, especially those of a streptococcal origin. Cultures of the infection site, usually the throat, should be obtained and antibiotic sensibility of the offending organism determined. Prompt medical assessment for necessary antibiotic therapy should be sought when infection is suspected. The use of prophylactic immunizations is recommended as appropriate.

ORGANIZATIONS

American Association of Kidney Patients, 3505 E. Frontage Road, Suite 315, Tampa, FL, 33607, (813) 636-8122, (800) 749-2257, info@aakp.org, http://www.aakp.org.

American Kidney Fund (AKF), 6110 Executive Boulevard, Suite 1010, Rockville, MD, 20852, (800) 638-8299, http://www.kidneyfund.org.

National Institute of Diabetes and Digestive and Kidney Diseases, NIDDK, NIH Bldg 31, Rm 9A06 31 Center Drive, MSC 2560, Bethesda, MD, 20892-2560, (301) 496.3583, http://www2.niddk.nih.gov.

National Kidney Foundation, Inc. , 30 East 33rd Street, New York, NY, 10016, (212) 889-2210, (212) 689-9261, (800) 622-9010, http://www.kidney.org.

Kathleen D. Wright, RN

Glossopharyngeal neuralgia *see* **Neuralgia**

Glucose-6-phosphate dehydrogenase deficiency

Definition

Glucose-6-phosphate dehydrogenase deficiency is an inherited condition caused by a defect or defects in the gene that codes for the enzyme, glucose-6-phosphate dehydrogenase (G6PD). It can cause **hemolytic anemia**, varying in severity from life-long anemia, to rare bouts of anemia to total unawareness of the condition. The episodes of hemolytic anemia are usually triggered by oxidants, infection, or by eating fava beans.

Description

G6PD deficiency is the most common enzyme deficiency in the world, with about 400 million people living with it. It is most prevalent in people of African, Mediterranean, and Asian ancestry. The incidence in different populations varies from zero in South American Indians to less than 0.1% of Northern Europeans to about 50% of Kurdish males. In the United States, it is most common among African American males; about 11 to 14% are G6PD-deficient.

G6PD deficiency is a recessive sex-linked trait. Thus, males have only one copy of the G6PD gene, but females have two copies. Recessive genes are masked in the presence of a gene that encodes normal G6PD. Accordingly, females with one copy of the gene for G6PD deficiency are usually normal, while males with one copy have the trait.

G6PD is present in all human cells but is particularly important to red blood cells. It is required to make NADPH in red blood cells but not in other cells. It is also required to make glutathione. Glutathione and NADPH both help protect red blood cells against oxidative damage. Thus, when G6PD is defective, oxidative damage to red blood cells readily occurs, and they break open as a result. This event is called hemolysis, and multiple hemolyses in a short time span constitute an episode of hemolytic anemia.

There are almost 100 different known forms of G6PD enzyme molecules encoded by defective G6PD genes, yet not one of them is completely inactive. This suggests that G6PD is indispensable. Many G6PD defective enzymes are deficient in their stability rather than their initial ability to function. Since red blood cells lack nuclei, they, unlike other cells, cannot synthesize new enzyme molecules to replace defective ones. Hence, we expect young red blood cells to have new, functional G6PD and older cells to have nonfunctioning G6PD. This explains why episodes of hemolytic anemia are frequently self-limiting; new red blood cells are generated with enzymes able to afford protection from oxidation.

The geographic distribution of G6PD deficiency, allowing for migration, coincides with the geographic distribution of **malaria**. This fact and survival statistics suggest that G6PD deficiency protects against malaria.

Glucose-6-phosphate dehydrogenase deficiency is also known as G6PD deficiency, favism, and primaquine sensitivity.

Causes and symptoms

Causes

G6PD deficiency is caused by one copy of a defective G6PD gene in males or two copies of a defective G6PD gene in females. Hemolytic anemic attacks can be caused by oxidants, infection, and or by eating fava beans.

Symptoms

The most significant consequence of this disorder is hemolytic anemia, which is usually episodic, but the vast majority of people with G6PD deficiency have no symptoms.

The many different forms of G6PD deficiency have been divided into five classes according to severity.

- Class 1–enzyme deficiency with chronic hemolytic anemia
- Class 2–severe enzyme deficiency with less than 10% of normal activity
- Class 3–moderate to mild enzyme deficiency with 10–60% of normal activity
- Class 4–very mild or no enzyme deficiency
- Class 5–increased enzyme activity

KEY TERMS

Bilirubin—A breakdown product derived from hemoglobin; removed from the blood by the liver.

Enzyme—A protein catalyst; one of the two kinds of biological catalysts, which are exceedingly specific; each different enzyme only catalyzes one or two specific reactions.

Enzyme activity—A measure of the ability of an enzyme to catalyze a specific reaction.

Glutathione—A molecule that acts as a co-enzyme in cellular oxidation-reduction reactions.

Hemolysis—Lysis (opening) of red blood cells, with concomitant leakage of cell contents from the cells.

Hemolytic anemia—Anemia due to hemolysis.

Jaundice—Yellowish skin color due to liver disease.

Neonatal—Describes babies just after they are born.

Recessive trait—An inherited trait that is outwardly obvious only when two copies of the gene for that trait are present–as opposed to a dominant trait where one copy of the gene for the dominant trait is sufficient to display the trait. The recessive condition is said to be masked by the presence of the dominant gene when both are present; i.e., the recessive condition is seen only in the absence of the dominant gene.

Sex-linked—Refers to genes or traits carried on one of the sex chromosomes, usually the X.

X chromosome—One of the two types of sex chromosomes, present twice in female cells and once in male cells.

The major symptoms of hemolytic anemia are **jaundice**, dark urine, abdominal **pain**, back pain, lowered red blood cell count, and elevated bilirubin. People who suffer from severe and chronic forms of G6PD deficiency in addition may have **gallstones**, enlarged spleens, defective white blood cells, and **cataracts**.

Attacks of hemolytic anemia are serious for infants. Brain damage and **death** are possible but preventable outcomes. Newborns with G6PD deficiency are about 1.5 times as likely to get **neonatal jaundice** than newborns without G6PD deficiency.

Diagnosis

Blood tests can detect G6PD deficiency, either by measuring the G6PD enzyme activity between episodes or by measuring bilirubin during an episode. Such tests cost about $50.00. Family histories are helpful, too.

Treatment

In a typical attack of hemolytic anemia, no treatment is needed; the patient will recover in about eight days. However, blood transfusions are necessary in severe cases. Recent success treating elevated bilirubin in newborns by exposing them to bright light has decreased the need for neonatal transfusions.

Alternative treatment

Vitamin E and **folic acid** (both anti-oxidants) may help decrease hemolysis in G6PD-deficient individuals.

Prognosis

The prognosis for almost everyone with G6PD deficiency is excellent. Large studies have shown that G6PD-deficient individuals do not acquire any illnesses more frequently than the rest of the population. In fact the opposite may be true for some diseases like ischemic heart disease and cerebrovascular disease.

Prevention

Most episodes of hemolytic anemia can be prevented by avoiding fava beans, oxidant drugs, and oxidant chemicals. All of the following oxidants can trigger attacks: acetanilid, dapsone, doxorubicin, furazolidone, methylene blue, nalidixic acid, napthalene, niridazole, nitrofurantoin, phenazopyridine, phenylhydrazine, primaquine, quinidine, quinine, sulfacetamide, sulfamethoxazole, sulfonamide, sulfapyridine, thiazolesulfone, toluidine blue, and trinitrotoluene. Since infections also trigger hemolytic attacks and have other dire consequences, sometimes it is advisable to use one of the listed drugs.

It is especially important to screen newborns who are likely to have G6PD deficiency to ensure that G6PD-deficient babies won't be subjected to any of the triggers of hemolytic anemia. Pregnant women, especially in areas where G6PD deficiency is prevalent, should avoid eating fava beans.

Resources

OTHER

G6PD Deficiency Favism Association. http://www.g6pd.org/favism/english/index.mvc.

ORGANIZATIONS

Genetic Alliance, Inc., 4301 Connecticut Ave., NW, Suite 404, Washington, DC, 20008-2369, (202) 966-5557, (202) 966-8553, info@geneticalliance.org, http://www.geneticalliance.org.

Lorraine Lica, PhD

Glucosylcerebroside lipidosis *see* **Gaucher disease**

Gluten-free diet

Definition

A gluten-free diet is a diet that is completely free of gluten, which is a generic name for storage protein found in certain grains. In **celiac disease** (also referred to as celiac sprue), individuals develop an inflammatory immune system response to gluten that results in damage to the small intestine. This damage inhibits absorption of nutrients. Some individuals also develop **dermatitis** herpetiformis, an itchy and blistering skin condition. To control symptoms of gluten intolerance, affected individuals must completely avoid foods that contain gluten.

Origins

Guidelines for this diet have been developed by dietitians for several organizations associated with celiac disease and dermatitis herpetiformis, including the Gluten Intolerance Group, the Celiac Sprue Association, and the Celiac Disease Foundation. The American Dietetic Association also sponsored the development of a gluten-free diet through a cooperative effort of

Gluten-free diet

Ingredients/foods to avoid	May contain gluten	Foods allowed
Barley	Baking powder	Amaranth
Bran (wheat or oat)	Beans, baked	Beans, dried, unprocessed
Bulgur	Bouillon cubes	Buckwheat
Cake meal	Candy	Cassava
Couscous	Cheese sauces and spreads	Cheese, aged
Emulsifier	Chips, potato and tortilla	Corn
Farina	Chocolate drinks and mixes	Eggs, unprocessed
Flavoring	Coffee substitutes	Fish, unprocessed
Flour, enriched, durum, graham, semolina	Cold cuts	Flax
Gluten	Communion wafers	Fruits and juices, fresh, frozen or canned
Hydrolyzed plant protein	Corn cakes, popped	Herbs and spices, pure
Kamut	Egg substitutes, dried eggs	Ketchup
Malt and malt flavoring	French fries	Legumes
Matzo meal	Fruits, dried	Meats, unprocessed
Oatmeal and oat bran	Fruit-flavored drinks	Milk
Oats, rolled	Fruit pie fillings	Millet
Rye	Gravy	Mustard
Semolina	Hot dogs and other processed meats	Nuts, unprocessed, and nut flours
Seitan	Matzo	Olives
Soy sauce or soy sauce solids	Mayonnaise	Pickles, plain
Soy	Milk drinks	Potatoes and sweet potatoes
Spelt	Nuts, dry roasted	Quinoa
Stablizer	Peanut butter	Rice, wild rice, Indian rice
Starch, modified, or modified food starch	Pudding mixes	Sago
Triticale	Rice, brown	Seeds, unprocessed
Vegetable gum	Rice crackers and cakes	Soy flour
Vegetable protein	Rice mixes	Soy sauce, gluten-free
Vinegar, malt	Salad dressings	Sorghum
Wheat	Sauces	Tapioca
Wheat berries	Seasoning mixes	Tomato paste
Wheat bran	Sour cream	Vegetables without gluten-containing additives
Wheat, cracked	Soy nuts	Vinegar, apple, cider, and distilled white
Wheat germ	Syrup	Yucca
Wheat protein and hydrolyzed wheat protein	Teas, flavored and herbal	
Wheat starch	Turkey, self-basting	
Whole wheat	Vegetables in sauces	
	Yogurt, flavored or frozen	

(Table by PreMediaGlobal. Reproduced by permission of Gale, a part of Cengage Learning.)

dietitian experts in celiac disease in Canada and the United States. This diet was published in October 2000.

Description

The gluten-free diet is the prescribed medical treatment for gluten intolerance diseases, including celiac disease and dermatitis herpetiformis. Celiac disease is a genetically inherited, chronic digestive disease that results in damage to parts of the small intestine that are responsible for absorption of nutrients. Celiac disease affects almost three million people in the United States, about one percent of the population. Another 3 million Europeans are affected. Celiac disease is found among North American and European populations where wheat is a staple food, but it is found infrequently among people of Chinese and Japanese heritage and individuals with an African-Caribbean background, where wheat is not as widely consumed.

In addition, dermatitis herpetiformis is an important disorder or complication of gluten-sensitivity. It manifests in the form of a skin rash. Approximately 10% of individuals with celiac disease have dermatitis herpetiformis, but about 85% of individuals with dermatitis herpetiformis also have celiac disease.

When a person with celiac disease consumes gluten, the villi of the small intestine, where absorption of key nutrients takes place, become damaged, resulting in nutrients passing through the digestive system without being absorbed. The person exhibits gastrointestinal distress and eventually **malnutrition**. In infancy, celiac disease can manifest as **failure to thrive**, **diarrhea**, abdominal distention, developmental delay, and in some infants, as severe malnutrition.

After infancy, the symptoms of celiac disease are less dramatic. Older children may be short or exhibit dental enamel defects. Women comprise about 75% of newly diagnosed adult cases of celiac disease. Symptoms of celiac disease include diarrhea, **constipation** alternating with diarrhea, intestinal gas, fatty, greasy, foul-smelling stools, bloating, **nausea**, **vomiting**, skin irritation, weight loss, anemia, neurological effects (including seizures, and possibly migraine headaches), **fatigue**, concentration and memory problems. In some cases, there may be intestinal damage without significant gastrointestinal symptoms. Celiac disease is diagnosed by blood tests for certain antibodies and a **small intestine biopsy**. A positive small intestine biopsy, followed by an improvement in health after following a gluten-free diet, is confirmation of celiac disease. A gluten-free diet should not be started before diagnosis is confirmed.

Some individuals may exhibit gluten intolerance, with gastrointestinal symptoms similar to those seen with celiac disease, but without its resulting intestinal damage. Gluten intolerance is diagnosed by following a gluten-free diet, followed by reintroduction of gluten-containing foods, to evaluate health improvement associated with elimination or reduction of gluten from the diet. Some individuals with gluten intolerance may be able to tolerate a low-gluten diet under the supervision of a physician or dietitian.

A gluten-free diet also may be helpful for individuals with **multiple sclerosis** and other **autoimmune disorders**, as well as for individuals with **autism** spectrum disorders, **attention deficit hyperactivity disorder (ADHD)**, and some behavioral problems.

The foods of concern for individuals with, or susceptible to, celiac disease are the cereal grains that contain the storage proteins prolamin and glutelin (commonly referred to as glutens in wheat), including all varieties of wheat (e.g., durum, spelt, kamut), barley (where the storage proteins are called hordiens), rye (where the storage proteins are called secalins), and their cross-bred hybrids (e.g., triticale).

Grains and starches that are allowed in a gluten-free diet include: rice, corn, soy, potato, sweet potato, tapioca, beans, garfava, sorghum, quinoa, millet, arrowroot, amaranth, tef, nut flours, and buckwheat. However, some commercial buckwheat products are mixtures of wheat and buckwheat flours and should be avoided. Other foods that are allowed (only a partial list) include fresh, canned, and frozen fruit or fruit juices, fresh vegetables, canned and frozen vegetables without gluten-containing additives, milk, aged cheese, all unprocessed meats, poultry, fish, eggs, dried beans, nuts, and seeds. A dietitian should be consulted to develop and monitor a gluten-free diet.

Gluten-free foods can be found in health food stores, through mail order sources, and in some supermarkets. Cookbooks are available to help in food preparation. Many food manufacturers maintain lists of gluten-free products. The Gluten-Free Certification Organization (GFCO) of the Gluten Intolerance Group, in cooperation with the Food Services, Inc., a subsidiary of the Orthodox Union, a kosher certification agency, has developed a gluten-free certification program. This program benefits consumers by giving them confidence that a product is gluten-free through a process whereby products have been tested and the manufacturing site inspected. The program also saves the consumer time that would have been spent calling the manufacturer for the gluten-free status of the product. Certification is a yearly process based on ingredient review, on-site

KEY TERMS

Anemia—A condition in which there are too few red blood cells, too many abnormal red blood cells, or too little iron-containing hemoglobin for normal oxygen transport in the body.

Attention deficit hyperactivity disorder (ADHD)—A learning and behavioral disorder characterized by difficulty in sustaining attention, impulsive behavior, and excessive activity.

Autoimmunity—A condition in which the body's immune system produces antibodies in response to its own tissues or blood components instead of foreign particles or microorganisms.

Corticosteroids —Medication that acts like a type of hormone (cortisol) produced by the adrenal gland of the body. Corticosteroids produced by the body stimulate specific types of functional activity. As a drug, a corticosteroid (sometimes just called steroid) provides extra cortisol, which helps treat infection or trauma to the body.

Immunosuppressant—Any agent that decreases the response of the immune response of an individual.

Kosher—Conforming to Jewish dietary laws.

Osteomalacia—A softening of bones caused by lack of vitamin D and/or calcium in the diet.

Osteoporosis—A condition found in older individuals in which bones decrease in density and become fragile and more likely to break. It can be caused by lack of vitamin D and/or calcium in the diet.

Type 1 diabetes—A chronic immune system disorder in which the pancreas does not produce sufficient amounts of insulin, a hormone that enables cells to use glucose for energy. Also called juvenile diabetes, it must be treated with insulin injections.

inspection, and product testing. The Celiac Sprue Association (CSA) also has the CSA Recognition Seal Program that certifies gluten-free products. Requirements for obtaining the CSA Seal for products include:

- Ingredient review and verification by testing to assure products are free of wheat, barley, rye and oats
- Provision of written facility procedures and on-site facility audits to assure that procedures are in place to control any cross or outside contamination in processing and packaging

Foods may contain gluten, although gluten will not be indicated on the ingredient list, because it was not included in the formulation of the product. For example, a conveyer belt may be dusted with a gluten-containing material to prevent foods from sticking and may contaminate the finished food product.

Function

The gluten-free diet is used by individuals who are gluten-sensitive to prevent damage to their small intestines and to prevent serious complications such as gastrointestinal cancers, iron-deficiency anemia, and decreased bone mineral density.

Benefits

A gluten-free diet has been shown to greatly reduce the risk for **cancer** and overall mortality for individuals with symptomatic celiac disease.

For many people with celiac disease, following a gluten-free diet will stop the symptoms of the disease and result in improved health, usually within several months, although for some individuals, recovery may take up to one year. However, the health of some people with extensive damage to their small intestine may not improve. Refractory celiac disease (RCD), that is celiac disease that fails to respond to treatment, is a rare syndrome with a poor prognosis, defined by malabsorption due to gluten-related intestinal damage after initial or subsequent failure of a strict gluten-free diet and after exclusion of any other disease or disorder mimicking celiac disease. Other treatments may be necessary to treat the RCD, such as the use of **corticosteroids** and **immunosuppressant drugs**, but data on their effectiveness is lacking.

Precautions

In addition to gluten-containing grains, gluten can be found in a large variety of foods including soups, salad **dressings**, processed foods, candy, imitation bacon and seafood, marinades, processed luncheon meats, sauces and gravies, self-basting poultry, soy sauce or soy sauce solids, thickeners, communion wafers, and natural flavorings. Unidentified starch, binders, and fillers in medications, supplements, or **vitamins** and adhesives in stamps and stickers can also be unsuspected sources of gluten. Play dough, which contains wheat, can be harmful if hands are put on or in the mouth after contact or hands are not washed after play.

An individual following a gluten-free diet must read labels every time a food item purchased or consumed. Ingredients that may contain hidden sources of gluten include unidentified starch, modified food starch, hydrolyzed vegetable or plant protein (HVP or HPP), texturized vegetable protein (TVP), and binders, fillers, and extenders. In addition, manufacturers can change ingredients at any time, and a product may no longer be gluten-free. Ingredients may be verified by contacting a manufacturer and specifying the ingredient and lot number of a food item. If a person cannot verify ingredients in a food product or if the ingredient list is unavailable, the food should not be eaten, to avoid damage to the small intestine that occurs every time gluten is consumed.

Gluten-free recommendations can be difficult to follow. It is recommended that an affected person keeps the diet simple at the beginning by eating fresh fruits and vegetables, milk, unprocessed protein foods such as fresh beef, pork, poultry, fish, and eggs, natural nuts, seeds, and vegetable oils without additives.

Pure, uncontaminated oats eaten in moderation (about one cup cooked daily) may be safe for individuals with celiac disease. However, in many cases oats can become cross contaminated with grains containing gluten during growth, harvest, transport, storage, or processing. Some individuals with celiac disease who introduce oats to their diet may experience abdominal discomfort, gas, and stool changes until they become accustomed to the increased fiber levels from the oats. Others with celiac disease may exhibit a hypersensitivity to oats and should avoid their consumption. Research published in the early 2000s (2000 to 2004) indicated that oats may contain a protein similar to gluten that causes intestinal inflammation in some individuals with celiac disease. Individuals with celiac disease should consult their health care provider or dietitian before including oats in their diet and should have their antibody levels monitored regularly.

Most all beers are brewed with barley and some are brewed with wheat, and thus should not be consumed by a person following a gluten-free diet. Sorghum and buckwheat beers are available but are a specialty product. Most distilled forms of alcohol are gluten-free unless additives and colorings containing gluten have been added. Wines also usually are gluten-free.

Since celiac disease is an inherited autoimmune disease, screening of family members is recommended. The chances of developing symptoms of gluten-sensitivity increases to 10–20% in individuals who have a first-degree relative (parent, sibling, child) with celiac disease. Celiac disease is also associated with other autoimmune syndromes such as Type 1 diabetes.

Risks

A gluten-free diet is difficult to follow, and continued health problems usually are associated with problems with adhering to the diet. A person can exhibit celiac-related symptoms for months after a single intake of gluten. Individuals with gluten-sensitivity who do not treat their disease are at a higher risk for gastrointestinal T-cell lymphoma and other gastrointestinal cancers. However, the maintenance of a long-term gluten-free state reduces the risk of lymphoma to the level seen in the general population. Other complications of gluten-sensitivity include decreased mineral bone density and iron-deficiency. Individuals with celiac disease and dermatitis herpetiformis must maintain a gluten-free diet for the rest of their lives, for these diseases cannot be cured.

Individuals are more likely to adhere to the diet if a dietitian and support groups are involved. If a person is not responding well to a gluten-free diet, the doctor may:

- Investigate whether the initial diagnosis of celiac disease was correct
- Check for other conditions that can be causing symptoms, such as pancreatic insufficiency, irritable bowel syndrome, bacterial overgrowth, lymphocytic colitis, T-cell lymphoma, fructose intolerance, or tropical sprue
- Refer the person to a dietician to check for errors in the diet or for compliance with the diet

To monitor dietary adherence to the gluten-free diet, the dietitian will examine the person's dietary history and habits. Blood tests will be conducted to see if gluten antibody levels have returned to normal levels. If there is clinical concern that a person is not adhering to the gluten-free diet or that the diet is not effective, a biopsy of the small intestine may be conducted.

The gluten-free diet is complex, and it cannot be assumed that chefs in restaurants or others who prepare food (including friends and family) are aware of potential sources of gluten contamination. Education of family and friends is important in accomplishing a lifestyle change. In restaurants simple dishes without sauces should be ordered, and the person should inquire whether grain products are prepared with the same equipment or utensils used to prepare other foods. Although a food may meet labeling standards to be called gluten-free, it may be gluten-contaminated by the way in which it is prepared or stored. Other difficulties associated with following a gluten-free diet include lifestyle changes such as avoiding travel, finding gluten-free foods, especially those of good quality, determining whether foods are gluten-free, not being invited out because of the diet, with resulting social isolation, and maintaining a gluten-free diet when in the hospital.

As with any restrictive diet, the gluten-free diet has potential for nutritional inadequacy. Individuals who are sensitive to gluten are at increased risk for **osteoporosis** and osteomalacia due to malabsorption of **calcium** and vitamin D. Most individuals with celiac disease have some degree of osteopenia or osteoporosis. Calcium and vitamin D supplementation along with strict adherence to a gluten-free diet usually results in remineralization of the skeleton. Iron or other vitamin deficiencies may also be present and must be treated appropriately. The consumption of gluten-free fiber-rich foods (for example, brown rice, fruits, and vegetables) and adequate fluid intake is recommended to assist in the prevention of constipation.

Women with untreated celiac disease often exhibit a history of miscarriages, anemia, low birth weight babies, and unfavorable outcome of **pregnancy**. It is suggested that testing for celiac disease be included in the battery of tests prescribed for pregnant women. Celiac disease is considerably more common than most of the diseases for which pregnant women are routinely screened. Unfavorable events associated with celiac disease may be prevented by a gluten-free diet.

Research and general acceptance

The gluten-free diet is recognized by the medical community as the required treatment for individuals exhibiting gluten-sensitivity.

The National Institutes of Health has noted that the strict definition of a gluten-free diet remains controversial due to the lack of an accurate method to detect gluten in food products and the lack of scientific evidence for what constitutes a safe amount of gluten ingestion. No international agreement has yet been developed on how much gluten a person with gluten-sensitivity can tolerate. Research is on going to better identify levels that are acceptable, and health professionals involved in the therapy of celiac disease should keep up-to-date on the latest research. On January 23, 2007, the United States Food and Drug Administration proposed to set a standard of 20 part per million as the maximum acceptable level of gluten allowed for a product to be labeled as gluten-free. Labeling is voluntary. European standards for labeling a food gluten-free are more strict than those in the United States.

Research continues on the benefits of a gluten-free diet for individuals with multiple sclerosis and other autoimmune disorders, as well as for individuals with autism spectrum disorders, **ADHD**, and some behavioral problems.

In addition, a new enzyme that was being developed for commercial food processing has been found to break down gluten molecules quickly and almost completely. The enzyme is made from *Aspergillis niger*, a common fungus that is the source of other food grade enzymes already being manufactured for human consumption. Fritz Koning of Leiden University Medical Center in the Netherlands is leading the research. He stated that if the enzyme proves itself in clinical trials to eliminate the need for a gluten-free diet, it could be mass produced at a reasonable cost.

Resources

BOOKS

Hasselbeck, Elisabeth. *The G-Free Diet: A Gluten-Free Survival Guide*. New York: Center Street, 2009.

Korn, Danna. *Living Gluten-Free for Dummies*. Hoboken, NJ: Wiley Publishing, Inc., 2006.

Korn, Danna and Connie Sarros. *Gluten-free Cooking for Dummies*. Indianapolis, IN : Wiley Pub., Inc., 2008.

OTHER

Celiac Disease. MedlinePlus January 6, 2010. http://www.nlm.nih.gov/medlineplus/celiacdisease.html

Celiac Disease. FamilyDoctor.org December 2009. http://familydoctor.org/online/famdocen/home/common/digestive/disorders/236.printerview.html

Glutenfree.com (accessed January 2010). http://www.glutenfree.com/home.aspx

ORGANIZATIONS

American Dietetic Association, 120 South Riverside Plaza, Suite 2000, Chicago, IL, 60606-6995, (800) 877-1600, http://www.eatright.org.

Gluten Intolerance Group, 31214 124th Ave SE, Auburn, WA, 98092, 253-833-6655, 253-833-6675, info@gluten.net, http://www.gluten.net.

Celiac Sprue Association, P.O. Box 31700, Omaha, NE, (402) 558-0600, (877) 272-4272, celiacs@csaceliacs.org, http://www.csaceliacs.org.

Celiac Disease Foundation, 13251 Ventura Boulevard, Studio City , CA, 91604-1838, (818) 990-2354, (818) 990-2379, cdf@celiac.org, http://www.celiac.org.

Judith L. Sims
Tish Davidson, AM

Gluten enteropathy *see* **Celiac disease**

Glyburide *see* **Antidiabetic drugs**

Glycogen storage diseases

Definition

Glycogen serves as the primary fuel reserve for the body's energy needs. Glycogen storage diseases, also known as glycogenoses, are genetically linked metabolic disorders that involve the enzymes regulating glycogen metabolism. Symptoms vary by the glycogen storage disease (GSD) type and can include **muscle cramps** and wasting, enlarged liver, and low blood sugar. Disruption of glycogen metabolism also affects other biochemical pathways as the body seeks alternative fuel sources. Accumulation of abnormal metabolic by-products can damage the kidneys and other organs. GSD can be fatal, but the risk hinges on the type of GSD.

Description

Most of the body's cells rely on glucose as an energy source. Glucose levels in the blood are very stringently controlled within a range or 70–100 mg/dL, primarily by hormones such as insulin and glucagon. Immediately after a meal, blood glucose levels rise and exceed the body's immediate energy requirements. In a process analogous to putting money in the bank, the body bundles up the extra glucose and stores it as glycogen in the liver and muscles. Later, as the blood glucose levels begin to dip, the body makes a withdrawal from its glycogen savings.

The system for glycogen metabolism relies on a complex system of enzymes. These enzymes are responsible for creating glycogen from glucose, transporting the glycogen to and from storage areas within cells, and extracting glucose from the glycogen as needed. Both creating and tearing down the glycogen macromolecule are multistep processes requiring a different enzyme at each step. If one of these enzymes is defective and fails to complete its step, the process halts. Such enzyme defects are the underlying cause of GSDs.

The enzyme defect arises from an error in its gene. Since the error is in the genetic code, GSDs can be passed down from generation-to-generation. However, all but one GSD are linked to autosomal genes, which means a person inherits one copy of the gene from each parent. Following a Mendelian inheritance pattern, the normal gene is dominant and the defective gene is recessive. As long as a child receives at least one normal gene, there is no risk for a GSD. GSDs appear only if a person inherits a defective gene from both parents.

The most common forms of GSD are Types I, II, III, and IV, which may account for more than 90% of all cases. The most common form is Type I, or von Gierke's disease, which occurs in one out of every 100,000 births. Other forms, such as Types VI and IX, are so rare that reliable statistics are not available. The overall frequency of all forms of glycogen storage disease is approximately one in 20,000–25,000 live births.

Causes and symptoms

GSD symptoms depend on the enzyme affected. Since glycogen storage occurs mainly in muscles and the liver, those sites display the most prominent symptoms.

There are at least 10 different types of GSDs which are classified according to the enzyme affected:

- Type Ia, or von Gierke's disease, is caused by glucose-6-phosphatase deficiency in the liver, kidney, and small intestine. The last step in glycogenolysis, the breaking down of glycogen to glucose, is the transformation of glucose-6-phosphate to glucose. In GSD I, that step does not occur. As a result, the liver is clogged with excess glycogen and becomes enlarged and fatty. Other symptoms include low blood sugar and elevated levels of lactate, lipids, and uric acid in the blood. Growth is impaired, puberty is often delayed, and bones may be weakened by osteoporosis. Blood platelets are also affected and frequent nosebleeds and easy bruising are common. Primary symptoms improve with age, but after age 20–30, liver tumors, liver cancer, chronic renal disease, and gout may appear.
- Type Ib is caused by glucose-6-phosphatase translocase deficiency. In order to carry out the final step of glycogenolysis, glucose-6-phosphate has to be transported into a cell's endoplasmic reticulum. If translocase, the enzyme responsible for that movement, is missing or defective, the same symptoms occur as in Type Ia. Additionally, the immune system is weakened and victims are susceptible to bacterial infections, such as pneumonia, mouth and gum infections, and inflammatory bowel disease. Types Ic and Id are also caused by defects in the translocase system.
- Type II, or Pompe's disease or acid maltase deficiency, is caused by lysosomal alpha-D-glucosidase deficiency in skeletal and heart muscles. GSD II is subdivided according to the age of onset. In the infantile form, infants seem normal at birth, but within a few months they develop muscle weakness, trouble breathing, and an enlarged heart. Cardiac failure and death usually occur before age 2, despite medical treatment. The juvenile and adult forms of GSD II affect mainly the skeletal muscles in the body's limbs and torso. Unlike the infantile form, treatment can extend life, but there is no cure. Respiratory failure is the primary cause of death.

- Type III, or Cori's disease, is caused by glycogen debrancher enzyme deficiency in the liver, muscles, and some blood cells, such as leukocytes and erythrocytes. About 15% of GSD III cases only involve the liver. The glycogen molecule is not a simple straight chain of linked glucose molecules, but rather an intricate network of short chains that branch off from one another. In glycogenolysis, a particular enzyme is required to unlink the branch points. When that enzyme fails, symptoms similar to GSD I occur; in childhood, it may be difficult to distinguish the two GSDs by symptoms alone. In addition to the low blood sugar, retarded growth, and enlarged liver causing a swollen abdomen, GSD III also causes muscles prone to wasting, an enlarged heart, and heightened levels of lipids in the blood. The muscle wasting increases with age, but the other symptoms become less severe.
- Type IV, or Andersen's disease, is caused by glycogen brancher enzyme deficiency in the liver, brain, heart, skeletal muscles, and skin fibroblasts. The glycogen constructed in GSD IV is abnormal and insoluble. As it accumulates in the cells, cell death leads to organ damage. Infants born with GSD IV appear normal at birth, but are diagnosed with enlarged livers and failure to thrive within their first year. Infants who survive beyond their first birthday develop cirrhosis of the liver by age 3–5 and die as a result of chronic liver failure.
- Type V, or McArdle's disease, is caused by glycogen phosphorylase deficiency in skeletal muscles. Under normal circumstances, muscles cells rely on oxidation of fatty acids during rest or light activity. More demanding activity requires that they draw on their glycogen stockpile. In GSD V, this form of glycogenolysis is disabled and glucose is not available. The main symptoms are muscle weakness and cramping brought on by exercise, as well as burgundy-colored urine after exercise due to myoglobin (a breakdown product of muscle) in the urine.
- Type VI, or Hers' disease, is caused by liver phosphorylase deficiency, which blocks the first step of glycogenolysis. In contrast to other GSDs, Type VI seems to be linked to the X chromosome. Low blood sugar is one of the key symptoms, but it is not as severe as in some other forms of GSD. An enlarged liver and mildly retarded growth also occur.
- Type VII, or Tarui's disease, is caused by muscle phosphofructokinase deficiency. Although glucose may be available as a fuel in muscles, the cells cannot metabolize it. Therefore, abnormally high levels of glycogen are stockpiled in the muscle cells. The symptoms are similar to GSD V, but also include anemia and increased levels of uric acid.
- Types VIII and XI are caused by defects of enzymes in the liver phosphorylase activating-deactivating cascade and have symptoms similar to GSD VI.
- Type IX is caused by liver glycogen phosphorylase kinase deficiency and, symptom-wise, is very similar to GSD VI. The main differences are that the symptoms may not be as severe and may also include exercise-related problems in the muscles, such as pain and cramps. The symptoms abate after puberty with proper treatment. Most cases of GSD IX are linked to the X chromosome and therefore affect males.
- Type X is caused by a defect in the cyclic adenosine monophosphate-dependent (AMP) kinase enzyme and presents symptoms similar to GSDs VI and IX.

Diagnosis

Diagnosis usually occurs in infancy or childhood, although some milder types of GSD go unnoticed well into adulthood and old age. It is even conceivable that some of the milder GSDs are never diagnosed.

The four major symptoms that typically lead a doctor to suspect GSDs are low blood sugar, enlarged liver, retarded growth, and an abnormal blood biochemistry profile. A definitive diagnosis is obtained by biopsy of the affected organ or organs. The biopsy sample is tested for its glycogen content and assayed for enzyme activity. There are DNA-based techniques for diagnosing some GSDs from more easily available samples, such as blood or skin. These DNA techniques can also be used for prenatal testing.

Treatment

Some GSD types cannot be treated, while others are relatively easy to control through symptom management. In more severe cases, receiving an organ transplant is the only option. In the most severe cases, there are no available treatments and the victim dies within the first few years of life.

Of the treatable types of GSD, many are treated by manipulating the diet. The key to managing GSD I is to maintain consistent levels of blood glucose through a combination of nocturnal intragastric feeding (usually for infants and children), frequent high-carbohydrate meals during the day, and regular oral doses of cornstarch (people over age 2). Juvenile and adult forms of GSD II can be managed somewhat by a high protein diet, which also helps in cases of GSD III, GSD VI, and GSD IX. GSD V and GSD VII can also be managed with a high protein diet and by avoiding strenuous **exercise**.

KEY TERMS

Amniocentesis—A medical test done during pregnancy in which a small sample of the amniotic fluid is taken from around the fetus. The fluid contains fetal cells that can be examined for genetic abnormalities.

Autosomal gene—A gene found on one of the 22 autosomal chromosome pairs; i.e., not on a sex (X or Y) chromosome.

Chorionic villus sampling—A medical test done during pregnancy in which a sample of the membrane surrounding the fetus is removed for examination. This examination can reveal genetic fetal abnormalities.

Glucose—A form of sugar that serves as the body's main energy source.

Glycogen—A macromolecule composed mainly of glucose that serves as the storage form of glucose that is not immediately needed by the body.

Glycogenolysis—The process of tearing-down a glycogen molecule to free up glucose.

Glycogenosis—An alternate term for glycogen storage disease. The plural form is glycogenoses.

Gout—A painful condition in which uric acid precipitates from the blood and accumulates in joints and connective tissues.

Mendelian inheritance—An inheritance pattern for autosomal gene pairs. The genetic trait displayed results from one parent's gene dominating over the gene inherited from the other parent.

Osteoporosis—A disease in which the bones become weak and brittle.

Renal disease—Kidney disease.

Transgenic animal—Animals that have had genes from other species inserted into their genetic code.

For GSD cases in which dietary therapy is ineffective, organ transplantation may be the only viable alternative. Liver transplants have been effective in reversing the symptoms of GSD IV.

Advances in genetic therapy offer hope for effective treatment in the future. This therapy involves using viruses to deliver a correct form of the gene to affected cells.

Prognosis

People with well-managed, treatable types of GSD can lead long, relatively normal lives. This goal is accomplished with the milder types of GSD, such as Types VI, IX, and X. As the GSD type becomes more severe, a greater level of vigilance against infections and other complications is required. Given current treatment options, complications such as **liver disease**, **heart failure**, and **respiratory failure** may not be warded-off indefinitely. Quality of life and life expectancy are substantially decreased.

Prevention

Because GSD is an inherited condition, it is not preventable. If both parents carry the defective gene, there is a one-in-four chance that their offspring will inherit the disorder. Other children may be carriers or they may miss inheriting the gene altogether.

Through chorionic villi sampling and **amniocentesis**, the disorder can be detected prior to birth. Some types of GSD can be detected even before conception occurs, if both parents are tested for the presence of the defective gene. Before undergoing such testing, the prospective parents should meet with a genetic counselor and other professionals in order to make an informed decision.

ORGANIZATIONS

Acid Maltase Deficiency Association, PO Box 700248, San Antonio, TX, 8270-0248, (210) 494-6144, tianrama@aol.com, http://www.amda-pompe.org.

American Liver Foundation, 75 Maiden Lane, Suite 603, New York, NY, 10038, (212) 668-1000, (212) 483-8179, http://www.liverfoundation.org.

Association for Glycogen Storage Disease, PO Box 896, Durant, IA, 52747-9769, (563) 514-4022, maryc@agsdus.org, http://www.agsdus.org.

Julia Barrett

Glycosylated hemoglobin test

Definition

Glycosylated hemoglobin is a test that indicates how much sugar has been in a person's blood during the past two to four months. It is used to monitor the effectiveness of diabetes treatment.

Purpose

Diabetes is a disease in which a person cannot effectively use sugar in the blood. Left untreated, blood sugar levels can be very high. High sugar levels increase risk of complications, such as damage to eyes, kidneys, heart, nerves, blood vessels, and other organs.

A routine blood sugar test reveals how close to normal a sugar level is at the time of the test. The glycosylated **hemoglobin test** reveals how close to normal it has been during the past several months.

This information helps a physician evaluate how well a person is responding to diabetes treatment and to determine how long sugar levels have been high in a person newly diagnosed with diabetes.

Description

The Diabetes Control and Complications Trial (DCCT) demonstrated that people with diabetes who maintained blood glucose (sugar) and total fasting hemoglobin levels at or close to a normal range decreased their risk of complications by 50–75%. Based on results of this study, the American Diabetes Association (ADA) recommends routine glycosylated hemoglobin testing to measure long-term control of blood sugar.

Glycosylated hemoglobin measures the percentage of hemoglobin bound to glucose. Hemoglobin is a protein found in every red blood cell. As hemoglobin and glucose are together in the red blood cell, the glucose gradually binds to the A1c form of hemoglobin in a process called glycosylation. The amount bound reflects how much glucose has been in the blood during the past average 120-day lifespan of red cells.

Several methods are used to measure the amount of bound hemoglobin and glucose. They are electrophoresis, chromatography, and immunoassay. All are based on the separation of hemoglobin bound to glucose from that without glucose.

The ADA recommends glycosylated hemoglobin be done during a person's first diabetes evaluation, again after treatment is begun and sugar levels are stabilized, then repeated at least semiannually. If the person does not meet treatment goals or sugar levels have not stabilized, the test should be repeated quarterly.

Other names for the test include: Hemoglobin A1c, HbA1c, Diabetic control index, GHb, glycosylated hemoglobin, and glycated hemoglobin. The test is covered by insurance. Results usually are available the following day.

KEY TERMS

Diabetes mellitus—A disease in which a person can't effectively use sugar in the blood to meet the needs of the body. It is caused by a lack of the hormone insulin.

Glucose—The main form of sugar used by the body for energy.

Glycosylated hemoglobin—A test that measures the amount of hemoglobin bound to glucose. It is a measure of how much glucose has been in the blood during the past two to four months.

Preparation

A person does not need to fast before this test. A healthcare worker ties a tourniquet on the person's upper arm, locates a vein in the inner elbow region, and inserts a needle into the vein. Vacuum action draws the blood through the needle into an attached tube. Collection of the sample takes only a few minutes. This test requires 5 mL of blood.

While home HbA1c tests are available, they should only be used with a doctor's guidance.

Aftercare

Discomfort or bruising may occur at the puncture site, or the person may feel dizzy or faint. Pressure to the puncture site until bleeding stops reduces bruising. Warm packs relieve discomfort.

Normal results

Diabetes treatment should achieve glycosylated hemoglobin levels of less than 7.0%. Normal value for a non-diabetic person is 4.0–6.0%.

Because laboratories use different methods, results from different laboratories can not always be compared. The National Glycosylation Standardization Program gives a certification to laboratories using tests standardized to those used in the DCCT study.

Abnormal results

Results require interpretation by a physician with knowledge of the person's clinical condition, as well as the test method used. Some methods give false high or low results if the person has an abnormal hemoglobin, such as hemoglobin S or F.

Conditions that increase the lifespan of red cells, such as a **splenectomy** (removal of the spleen), falsely increase levels. Conditions that decrease the lifespan, such as hemolysis (disruption of the red blood cell membrane), falsely decrease levels.

Resources

PERIODICALS

"Simple Choice A1c." *Diabetes Forecast* January 2004: RG7.

ORGANIZATIONS

American Diabetes Association, 1701 North Beauregard Street, Alexandria, VA, 22311, (800) 342-2383, AskADA@diabetes.org, http://www.diabetes.org.

Centers for Disease Control and Prevention (CDC), 1600 Clifton Road, Atlanta, GA, 30333, (800) 232-4636, cdcinfo@cdc.gov, http://www.cdc.gov.

National Diabetes Information Clearinghouse (NDIC), 1 Information Way, Bethesda, MD, 20892-3560, (703) 738-4929, (800) 860-8747, ndic@info.niddk.nih.gov, http://diabetes.niddk.nih.gov.

Nancy J. Nordenson
Teresa G. Odle

Goiter

Definition

Goiter refers to any visible enlargement of the thyroid gland.

Description

The thyroid gland sits astride the trachea (windpipe) and is shaped like a butterfly. It makes thyroxin, a hormone that regulates the metabolic activity of the body, rather like the gas pedal on a car. Too much thyroxin increases the metabolism, causing weight loss, temperature elevation, nervousness, and irritability. Too little thyroxin slows the metabolism down, deepens the voice, causes weight gain and water retention, and retards growth and mental development in children. Both conditions also alter hair and skin growth, bowel function, and menstrual flow.

Curiously, the thyroid gland is often enlarged whether it is making too much hormone, too little, or sometimes even when it is functioning normally. The thyroid is controlled by the pituitary gland, which secretes thyroid stimulating hormone (TSH) in response to the amount of thyroxin it finds in the blood. TSH increases the amount of thyroxin secreted by the thyroid and also causes the thyroid gland to grow.

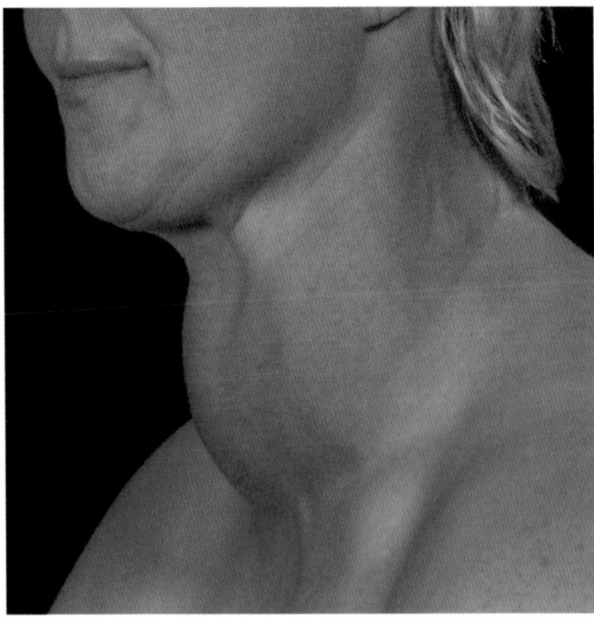

This woman's goiter may have been caused by an insufficient intake of iodine. *(Custom Medical Stock Photo, Inc. Reproduced by permission.)*

- Hyperthyroid goiter–If the amount of stimulating hormone is excessive, the thyroid will both enlarge and secrete too much thyroxin. The result–hyperthyroidism with a goiter. Graves' disease is the most common form of this disorder.
- Euthyroid goiter–The thyroid is the only organ in the body to use iodine. If dietary iodine is slightly inadequate, too little thyroxin will be secreted, and the pituitary will sense the deficiency and produce more TSH. The thyroid gland will enlarge enough to make sufficient thyroxin.
- Hypothyroid goiter–If dietary iodine is severely reduced, even an enlarged gland will not be able to make enough thyroxin. The gland will keep growing under the influence of TSH, but it may never be able to make enough thyroxin.

Causes and symptoms

Excess TSH (or similar hormones), cysts, and tumors will enlarge the thyroid gland. Of these, TSH enlarges the entire gland while cysts and tumors enlarge only a part of it.

The only symptom from a goiter is the large swelling just above the breast bone. Rarely, it may constrict the trachea (windpipe) or esophagus and cause

KEY TERMS

Cyst—A liquid-filled structure developing abnormally in the body.

Euthyroid—Having the right amount of thyroxin stimulation.

Hyperthyroid—Having too much thyroxin stimulation.

Hypothyroid—Having too little thyroxin stimulation.

Pituitary gland—The master gland, located in the middle of the head, that controls most of the other glandss by secreting stimulating hormones.

Radiotherapy—The use of ionizing radiation, either as x rays or radioactive isotopes, to treat disease.

Thyroxin—The hormone secreted by the thyroid gland.

difficulty breathing or swallowing. The rest of the symptoms come from thyroxin or the lack of it.

Diagnosis

The size, shape, and texture of the thyroid gland help the physician determine the cause. A battery of blood tests are required to verify the specific thyroid disease. Functional imaging studies using radioactive iodine determine how active the gland is and what it looks like.

Treatment

Goiters of all types will regress with treatment of the underlying condition. Dietary iodine may be all that is needed. However, if an iodine deficient thyroid that has grown in size to accommodate its deficiency is suddenly supplied an adequate amount of iodine, it could suddenly make large amounts of thyroxin and cause a thyroid storm, the equivalent of racing your car motor at top speed.

Hyperthyroidism can be treated with medications, therapeutic doses of radioactive iodine, or surgical reduction. Surgery is much less common now than it used to be because of progress in drugs and radiotherapy.

Prognosis

Although goiters diminish in size, the thyroid may not return to normal. Sometimes thyroid function does not return after treatment, but thyroxin is easy to take as a pill.

Prevention

Euthyroid goiter and hypothyroid goiter are common around the world because many regions have inadequate dietary iodine, including some places in the United States. International relief groups are providing iodized salt to many of these populations. Because **mental retardation** is a common result of **hypothyroidism** in children, this is an extremely important project.

ORGANIZATIONS

International Council for the Control of Iodine Deficiency Disorders, P.O. Box 51030, 375 des Epinettes, Ottawa, Ontario, Canada, K1E 3E), http://www.iccidd.org.

J. Ricker Polsdorfer, MD

Gonadal dysgenesis *see* **Turner syndrome**

Gonorrhea

Definition

Gonorrhea is a highly contagious sexually transmitted infection (STI) or disease (STD) caused by the bacterium *Neisseria gonorrhoeae*. These bacteria grow in the urethra and in warm, moist parts of the reproductive tract, including the cervix, uterus, and fallopian tubes of women. The bacteria also can infect the anus, mouth, throat, and eyes. Untreated gonorrhea can cause serious medical complications.

Demographics

For most of the twentieth century gonorrhea was the most common STD worldwide. The incidence of gonorrhea has declined steadily in the developed world since the mid-1970s, reaching an all-time low in 2004. This decline is largely due to increased public awareness of the risks and prevention of STDs such as herpes and HIV/AIDS. However there are still about 200 million new cases of gonorrhea annually throughout the world and gonorrhea rates in certain urban areas of the United States are once again on the rise.

Gonorrhea is the second most common reportable disease in the United States. More than 350,000 newly

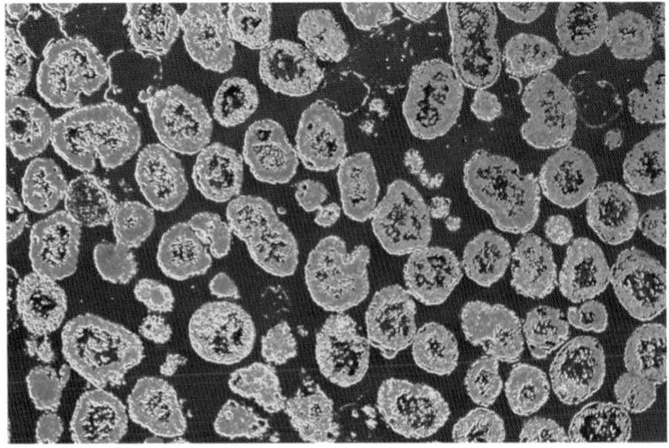

A transmission electron microscopy (TEM) image of *Neisseria gonorrhoeae*. *(Custom Medical Stock Photo, Inc. Reproduced by permission.)*

diagnosed cases were reported in 2007. Experts believe that the actual number is much higher since gonorrhea tends to be both under-diagnosed and underreported. Estimates of the actual number of annual cases in the United States range from 400,000 to one million. An estimated 40,000 pregnant women are infected with gonorrhea each year in the United States. **Pelvic inflammatory disease** (PID), the most common complication of gonorrhea, affects one million American women annually.

Although gonorrhea affects people of all ages, races, and socioeconomic levels, adolescents and young adults are at the highest risk. More than 80% of cases occur in those aged 15 to 29. Gonorrhea is most common among females aged 15–19 and males aged 20–24. Infection rates are higher in men than in women and highest in men who have sex with other men. African Americans and those living in urban areas and having multiple sex partners are at the greatest risk for infection.

Description

Commonly called "the clap," gonorrhea is transmitted through sexual contact, including oral, anal, and vaginal intercourse. The risk of contracting gonorrhea from a single sexual encounter with an infected partner is 60–90%. Gonorrhea also can be spread through contact with the bodily fluids of an infected person. There is some evidence for transmission of gonorrhea among children and from adults to children via unclean hands. However gonorrhea infection in children is considered a warning flag for **sexual abuse**.

Gonorrhea usually affects the genitourinary tract, but can also spread to the rectum, throat, and eyes. Left untreated, gonorrhea can spread through the bloodstream and infect the reproductive system, joints, heart valves, skin, liver, and brain. As many as 10% of women infected with gonorrhea experience a **pregnancy** in a fallopian tube (**ectopic pregnancy**) or become infertile as a result of PID. Gonorrhea also increases the risk of contracting and transmitting HIV/AIDS. Being cured of gonorrhea does not protect a person against re-infection.

Pregnant women with untreated gonorrhea are at increased risk for **miscarriage**, preterm birth, or membranes that rupture prematurely. An infected mother can transmit the disease to her infant as it passes through the birth canal during delivery, causing newborn conjunctivitis—an eye infection that can lead to blindness. The infant also is at risk for joint infection or a life-threatening blood infection.

Risk factors

Risk factors for gonorrhea are similar to those for other STDs. The primary risk factors are unprotected sex (without a condom) with multiple partners.

Causes and symptoms

Gonnorrhea is caused by the bacterium *N. gonorrhoeae*, which is transmitted through sexual contact. It can be transmitted to the eyes by touching an infected organ and then touching the eyes. *N. gonorrhoeae* cannot survive for any length of time outside of the human body. It cannot be transmitted via a toilet seat or by shaking hands.

Although most gonorrhea-infected males have symptoms, as many as 80% of infected females do not. Symptoms usually appear between one and 14 days following infection, but the incubation period can be as long as 30 days. Often the only symptom of gonorrhea is inflammation of mucous membranes in the genital region. Some people experience **nausea**, **vomiting**, **fever**, and chills, and **pain** during intercourse.

In males the infection usually appears first in the urethra—the tube that carries urine and sperm to the outside of the body. About 95% of infected men have thick, cloudy, white, yellowish, green, or bloody discharge from the penis. Other common symptoms in males include frequent urination and burning or pain during urination. Complications of gonorrhea in males can affect the prostate, testicles, and surrounding glands. **Epididymitis** is a painful condition of the testicles that can lead to sterility if untreated.

In females gonorrhea usually infects the cervix—the lower narrow portion of the uterus that opens to

KEY TERMS

Cervix—The lower, narrow part—or neck—of the uterus.

Chlamydia—The most common sexually transmitted bacterial infection in the United States. It often occurs along with gonorrhea. The majority of infected women have no symptoms.

Conjunctivitis—An inflammation of the eye that can be caused by gonorrhea or chlamydia.

Ectopic pregnancy—A pregnancy that develops outside of the uterus, such as in the fallopian tubes. The fetus dies and the mother's life may be threatened.

ELISA—Enzyme-linked immunosorbent assay; a screening test that uses antibodies to detect infections such as gonorrhea and HIV.

HIV/AIDS—Human immunodeficiency virus/acquired immunodeficiency syndrome; a sexually transmitted viral disease that is more likely to be transmitted or acquired in the presence of gonorrhea or another STD.

Neisseria gonorrhoeae—The bacterium that causes gonorrhea.

Nucleic acid amplification test (NAAT)—A screening test for gonorrhea that detects bacterial DNA in a urine sample or cervical swab.

Pelvic inflammatory disease (PID)—An infection of the female upper genital tract that can be a complication of gonorrhea. At least 25% of women with PID suffer long-term consequences such as infertility or an ectopic pregnancy.

Sexually transmitted disease (STD)—A disease that is transmitted by sexual contact, including gonorrhea, chlamydia, HIV/AIDS, genital herpes, syphilis, and genital warts.

Sexually transmitted infection (STI)—An infectious disease, such as gonorrhea, that is transmitted through sexual activity.

Sterility—Inability to conceive a child.

Urethra—The urine channel leading from the bladder to the outside of the body and, in men, the channel for semen.

Urethritis—Inflammation of the urethra.

the vagina—as well as the uterus and fallopian tubes. Symptoms can include:

- vaginal discharge that may be cloudy and yellow
- frequent, painful, or burning urination
- bleeding between menstrual periods
- pain or bleeding during vaginal intercourse
- heavy bleeding during menstrual periods
- chronic abdominal pain

Women are more likely than men to suffer from complications of gonorrhea because the disease often progresses without symptoms. The most common complication of untreated gonorrhea is PID, which can occur in as many as 40% of infected women. PID can damage the ovaries and fallopian tubes, resulting in a pregnancy developing outside of the uterus or sterility. A less common complication is disseminated gonococcal infection (DGI), in which the bacteria travels through the blood to distant sites such as the skin or joints.

Newborn **conjunctivitis** caused by gonorrhea usually appears two–seven days after birth. Symptoms of eye infection include redness, **itching**, or discharge from the eye. Other symptoms of gonorrhea in infants and children include irritation, redness, swelling, or a pus-like discharge from the urethra and possibly painful urination.

Anal gonorrheal infection may cause rectal itching, discharge, a constant urge to move the bowels, painful bowel movements, or blood in the stool. However about 90% of anal infections are without symptoms. Oral gonorrheal infection may cause a **sore throat** or painful swallowing.

Diagnosis

Examination

An initial diagnosis of gonorrhea is based on symptoms, sexual history, and at-risk behavior. The diagnosis may be made by a family physician or STD specialist or at a public health clinic. Women may be diagnosed by an obstetrician/gynecologist, particularly if there are gynecological complications. Men may be diagnosed by a urologist. Physicians are required to report cases of gonorrhea to public health officials. Patients are asked to provide the names of all sexual partners who may have been exposed to the infection, so that they can be notified and tested for gonorrhea.

Tests

Many physicians use more than one test to confirm a diagnosis of gonorrhea:

- A nucleic acid amplifications test (NAAT) that detects bacterial DNA in a urine or cervical sample is the fastest and most accurate diagnostic test.
- An enzyme-linked immunosorbent assay (ELISA) that uses antibodies specific for *N. gonorrhoeae* is also fast and sensitive.
- Culturing bacteria from a discharge or sample obtained with a cotton swab can diagnose gonorrhea and determine whether the bacteria are drug resistant. Culturing takes for up to two days.
- Discharge from an infected area can Gram stained and examined under a microscope for the presence of *N. gonorrhoeae*; however this test is only about 70% accurate in men and about 50% accurate in women.
- Since other STDs, such as chlamydia and syphilis, often occur along with gonorrhea, patients also may be tested for these infections.

Treatment

Traditional

Gonorrhea is treated with **antibiotics**. Patients should refrain from sexual intercourse until they and their partners have completed treatment and had follow-up testing to ensure that the infection has been completely eradicated.

Drugs

In the past gonorrhea was usually treated with penicillin, a penicillin derivative, or tetracycline. However since the 1940s *N. gonorrhoeae* has become increasingly resistant to these antibiotics. Resistance to fluoroquinolone antibiotics also has increased rapidly over the past decade. Therefore as of 2009, the recommended treatments for gonorrhea are:

- a single 125-mg injection of ceftriaxone
- a single 400-mg dose of oral cefixime
- another single-dose cephalosporin antibiotic

Infants born to gonorrhea-infected mothers may be treated with intravenous ceftriaxone or another antibiotic. Infant conjunctivitis caused by gonorrhea is treated with an eye ointment containing polymyxin and bacitracin, erythromycin, or tetracycline.

If chlamydial infection is also present, a combination of antibiotics—such as ceftriaxone and doxycycline or azithromycin—is used to treat both infections simultaneously. Erythromycin is used to treat chlamydia in pregnant women.

Alternative

Antibiotic treatment for gonorrhea may be complemented with various alternative therapies:

- *Lactobacillus acidophilus* or live-culture yogurt can help replace gastrointestinal flora that are killed by the antibiotics.
- Zinc, multivitamin/mineral complexes, vitamin C, and garlic (*Allium sativum*) may help improve immune system function.
- Kelp (*Macrocystis pyrifera* and related species) can supply vitamins and minerals.
- Teas or douches made with calendula (*Calendula officinalis*), myrrh (*Commiphora molmol*), and thuja (*Thuja occidentalis*) may reduce discharge and inflammation.
- The Chinese herb *Coptis chinensis*, used for "damp-heat;" infections, can be helpful for treating the genitourinary tract, especially if PID develops.
- Various other herbs can help treat reproductive and urinary system symptoms.
- With physician approval, a three-day juice fast may help cleanse the urinary and gastrointestinal systems and support healing.
- Acupuncture or acupressure can help cleanse body systems.

Home remedies

Antibiotic treatment is absolutely essential for gonorrhea. Hot baths can help reduce pain and inflammation.

Prognosis

Gonorrhea is curable with cephalosporin antibiotics and the prognosis is excellent with prompt treatment. However many people, especially women, have no symptoms of the disease and are unaware that they are infected. Adolescent girls are at particular risk for untreated gonorrhea. Up to 40% of women who do not receive early treatment may develop PID, which can damage the fallopian tubes and result in sterility. Women who have had PID are six–ten times more likely to have an ectopic pregnancy. Although the risk of **infertility** is higher for women than for men, men also can become sterile if untreated gonorrhea causes inflammation of the urethra (**urethritis**).

Untreated gonorrhea can cause inflammation, abscesses, and scarring. In about 2% of patients with untreated gonorrhea, the infection spreads throughout the body, causing fever, arthritis-like joint pain, and **skin lesions**. The bacterium also can infect the heart valves and brain. In men, untreated gonorrhea can affect the prostate, testicles, and surrounding glands.

Prevention

The best prevention for gonorrhea is sexual abstinence or sexual activity that is confined to a mutually monogamous relationship in which both partners have been tested for gonorrhea and other STDs. If used properly and consistently for vaginal and anal sex, latex male **condoms** and polyurethane female condoms can reduce the risk of *N. gonorrhoeae* transmission. A dental dam may reduce the risk of transmission during oral sex. However anyone who has multiple sexual partners should be tested regularly for gonorrhea and other STDs. It is recommended that all sexually active teenagers and young adults be screened regularly for gonorrhea. All pregnant women should be screened at their first prenatal visit.

All newborns are treated under the eyelids with an antibiotic ointment, such as silver nitrate or erythromycin, to prevent gonorrhea. Infants born to mothers with untreated gonorrhea are given a prophylactic dose of ceftriaxone.

Resources

BOOKS

Grimes, Jill. *Seductive Delusions: How Everyday People Catch STDs.* Baltimore: Johns Hopkins University Press, 2008.

Marr, Lisa. *Sexually Transmitted Diseases: A Physician Tells You What You Need to Know*, 2nd ed. Baltimore: Johns Hopkins University Press, 2007.

Michaud, Christopher. *Gonorrhea.* New York: Rosen, 2006.

Sutton, Amy. *Sexually Transmitted Diseases Sourcebook*, 3rd ed. Detroit: Omnigraphics, 2006.

PERIODICALS

Du, Ping, et al. "Changes in Community Economic Status and Racial Distribution Associated with Gonorrhea Rates: An Analysis at the Community Level." *Sexually Transmitted Diseases* 36, no. 7 (July 2009): 430-438.

Hosenfeld, Christina B., et al. "Repeat Infection with Chlamydia and Gonorrhea Among Females: A Systematic Review of the Literature." *Sexually Transmitted Diseases* 36, no. 8 (August 2009): 478-489.

Workowski, K. A., S. M. Berman, and J. M. Douglas, Jr. "Emerging Antimicrobial resistance in *Neisseria gonorrhoeae*: Urgent Need to Strengthen Prevention Strategies." *Annals of Internal Medicine* 148, no. 9 (April 15, 2008): 606-613.

OTHER

Behrman, Amy J., and William H. Shoff. "Gonorrhea." *eMedicine*.http://emedicine.medscape.com/article/782913-overview

"Gonorrhea." *National Institute of Allergy and Infectious Diseases*.http://www3.niaid.nih.gov/topics/gonorrhea

"Gonorrhea." *Sexually Transmitted Diseases Surveillance, 2007*.http://www.cdc.gov/std/stats07/gonorrhea.htm

"Gonorrhea: Frequently Asked Questions." *womenshealth.gov*http://www.womenshealth.gov/faq/gonorrhea.cfm

Gonorrhea: Questions and Answers. *American Social Health Association*.http://www.ashastd.org/learn/learn_gonorrhea.cfm

"Updated Recommended Treatment Regimens for Gonococcal Infections and Associated Conditions—United States, April 2007." *Centers for Disease Control and Prevention*.http://www.cdc.gov/std/treatment/2006/updated-regimens.htm

ORGANIZATIONS

American Social Health Association, P.O. Box 13827, Research Triangle Park, NC, 27709, (919) 361-8400, (800) 227-8922, (919) 361-8425, info@ashastd.org, http://www.ashastd.org.

National Institute of Allergy and Infectious Diseases (NIAID), Office of Communications and Public Liaison, 6610 Rockledge Drive, Bethesda, MD, 20892-66123, (866) 284-4107, http://www3.niaid.nih.gov.

U.S. Centers for Disease Control and Prevention (CDC), 1600 Clifton Road, Atlanta, GA, 30333, 800-CDC-INFO (232-4636), cdcinfo@cdc.gov, http://www.cdc.gov.

Teresa G. Odle
Margaret Alic, PhD

Goodpasture's syndrome

Definition

An uncommon and life-threatening hypersensitivity disorder believed to be an autoimmune process related to antibody formation in the body. Goodpasture's syndrome is characterized by renal (kidney) disease and lung hemorrhage.

Demographics

Goodpasture's syndrome is a rare autoimmune disorder, with a predominance in young males typically between the ages of 20 and 30 years. It occurs more often in African Americans than Caucasians, and has also been observed in the Maori ethnic group of New Zealand.

Risk factors

There are no known risk factors for Goodpasture's syndrome however in some cases, affected individuals have been known to be ill with an upper respiratory tract infection before the development of the disorder. There may also be a connection between substances such as hydrocarbon solvents and some chemicals found in certain weed killers, however, the exact cause of Goodpasture's syndrome remains unknown.

Description

The disorder is characterized by an autoimmune reaction which deposits antibodies in the membranes of both the lung and kidneys, causing both inflammation of kidney (**glomerulonephritis**) and lung bleeding.

Causes and symptoms

The exact cause is unknown. It is an autoimmune disorder; that is, the immune system is fighting the body's own normal tissues through creating antibodies that attack the lungs and kidneys. Sometimes the disorder is triggered by a viral infection, or by the inhalation of gasoline or other hydrocarbon solvents. An association also exists between cigarette **smoking** and the syndrome. The target antigen of the Goodpasture's antibodies has been localized to a protein chain (type IV collagen).

Symptoms include foamy, bloody, or dark colored urine, decreased urine output, **cough** with bloody sputum, difficulty breathing after exertion, weakness, **fatigue**, **nausea** or **vomiting**, weight loss, nonspecific chest **pain** and/or pale skin.

Diagnosis

The clinician will perform a battery of tests to confirm a diagnosis. These tests include a **complete blood count** (CBC) to confirm anemia, iron levels to check for blood loss and blood urea nitrogen (BUN) and creatinine levels to test the kidney function. A **urinalysis** will be done to check for damage to the kidneys. A sputum test will be done to look for specific antibodies. A **chest x ray** will be done to assess the amount of fluid in the lung tissues. A lung needle biopsy and a **kidney biopsy** will show immune system deposits. The kidney biopsy can also show the presence of the harmful antibodies that attack the lungs and kidneys.

Treatment

Treatment is focused on slowing the progression of the disease. Treatment is most effective when begun early, before kidney function has deteriorated to a point where the kidney is permanently damaged, and dialysis is necessary. **Corticosteroids**, such as prednisone, or other anti-inflammatory medications may be used to reduce the immune response. Immune suppressants such as cyclophosphamide or azathioprine are used aggressively to reduce immune system effects.

A procedure whereby blood plasma, which contains antibodies, is removed from the body and replaced with fluids or donated plasma (**plasmapheresis**) may be performed daily for two or more weeks to remove circulating antibodies. It is fairly effective in slowing or reversing the disorder. Dialysis to clean the blood of wastes may be required if kidney function is poor. A kidney transplant may be successful, especially if performed after circulating antibodies have been absent for several months.

Prognosis

The probable outcome is variable. Most cases progress to severe renal failure and end-stage renal disease within months. Early diagnosis and treatment makes the probable outcome more favorable.

Prevention

No known prevention of Goodpasture's syndrome exists. Smoking cessation can reduce further

KEY TERMS

Antibody—A protein molecule produced by the immune system in response to a protein that is not recognized as belonging in the body.

Antigen—Any substance that, as a result of coming in contact with appropriate cells, induces a state of sensitivity and/or immune responsiveness after a period of time and that reacts in a demonstrable way with antibodies.

Autoimmune disorder—An abnormality within the body whereby the immune system incorrectly attacks the body's normal tissues, thereby causing disease or organ dysfunction.

Blood urea nitrogen (BUN)—A test used to measure the blood level of urea nitrogen, a waste that is normally filtered from the kidneys.

Creatinine—A test used to measure the blood level of creatinine, a waste product filtered out of the blood by the kidneys. Higher than usual levels of this substance may indicate kidney disease.

Glomerulus (glomeruli)—A small tuft of blood capillaries in the kidney, responsible for filtering out waste products.

damage to the lungs. Early diagnosis and treatment may slow progression of the disorder.

Resources

BOOKS

Clatworthy, Menna. *Nephrology: Clinical Cases Uncovered.* New York, NY: Wiley-Blackwell, 2010.

O'Callaghan, Chris. *The Renal System at a Glance,* 3rd ed. New York, NY: Wiley-Blackwell, 2009.

Stam, Lawrence, E.*100 Questions & Answers About Kidney Dialysis.*Sudbury, MA: Jones and Bartlett Publishers, 2009.

ORGANIZATIONS

American Association of Kidney Patients, 100 S. Ashley Dr., #280, Tampa, FL, 33602, (800) 749-2257, http://www.aakp.org.

American Kidney Fund (AKF), Suite 1010, 6110 Executive Boulevard, Rockville, MD, 20852, (800) 638-8299, http://www.kidneyfund.org.

National Kidney Foundation, 30 East 33rd St., New York, NY, 10016, (800) 622-9010, http://www.kidney.org.

National Organization for Rare Diseases, P.O. Box 8923, Fairfield, CT, 06812, (213) 745-6518, http://www.rarediseases.org.

Kim A. Sharp, M.Ln.
Laura Jean Cataldo, RN, Ed.D.

Gout

Definition

Gout is a form of acute arthritis that causes severe **pain** and swelling in the joints. It most commonly affects the big toe, but may also affect the heel, ankle, hand, wrist, or elbow. It affects the spine often enough to be a factor in back pain. Gout usually comes on suddenly, goes away after 5–10 days, and can keep recurring. Gout is different from other forms of arthritis because it occurs when there are high levels of uric acid circulating in the blood, which can cause urate crystals to settle in the tissues of the joints.

Description

Uric acid, which is found naturally in the bloodstream, is formed as the body breaks down waste products, mainly those containing purine, a substance that is produced by the body and is also found in high concentrations in some foods, including brains, liver, sardines, anchovies, and dried peas and beans. Normally, the kidneys filter uric acid out of the blood and excrete it in the urine. Sometimes, however, the body produces too much uric acid or the kidneys aren't efficient enough at filtering it from the blood, and it builds up in the blood stream, a condition known as hyperuricemia. A person's susceptibility to gout may increase because of the inheritance of certain genes or from being overweight and eating a rich diet. In some cases, another disease (such as lymphoma, leukemia, or **hemolytic anemia**) may be the underlying cause of the uric acid buildup that results in gout. An additional factor is occupational or environmental; it is now known that chronic exposure to high levels of lead decreases the body's excretion of urates, allowing uric acid to accumulate in the blood.

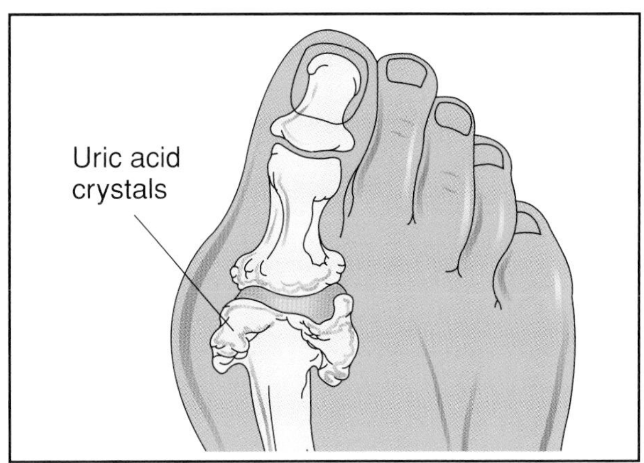

Gout, a form of acute arthritis, most commonly occurs in the big toe. It is caused by high levels of uric acid in the blood, in which urate crystals settle in the tissues of the joints and produce severe pain and swelling. *(Illustration by Electronic Illustrators Group. Reproduced by permission of Gale, a part of Cengage Learning.)*

Hyperuricemia does not always cause gout. Over the course of years, however, sharp urate crystals build up in the synovial fluid of the joints. Often, some precipitating event, such as an infection, surgery, the **stress** of hospitalization, a stubbed toe, or even a heavy drinking binge can cause inflammation. White blood cells, mistaking the urate crystals for a foreign invader, flood into the joint and surround the crystals, causing inflammation—in other words, the redness, swelling, and pain that are the hallmarks of a gout attack.

Causes and symptoms

As a result of high levels of uric acid in the blood, needle-like urate crystals gradually accumulate in the joints. Urate crystals may be present in the joint for a long time without causing symptoms. Infection, injury

KEY TERMS

Allopurinol—A drug that corrects hyperuricemia by inhibiting urate production.

Colchicine—A drug used to treat painful flare-ups of gout.

Corticosteroids—Medications related to a natural body hormone called hydrocortisone, which are used to treat inflammation.

Hyperuricemia—High levels of a waste product called uric acid in the blood.

Probenecid—A drug that corrects hyperuricemia by increasing the urinary excretion of urate.

Purine—A substance found in foods that is broken down into urate and may contribute to hyperuricemia and gout.

Sulfinpyrazone—A drug that corrects hyperuricemia by increasing the urinary excretion of urate.

Synovial fluid—Fluid surrounding the joints which acts as a lubricant, reducing the friction between the joints.

Tophus (plural, tophi)—A chalky deposit of a uric acid compound found in gout. Tophi occur most frequently around joints and in the external ear.

Urate crystals—Crystals formed by high levels of uric acid in the blood.

to the joint, surgery, drinking too much, or eating the wrong kinds of foods may suddenly bring on the symptoms, which include pain, tenderness, redness, warmth, and swelling of the joint. In many cases, the gout attack begins in the middle of the night. The pain is often so excruciating that the sufferer cannot bear weight on the joint or tolerate the pressure of bed-covers. The inflamed skin over the joint may be red, shiny, and dry, and the inflammation may be accompanied by a mild **fever**. These symptoms may go away in about a week and disappear for months or years at a time. However, over the course of time, attacks of gout recur more and more frequently, last longer, and affect more joints. Eventually, stone-like deposits known as tophi may build up in the joints, ligaments, and tendons, leading to permanent joint deformity and decreased motion. (In addition to causing the tophi associated with gout, hyperuricemia can also cause **kidney stones**, also called renal calculi or uroliths.)

Gout affects an estimated one million Americans; according to the National Institutes of Health, it accounts for about 5% of all cases of arthritis. It occurs more often in men than in women; the sex ratio is about 4:1. Uric-acid levels tend to increase in men at **puberty**, and, because it takes 20 years of hyperuricemia to cause gout symptoms, men commonly develop gout in their late 30s or early 40s. Women more typically develop gout later in life, starting in their 60s. According to some medical experts, estrogen protects against hyperuricemia, and when estrogen levels fall during **menopause**, urate crystals can begin to build up in the joints. Excess body weight, regular excessive alcohol intake, the use of blood pressure medications called **diuretics**, and high levels of certain fatty substances in the blood (serum **triglycerides**) associated with an increased risk of heart disease can all increase a person's risk of developing gout.

Gout appears to be on the increase in the American population. According to a study published in November 2002, there was a twofold increase in the incidence of gout over the 20 years between 1977 and 1997. It is not yet known whether this increase is the result of improved diagnosis or whether it is associated with risk factors that have not yet been identified.

Diagnosis

Usually, physicians can diagnose gout based on the **physical examination** and medical history (the patient's description of symptoms and other information). Doctors can also administer a test that measures the level of uric acid in the blood. While normal uric acid levels don't necessarily rule out gout and high levels don't confirm it, the presence of hyperuricemia increases the likelihood of gout. The development of a tophus can confirm the diagnosis of gout. The most definitive way to diagnose gout is to take a sample of fluid from the joint and test it for urate crystals.

Treatment

The goals of treatment for gout consist of alleviating pain, avoiding severe attacks in the future, and preventing long-term joint damage. In addition to taking pain medications as prescribed by their doctors, people having gout attacks are encouraged to rest and to increase the amount of fluids that they drink.

Acute attacks of gout can be treated with nonaspirin, **nonsteroidal anti-inflammatory drugs** (NSAIDs) such as naproxen **sodium** (Aleve), ibuprofen (Advil), or indomethacin (Indocin). In some cases, these drugs can aggravate a peptic ulcer or existing **kidney disease** and cannot be used. Doctors may also use colchicine (Colbenemid), especially in cases where nonsteroidal anti-inflammatory drugs cannot be used. Colchicine may cause **diarrhea**, which tends to go away once the patient stops taking it. **Corticosteroids** such as prednisone (Deltasone) and adrenocorticotropic hormone (Acthar) may be given orally or may be injected directly into the joint for a more concentrated effect. While all of these drugs have the potential to cause side effects, they are used for only about 48 hours and are not likely to cause major problems. However, **aspirin** and closely related drugs (salicylates) should be avoided because they can ultimately worsen gout.

Once an acute attack has been successfully treated, doctors try to prevent future attacks of gout and long-term joint damage by lowering uric acid levels in the blood. There are two types of drugs for correcting hyperuricemia. Such uricosuric drugs as probenecid (Benemid) and sulfinpyrazone (Anturane) lower the levels of urate in the blood by increasing its removal from the body (excretion) through the urine. These drugs may promote the formation of kidney stones, however, and they may not work for all patients, especially those with kidney disease. Allopurinol (Zyloprim), a type of drug called a xanthine-oxidase inhibitor, blocks the production of urate in the body, and can dissolve kidney stones as well as treating gout. The potential side effects of allopurinol include rash, a skin condition known as **dermatitis**, and liver dysfunction. In 2004, the FDA was seeking trial data on a new drug called oxypurinol (Oxyprim) for treating chronic gout. These medications may have to be taken for life to prevent further gout attacks.

Alternative treatment

Alternative approaches to gout focus on correcting hyperuricemia by encouraging weight loss and limiting the intake of alcohol and purine-rich foods. In addition, consuming garlic (*Allium sativum*) has been recommended to help prevent gout. Increasing fluid intake, especially by drinking water, is also recommended. During an acute attack, contrast **hydrotherapy** (alternating three-minute hot compresses with 30–second cold compresses) can help dissolve the crystals and resolve the pain faster.

Prognosis

Gout cannot be cured but usually it can be managed successfully. As tophi dissolve, joint mobility generally improves. (In some cases, however, medicines alone do not dissolve the tophi and they must be removed surgically.) Lowering uric acid in the blood also helps to prevent or improve the kidney problems that may accompany gout.

Prevention

For centuries, gout has been known as a "rich man's disease" or a disease caused by overindulgence in food and drink. While this view is perhaps a little overstated and oversimplified, lifestyle factors clearly influence a person's risk of developing gout. Since **obesity** and excessive alcohol intake are associated with hyperuricemia and gout, losing weight and limiting alcohol intake can help ward off gout. **Dehydration** may also promote the formation of urate crystals, so people taking diuretics or "water pills" may be better off switching to another type of blood pressure medication. Everyone should be sure to drink at least six to eight glasses of water each day. Since purine is broken down in the body into urate, it may also be helpful to avoid foods high in purine, such as organ meats, sardines, anchovies, red meat, gravies, beans, beer, and wine. A 2004 study revealed that eating more low-fat dairy products could reduce risk of developing gout.

Resources

BOOKS

Konshin, Victor. *Beating Gout: A Sufferer's Guide to Living Pain Free*. Williamsville, NY: Ayerware Publications, 2009.

Parker, James N., M.D., and Philip M. Parker, Ph. D. *The Official Patient's Sourcebook on Gout: A Revised and Updated Directory for the Internet Age*. San Diego, CA: ICON Health Publications, 2005.

PERIODICALS

Arromdee, E., C. J. Michet, C. S. Crowson, et al. "Epidemiology of Gout: Is the Incidence Rising?" *Journal of Rheumatology*29 (November 2002): 2403–2406.

Coghill, Kim. "FDA Panel Discusses Endpoints for Approval of Gout Products." *Bioworld Today* (June 3, 2004).

"Dairy-rich Diet May Help Prevent Gout." *Tufts University Health & Nutrition Letter* (June 2004): 2.

MacReady, Norma. "New Gout Quality-of-care Standards Take Aim at Medication-related Errors." *Internal Medicine News* (June 1, 2004): 18.

OTHER

National Institute of Arthritis and Musculoskeletal and Skin Diseases (NIAMS). *Questions and Answers About Gout*. Bethesda, MD: NIAMS, 2002. NIH Publication No. 02-5027. http://www.niams.nih.gov/hi/topics/gout/gout/htm.

Rebecca Frey, Ph.D
Teresa G. Odle
Laura Jean Cataldo, RN, Ed.D.

Gout drugs

Definition

Gout drugs are medicines that prevent or relieve the symptoms of gout, a disease that affects the joints and kidneys.

Purpose

Gout is a disease in which uric acid, a waste product that normally passes out of the body in urine, collects and forms crystals in the joints and the kidneys. When uric acid crystals build up in the joints, the tissue around the joint becomes inflamed, and nerve endings in the area become irritated, causing extreme **pain**. Uric acid crystals in the kidneys can lead to **kidney stones** and eventually to kidney failure.

The symptoms of gout–severe pain, usually in the hand or foot (often at the base of the big toe), but sometimes in the elbow or knee–should be reported to a health care professional. If not treated, gout can lead to high blood presssure, deformed joints, and even **death** from kidney failure. Fortunately, the condition is easily treated. For patients who have just had their first attack, physicians may prescribe only medicine to reduce the pain and inflammatin, such as **nonsteroidal anti-inflammatory drugs**, **corticosteroids**, or colchicine. Patients may also be advised to change their eating and drinking habits, avoiding organ meats and other protein-rich foods, cutting out alcoholic beverages, and drinking more water. Some people never have another gout attack after the first. For those who do, physicians may prescribe additional drugs that either help the body get rid of uric acid or reduce the amount of uric acid the body produces. These drugs will not relieve gout attacks that already have started, but will help prevent attacks when taken regularly.

Description

Three main types of drugs are used in treating gout. Colchicine helps relieve the symptoms of gout by reducing inflammation. Allopurinol (Lopurin, Zyloprim) reduces the amount of uric acid produced in the body. Probenecid (Benemid, Probalan) and sulfinpyrazone (Anturane) help the body get rid of excess uric acid. Physicians may recommend that patients take more than one type of gout drug at the same time. Some of these medicines may also be prescribed for other medical conditions that are caused by too much uric acid in the body.

Recommended dosage

The recommended dosage depends on the type of gout drug. Check with the physician who prescribed the drug or the pharmacist who filled the prescription for the correct dosage.

Always take gout drugs exactly as directed. Never take larger or more frequent doses than recommended. Patients who are told to take more than one gout drug should carefully follow the physician's directions for taking all medicines.

Gout drugs such as allopurinol, probenecid, and sulfinpyrazone must be taken regularly to prevent gout attacks. The medicine may take some time to begin working, so gout attacks may continuee for awhile after starting to take the drug. Continuing to take the drug is important, even if it does not seem to be working at first.

Colchicine may be taken regularly in low doses to help prevent gout attacks or in high doses for only a few hours at a time to relieve an attack. The chance of serious side effects is greater when this medicine is taken in high doses for short periods.

Precautions

Seeing a physician regularly while taking gout drugs is important. The physician will check to make sure the medicine is working as it should and will watch for unwanted side effects. Blood tests may be ordered to help the physician monitor how well the drug is working.

Drinking alcohol, including beer and wine, may increase the amount of uric acid in the body and may interfere with the effects of gout medicine. People with gout (or other conditions that result from excess uric acid) may need to limit the amount of alcohol they drink or stop drinking alcohol altogether.

Some people feel drowsy or less alert when taking gout drugs. Anyone who takes this type of medicine should not drive, use machines or do anything else that might be dangerous until they have found out how the drugs affect them.

Some gout drugs may change the results of certain medical tests. Before having medical tests, anyone taking this medicine should alert the health care professional in charge.

Older people may be especially sensitive to the effects of colchicine. The drug may also stay in their bodies longer than it does in younger people. Both the increased sensitivity to the drug and the longer time for the drug to leave the body may increase the chance of side effects.

Special conditions

People who have certain medical conditions or who are taking certain other medicines can have problems if they take gout drugs. Before taking these drugs, be sure to let the physician know about any of these conditions:

ALLERGIES. Anyone who has ever had unusual reactions to gout drugs or to medicines used to relieve pain or inflammation should let his or her physician know before taking gout drugs. The physician should also be told about any **allergies** to foods, dyes, preservatives, or other substances.

DIABETES. Some gout drugs may cause false results on certain urine sugar tests, but not on others. Diabetic patients who take gout drugs should check with their physicians to find out if their medicine will affect the results of their urine sugar tests.

PREGNANCY. The effects of taking gout drugs during **pregnancy** are not fully understood. Women who are pregnant or who may become pregnant should check with their physicians before using gout drugs.

BREASTFEEDING. Gout drugs may pass into breast milk. Women who are taking this medicine and want to breastfeed their babies should check with their physicians.

OTHER MEDICAL CONDITIONS. Gout drugs may cause problems for people with certain medical conditions. For example, the risk of severe allergic reactions or other serious side effects is greater when people with these medical conditions take certain gout drugs:

- congestive heart disease
- high blood pressure
- blood disease
- diabetes
- kidney disease or kidney stones
- cancer being treated with drugs or radiation
- stomach or intestinal problems, including stomach ulcer (now or in the past)

Before using gout drugs, people with any of medical problems listed above should make sure their physicians are aware of their conditions.

USE OF CERTAIN MEDICINES. Taking gout drugs with certain other drugs may affect the way the drugs work or may increase the chance of side effects.

Side effects

A skin rash that develops during treatment with gout drugs may be a sign of a serious and possibly life-threatening reaction. If any of these symptoms occur, stop taking the medicine and check with a physician immediately:

- skin rash, itching, or hives
- scaly or peeling skin
- chills, fever, sore throat, nausea and vomiting, yellow skin or eyes, joint pain, muscle aches or pains–especially if these symptoms occur at the same time or shortly after a skin rash

Patients taking colchicine should stop taking it immediately if they have **diarrhea**, stomach pain, **nausea**, or **vomiting**. If these symptoms continue for 3 hours or more after the medicine is stopped, check with a physician.

Other side effects may also need medical attention. If any of the following symptoms occur while taking gout drugs, check with the physician who prescribed the medicine as soon as possible:

- pain in the side or lower back
- painful urination
- blood in the urine

Less serious side effects, such as **headache**, loss of appetite, and joint pain and inflammation usually go away as the body adjusts to the drug and do not need medical treatment.

Other side effects may occur. Anyone who has unusual symptoms while taking gout drugs should get in touch with his or her physician.

INTERACTIONS. Gout drugs may interact with other medicines. When this happens, the effects of one or both of the drugs may change or the risk of side effects may be greater. Anyone who takes gout drugs should let the physician know all other medicines he or she is taking. Among the drugs that may interact with gout drugs are:

- **Aspirin** or other salicylates. These drugs may keep gout drugs from working properly.
- Nonsteroidal anti-inflammatory drugs such as indomethacin (Indocin) and ketoprofen (Orudis). Taking these medicines with probenecid may increase the chance of side effects from the nonsteroidal anti-inflammatory drugs.
- Blood thinners. When taken with blood thinners, such as warfarin (Coumadin), gout drugs may increase the chance of bleeding. A lower blood thinner dose may be necessary.

- Blood viscosity reducing medicines such as pentoxifylline (Trental). Taking this medicine with blood thinners may increase the chance of bleeding.
- Medicine for infections. Probenecid may increase the levels of these medicines in the blood. This may make the other medicine work better, but may also increase the risk of side effects.
- The immunosuppressant drug azathioprine (Imuran), used to prevent organ rejection in transplant patients and to treat **rheumatoid arthritis**. Taking this medicine with allopurinol can increase the risk of side effects from the azathioprine.
- Anticancer drugs such as mercaptopurine (Purinethol), plicamycin (Mithracin), and methotrexate (Rheumatrex). Taking this medicine with gout drugs may increase the risk of side effects from the anticancer drug.
- Antiretroviral drugs such as zidovudine (Retrovir). Probenecid may increase the level of this medicine in the blood. This may make side effects more likely.
- Antiseizure medicines such as Depakote (divalproex) and Depakene (valproic acid). Using these medicines with sulfinpyrazone may increase the chance of bleeding.

The list above does not include every drug that may interact with gout drugs. Be sure to check with a physician or pharmacist before combining gout drugs with any other prescription or nonprescription (over-the-counter) medicine.

Nancy Ross-Flanigan

Gouty arthritis *see* **Gout**

Graft-vs.-host disease

Definition

Graft-vs.-host disease is an immune attack on the recipient by cells from a donor.

Description

The main problem with transplanting organs and tissues is that the recipient host does not recognize the new tissue as its own. Instead, it attacks it as foreign in the same way it attacks germs, to destroy it.

If immunogenic cells from the donor are transplanted along with the organ or tissue, they will attack the host, causing graft vs. host disease.

The only transplanted tissues that house enough immune cells to cause graft vs. host disease are the blood and the bone marrow. Blood transfusions are used every day in hospitals for many reasons. Bone marrow transplants are used to replace blood forming cells and immune cells. This is necessary for patients whose **cancer** treatment has destroyed their own bone marrow. Because bone marrow cells are among the most sensitive to radiation and **chemotherapy**, it often must be destroyed along with the cancer. This is true primarily of leukemias, but some other cancers have also been treated this way.

Causes and symptoms

Even if the donor and recipient are well matched, graft-vs.-host disease can still occur. There are many different elements involved in generating immune reactions, and each person is different, unless they are identical twins. Testing can often find donors who match all the major elements, but there are many minor ones that will always be different. How good a match is found also depends upon the urgency of the need and some good luck.

Blood **transfusion** graft-vs.-host disease affects mostly the blood. Blood cells perform three functions: carrying oxygen, fighting infections, and clotting. All of these cell types are decreased in a transfusion graft-vs.-host reaction, leading to anemia (lack of red blood cells in the blood), a decrease in resistance to infections, and an increase in bleeding. The reaction occurs between four to 30 days after the transfusion.

The tissues most affected by bone marrow graft-vs.-host disease are the skin, the liver, and the intestines. One form or the other occurs in close to half of the patients who receive bone marrow transplants.

Bone marrow graft-vs.-host disease comes in an acute and a chronic form. The acute form appears within two months of the transplant; the chronic form usually appears within three months. The acute disease produces a skin rash, liver abnormalities, and **diarrhea** that can be bloody. The skin rash is primarily a patchy thickening of the skin. Chronic disease can produce a similar skin rash, a tightening or an inflammation of the skin, lesions in the mouth, drying of the eyes and mouth, hair loss, liver damage, lung damage, and **indigestion**. The symptoms are similar to an autoimmune disease called **scleroderma**.

Both forms of graft-vs.-host disease bring with them an increased risk of infections, either because of the process itself or its treatment with cortisone-like drugs and immunosuppressives. Patients can die of liver failure, infection, or other severe disturbances of their system.

KEY TERMS

Anemia—Too few red blood cells, or too little hemoglobin in them.

Immunoglobulin—Chemicals in the blood that defend against infections.

Immunosuppressive—A chemical which suppresses an immune response.

Inflammation—The body's immune reaction to presumed foreign substances like germs. Inflammation is characterized by increased blood supply and activation of defense mechanisms. It produces redness, swelling, heat, and pain.

Lesion—Localized disease or damage.

Scleroderma—Progressive disease of the connective tissue of the skin and internal organs.

Treatment

Both the acute and the chronic disease are treated with cortisone-like drugs, immunosuppressive agents like cyclosporine, or with **antibiotics** and immune chemicals from donated blood (**gamma globulin**). Infection with one particular virus, called cytomegalovirus (CMV) is so likely a complication that some experts recommend treating it ahead of time.

Prognosis

Children with **acute leukemias** have greatly benefited from the treatment made possible by **bone marrow transplantation**. Survival rates have climbed by 15–50%. It is an interesting observation that patients who develop graft-vs.-host disease are less likely to have a recurrence of the leukemia that was being treated. This phenomenon is called graft-vs.-leukemia.

Bone marrow transplant patients who do not have a graft-vs.-host reaction gradually return to normal immune function in a year. A graft-vs.-host reaction may prolong the diminished immune capacity indefinitely, requiring supplemental treatment with immunoglobulins (gamma globulin).

Somehow the grafted cells develop a tolerance to their new home after six to 12 months, and the medications can be gradually withdrawn. Graft-vs.-host disease is not the only complication of blood transfusion or bone marrow transplantation. Host-vs.-graft or rejection is also common and may require a repeat transplant with another donor organ. Infections are a constant threat in bone marrow transplant because of the disease being treated, the prior radiation or chemotherapy and the medications used to treat the transplant.

Prevention

For recipients of blood transfusions who are especially likely to have graft-vs.-host reactions, the red blood cells can safely be irradiated (using x rays) to kill all the immune cells. The red blood cells are less sensitive to radiation and are not harmed by this treatment.

Much current research is directed towards solving the problem of graft-vs.-host disease. There are efforts to remove the immunogenic cells from the donor tissue, and there are also attempts to extract and purify bone marrow cells from the patient before treating the cancer. These cells are then given back to the patient after treatment has destroyed all that were left behind.

Resources

BOOKS

Fauci, Anthony S., et al., eds. *Harrison's Principles of Internal Medicine*. 17th ed. New York: McGraw–Hill Professional, 2008.

J. Ricker Polsdorfer, MD

Grafts and grafting *see* **Bone grafting; Coronary artery bypass graft surgery; Graft-vs.-host disease; Skin grafting**

Granular conjunctivitis *see* **Trachoma**

Granulocytic ehrlichiosis *see* **Ehrlichiosis**

Granulocytopenia *see* **Neutropenia**

Granuloma inguinale

Definition

Granuloma inguinale is a sexually transmitted infection that affects the skin and mucous membranes of the anal and genital areas. Its name is derived from granuloma, a medical term for a mass or growth of granulation tissue, and *inguinale*, a Latin word that means located in the groin. Granulation tissue is tissue formed during wound healing that is rich in blood capillaries and has a rough or lumpy surface.

Description

Granuloma inguinale is a chronic infection with frequent relapses caused by a rod-shaped bacterium. It occurs worldwide but is most common in tropical or

KEY TERMS

Donovan bodies—Rod-shaped oval organisms found in tissue samples from patients with granuloma inguinale. Donovan bodies appear deep purple when stained with Wright's stain.

Granulation tissue—A kind of tissue formed during wound healing, with a rough or irregular surface and a rich supply of blood capillaries.

Granuloma—An inflammatory swelling or growth composed of granulation tissue, as in granuloma inguinale.

Keloid—An unusual or abnormal growth of scar tissue, as in the third stage of granuloma inguinale.

Punch biopsy—A method of obtaining skin samples under local anesthesia using a surgical skin punch.

Superinfection—A condition in which a patient with a contagious disease acquires a second infection, as when a patient with granuloma inguinale is also infected with syphilis.

Wright's stain—A chemical used to stain tissue samples for laboratory analysis.

subtropical countries, where it is associated with poverty and poor hygiene. As many as 20% of male patients with **sexually transmitted diseases** (STDs) in tropical countries have granuloma inguinale. The disease is less common in the United States, with fewer than 100 reported cases per year. Most patients are between the ages of 20 and 40 years, with a 2:1 male-to-female ratio.

Although granuloma inguinale is relatively uncommon in the United States in comparison with other STDs, it is still a significant public health problem. It can be acquired through casual sexual contacts when traveling abroad. Moreover, patients with granuloma inguinale are vulnerable to superinfection (infection by other disease agents) with other STDs, especially **syphilis**. Patients with granuloma inguinale are also a high-risk group for Acquired Immune Deficiency Syndrome (**AIDS**) transmission, because the disease causes open genital ulcers that can be easily invaded by the AIDS virus.

Granuloma inguinale is spread primarily through heterosexual and male homosexual contact; however, its occurrence in children and sexually inactive adults indicates that it may also be spread by contact with human feces. Granuloma inguinale is not highly contagious; however, persons with weakened immune systems are at greater risk of infection.

Causes and symptoms

Granuloma inguinale, which is sometimes called donovanosis, is caused by *Calymmatobacterium granulomatis*, a rod-shaped bacterium formerly called *Donovania granulomatis*. The bacterium has an incubation period ranging from eight days to 12 weeks, with an average of two to four weeks. The disease has a slow and gradual onset, beginning with an inconspicuous pimple or lumpy eruption on the skin. In 90% of patients, the initial sign of infection is in the genital region, but a minority of patients will develop the sore in their mouth or anal area if their sexual contact involved those parts of the body. Many patients do not notice the sore because it is small and not usually painful. In some women, the first symptom of granuloma inguinale is bleeding from the genitals.

The initial pimple or sore is typically followed by three stages of disease. In the first stage, the patient develops a mass of pink or dull red granulation tissue in the area around the anus. In the second stage, the bacteria erode the skin to form shallow, foul-smelling ulcers which spread from the genital and anal areas to the thighs and lower abdomen. The edges of the ulcers are marked by granulation tissue. In the third stage, the ulcerated areas form deep masses of keloid or scar tissue that may spread slowly for many years.

Patients with long-term infections are at risk for serious complications. The ulcers in second-stage granuloma inguinale often become superinfected with syphilis or other STD organisms. Superinfected ulcers become painful to touch, filled with pus and dead tissue, and are much more difficult to treat. There may be sizable areas of tissue destruction in superinfected patients. In addition, the scar tissue produced by third-stage infection can grow until it closes off parts of the patient's urinary tract. It is also associated with a higher risk of genital **cancer**.

Diagnosis

The most important aspect of diagnosis is distinguishing between granuloma inguinale and other STDs, particularly since many patients will be infected with more than one STD. Public health officials recommend that patients tested for granuloma inguinale be given a blood test for syphilis as well. In addition, the doctor will need to distinguish between granuloma inguinale and certain types of skin cancer, **amebiasis**, fungal infections, and other bacterial ulcers. The most significant distinguishing characteristic of granuloma inguinale is the skin ulcer, which is larger than in most other diseases, painless, irregular in shape, and likely to bleed when touched.

The diagnosis of granuloma inguinale is made by finding Donovan bodies in samples of the patient's skin tissue. Donovan bodies are oval rod-shaped organisms that appear inside infected tissue cells under a microscope. The doctor obtains a tissue sample either by cutting a piece of tissue from the edge of an skin ulcer with a scalpel or by taking a punch biopsy. To make a punch biopsy, the doctor will inject a local anesthetic into an ulcerated area and remove a piece of skin about 1/16 of an inch in size with a surgical skin punch. The tissue sample is then air-dried and stained with Wright's stain, a chemical that will cause the Donovan bodies to show up as dark purple safety pin-shaped objects inside lighter-staining capsules.

Treatment

Granuloma inguinale is treated with oral **antibiotics**. Three weeks of treatment with erythromycin, streptomycin, or tetracycline, or 12 weeks of treatment with ampicillin are standard forms of therapy. Although the skin ulcers will start to show signs of healing in about a week, the patient must take the full course of medication to minimize the possibility of relapse.

Prognosis

Most patients with granuloma inguinale recover completely, although superinfected ulcers may require lengthy courses of medication. Early treatment prevents the complications associated with second- and third-stage infection.

Prevention

Prevention of granuloma inguinale has three important aspects:

- Avoidance of casual sexual contacts, particularly among homosexual males, in countries with high rates of the disease
- Tracing and examination of an infected person's recent sexual contacts
- Monitoring the patient's ulcers or scar tissue for signs of reinfection for a period of six months after antibiotic treatment

Resources

BOOKS

McPhee, Stephen, and Maxine Papadakis.*Current Medical Diagnosis and Treatment, 2010*, 49th ed. New York: McGraw–Hill Medical, 2009.

Rebecca J. Frey, PhD

Granulomatous ileitis *see* **Crohn's disease**

Graves' disease *see* **Hyperthyroidism**

Greenfield filter *see* **Vena cava**

Grippe *see* **Influenza**

Group A streptococcus infection *see* **Streptococcal infections**

Group B streptococcus infection *see* **Streptococcal infections**

Group therapy

Definition

Group therapy is a form of psychosocial treatment where a small group of patients meet regularly to talk, interact, and discuss problems with each other and the group leader (therapist).

Purpose

Group therapy attempts to give individuals a safe and comfortable place where they can work out problems and emotional issues. Patients gain insight into their own thoughts and behavior, and offer suggestions and support to others. In addition, patients who have a difficult time with interpersonal relationships can benefit from the social interactions that are a basic part of the group therapy experience.

Precautions

Patients who are suicidal, homicidal, psychotic, or in the midst of a major acute crisis are typically not referred for group therapy until their behavior and emotional state have stabilized. Depending on their level of functioning, cognitively impaired patients (like patients with organic brain disease or a traumatic brain injury) may also be unsuitable for group therapy intervention. Some patients with sociopathic traits are not suitable for most groups.

Description

A psychologist, psychiatrist, social worker, or other healthcare professional typically arranges and conducts group therapy sessions. In some therapy groups, two co-therapists share the responsibility of group leadership. Patients are selected on the basis of what they might gain from group therapy interaction and what they can contribute to the group as a whole.

Therapy groups may be homogeneous or heterogeneous. Homogeneous groups have members with similar diagnostic backgrounds (for example, they may all suffer from depression). Heterogeneous groups have a mix of individuals with different emotional issues. The number of group members varies widely, but is typically no more than 12. Groups may be time limited (with a predetermined number of sessions) or indefinite (where the group determines when therapy ends). Membership may be closed or open to new members once sessions begin.

The number of sessions in group therapy depends on the makeup, goals, and setting of the group. For example, a therapy group that is part of a **substance abuse** program to rehabilitate inpatients would be called short-term group therapy. This term is used because, as patients, the group members will only be in the hospital for a relatively short period of time. Long-term therapy groups may meet for six months, a year, or longer. The therapeutic approach used in therapy depends on the focus of the group and the psychological training of the therapist. Some common techniques include psychodynamic, cognitive-behavioral, and **Gestalt therapy**.

In a group therapy session, group members are encouraged to openly and honestly discuss the issues that brought them to therapy. They try to help other group members by offering their own suggestions, insights, and empathy regarding their problems. There are no definite rules for group therapy, only that members participate to the best of their ability. However, most therapy groups do have some basic ground rules that are usually discussed during the first session. Patients are asked not to share what goes on in therapy sessions with anyone outside of the group. This protects the confidentiality of the other members. They may also be asked not to see other group members socially outside of therapy because of the harmful effect it might have on the dynamics of the group.

The therapist's main task is to guide the group in self-discovery. Depending on the goals of the group and the training and style of the therapist, he or she may lead the group interaction or allow the group to take their own direction. Typically, the group leader does some of both, providing direction when the group gets off track while letting them set their own agenda. The therapist may guide the group by simply reinforcing the positive behaviors they engage in. For example, if a group member shows empathy to another member, or offers a constructive suggestion, the therapist will point this out and explain the value of these actions to the group. In almost all group therapy situations, the therapist will attempt to emphasize the common traits among group members so that members can gain a sense of group identity. Group members realize that others share the same issues they do.

The main benefit group therapy may have over individual **psychotherapy** is that some patients behave and react more like themselves in a group setting than they would one-on-one with a therapist. The group therapy patient gains a certain sense of identity and social acceptance from their membership in the group. Suddenly, they are not alone. They are surrounded by others who have the same anxieties and emotional issues that they have. Seeing how others deal with these issues may give them new solutions to their problems. Feedback from group members also offers them a unique insight into their own behavior, and the group provides a safe forum in which to practice new behaviors. Lastly, by helping others in the group work through their problems, group therapy members can gain more self-esteem. Group therapy may also simulate family experiences of patients and will allow family dynamic issues to emerge.

Self-help groups like Alcoholics Anonymous and Weight Watchers fall outside of the psychotherapy realm. These self-help groups do offer many of the same benefits of social support, identity, and belonging that make group therapy effective for many. Self-help group members meet to discuss a common area of concern (like **alcoholism**, **eating disorders**, **bereavement**, parenting). Group sessions are not run by a therapist, but by a nonprofessional leader, group member, or the group as a whole. Self-help groups are sometimes used in addition to psychotherapy or regular group therapy.

Preparation

Patients are typically referred for group therapy by a psychologist or psychiatrist. Some patients may need individual therapy first. Before group sessions begin, the therapist leading the session may conduct a short intake interview with the patient to determine if the group is right for the patient. This interview will also allow the therapist to determine if the addition of the patient will benefit the group. The patient may be

KEY TERMS

Cognitive-behavioral—A therapy technique that focuses on changing beliefs, images, and thoughts in order to change maladjusted behaviors.

Gestalt—A humanistic therapy technique that focuses on gaining an awareness of emotions and behaviors in the present rather than in the past.

Psychodynamic—A therapy technique that assumes improper or unwanted behavior is caused by unconscious, internal conflicts and focuses on gaining insight into these motivations.

given some preliminary information on the group before sessions begin. This may include guidelines for success (like being open, listening to others, taking risks), rules of the group (like maintaining confidentiality), and educational information on what group therapy is about.

Aftercare

The end of long-term group therapy may cause feelings of grief, loss, abandonment, anger, or rejection in some members. The group therapist will attempt to foster a sense of closure by encouraging members to explore their feelings and use newly acquired coping techniques to deal with them. Working through this termination phase of group therapy is an important part of the treatment process.

Risks

Some very fragile patients may not be able to tolerate aggressive or hostile comments from group members. Patients who have trouble communicating in group situations may be at risk for dropping out of group therapy. If no one comments on their silence or makes an attempt to interact with them, they may begin to feel even more isolated and alone instead of identifying with the group. Therefore, the therapist usually attempts to encourage silent members to participate early on in treatment.

Normal results

Studies have shown that both group and individual psychotherapy benefit about 85% of the patients that participate in them. Optimally, patients gain a better understanding of themselves, and perhaps a stronger set of interpersonal and coping skills through the group therapy process. Some patients may continue therapy after group therapy ends, either individually or in another group setting.

Resources

BOOKS

Bieling, Peter J., Randi E. McCabe, and Martin M. Antony. *Cognitive-Behavioral Therapy in Groups*. New York: Guilford Press, 2006.

Yalom, Irvin D., and Molyn Leszcz. *Theory and Practice of Group Psychotherapy*, 5th ed. New York: Basic Books, 2005.

ORGANIZATIONS

American Psychiatric Association, 1000 Wilson Boulevard, Suite 1825, Arlington, VA, 22209-3901, (703) 907-7300, apa@psych.org, http://www.psych.org.

American Psychological Association (APA), 750 First Street NE, Washington, DC, 20002-4242, (202) 336-5500, (800) 374-2721, http://www.apa.org.

Paula Anne Ford-Martin
brenda w. lerner

Growth hormone suppression test *see* **Growth hormone tests**

Growth hormone tests

Definition

Growth hormone (hGH), or somatotropin, is a hormone responsible for normal body growth and development by stimulating protein production in muscle cells and energy release from the breakdown of fats. Tests for growth hormone include Somatotropin hormone test, Somatomedin C, Growth hormone suppression test (glucose loading test), and Growth hormone stimulation test (Arginine test or Insulin tolerance test).

Purpose

Growth hormone tests are ordered for the following reasons:

- to identify growth deficiencies, including delayed puberty and small stature in adolescents that result from pituitary or thyroid malfunction
- to aid in the diagnosis of hyperpituitarism that is evident in gigantism or acromegaly
- to screen for inadequate or reduced pituitary gland function

- to assist in the diagnosis of pituitary tumors or tumors related to the hypothalamus, an area of the brain
- to evaluate hGH therapy

Precautions

Taking certain drugs such as amphetamines, dopamine, **corticosteroids**, and phenothiazines may increase and decrease growth hormone secretion, respectively. Other factors influencing hGH secretion include **stress**, **exercise**, diet, and abnormal glucose levels. These tests should not be done within a week of any radioactive scan.

Description

Several hormones play important roles in human growth. The major human growth hormone (hGH), or somatotropin, is a protein made up of 191 amino acids that is secreted by the anterior pituitary gland and coordinates normal growth and development. Human growth is characterized by two spurts, one at birth and the other at **puberty**. hGH plays an important role at both of these times. Normal individuals have measurable levels of hGH throughout life. Yet levels of hGH fluctuate during the day and are affected by eating and exercise. Receptors that respond to hGH exist on cells and tissues throughout the body. The most obvious effect of hGH is on linear skeletal development. But the metabolic effects of hGH on muscle, the liver, and fat cells are critical to its function. Surprisingly, a 2004 study reported that obese people have lower-than-normal levels of human growth hormone in their bodies. Humans have two forms of hGH, and the functional difference between the two is unclear. They are both formed from the same gene, but one lacks the amino acids in positions 32–46.

GH is produced in the anterior portion of the pituitary gland by somatotrophs under the control of hormonal signals in the hypothalamus. Two hypothalamic hormones regulate hGH; they are growth hormone-releasing hormone (GHRH) and growth hormone—inhibiting hormone (GHIH). When blood glucose levels fall, GHRH triggers the secretion of stored hGH. As blood glucose levels rise, GHRH release is turned off. Increases in blood protein levels trigger a similar response. As a result of this hypothalamic feedback loop, hGH levels fluctuate throughout the day. Normal plasma hGH levels average 1–3 ng/ML with peaks as high as 60 ng/ML. In addition, plasma glucose and amino acid availability for growth is also regulated by the hormones adrenaline, glucagon, and insulin.

Most hGH is released at night. Peak spikes of hGH release occur around 10 p.m., midnight, and 2 a.m. The logic behind this night-time release is that most of hGH's effects are controlled by other hormones, including the somatomedins, IGH-I and IGH-II. As a result, the effects of hGH are spread out more evenly during the day.

A number of hormonal conditions can lead to excessive or diminished growth. Because of its critical role in producing hGH and other hormones, an abnormal pituitary gland will often yield altered growth. Dwarfism (very small stature) can be due to underproduction of hGH, lack of IGH-I, or a flaw in target tissue response to either of these growth hormones. Overproduction of hGH or IGH-I, or an exaggerated response to these hormones can lead to **gigantism** or acromegaly, both of which are characterized by a very large stature.

Gigantism is the result of hGH overproduction in early childhood leading to a skeletal height up to 8 feet (2.5m) or more. Acromegaly results when hGH is overproduced after the onset of puberty. In this condition, the epiphyseal plates of the long bone of the body do not close, and they remain responsive to additional stimulated growth by hGH. This disorder is characterized by an enlarged skull, hands and feet, nose, neck, and tongue.

Somatotropin

Somatotropin is used to identify hGH deficiency in adolescents with short stature, delayed sexual maturity, and other growth deficiencies. It also aids in documenting excess hGH production that is responsible for gigantism or acromegaly, and confirms underactivity or overproduction of the pituitary gland (**hypopituitarism** or hyperpituitarism). However, due to the episodic secretion of hGH, as well as hGH production in response to stress, exercise, or other factors, random assays are not an adequate determination of hGH deficiency. To negate these variables and obtain more accurate readings, a blood sample can be drawn one to 1.5 hours after sleep (hGH levels increase during sleep), or strenuous exercise can be performed for 30 minutes before blood is drawn (hGH levels increase after exercise). The hGH levels at the end of an exercise period are expected to be maximal.

Somatomedin C

The somatomedin C test is usually ordered to detect pituitary abnormalities, hGH deficiency, and acromegaly. Also called insulin-like growth factor (IGF-1), somatomedin C is considered a more accurate reflection of the blood concentration of hGH because such variables as time of day, activity levels, or diet do not influence the results. Somatomedin C is part of a group of peptides, called somatomedins, through which hGH exerts its effects. Because it circulates in the bloodstream bound to long-lasting proteins, it is more stable than hGH. Levels of somatomedin C depend on hGH levels, however. As a result, somatomedin C levels are low when hGH levels are deficient. Abnormally low test results of somatomedin C require an abnormally reduced or absent hGH during an hGH stimulation test in order to diagnose hGH deficiency. Nonpituitary causes of reduced somatomedin C include **malnutrition**, severe chronic illness, severe **liver disease**, **hypothyroidism**, and Laron's dwarfism.

Growth hormone stimulation test

The hGH stimulation test, also called hGH Provocation test, Insulin Tolerance, or Arginine test, is performed to test the body's ability to produce human growth hormone, and to identify suspected hGH deficiency. A normal patient can have low hGH levels, but if hGH is still low after stimulation, a diagnosis can be more accurately made.

Insulin-induced **hypoglycemia** (via intravenous injection of insulin) stimulates hGH and corticotropin secretion as well. If such stimulation is unsuccessful, then there is a malfunction of the anterior pituitary gland. Blood samples may be obtained following an energetic exercise session lasting 20 minutes.

A substance called hGH-releasing factor has recently been used for hGH stimulation. This approach promises to be more accurate and specific for hGH deficiency caused by the pituitary. Growth hormone deficiency is also suspected when x-ray determination of bone age indicates retarded growth in comparison to chronologic age. At present, the best method to identify hGH-deficient patients is a positive stimulation test followed by a positive response to a therapeutic trial of hGH.

Growth hormone suppression test

Also called the glucose loading test, this procedure is used to evaluate excessive baseline levels of human growth hormone, and to confirm diagnosis of gigantism in children and acromegaly in adults. The procedure requires two different blood samples, one drawn before the administration of 100 g of glucose (by mouth), and a second sample two hours after glucose ingestion.

Normally, a glucose load suppresses hGH secretion. In a patient with excessive hGH levels, failure of suppression indicates anterior pituitary dysfunction and confirms a diagnosis of **acromegaly and gigantism**.

Preparation

Somatotropin: This test requires a blood sample. The patient should be **fasting** (nothing to eat or drink from midnight the night before the test). Stress and/or exercise increases hGH levels, so the patient should be at complete rest for 30 minutes before the blood sample is drawn. If the physician has requested two samples, they should be drawn on consecutive days at approximately the same time on both days, preferably between 6 a.m. and 8 a.m.

Somatomedin C: This test requires a blood sample. The patient should have nothing to eat or drink from midnight the night before the test.

Growth hormone stimulation: This test requires intravenous administration of medications and the withdrawal of frequent blood samples, which are obtained at 0, 60, and 90 minutes after injection of arginine and/or insulin. The patient should have nothing to eat or drink after midnight the night before the test.

Growth hormone suppression: This test requires two blood samples, one before the test and another two hours after administration of 100 g of glucose solution by mouth. The patient should have nothing to eat or drink after midnight, and physical activity should be limited for 10–12 hours before the test.

Risks

Growth hormone stimulation: Only minor discomfort is associated with this test, and results from the insertion of the IV line and the low blood sugar (hypoglycemia) induced by the insulin injection. Some patients may experience sleepiness, sweating and/or nervousness, all of which can be corrected after the test by ingestion of cookies, juice, or a glucose infusion. Severe cases of hypoglycemia may cause ketosis (excessive amounts of fatty acid byproducts in the body), acidosis (a disturbance of the body's acid-base balance), or **shock**. With the close observation required for the test, these are unlikely.

Growth hormone suppression: Some patients experience **nausea** after the administration of this amount of glucose. Ice chips can alleviate this symptom.

Normal results

Normal results may vary from laboratory to laboratory but are usually within the following ranges:

KEY TERMS

Acromegaly—A rare disease resulting from excessive growth hormone caused by a benign tumor. If such a tumor develops within the first 10 years of life, the result is gigantism (in which growth is accelerated) and not acromegaly. Symptoms include coarsening of the facial features, enlargement of the hands, feet, ears, and nose, jutting of the jaw, and a long face.

Dwarfism, pituitary—Short stature. When caused by inadequate amounts of growth hormone (as opposed to late growth spurt or genetics), hGH deficiency results in abnormally slow growth and short stature with normal proportions.

Gigantism—Excessive growth, especially in height, resulting from overproduction during childhood or adolescence of growth hormone by a pituitary tumor. Untreated, the tumor eventually destroys the pituitary gland, resulting in death during early adulthood. If the tumor develops after growth has stopped, the result is acromegaly, not gigantism.

Pituitary gland—The pituitary is the most important of the endocrine glands (glands that release hormones directly into the bloodstream). Sometimes referred to as the "master gland," the pituitary regulates and controls the activities of other endocrine glands and many body processes.

Somatotropin:

- men: 5 ng/mL
- women: less than 10 ng/mL
- children: 0–10 ng/mL
- newborn: 10–40 ng/mL

Somatomedin C:

- adult: 42–110 ng/mL
- Child:
- 0–8 years: Girls 7–110 ng/ml; Boys 4–87 ng/mL
- 9–10 years: Girls 39–186 ng/ml; Boys 26–98 ng/mL
- 11–13 years: Girls 66–215 ng/ml; Boys 44–207 ng/mL
- 14–16 years: Girls 96–256 ng/ml; Boys 48 255 ng/mL

Growth hormone stimulation: greater than 10 ng/mL.

Growth hormone suppression: Normally, glucose suppresses hGH to levels of undetectable to 3 ng/mL in 30 minutes to two hours. In children, rebound stimulation may occur after two to five hours.

Abnormal results

Somatotropin hormone: Excess hGH is responsible for the syndromes of gigantism and acromegaly. Excess secretion is stimulated by **anorexia nervosa**, stress, hypoglycemia, and exercise. Decreased levels are seen in hGH deficiency, dwarfism, hyperglycemia, **failure to thrive**, and delayed sexual maturity.

Somatomedin C: Increased levels contribute to the syndromes of gigantism and acromegaly. Stress, major surgery, hypoglycemia, **starvation**, and exercise stimulate hGH secretion, which in turn stimulates somatomedin C.

Growth hormone stimulation: Decreased levels are seen in pituitary deficiency and hGH deficiency. Diseases of the pituitary can result in failure of the pituitary to secrete hGH and/or all the pituitary hormones. As a result, the hGH stimulation test will fail to stimulate hGH secretion.

Growth hormone suppression: The acromegaly syndrome elevates base hGH levels to 75 ng/mL, which in turn are not suppressed to less than 5 ng/mL during the test. Excess hGH secretion may cause unchanged or rising hGH levels in response to glucose loading, confirming a diagnosis of acromegaly or gigantism. In such cases, verification of results is required by repeating the test after a one-day rest.

Resources

PERIODICALS

"Weight-loss Hormone." *Better Nutrition* (May 2004): 32.

Janis O. Flores
Teresa G. Odle

Guaifenesin *see* **Expectorants**

Guided imagery

Definition

Guided imagery is the use of relaxation and mental visualization to improve mood and/or physical well-being.

Purpose

The connection between the mind and physical health has been well documented and extensively studied. Positive mental imagery can promote relaxation and reduce **stress**, improve mood, control high blood pressure, alleviate **pain**, boost the immune system, and lower cholesterol and blood sugar levels. Through guided imagery techniques, patients can learn to control functions normally controlled by the autonomic nervous system, such as heart rate, blood pressure, respiratory rate, and body temperature.

One of the biggest benefits of using guided imagery as a therapeutic tool is its availability. Imagery can be used virtually anywhere, anytime. It is also an equal opportunity therapy. Although some initial training in the technique may be required, guided imagery is accessible to virtually everyone regardless of economic status, education, or geographical location.

Guided imagery also gives individuals a sense of empowerment, or control. The technique is induced by a therapist who guides the patient. The resulting mental imagery used is solely a product of the individual's imagination. Some individuals have difficulty imagining. They may not get actual clear images but perhaps vague feelings about the guided journey. However these individuals' brains and nervous systems responses seem to be the same as those with more detailed imaginings.

Patients who feel uncomfortable "opening up" in a traditional therapist-patient session may feel more at ease with a self-directed therapy like guided imagery.

Description

Guided imagery is simply the use of one's imagination to promote mental and physical health. It can be self-directed, where the individual puts himself into a relaxed state and creates his own images, or directed by others. When directed by others, an individual listens to a therapist, video, or audiotaped exercise that leads him through a relaxation and imagery exercise. Some therapists also use guided imagery in group settings.

Guided imagery is a two-part process. The first component involves reaching a state of deep relaxation through breathing and muscle relaxation techniques. During the relaxation phase, the person closes her eyes and focuses on the slow, in and out sensation of breathing. Or, she might focus on releasing the feelings of tension from her muscles, starting with the toes and working up to the top of the head. Relaxation tapes often feature soft music or tranquil, natural sounds such as rolling waves and chirping birds in order to promote feelings of relaxation.

Once complete relaxation is achieved, the second component of the exercise is the imagery, or visualization, itself. There are a number of different types of guided imagery techniques, limited only by the imagination. Some commonly used types include relaxation imagery, healing imagery, pain control imagery, and mental rehearsal.

Relaxation imagery

Relaxation imagery involves conjuring up pleasant, relaxing images that rest the mind and body. These may be experiences that have already happened, or new situations.

Healing imagery

Patients coping with diseases and injuries can imagine **cancer** cells dying, **wounds** healing, and the body mending itself. Or, patients may picture themselves healthy, happy, and symptom-free. Another healing imagery technique is based on the idea of *qi*, or energy flow, an idea borrowed from **traditional Chinese medicine**. Chinese medicine practitioners believe that illness is the result of a blockage or slowing of energy flow in the body. Individuals may use guided imagery to imagine energy moving freely throughout the body as a metaphor for good health.

Pain control imagery

Individuals can control pain through several imagery techniques. One method is to produce a mental image of the pain and then transform that image into something less frightening and more manageable. Another is to imagine the pain disappearing, and the patient as completely pain-free. Or, one may imagine the pain as something over which he has complete control. For example, patients with back problems may imagine their pain as a high voltage electric current surging through their spine. As they use guided imagery techniques, they can picture themselves reaching for an electrical switch and turning down the power on the current to alleviate the pain.

Mental rehearsal

Mental rehearsal involves imagining a situation or scenario and its ideal outcome. It can be used to reduce **anxiety** about an upcoming situation, such as labor and delivery, surgery, or even a critical life event such as an important competition or a job interview. Individuals picture themselves going through each step of the anxiety-producing event and then successfully completing it.

KEY TERMS

Aromatherapy—The therapeutic use of plant-derived, aromatic essential oils to promote physical and psychological well-being.

Autonomic nervous system—The part of the nervous system that controls so-called involuntary functions such as heart rate, salivary gland secretion, respiratory function, and pupil dilation.

Preparations

For a successful guided imagery session, individuals should select a quiet, relaxing location where there is a comfortable place to sit or recline. If the guided imagery session is to be prompted with an audiotape or videotape, a stereo, VCR, or portable tape player should be available. Some people find that quiet background music improves their imagery sessions.

The session, which can last anywhere from a few minutes to an hour, should be uninterrupted. Taking the phone off the hook and asking family members for solitude can ensure a more successful and relaxing session.

Imagery combined with other relaxation techniques such as **yoga**, massage, or **aromatherapy** can greatly enhance the effects of these therapies. It can be done virtually anywhere.

Precautions

Because of the state of extreme relaxation involved in guided imagery, individuals should never attempt to use guided imagery while driving or operating heavy machinery.

Side effects

Guided imagery can induce sleepiness, and some individuals may fall asleep during a session. Other than this, there are no known adverse side effects to guided imagery.

Research and general acceptance

Use of guided imagery is a widely accepted practice among mental healthcare providers and is gaining acceptance as a powerful pain control tool across a number of medical disciplines. Results of a study conducted at The Cleveland Clinic Foundation and published in 1999 found that cardiac surgery patients who used a guided imagery tape prior to surgery experienced less pain and anxiety. These patients also left the hospital earlier following surgery than patients who used pain medication only.

Another study conducted by Harvard Medical School researchers found that for more than 200 patients undergoing invasive vascular or renal surgery, guided imagery controlled pain and anxiety more effectively than medication alone.

Resources

BOOKS

Hall, Eric, et al. *Guided Imagery: Creative Interventions in Counselling & Psychotherapy*. London; Thousand Oaks, CA: SAGE, 2006.

OTHER

Brennan, Patricia. "Stress First Aid Kit." (Guided imagery audiotape set.) Available from Inside Out Publishing at (888) 727-3296 or http://www.facingthedawn.com.

ORGANIZATIONS

The Academy for Guided Imagery, 30765 Pacific Coast Highway, Suite 359, Malibu, CA, 90265, (800) 727-2070, (800) 726-2070, info@acadgi.com, http://www.academyforguidedimagery.com.

Paula Anne Ford-Martin

Guillain-Barré syndrome

Definition

Guillain-Barré syndrome (GBS), also called acute idiopathic polyneuritis, acute inflammatory polyneuropathy, infectious polyneuritis, and Landry-Guillain-Barré syndrome, causes progressive muscle weakness and **paralysis**, which develops over days or up to four weeks and lasts several weeks to several months.

Demographics

Guillain-Barré syndrome is found worldwide in all races. It is a rare disorder. In the United States, there are about 3 cases per 100,000 population. Risk increases with age, with infant at least risk, young adults accounting for about 1.5 cases per 100,000 population, and people over age 70 for 8.6 cases per 100,000 population.

Description

Guillain-Barré syndrome is a disorder characterized by progressive symmetrical paralysis and loss of reflexes, usually beginning in the legs. The paralysis characteristically involves more than one limb, is

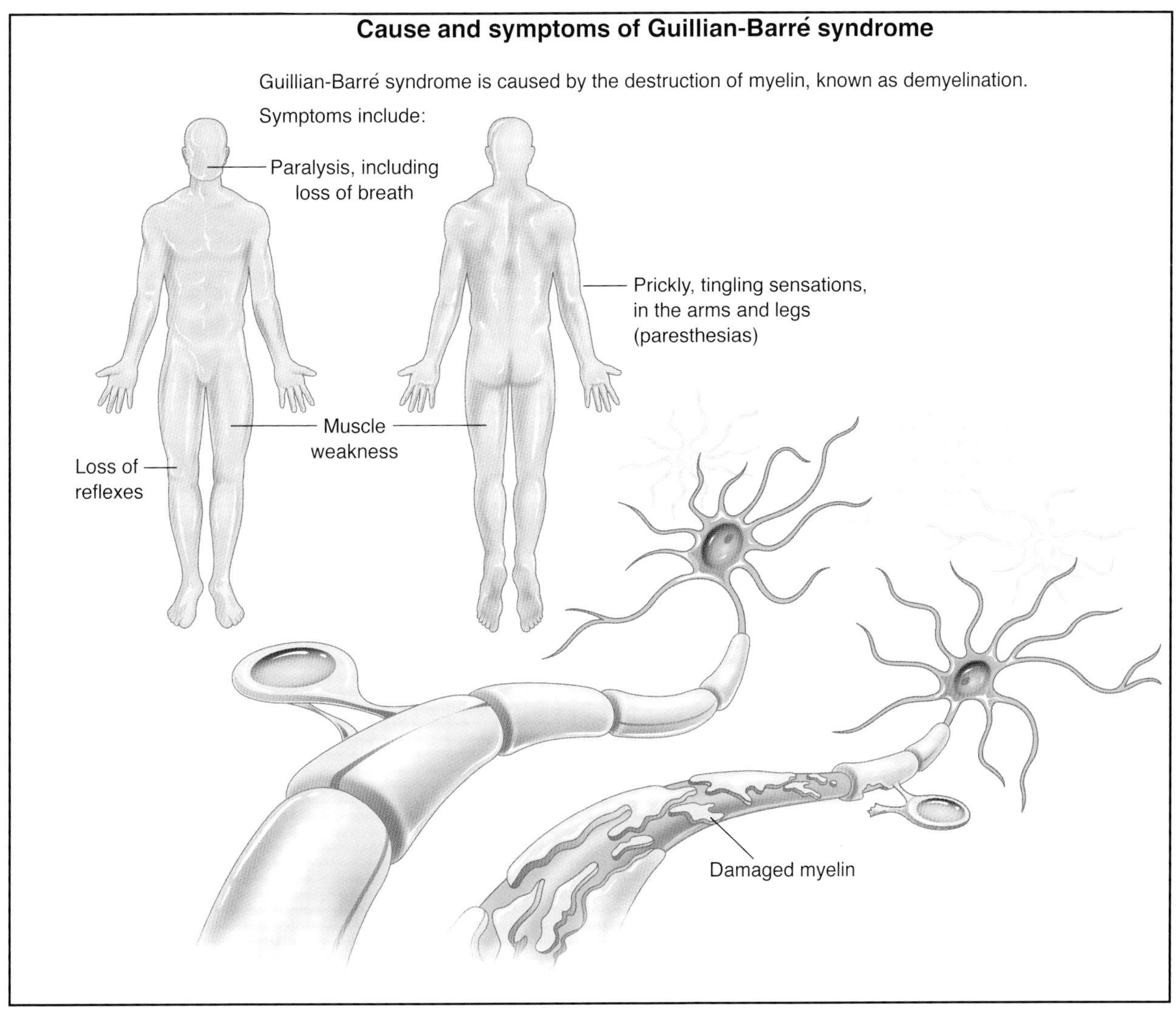

(Illustration by Electronic Illustrators Group. Reproduced by permission of Gale, a part of Cengage Learning.)

progressive, and usually proceeds from the end of an extremity toward the torso. The classic scenario in GBS involves a patient who has just recovered from a typical, seemingly uncomplicated viral infection. Symptoms of muscle weakness appear one to four weeks later. The most common preceding infections are cytomegalovirus, herpes, **Epstein-Barr virus**, and viral hepatitis. A gastrointestinal infection with the bacteria *Campylobacter jejuni* is also common and may cause a severe type of GBS from which it is particularly difficult to recover. About 5% of GBS patients have a surgical procedure as a preceding event. GBS appears to be an autoimmune disorder, apparently caused by a misdirected immune response that results in the direct destruction of the myelin sheath surrounding the peripheral nerves or of the axon of the nerve itself.

Patients with lymphoma, **systemic lupus erythematosus**, or **AIDS** have a higher than normal risk of GBS. Other GBS patients have recently received an immunization, while still others have no known preceding event. In 1976–77, there was a vastly increased number of GBS cases among people who had been recently vaccinated against the Swine flu. The reason for this phenomenon has never been identified, and no other flu vaccine has caused such an increase in GBS cases.

Causes and symptoms

The cause of the weakness and paralysis of GBS is the loss of myelin, which is the material that coats nerve cells. (The loss of myelin is called demyelination.) Myelin is an insulating substance that is wrapped around all nerves in the body. Its function is to speed conduction

KEY TERMS

Autoimmune disorder—A disorder in which the body's immune system produces antibodies that attack its own healthy tissues or blood components.

Demyelination—Disruption or destruction of the myelin sheath, leaving a bare nerve. Results in a slowing or stopping of impulses traveling along that nerve.

Idiopathic—Of unknown origin; without a known cause.

Inflammation—The body's response to tissue damage. Includes warmth, swelling, redness, and pain in the affected part.

Myelin—The substance that is wrapped around nerves. Myelin is responsible for speed and efficiency of impulses traveling through those nerves. When the myelin sheath is damaged, nerve communication is disrupted.

Peripheral nervous system—Nerves that are not part of the brain of spinal cord.

Systemic lupus erythematosus (SLE)—A chronic, inflammatory, autoimmune disorder in which the individual's immune system attacks, injures, and destroys the body's own organs and tissues. It may affect many organ systems including the skin, joints, lungs, heart, and kidneys.

of nerve impulses. Without myelin, nerve conduction slows or stops. GBS has a short, severe course. It causes inflammation and destruction of the myelin sheath, and it disturbs multiple nerves. Therefore, it is considered an acute inflammatory demyelinating polyneuropathy.

The reason for the destruction of myelin in GBS is not completely understood, although it is thought that the underlying problem is autoimmune in nature and is triggered in most cases by infection. An autoimmune disorder is one in which the body's immune system, trained to fight against such foreign invaders as viruses and bacteria, somehow becomes improperly programmed. The immune system becomes confused and is not able to distinguish between foreign invaders and the body itself. Elements of the immune system are unleashed against areas of the body, resulting in damage and destruction. For some reason, in the case of GBS, the myelin sheath appears to become a target for the body's own immune system.

The first symptoms of GBS consist of muscle weakness (legs first, then arms, then face), accompanied by prickly, **tingling** sensations (paresthesias). Symptoms affect both sides of the body simultaneously, a characteristic that helps distinguish GBS from other causes of weakness and paresthesias. Normal reflexes are first diminished, then lost. The weakness eventually affects all the voluntary muscles, resulting in paralysis. When those muscles necessary for breathing become paralyzed, the patient must be placed on a mechanical ventilator, which takes over the function of breathing. This occurs about 30% of the time. Very severely ill GBS patients may have complications stemming from other nervous system abnormalities that can result in problems with fluid balance in the body, severely fluctuating blood pressure, and heart rhythm irregularities.

Diagnosis

Diagnosis of GBS is made by looking for a particular cluster of symptoms (progressively worse muscle weakness and then paralysis), and by analyzing the cerebrospinal fluid (CSF) that bathes the brain and spinal canal. This fluid is obtained by a **lumbar puncture**, which consists of inserting a needle into the lower back (lumbar region) and withdrawing a small amount of CSF. When examined in a laboratory, the CSF of a person with GBS will reveal a greater-than-normal quantity of protein, normal numbers of white blood cells, and a normal amount of sugar. Electrodiagnostic studies may show slowing or block of conduction in nerve endings in parts of the body other than the brain. Minor abnormalities will be present in 90% of patients.

Treatment

There is no direct treatment for GBS. Instead, treatments are used that support the patient with the disabilities caused by the disease. The progress of paralysis must be carefully monitored, in order to provide mechanical assistance for breathing if it becomes necessary. Careful attention must also be paid to the amount of fluid the patient is taking in by drinking and eliminating by urinating. Blood pressure, heart rate, and heart rhythm also must be monitored.

A procedure called **plasmapheresis**, performed early in the course of GBS, has been shown to shorten the course and severity of GBS. Plasmapheresis consists of withdrawing the patient's blood, passing it through an instrument that separates the different types of blood cells, and returning all the cellular components (red and white blood cells and platelets) along with either donor plasma or a manufactured replacement solution. This is thought to rid the blood of the substances that are attacking the patient's myelin.

It has also been shown that the use of high doses of immunoglobulin given intravenously (by drip through a needle in a vein) may be just as helpful as plasmapheresis. Immunoglobulin is a substance naturally manufactured by the body's immune system in response to various threats. It is interesting to note that corticosteroid drugs (such as prednisone), often the mainstay of anti-autoimmune disease treatment, are not only unhelpful, but may in fact be harmful to patients with GBS.

Physical therapy and **occupational therapy** may be used to help restore function as the patient begins to recover.

Prognosis

About 85% of GBS patients make reasonably good recoveries. However, 30% of adult patients, and a greater percentage of children, never fully regain their previous level of muscle strength. Some of these patients suffer from residual weakness, others from permanent paralysis. About 10% of GBS patients begin to improve, then experience a relapse; these patients suffer chronic GBS symptoms. Between 2% and 12% of all GBS patients die from complications of the disorder, with patients over age 60 most at risk for **death**. Cause of death most often is either from cardiac rhythm disturbances or from ventilator-related complications such as **pneumonia**.

Patients with certain characteristics tend to have a worse outcome. These include people of older age, those who required breathing support with a mechanical ventilator, and those who had their worst symptoms within the first seven days.

Prevention

Because so little is known about what causes GBS to develop, there are no known methods of prevention.

Resources

BOOKS

Parry, Gareth J. and Joel S. Steinberg. *Guillain-Barré Syndrome: From Diagnosis to Recovery*. Saint Paul, MN: AAN Press, 2007.

OTHER

Guillain-Barré Syndrome. MedlinePlus. February 4, 2010. http://www.nlm.nih.gov/medlineplus/guillainbarresyndrome.html

Guillain-Barré Syndrome. Mayo Foundation for Medical Research and Education. May 30, 2009. http://www.mayoclinic.com/print/guillain-barre-syndrome/DS00413

LoGuidice, Michael A. and Mark Persin. Guillain-Barré Syndrome. eMedicineHealth August 10, 2005. /www.emedicinehealth.com/guillain-barre_syndrome/article_em.htm

ORGANIZATIONS

American Autoimmune Diseases Association, 22100 Gratiot Avenue, East Detroit, MI, 48021, (586) 776-3900, (800) 598-4668, (586) 776-3903, http://www.aarda.org.

GBS/CIDP Foundation International, 04 1/2 Forrest Avenue, NarberthPA, USA, 19079, (610) 667-0131, (866) 224-3301, (610) 667-7036, http://gbs-cidp.org.

National Institute of Neurological Disorders and Stroke (NINDS), P.O. Box 5801, Bethesda, MD, 20828, (301) 496-5751. TTY: (301) 468-5981, (800) 352-9424, http://www.ninds.nih.gov.

Rosalyn Carson-DeWitt, MD
Tish Davidson, AM

Guinea worm infection

Definition

Infection occurs when the parasitic guinea worm resides within the body. Infection is not apparent until a pregnant female worm prepares to expel embryos. The infection is rarely fatal, but the latter stage is painful. The infection is also referred to as dracunculiasis, and less commonly as dracontiasis.

Description

Before the early 1980s, guinea worms infected 10–15 million people annually in central Africa and parts of Asia. By 1996, worldwide incidence of infection fell to fewer than 153,000 cases per year. Complete eradication of guinea worm infection is a goal of international water safety programs.

To survive, guinea worms require three things: water during the embryo stage, an intermediate host during early maturation, and a human host during adulthood. In bodies of water, such as ponds, guinea worm embryos are eaten by tiny, lobster-like water fleas. Once ingested, the embryos mature into larvae.

Humans become hosts by consuming water containing infected water fleas. Once in the human intestine, larvae burrow into surrounding tissue. After three to

KEY TERMS

Guinea worm embryo—The guinea worm at its earliest life stage prior to or shortly after being expelled from an adult female worm.

Guinea worm larvae—The guinea worm during its middle life stage as it matures within a water flea. The larvae can only grow to adulthood within a human host.

Host—With regard to guinea worm infection, either the water flea or human from which the worm gets nourishment and shelter as it matures.

Secondary infection—An illness–typically caused by bacteria–that follows from a guinea worm infection.

four, the worms mate. Males die soon after, but pregnant females continue to grow. As adults, each thread-like worm can be three feet long and harbor three million embryos. More than one guinea worm can infect a person at the same time.

About eight months later, the female prepares to expel mature embryos by migrating toward the skin surface. Until this point, most people are unaware that they are infected. Extreme **pain** occurs as the worm emerges from under the skin, often around the infected person's ankle. The pain is temporarily relieved by immersing the area in water, an act that contaminates the water and starts the cycle again.

Causes and symptoms

Dracunculus medinensis, or guinea worm, causes infection. Symptoms are commonly absent until a pregnant worm prepares to expel embryos. By secreting an irritating chemical, the worm causes a blister to form on the skin surface. This chemical also causes **nausea**, **vomiting**, **dizziness**, and **diarrhea**. The blister is accompanied by a burning, stabbing pain and can form anywhere on the body; but, the usual site is the lower leg or foot. Once the blister breaks, an open sore remains until the worm has expelled all the embryos.

Diagnosis

Guinea worm infection is identified by the symptoms.

Treatment

Most people infected with guinea worm rely on traditional medicine. The worm is extracted by gently and gradually pulling the worm out and winding it around a small strip of wood. Surgical removal is possible, but rarely done in rural areas. Extraction is complemented by herbs and oils to treat the wound site. Such treatment can ease extraction and may help prevent secondary infections.

Modern medicine offers safe surgical removal of the guinea worm, and drug therapy can prevent infection and pain. Using drugs to combat the worms has had mixed results.

Prognosis

If the worm is completely removed, the wound heals in approximately two to four weeks. However, if a worm emerges from a sensitive area, such as the sole of a foot, or if several worms are involved, healing requires more time. Recovery is also complicated if the worm breaks during extraction. Serious secondary infections frequently occur in such situations. There is the risk of permanent disability in some cases, and having one guinea worm infection does not confer immunity against future infections.

Prevention

Guinea worm infection is prevented by disrupting transmission. Wells and other protected water sources are usually safe from being contaminated with worm embryos. In open water sources, poisons may be used to kill water fleas. Otherwise, water must be boiled or filtered.

Resources

OTHER

Centers for Disease Control & Prevention, Center for Global Health. July 7, 2009 (accessed November 2010). http://www.dpd.cdc.gov/dpdx/HTML/Dracunculiasis.htm

Julia Barrett

Gulf War syndrome

Definition

Gulf War syndrome describes a wide spectrum of illnesses and symptoms ranging from **asthma** to **sexual dysfunction** that have been reported by U.S. and U.S. allied soldiers who served in the Persian Gulf War in 1990–1991.

Description

Between 1994 and 1999, 145 federally funded research studies on Gulf War-related illnesses were undertaken at a cost of over $133 million. Despite this investment and the data collected from over 100,000 veterans who have registered with the Department of Defense (DOD) and/or Veterans Administration (VA) as having Gulf War-related illnesses, there is still much debate over the origin and nature of Gulf War syndrome. A 2006 study for the U.S. Department of Veterans Affairs concluded Gulf War Syndrome does not constitute a single illness and as of 2007, the DOD has failed to establish a definite cause for the disorder. Veterans who have the illness experience a wide range of debilitating symptoms that elude a single diagnosis. Common symptoms include **fatigue**, trouble breathing, headaches, disturbed sleep, **memory loss**, and lack of concentration. Similar experiences among Gulf War veterans have been reported in the United Kingdom and Canada.

Causes and symptoms

There is much current debate over a possible causative agent for Gulf War syndrome other than the **stress** of warfare. Intensive efforts by the Veterans Administration and other public and private institutions have investigated a wide range of potential factors. These include chemical and biological weapons, the immunizations and preventive treatments used to protect against them, smoke from oil well fires, exposure to depleted uranium, and diseases endemic to the Arabian peninsula. So far investigators have not approached a consensus. In its final report released in December 2000, the Presidential Special Oversight Board for Department of Defense Investigations of Gulf War Chemical and Biological Incidents cited combat stress as a possible causative factor, but called for further research. There is also a likelihood that U.S. and allied forces were exposed to low levels of sarin and/or cyclosarin (nerve gases) released during the destruction of Iraqi munitions at Kharnisiyah, Iraq, and that these chemicals might be linked to the syndrome. In July 1997, the VA informed approximately 100,000 U.S. servicemen of their possible exposure to the nerve agents.

In October 1999, the U.S. Pentagon released a report that hypothesized that an experimental drug known as pyriostigmine bromide (PB) might be linked to the physical symptoms manifested in Gulf War Syndrome. The experimental drug was given to U.S. and Canadian troops during the war to protect soldiers against the effects of the chemical nerve agent soman. It has also been suggested that botulinum toxoid and **anthrax** vaccinations administered to soldiers during the conflict may be responsible for some manifestations of the syndrome.

Some studies have shown that Gulf War veterans have a higher incidence of positive tests for *Mycoplasma fermentans*, a bacteria, in their bloodstream. However, other clinical studies have not found a link between the bacterial infection and Gulf War-related illnesses.

Statistical analysis tells us that the following symptoms are about twice as likely to appear in Gulf War veterans than in their non-combat peers: depression, posttraumatic stress disorder (PTSD), chronic fatigue, cognitive dysfunction (diminished ability to calculate, order thoughts, evaluate, learn, and remember), **bronchitis**, asthma, fibromyalgia, alcohol **abuse**, **anxiety**, and sexual discomfort. PTSD is the modern equivalent of shell shock (World War I) and battle fatigue (World War II). It encompasses most of the psychological symptoms of war veterans, including nightmares, panic at sudden loud noises, and inability to adjust to peacetime living. **Chronic fatigue syndrome** has a specific medical definition that attempts to separate common fatigue from a more disabling illness in hope of finding a specific cause. Fibromyalgia is another newly defined syndrome, and as such it has arbitrarily rigid defining characteristics. These include a certain duration of illness, a specified minimum number of joint and muscle **pain** located in designated areas of the body, sleep disturbances, and other associated symptoms and signs.

Researchers have identified three distinct syndromes and several variations in Gulf War veterans. Type one patients suffer primarily from impaired thinking. Type two patients have a greater degree of confusion and ataxia (loss of coordination). Type three patients were the most affected by joint pains, muscle pains, and extremity paresthesias (unnatural sensations like burning or **tingling** in the arms and legs). In each of the three types, researchers found different but measurable impairments on objective testing of neurological function. The business of the nervous system is much more complex and subtle than other body functions. Measuring it requires equally complex effort. The tests used in this study carefully measured and compared localized nerve performance at several different tasks against the same values in normal subjects. Brain wave response to noise and touch, eye muscle response to spinning, and caloric testing (stimulation of the ear with warm and cold water, which causes vertigo) were clearly different between the normal and the test subjects. The researchers concluded that there was "a generalized injury to the

KEY TERMS

Ataxia—Lack of coordination.

Caloric testing—Flushing warm and cold water into the ear stimulates the labyrinth and causes vertigo and nystagmus if all the nerve pathways are intact.

Endemic—Always there.

Paresthesia—An altered sensation often described as burning, tingling, or pin pricks.

Syndrome—Common features of a disease or features that appear together often enough to suggest they may represent a single, as yet unknown, disease entity. When a syndrome is first identified, an attempt is made to define it as strictly as possible, even to the exclusion of some cases, in order to separate out a pure enough sample to study. This process is most likely to identify a cause, a positive method of diagnosis, and a treatment. Later on, less typical cases can be considered.

nervous system." Another research group concluded their study by stating that there was "a spectrum of neurologic injury involving the central, peripheral, and autonomic nervous systems."

Diagnosis

Until there is a clear definition of the disease, diagnosis is primarily an exercise in identifying those Gulf War veterans who have undefined illness in an effort to learn more about them and their symptoms. Both the Department of Defense and the Veterans Administration currently have programs devoted to this problem. Both the DOD's Comprehensive Clinical Evaluation Program and the VA's Persian Gulf Registry provide free, in-depth medical evaluations to Gulf War veterans and their families. In addition to providing individual veterans with critical medical care, these organizations use the cumulative data from these programs to advance research on Gulf War Syndrome itself.

Treatment

Specific treatment awaits specific diagnosis and identification of a causative agent. Meanwhile, veterans can benefit from the wide variety of supportive and non-specific approaches to this and similar problems. There are many drugs available for symptomatic relief. Psychological counseling by those specializing in this area can be immensely beneficial, even life-saving for those contemplating **suicide**. Veterans' benefits are available for those who are impaired by their symptoms.

Alternative treatment

The symptoms can be worked with using many modalities of alternative health care. The key to working successfully with people living their lives with Gulf War syndrome is long-term, ongoing care, whether it be **hypnotherapy**, **acupuncture**, homeopathy, **nutrition**, vitamin/mineral therapy, or bodywork.

Experimental treatment with **antibiotics** is advocated by some healthcare professionals who believe that Gulf War illness is related to a *Mycoplasma fermentans* bacterial infection. However, a conclusive link has not been clinically proven.

Prognosis

The outlook for Persian Gulf War veterans is unclear, but will hopefully improve as more information is gathered about the illness. Gradual return to a functioning life may take many years of work and much help. It is important to note that even in the absence of an identifiable and curable cause, recovery is possible.

Resources

BOOKS

Gulf War Syndrome: A Medical Dictionary, Bibliography, and Annotated Research Guide to Internet References. San Diego: ICON Health Publications, 2004.

Pall, Martin L.*Explaining 'Unexplained Illnesses': Disease Paradigm for Chronic Fatigue Syndrome, Multiple Chemical Sensitivity, Fibromyalgia, Post–Traumatic Stress Disorder, and Gulf War Syndrome*. Binghamton, NY: Harrington Park Press, 2007.

PERIODICALS

Duff, Katherine. "Unexplained Illnesses Emerge From the Dark Ages."*Townsend Letter: The Examiner of Alternative Medicine*(June 2007): 146–147.

"National Briefing Washington: No Single Gulf War Syndrome, Study Says."*New York Times*(September 13, 2006): A-19.

"Parasympathetic Nervous System at Risk."*USA Today Magazine*(February 2005): 13.

Radford, Benjamin. "New Report Casts Doubt on Gulf War Syndrome."*Skeptical Inquirer*(January-February 2007): 13–14.

ORGANIZATIONS

Office of the Special Assistant for Gulf War Illnesses, Force Health Protection & Readiness Policy & Programs Four Skyline Place, 5113 Leesburg Pike, Suite 901, Falls Church, VA, 22041, (800) 497-6261, http://www.gulflink.osd.mil.

The American Legion, 700 North Pennsylvania St., Indianapolis, IN, 46206, (800) 433-3318, http://www.legion.org.

Veterans Administration. Persian Gulf Medical Information Helpline, 400 South 18th Street, St. Louis, MO, 63103-2271, http://www.publichealth.va.gov/exposures/gulfwar.

Paula Anne Ford-Martin
Ken R. Wells

Gum disease *see* **Periodontal disease**

Günther's disease *see* **Porphyrias**

Gynecomastia (male breast enlargement)

Definition

Gynecomastia is a benign (noncancerous) condition caused by the development of unusually large mammary glands in the male resulting in enlargement of the male breast. The English word comes from two Greek words meaning "woman" and "breast." Enlargement of the male breast caused solely by deposits of fat associated with **obesity** is called pseudogynecomastia or lipomastia.

Demographics

Gynecomastia by definition is a condition found only in males. It occurs in three different age groups: infants, adolescents, and older men. Between 60% and 90% of male infants have temporary gynecomastia resulting from exposure to the mother's high estrogen levels during **pregnancy**. Various studies report the rate of gynecomastia in male adolescents as being between four and 69%.

In older men, the rate of gynecomastia is between 24% and 65%. The condition is thought to be equally common in all races and ethnic groups.

Description

The enlargement of the male breast that characterizes gynecomastia is caused by the growth of glandular tissue directly under the areola (the pigmented skin surrounding the nipple), usually in a symmetrical fashion just below the nipple. In most cases the extra glandular tissue is less than two inches across. In older men there may be extra fibrous tissue accumulating below the areola along with the increased growth of glandular tissue. Mild gynecomastia may take the form of puffy nipples, while severe gynecomastia—particularly in older men— may take the form of large sagging breasts, often referred to informally as "man boobs." The enlarged lump of glandular tissue under the nipple typically feels rubbery in texture.

In most cases the swelling of the breast is bilateral (affects both breasts) but it may also be unilateral, occurring in only one breast. In some cases the gynecomastia affects both breasts but not to the same extent, so that one is noticeably larger than the other.

Doctors divide gynecomastia into two major categories: physiologic and pathologic. Physiologic gynecomastia is caused by an imbalance in the amounts of estrogen and androgen in the man's body in favor of estrogen. Although estrogen is usually thought of as a female sex hormone, men's bodies also produce small amounts of it. Normally, the male body produces much more testosterone, a male sex hormone, than estrogen; the usual ratio is 100:1. But if the testosterone level in the male body is low for some reason or the estrogen level unusually high, gynecomastia can occur. In male infants, the imbalance between estrogen and testosterone results from exposure to the estrogen in the mother's circulation before birth; gynecomastia in infants typically goes away between two and three weeks after birth. In adolescent boys, the imbalance between the two sex hormones leads to gynecomastia lasting anywhere from six months to two or three years. Gynecomastia in older males typically results from a combination of causes: lowered levels of testosterone secretion; the conversion of some of the testosterone that is produced to estradiol, a female sex hormone; and the side effects of certain drugs that are frequently prescribed for older men.

Pathologic gynecomastia differs from physiologic gynecomastia in that it is associated with other diseases and disorders. These may include diseases that result in lowered testosterone production or increased estrogen production. Disorders associated with low testosterone production include genetic disorders like **Klinefelter syndrome** and Kallmann syndrome; trauma to or viral infection of the testicles; tumors of the pituitary gland; **hyperthyroidism**; kidney failure; malnutrition; or **small cell lung cancer**, gastric carcinoma, renal cell carcinoma, or kidney failure. Disorders associated with increased production of estrogen or increased conversion of testosterone to estradiol include cancers of the lung, kidney, and digestive tract; and chronic **liver disease**, malnutrition, hyperthyroidism, and tumors of the adrenal glands.

KEY TERMS

Areola—The area of pigmented skin surrounding the human nipple in both males and females. It is roughly circular in shape.

Bilateral—Located on or affecting both sides of the body.

Hyperthyroidism—A condition in which the thyroid gland in the throat is overactive and produces too much thyroid hormone.

Idiopathic—Of unknown cause or spontaneous origin.

Kallmann syndrome—A rare genetic disorder in which the hypothalamus does not produce enough gonadotropin–releasing hormone, leading to underfunctioning of the testes in males and the ovaries in females.

Klinefelter syndrome—A genetic disorder in which a male has an extra X chromosome, making his genetic sex classification 47, XXY. About a third of males with Klinefelter syndrome develop gynecomastia.

Liposuction—A cosmetic surgery technique for removing unwanted fat cells from the abdomen, hips, thighs, or male breast while doing as little damage as possible to nearby connective tissue and blood vessels.

Pseudogynecomastia—Enlargement of the male breast caused solely by fat accumulation. It is also called lipomastia.

Unilateral—Located on or affecting only one side of the body.

Risk factors

Risk factors for gynecomastia include:

- Age. Infants, boys undergoing puberty, and men over 50 are at increased of gynecomastia.
- Family history of gynecomastia.
- Use of anabolic steroids or injected androgens to improve athletic performance.
- Diagnosis with Klinefelter syndrome, Kallmann syndrome, or other genetic disorders that affect the size of the testes or their ability to produce testosterone.
- Kidney disease, liver disease, or thyroid disease.
- Cancers that are hormonally active, including cancers of the kidneys, digestive tract, and lungs.
- Having to take prescription drugs that stimulate estrogen synthesis, lower testosterone production, or are otherwise known to cause gynecomastia as a side effect.

Causes and symptoms

Causes

As has been noted, gynecomastia can be caused by a number of conditions, ranging from normal shifts in hormone balance at certain points in the male life cycle to genetic conditions, medication side effects, and **cancer**. The causes for which males seek help with gynecomastia are as follows in order of frequency:

- Persistent (two years or longer) gynecomastia of puberty: 25%
- Drug–related gynecomastia: 10% to 25%
- Idiopathic (no detectable disease or disorder): 25%
- Cirrhosis of the liver or malnutrition: 8%
- Underdeveloped testicles: 8%
- Testicular tumors: 3%
- Hyperthyroidism: 1.5%
- Kidney disease: 1%

Symptoms

The symptoms of gynecomastia are visible enlargement of the breast. Most boys and men will also feel some **pain** or tenderness around the areola. A discharge from the nipple is not normal with gynecomastia, however, and may indicate **breast cancer**, as one percent of all cancers of the breast occur in males.

Diagnosis

A formal diagnosis is not usually necessary for male infants as the condition is temporary in infancy and does not require treatment.

In adolescent boys and older men, diagnosis is based on a combination of patient and family history, an office examination, imaging studies, and a blood test. In terms of patient history, the doctor will ask the patient's age at the time the gynecomastia first appeared, how long it has been present, whether the patient is using **steroids**, whether the patient is consuming alcohol or drugs of **abuse**, what prescription medications the patient is taking, and whether there is a family history of gynecomastia.

Examination

The office examination is intended to check for abnormally small testicles, testicular tumors, and other abnormalities of the male genitals, and to distinguish between gynecomastia and pseudogynecomastia. To tell whether the breast is enlarged by glandular tissue or only by fat, the doctor will ask the patient to lie flat on the examination table with arms raised above the head. The doctor will then place his or her thumbs on either side of the nipple and slowly bring the thumbs together. If the patient has gynecomastia, the doctor will feel a ridge of glandular tissue. If only fat is present, no such ridge will be felt.

The doctor will also check to see whether there is any discharge from the patient's nipple, and for signs of thyroid, kidney, or liver disease.

Tests

The tests most commonly performed are a mammogram and a blood test to check for abnormalities in thyroid, liver, or kidney function. If the doctor suspects an underlying cancer, the patient may also be given an MRI, ultrasound of the testicles, a chest x ray, or a tissue biopsy.

Treatment

Treatment for gynecomastia ranges from none at all to drugs or surgery. Adolescents may also be referred to **psychotherapy** to help them cope with the social embarrassment caused by the disorder and their psychological reactions to it.

Traditional

Gynecomastia by itself is not a danger to health, although its underlying cause may require treatment. In many cases, treatment of that cause relieves the gynecomastia as well. In the case of adolescents, most doctors recommend simple observation of the condition (a checkup every three to six months), as it usually goes away by itself in two to three years. If the adolescent is having significant pain in the enlarged breasts, if the condition persists beyond three years, or if the teenager is having serious psychological problems related to the gynecomastia, the doctor may recommend breast surgery. Surgical treatment may consist either of **mastectomy** (surgical removal of the glandular tissue in the breast) or **liposuction** (removal of the fat surrounding the glandular tissue while leaving the glandular tissue intact).

Pseudogynecomastia can be helped somewhat by encouraging the patient to lose weight; however, it is not possible as of 2010 to target a specific area of the body for fat loss, and the patient may still have larger breasts than he would like. Liposuction can also be used successfully to treat pseudogynecomastia.

Drugs

Some older men can be treated with tamoxifen or raloxifene, drugs used to treat breast cancer in women; between 70% and 80% report complete reduction of the gynecomastia after taking these drugs. In addition, men whose gynecomastia is caused by prescription medications for other conditions may be helped by having their doctor switch them to another drug. Drugs known to cause gynecomastia as a side effect include methyldopa, busulfan, tricyclic antidepressants, diazepam, penicillamine, omeprazole, phenothiazines, calcium channel blockers, angiotensin–converting enzyme (ACE) inhibitors, ketoconazole, metronidazole, alkylating agents, cisplatin, spironolactone, cimetidine, flutamide, **finasteride**, and etomidate.

Patients abusing alcohol, heroin, or **marijuana** may be helped by stopping their use of these substances, as all three are known to cause gynecomastia.

Prognosis

In 90% of cases, gynecomastia will eventually go away by itself. For those patients with persistent gynecomastia, drug therapy or **plastic surgery** will usually relieve the condition. Men with Klinefelter syndrome, however, have a 10– to 20–fold increased risk of breast cancer, and should be checked for any abnormalities in their breasts during every routine office physical.

Prevention

There is no known way to prevent gynecomastia in male infants as of 2010, whether physiologic or pathologic. Male adolescents can lower their risk of gynecomastia by avoiding steroids for muscle building, illicit drugs, and heavy alcohol consumption. Older men should ask their doctor whether any of the medications currently prescribed for them are known to cause gynecomastia, and if so, whether other drugs can be substituted.

Resources

BOOKS

Judd, Sandra J., editor. *Men's Health Concerns Sourcebook*, 3rd ed. Detroit, MI: Omnigraphics, 2009.

Neinstein, Lawrence S., editor–in–chief. *Handbook of Adolescent Health Care*. Philadelphia: Wolters Kluwer Health/Lippincott Williams and Wilkins, 2009.

Sabel, Michael S. *Surgical Foundations: Essentials of Breast Surgery*. Philadelphia: Mosby/Elsevier, 2009.

PERIODICALS

Basaria, S. "Androgen Abuse in Athletes: Detection and Consequences." *Journal of Clinical Endocrinology and Metabolism* 95 (April 2010): 1533–1543.

Devalia, H.L., and G.T. Layer. "Current Concepts in Gynaecomastia." *Surgeon* 7 (April 2009): 114–19.

Johnson, R.E., and M.H. Murad. "Gynecomastia: Pathophysiology, Evaluation, and Management." *Mayo Clinic Proceedings* 84 (November 2009): 1010–1015.

Kapoor, S. "Cutaneous Manifestations of Systemic Conditions Associated with Gynecomastia." *Skinmed* 8 (March–April 2010): 87–92.

Wauters, C.A., et al. "Is Cytology Useful in the Diagnostic Workup of Male Breast Lesions? A Retrospective Study over a 16–year Period and Review of the Recent Literature." *Acta Cytologica* 54 (May–June 2010): 259–64.

OTHER

Allee, Mark R., and Mary Zoe Baker. "Gynecomastia." eMedicine, March 22, 2010. http://emedicine.medscape.com/article/120858–overview (accessed September 4, 2010).

Children's Hospital Boston. "My Child Has Gynecomastia," http://www.childrenshospital.org/az/Site978/mainpageS978P0.html (accessed September 4, 2010).

Mayo Clinic. "Gynecomastia (Enlarged Breasts in Men)." http://www.mayoclinic.com/health/gynecomastia/DS00850 (accessed September 4, 2010).

TeensHealth. "I'm a Guy . . . So How Come I'm Developing Breasts?" http://kidshealth.org/teen/sexual_health/guys/boybrst.html (accessed September 4, 2010).

ORGANIZATIONS

American Academy of Child and Adolescent Psychiatry (AACAP), 3615 Wisconsin Avenue, NW, Washington, DC, 20016–3007, (202) 966-7300, (202) 966-2891, http://www.aacap.org.

American Association of Clinical Endocrinologists (AACE), 245 Riverside Ave., Suite 200, Jacksonville, FL, 32202, (904) 353-7878, http://www.aace.com/college.

American Society of Plastic Surgeons (ASPS), 444 East Algonquin Rd., Arlington Heights, IL, 60005, (847) 228-9900, http://www.plasticsurgery.org.

National Adolescent Health Information Center (NAHIC), LHTS Suite 245, Box 0503, San Francisco, CA, 94143, (415) 502-4856, (415) 502-4858, nahic@ucsf.edu, http://nahic.ucsf.edu.

Society for Adolescent Health and Medicine (SAHM), 111 Deer Lake Rd., Suite 100, Deerfield, IL, 60015, (847) 753-5226, (847) 480-9282, info@adolescenthealth.org, http://www.adolescenthealth.org/AM/Template.cfm?Section = Home.

Gale B. Slap, MD
Rebecca J. Frey, PhD

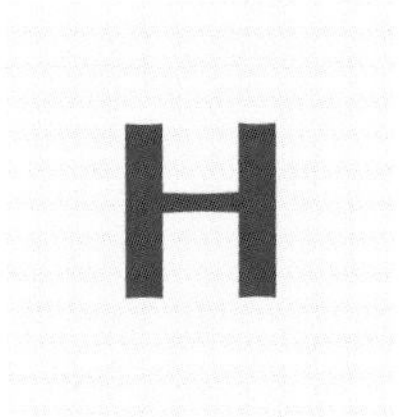

H1N1 influenza

Definition

Pandemic 2009 H1N1 **influenza**, initially termed a swine flu, is an infectious respiratory disease caused by a subtype of the influenza A virus first identified in April 2009. The virus and associated influenza spread rapidly around the globe, and on June 11, 2009, World Health Organization (WHO) officials declared H1N1 influenza to be a global pandemic, the first new pandemic of the twenty-first century. According to the Centers for Disease Control (CDC), the U.S. Public Health Emergency for 2009 H1N1 Influenza expired on June 23, 2010.

Demographics

As of July 2009, the World Health Organization (WHO) offices reported more than 94,000 laboratory-confirmed cases of 2009 H1N1 influenza in 135 countries. At least 700 deaths were already attributed to the novel virus, and WHO officials characterized the 2009 H1N1 flu as the fastest spreading pandemic on record.

Despite high initial estimates, by June 24, 2009, Mexico had reported 7,847 confirmed cases and 115 laboratory-confirmed deaths. The United States reported 21,449 confirmed cases and 87 deaths, and Canada reported 6,457 cases and 15 deaths. Deaths were also reported in Colombia Costa Rica, Dominican Republic, Guatemala, the Philippines, and the United Kingdom. The spread of the virus into the Southern Hemisphere was evidenced by Australia's reporting of 2,857 cases including 2 deaths, Argentina's reporting of 1,213 cases including 7 deaths, and Chile's reporting 4,315 cases including 4 deaths. As with all reports related to a developing outbreak, daily reports of cases and deaths are simply considered by experts to be a snapshot of data; both the number of countries reporting and cases confirmed will increase until the pandemic subsides. In July 2009, with the pandemic well established in both the Northern and Southern Hemispheres, WHO officials stopped accumulating individual case counts in favor of concentrating on pandemic flu mitigation strategies such as vaccine and anti-viral medication development and delivery. Especially in developing countries with established outbreaks, data would be difficult to collect and prone to error. Counting individual cases is also difficult because many are mild and go unreported.

Newswires are often filled with unverified reports, and even the time difference between offices reporting laboratory-confirmed results can seemingly swing figures rapidly. In addition, there is often a delay or backlog in such reporting. Uncertainties in the number of cases and confirmed deaths create a degree of uncertainty in assessments of the lethality of the virus and course of the outbreak. As of August 2009, there was no evidence that the H1N1 pandemic would be more lethal on a case-by-case basis than a typical seasonal flu. However, pandemic flu viruses often cause significant global deaths because so many more people are infected than in normal influenza seasons.

Common seasonal influenza (the type for which vaccinations are offered each year) normally accounts for about 200,000 hospitalizations and 36,000 deaths annually in the United States. Globally, WHO officials estimate that between 300,000 and 500,000 people die from flu complications each year. Although people of all ages can contract influenza, young children and the elderly, along with those with compromised immune systems (e.g., **cancer** patients or those with HIV/AIDS) are most at risk during a normal seasonal flu. Most deaths are caused by **pneumonia**, a common complication of seasonal flu. During the initial outbreak of 2009 H1N1 flu in Mexico, reports indicated that otherwise healthy adults aged 20 to 44 years were dying of the disease in higher than expected numbers. By the end of July 2009, in the United States, approximately 50 percent of the reported cases of pandemic H1N1 flu occurred in young people from 5 to 24 years old, and the highest rate

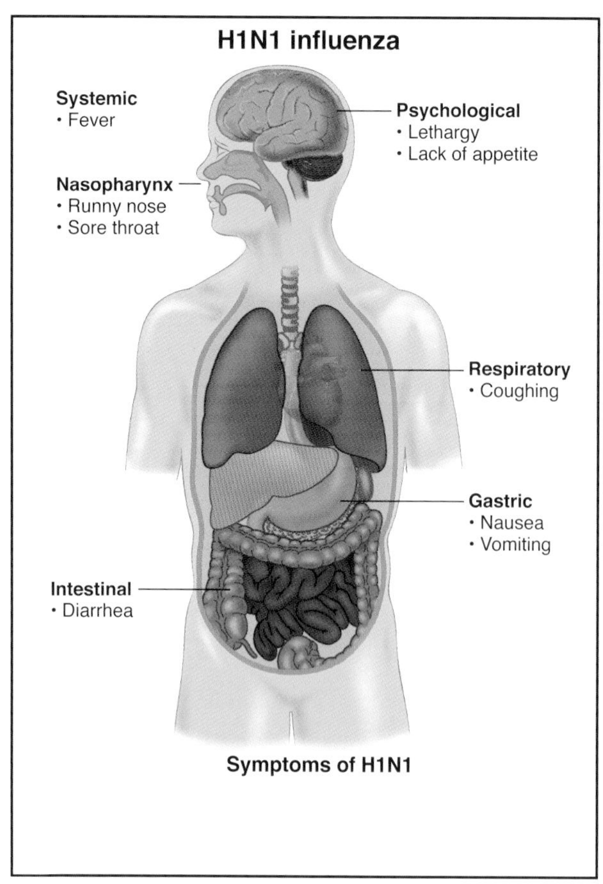

(Illustration by Electronic Illustrators Group. Reproduced by permission of Gale, a part of Cengage Learning.)

of hospitalization was among infants and young children under four years of age. Although there is no definitive cause, the pattern of illness differs from normal seasonal flu, which usually results in a greater number of cases in the elderly. A report published in the medical journal *The Lancet* showed that early in the pandemic, pregnant women were four times as likely as other people who contract swine flu to require hospitalization. The physiological reasons remain under study.

Description

In April 2009, scientists at the U.S. Centers for Disease Control and Prevention (CDC) and at a research laboratory in Winnipeg, Canada, confirmed that a new strain of influenza was causing illness in humans. Genetic analysis showed that although the H1N1 virus is a novel genetic reassortment of genes of swine, human, and avian origin, the majority of the H1N1 genome is traceable and comparable to other viruses that cause seasonal influenza.

It remains a subject of intense research as to when and where the 2009 H1N1 flu virus may have entered the human population. Although the first cases erupted in Mexico and the United States in March and April 2009, this does not mean that the genetic reassortment of the virus took place in Mexico or the United States, or that the virus entered the human population in either country.

The 2009 H1N1 influenza virus was initially classified as a swine flu because it contains swine flu genes. This means only that the virus passed through swine at some point in its evolution. When and where the virus passed through swine is a subject of continued investigation. Although probable, it is not a certainty that the virus was most recently transmitted from swine to humans. Based on preliminary genetic analysis, experts conjecture such a transfer might have taken place in late 2008. As of June 12, 2009, however, none of the cases encountered in the 2009 H1N1 flu outbreak could be definitively traced to contact with pigs. In fact, the first confirmed outbreak of H1N1 recorded in swine was on a Canadian farm. Experts strongly suspect that a human farm worker who had traveled from Mexico infected the swine.

H1N1 strains of influenza are common in pigs, and swine flu viruses can be transmitted from pigs to humans who are in close contact with infected animals. However, before the 2009 H1N1 outbreak, documented transmission of recent swine flu viruses from person to person was extremely limited and had not resulted in documented outbreaks of human disease.

What made health experts in 2009 so concerned about the new H1N1 virus was that it was a novel virus of unknown lethality that had gained the ability to efficiently pass from person to person (human transmission). Because 2009 H1N1 flu was new, humans had no immunity to it. As a result, the resources of the WHO, the CDC, state public health departments, and various international organizations charged with protecting public health were mobilized to attempt to mitigate a worldwide influenza pandemic.

Understanding the influenza virus

Viruses are simple organisms consisting of a protein matrix containing genetic information. They are so small that they can be seen only with an electron microscope. Because they are metabolically inert outside of a host cell, viruses cannot reproduce on their own. They are parasites and must enter a host cell and take over the host cell's resources in order to make millions of new virus particles.

Influenza is caused by a hardy group of viruses belonging to the Orthomyxoviridae family. There are three types of influenza viruses: types A, B, and C. Type A influenza virus is the most threatening to humans. The type B virus is stable, changing little from year to year, and can be effectively controlled through **vaccination**. Type C influenza viruses cause only mild illness in humans. The type A virus, however, easily changes, or mutates, into new strains or subtypes. Each strain contains slightly different genetic information. Because of this, no single vaccine is completely effective against all type A viruses, and whenever a new strain arises, as in the case of the 2009 H1N1, the body's immune system treats the virus as a completely new antigen.

How new strains develop

Humans are not the only animals vulnerable to influenza A infections. Different strains of influenza A cause disease in other animals, including wild birds, chickens, ducks, and turkeys (collectively called avian or bird flu), pigs, horses, ferrets, whales, seals, and dogs. Pigs and birds are the critical species in the development of new flu strains that can infect humans. Wild birds serve as a reservoir for the influenza A viruses; some strain of **avian flu** is always present in the world bird population. Birds shed live virus in their droppings (feces), and because many species of bird migrate long distances, they can infect large areas. Pigs carry their own strains of influenza A, but they also can become infected with avian influenza if they are exposed to infected bird droppings or contaminated water. If a pig simultaneously becomes infected with a strain of swine influenza and a strain of avian influenza, when the virus reproduces, genetic information can be exchanged so that new strains of influenza A develop that incorporate some genetic material from the avian virus and some genetic material from the swine virus.

Most new strains of influenza that result from a recombination or reassortment of avian and swine flu viruses do not survive, cannot infect humans, or die out quickly. Occasionally, however, a strain develops that can infect humans and that has the ability not only to pass from pig to human, but also from person to person. Because the virus is new to humans, the body has few defenses against it, and the vaccines included in seasonal flu shots are ineffective against it. When a new strain of flu arises that can pass easily from person to person, it has the potential to cause a pandemic, rapidly infecting and sometimes killing millions of people across the world.

Influenza pandemics have occurred during thousands of years of recorded history. The worst influenza pandemic in modern history occurred in 1918–1919 and killed an estimated 20 to 40 million people. In 1957, another pandemic known as the Asian flu killed about 70,000 Americans. This was followed by the pandemic Hong Kong flu in 1968. Then in 1976, Americans experienced a swine flu scare. During February 1976, several recruits at the Army Fort Dix in New Jersey developed unusually severe flu symptoms. When samples from some of the sick men were sent to the CDC for analysis, four samples showed a previously unknown flu virus that appeared to be similar to the virus that caused the 1918–1919 pandemic. After one soldier died of the flu, the United States began a $135 million emergency immunization program. However, the virus 1976 proved to be much less dangerous than the 1918 virus. In the end, the 1976 swine flu never spread beyond Fort Dix. About 500 people became sick and only one person died.

People who are most likely to become infected with the H1N1 influenza are those who are in close contact with someone who is infected. The incubation period is uncertain, although it is most likely less than seven days. The disease is passed to others through infected droplets that are spread by coughing, sneezing, kissing, and close physical contact. The virus can also spread indirectly. Tests of other viral strains typically show that Type A viruses can live up to two hours on hard surfaces such as door knobs, telephones, or children's toys. This means that an infected person can leave the flu virus on objects where it can be picked up by another person who then touches his or her own mouth, nose, or eyes and becomes infected. People are contagious for about one day before symptoms appear. Adults remain contagious for about seven days after they begin to show symptoms; children can remain contagious for up to 10 days.

Causes and symptoms

The H1N1 flu is caused by a newly identified strain of influenza virus. Genetic tests established that H1N1 strains encountered thus far are consistent (nearing 99 percent genetic matches among viruses examined from patient samples taken from six countries). Of particular interest to **infectious disease** research are the genes that control hemagglutinin (H), neuraminidase (N), two surface proteins with subtypes that are numbered, hence H1N1 flu or H5N1 avian flu virus, genes that control the nucleoprotein, the surrounding matrix, and three key polymerase enzymes (designated PA, PB1, and PB2) that the virus must have to reproduce. Genetically, the 2009 H1N1 presents a mixed background, with these key genes derived from human, swine, and avian sources (a triple reassortment). The hemagglutinin [H] produced is equidistant to the swine flu sequences found in the North America, Europe, and Asia. The neuraminidase and matrix genes sequences are close to genes found in swine flu strains found in Asia. Early evidence indicates similarities to influenza strains where the PB1 gene is of human origin and the PA and PB2 genes are from avian sources.

Symptoms of H1N1 flu are similar to the symptoms of seasonal influenza. These include **fever**, **cough**, **sore**

KEY TERMS

Incubation period—The time between when an individual becomes infected with a disease-causing agent and when symptoms begin to appear.

Pandemic—The occurrence of a disease that in a short time infects a large percentage of the population over a wide geographical area.

Parasite—An organism that lives in or with another organism, called the host, in parasitism, a type of association characterized by the parasite obtaining benefits from the host, such as food, and the host being injured as a result.

throat, runny nose, body aches, **headaches**, chills, loss of appetite, and exhaustion. Some people experience **nausea**, **vomiting**, and **diarrhea**. Although most cases of H1N1 flu are mild to moderate, complications such as severe pneumonia can result in **respiratory failure** and **death**. Neurological complications including seizures have also been linked to H1N1 flu in children.

Diagnosis

Normally influenza is diagnosed on the basis of symptoms and the health care provider's knowledge of whether influenza is prevalent in the local area. An influenza test can be performed in the doctor's office that is about 75% accurate. However, this test cannot distinguish between strains of influenza A and, therefore, is not useful in determining if the patient has H1N1. To make this determination, a mucus sample must be sent to laboratory capable of rapid PCR analysis. Prior to May 1, 2009, only two laboratories in North America, the CDC laboratories in Atlanta and Canadian research laboratories in Winnipeg, were capable of definitively diagnosing the 2009 H1N1 flu. However, PCR machines are being installed in labs in Mexico that will allow rapid definitive diagnosis.

Tests

The most accurate test for influenza is done by taking a mucus sample from the throat of an infected person. Because of the time delay involved in testing, knowing the strain of flu does not provide much help to the patient, but this information helps the CDC and WHO understand how and where flu is spreading. During an influenza pandemic, physicians often forgo laboratory confirmation of influenza, relying on signs and symptoms for diagnosis. In the United Kingdom, persons with flu symptoms are given access to **antiviral drugs** after answering questions that indicate an influenza diagnosis on a government-sponsored public health website. This saves physician resources for handling severe or emergent cases, provides quick access to treatment, and helps the person with symptoms to stay home, thereby reducing the pool of infected persons in public available to infect others.

Treatment

Supportive treatment for H1N1 appears to be the same as for all influenza viruses and includes drinking plenty of fluids, extended bed rest, and use of **acetaminophen** to treat aches and fever. H1N1 influenza A virus also responds to two antiviral drugs, oseltamivir (Tamiflu) and zanamivir (Relenza). These drugs do not prevent or cure flu, but if taken within 48 hours of the start of symptoms, they reduce the severity and duration of the disease. In late April 2009, the United States government released stockpiled supplies of these antiviral drugs to combat H1N1 flu. Initial tests show that H1N1 is resistant to two other antiviral drugs, amantadine (Symmetrel, Symadine) and rimantadine (Flumandine), making these drugs ineffective. **Antibiotics** also are ineffective against all viruses, including H1N1, but can be used to treat bacterial complications of influenza, such as pneumonia.

In late June 2009, public health officials in Denmark reported the first case of A/H1N1 influenza that was resistant to oseltamivir. Although some cases of resistance normally occur and develop with seasonal influenzas, any emergence of Tamiflu-resistant 2009 A/H1N1 influenza virus puts public health officials on alert for appearance of the resistant virus elsewhere. Isolated cases of Tamiflu-resistant H1N1 have also been identified in Japan, Hong Kong (Special Administrative Region of China), and Canada. Thus far, the Tamiflu-resistant viral influenza remains treatable with zanamivir (Relenza), the other antiviral drug usually effective against the A/H1N1 virus.

Alternative treatment

No scientific testing exists to validate any claim of effectiveness of any alternative medical treatments specific to H1N1 flu. Although claims of effectiveness (and/or potential harm) for any alternative medical treatment should be carefully scrutinized for supporting scientific evidence, there are a number of alternative treatments commonly used to support relief of symptoms. Because there is no scientifically validated antiviral treatment, if flu is suspected, persons should consult with a physician to determine if they are in need of antiviral medicines.

Alternative practitioners recommend herbal teas to soothe the throat and allegedly "boost" the immune system. Other herbal treatments recommended by alternative practitioners for seasonal flu routinely include:

- Ginger (*Zingiber officinalis*) to reduce fever and pain, settle the stomach, and suppress cough
- Echinacea (*Echinacea purpurea* or *angustifolia*) to reduce flu symptoms, including sore throat, chills, sweating, fatigue, weakness, body aches, and headaches
- Cordyceps (*Cordyceps sinensis*) to modulate and allegedly "boost" the immune system and improve respiration
- Eucalyptus (*Eucalyptus globulus*) or peppermint (*Mentha piperita*) essential oils added to a steam vaporizer to help clear chest and nasal congestion

Prognosis

Because 2009 H1N1 is a new strain of influenza, it is difficult to predict the course of the disease. Generally cases have been mild, but as with all flu, cases can be life-threatening if complications develop. Underlying health conditions may be worsened by the disease, and pneumonia, a common and sometimes fatal complication of seasonal flu, may develop.

Prevention

The best ways to prevent H1N1 infection include the following:

- Wash hands well and often. Hands should be washed with soap and warm water to above the wrists for 15–20 seconds or about the time it takes to sing the happy birthday song slowly. If soap and water are not available, use an alcohol-based hand sanitizer.
- Cover the mouth when coughing; dispose of used tissues in a covered container.
- Avoid touching the nose, mouth, and eyes.
- Stay home if flu symptoms appear.
- Avoid crowded places such as movie theaters.

Note that surgical masks are unlikely to protect against the influenza virus, but are effective in reducing dissemination of droplets that can contain viral particles. Also, antiviral medications do not prevent influenza; they simply help shorten the intensity and duration of the illness.

Vaccination

World public health officials have recommended prioritizing vaccine recipients according to individual risk, as well as to ensure the greatest benefit for overall public health. Pregnant women and people caring for infants, children, young people under 25 years of age, and persons with underlying health conditions such as **asthma** or diabetes are recommended to receive priority vaccination against pandemic H1N1 influenza. In addition, healthcare workers are suggested to be among the first immunized in order to keep hospitals, doctors' offices, and other critical healthcare infrastructure functional during a pandemic flu.

Public health officials acknowledged that production of the H1N1 vaccine fell far short of global demand. At current rates of production, 900 million doses of the new H1N1 vaccine can be produced each year (as two doses are required per person, enough to vaccinate 450 million people). The vaccine is produced in only a handful of countries and there are concerns these countries, along with wealthier nations will obtain the vast majority of vaccine produced. The shortages may also hinder WHO efforts to secure donations of vaccine or agreements that will enable poorer countries to purchase vaccine at a lower price. The current seasonal influenza vaccine protects against an H3N2 virus, an influenza B virus, and the H1N1 virus.

Resources

BOOKS

Hays, J. N. *Epidemics and Pandemics: Their Impacts on Human History*. Santa Barbara, CA: ABC–CLIO, 2005.

Ryan, Jeffrey R. *Pandemic Influenza: Emergency Planning and Community Preparedness*. Boca Raton, FL: CRC Press, 2009.

Shors, Teri. *Understanding Viruses*. Sudbury, MA: Jones and Bartlett Publishers, 2009.

PERIODICALS

Barry, John M. "The Site of Origin of the 1918 Influenza Pandemic and its Public Health Implications." *Journal of Translational Medicine* 2004.

Kaiser, Jocelyn. "Resurrected Influenza Virus Yields Secrets of Deadly 1918 Pandemic." *Science*. 310 (2005): 28029.

Loo, Yueh-Ming, and Michael Gale Jr. "Fatal Immunity and the 1918 Virus." *Nature*. 445 (2007): 18–19.

Mills, Christina E., James M. Robins, and March Lipsitch. "Transmissibility of 1918 Pandemic Influenza." *Science*. 432 (2004): 904–906.

Monto, Arnold S. "Vaccines and Antiviral Drugs in Pandemic Preparedness." *Emerging Infectious Diseases* 12 (January 2006): 55–61.

OTHER

Centers for Disease Control and Prevention (CDC). Flu.gov: Know What to Do About the Flu. http://www.pandemicflu.gov.

Centers for Disease Control and Prevention (CDC). H1N1 Flu (Swine Flu). http://www.cdc.gov/h1n1flu/.

Centers for Disease Control and Prevention (CDC). Influenza. http://www.cdc.gov/flu.

National Geographic Society. Influenza. http://science.nationalgeographic.com/science/health-and-human-body/human-diseases/influenza-article.html.

National Institutes of Health (NIH). Influenza. http://health.nih.gov/topic/Influenza.

PandemicFlu.gov (United States). Individuals and Families Planning. http://www.pandemicflu.gov/plan/individual/index.html.

World Health Organization (WHO). Global Alert and Response (EPR). WHO Programs and Projects. http://www.who.int/entity/csr/en.

World Health Organization (WHO). Influenza. http://www.who.int/entity/mediacentre/factsheets/fs211/en/index.html.

ORGANIZATIONS

United States Centers for Disease Control and Prevention (CDC), 1600 Clifton Road, Atlanta, GA, 30333, (779) 488-7100, (800) 232-4636, cdcinfo@cdc.gov, http://www.cdc.gov.

World Health Organization. Regional Office for the Americas, 525 23rd Street N.W., Washington, DC, 20037, (202) 974-3000, postmaster@paho.org, http://new.paho.org/hq/.

Brenda Wilmoth Lerner
Tish Davidson, A.M.

H-2 blockers

Definition

Histamine H-2 receptor blockers act by stopping the pathway that leads to the secretion of stomach acid. There are two kinds of pathways that react to stimulation by histamine. Histamine is produced in the body and released by mast cells in response to some types of injury or to the presence of an antigen. When histamine reaches the H-1 receptors, the reaction results in dilation of capillaries, leading to redness and swelling, along with **itching**. These reactions can be controlled with traditional **antihistamines**.

Histamine that reaches the H-2 receptors causes increased secretion of stomach acid.

Purpose

H2 receptor blockers are used to treat conditions associated with excess amounts of stomach acid, although in some cases they have been replaced by the **proton pump inhibitors**, which have a greater effect on reducing acid secretions.

H2 receptor blockers are used to treat the following conditions:

- duodenal ulcer, as short term therapy and maintenance
- gastric ulcer, as short term therapy and maintenance
- gastroesophageal reflux disease (GERD), including endoscopically diagnosed erosive esophagitis
- pathological hypersecretory conditions such as Zollinger-Ellison syndrome, systemic mastocytosis, and multiple endocrine adenomas
- upper GI bleeding
- heartburn, acid indigestion, and sour stomach

None of the drugs in this class has been approved for use by children under the age of 12 years. However, standard pediatric texts have reported use by infants and children.

Description

There are four H2 receptor blockers on the market. Although they all work in the same manner and have similar effects, they are not all approved for the same uses.

Cimetidine (Tagamet) is available in both prescription and over-the-counter forms. The oldest of the group and the most studied, this drug is the least potent of the H2 receptor blockers, which means that higher dosages are required to provide comparable effects. There is no evidence that higher potency improves therapeutic results.

Cimetidine is the only drug in its class which is approved for prevention of upper gastro-intestinal bleeding. It has been reported on for a number of uses, with varying degrees of success. Cimetidine, like ranitidine, has shown some benefit in treatment of colorectal **cancer**. Although some claims have been made that cimetidine is useful in treatment of **acetaminophen** overdose, the evidence for this use is lacking, and cimetidine should not be used. Because cimetidine is a mild antiandrogen, it has been of some use in treatment of **hirsutism** (abnormal growth of hair on a woman's face and body).

The three other H2 receptor blockers, famotidine (Pepcid, Pepcid AC), nizatidine (Axid), and ranitidine (Zantac), are similar in their uses. All are approved for treatment of duodenal ulcer both acute treatment and maintenance therapy, gastro-esophageal reflux disease, including erosive esophagitis and gastric ulcer short term treatment, although in this group ranitidine alone is approved for maintenance treatment.

In their over-the-counter (non-prescription) forms, cimetidine and famotidine are approved for treatment of **heartburn**, acid **indigestion**, and sour stomach.

Drugs in this class are similar in other respects as well. Although study results vary, cimetidine will usually show its effects within one hour and last for about five hours after a single dose; famotidine and nizatidine also show effects within one hour but may act for up to 12 hours at maximum dosing. Ranitidine has a comparable onset of action and duration in adults but may be slower in the elderly. Onset and duration of action will vary with the individual, the dose of medication, and the presence or absence of food or **antacids** in the stomach.

When *Facts and Comparisons*, a widely used on-line drug information resource, compared the published reports on cure rates for duodenal ulcers, it found that after eight weeks of treatment, all drugs showed healing rates in the range of 82% to 95%. These results were based on comparing separate studies and did not represent comparative trials of the drugs against each other.

Recommended dosage

Cimetidine doses for patients over the age of 12 years, for oral administration.

- Short-term treatment of active duodenal ulcer: 800 mg at bedtime. Other dose regimens are sometimes used.
- Heartburn, acid indigestion, and sour stomach using the over-the-counter product: 100 to 200 mg with water when symptoms start. The dose may be repeated once in 24 hours.
- Prevention of heartburn, acid indigestion, and sour stomach using the over-the-counter product: 100 to 200 mg with water up to one hour before eating food or drinking beverages expected to cause symptoms. Dose should not exceed 400 mg in 24 hours.
- Treatment of hypersecretory conditions: 300 mg four times a day, with meals and at bedtime.
- Gastroesophageal reflux disease: 800 to 1600 mg a day, divided into smaller doses. Treatment usually lasts 12 weeks.

Famotidine doses for patients over the age of 12 years, for oral administration.

- Treatment of duodenal ulcers: 40 mg once a day at bedtime. If necessary, 20 milligrams two times a day may be used.
- Prevention of duodenal ulcers: 20 mg once a day at bedtime.
- Gastric ulcers: 40 mg once a day at bedtime.
- To treat heartburn, acid indigestion, and sour stomach using the over-the-counter product: 10 mg with water when symptoms start. The dose may be repeated once in 24 hours.
- Hypersecretory conditions: 20 mg every six hours.
- Gastroesophageal reflux disease: 20 mg two times a day, usually for up to six weeks.

Nizatidine doses for patients over the age of 12 years, for oral administration.

- Treatment of duodenal or gastric ulcers: 300 mg once a day at bedtime. Alternately, 150 mg two times a day.
- Prevention of duodenal ulcers: 150 mg once a day at bedtime.
- Prevention of heartburn, acid indigestion, and sour stomach: 75 mg taken 30 to 60 minutes before meals which may cause symptoms. The dose may be repeated once in 24 hours.
- Gastroesophageal reflux disease: 150 mg two times a day.

Ranitidine doses for patients over the age of 12 years, for oral administration.

- Duodenal ulcers, treatment: 150 mg two times a day. Alternately, 300 mg once a day at bedtime.
- Duodenal ulcers, prevention: 150 mg at bedtime.
- Gastric ulcers, treatment: 150 mg two times a day.
- Heartburn, acid indigestion, and sour stomach, treatment: 75 mg with water when symptoms start. The dose may be repeated once in 24 hours.
- Heartburn, acid indigestion, and sour stomach, prevention: 75 mg with water taken 30 to 60 minutes before meals or beverages which may cause symptoms. The dose may be repeated once in 24 hours.
- Hypersecretory conditions: 150 mg two times a day.
- Gastroesophageal reflux disease: 150 mg two times a day. The dose may be increased as needed.

Precautions

Overall, the histamine H2 receptor blockers are a safe class of drugs. However, some patients may be particularly susceptible to adverse effects of these drugs. H2 receptor blockers are metabolized in the liver and excreted through the kidneys. Therefore, patients with kidney or liver problems may require reduced doses in order to maintain safe blood levels of the drugs.

Although the safety and effectiveness of H2 receptor blockers in patients over the age of 65 appears to be similar to that seen in younger patients, age-associated reductions in kidney function may lead to elevated blood levels.

Allergic reactions to these drugs are rare but have been reported.

The histamine H2 receptor blockers are **Pregnancy** category B. There are no adequate and well-controlled studies with these agents in pregnant women. Women should use them only when clearly needed and when the potential benefits outweigh the potential hazards to the fetus. Cimetidine is known to cross the placenta.

All drugs in this class are excreted into breast milk and should not be taken by nursing women. Decide whether to discontinue nursing, or discontinue the drug, taking into account the importance of the drug to the mother.

These drugs may mask the symptoms of **stomach cancer**.

Side effects

Although side effects due to the H2 receptor blockers are relatively rare and usually mild, a large number of adverse effects have been reported, in part because of the high use of these drugs. For example, the most common single adverse effect of cimetidine has been a 4% incidence of breast enlargement among males taking the drug in high doses for hypersecretory conditions. Similarly, the incidence of **headache** among high-dose cimetidine patients was 3.5%. Among patients taking lower doses, the frequency of headache was 2.1% compared to 2.3% in a placebo control group. Decreased **white blood cell count** was reported in 1 in 1,000,000 patients.

The reported side effects from the H2 receptor blocks are:

- abdominal pain
- back, leg, or stomach pain
- bleeding or crusting sores on lips
- blistering, burning, redness, scaling, or tenderness of skin
- blisters on palms of hands and soles of feet
- changes in vision or blurred vision
- coughing or difficulty in swallowing
- dark-colored urine
- dizziness
- fainting
- fast, pounding, or irregular heartbeat
- fever and/or chills
- flu-like symptoms
- general feeling of discomfort or illness
- hives
- inflammation of blood vessels
- joint pain
- light-colored stools
- mood or mental changes, including anxiety, agitation, confusion, hallucinations (seeing, hearing, or feeling things that are not there), mental depression, nervousness, or severe mental illness
- muscle cramps or aches
- nausea, vomiting, or loss of appetite
- pain
- peeling or sloughing of skin
- red or irritated eyes
- shortness of breath
- skin rash or itching
- slow heartbeat
- sore throat
- sores, ulcers, or white spots on lips, in mouth, or on genitals
- sudden difficult breathing
- swelling of face, lips, mouth, tongue, or eyelids
- swelling of hands or feet
- swollen or painful glands
- tightness in chest
- troubled breathing, unusually slow or irregular breathing
- unusual bleeding or bruising
- unusual tiredness or weakness
- wheezing
- yellow eyes or skin

Less frequently reported are

- constipation
- decreased sexual ability (especially in patients with Zollinger-Ellison disease who have received high doses of cimetidine for at least 1 year)
- decrease in sexual desire
- diarrhea
- difficult urination
- dizziness
- drowsiness
- dryness of mouth or skin
- headache
- increased or decreased urination
- increased sweating
- loss of hair
- ringing or buzzing in ears
- runny nose
- swelling of breasts or breast soreness in females and males
- trouble in sleeping

Not all of these adverse effects have been reported with all of the H2 receptor blockers, and some of the adverse effects may not have been drug related. However, because of the high similarity between drugs in this class, any of the reported adverse effects may be considered a possible result of therapy.

KEY TERMS

Duodenal—Pertaining to the first part of the small intestine.

Gastric—Pertaining to the stomach.

Hirsutism—Abnormal growth of hair on a woman's face and body.

Histamine—A physiologically active compound found in plant and animal tissue and released from mast cells as part of an allergic reaction in humans. It stimulates gastric secretion and causes dilation of capillaries, constriction of bronchial smooth muscle, and decreased blood pressure.

Hypersecretory—Excessive secretions, overproduction of stomach acid.

Mast cell—A cell found in connective tissue that releases substances such as heparin and histamine in response to injury or inflammation of bodily tissues.

Peptic—Induced by or associated with the action of digestive secretions.

Ulcer—A slow-healing sore on the surface of a mucous membrane, especially the membrane lining the stomach or other part of the digestive tract.

Zollinger-Ellizon syndrome—Severe peptic ulceration from excessive stomach acid production stimulated by one or more tumors that produce a powerful acid secretion.

Interactions

Cimetidine and ranitidine are both metabolized in the liver using the cytochrome P450 oxidase enzyme system. Since the same enzymes metabolize many drugs, taking two or more drugs that affect the same group of enzymes may cause one of the drugs to be retained in the body longer than would have been expected. The following is a partial list of drugs which may interact with cimetidine, or to a lesser extent with ranitidine.

- benzodiazepines, including Valium, Librium and Xanax
- caffeine
- calcium channel blockers, including Adalat, Calan, Procadia, and others
- carbamazepine
- chloroquine
- labetolol
- lidocaine
- metoprolol
- metronidazole
- phenytoin
- propranolol
- quinidine
- quinine
- sulfonylureas (includes many of the drugs used to treat diabetes)
- theophyllines (used to treat asthma; Dyphylline, a member of this group, does not interact with cimetidine)
- triamterene (a diuretic drug rarely used alone but may be found in fixed combinations, including Dyazide and Maxzide)
- tricyclic antidepressants (a group that includes amitriptyline, imipramine, and others)
- valproic acid
- warfarin

Additional drugs may also interact with the H2 receptor blockers, particularly those which might have a similar mechanism or action or adverse effects.

Resources

BOOKS

Beers, Mark H., Robert S. Porter, and Thomas V. Jones, eds. *The Merck Manual of Diagnosis and Therapy*. 18th ed. Whitehouse Station, NJ: Merck Research Laboratories, 2006.

Physicians' Desk Reference 2005. Montvale, NJ: Thomson Healthcare, 2004.

Robertson, Jason, et al. *The Harriet Lane Handbook: A Manual for Pediatric House Officers*. Orlando, FL: Mosby, 2005.

PERIODICALS

Black, R. A., and D. A. Hill. "Over-the-counter medications in pregnancy." *American Family Physician* 67, no. 12 (June 15, 2003): 2517–24.

Chandramouli, J. "What is the most effective therapy for preventing NSAID-induced gastropathy?" *Journal of Pain and Palliative Care Pharmacotherapy* 16, no. 2 (2002): 23–36.

ORGANIZATIONS

American College of Gastroenterology, PO Box 342260, Bethesda, MD, 20827-2260, (301) 263-9000, http://www.acg.gi.org.

American Gastroenterological Association (AGA), 4930 Del Ray Avenue, Bethesda, MD, 20814, (301) 654-2055, (301) 654-5920, member@gastro.org, http://www.gastro.org.

Samuel D. Uretsky, Pharm.D.

Habitual abortion *see* **Recurrent miscarriage**

Hair transplantation

Definition

Hair transplantation is a surgical procedure used to treat baldness or hair loss. Typically, tiny patches of scalp are removed from the back and sides of the head and implanted in the bald spots in the front and top of the head.

Purpose

Hair transplantation is a cosmetic procedure performed on men (and occasionally on women) who have significant hair loss, thinning hair, or bald spots where hair no longer grows. In men, hair loss and baldness are most commonly due to genetic factors (a tendency passed on in families) and age. Male pattern baldness, in which the hairline gradually recedes to expose more and more of the forehead, is the most common form. Men may also experience a gradual thinning of hair at the crown or very top of the skull. For women, hair loss is more commonly due to hormonal changes and is more likely to be a thinning of hair from the entire head. An estimated 50,000 men get transplants each year. Transplants can also be done to replace hair lost due to **burns**, injury, or diseases of the scalp.

Precautions

Although hair transplantation is a fairly simple procedure, some risks are associated with any surgery. It is important to inform the physician about any medications currently being used and about previous allergic reactions to drugs or anesthetic agents. Patients with blood clotting disorders also need to inform their physician before the procedure is performed.

Description

Hair transplantation surgery is performed by a physician in an office, clinic, or hospital setting. Each surgery lasts two to three hours during which approximately 250 grafts will be transplanted. A moderately balding man may require up to 1,000 grafts to get good coverage of a bald area, so a series of surgeries scheduled three to four months apart is usually required. The patient may be completely awake during the procedure with just a local anesthetic drug applied to numb the areas of the scalp. Some patients may be given a drug to help them relax or may be given an anesthetic drug that puts them to sleep.

The most common transplant procedure uses a thin strip of hair and scalp from the back of the head. This strip is cut into smaller clumps of five or six hairs. Tiny cuts are made in the balding area of the scalp and a clump is implanted into each slit. The doctor performing the surgery will attempt to recreate a natural looking hairline along the forehead. Mini-grafts, micrografts, or implants of single hair follicles can be used to fill in between larger implant sites and can provide a more natural-looking hairline. The implants will also be arranged so that thick and thin hairs are interspersed and the hair will grow in the same direction.

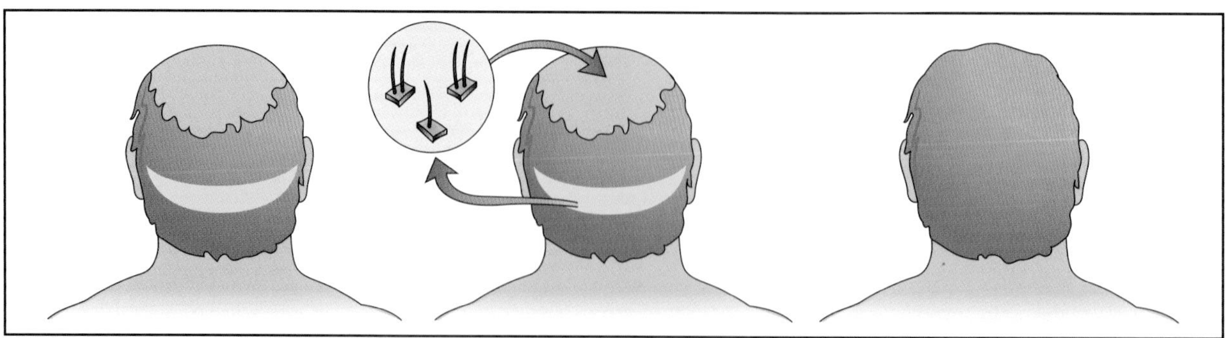

The most common hair transplant procedure involves taking small strips of scalp containing hair follicles from the donor area, usually at the sides or back of the head. These strips are then divided into several hundred smaller grafts. The surgeon relocates these grafts containing skin, follicle, and hair to tiny holes in the balding area by using microsurgical instruments or lasers. *(Illustration by Electronic Illustrators Group. Reproduced by permission of Gale, a part of Cengage Learning.)*

KEY TERMS

Anesthetic agents—Medication or drugs that can be injected with a needle or rubbed onto and area to make it numb before a surgical procedure. Anesthesia drugs may also be given by mouth, breathed in as a gas, or injected into a vein or muscle to make a patient relaxed or unconscious.

Hair follicle—A tube-like indentation in the skin from which a single hair grows.

Minigraft or micrograft—Transplantation of a small number of hair follicles, as few as one to three hairs, into a transplant site.

Transplantation—Surgically cutting out hair follicles and replanting them in a different spot on the head.

Another type of hair replacement surgery is called scalp reduction. This involves removing some of the skin from the hairless area and "stretching" some of the nearby hair-covered scalp over the cut-away area.

Health insurance will not pay for hair transplants that are done for cosmetic reasons. Insurance may pay for hair replacement surgery to correct hair loss due to accident, burn, or disease.

It is important to be realistic about what the final result of a hair transplant will look like. This procedure does not create new hair, it simply redistributes the hair that the patient still has. Some research has been conducted where chest hair has been transplanted to the balding scalp, but this procedure is not widely practiced.

Preparation

It is important to find a respected, well-established, experienced surgeon and discuss the expected results prior to the surgery. The patient may need blood tests to check for bleeding or clotting problems and may be asked not to take **aspirin** products before the surgery. The type of anesthesia used will depend on how extensive the surgery will be and where it will be performed. The patient may be awake during the procedure, but may be given medication to help them relax. A local anesthetic drug which numbs the area will be applied or injected into the skin at the surgery sites.

Aftercare

The area may need to be bandaged overnight. The patient can return to normal activities; however, strenuous activities should be avoided in the first few days after the surgery. On rare occasions, the implants can be "ejected" from the scalp during vigorous **exercise**. There may be some swelling, bruising, **headache**, and discomfort around the graft areas and around the eyes. These symptoms can usually be controlled with a mild **pain** reliever like aspirin. Scabs may form at the graft sites and should not be scraped off. There may be some **numbness** at the sites, but it will diminish within two to three months.

Risks

Although there are rare cases of infection or scarring, the major risk is probably that the grafted area does not look the way the patient expected it to look.

Normal results

The transplanted hair will fall out within a few weeks, however, new hair will start to grow in the graft sites within about three months. A normal rate of hair growth is about 0.25–0.5 in (6–13 mm) per month.

Abnormal results

Major complications as a result of hair transplantation are extremely rare. Occasionally, a patient may have problems with delayed healing, infection, scarring, or rejection of the graft, but this is uncommon.

Resources

OTHER

"Hair Transplant." Ienhance. http://www.ienhance.com.

"Transplants; Flap Surgery; and The Perfect Candidate." Transplant Network. http://www.hair-transplants.net.

ORGANIZATIONS

American Academy of Cosemetic Surgery, 737 North Michigan Ave., Suite 2100, Chicago, IL, 60611-5641, (312) 981-6760, (312) 981-6787, info@cosmeticsurgery.org, http://www.cosmeticsurgery.org.

American Academy of Facial Plastic and Reconstructive Surgery (AAFPRS), 310 South Henry Street, Alexandria, VA, 22314, (703) 299-9291, info@aafprs.org, http://www.aafprs.org/.

Altha Roberts Edgren

Hairy cell leukemia

Definition

Hairy cell leukemia is a disease in which a type of white blood cell called the lymphocyte, present in the blood and bone marrow, becomes malignant and proliferates. It is called hairy cell leukemia because the cells have tiny hair-like projections when viewed under the microscope.

Description

Hairy cell leukemia (HCL) is a rare **cancer**. It was first described in 1958 as *leukemic reticuloendotheliosis*, erroneously referring to a red blood cell because researchers were unsure of the cell of origin. It became more easily identifiable in the 1970s. There are approximately 600 new cases diagnosed every year in the United States, making up about 2% of the adult cases of leukemia each year.

HCL is found in cells located in the blood. There are three types of cells found in the blood: the red blood cells that carry oxygen to all the parts of the body; the white blood cells that are responsible for fighting infection and protecting the body from diseases; and the platelets that help in the clotting of blood. Hairy cell leukemia affects a type of white blood cell called the lymphocyte. Lymphocytes are made in the bone marrow, spleen, lymph nodes, and other organs. It specifically affects B-lymphocytes, which mature in the bone marrow. However, extremely rare variants of HCL have been discovered developing from T-lymphocytes, which mature in the thymus.

When hairy cell leukemia develops, the white blood cells become abnormal both in the way they appear (by acquiring hairy projections) and in the way they act (by proliferating without the normal control mechanisms).

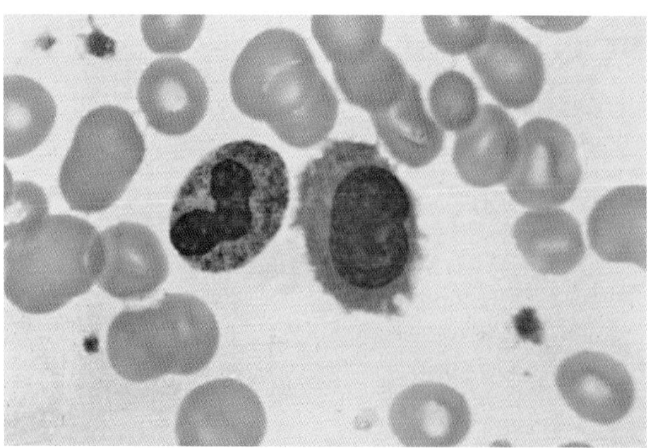

A magnified image of white blood cells with "hairy" projections. *(M. Abbey/Photo Researchers, Inc.)*

Further, the cells tend to accumulate in the spleen, causing it to become enlarged. The cells may also collect in the bone marrow and prevent it from producing normal blood cells. As a result, there may not be enough normal white blood cells in the blood to fight infection.

The median age at which people develop HCL is 52 years. Though it occurs in all ages, HCL more commonly develops in the older population. Men are four times more likely to develop HCL than women. There have been reports of familial aggregation of disease, with higher occurrences in Ashkenazi Jewish men. A potential genetic link is undergoing further investigation.

Causes and symptoms

The cause of hairy cell leukemia is not specifically known. However, exposure to radiation is a known cause of leukemia in general. Familial involvement is another theory, suggesting that there is a genetic component associated with this disease.

HCL is a chronic (slowly progressing) disease, and the patients may not show any symptoms for many years. As the disease advances, the patients may suffer from one or more of the following symptoms:

- weakness
- fatigue
- recurrent infections
- fever
- anemia
- bruising
- pain or discomfort in the abdominal area
- weight loss (uncommon)
- night sweats (uncommon)

Pain and discomfort are caused by an enlarged spleen, which results from the accumulation of the abnormal hairy cells in the spleen. Blood tests may show abnormal counts of all the different types of cells. This happens because the cancerous cells invade the bone marrow as well and prevent it from producing normal blood cells. Because of the low white cell count in the blood, the patient may have frequent infections. **Fever** often accompanies the infections. The patient is most susceptible to bacterial infections, but infections of any kind are the major cause of **death**. The low red cell count may cause anemia, **fatigue**, and weakness, and the low **platelet count** may cause the person to bruise and bleed easily.

Diagnosis

When a patient suffers from the above symptoms, the doctor will palpate the abdomen and may order

KEY TERMS

Anemia—A condition in which there is low iron in the blood due to a deficiency of red blood cells.

Bone marrow—The spongy tissue inside the large bones in the body that is responsible for making the red blood cells, white blood cells, and platelets.

Bone marrow aspiration and biopsy—A procedure in which a needle is inserted into the large bones of the hip or spine and a small piece of marrow is removed for microscopic examination.

Immunotherapy—A mode of cancer treatment in which the immune system is stimulated to fight the cancer.

Leukemia—A disease in which the cells that constitute the blood become cancerous or abnormal.

Lymph nodes—Oval-shaped organs that are the size of peas, located throughout the body, and contain clusters of cells called lymphocytes. They filter out and destroy the bacteria, foreign particles, and cancerous cells from the blood.

Malignant—Cells that have the ability to invade locally, cause destruction of surrounding tissue, and travel to other sites in the body.

Keratoconjunctivitis—Inflammation of the conjunctiva and cornea of the eye.

Spleen—An organ that lies next to the stomach. Its function is to remove the worn-out blood cells and foreign materials from the blood stream.

Splenectomy—A surgical procedure that involves the surgical removal of the spleen.

scans to see if the spleen is enlarged (splenomegaly). An enlarged spleen is present in 80% of patients. An enlarged liver is less common, but can occur.

If the spleen is enlarged, the doctor may order several blood tests. In these tests, the total numbers of each of the different types of blood cells (CBC) are reported. Sixty to eighty percent of patients suffer from pancytopenia, which is a dramatic reduction in the number of red blood cells, white blood cells, and platelets circulating in the blood.

If the blood tests are abnormal, the doctor may order a **bone marrow aspiration and biopsy**. In order to establish a diagnosis, hairy cells must be present in the bone marrow.

Treatment

When physicians perform blood tests, they will determine the level of hemoglobin (the oxygen-transporting molecule of red blood cells). Serum hemoglobin levels and the size of the spleen, which can be measured on exam and by using an x ray, are proposed criteria for determining the stage of HCL. The following are the three proposed stages and their criteria:

- Stage I: Hemoglobin greater than 12 g/dL (1 g = approximately 0.02 pint and 1 dL = approximately 0.33 ounce) and spleen less than or equal to 10 cm (3.9 inches).
- Stage II: Hemoglobin between 8.5 and 12 g/dL and spleen greater than 10 cm (3.9 inches).
- Stage III: Hemoglobin less than 8.5 g/dL and spleen greater than 10 cm (3.9 inches).

Since there is generally no accepted staging system, another method for evaluating the progression of HCL is to group patients into two categories: untreated HCL and progressive HCL, in which hairy cells are present after therapy has been administered.

Some people with hairy cell leukemia have very few or no symptoms at all, and it is reasonable to expect that 10% of patients may not need any treatment. However, if the patient is symptomatic and needs intervention, HCL is especially responsive to treatment.

There are three main courses of treatment: **chemotherapy**, **splenectomy** (surgical removal of the spleen), and immunotherapy. Once a patient meets treatment criteria, purine analogues, particularly the drugs pentostatin and cladribine, are the first-line therapy. Pentostatin is administered at 5mg/m^2 for two days every other week until total remission is achieved. Patients may experience side effects such as fever, **nausea**, **vomiting**, **photosensitivity**, and keratoconjuctivitis. However, follow-up studies estimate a relapse-free survival rate at 76%. Cladribine (2-CdA) taken at 0.1mg/kg/day for seven days also has an impressive response. Eighty-six percent of patients experience complete remission after treatment, while 16% experience partial remission. Fever is the principal side effect of 2-CdA.

Biological therapy or immunotherapy, where the body's own immune cells are used to fight cancer, is also being investigated in clinical trials for hairy cell leukemia. A substance called interferon that is produced by the white blood cells of the body was the first systemic treatment that showed consistent results in fighting

HCL. The FDA approved interferon-alpha (INF-alpha) to fight HCL. The mechanism by which INF-alpha works is not clearly understood. However, it is known that interferon stimulates the body's natural killer cells that are suppressed during HCL. The standard dosage is 2 MU/m^2 three times a week for 12 months. Side effects include fever, myalgia, malaise, **rashes**, and gastrointestinal complaints.

If the spleen is enlarged, it may be removed in a surgical procedure known as splenectomy. This usually causes a remission of the disease. However, 50% of patients that undergo splenectomy require some type of systemic treatment such as chemotherapy or immunotherapy. Splenectomy is not the most widely used course of treatment as it was many years ago. Although the spleen is not an indispensable organ, it is responsible for helping the body fight infection. Therefore, other therapies are preferred in order to salvage the spleen and its functions.

Most patients have excellent prognosis and can expect to live 10 years or longer. The disease may remain silent for years with treatment. Continual follow-up is necessary to monitor the patient for relapse and determine true cure rates.

Alternative treatment

Many individuals choose to supplement traditional therapy with complementary methods. Often, these methods improve the tolerance of side effects and symptoms as well as enrich the quality of life. The American Cancer Society recommends that patients talk to their doctor to ensure that the methods they are using are safely supplementing traditional therapy. Some complementary treatments include the following:

- yoga
- meditation
- religious practices and prayer
- music therapy
- art therapy
- massage therapy
- aromatherapy

Prevention

Since the cause for the disease is unknown and there are no specific risk factors, there is no known prevention.

Resources

BOOKS

Abeloff, Martin D., et al. *Clinical Oncology*. 4th ed. New York: Churchill Livingstone/Elsevier, 2008.

Saven, A. *Hairy Cell Leukemia, An Issue of Hematology/Oncology Clinics*. Philadelphia: Saunders, 2006.

OTHER

"Coping With Side Effects." National Cancer Institute. July 2, 2001. http://cancernet.nci.nih.gov/chemotherapy/chemoside.html.

NCI/PDQ Patient Statement, "Hairy cell leukemia." National Cancer Institute, 2001.

ORGANIZATIONS

American Cancer Society, 1599 Clifton Rd. NE, Atlanta, GA, 30329, (800) 227-2345, http://www.cancer.org.

Cancer Research Institute (National Headquarters), One Exchange Plaza, 55 Broadway, Suite 1802, New York, NY, (212) 688-7515, (212) 832-9376, (800) 992-2623, http://www.cancerresearch.org/.

Hairy Cell Leukemia Research Foundation, 790 Estate Drive, Suite 180, Deerfield, IL, 60015, (866) 376-0046, hairycellpatientservices@hotmail.com, http://www.hairycellleukemia.org/.

Leukemia and Lymphoma Society, 1311 Mamaroneck Avenue, Suite 310, White Plains, NY, 10605, (800) 955-4572, http://www.leukemia-lymphoma.org.

National Cancer Institute (National Institutes of Health), NCI Office of Communications and Education, 6116 Executive Blvd., Suite 300, Bethesda, MD, 20892-8322, (800) 4-CANCER (422-6237), cancergovstaff@mail.nih.gov, http://www.cancer.gov/.

Oncolink. University of Pennsylvania Cancer Center, 3400 Spruce Street, 2 Donner, Philadelphia, PA, 19104, (215) 349-8895, (215) 349-5445, hampshire@uphs.upenn.edu, http://oncolink.org.

Lata Cherath, PhD
Sally C. McFarlane-Parrott

Halitosis *see* **Bad breath**

Hallucinations

Definition

Hallucinations are false or distorted sensory experiences that appear to be real perceptions. These sensory impressions are generated by the mind rather than by any external stimuli, and may be seen, heard, felt, and even smelled or tasted.

Description

A hallucination occurs when environmental, emotional, or physical factors such as **stress**, medication, extreme **fatigue**, or mental illness cause the mechanism within the brain that helps to distinguish conscious perceptions from internal, memory-based perceptions to

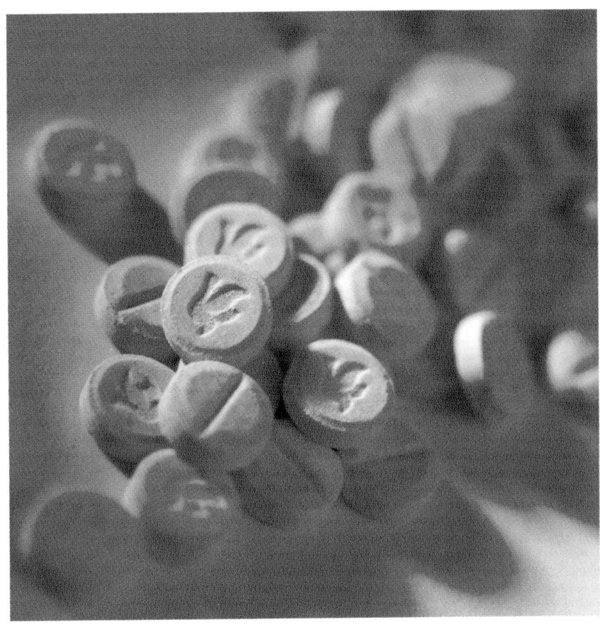

Ecstasy tablets. *(© Andrew Brookes/Corbis.)*

misfire. As a result, hallucinations occur during periods of consciousness. They can appear in the form of visions, voices or sounds, tactile feelings (known as haptic hallucinations), smells, or tastes.

Patients suffering from **dementia** and psychotic disorders such as **schizophrenia** frequently experience hallucinations. Hallucinations can also occur in patients who are not mentally ill as a result of stress overload or exhaustion, or may be intentionally induced through the use of drugs, **meditation**, or sensory deprivation. A 1996 report published in the *British Journal of Psychiatry* noted that 37% of 4,972 people surveyed experienced hypnagogic hallucinations (hallucinations that occur as a person is falling to sleep). Hypnopomic hallucinations (hallucinations that occur just upon waking) were reported by 12% of the sample.

Causes and symptoms

Common causes of hallucinations include:

- Drugs. Hallucinogenics such as ecstasy (3,4-methylenedioxymethamphetamine, or MDMA), LSD (lysergic acid diethylamide, or acid), mescaline (3,4,5-trimethoxyphenethylamine, or peyote), and psilocybin (4-phosphoryloxy-N, N-dimethyltryptamine, or mushrooms) trigger hallucinations. Other drugs, such as marijuana and PCP, have hallucinatory effects. Certain prescription medications may also cause hallucinations. In addition, drug withdrawal may induce tactile and visual hallucinations as in an alcoholic suffering from delirium tremens (DTs).
- Stress. Prolonged or extreme stress can impede thought processes and trigger hallucinations.
- Sleep deprivation and/or exhaustion. Physical and emotional exhaustion can induce hallucinations by blurring the line between sleep and wakefulness.
- Meditation and/or sensory deprivation. When the brain lacks external stimulation to form perceptions, it may compensate by referencing the memory and form hallucinatory perceptions. This condition is commonly found in blind and deaf individuals.
- Electrical or neurochemical activity in the brain. A hallucinatory sensation—usually involving touch—called an aura, often appears before, and gives warning of, a migraine. Also, auras involving smell and touch (tactile) are known to warn of the onset of an epileptic attack.
- Mental illness. Up to 75% of schizophrenic patients admitted for treatment report hallucinations.
- Brain damage or disease. Lesions or injuries to the brain may alter brain function and produce hallucinations.

Diagnosis

Aside from hypnogogic and hypnopompic hallucinations, more than one event suggests a person should seek evaluation. A general physician, psychologist, or psychiatrist will try to rule out possible organic, environmental, or psychological causes through a detailed medical examination and social history. If a psychological cause such as schizophrenia is suspected, a psychologist will typically conduct an interview with the patient and his family and administer one of several clinical inventories, or tests, to evaluate the mental status of the patient.

Occasionally, people who are in good mental health will experience a hallucination. If hallucinations are infrequent and transitory and can be accounted for by short-term environmental factors such as **sleep deprivation** or meditation, no treatment may be necessary. However, if hallucinations are hampering an individual's ability to function, a general physician, psychologist, or psychiatrist should be consulted to pinpoint their source and recommend a treatment plan.

Treatment

Hallucinations that are symptomatic of a mental illness such as schizophrenia should be treated by a psychologist or psychiatrist. Antipsychotic medication

KEY TERMS

Aura—A subjective sensation or motor phenomenon that precedes and indicates the onset of a neurological episode, such as a migraine or an epileptic seizure.

Hypnogogic hallucination—A hallucination, such as the sensation of falling, that occurs at the onset of sleep.

Hypnopompic hallucination—A hallucination that occurs as a person is waking from sleep.

Sensory deprivation—A situation where an individual finds himself in an environment without sensory cues. Also, (used here) the act of shutting one's senses off to outside sensory stimuli to achieve hallucinatory experiences and/or to observe the psychological results.

such as thioridazine (Mellaril), haloperidol (Haldol), chlorpromazine (Thorazine), clozapine (Clozaril), or risperidone (Risperdal) may be prescribed.

Prognosis

In many cases, chronic hallucinations caused by schizophrenia or some other mental illness can be controlled by medication. If hallucinations persist, psychosocial therapy can be helpful in teaching the patient the coping skills to deal with them. Hallucinations due to sleep deprivation or extreme stress generally stop after the cause is removed.

ORGANIZATIONS

American Psychological Association (APA), 750 First St. NE, Washington, DC, 20002-4242, (202) 336-5500, (800) 374-2721, http://www.apa.org/.

National Alliance for the Mentally Ill (NAMI), 3803 N. Fairfax Dr., Ste. 100, Arlington, VA, 22203, (703) 524-7600, (703) 524-9094, (800) 950-6264, http://www.nami.org.

Paula Anne Ford-Martin

Hallucinogen *see* **Lysergic acid diethylamide**

Hallux valgus *see* **Bunion**

Haloperidol *see* **Antipsychotic drugs**

Hammertoe

Definition

Hammertoe is a condition in which the toe is bent in a claw-like position. It can be present in more than one toe but is most common in the second toe.

Description

Hammertoe is described as a deformity in which the toes bend downward with the toe joint usually enlarged. Over time, the joint enlarges and stiffens as it rubs against shoes. Other foot structures involved include the overlying skin and blood vessels and nerves connected to the involved toes.

Causes and symptoms

The shortening of tendons responsible for the control and movement of the affected toe or toes cause hammertoe. Top portions of the toes become callused from the friction produced against the inside of shoes. This common foot problem often results from improper fit of footwear. This is especially the case with high-heeled shoes placing pressure on the front part of the foot that compresses the smaller toes tightly together. The condition frequently stems from muscle imbalance, and usually leaves the affected individual with impaired balance.

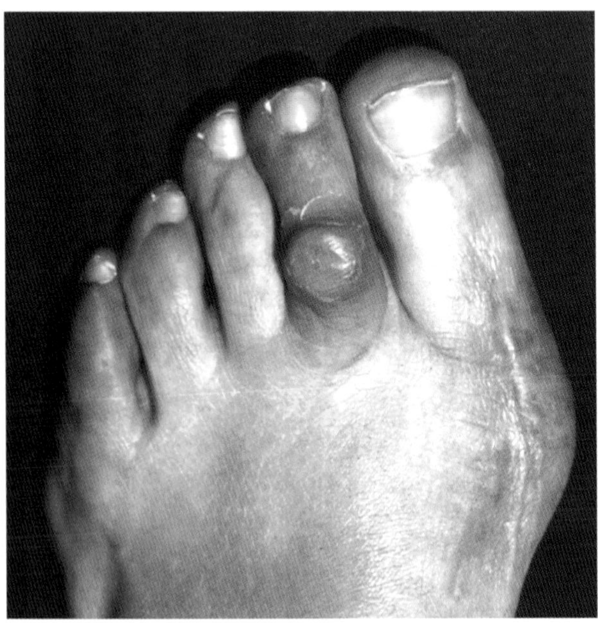

Hammertoe most commonly affects the second toe which, as shown, often develops a corn over the deformity. *(Custom Medical Stock Photo, Inc. Reproduced by permission.)*

Diagnosis

A thorough medical history and physical exam by a physician is always necessary for the proper diagnosis of hammertoe and other foot conditions. Because the condition involves bony deformity, x rays can help to confirm the diagnosis.

Treatment

Conservative

Wearing proper footwear and stockings with plenty of room in the toe region can provide treatment for hammertoe. Stretching exercises may be helpful in lengthening the excessively tight tendons.

Surgery

In advanced cases where conservative treatment is unsuccessful, surgery may be recommended. The tendons that attach to the involved toes are located and an incision is made to free the connective tissue to the foot bones. Additional incisions are made so the toes no longer bend in a downward fashion. The middle joints of the affected toes are connected permanently with surgical hardware such as pins and wire sutures. The incision is then closed with fine sutures. These sutures are removed approximately 7 to 10 days after surgery.

Alternative treatment

Various soft tissue and joint treatments offered by **chiropractic** and **massage therapy** may be useful to decrease the tightness of the affected structures.

Prognosis

If detected early, hammertoe can be treated nonsurgically. If surgery becomes necessary, surgical risks are minimal with the overall outcome providing good results.

Prevention

Wearing comfortable shoes that fit well can prevent many foot ailments. Foot width may increase with age. Feet should always be measured before buying shoes. The upper part of the shoes should be made of a soft, flexible material to match the shape of the foot. Shoes made of leather can reduce the possibility of skin irritations. Soles should provide solid footing and not be slippery. Thick soles lessen pressure when walking on hard surfaces. Low-heeled shoes are more comfortable, safer, and less damaging than high-heeled shoes.

ORGANIZATIONS

American Orthopaedic Foot and Ankle Society, 6300 N. River Road, Suite 510, Rosemont, IL, 60018, (847) 698-4654, (800) 235-4855.

American Podiatric Medical Association, 9312 Old George town Road, Bethesda, MD, 20814-1621, (301) 581-9200, http://www.apma.org.

Jeffrey P. Larson, RPT

Hand–foot–and–mouth disease

Definition

Hand–foot–and–mouth disease is an infection of young children in which characteristic fluid–filled blisters appear on the hands, feet, and inside the mouth.

Demographics

Hand–foot–and-mouth disease is very common among young children and often occurs in clusters of children who are in daycare together.

An outbreak of hand–foot–and–mouth disease occurred in Singapore in 2000, with more than 1,000 diagnosed cases, all in children, resulting in four deaths. A smaller outbreak occurred in Malaysia in 2000. In 1998, a serious outbreak of enterovirus 71 in Taiwan resulted in more than one million cases of hand–foot–and–mouth disease. Of these, there were 405 severe cases

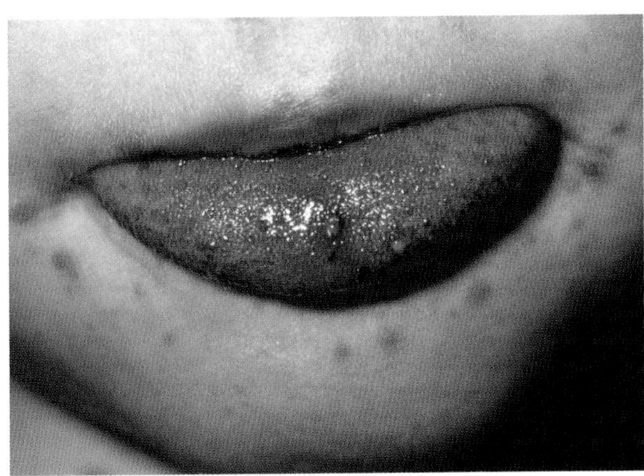

Skin lesions on the tongue and around the mouth of a five-year-old boy due to hand-foot-mouth disease. *(Dr. P. Marazzi/ Photo Researchers, Inc.)*

and 78 deaths, 71 of which were children younger than five years of age.

Hand–foot–and–mouth should not be confused with foot and mouth disease, which infects cattle but is extremely rare in humans. An outbreak of foot and mouth disease swept through Great Britain and into other parts of Europe and South America in 2001.

Description

Coxsackie viruses belong to a family of viruses called enteroviruses. These viruses live in the gastrointestinal tract and are therefore present in feces. They can be spread easily from one person to another when poor hygiene allows the virus within the feces to be passed from person to person. After exposure to the virus, development of symptoms takes only four to six days. Hand–foot–and–mouth disease can occur year–round, although the largest number of cases are in summer and fall months.

Causes and symptoms

Hand–foot–and–mouth disease is very common among young children and often occurs in clusters of children who are in daycare together. It is spread when poor hand–washing after a diaper change or contact with saliva (drool) allows the virus to be passed from one child to another.

Within about four to six days of acquiring the virus, an infected child may develop a relatively low–grade **fever**, ranging from 99–102°F (37–38.9°C). Other symptoms include **fatigue**, loss of energy, decreased appetite, and a sore sensation in the mouth that may interfere with feeding. After one to two days, fluid–filled bumps (vesicles) appear on the inside of the mouth, along the surface of the tongue, on the roof of the mouth, and on the insides of the cheeks. These are tiny blisters, about three to seven millimeters in diameter. Eventually, they may appear on the palms of the hands and on the soles of the feet. Occasionally, these vesicles may occur in the diaper region.

The vesicles in the mouth cause the majority of discomfort, and the child may refuse to eat or drink due to **pain**. This phase usually lasts for an average of a week. As long as the bumps have clear fluid within them, the disease is at its most contagious. The fluid within the vesicles contains large quantities of the causative viruses. Extra care should be taken to avoid contact with this fluid.

KEY TERMS

Enteroviruses—Viruses which live in the gastrointestinal tract. Coxsackie viruses, viruses that cause hand–foot–mouth disease, are an enterovirus.

Vesicle—A bump on the skin filled with fluid.

Diagnosis

Diagnosis is made by most practitioners solely on the basis of the unique appearance of blisters of the mouth, hands, and feet in a child not appearing very ill.

Treatment

There are no treatments available to cure or decrease the duration of the disease. Medications like **acetaminophen** or ibuprofen may be helpful for decreasing pain, and allowing the child to eat and drink. It is important to try to encourage the child to take in adequate amounts of fluids, in the form of ice chips or popsicles if other foods or liquids are too uncomfortable.

Alternative treatment

There are no effective alternative treatments for hand–foot–and–mouth disease.

Prognosis

The prognosis for a child with hand–foot–and–mouth disease is excellent. The child is usually completely better within about a week of the start of the illness.

Prevention

Prevention involves careful attention to hygiene. Thorough, consistent hand–washing practices and discouraging the sharing of clothes, towels, and stuffed toys are all helpful. The virus continues to be passed in the feces for several weeks after infection, so good hygiene should be practiced long after all signs of infection have passed.

Resources

BOOKS

Morag, Abraham, and Pearay L. Ogra. "Viral Infections." In Behrman, Richard, editor. *Nelson Textbook of Pediatrics*, 16th ed. Philadelphia: W.B. Saunders Co., 2000.

PERIODICALS

Lee T.C., et al. "Diseases Caused by Enterovirus 71 Infection." *The Pediatric Infectious Disease Journal*. 28(10) (October 2009): 904–10.

Ooi M.H., et al. "Identification and Validation of Clinical Predictors for the risk of Neurological Involvement in

Children with Hand, Foot, and Mouth Disease in Sarawak." *BMC Infectious Diseases*. 9 (January 19 2009): 3.

Rosalyn Carson–DeWitt, MD
Ken R. Wells
Karl Finley

Hand-Schüller-Christian syndrome *see* **Histiocytosis X**

Hansen's disease *see* **Leprosy**

Hantavirus infections

Definition

Hantavirus infection is caused by a group of viruses that can infect humans with two serious illnesses: hemorrhagic **fever** with renal syndrome (HFRS), and Hantavirus pulmonary syndrome (HPS).

Description

Hantaviruses are found without causing symptoms within various species of rodents and are passed to humans by exposure to the urine, feces, or saliva of those infected rodents. Ten different hantaviruses have been identified as important in humans. Each is found in specific geographic regions and therefore is spread by different rodent carriers. Further, each type of virus causes a slightly different form of illness in its human hosts:

- Hantaan virus is carried by the striped field mouse and exists in Korea, China, Eastern Russia, and the Balkans. Hantaan virus causes a severe form of hemorrhagic fever with renal syndrome (HFRS).
- Puumula virus is carried by bank voles and exists in Scandinavia, western Russia, and Europe. Puumula virus causes a milder form of HFRS, usually termed *nephropathia epidemica*.
- Seoul virus is carried by a type of rat called the Norway rat and exists worldwide, but causes disease almost exclusively in Asia. Seoul virus causes a form of HFRS that is slightly milder than that caused by Hantaan virus, but results in liver complications.
- Prospect Hill virus is carried by meadow voles and exists in the United States, but has not been found to cause human disease.
- Sin Nombre virus, the most predominant strain in the United States, is carried by the deer mouse. This virus was responsible for severe cases of HPS that occurred in the southwestern United States in 1993.
- Black Creek Canal virus has been found in Florida. It is predominantly carried by cotton rats.
- New York virus strain has been documented in New York State. The vectors for this virus seem to be deer mice and white-footed mice.
- Bayou virus has been reported in Louisiana and Texas and is carried by the marsh rice rat.
- Blue River virus has been found in Indiana and Oklahoma and seems to be associated with the white-footed mouse.
- Monongahela virus, discovered in 2000, has been found in Pennsylvania and is transmitted by the white-footed mouse.

Causes and symptoms

Hemorrhagic fever with renal syndrome (HFRS)

Hantaviruses that produce forms of hemorrhagic fever with renal syndrome (HFRS) cause a classic group of symptoms, including fever, malfunction of the kidneys, and low **platelet count**. Because platelets are blood cells important in proper clotting, low numbers of circulating platelets can result in spontaneous bleeding, or hemorrhage.

Patients with HFRS have **pain** in the head, abdomen, and lower back and may report bloodshot eyes and blurry vision. Tiny pinpoint hemorrhages, called petechiae, may appear on the upper body and the soft palate in the mouth. The patient's face, chest, abdomen, and back often appear flushed and red, as if sunburned.

After about five days, the patient may have a sudden drop in blood pressure; often it drops low enough to cause the clinical syndrome called **shock**. Shock is a state in which blood circulation throughout the body is insufficient to deliver proper quantities of oxygen. Lengthy shock can result in permanent damage to the body's organs, particularly the brain, which is very sensitive to oxygen deprivation.

Around day eight of HFRS, kidney involvement results in multiple derangements of the body chemistry. Simultaneously, the hemorrhagic features of the illness begin to cause spontaneous bleeding, as demonstrated by bloody urine, bloody vomit, and in very serious cases, brain hemorrhages with resulting changes in consciousness.

Day 11 often brings further chemical derangements, with associated confusion, **hallucinations**, seizures, and lung complications. Those who survive this final phase usually begin to turn the corner toward recovery at this time, although recovery takes approximately six weeks.

KEY TERMS

Hemodialysis—A method of mechanically cleansing the blood outside of the body, in order to remove various substances that would normally be cleared by the kidneys. Hemodialysis is used when an individual is in relative, or complete, kidney failure.

Hemorrhagic—A condition resulting in massive, difficult-to-control bleeding.

Petechiae—Pinpoint size red spots caused by hemorrhaging under the skin.

Platelets—Circulating blood cells that are crucial to the mechanism of clotting.

Prodrome—Early symptoms or warning signs

Pulmonary—Referring to the lungs.

Renal—Referring to the kidneys.

Shock—Shock is a state in which blood circulation is insufficient to deliver adequate oxygen to vital organs.

Hantavirus pulmonary syndrome (HPS)

Hantavirus pulmonary syndrome (HPS) develops in four stages. They are:

- The incubation period. This lasts from one to five weeks from exposure. Here, the patient may exhibit no symptoms.
- The prodrome, or warning signs, stage. Symptoms begin with a fever, muscle aches, headache, dizziness, and abdominal pain and upset. Sometimes there is vomiting and diarrhea.
- The cardiopulmonary stage. The patient slips into this stage rapidly, sometimes within a day or two of initial symptoms, sometimes as long as 10 days later. There is a drop in blood pressure, shock, and leaking of the blood vessels of the lungs, which results in fluid accumulation in the lungs, and subsequent shortness of breath. The fluid accumulation can be so rapid and so severe as to put the patient in respiratory failure within only a few hours. Some patients experience severe abdominal tenderness.
- The convalescent stage. If the patient survives the respiratory complications of the previous stage, there is a rapid recovery, usually within a day or two. However, abnormal liver and lung functioning may persist for six months.

Diagnosis

Serologic techniques help diagnose a hantavirus infection. The patient's blood is drawn, and the ELISA (enzyme-linked immunosorbent assay) is done in a laboratory to identify the presence of specific immune substances (antibodies)—substances which an individual's body would only produce in response to the hantavirus.

It is very difficult to demonstrate the actual virus in human tissue or to grow cultures of the virus within the laboratory, so the majority of diagnostic tests use indirect means to demonstrate the presence of the virus.

Treatment

Treatment of hantavirus infections is primarily supportive because there are no agents available to kill the viruses and interrupt the infection. Broad-spectrum **antibiotics** are given until the diagnosis is confirmed. Supportive care consists of providing treatment in response to the patient's symptoms. Because both HFRS and HPS progress so rapidly, patients must be closely monitored so that treatment may be started at the first sign of a particular problem. Low blood pressure is treated with medications. Blood transfusions are given for both hemorrhage and shock states. Hemodialysis is used in kidney failure. (Hemodialysis involves mechanically cleansing the blood outside of the body, to replace the kidney's normal function of removing various toxins form the blood.) Rapid respiratory assistance is critical, often requiring intubation.

The anti-viral agent ribavirin has been approved for use in early treatment of hantavirus infections.

Prognosis

The diseases caused by hantaviruses are extraordinarily lethal. About 6–15% of people who contract HFRS have died. Almost half of all people who contract HPS will die. This gives HPS one of the highest fatality rates of any acute viral disease. It is essential that people living in areas where the hantaviruses exist seek quick medical treatment should they begin to develop an illness that might be due to a hantavirus.

Prevention

There are no immunizations currently available against any of the hantaviruses. In 2003, developments in genetic science were helping researchers work on a possible **vaccination** and therapy for several versions of hantavirus, including the Sin Nombre virus that causes HPS. With further work, a gene-based vaccine could become available in the future. However, the only known forms of hantavirus prevention involve rodent control within the community and within individual households. The following is a list of preventive measures:

- Avoiding areas known to be infested by rodents is essential.
- Keeping a clean home and keeping food in rodent-proof containers.
- Disposing of garbage and emptying pet food dishes at night.
- Setting rodent traps around baseboards and in tight places. Disposing of dead animals with gloves and disinfecting the area with bleach.
- Using rodenticide as necessary.
- Sealing any entry holes 0.25 inch wide or wider around foundations with screen, cement, or metal flashing.
- Clearing brush and junk from house foundations.
- Putting metal flashing around house foundations.
- Elevating hay, woodpiles, and refuse containers.
- Airing out all sealed outbuildings or cabins 30 minutes before cleaning for the season.
- When camping, avoiding sleeping on the bare ground. It is advised to sleep on a cot or in a tent with a floor.

Resources

BOOKS

Fong, I.W., and Ken Alibek. *New and Evolving Infections of the 21st Century*. New York: Springer, 2007.

PERIODICALS

"DNA Vaccine Protects Against Hantavirus Pulmonary Syndrome." *Heart Disease Weekly*. November 2, 2003: 31.

Janie F. Franz
Teresa G. Odle

Haptoglobin test

Definition

This test is done to help evaluate a person for **hemolytic anemia**.

Purpose

Haptoglobin is a blood protein made by the liver. The haptoglobin levels decrease in hemolytic anemia. Hemolytic **anemias** include a variety of conditions that result in hemolyzed, or burst, red blood cells.

Decreased values can also indicate a slower type of red cell destruction unrelated to anemia. For example, destruction can be caused by mechanical heart valves or abnormal hemoglobin, such as **sickle cell disease** or **thalassemia**.

Haptoglobin is known as an acute phase reactant. Its level increases during acute conditions such as infection, injury, tissue destruction, some cancers, **burns**, surgery, or trauma. Its purpose is to remove damaged cells and debris and rescue important material such as iron. Haptoglobin levels can be used to monitor the course of these conditions.

Description

Hemoglobin is the protein in the red blood cell that carries oxygen throughout the body. Iron is an essential part of hemoglobin; without iron, hemoglobin can not function. Haptoglobin's main role is to save iron by attaching itself to any hemoglobin released from a red cell.

When red blood cells are destroyed, the hemoglobin is released. Haptoglobin is always present in the blood waiting to bind to released hemoglobin. White blood cells (called macrophages) bring the haptoglobin-hemoglobin complex to the liver, where the haptoglobin and hemoglobin are separated and the iron is recycled.

In hemolytic anemia, so many red cells are destroyed that most of the available haptoglobin is needed to bind the released hemoglobin. The more severe the hemolysis, the less haptoglobin remains in the blood.

Haptoglobin is measured in several different ways. One way is called rate nephelometry. A person's serum is mixed with a substance that will bind to haptoglobin. The amount of bound haptoglobin is measured using a rate nephelometer, which measures the amount of light scattered by the bound haptoglobin. Another way of measuring haptoglobin is to measure it according to how much hemoglobin it can bind.

Preparation

This test requires 5 mL of blood. The person being tested should avoid taking **oral contraceptives** or androgens before this test. A healthcare worker ties a tourniquet on the person's upper arm, locates a vein in the inner elbow region, and inserts a needle into that vein. Vacuum action draws the blood through the needle into an attached tube. Collection of the sample takes only a few minutes.

KEY TERMS

Acute phase reactant—A substance in the blood that increases as a response to an acute condition such as infection, injury, tissue destruction, some cancers, burns, surgery, or trauma.

Haptoglobin—A blood protein made by the liver. Its main role is to save iron by attaching itself to any hemoglobin released from a red cell.

Hemoglobin—The protein in the red blood cell that carries oxygen.

Hemolytic anemia—A variety of conditions that result in hemolyzed, or burst, red blood cells.

Aftercare

Discomfort or bruising may occur at the puncture site or the person may feel dizzy or faint. Pressure to the puncture site until the bleeding stops reduces bruising. Warm packs to the puncture site relieve discomfort.

Normal results

Normal results vary based on the laboratory and test method used. Haptoglobin is not present in newborns at birth, but develop adult levels by six months.

Abnormal results

Decreased haptoglobin levels usually indicates hemolytic anemia. Other causes of red cell destruction also decrease haptoglobin: a blood **transfusion** reaction; mechanical heart valve; abnormally shaped red cells; or abnormal hemoglobin, such as thalassemia or sickle cell anemia.

Haptoglobin levels are low in **liver disease**, because the liver can not manufacture normal amounts of haptoglobin. Low levels may also indicate an inherited lack of haptoglobin, a condition found particularly in African Americans.

Haptoglobin increases as a reaction to illness, trauma, or rheumatoid disease. High haptoglobin values should be followedup with additional tests. Drugs can also effect haptoglobin levels.

Normal results vary widely from person to person. Unless the level is very high or very low, haptoglobin levels are most valuable when the results of several tests done on different days are compared.

Nancy J. Nordenson

Hardening of the arteries *see* **Atherosclerosis**

Harelip *see* **Cleft lip and palate**

Hartnup disease

Definition

Hartnup disease is an inherited nutritional disorder with primary symptoms including a red, scaly rash and sensitivity to sunlight.

Description

Hartnup disease was first identified in the 1950s in the Hartnup family in London. A defect in intestines and kidneys makes it difficult to break down and absorb protein in the diet. This causes a condition very similar to pellegra (niacin deficiency). The condition occurs in about one of every 26,000 live births.

Causes and symptoms

Hartnup disease is an in-born error of metabolism, that is, a condition where certain nutrients cannot be digested and absorbed properly. The condition is passed on genetically in families. It occurs when a person inherits two recessive genes for the disease, one from each parent. People with Hartnup disease are not able to absorb some of the amino acids (the smaller building blocks that make up proteins) in their intestines. One of the amino acids that is not well absorbed is tryptophan, which the body uses to make its own form of niacin.

The majority of people with this disorder do not show any symptoms. About 10–20% of people with Hartnup disease do have symptoms. The most prominent symptom is a red, scaly rash that gets worse when the patient is exposed to sunlight. **Headache**, **fainting**, and **diarrhea** may also occur. **Mental retardation**, cerebral ataxia (muscle weakness), and **delirium** (a confused, agitated, delusional state) are some of the more serious complications that can occur. Short stature has also been noted in some patients. Although this is an inherited disease, the development of symptoms depends on a variety of factors including diet, environment, and other genetic traits controlling amino acid levels in the body. Symptoms can be brought on by exposure to sunlight, **fever**, drugs, or other stresses. Poor **nutrition** frequently precedes an attack of symptoms. The frequency of attacks usually decreases as the patient gets older.

KEY TERMS

Amino acids—Proteins are made up of organic compounds called amino acids. The human body uses amino acids to build and repair body tissue. The body can make some of its own amino acids from other nutrients in the diet; these are called nonessential amino acids. Essential amino acids are those that cannot be made by the body but must be consumed in the diet. Animal proteins (like meat, eggs, fish, and milk) provide all of the amino acids.

Aminoaciduria—A condition confirmed by laboratory tests where high levels of amino acids are found in the urine.

Pellegra—A condition caused by a dietary deficiency of one of the B vitamins called niacin.

Tryptophan—An essential amino acid that has to consumed in the diet because it cannot be manufactured by the body. Tryptophan is converted by the body to niacin, one of the B vitamins.

Diagnosis

The symptoms of this disease suggest a deficiency of a B vitamin called niacin. A detailed diet history can be used to assess if there is adequate protein and **vitamins** in the diet. The diagnosis of Hartnup disease is confirmed by a laboratory test of the urine which will contain an abnormally high amount of amino acids (aminoaciduria).

Treatment

The vitamin niacin is given as a treatment for Hartnup disease. The typical dosage ranges from 40–200 mg of nicotinamide (a form of niacin) per day to prevent pellagra-like symptoms. Some patients may require dietary supplements of tryptophan.

Eating a healthy, high protein diet can relieve the symptoms and prevent them from recurring.

Prognosis

The prognosis for a healthy life is good once the condition has been identified and treated.

Prevention

Hartnup disease is an inherited condition. Parents may not have the disease themselves, but may pass the genes responsible for it on to their children. **Genetic testing** can be used to identify carriers of the genes. Symptoms can usually be controlled with a high protein diet, vitamin supplements of niacin, and by avoiding the stresses that contribute to attacks of symptoms.

Resources

OTHER

"Hartnup disorder." OMIM Homepage, Online Mendelian Inheritance in Man. http://www.ncbi.nlm.nih.gov/Omim.

"Nephrology: Hartnup disease." Medstudents.com. http://www.medstudents.com.

ORGANIZATIONS

National Institute of Diabetes and Digestive and Kidney Diseases, NIDDK, NIH Bldg 31, Rm 9A06 31 Center Drive, MSC 2560, Bethesda, MD, 20892-2560, (301) 496-3583, http://www2.niddk.nih.gov.

National Organization for Rare Disorders, P.O. Box 8923, New Fairfield, CT, 06812-8923, (800) 999-6673, http://www.rarediseases.org.

Altha Roberts Edgren

Hashimoto's disease *see* **Thyroiditis**

Hatha yoga

Definition

Hatha **yoga** is the most widely practiced form of yoga in the United States. It is the branch of yoga which concentrates on physical health and mental well-being. Hatha yoga uses bodily postures (*asanas*), breathing techniques (*pranayama*), and **meditation** (*dyana*) with the goal of bringing about a sound, healthy body and a clear, peaceful mind. There are nearly 200 hatha yoga postures, with hundreds of variations, which work to make the spine supple and to promote circulation in all the organs, glands, and tissues. Hatha yoga postures also stretch and align the body, promoting balance and flexibility.

Purpose

In a celebrated 1990 study, *Dr. Dean Ornish's Program for Reversing Heart Disease* (Random House), a cardiologist showed that yoga and meditation combined with a low-fat diet and group support could significantly reduce the blockage of coronary arteries. Other studies have shown yoga's benefit in reducing stress-related problems such as high blood pressure and cholesterol. Meditation has been adopted by medical schools and clinics as an effective **stress** management technique. Hatha yoga is also used by physical therapists to improve many injuries and disabilities, as the gentleness and adaptability of yoga make it an excellent **rehabilitation** program.

Yoga has been touted for its ability to reduce problems with such varying conditions as **asthma**, backaches, diabetes, **constipation**, **menopause**, **multiple sclerosis**, **varicose veins**, and **carpal tunnel syndrome**. A vegetarian diet is the dietary goal of yoga, and this change of lifestyle has been shown to significantly increase longevity and reduce heart disease.

Yoga as a daily **exercise** program can improve fitness, strength, and flexibility. People who practice yoga correctly every day report that it can promote high levels of overall health and energy. The mental component of yoga can clarify and discipline the mind, and yoga practitioners say its benefits can permeate all facets of a person's life and attitude, raising self-esteem and self-understanding.

Description

Origins

Yoga was developed in ancient India as far back as 5,000 years ago; sculptures detailing yoga positions have been found in India which date back to 3000 B.C. Yoga is derived from a Sanskrit word which means "union." The goal of classical yoga is to bring self-transcendence, or enlightenment, through physical, mental and spiritual health. Many people in the West mistakenly believe yoga to be a religion, but its teachers point out that it is a system of living designed to promote health, peace of mind, and deeper awareness of ourselves. There are several branches of yoga, each of which is a different path and philosophy toward self-improvement. Some of these paths include service to others, pursuit of wisdom, non-violence, devotion to God, and observance of spiritual rituals. Hatha yoga is the path which has physical health and balance as a primary goal, for its practitioners believe that greater mental and spiritual awareness can be brought about with a healthy and pure body.

The origins of hatha yoga have been traced back to the eleventh century A.D. The Sanskrit word *ha* means "sun" and *tha* means "moon," and thus hatha, or literally sun-moon yoga, strives to balance opposing parts of the physical body, the front and back, left and right, top and bottom. Some yoga masters (*yogis*) claim that hatha yoga was originally developed by enlightened teachers to help people survive during the Age of Kali, or the spiritual dark ages, in which Hindus believe we are now living.

The original philosophers of yoga developed it as an eight-fold path to complete health. These eight steps include moral and ethical considerations (such as honesty, non-aggression, peacefulness, non-stealing, generosity, and sexual propriety), self-discipline (including purity, simplicity, devotion to God, and self-knowledge), posture, breath control, control of desires, concentration, meditation, and happiness. According to yogis, if these steps are followed diligently, a person can reach high levels of health and mental awareness.

As it has subsequently developed, hatha yoga has concentrated mainly on two of the eight paths, breathing and posture. Yogis believe breathing to be the most important metabolic function; we breathe roughly 23,000 times per day and use about 4,500 gallons of air, which increases during exercise. Thus, breathing is extremely important to health, and *prana*, or life-force, is found most abundantly in the air and in the breath. If we are breathing incorrectly, we are hampering our potential for optimal health. *Pranayama*, literally the "science of breathing" or "control of life force," is the yogic practice of breathing correctly and deeply.

In addition to breathing, hatha yoga utilizes asanas, or physical postures, to bring about flexibility, balance and strength in the body. Each of these postures has a definite form and precise steps for achieving the desired position and for exiting it. These postures, yogis maintain, have been scientifically developed to increase circulation and health in all parts of the body, from the muscular tissues to the glands and internal organs. Yogis claim that although hatha yoga can make the body as strong and fit as any exercise program, its real benefits come about because it is a system of maintenance and balance for the whole body.

Yoga was brought to the United States in the late 1800s, when Swami Vivekananda, an Indian yogi, presented a lecture on yoga in Chicago. Hatha yoga captured the imagination of the Western mind, because accomplished yogis could demonstrate incredible levels of fitness, flexibility, and control over their bodies and metabolism. Yoga has flourished in the West. Americans have brought to yoga their energy and zest for innovation, which troubles some Indian yogis and encourages others, as new variations and schools of yoga have developed. For instance, power yoga is a recent Americanized version of yoga which takes hatha yoga principles and speeds them up into an extremely rigorous aerobic workout, and many strict hatha yoga teachers oppose this sort of change to their philosophy. Other variations of hatha yoga in the United States now include Iyengar, Ashtanga, Kripalu, Integral, Viniyoga, Hidden Language, and Bikram yoga, to name a few. Sivananda yoga was practiced by Lilias Folen, who was responsible for introducing many Americans to yoga through public television.

Iyengar yoga was developed by B.K.S. Iyengar, who is widely accepted as one of the great living yogis. Iyengar uses classical hatha yoga asanas and breathing techniques, but emphasizes great precision and strict form in the poses and uses many variations on a few postures. Iyengar allows the use of props such as belts, ropes, chairs, and blocks to enable students to get into postures they otherwise couldn't. In this respect, Iyengar yoga is good for **physical therapy** because it assists in the manipulation of inflexible or injured areas.

Ashtanga yoga, made popular by yogi K. Patabhi Jois, also uses hatha yoga asanas, but places an emphasis on the sequences in which these postures are performed. Ashtanga routines often unfold like long dances with many positions done quickly one after the other. Ashtanga is thus a rigorous form of hatha yoga, and sometimes can resemble a difficult aerobic workout. Ashtanga teachers claim that this form of yoga uses body heat, sweating, and deep breathing to purify the body.

Kripalu yoga uses hatha yoga positions but emphasizes the mental and emotional components of each asana. Its teachers believe that tension and long-held emotional problems can be released from the body by a deep and meditative approach to the yoga positions. Integral yoga seeks to combine all the paths of yoga and is generally more meditative than physical, emphasizing spirituality and awareness in everyday life. Viniyoga tries to adapt hatha yoga techniques to each individual body and medical problem. Hidden Language yoga was developed by Swami Sivananda Radha, a Western man influenced by Jungian psychology. It emphasizes the symbolic and psychological parts of yoga postures and techniques. Its students are encouraged to write journals and participate in group discussions as part of their practice. Bikram yoga has became very popular in the late 1990s, as its popular teacher, Bikram Choudury, began teaching in Beverly Hills and has been endorsed by many famous celebrities. Bikram yoga uses the repetition of 26 specific poses and two breathing techniques to stretch and tone the whole body.

A hatha yoga routine consists of a series of physical postures and breathing techniques. Routines can take anywhere from 20 minutes to two hours, depending on the needs and ability of the practitioner. Yoga should always be adapted to one's state of health; that is, a shorter and easier routine should be used when a person is fatigued. Yoga is ideally practiced at the same time every day, to encourage the discipline of the practice. It can be done at any time of day; some prefer it in the morning as a wake-up routine, while others like to wind down and de-stress with yoga at the end of the day.

Yoga asanas consist of three basic movements: backward bends, forward bends, and twisting movements. These postures are always balanced; a back bend should be followed with a forward bend, and a leftward movement should be followed by one to the right. Diaphragm breathing is important during the poses, where the breath begins at the bottom of the lungs. The stomach should move outward with the inhalation and relax inward during exhalation. The breath should be through the nose at all times during hatha asanas. Typically, one inhales during backward bends and exhales during forward bending movements.

The mental component in yoga is as important as the physical movements. Yoga is not a competitive sport, but a means to self-awareness and self-improvement. An attitude of attention, care, and non-criticism is important; limitations should be acknowledged and calmly improved. Patience is important, and yoga stretches should be slow and worked up to gradually. The body should be worked with, and never against, and a person should never overexert. A yoga stretch should be done only so far as proper form and alignment of the whole body can be maintained. Some yoga stretches can be uncomfortable for beginners, and part of yoga is learning to distinguish between sensations that are beneficial and those that can signal potential injury. A good rule is that positions should be stopped when there is sharp **pain** in the joints, muscles, or tendons.

Preparations

All that is needed to perform hatha yoga is a flat floor and adequate space for stretching out. A well-ventilated space is preferable, for facilitating proper breathing technique. Yoga mats are available which provide non-slip surfaces for standing poses. Loose, comfortable clothing should be worn. Yoga should be done on an empty stomach; a general rule is to wait three hours after a meal.

Yoga is an exercise that can be done anywhere and requires no special equipment. Yoga uses only gravity and the body itself as resistance, so it is a low-impact activity excellent for those who don't do well with other types of exercise. The mental component of yoga can

KEY TERMS

Asana—Yoga posture or stance.

Diaphragm breathing—Method of deep breathing using the entire lungs.

Dyana—Yoga meditation.

Meditation—Technique of mental relaxation.

Prana—Yoga term for life-enhancing nutrient found in air, food, and water.

Pranayama—Yoga method of breathing.

appeal to those who get bored easily with exercise. By the same token, yoga can be a good stress management tool for those who prefer movement to sitting meditation.

Precautions

As with any exercise program, people should check with their doctors before starting yoga practice for the first time. Those with medical conditions, injuries, or spinal problems should find a yoga teacher familiar with their conditions before beginning yoga. Pregnant women, particularly after the third month of **pregnancy**, should only perform a few yoga positions with the supervision of an experienced teacher. Some yoga asanas can be very difficult, and potentially injurious, for beginners, so teachers should always be consulted as preparation for advanced yoga positions. Certain yoga positions should not be performed by those with fevers or during menstruation.

Side effects

Those just beginning hatha yoga programs often report **fatigue** and soreness throughout the body, as yoga stretches and exercises muscles and tendons which are often long-neglected. Some yogic breathing and meditation techniques can be difficult for beginners and can cause **dizziness** or disorientation; these are best performed under the guidance of a teacher.

Resources

BOOKS

Feuerstein, Georg, and Larry Payne. *Yoga for Dummies*. New York: For Dummies, 2010.

ORGANIZATIONS

International Association of Yoga Therapists (IAYT), P.O. Box 12890, Prescott, AZ, 86304, (928) 541-0004, http://www.iayt.org/.

Douglas Dupler, MA

Haverhill fever *see* **Rat-bite fever**

Hay fever *see* **Allergic rhinitis**

HBF test *see* **Fetal hemoglobin test**

HCG *see* **Infertility drugs**

Head and neck cancer

Definition

The term head and neck cancers refers to a group of cancers found in the head and neck region. This includes tumors found in:

- The oral cavity (mouth). The lips, the tongue, the teeth, the gums, the lining inside the lips and cheeks, the floor of the mouth (under the tongue), the roof of

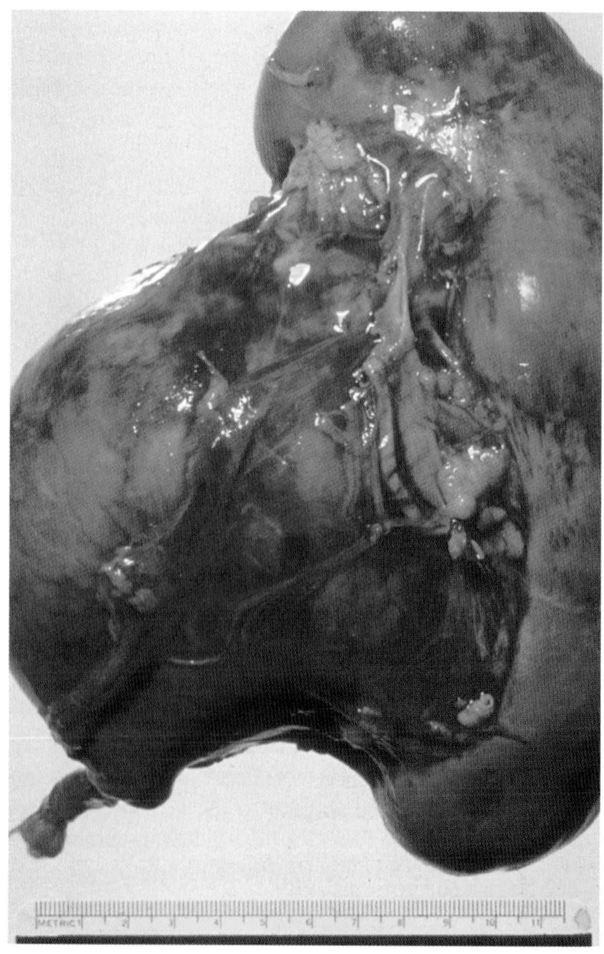

A specimen of a squamous cell carcinoma of the tongue and jaw. *(Custom Medical Stock Photo, Inc. Reproduced by permission.)*

the mouth and the small area behind the wisdom teeth are all included in the oral cavity.

- The oropharynx (which includes the back one-third of the tongue, the back of the throat and the tonsils).
- Nasopharynx (which includes the area behind the nose).
- Hypopharynx (lower part of the throat).
- The larynx (voice box, located in front of the neck, in the region of the Adam's apple). In the larynx, the cancer can occur in any of the three regions: the glottis (where the vocal cords are); the supraglottis (the area above the glottis); and the subglottis (the area that connects the glottis to the windpipe).

The most frequently occurring cancers of the head and neck area are oral cancers and laryngeal cancers. Almost half of all the head and neck cancers occur in the oral cavity, and a third of the cancers are found in the larynx. By definition, the term "head and neck cancers" usually excludes tumors that occur in the brain.

Description

Head and neck cancers involve the respiratory tract and the digestive tract; and they interfere with the functions of eating and breathing. Laryngeal cancers affect speech. Loss of any of these functions is significant. Hence, early detection and appropriate treatment of head and neck cancers is of utmost importance.

Roughly 10% of all cancers are related to the head and the neck. In 2005, 39,000 men and women developed head and neck cancers and nearly 13,000 die each year from the disease. The American Cancer Society estimates that approximately, 12,100 new cases of laryngeal cancer alone will be diagnosed yearly and 3,600 people (2,870 men and 730 women) will die from this disease. Oral cancer is the sixth most common cancer in the United States. Approximately 35,000 new cases are diagnosed each year, and it causes at least 7,600 deaths. Among the major cancers, the survival rate for head and neck cancers is one of the poorest. Less than 50% of patients survive five years or more after initial diagnosis. This is because the early signs of head and neck cancers are frequently ignored. Hence, when it is first diagnosed, it is often in an advanced stage and not very amenable to treatment.

The risk for both oral cancer and laryngeal cancer seems to increase with age. Most of the cases occur in individuals over 40 years of age, the average age at diagnosis being 60. While oral cancer strikes men twice as often as it does women, laryngeal cancer is four times more common in men than in women. Both diseases are more common in African Americans than among whites.

Causes and symptoms

Although the exact cause for these cancers is unknown, tobacco is regarded as the single greatest risk factor: 75-80% of the oral and laryngeal cancer cases occur among smokers. Heavy alcohol use has also been included as a risk factor. A combination of tobacco and alcohol use increases the risk for oral cancer by 6–15 times more than for users of either substance alone. In rare cases, irritation to the lining of the mouth, due to jagged teeth or ill-fitting dentures, has been known to cause oral cancer. Exposure to asbestos appears to increase the risk of developing laryngeal cancer.

In the case of lip cancer, just like skin cancer, exposure to sun over a prolonged period has been shown to increase the risk. In Southeast Asian countries (India and Sri Lanka), chewing of betel nuts has been associated with cancer of the lining of the cheek. An increased incidence of nasal cavity cancer has been observed among furniture workers, probably due to the inhalation of wood dust. A virus (Epstein-Barr) has been shown to cause nasopharyngeal cancer.

Head and neck cancers are one of the easiest to detect. The early signs can be both seen and felt. The signs and symptoms depend on the location of the cancer:

- Mouth and oral cavity: a sore that does not heal within two weeks, unusual bleeding from the teeth or gums, a white or red patch in the mouth, a lump or thickening in the mouth, throat, or tongue.
- Larynx: persistent hoarseness or sore throat, difficulty breathing, or pain.
- Hypopharynx and oropharynx: difficulty in swallowing or chewing food, ear pain.
- Nose, sinuses, and nasopharyngeal cavity: pain, bloody discharges from the nose, blocked nose, and frequent sinus infections that do not respond to standard antibiotics.

When detected early and treated appropriately, head and neck cancers have an excellent chance of being cured completely.

Diagnosis

Specific diagnostic tests used depend on the location of the cancer. The standard tests are:

Physical examination

The first step in diagnosis is a complete and thorough examination of the oral and nasal cavity, using mirrors and other visual aids. The tongue and the back of the throat are examined as well. Any suspicious looking lumps or lesions are examined with fingers (palpation). In order to look inside the larynx, the doctor may sometimes perform a procedure known as **laryngoscopy**. In indirect laryngoscopy, the doctor looks down the throat with a small, long handled mirror. Sometimes the doctor inserts a lighted tube (laryngoscope or a fiberoptic scope) through the patient's nose or mouth. As the tube goes down the throat, the doctor can observe areas that cannot be seen by a simple mirror. This procedure is called a direct laryngoscopy. Some-times patients may be given a mild sedative to help them relax, and a local anesthetic to ease any discomfort.

Blood tests

The doctor may order blood or other immunological tests. These tests are aimed at detecting antibodies to the **Epstein-Barr virus**, which has been known to cause cancer of the nasopharynx.

Imaging tests

X rays of the mouth, the sinuses, the skull, and the chest region may be required. A computed tomography scan (CT scan), a procedure in which a computer takes a series of x ray pictures of areas inside the body, may be done. Ultrasonograms (images generated using sound waves) or an MRI (**magnetic resonance imaging**, a procedure in which a picture is created using magnets linked to a computer), are alternate procedures which a doctor may have done to get detailed pictures of the areas inside the body.

Biopsy

When a sore does not heal or a suspicious patch or lump is seen in the mouth, larynx, nasopharynx, or throat, a biopsy may be performed to rule out the possibility of cancer. The biopsy is the most definitive diagnostic tool for detecting the cancer. If cancerous cells are detected in the biopsied sample, the doctor may perform more extensive tests in order to find whether, and to where, the cancer may have spread.

Treatment

The cancers can be treated successfully if diagnosed early. The choice of treatment depends on the size of the tumor, its location, and whether it has spread to other parts of the body.

In the case of lip and mouth cancers, sometimes surgery is performed to remove the cancer. **Radiation therapy**, which destroys the cancerous cells, is also one of the primary modes of treatment and may be used alone or in combination with surgery. If lip surgery is drastic, **rehabilitation** cosmetic or **reconstructive surgery** may have to be considered.

Cancers of the nasal cavity are often diagnosed late because they have no specific symptoms in their early stages or the symptoms may just resemble chronic **sinusitis**. Hence, treatment is often complex, involving a combination of radiotherapy and surgery. Surgery is generally recommended for small tumors. If the cancer cannot be removed by surgery, radiotherapy is used alone.

Treatment of oropharynx cancers (cancers that are either in the back of the tongue, the throat, or the tonsils) generally involves radiation therapy and/or surgery. After aggressive surgery and radiation, rehabilitation is often necessary and is an essential part of the treatment. The patient may experience difficulties with swallowing, chewing, and speech and may require a team of health care workers, including speech therapists, prosthodontists, occupational therapists, etc.

Cancers of the nasopharynx are different from the other head and neck cancers in that there does not appear to be any association between alcohol and tobacco use and the development of the cancer. In addition, the incidence is seen primarily in two age groups: young adults and 50–70 year-olds. The Epstein-Barr virus has been implicated as the causative agent in most patients. While 80–90% of small tumors are curable by radiation therapy, advanced tumors that have spread to the bone and cranial nerves are difficult to control. Surgery is not very helpful and, hence, is rarely attempted. Radiation remains the only treatment of choice to treat the cancer that has metastasized (traveled) to the lymph nodes in the neck.

In the case of cancer of the larynx, radiotherapy is the first choice to treat small lesions. This is done in an attempt to preserve the voice. If the cancer recurs later, surgery may be attempted. If the cancer is limited to one of the two vocal cords, laser excision surgery is used. In order to treat advanced cancers, a combination of surgery and radiation therapy is often used. Because the chances of a cure in the case of advanced laryngeal cancers are rather low with current therapies, the patient may be advised to participate in clinical trials so they may get access to new experimental drugs and procedures, such as **chemotherapy**, that are being evaluated.

When only part of the larynx is removed, a relatively slight change in the voice may occur—the patient may sound slightly hoarse. However, in a total **laryngectomy**, the entire voice box is removed. The patients then have to

KEY TERMS

Biopsy—The surgical removal and microscopic examination of living tissue for diagnostic purposes.

Chemotherapy—Treatment of cancer with synthetic drugs that destroy the tumor either by inhibiting the growth of the cancerous cells or by killing the cancer cells.

Clinical trials—Highly regulated and carefully controlled patient studies, where either new drugs to treat cancer or novel methods of treatment are investigated.

Computerized tomography scan (CT scan)—A medical procedure where a series of X-rays are taken and put together by a computer in order to form detailed pictures of areas inside the body.

Laryngoscopy—A medical procedure that uses flexible, lighted, narrow tubes inserted through the mouth or nose to examine the larynx and other areas deep inside the neck.

Magnetic resonance imaging (MRI)—A medical procedure used for diagnostic purposes where pictures of areas inside the body can be created using a magnet linked to a computer.

Radiation therapy—Treatment using high energy radiation from x-ray machines, cobalt, radium, or other sources.

Stoma—When the entire larynx must be surgically removed, an opening is surgically created in the neck so that the windpipe can be brought out to the neck. This opening is called the stoma.

Ultrasonogram—A procedure where high-frequency sound waves that cannot be heard by human ears are bounced off internal organs and tissues. These sound waves produce a pattern of echoes which are then used by the computer to create sonograms, or pictures, of areas inside the body.

X rays—High energy radiation used in high doses, either to diagnose or treat disease.

re-learn to speak using different approaches, such as esophageal speech, tracheo-esophageal (TE) speech, or by means of an artificial larynx.

In esophageal speech, the patients are taught how to create a new type of voice by forcing air through the esophagus (food pipe) into the mouth. This method has a high success rate of approximately 65% and patients are even able to go back to jobs that require a high level of verbal communication, such as telephone operators and salespersons.

In the second approach, TE speech, a small opening, called a **fistula**, is created surgically between the trachea (breathing tube to the lungs) and the esophagus (tube into the stomach) to carry air into the throat. A small tube, known as the "voice prosthesis," is placed in the opening of the fistula to keep it open and to prevent food and liquid from going down into the trachea. In order to talk, the stoma (or the opening made at the base of the neck) must be covered with one's thumb during exhalation. As the air is forced out from the trachea into the esophagus, it vibrates the walls of the esophagus. This produces a sound that is then modified by the lips and tongue to produce normal sounding speech.

In the third approach, an artificial larynx, a battery driven vibrator, is placed on the outside of the throat. Sound is created as air passes through the stoma (opening made at the base of the neck) and the mouth forms words.

Prognosis

Oral cavity

With early detection and immediate treatment, survival rates can be dramatically improved. For lip and oral cancer, if detected at its early stages, almost 80% of the patients survive five years or more. However, when diagnosed at the advanced stages, the five year survival rate drops to a mere 18%.

Nose and sinuses

Cancers of the nasal cavity often go undetected until they reach an advanced stage. If diagnosed at the early stages, the five-year survival rates are 60–70%. However, if cancers are more advanced, only 10–30% of the patients survive five years or more.

Oropharynx

In cancer of the oropharynx, 60–80% of the patients survive five years or more if the cancer is detected in the early stages. As the cancer advances, the survival rate drops to 15–30%.

Nasopharynx

Patients who are diagnosed with early stage cancers that have originated in the nasopharynx have an excellent chance of a complete cure (almost 95%).

Unfortunately, most of the time, the patients are in an advanced stage at the time of initial diagnosis. With the new chemotherapy drugs, the five year survival rate has improved and 5–40% of the patients survive five years or longer.

Larynx

Small cancers of the larynx have an excellent five-year survival rate of 75–95%. However, as with most of the head and neck cancers, the survival rates drop dramatically as the cancer advances. Only 15–25% of the patients survive five years or more after being initially diagnosed with advanced laryngeal cancer.

Prevention

Refraining from the use of all tobacco products (cigarettes, cigars, pipe tobacco, chewing tobacco), consuming alcohol in moderation, and practicing good **oral hygiene** are some of the measures that one can take to prevent head and neck cancers. Since there is an association between excessive exposure to the sun and lip cancer, people who spend a lot of time outdoors in the sun should protect themselves from the sun's harmful rays. Regular physical examinations, or mouth examination by the patient himself, or by the patient's doctor or dentist, can help detect oral cancer in its very early stages.

Since working with asbestos has been shown to increase one's risk of getting cancer of the larynx, asbestos workers should follow safety rules to avoid inhaling asbestos fibers. Also, **malnutrition** and vitamin deficiencies have been shown to have some association with an increased incidence of head and neck cancers. The American Cancer Society, therefore, recommends eating a healthy diet, consisting of at least five servings of fruits and vegetables every day, and six servings of food from other plant sources such as cereals, breads, grain products, rice, pasta, and beans. Reducing one's intake of high-fat food from animal sources is advised.

ORGANIZATIONS

American Association of Oral & Maxillofacial Surgeons, 9700 West Bryn Mawr Avenue, Rosemont, IL, 60018-5701, (847) 678-6200, (847) 678-6286, (800) 822-6637, http://www.aaoms.org.

National Cancer Institute (National Institutes of Health), NCI Office of Communications and Education, 6116 Executive Blvd. Suite 300, Bethesda, MD, 20892-8322, (800) 4-CANCER (422-6237), cancergovstaff@mail.nih.gov, http://www.cancer.gov/.

National Institute of Dental and Craniofacial Research, National Institutes of Health, Bethesda, MD, (301) 470-4098, (866) 232-4528, nidcrinfo@mail.nih.gov, http://www.nidcr.nih.gov.

The International Association of Laryngectomees (IAL), 925B Peachtree Street - NE Suite 316 , Atlanta, GA, 30309, (866) 425-3678, http://www.theial.com/ial/.

Thyroid, Head and Neck Cancer Foundation, 10 Union Square East, Suite 5B, New York, NY, 10003, (212) 844-6832, (212) 844-8465, info@thancfoundation.org, http://www.thancfoundation.org.

Lata Cherath, PhD

Head injury

Definition

Injury to the head may damage the scalp, skull, or brain. The most important consequence of head trauma is traumatic brain injury. Head injury may occur either as a closed head injury, such as the head hitting a car's windshield, or as a penetrating head injury, as when a bullet pierces the skull. Both may cause damage that ranges from mild to profound. Very severe injury can be fatal because of profound brain damage.

Description

External trauma to the head is capable of damaging the brain, even if there is no external evidence of damage. More serious injuries can cause skull fracture, **blood clots** between the skull and the brain, or bruising and tearing of the brain tissue itself.

Injuries to the head can be caused by traffic accidents, **sports injuries**, falls, workplace accidents, assaults, or bullets. Most people have had some type of head injury at least once in their lives, but rarely do they require a hospital visit.

Each year about two million people have a serious head injury and up to 750,000 of them are severe enough to require hospitalization. Brain injury is most likely to occur in males between ages 15 and 24, usually as a result of car and motorcycle accidents. About 70% of all accidental deaths are due to head injuries, as are most of the disabilities that occur after trauma.

A person who has had a head injury and who is experiencing the following symptoms should seek medical care immediately:

- serious bleeding from the head or face
- loss of consciousness, however brief
- confusion and lethargy
- lack of pulse or breathing
- clear fluid drainage from the nose or ear

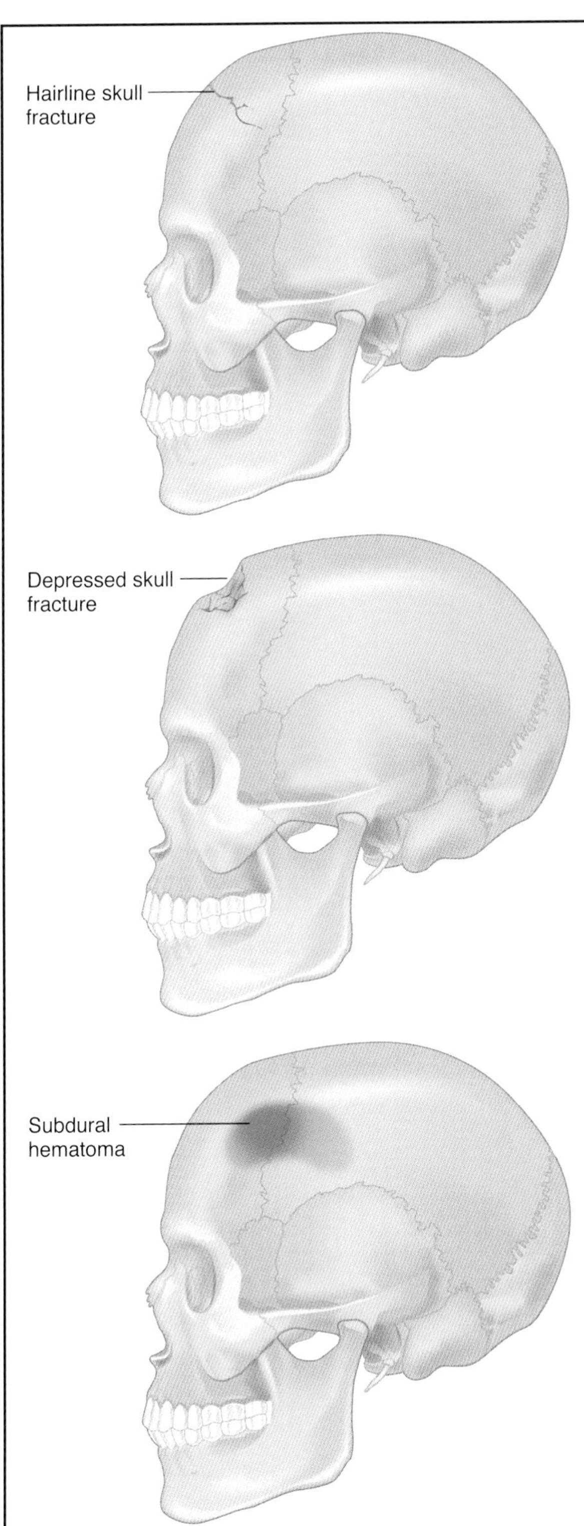

Illustration depicting three types of head injury: hairline fracture, depressed fracture, and subdural hematoma. *(Illustration by Electronic Illustrators Group. Reproduced by permission of Gale, a part of Cengage Learning.)*

Causes and symptoms

A head injury may cause damage both from the direct physical injury to the brain and from secondary factors, such as lack of oxygen, brain swelling, and disturbance of blood flow. Both closed and penetrating head injuries can cause swirling movements throughout the brain, tearing nerve fibers and causing widespread bleeding or a blood clot in or around the brain. Swelling may raise pressure within the skull (intracranial pressure) and may block the flow of oxygen to the brain.

Head trauma may cause a **concussion**, in which there is a brief loss of consciousness without visible structural damage to the brain. In addition to loss of consciousness, initial symptoms of brain injury may include:

- memory loss and confusion
- vomiting
- dizziness
- partial paralysis or numbness
- shock
- anxiety

After a head injury, there may be a period of impaired consciousness followed by a period of confusion and impaired memory with disorientation and a breakdown in the ability to store and retrieve new information. Others experience temporary **amnesia** following head injury that begins with **memory loss** over a period of weeks, months, or years before the injury (retrograde amnesia). As the patient recovers, memory slowly returns. Post-traumatic amnesia refers to loss of memory for events during and after the accident.

Epilepsy occurs in 2–5% of people who have had a head injury; it is much more common in people who have had severe or penetrating injuries. Most cases of epilepsy appear right after the accident or within the first year and become less likely with increased time following the accident.

Closed head injury

Closed head injury refers to brain injury without any penetrating injury to the brain. It may be the result of a direct blow to the head; of the moving head being rapidly stopped, such as when a person's head hits a windshield in a car accident; or by the sudden deceleration of the head without its striking another object. The kind of injury the brain receives in a closed head injury is determined by whether or not the head was unrestrained upon impact and the direction, force, and velocity of the blow. If the head is resting on impact, the maximum damage will be found at the impact site. A moving head will cause a "contrecoup injury" where

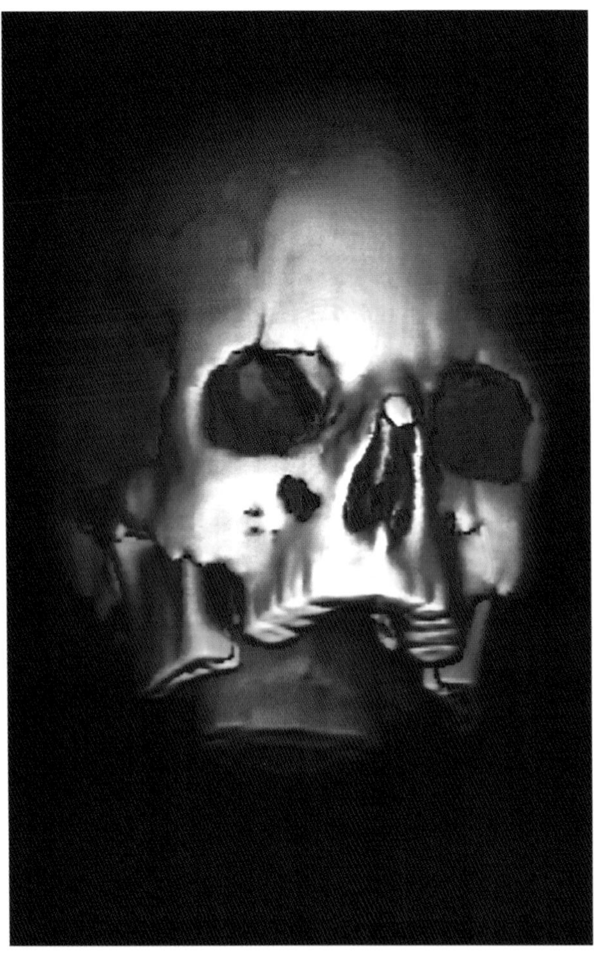

A three-dimensional computed tomography (CT) scan of a human skull showing a depressed skull fracture above the right eye. *(Custom Medical Stock Photo, Inc. Reproduced by permission.)*

the brain damage occurs on the side opposite the point of impact, as a result of the brain slamming into that side of the skull. A closed head injury also may occur without the head being struck, such as when a person experiences **whiplash**. This type of injury occurs because the brain is of a different density than the skull and can be injured when delicate brain tissues hit against the rough, jagged inner surface of the skull.

Penetrating head injury

If the skull is fractured, bone fragments may be driven into the brain. Any object that penetrates the skull may implant foreign material and dirt into the brain, leading to an infection.

Skull fracture

A skull fracture is a medical emergency that must be treated promptly to prevent possible brain damage. Such an injury may be obvious if blood or bone fragments are visible, but it is possible for a fracture to have occurred without any apparent damage. A skull fracture should be suspected if there is:

- blood or clear fluid leaking from the nose or ears
- unequal pupil size
- bruises or discoloration around the eyes or behind the ears
- swelling or depression of part of the head

Intracranial hemorrhage

Bleeding (hemorrhage) inside the skull may accompany a head injury and cause additional damage to the brain. A blood clot (hematoma) may occur if a blood vessel between the skull and the brain ruptures; when the blood leaks out and forms a clot, it can press against brain tissue, causing symptoms from a few hours to a few weeks after the injury. If the clot is located between the bones of the skull and the covering of the brain (dura), it is called an epidural hematoma. If the clot is between the dura and the brain tissue itself, the condition is called a **subdural hematoma**. In other cases, bleeding may occur deeper inside the brain. This condition is called intracerebral hemorrhage or intracerebral contusion (from the word for bruising).

In any case, if the blood flow is not stopped, it can lead to unconsciousness and **death**. The symptoms of bleeding within the skull include:

- nausea and vomiting
- headache
- loss of consciousness
- unequal pupil size
- lethargy

Post-concussion syndrome

If the head injury is mild, there may be no symptoms other than a slight **headache**. There also may be confusion, **dizziness**, and blurred vision. While the head injury may seem to have been quite mild, in many cases symptoms persist for days or weeks. Up to 60% of patients who sustain a mild brain injury continue to experience a range of symptoms called "post-concussion syndrome," as long as six months or a year after the injury.

The symptoms of **post-concussion syndrome** can result in a puzzling interplay of behavioral, cognitive, and emotional complaints that can be difficult to diagnose, including:

- headache
- dizziness
- mental confusion

- behavior changes
- memory loss
- cognitive deficits
- depression
- emotional outbursts

Diagnosis

The extent of damage in a severe head injury can be assessed with computed tomography (CT) scan, **magnetic resonance imaging** (MRI), **positron emission tomography (PET)** scans, electroencephalograms (EEG), and routine neurological and neuropsychological evaluations.

Doctors use the Glasgow **Coma** Scale to evaluate the extent of brain damage based on observing a patient's ability to open his or her eyes, respond verbally, and respond to stimulation by moving (motor response). Patients can score from 3 to 15 points on this scale. People who score below eight when they are admitted usually have suffered a severe brain injury and will need rehabilitative therapy as they recover. In general, higher scores on the Glasgow Coma Scale indicate less severe brain injury and a better prognosis for recovery.

Patients with a mild head injury who experience symptoms are advised to seek out the care of a specialist; unless a family physician is thoroughly familiar with medical literature in this newly emerging area, experts warn that there is a good chance that patient complaints after a mild head injury will be downplayed or dismissed. In the case of mild head injury or post-concussion syndrome, CT and MRI scans, electroencephalograms (EEG), and routine neurological evaluations all may be normal because the damage is so subtle. In many cases, these tests cannot detect the microscopic damage that occurs when fibers are stretched in a mild, diffuse injury. In this type of injury, the axons lose some of their covering and become less efficient. This mild injury to the white matter reduces the quality of communication between different parts or the brain. A **PET** scan, which evaluates cerebral blood flow and brain metabolism, may be of help in diagnosing mild head injury.

Patients with continuing symptoms after a mild head injury should call a local chapter of a head-injury foundation that can refer patients to the best nearby expert.

Treatment

If a concussion, bleeding inside the skull, or skull fracture is suspected, the patient should be kept quiet in a darkened room, with head and shoulders raised slightly on a pillow or blanket.

After initial emergency treatment, a team of specialists may be needed to evaluate and treat the problems that result. A penetrating wound may require surgery. Those with severe injuries or with a deteriorating level of consciousness may be kept hospitalized for observation. If there is bleeding inside the skull, the blood may need to be surgically drained; if a clot has formed, it may need to be removed. Severe skull **fractures** also require surgery.

Supportive care and specific treatments may be required if the patient experiences further complications. People who experience seizures, for example, may be given **anticonvulsant drugs**, and people who develop fluid on the brain (**hydrocephalus**) may have a shunt inserted to drain the fluid.

In the event of long-term disability as a result of head injury, there are a variety of treatment programs available, including long-term **rehabilitation**, coma treatment centers, transitional living programs, behavior management programs, life-long residential or day treatment programs and independent living programs.

Prognosis

Prompt, proper diagnosis and treatment can help alleviate some of the problems after a head injury. It usually is difficult to predict the outcome of a brain injury in the first few hours or days; a patient's prognosis may not be known for many months or even years.

The outlook for someone with a minor head injury generally is good, although recovery may be delayed and symptoms such as headache, dizziness, and cognitive problems can persist for up to a year or longer after an accident. This can limit a person's ability to work and cause strain in personal relationships.

Serious head injuries can be devastating, producing permanent mental and physical disability. Epileptic seizures may occur after a severe head injury, especially a penetrating brain injury, a severe skull fracture, or a serious brain hemorrhage. Recovery from a severe head injury can be very slow, and it may take five years or longer to heal completely. Risk factors associated with an increased likelihood of memory problems or seizures after head injury include age, length and depth of coma, duration of post-traumatic and retrograde amnesia, presence of focal brain injuries, and initial Glasgow Coma Scale score.

As researchers learn more about the long-term effects of head injuries, they have started to uncover links to later conditions. A 2003 report found that mild

KEY TERMS

Computed tomography scan (CT)—A diagnostic technique in which the combined use of a computer and x rays produce clear cross-sectional images of tissue. It provides clearer, more detailed information than x rays alone.

Electroencephalogram (EEG)—A record of the tiny electrical impulses produced by the brain's activity. By measuring characteristic wave patterns, the EEG can help diagnose certain conditions of the brain.

Magnetic resonance imaging (MRI)—A diagnostic technique that provides high quality cross-sectional images of organs within the body without x rays or other radiation.

Positron emission tomography (PET) scan—A computerized diagnostic technique that uses radioactive substances to examine structures of the body. When used to assess the brain, it produces a three-dimensional image that reflects the metabolic and chemical activity of the brain.

brain injury during childhood could speed up expression of **schizophrenia** in those who were already likely to get the disorder because of genetics. Those with a history of a childhood brain injury, even a minor one, were more likely to get familial schizophrenia than a sibling and to have earlier onset. Another study in 2003 found that people who had a history of a severe head injury were four times more likely to develop Parkinson's disease than the average population. Those requiring hospitalization for their head injuries were 11 times as likely. The risk did not increase for people receiving mild head injuries.

Prevention

Many severe head injuries could be prevented by wearing protective helmets during certain sports or when riding a bike or motorcycle. Seat belts and airbags can prevent many head injuries that result from car accidents. Appropriate protective headgear always should be worn on the job where head injuries are a possibility.

Resources

BOOKS

Daisley, Audrey, Rachel Tams, and Udo Kischka. *Head Injury*. New York: Oxford University Press, 2009.

Huff, Eane. *Heads Up: Finding Possibility and Purpose with Head Injury*. Parker, CO: Outskirts Press, 2009.

Mason, Michael Paul. *Head Cases: Stories of Brain Injury and Its Aftermath*. New York: Farrar, Straus and Giroux, 2009.

Smith, Terry. *Surviving Head Trauma: A Guide to Recovery Written by a Traumatic Brain Injury Patient*. Bloomington, IN: iUniverse, 2009.

PERIODICALS

"Childhood Head Injury Tied to Later Schizophrenia." *The Brown University Child and Adolescent Behavior Letter* (June 2003): 5.

"Link to Head Injury Found." *Pain & Central Nervous System Week* (June 9, 2003): 3.

ORGANIZATIONS

American Epilepsy Society, 342 N. Main St., West Hartford, CT, 06117-2507, (860) 586-7505, http://www.aesnet.org.

Brain Injury Association of America, 1608 Spring Hill Road, Suite 110, Vienna, VA, 22182, (703) 761-0750, http://www.biausa.org.

Brain Injury Resource Center, P.O. Box 84151, Seattle, WA, 98124, (206) 621-8558, http://www.headinjury.com.

Family Caregiver Alliance, 425 Bush St., Ste. 500, San Francisco, CA, 94108, (800) 445-8106, http://www.caregiver. org.

Head Trauma Support Project, Inc, 2500 Marconi Ave., Ste. 203, Sacramento, CA, 95821, (916) 482-5770

National Head Injury Foundation, 333 Turnpike Rd., Southboro, MA, 01722, (617) 485-9950

National Institute of Neurological Disorders and Stroke (NINDS), P.O. Box 5801, Bethesda, MD, 20824, (301) 496-5751, (800) 352-9424, http://www.ninds.nih.gov.

Carol A. Turkington
Teresa G. Odle
Laura Jean Cataldo, RN, EdD

Head lice *see* **Lice infestation**
Head trauma *see* **Head injury**

Headache

Definition

A headache involves **pain** in the head which can arise from many disorders or may be a disorder in and of itself.

Description

There are three types of primary headaches: tension-type (muscular contraction headache), migraine (vascular headaches), and cluster. Virtually everyone experiences a tension-type headache at some point. An estimated 18% of American women suffer migraines, compared to 6% of men. Cluster headaches affect fewer than 0.5% of the population, and men account for approximately 80% of all cases. Headaches caused by illness are secondary headaches and are not included in these numbers.

Approximately 40–45 million people in the United States suffer chronic headaches. Headaches have an enormous impact on society due to missed workdays and productivity losses.

Causes and symptoms

Traditional theories about headaches link tension-type headaches to muscle contraction, and migraine and cluster headaches to blood vessel dilation (swelling). Pain-sensitive structures in the head include blood vessel walls, membranous coverings of the brain, and scalp and neck muscles. Brain tissue itself has no sensitivity to pain. Therefore, headaches may result from contraction of the muscles of the scalp, face or neck; dilation of the blood vessels in the head; or brain swelling that stretches the brain's coverings. Involvement of specific nerves of the face and head may also cause characteristic headaches. Sinus inflammation is a common cause of headache. Keeping a headache diary may help link headaches to stressful occurrences, menstrual phases, food triggers, or medication.

Tension-type headaches are often brought on by **stress**, overexertion, loud noise, and other external factors. The typical tension-type headache is described as a tightening around the head and neck, and an accompanying dull ache.

Migraines are intense throbbing headaches occurring on one or both sides of the head, usually on one side. The pain is accompanied by other symptoms such as **nausea**, **vomiting**, blurred vision, and aversion to light, sound, and movement. Migraines often are triggered by food items, such as red wine, chocolate, and aged cheeses. For women, a hormonal connection is likely, since headaches occur at specific points in the menstrual cycle, with use of **oral contraceptives**, or the use of **hormone replacement therapy** after **menopause**. Research shows that a complex interaction of nerves and neurotransmitters in the brain act to cause migraine headaches.

Cluster headaches cause excruciating pain. The severe, stabbing pain centers around one eye, and eye tearing and nasal congestion occur on the same side. The headache lasts from 15 minutes to four hours and may recur several times in a day. Heavy smokers are more likely to suffer cluster headaches, which also are associated with alcohol consumption.

Diagnosis

Since headaches arise from many causes, a physical exam assesses general health and a neurologic exam evaluates the possibility of neurologic disease as a cause for the headache. If the headache is the primary illness, the doctor asks for a thorough history of the headache. Questions revolve around its frequency and duration, when it occurs, pain intensity and location, possible triggers, and any prior symptoms. This information aids in classifying the headache.

Warning signs that should point out the need for prompt medical intervention include:

- "Worst headache of my life." This may indicate subarachnoid hemorrhage from a ruptured aneurysm (swollen blood vessel) in the head or other neurological emergency.
- Headache accompanied by one-sided weakness, numbness, visual loss, speech difficulty, or other signs. This may indicate a stroke. Migraines may include neurological symptoms.
- Headache that becomes worse over a period of six months, especially if most prominent in the morning or if accompanied by neurological symptoms. This may indicate a brain tumor.
- Sudden onset of headache. If accompanied by fever and stiff neck, this can indicate meningitis.

Headache diagnosis may include neurological imaging tests such as computed tomography scan (CT scan) or **magnetic resonance imaging** (MRI).

Treatment

Headache treatment is divided into two forms: abortive and prophylactic. Abortive treatment addresses a headache in progress, and prophylactic treatment prevents headache occurrence.

Tension-type headaches can be treated with **aspirin**, **acetaminophen**, ibuprofen, or naproxen. In early 1998, the FDA approved extra-strength Excedrin, which includes **caffeine**, for mild migraines. Physicians continue to investigate and monitor the best treatment for migraines and generally prefer a stepped approach, depending on headache severity, frequency, and impact on the patient's quality of life. A group of drugs called triptans are usually preferred for abortive treatment. About seven triptans are available in the United States, and the pill forms are considered most effective. They should be taken as early as possible during the typical migraine attack. The most common prophylactic

KEY TERMS

Abortive—Referring to treatment that relieves symptoms of a disorder.

Analgesics—A class of pain-relieving medicines, including aspirin and Tylenol.

Biofeedback—A technique in which a person is taught to consciously control the body's response to a stimulus.

Chronic—Referring to a condition that occurs frequently or continuously or on a regular basis.

Prophylactic—Referring to treatment that prevents symptoms of a disorder from appearing.

Transcutaneous electrical nerve stimulation—A method that electrically stimulates nerve and blocks the transmission of pain signals, called TENS.

therapies include antidepressants, **beta blockers**, **calcium channel blockers**, and antiseizure medications. Antiseizure medications have proven particularly effective at blocking the actions of neurotransmitters that start migraine attacks. Topiramate (Topamax) was shown effective in several combined clinical trials in 2004 at 50 to 200 mg per day.

In 2004, a new, large study added evidence to show the effectiveness of botulinum toxin type A (Botox) treatment to prevent headache pain for those with frequent, untreatable tension and migraine headaches. Patients were treated every three months, with two to five injections each time. They typically received relief within two to three weeks.

Cluster headaches may also be treated with ergotamine and sumatriptan, as well as by inhaling pure oxygen. Prophylactic treatments include prednisone, **calcium** channel blockers, and methysergide.

Alternative treatment

Alternative headache treatments include:

- acupuncture or acupressure
- biofeedback
- chiropractic
- herbal remedies using feverfew (*Chrysanthemum parthenium*), valerian (*Valeriana officinalis*), white willow (*Salix alba*), or skullcap (*Scutellaria lateriflora*), among others
- homeopathic remedies chosen specifically for the individual and his/her type of headache
- hydrotherapy
- massage
- magnesium supplements
- regular physical exercise
- relaxation techniques, such as meditation and yoga
- transcutaneous electrical nerve stimulation (TENS) (A procedure that electrically stimulates nerves and blocks the signals of pain transmission.)

Prognosis

Headaches are typically resolved through the use of **analgesics** and other treatments. Research in 2004 showed that people who have migraine headaches more often than once a month may be at increased risk for **stroke**.

Prevention

Some headaches may be prevented by avoiding triggering substances and situations, or by employing alternative therapies, such as **yoga** and regular **exercise**. Since **food allergies** often are linked with headaches, especially cluster headaches, identification and elimination of the allergy-causing food(s) from the diet can be an important preventive measure.

Resources

PERIODICALS

Kruit, Mark C., et al. "Migraine as a Risk Factor for Subclinical Brain Lesions." *JAMA, Journal of the American Medical Association*. January 28, 2004: 427–435.

Norton, Patrice G. W. "Botox Stops Headache Pain in Recalcitrant Cases." *Clinical Psychiatry News*. March 2004: 72.

Taylor, Frederick, et al. "Diagnosis and Management of Migraine in Family Practice." *Journal of Family Practice*. January 2004: S3–S25.

ORGANIZATIONS

American Council for Headache Education (ACHE), 19 Mantua Road, Mount Royal, NJ, 08061, (856) 423-0043, (858) 423-0082, achehq@talley.com, http://www.achenet.org.

National Headache Foundation, 820 N. Orleans, Suite 217, Chicago, IL, 60610, (312) 274-2650, (888) NHF-5552, info@headaches.org, http://www.headaches.org.

Julia Barrett
Teresa G. Odle

Hearing aids

Definition

A hearing aid is a device that can amplify sound waves in order to help a deaf or hard-of-hearing person hear sounds more clearly.

Purpose

Recent technology can help most people with **hearing loss** understand speech better and achieve better communication.

Precautions

It's important that a person being fitted for a hearing aid understand what an aid can and can't do. An aid can help a person hear better, but it won't return hearing to normal levels. Hearing aids boost all sounds, not just those the person wishes to hear. Especially when the source of sound is far away (such as up on a stage), environmental noise can interfere with good speech perception. In addition, while the aid amplifies sound, it doesn't necessarily improve the clarity of the sound. A hearing aid is a machine and can never duplicate the true sound that people with normal hearing experience, but it will help the person take advantage of the hearing that remains.

Description

More than 1,000 different models are available in the United States. All of them include a microphone (to pick up sound), amplifier (to boost sound strength), a receiver or speaker (to deliver sound to the ear), and are powered by a battery. Depending on the style, it's possible to add features to filter or block out background noise, minimize feedback, lower sound in noisy settings, or boost power when needed.

Hearing aids are either "monaural" (a hearing aid for one ear), or "binaural" (for two ears); more than 65% of all users have binaural aids. Hearing aids are divided into several different types:

- digital
- in-the-ear
- in-the-canal
- behind-the-ear
- on-the-body

Digital aids are sophisticated, very expensive aids that borrow computer technology to allow a person to tailor an aid to a specific hearing loss pattern. Using miniature computer chips, the aids can selectively boost certain frequencies while leaving others alone. This means a person could wear such an aid to a loud party and screen out unwanted background noise, while tuning in on one-on-one conversations. The aid is programmed by the dealer to conform to the patient's

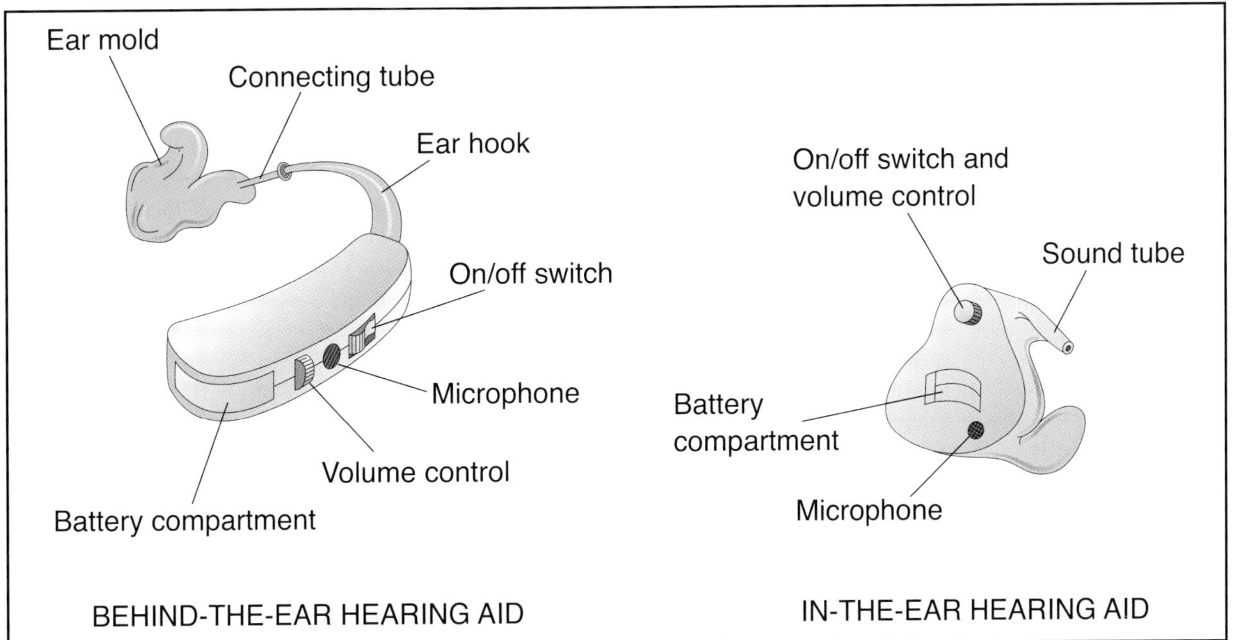

Hearing aids are devices that can amplify sound waves to help a deaf or hard-of-hearing person hear sounds more clearly. *(Illustration by Electronic Illustrators Group. Reproduced by permission of Gale, a part of Cengage Learning.)*

specific hearing loss. Some models can be programmed to allow the wearer to choose different settings depending on the noise of the environment.

In-the-ear aids are lightweight devices whose custom-made housings contain all the components; this device fits into the ear canal with no visible wires or tubes. It's possible to control tone but not volume with these aids, so they are helpful only for people with mild hearing loss. Some people find these aids are easier to put on and take off than behind-the-ear aids. However, because they are custom-fit to a person's ear, it is not possible to try on before ordering. Some people find them uncomfortable in hot weather.

In-the-canal aids fit far into the ear canal, with only a small bit extending into the external ear. The smallest is the MicroCanal, which fits out of sight down next to the eardrum and is removed with a small transparent wire. These are extremely expensive, but they are not visible, offer better acoustics, and are easier to maintain. They can more closely mimic natural sound because of the position of the microphone, this position also cuts down on wind noise. However, their small size makes them harder to handle, and their battery is especially small and difficult to insert. Adjusting the volume may be hard, since a person must stick a finger down into the ear to adjust volume, and this very tiny aid doesn't have the power of other, larger aids.

Behind-the-ear aids include a microphone, amplifier, and receiver inside a small curved case worn behind the ear; the case is connected to the earmold by a short plastic tube. The earmold extends into the ear canal. Some models have both tone and volume control plus a telephone pickup device. However, many users think them unattractive and out of date, and people who wear glasses find that the glasses interfere with the aid's fit. Others don't have space behind the ear for the mold to fit comfortably. However, they do offer a few advantages.

Behind-the-ear aids:

- don't require as much maintenance
- are easily interchangeable if they need to be serviced
- are more powerful
- are easier to handle than smaller aids
- can provide better sound quality
- tend to be more reliable

Eyeglass models are the same as behind-the-ear devices, except that the case fits into an eyeglass frame instead of resting behind the ears. Not many people buy this type of aid, but those who do believe it's less obvious, although there is a tube that travels from the temple of the glasses to the earmold. However, it can be hard to fit this type of aid, and repairs can be problematic. Also, if the aid breaks, the person also loses the benefit of the glasses.

CROS or the crossover system type of hearing aid is often used in conjunction with the eyeglass model. The CROS (contralateral routing of signal) system features a microphone behind the ear that feeds the amplified signal to the better ear, eliminating "head shadow," which occurs when the head blocks sound from the better ear. This type may help make speech easier to understand for people with a high-frequency loss in both ears.

A BI-CROS system uses two microphones (one above each ear) that send signals to a single amplifier. Sound then travels to a single receiver, which transfers it to the better ear via a conventional earmold.

On-the-body aids feature a larger microphone, amplifier, and power supply inside a case carried inside the pocket, or attached to clothing. The receiver attaches directly to the earmold; its power comes through a flexible wire from the amplifier. Although larger than other aids, the on-the-body aids are more powerful and easier to adjust than other devices. While not popular for everyone, they are often used by those with a profound hearing loss, or by very young children. Some people who are almost totally deaf find they need the extra power boost available only from a body aid.

The latest aids on the market may eliminate the amplifier and speaker in favor of a tiny magnet mounted on a silicone disk, similar to a contact lens, which rests right on the eardrum. Called the Earlens, it is designed to be held in place by a thin film of oil. Users wear a wireless microphone, either in the ear or on a necklace, that picks up sounds and converts them into magnetic signals, making the magnet vibrate. As the Earlens vibrates, so does the eardrum, transmitting normal-sounding tones to the middle and inner ears.

Other researchers are bypassing the middle ear completely; they surgically implant a tiny magnet in the inner ear. By attaching a magnet to the round window, they open a second pathway to the inner ear. An electromagnetic coil implanted in bone behind the ear vibrates the implanted magnet. Unlike the Earlens, this magnetic implant would not block the normal hearing pathway.

Preparation

The fist step in getting a hearing aid is to have a medical exam and a hearing evaluation. (Most states prohibit anyone selling a hearing aid until the patient has been examined by a physician to rule out medical problems.) After performing a hearing evaluation, an audiologist should be able to determine whether a

KEY TERMS

Audiologist—A person with a degree and/or certification in the areas of identification and measurement of hearing impairments and rehabilitation of those with hearing problems.

Eardrum—A paper-thin covering stretching across the ear canal that separates the middle and outer ears.

Middle ear—The small cavity between the eardrum and the oval window that houses the three tiny bones of hearing.

Oval window—A tiny opening at the entrance to the inner ear.

hearing aid will help, and which one will do the most good. This is especially important because aids can be very expensive (between $500 and $4,000) and are often not covered by health insurance. Hearing aids come in a wide range of styles and types, requiring careful testing to make sure the aid is the best choice for a particular hearing loss.

Some audiologists sell aids; others can make a recommendation, or give one a list of competent dealers in one's area. Patients should shop around and compare prices. In all but three states, hearing aids must be fitted and sold only by licensed specialists called dealers, specialists, dispensers, or dispensing audiologists.

The hearing aid dealer will make an impression of the consumer's ears using a putty-like material, from which a personalized earmold will be created. It's the dealer's job to make sure the aid fits properly. The person may need several visits to find the right hearing aid and learn how to use it. The dealer will help the consumer learn how to put the aid on, adjust the controls, and maintain the device. The dealer should be willing to service the aid and provide information about what to do if sensitivity to the earmold develops. (Some people are allergic to the materials in the mold.)

Aftercare

Within several weeks, the wearer should return to the dealer to have the aid checked, and to discuss the progress in wearing the aid. About 40% of all aids need some modification or adjustment in the beginning.

Within the first month of getting an aid, the patient should make an appointment for a full hearing examination to determine if the aid is functioning properly.

Risks

While there are no medical risks to hearing aids, there is a risk associated with hearing aids: many people end up not wearing their aids because they say everything seems loud when wearing them. This is because they have lived for so long with a hearing problem that they have forgotten how loud "normal" sound can be. Other potential problems with hearing aids include earmold discomfort and a build up of excess ear wax after getting a hearing aid.

Normal results

A hearing aid will boost the loudness of sound, which can improve a person's ability to understand speech.

ORGANIZATIONS

American Academy of Otolaryngology—Head and Neck Surgery, 1650 Diagonal Road, Alexandria, VA, 22314-2857, (703) 836-4444, http://www.entnet.org.

Better Hearing Institute, 1444 I Street, NW, Suite 700, Washington, DC, 20005, (202) 449-1100, (800) 327-9355, mail@betterhearing.org, http://www.betterhearing.org/, http://www.betterhearing.org/

Hearing Industries Association, 1444 I Street, N.W., Suite 700, Washington, DC, 20005, (202))449-1090, (202) 216-9646, mspangler@bostrom.com, http://www.hearing.org.

Hearing Loss Association of America, 7910 Woodmont Ave., Suite 1200, Behtesda, MD, 20814, (301) 657-2248, http://www.hearingloss.org.

National Institute on Deafness and Other Communication Disorders, 31 Center Drive, MSC 2320, Bethesda, MD, 20892-2320, (800) 241-1044 , nidcdinfo@nidcd.nih.gov, http://www.nidcd.nih.gov.

Starkeu Hearing Foundation, 6700 Washington Ave South, Eden Prairie, MN, 55344, (866) 354-3254 , http://www.starkeyhearingfoundation.org.

Carol A. Turkington

Hearing loss

Definition

Hearing loss is any degree of impairment of the ability to apprehend sound. Such impairment occurs primarily due to natural causes (heredity) and environmental factors (extended exposure to loud sounds). Secondary factors of hearing loss include obstructions

Decibel ratings and hazardous levels of noise

Decibel level	Examples of sounds
30	Soft whisper
35	Noise may prevent listener from falling asleep
40	Quiet office noise level
50	Quiet conversation
60	Average television volume, sewing machine, lively conversation
70	Busy traffic, noisy restaurant
80	Heavy city traffic, factory noise, alarm clock
90	Cocktail party, lawn mower
100	Pneumatic drill
120	Sandblasting, thunder
140	Jet airplane
180	Rocket launching pad

At volumes above 110 decibels, hearing may become painful.
A volume above 120 decibels is considered deafening.
At volumes above 135 decibels, hearing will become extremely painful and hearing loss may result if exposure is prolonged.
At volumes above 180 decibels, hearing loss is almost certain with any exposure.

(Table by PreMediaGlobal. Reproduced by permission of Gale, a part of Cengage Learning.)

within the ear canal, primarily ear wax but sometimes also other natural or foreign materials.

Demographics

Generally, some hearing loss occurs gradually as humans get older. According to the National Institutes of Health, about one out of three older Americans between the ages of 65 and 75 years has hearing loss. Over the age of 75 years, hearing loss occurs in about one out two people in the United States. However, hearing loss can happen to any person regardless of age.

Description

Sound can be measured accurately. The term decibel (dB) refers to an amount of energy moving sound from its source to one's ears or to a microphone. For instance, a whisper is equivalent to about 30 dB and a washing machine is around 70 dB, both well within the range that will not produce hearing loss. However, heavy traffic and a hair dryer each produce about 85 to 90 dB, which is within the range that is considered risky for producing a loss of hearing. Even worse, a jet taking off and a shotgun blast each produce between 140 and 165 dB, which is within the range that can cause considerable degradation to one's hearing. In fact, a drop of more than 10 dB in the level of sound a person can hear is significant.

Sound travels through a medium like air or water as waves of compression and rarefaction. These waves are collected by the external ear and cause the tympanic membrane (ear drum) to vibrate. The chain of ossicles connected to the ear drum—the incus, malleus, and stapes—carry the vibration to the oval window, increasing its amplitude 20 times on the way. There the energy causes a standing wave in the watery liquid (endolymph) inside the Organ of Corti. (A standing wave is one that does not move. A vibrating cup of coffee, for instance, will demonstrate standing waves.) The configuration of the standing wave is determined by the frequency of the sound. Many thousands of tiny nerve fibers detect the highs and lows of the standing wave and transmit their findings to the brain, which interprets the signals as sound.

To summarize, sound energy passes through the air of the external ear, the bones of the middle ear and the liquid of the inner ear. It is then translated into nerve impulses, sent to the brain through nerves and understood there as sound. It follows that there are five steps in the hearing process:

- air conduction through the external ear to the ear drum
- bone conduction through the middle ear to the inner ear
- water conduction to the Organ of Corti
- nerve conduction into the brain
- interpretation by the brain.

Hearing can be interrupted (that is, hearing loss can result) in several ways at each of the five steps.

Risk factors

Some of the risk factors that can lead to hearing loss include:

- Age: Exposure to loud sounds over many years
- Heredity: Being born within a family that is prone to hearing loss
- Occupation: A person's place of work or employment—one that involves loud noises on a regular basis (such as construction workers using pneumatic hammers or loggers using chain saws)
- Recreation: Exposure to loud noises during recreational activities, such as rock concerts, snowmobiling, and automobile races, along with the use of musical and other sound-generating devices hooked up directly to the ear
- Illnesses: Medical conditions that involve exceptionally high fevers, such as meningitis
- Medications: Continual use of drugs, such as pain relievers and nonsteroidal anti-inflammatory drugs

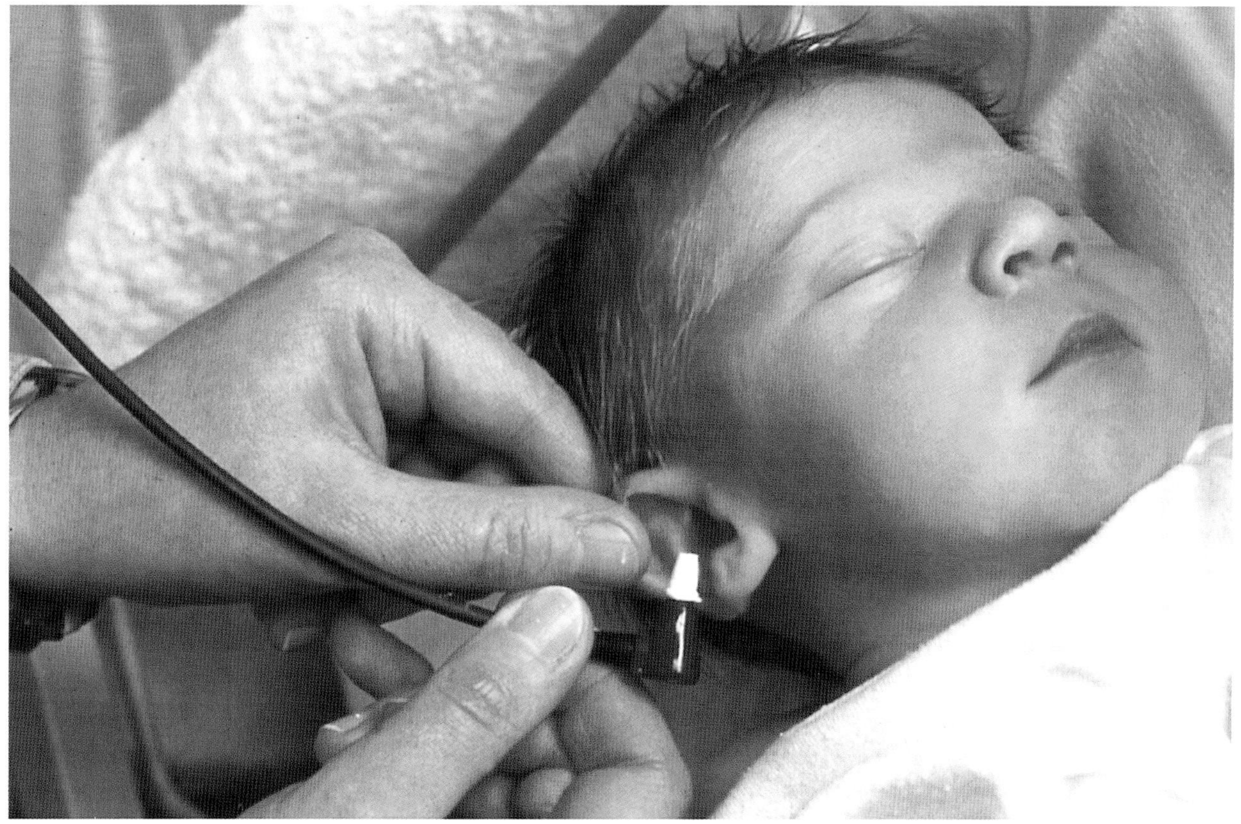

An Oto-Acoustic Emission (OAE) hearing test being performed on a newborn baby. The probe emits harmless sound into the baby's ear, and the response of the inner ear is detected and registered on a computer. Early diagnosis of a hearing disorder is important in young children, who may experience difficulties in speech and language development. *(James King-Holmes/Photo Researchers, Inc.)*

Causes and Symptoms

The external ear canal can be blocked with ear wax, **foreign objects**, infection, and tumors. Wax build-up can cause hearing loss in people of any age. Overgrowth of the bone, a condition that occurs when the ear canal has been flushed with cold water repeatedly for years, can also narrow the passageway, making blockage and infection more likely. This condition occurs often in Northern Californian surfers and is therefore called "surfer's ear."

The ear drum is so thin a physician can see through it into the middle ear. Sharp objects, pressure from an infection in the middle ear, or even a firm cuffing or slapping of the ear, can rupture it. It is also susceptible to pressure changes during scuba diving.

Several conditions can diminish the mobility of the ossicles (small bones) in the middle ear. **Otitis media** (an infection in the middle ear) occurs when fluid cannot escape into the throat because of blockage of the eustachian tube. The fluid then accumulates—whether it is pus or just mucus—which dampens the motion of the ossicles. A disease called **otosclerosis** can bind the stapes in the oval window and thereby cause deafness.

All of the conditions mentioned so far that occur in the external and middle ear are causes of conductive hearing loss.

The second category, sensory hearing loss, refers to damage to the Organ of Corti and the acoustic nerve. Prolonged exposure to loud noise is the leading cause of sensory hearing loss. At least one million people have this condition in the United States, many of whom were identified during the military draft and rejected as being unfit for duty. The cause is often believed to be prolonged exposure to rock music. Occupational noise exposure is the other leading cause of noise induced hearing loss (NIHL) and is ample reason for wearing ear protection on the job. A third of people over 65 years of age have presbycusis—sensory hearing loss due to **aging**. Both NIHL and presbycusis are primarily high frequency losses. In most languages, the high frequency sounds define speech, so these people hear plenty of noise. They just cannot easily make out what it means. They have particular trouble selecting out speech from background noise.

Brain infections like **meningitis**, drugs such as the aminoglycoside **antibiotics** (streptomycin, gentamycin, kanamycin, tobramycin), and Meniere's disease also cause permanent sensory hearing loss. Meniere's disease combines attacks of hearing loss with attacks of vertigo. The symptoms may occur together or separately. High doses of salicylates like **aspirin** and quinine can cause a temporary high-frequency loss. Prolonged high doses can lead to permanent deafness. There is an hereditary form of sensory deafness and a congenital form most often caused by **rubella** (German **measles**).

The general symptoms of hearing loss include the following:

- Unclear (muffled) voices and noises
- Difficulty with the understanding of spoken words, especially when background noises are present
- Requests for people to talk slowly or more distinctly
- Inability to participate in conversations
- Reluctance to attend social events.

Sudden hearing loss—at least 30dB in less than three days—is most commonly caused by cochleitis, a mysterious viral infection.

The final category of hearing loss is neural. Damage to the acoustic nerve and the parts of the brain that perform hearing are the most likely to produce permanent hearing loss. Strokes, **multiple sclerosis**, and acoustic neuromas are all possible causes of neural hearing loss.

Hearing can also be diminished by extra sounds generated by the ear, most of them from the same kinds of disorders that cause diminished hearing. These sounds are referred to as **tinnitus** and can be ringing, blowing, clicking, or anything else that no one but the patient hears.

Diagnosis

An examination of the ears and nose combined with simple hearing tests done in the physician's office can detect many common causes of hearing loss. An audiogram often concludes the evaluation, since this simple means often produces a diagnosis. If the defect is in the brain or the acoustic nerve, further neurological testing and imaging will be required.

The audiogram has many uses in diagnosing hearing deficits. The pattern of hearing loss across the audible frequencies gives clues to the cause. Several alterations in the testing procedure can give additional information. For example, speech is perceived differently than pure tones. Adequate perception of sound combined with inability to recognize words points to a brain problem rather than a sensory or conductive deficit. Loudness perception is distorted by disease in certain areas but not in others. Acoustic neuromas often distort the perception of loudness.

Treatment

Conductive hearing loss can almost always be restored to some degree, if not completely. Some ways to restore hearing loss are:

- matter in the ear canal can be easily removed with a dramatic improvement in hearing.
- surfer's ear gradually regresses if cold water is avoided or a special ear plug is used. In advanced cases, surgeons can grind away the excess bone.
- middle ear infection with fluid is also simple to treat. If medications do not work, surgical drainage of the ear is accomplished through the ear drum, which heals completely after treatment.
- traumatically damaged ear drums can be repaired with a tiny skin graft.
- surgical repair of otosclerosis through an operating microscope is one of the most intricate of procedures, substituting tiny artificial parts for the original ossicles.

Sensory and neural hearing loss, on the other hand, cannot readily be cured. Fortunately the loss is not often complete, so that **hearing aids** can fill the deficit.

In-the-ear hearing aids can boost the volume of sound by up to 70 dB. (Normal speech is about 60 dB.) Federal law now requires that they be dispensed only with a physician's prescription. For complete conduction hearing loss there are now available bone conduction hearing aids and even devices that can be surgically implanted in the cochlea.

Tinnitus can sometimes be relieved by adding white noise (like the sound of wind or waves crashing on the shore) to the environment.

Decreased hearing is such a common problem that there are legions of organizations to provide assistance. Special language training, both in lip reading and signing, special schools, and special camps for children are all available in most regions of the United States.

Alternative treatment

Conductive hearing loss can be treated with alternative therapies that are specific to the particular condition. Sensory hearing loss may be helped by homeopathic therapies. Oral supplementation with essential fatty

KEY TERMS

Decibel—A unit of the intensity of sound, a measure of loudness.

Meniere's disease—The combination of vertigo and decreased hearing caused by abnormalities in the inner ear.

Multiple sclerosis—A progressive disease of brain and nerve tissue.

Otosclerosis—A disease that scars and limits the motion of the small conducting bones in the middle ear.

Stroke—Sudden loss of blood supply to part of the brain.

acids such as flax oil and omega 3 oil can help alleviate the accumulation of wax in the ear.

Prognosis

The prognosis for reducing or eliminating hearing loss widely varies. Whether hearing loss can be solved is generally dependent on the cause. Conductive hearing loss is usually able to be cured. However, sensory hearing loss is more complicated to treat and is usually not curable. People can regain a majority of their hearing with the use of hearing aids.

Prevention

Prompt treatment and attentive follow-up of middle ear infections in children will prevent this cause of conductive hearing loss. Control of infectious childhood diseases, such as measles, has greatly reduced sensory hearing loss as a complication of epidemic diseases. Laws that require protection from loud noise in the workplace have achieved substantial reduction in noise induced hearing loss. Surfers should use the right kind of ear plugs.

Resources

BOOKS

Brookshire, Robert H. *Introduction to Neurogenic Communication Disorders (7th edition)*. St. Louis, MO: Mosby, 2007.

OTHER

Hearing Disorders and Deafness. MedlinePlus, National Library of Medicine and National Institutes of Health. (September 1, 2010), http://www.nlm.nih.gov/medlineplus/hearingdisordersanddeafness.html (accessed September 15, 2010).

Hearing Loss. Mayo Clinic. (August 22, 2009), http://www.mayoclinic.com/health/hearing-loss/DS00172 (accessed September 14, 2010).

ORGANIZATIONS

Alexander Graham Bell Academy for Listening and Spoken Language, 3417 Volta Place NW, Washington, DC, 20007, (202) 204-4700, (202) 337-8314, academy@agbell.org, http://agbell.org/NetCommunity/Page.aspx?pid=330.

Alexander Graham Bell Association for the Deaf and Hard of Hearing, 3417 Volta Place NW, Washington, DC, 20007, (202) 337-5220, http://nc.agbell.org/.

Better Hearing Institute, 1444 I Street NW; Suite 700, Washington, DC, 20005, (202) 449-1100, mail@betterhearing.org, http://www.betterhearing.org/.

Center for Hearing and Communications, 50 Broadway, Sixth Floor, New York City, NY, 10004, (917) 305-7700, http://www.chchearing.org/.

Central Institute for the Deaf, 825 South Taylor Avenue, St. Louis, MO, 63110, (314) 977-0132, (877) 444-4574, (314) 977-0023, http://www.cid.edu/home.aspx.

Hearing Loss Association of America, 7910 Woodmont Avenue, Suite 1200, Bethesda, MD, 20814, (301) 657-2248, http://www.hearingloss.org/.

National Association of the Deaf, 8630 Fenton Street, Suite 820, Silver Spring, MD, 20910-3819, (301) 587-1788, (301) 587-1791, http://www.nad.org/.

The Sight & Hearing Association, 1246 University Avenue West, Suite 226, St. Paul, MN, 55104-4125, (651) 645-2546, (800) 992-0424, (651) 645-2742, mail@sightandhearing.org, http://www.sightandhearing.org/.

World Recreation Association of the Deaf, Post Office Box 3211, Quartz Hill, CA, 93586, (661) 952-7752, wradceo@aol.com, http://www.wrad.org/.

J. Ricker Polsdorfer, MD

Hearing test with an audiometer *see* **Audiometry**

Hearing tests with a tuning fork

Definition

A tuning fork is a metal instrument with a handle and two prongs or tines. Tuning forks, made of steel, aluminum, or magnesium-alloy will vibrate at a set frequency to produce a musical tone when struck. The vibrations produced can be used to assess a person's ability to hear various sound frequencies.

Purpose

A vibrating tuning fork held next to the ear or placed against the skull will stimulate the inner ear to vibrate and can help determine if there is **hearing loss**.

KEY TERMS

Mastoid process—The protrusions of bone behind the ears at the base of the skull.

Rinne test—A hearing test using a vibrating tuning fork which is held near the ear and held at the back of the skull.

Weber test—A hearing test using a vibrating tuning fork which is held at various points along the midline of the skull and face.

Precautions

No special precautions are necessary when tuning forks are used to conduct a hearing test.

Description

Two types of hearing tests with tuning forks are typically conducted. In the Rinne test, the vibrating tuning fork is held against the skull, usually on the bone behind the ear (mastoid process) to cause vibrations through the bones of the skull and inner ear. It is also held next to, but not touching, the ear, to cause vibrations in the air next to the ear. The patient is asked to determine which sound is louder, the sound heard through the bone or through the air. A second hearing test using a tuning fork is the Weber test. For this test, the stem or handle of the vibrating tuning fork is placed at various points along the midline of the skull and face. The patient is then asked to identify which ear hears the sound created by the vibrations. Tuning forks of different sizes produce different frequencies of vibrations and can be used to establish the range of hearing for an individual patient.

Preparation

No special preparation is required for a hearing test with tuning forks.

Aftercare

No special aftercare is required. If hearing loss is revealed during testing with tuning forks, the patient may require further testing to determine the extent of the hearing loss.

Risks

There are no risks associated with the use of tuning forks to screen for hearing loss.

Normal results

With the Rinne test, a person will hear the tone of the vibration longer and louder when the tuning fork is held next to the ear, rather than when it is held against the mastoid bone. For the Weber test, the tone produced when the tuning fork is placed along the center of the skull, or face, sounds about the same volume in each ear.

Abnormal results

The Rinne test detects a hearing loss when a patient hears a louder and longer tone when the vibrating tuning fork is held against the mastoid bone than when it is held next to the ear. The volume of sound vibrations conducted through parts of the skull and face in the Weber test can indicate which ear may have a hearing loss.

ORGANIZATIONS

American Academy of Otolaryngology—Head and Neck Surgery, 1650 Diagonal Road, Alexandria, VA, 22314-2857, (703) 836-4444, http://www.entnet.org.

EAR Foundation of Arizona, 668 North 44th Street, Suite 300, Phoenix, AZ, 85008 (602) 685-1050, (602) 239-5117, melissa@earfoundationaz.com, http://www.earfoundationaz.com.

Altha Roberts Edgren

Heart arrest *see* **Sudden cardiac death**
Heart arrhythmias *see* **Arrhythmias**

Heart attack

Definition

A heart attack is the **death** of or damage to heart muscle because the supply of blood to the heart is severely restricted or blocked. Heart attacks also are called myocardial infarctions (MIs).

Demographics

Heart attack is the leading cause of death in the United States. More than 1.5 million Americans experience a heart attack every year and between 500,000 and 700,000 die. Worldwide, heart attacks cause 12 million deaths each year. Most heart attacks are the result of years of silent but progressive **coronary artery disease** (CAD); a heart attack may be the first symptom of the disease. According to the American Heart Association,

63% of women and 48% of men who died suddenly of coronary artery disease had no previous symptoms.

Description

A heart attack occurs when one or more of the coronary arteries that supply blood to the heart are completely or substantially blocked and not enough oxygen reaches the heart (a condition called **ischemia**). The blockage usually is caused by **atherosclerosis**, the build-up of plaque in the artery walls, and/or by a blood clot in a coronary artery. Much less often, a healthy coronary artery has a spasm, and blood flow to part of the heart suddenly decreases or stops. Coronary artery spasm in young, healthy individuals is most often brought on by **methamphetamine** or **cocaine** use.

About half of all people who have heart attacks wait at least two hours before seeking help. This increases their chance of death or permanently disabled. The longer an artery remains blocked during a heart attack, the more damage will be done to the heart. Therefore, it is important to recognize the signs of a heart attack and seek prompt medical attention at the nearest hospital with 24-hour emergency cardiac care.

About one-fifth of all heart attacks are silent, that is, the individual does not know one has occurred. Although the person feels no **pain**, silent heart attacks still damage the heart.

The outcome of a heart attack depends on where the blockage is, whether heart rhythm is disturbed, and whether another coronary artery supplies blood to that part of the heart. Blockages in the left coronary artery usually are more serious than in the right coronary artery. Blockages that cause an arrhythmia, an irregular heartbeat, can cause sudden death.

Major risk factors

Major risk factors significantly increase the risk of coronary artery disease. Those which cannot be changed include:

- Heredity. People whose parents have coronary artery disease are more likely to develop it. The risk of heart attack is highest for those who have a male parent or sibling who has had a heart attack before age 45 or a female parent or sibling who has had a heart attack before age 55.
- Gender. Men under 60 years of age are more likely to have heart attacks than women of the same age.
- Age. Men over the age of 45 and women over the age of 55 are considered at risk. Older people (those over 65) are at increased risk of dying from a heart attack. Older women are twice as likely to die within a few weeks of a heart attack as men of the same age.

Major risk factors that can be modified through lifestyle changes include:

- Smoking. Smoking greatly increases both the chance of developing coronary artery disease and the change of dying from it. Smokers are more than twice as likely to have a heart attack and have two to four times the risk of non-smokers of sudden cardiac death. They also are more likely to die within an hour of a heart attack. Exposure to second-hand smoke also increases risk.
- High cholesterol. Cholesterol is a soft, waxy substance that is produced by the liver, as well as obtained from eating cholesterol-containing food, such as meat, eggs, and other animal products. Cholesterol level is affected by age, sex, heredity, and diet.
- Cholesterol does not dissolve in blood. Instead, it moves through the circulatory system in combination with carrier substances called lipoproteins. There are two types of carrier-cholesterol combinations, low-density lipoprotein (LDL) or "bad" cholesterol and high-density lipoprotein (HDL) or "good" cholesterol.
- LDL picks up cholesterol in the liver and carries it through the circulatory system. Most of the cholesterol in the body is LDL cholesterol. When too much LDL cholesterol is present, it begins to drop out of the blood and stick to the walls of the arteries. The sticky material on the artery walls is called cholesterol plaque. Plaque can reduce the amount of blood flowing through the arteries and encourage blood clots to form. Total cholesterol of 240 mg/dL and over poses a high risk, and 200–239 mg/dL a borderline high risk. For LDL cholesterol, high risk starts at 130–159 mg/dL, depending on other risk factors.
- Researchers believe that HDL works opposite LDL. HDL picks up cholesterol off the walls of the arteries and takes it back to the liver where it can be broken down and removed from the body. This helps to keep the blood vessels open. Cholesterol can be measured by a simple blood test. To reduce the risk of cardiovascular disease, adults should keep their HDL cholesterol above 40 mg/dL.
- High blood pressure (hypertension). High blood pressure makes the heart work harder and over time weakens it. It increases the risk of heart attack, stroke, kidney failure, and congestive heart failure. A blood pressure of 140 over 90 or above is considered high. As the numbers increase, high blood pressure goes from being categorized as Stage 1 (mild) to Stage 4 (very severe). African Americans are at increased risk of developing severe hypertension.

KEY TERMS

Angina—Chest pain that happens when diseased blood vessels restrict the flow of blood to the heart. Angina often is the first symptom of coronary artery disease.

Atherosclerosis—A process in which the walls of the coronary arteries thicken due to the accumulation of plaque in the blood vessels. Atherosclerosis is the cause of coronary artery disease.

Coronary arteries—The arteries that provide blood to the heart. The coronary arteries surround the heart like a crown, coming out of the aorta, arching down over the top of the heart and dividing into two branches. These are the arteries where coronary artery disease occurs.

Myocardial infarction—The technical term for heart attack. Myocardial means heart muscle and infarction means death of tissue from lack of oxygen.

Plaque—A deposit of fatty and other substances that accumulate in the lining of the artery wall.

- Obesity and lack of physical activity. The heart of an obese individual must work harder, while lack of physical activity increases the risk of coronary artery disease. Even modest physical activity is beneficial if done regularly.
- Use of certain drugs or supplements. In the late twentieth century, ephedra (ma huang) gained popularity as a weight-loss supplement. The herb can cause life-threatening side effects, including heart attack, stroke, and seizures. Since April 2004, sale of products containing ephedra have been banned in the United States, although it may still be obtained illegally over the Internet. Hormone replacement therapy (HRT) was once believed to help prevent heart disease in postmenopausal women. However, the Women's Health Initiative, a very large clinical trial, found the opposite to be true. Potential adverse effects of HRT include increased risk of heart attack, stroke and blood clots, and an increased risk of breast cancer.

Contributing risk factors

Contributing risk factors have been linked to coronary artery disease, but their significance or prevalence cannot always be demonstrated or quantified. Contributing risk factors include:

- Diabetes mellitus. The risk of developing coronary artery disease is seriously increased for individuals with diabetes. More than 80% of diabetics die of some type of heart or blood vessel disease.
- Emotional factors. Long-term stress, anger, and guilt are thought to contribute to the development of coronary artery disease. Stress, the mental and physical reaction to life's irritations and challenges, increases the heart rate and blood pressure and can injure the lining of the arteries. Evidence shows that anger increases the risk of dying from heart disease and more than doubles the risk of having a heart attack right after an episode of anger.

Causes and symptoms

Heart attacks generally are the result of severe coronary artery disease. Most heart attacks are caused by **blood clots** that form on atherosclerotic plaque. These may break lose and travel through the circulatory system causing heart attack or **stroke** (blockage of an artery to the brain). Certain major risk factors increase the chance of developing coronary artery disease. Some of these can be modified and some cannot. People with a greater number of risk factors are more likely to develop coronary artery disease.

More than 60% of people who have a heart attack experience symptoms before the heart attack occurs. These symptoms sometimes occur days or weeks before the heart attack. Sometimes, people do not recognize the symptoms of a heart attack or are in denial that they are having one. Typical symptoms include:

- Uncomfortable pressure, fullness, squeezing, or pain in the center of the chest (angina) that lasts more than 30 minutes. Warning pains before a heart attack may last a shorter time or may go away with rest and then return.
- Pain that spreads to the shoulders, neck, arms, or jaw.
- Chest discomfort accompanied by lightheadedness, fainting, sweating, nausea, or shortness of breath.

All of these symptoms do not occur with every heart attack, and most have other common causes. Nevertheless, person with any of these symptoms should immediately call an emergency rescue service (recommended) or be driven (but not drive themselves) to the nearest hospital with a 24-hour cardiac care unit. The advantage of calling an emergency rescue service is that life-saving treatment may begin while the individual is in transit to the hospital.

Diagnosis

Experienced emergency care personnel usually can diagnose a heart attack simply by looking at the patient.

Tests

To confirm this diagnosis, they talk with the patient, check heart rate and blood pressure, perform an electrocardiogram, and take a blood sample. The electrocardiogram shows whether damage has occurred to the heart. Electrodes covered with conducting jelly are placed on the patient's chest, arms, and legs. They send impulses of the heart's electrical activity through an oscilloscope (a monitor) to a recorder, which traces them on paper. Damaged hearts produce a different electrical pattern from healthy hearts. The blood test shows the leak of cardiac enzymes or other biochemical markers from damaged cells in the bloodstream.

Treatment

The goal of treatment is to restore adequate blood flow and oxygen delivery to the heart, relieve pain, and prevent complications. Heart attacks are treated with **cardiopulmonary resuscitation** (CPR) when necessary to start and keep the patient breathing and the heart beating. Beta-blocker drugs may be given to help control heart rate. Other drugs may be used to relieve pain and **anxiety**. These treatments may be started by trained emergency medical service personnel in the ambulance on the way to the hospital.

Traditional

Once at the hospital, certain patients may receive intravenous drug therapy to dissolve blood clots (**thrombolytic therapy**). If started within six hours after the start of the heart attack, these drugs are successful in dissolving blood clots in about 80% of patients. If these drugs are given in a window 6–12 hours after the start of pain, the success rate drops to 50%. Thrombolytic therapy is not used if more than 12 hours has passed since chest pain started. Throughout treatment, the patient is monitored closely.

Additional treatment can include, electric shock, additional drug therapy, revascularization procedures, percutaneous transluminal coronary **angioplasty**, and coronary artery bypass surgery. An electrical-shock device (defibrillator), may be used to restore a normal rhythm if the heart is fluttering and contracting uncontrollably (arrhythmia). Supplemental oxygen often is used to ease the heart's workload. If oxygen is used within hours of the heart attack, it may help limit damage to the heart. Additional drugs may be used to stabilize the patient and limit damage to the heart, including **aspirin**, anticoagulants, painkillers, tranquilizers, beta-blockers, ace-inhibitors, nitrates, rhythm-stabilizing drugs, and **diuretics**. Once the patient has been stabilized, he or she is usually moved to the cardiac care unit (CCU) for special monitoring.

Drugs

To prevent additional heart attacks, aspirin and an anticoagulant drug often follow the thrombolytic drug. These help to prevent new blood clots from forming and existing blood clots from growing. **Anticoagulant drugs** help prevent the blood from clotting. The most common anticoagulants are heparin and warfarin. Heparin, an anticoagulant, often is given intravenously while the patient is in the hospital. Warfarin (Coumadin), taken orally, often is given later, and sometimes must be taken for life. Aspirin helps to prevent the dissolved blood clots from reforming.

To relieve pain, a nitroglycerine tablet taken under the tongue may be given. If the pain continues, morphine sulfate may be prescribed. Tranquilizers such as diazepam (Valium) and alprazolam (Ativan) may be prescribed to lessen the trauma of a heart attack.

To slow the heart rate and give the heart a chance to heal, beta-blockers often are given intravenously right after the heart attack. These can also help prevent sometimes-fatal **ventricular fibrillation**. Beta-blockers include atenolol (Tenormin), metoprolol (Lopressor), nadolol, pindolol (Visken), propranolol (Inderal), and timolol (Blocadren).

Nitrates, a type of vasodilator, also are given right after a heart attack to help improve the delivery of blood to the heart and ease **heart failure** symptoms. Nitrates include isosorbide mononitrate (Imdur), isosorbide dinitrate (Isordil, Sorbitrate), and nitroglycerin (Nitrostat).

When a heart attack causes an abnormal heartbeat, arrhythmia drugs may be given to restore and maintain the heart's normal rhythm. These include amiodarone (Cordarone), atropine, bretylium, disopyramide (Nor Pace), lidocaine (Xylocaine), procainamide (Procan), propafenone (Rythmol), propranolol (Inderal), quinidine, and sotalol (Betapace).

Angiotensin-converting enzyme (ACE) inhibitors reduce the resistance against which the heart beats and are used to manage and prevent heart failure. They are used to treat heart attack patients whose hearts do not pump well or who have symptoms of heart failure.

Taken orally, they include Altace, Capoten, Lotensin, Monopril, Prinivil, Vasotec, and Zestril. Angiotensin receptor blockers, such as losartan (Cozaar), may be substituted.

Diuretics can help get rid of excess fluids that sometimes accumulate when the heart is not pumping effectively. They also help reduce **hypertension**. Usually taken orally, they cause the body to increase urine output. Common diuretics include: bumetanide (Bumex), chlorthalidone (Hygroton), chlorothiazide (Diuril), furosemide (Lasix), hydrochlorothiazide (HydroDIRUIL, Esidrix), spironolactone (Aldactone), and triamterene (Dyrenium).

Surgery

Percutaneous transluminal coronary angioplasty and coronary artery bypass surgery are invasive revascularization procedures that open blocked coronary arteries and improve blood flow. They usually are performed only on patients for whom clot-dissolving drugs do not work, who have poor **exercise** stress tests, poor left ventricular function, or ischemia. Generally, angioplasty is tried before coronary artery bypass surgery is attempted.

Percutaneous transluminal coronary angioplasty, usually called coronary angioplasty, is a procedure in which a catheter (a tiny plastic tube) tipped with a balloon is threaded from a blood vessel in the thigh or arm into the blocked artery. The balloon is inflated and compresses the plaque to enlarge the blood vessel and open the blocked artery. The balloon is then deflated and the catheter is removed. Coronary angioplasty is performed in a hospital and generally requires a two-day stay. It is successful about 90% of the time. For one-third of patients, the artery narrows again within six months after the procedure. The procedure can be repeated. It is less invasive and less expensive than coronary artery bypass surgery.

In coronary artery bypass surgery, a detour is built around the coronary artery blockage using a healthy leg or chest wall artery or vein. The healthy vein then supplies oxygen-rich blood to the heart. Bypass surgery is major surgery done most often only when patients have blockages in two or three coronary arteries or a severely narrowed left main coronary arteries, or who have not responded to other treatments. It is performed in a hospital under **general anesthesia** using a heart-lung machine to support the patient while the heart is stopped and a healthy vein is attached to the coronary artery. About 70% of patients who have bypass surgery experience full relief from **angina**; about 20% experience partial relief. Long term, symptoms recur in only about 3 or 4% of patients per year. Five years after bypass surgery, survival expectancy is 90%, at 10 years it is about 80%, at 15 years it is about 55%, and at 20 years it is about 40%.

There are several other surgical procedures for unblocking coronary arteries including: **atherectomy**, where the surgeon grinds out and removes strips of plaque from the blocked artery and laser angioplasty, where a catheter with a laser tip is inserted to burn or break down the plaque. After the artery is opened, a tiny metal tube called a stent may be implanted permanently to help the artery remain open.

Alternative

Alternative therapies aim at preventing the progression of heart disease that leads to a heart attack. Changes in lifestyle can also prevent second heart attacks.

Herbal medicine offers a variety of remedies that may have a beneficial effect on coronary artery disease. Oats *(Avena sativa)*, garlic *(Allium sativum)*, and guggul *(Commiphora mukul)*, may help reduce cholesterol; linden *(Tilia europaea)* and hawthorn *(Crataegus spp.)* are sometimes recommended to control high blood pressure, a risk factor for heart disease. Tea *(Camellia sinensis)*, especially green tea, is high in **antioxidants**, which studies have shown may have a preventive effect against atherosclerosis.

Nutritional therapies have been shown to prevent coronary artery disease and stop, or even reverse, the progression of atherosclerosis. A low-fat, high-fiber diet is often recommended. It is essential to reduce the amount of meat and animal products consumed, as they are high in saturated fats. Whole grains, fresh fruits and vegetables, legumes, and nuts are recommended. Vitamin and mineral supplements that reduce, reverse, or protect against coronary artery disease include chromium; **calcium** and magnesium; B complex **vitamins**; the antioxidant vitamins B and E; L-carnitine; and zinc.

Yoga and other bodywork, massage, relaxation therapies, **aromatherapy**, and **music therapy** may also help by reducing stress and promoting physical and mental well being. By evoking the body's relaxation response through **meditation** and deep breathing, blood pressure, metabolic rate, and heart rate can all be reduced.

Rehabilitation

Successful recovery from a heart attack requires a substantial amount of **rehabilitation**. Most patients follow a three-stage rehabilitation program. Phase 1 begins in the hospital with low-level exercise to prevent complications from prolonged bed rest. Phase 2 begins after hospital discharge and usually takes place in an outpatient rehabilitation setting. The goals of phase 2 are to increase physical endurance and to promote return to normal daily activities. Phase 3 continues in an outpatient setting, It begins 3–6 months after the heart attack and may last up to one year. In phase 3, the level of exercise is gradually increased, ideally to the point where swimming, light jogging, or bicycling is possible. The effectiveness of rehabilitation, however, may be limited by other medical conditions.

Prognosis

Early recognition of a heart attack substantially improves survival. More than half or all people who have heart attacks die before they reach the hospital. Another 10% die in the hospital. Of people who leave the hospital after a heart attack, 27% of men and 44% of women die within one year. Within six years, 23% of men and 31% of women have another heart attack, 13% of men and 6% of women experience sudden death, and about 20% have heart failure. People who survive a heart attack have a chance of sudden death that is four to six times greater than others and a chance of illness and death that is two to nine times greater.

Prevention

Many heart attacks can be prevented through a healthy lifestyle that reduces risk factors for developing coronary artery disease. For patients who have already had a heart attack, a healthy lifestyle, participation in a **cardiac rehabilitation** program, and carefully following doctor's orders may prevent another heart attack. A heart-healthy lifestyle includes eating a heart-healthy diet, regular exercise, maintaining a healthy weight, no **smoking**, moderate drinking, no illegal drugs, controlling high blood pressure, and managing stress.

A heart-healthy diet includes a variety of foods that are low in fat (especially saturated fat), low in cholesterol, and high in fiber; plenty of fruits and vegetables; and limited **sodium** (salt). Saturated fat raises cholesterol. Polyunsaturated and monounsaturated fats are relatively better for the heart. Fat should comprise no more than 30 percent of total daily calories. The American Heart Association has information on heart-healthy living on its Web site and publishes several heart-healthy cookbooks.

Cholesterol comes from eating foods such as meat, eggs, and other animal products. It also is produced in the liver. Soluble dietary fiber can help lower cholesterol. Cholesterol intake should be limited to about 300 mg per day. Many lipid-lowering drugs can reduce LDL-cholesterol by an average of 25–30% when combined with a low-fat, low-cholesterol diet. Fruits and vegetables are rich in fiber, vitamins, and **minerals**. They are also low in calories and nearly fat free. Vitamin C and beta-carotene, found in many fruits and vegetables, also are beneficial. Excess sodium increases the risk of high blood pressure. Many processed foods contain large amounts of sodium, which should be limited to a daily intake of 2,400 mg—about the amount in a teaspoon of salt. In the United States, cholesterol, fats, fiber, sodium, and calories are listed on nutritional labels of all processed foods.

Regular aerobic exercise can lower blood pressure, help control weight, increase HDL ("good") cholesterol, and reduce stress. Moderate intensity aerobic exercise lasting about 30 minutes four or more times per week is recommended for maximum heart health. Three 10-minute exercise periods also are beneficial. Aerobic exercise—activities such as walking, jogging, and cycling—uses the large muscle groups and forces the body to use oxygen more efficiently. It also can include everyday activities, such as active gardening, climbing stairs, or brisk housework. However, any regular exercise, no matter how mild, is better than not exercising.

Maintaining a desirable body weight also is important in preventing heart attacks. In 2009, about one-third of all adult Americans were overweight or obese. People who are 20% or more over their ideal body weight have an increased risk of developing coronary artery disease. Losing weight can help reduce total and LDL cholesterol, reduce **triglycerides**, and boost relative levels of HDL cholesterol. It also may reduce blood pressure.

Smoking has many adverse effects on the heart. It increases the heart rate, constricts major arteries, and can create irregular heartbeats. It also raises blood pressure, contributes to the development of plaque, increases the formation of blood clots, and causes blood platelets to cluster and impede blood flow. Quitting can repair heart damage caused by smoking; even heavy smokers can return to heart health, and the health of their lungs also improves. Several studies have shown that ex-smokers face the same risk of heart disease as non-smokers within 5 to 10 years of quitting.

Drinking alcohol should always be done in moderation. Modest consumption of alcohol may protect against coronary artery disease; however, even small amounts of alcohol may have other negative effects depending on the individual's health status and medications being taken. The American Heart Association defines moderate consumption as one ounce of alcohol per day—roughly one cocktail, one 8-ounce glass of wine, or two 12-ounce glasses of beer. Excessive alcohol use is always bad for the heart, and illegal drugs, such as methamphetamines and cocaine, can seriously harm the heart and cause a fatal heart attack.

High blood pressure, one of the most common and serious risk factors for coronary artery disease, can be controlled through lifestyle changes and medication. People with moderate hypertension may be able to lower it through dietary changes, such as reducing sodium intake combined with exercising regularly, managing stress, quitting smoking, and drinking alcohol in moderation. If these changes do not work, or if hypertension is severe, drugs that lower blood pressure may be prescribed.

Stress management means controlling mental and physical reactions to life's irritations and challenges. Techniques for controlling stress include taking life more slowly, spending time with family and friends, thinking positively, getting enough sleep, exercising, and practicing relaxation techniques.

Daily aspirin therapy has been proven to help reduce blood clots associated with atherosclerosis. It also can lower the risk of strokes.

Resources

BOOKS

American Heart Association. *American Heart Association Low-fat, Low-cholesterol Cookbook: Delicious Recipes to Help Lower your Cholesterol*. New York, NY: Clarkson Potter, 2004.

Kligfield, Paul. *The Cardiac Recovery Handbook: The Complete Guide to Life After Heart Attack or Heart Surgery*, 2nd ed. Long Island City, NY: Hatherleigh Press, 2006.

Siple, Molly. *Low-cholesterol Cookbook for Dummies*. Indianapolis, IN: Wiley Pub., Inc, 2004.

OTHER

"ABCs of Preventing Heart Disease, Stroke, and Heart Attack." *American Heart Association*. April 20, 2009 [September 14, 2009]. http://www.americanheart.org/presenter.jhtml?identifier = 3035374.

"Heart Attack." September 9, 2009 [September 14, 2009]. http://www.nlm.nih.gov/medlineplus/heartattack.html.

Mayo Clinic Staff. "Heart Attack." November 30, 2007 [September 14, 2009]. http://www. mayoclinic.com/health/heart-attack/DS00094.

ORGANIZATIONS

American Association of Cardiovascular and Pulmonary Rehabilitation, 401 North Michigan Avenue, Suite 2200, Chicago, IL, 60611, (312) 321-5146, (312) 673-6924, aacvpr@aacvpr.org, http://www.aacvpr.org.

American College of Cardiology, Heart House, 2400 N Street, NW, Washington, DC, 20037, (202) 375-6000, (800) 253-4636 x8603, (202) 375-7000, resource@acc.org, http://www.acc.org.

American Heart Association, 7272 Greenville Avenue, Dallas, TX, 75231, (800) 242-8721, http://www.americanheart.org.

National Heart Lung and Blood Institute Health Information Center, P.O. Box 30105, Bethesda, MD, 20824-0105, (301) 592-8573; TTY: (240) 629-3255, (240) 629-3246, nhlbiinfo@nhlbi.nih.gov, http://www.nhlbi.nih.gov.

Tish Davidson, A.M.

Heart block

Definition

Heart block refers to a delay in the normal flow of electrical impulses that cause the heart to beat. They are further classified as first-, second-, or third-degree block.

Description

The muscles of the heart contract in a rhythmic order for each heart beat, because electrical impulses travel along a specific route called the conduction system. The main junction of this system is called the atrioventricular node (AV node). Just as on a highway, there are occasionally some delays getting the impulse from one point to another. These delays are classified according to their severity.

In first-degree heart block, the signal is just slowed down a little as it travels along the defective part of the conduction system so that it arrives late traveling from the atrium to the ventricle.

In second-degree heart block, not every impulse reaches its destination. The block may affect every other beat, every second or third beat, or be very rare. If the blockage is frequent, it results in an overall slowing of the heart called bradycardia.

Third-degree block, also called complete heart block, is the most serious. When no signals can travel through the AV node, the heart uses its backup impulse generator in the lower portion of the heart. Though this impulse usually keeps the heart from stopping entirely, it is too slow to be an effective pump.

Causes and symptoms

First-degree heart block is fairly common. It is seen in teenagers, in young adults, and in well-trained athletes. The condition may be caused by **rheumatic fever**, some types of heart disease, and by some drugs. First-degree heart block produces no symptoms.

KEY TERMS

Atrioventricular node (AV node)—Highly specialized area of the heart muscle which transmits electrical impulses.

Bradycardia—A slow heart rate, usually under 60 beats per minute.

Some cases of second-degree heart block may benefit from an artificial pace-maker. Second-degree block can occasionally progress to third-degree.

Third-degree heart block is a serious condition that affects the heart's ability to pump blood effectively. Symptoms include **fainting**, **dizziness**, and sudden **heart failure**. If the ventricles beat more than 40 times per minute, symptoms are not as severe, but include tiredness, low blood pressure on standing, and **shortness of breath**.

Young children who have received a forceful blunt chest injury, can experience first- or second-degree heart block.

Diagnosis

Diagnosis of first- and second-degree heart block is made by observing it on an electrocardiograph (ECG).

Third-degree heart block usually results in symptoms, such as fainting, dizziness, and sudden heart failure, which require immediate medical care. A physical exam and ECG confirm the presence of heart block.

Treatment

Some second- and almost all third-degree heart blocks require an artificial pacemaker. In an emergency, a temporary pacemaker can be used until an implanted device is advisable. Most people need the pacemaker for the rest of their lives.

Prognosis

Most people with first- and second-degree heart block don't even know they have it. For people with third-degree block, once the heart has been restored to its normal, dependable rhythm, most people live full and comfortable lives.

ORGANIZATIONS

American Heart Association National Center, 7272 Greenville Avenue, Dallas, TX, 75231, (800) 242-8721, Review.personal.info@heart.org.

Dorothy Elinor Stonely

Heart catheterization *see* **Cardiac catheterization**

Heart disease

Definition

Heart disease is a group of conditions affecting the structure and functions of the heart. The four primary conditions that make up heart disease are **coronary artery disease**, **heart attack**, **congenital heart disease**, and rheumatic heart disease. Other diseases include **angina** (chest **pain**) and arrhythmia (irregular heartbeat).

Description

The heart is a muscle that gets energy from blood carrying oxygen and nutrients. Having a constant supply of blood keeps the heart working properly. Most people think of heart disease as one condition. However, heart disease is a group of conditions affecting the structure and functions of the heart and has many root causes. Coronary artery disease (CAD) is the most common of these conditions and occurs when blood vessels in the heart become blocked or narrowed. This blockage limits the flow of blood through the coronary arteries, the major arteries supplying oxygen-rich blood to the heart. The coronary arteries expand when the heart is working harder and needs more oxygen. If the arteries are unable to expand, the heart is deprived of oxygen (myocardial **ischemia**). When the blockage is limited, chest pain or pressure called angina may occur. When the blockage cuts off the blood flow, the result is heart attack (myocardial infarction or heart muscle death).

A normal heart is a strong muscular pump. It weighs between 200 and 425 grams (7–15 ounces) and is a little larger than the size of an adult fist. During an average lifetime, the human heart will beat more than 2.5 billion times. The average heart beats about 100,000 times each day and pumps about 7,200 liters (1,900 gallons) of blood. The heart sits between the lungs in the middle of the chest, behind and slightly to the left of the breastbone. A double-layered membrane called the pericardium surrounds the heart like a sac. Blood loaded with oxygen comes from the lungs and enters the heart. To function, the heart needs a continuous supply of oxygen and nutrients, which it gets from the blood that is pumped through the coronary arteries. The heart and circulatory system make up the cardiovascular system. The heart pumps blood to the organs, tissues, and cells of the body, delivering oxygen and nutrients to every cell

Prevalence of heart disease in the United States[1]

	African American		Caucasian	
	Females	Males	Females	Males
Coronary heart disease	8.8%	7.8%	6.9%	9.4%
Heart attack	2.9%	3.6%	2.6%	5.1%
Angina pectoris	5.4%	4.0%	4.5%	4.7%
Total cardiovascular disease	**46.9%**	**44.6%**	**34.4%**	**38.1%**

[1]All statistics are from 2006, the most recent year for which data was available.

SOURCE: American Heart Association, *Heart Disease and Stroke Statistics—2010 Update*. Available online at: http://www.americanheart.org (accessed September 23, 2010).

(Table by PreMediaGlobal. Reproduced by permission of Gale, a part of Cengage Learning.)

and removing carbon dioxide and waste products made by those cells. Oxygen-rich blood is carried from the heart to the rest of the body through a complex network of arteries, arterioles, and capillaries. Oxygen-poor blood is carried back to the heart through veins.

Coronary artery disease

Healthy coronary arteries are open, elastic, smooth, and slick. The artery walls are flexible and expand to let more blood through when the heart needs to work harder. The disease process is thought to begin with an injury to the linings and walls of the arteries. This injury makes them susceptible to **atherosclerosis** and production of **blood clots** (thrombosis).

Coronary artery disease (CAD) is a condition in which plaque builds up inside the coronary arteries. These arteries supply the heart muscle with oxygen-rich blood. Plaque is made up of fat, cholesterol, **calcium**, and other substances found in the blood. When plaque builds up in the arteries, the condition is called atherosclerosis, commonly called hardening of the arteries. Plaque narrows the arteries and reduces blood flow to the heart. It also makes it more likely that blood clots will form in arteries. Blood clots can partially or completely block blood flow. When coronary arteries are narrowed or blocked, oxygen-rich blood can't reach the heart. This can cause angina or a heart attack. Angina is chest pain or discomfort that occurs when not enough oxygen-rich blood is flowing to an area of the heart. Angina may feel like pressure or squeezing in the chest. The pain also may occur in the shoulders, arms, neck, jaw, or back. A heart attack occurs when blood flow to an area of the heart is completely blocked. This prevents oxygen-rich blood from reaching that area of heart and causes it to die. Without quick treatment, a heart attack can lead to serious problems and even death. Over time, CAD can weaken the heart and lead to **heart failure** and **arrhythmias**. Heart failure is a condition in which the heart can't pump enough blood throughout the body. Arrhythmias are irregularities with the speed or rhythm of the heartbeat.

Heart attack (myocardial infarction)

A heart attack (myocardial infarction) occurs when the blood supply to the heart is slowed or stopped because of a blockage. Atherosclerosis, the narrowing of coronary arteries due to plaque buildup, causes more than 90% of heart attacks. A heart attack may also occur when a coronary artery temporarily contracts or goes into a severe spasm, effectively shutting off the flow of blood to the heart. The length of time the blood supply is cut off will determine the amount of damage to the heart.

Congenital heart disease

Congenital means existing at birth. A congenital heart defect happens when the heart or the blood vessels near the heart don't develop normally before birth. Congenital heart defects are present in about 1% of live births and are the most frequent congenital malformations in newborns. In most cases, researchers don't know why they happen. Some causes include viral infections, certain conditions such as **Down Syndrome**, and drug **abuse** during **pregnancy**, especially of alcohol, **cocaine**, and methamphetamines.

Rheumatic heart disease

Rheumatic heart disease describes a group of acute (short-term) and chronic (long-term) heart disorders that can occur as a result of **rheumatic fever**. One common result of rheumatic **fever** is heart valve damage. Due to the control of rheumatic fever in the

United States and most developed countries, it is relatively rare in these regions but is still a significant heart disease in parts of Africa, Asia, and South America. Rheumatic fever is an inflammatory disease that may affect many connective tissues of the body, especially those of the heart, joints, brain or skin. It usually starts out as a **strep throat** (streptococcal) infection. Anyone can get acute rheumatic fever, but it usually occurs in children between the ages of 5 and 15 years. About 60% of people with rheumatic fever develop some degree of subsequent heart disease.

Demographics

Heart disease is the leading cause of death in the United States, and it is a major cause of disability. Almost 700,000 people die of heart disease in the United States each year, about 29% of all U.S. deaths. Statistics from the Centers for Disease Control (CDC) report that coronary heart disease is the principal type of heart disease, reponsible for about 68.3% of all heart disease deaths. In 2005, coronary heart disease killed more than 7.6 million people. Worldwide, heart disease and **stroke** kill 17 million people a year, almost one-third of all deaths globally, according to the World Health Organization (WHO). By 2020, heart disease and stroke will become the leading cause of both death and disability worldwide, with the number of fatalities projected to increase to over 20 million a year and by 2030 to over 24 million a year. Men are slightly more likely to develop heart disease than women. An increasing number of women are experiencing heart disease but they are under-diagnosed. For both sexes, the risk of heart disease increases with age. In the United States, the number of heart disease deaths per 100,000 people by race is: Hispanics, 72; Asians and Pacific Islanders, 78; Native Americans, 80; African Americans, 206; and Caucasians, 259. However, when adjusted for differences in age distributions, the death rate from heart disease was 30% higher among African Americans than whites. In 2004, the number of deaths per 100,000 people in the U.S. by age groups was: 55–64, 218.8; 65–74, 541.6; 75–84, 1,506; and 85 and older, 4,896.

Causes and symptoms

Coronary artery disease

Over many years, plaque builds up on artery walls. Plaque is a sticky, yellow substance made of fatty substances like cholesterol, as well as calcium and waste products from cells. It narrows and clogs the arteries, slowing the flow of blood. The process is called atherosclerosis. Atherosclerosis is a slow, progressive condition that may begin as early as childhood and occur anywhere in the body but it usually affects large and medium sized arteries. Atherosclerotic plaques often form blood clots that can also block the coronary arteries (coronary thrombosis). Sometimes plaque in an artery can rupture. The body's repair system in turn creates a blood clot to heal the wound. The clot, however, can block the artery, leading to a heart attack or stroke.

Congenital defects and **muscle spasms** of arteries or heart muscles also block blood flow. Some research indicates that infection from organisms such as chlamydia bacteria may be responsible for some cases of heart disease.

Early warning signs may include: **fatigue**, pain, and **dizziness**, as well as the symptoms associated with angina: a squeezing, suffocating, or burning feeling in the chest that tends to start in the center of the chest but may move to the arm, neck, back, throat, or jaw. Women are more likely to experience atypical symptoms, such as vague chest discomfort.

Heart attack (myocardial infarction)

A heart attack occurs when the blood supply to the heart is partially or completely blocked. Symptoms include pain in the chest, neck, jaw, shoulder, arms or back, sudden discomfort or pain (especially in the chest) that does not go away, difficulty breathing, **nausea**, sweating, and **anxiety**.

Congenital heart disease

Congenital heart disease is caused by a defect in the heart at birth. The most common symptoms of congenital heart defects are a heart murmur, a bluish tint to the skin, lips, or fingernails, fast breathing, **shortness of breath**, and fatigue, especially during **exercise** or physical activity.

Rheumatic heart disease

It may take several years after an episode of rheumatic fever for valve damage to develop or symptoms to appear. **Antibiotics** can prevent streptococcal infection from developing into rheumatic fever. Any child with a persistent **sore throat** should have a **throat culture** to check for strep infection. Penicillin or another antibiotic will usually prevent strep throat from developing into rheumatic fever. Symptoms of heart valve problems, which are often the result of rheumatic heart disease, can include chest pain, excessive fatigue, heart **palpitations** (when the heart flutters or misses beats), a thumping sensation in the chest, shortness of breath, and swollen ankles, wrists or stomach.

Major risk factors

A number of major contributing risk factors increase the chance of developing heart disease. Some of these can be changed and some cannot. The greater the number of risk factors, the greater the chance of developing heart disease. Major risk factors significantly increase the chance of developing heart disease. These include:

- Heredity. People whose parents have heart disease are more likely to develop it. African Americans are also at increased risk because they experience a high rate of severe hypertension.
- Gender. Men are more likely to have heart attacks than women and have them at a younger age. Above the age of 60, however, women have heart disease at a rate equal to that of men.
- Age. Men who are 45 years of age and older and women who are 55 years of age and older are more likely to have heart disease. Occasionally, heart disease may strike men or women in their 30s. People more than 65 years old are more likely to die from a heart attack. Older women are twice as likely as older men to die within a few weeks of a heart attack.
- Smoking. Smoking increases both the chance of developing heart disease and the chance of dying from it. Smokers are more than twice as likely as non-smokers to have a heart attack and are two to four times more likely die from it.
- High cholesterol levels. Dietary sources of cholesterol are meat, dairy food, eggs, and other animal-fat products. Cholesterol is also produced by the body. Age, body fat, diet, exercise, heredity, and sex affect one's blood cholesterol. For typical, healthy patients, the American Heart Association recommends a total blood cholesterol below 200 mg/dL, which puts the person at a comparatively low risk for coronary heart disease. For these individuals, a total cholesterol level of 200–239 mg/dL is considered borderline high-risk, and a level of 240 mg/dL or above is considered high risk and doubles the risk for coronary heart disease. Persons with such risk factors as elevated low-density lipoprotein (LDL cholesterol, or "bad" cholesterol) levels, low high-density lipoprotein (HDL or "good" cholesterol) levels, or high triglyceride levels should consult with their doctor about what their target cholesterol level should be.
- High blood pressure. High blood pressure makes the heart work harder and weakens it over time. It increases the risk of heart attack, stroke, kidney failure, and congestive heart failure. A blood pressure of 140 over 90 or above is considered high. The risk of heart attack or stroke is raised several times for people with high blood pressure combined with obesity, smoking, high cholesterol levels, or diabetes. Nearly one-third of American adults have high blood pressure.
- Lack of physical activity. Lack of exercise increases the risk of heart disease. Even modest physical activity, such as walking, is beneficial if done regularly.
- Diabetes mellitus. The risk of developing heart disease is seriously increased for diabetics. About two-thirds of people who have type I or type II diabetes die as the result of a heart attack or stroke.

Contributing risk factors

Contributing risk factors have been linked to heart disease. These include:

- Obesity. Excess weight increases the strain on the heart and increases the risk of developing heart disease even if no other risk factors are present. Obesity increases blood pressure and blood cholesterol and can lead to diabetes.
- Hormone replacement therapy (HRT). Even though physicians once believed that HRT could help prevent heart disease in women, the Women's Health Initiative (WHI) released information in 2002 and 2003 showing that use of combined hormones (estrogen and progestin) is harmful in women who already have coronary artery disease. As of 2007, it continued to be debated if HRT, and estrogen in particular, can provide some protection against heart disease when a woman takes it soon after going through menopause.
- Stress and anger. Some scientists believe that poorly managed stress and anger can contribute to the development of heart disease and increase the blood's tendency to form clots (thrombosis). Stress increases the heart rate and blood pressure and can injure the lining of the arteries.
- Chest pain (angina). Angina is the main symptom of coronary heart disease, but it is not always present. Other symptoms include shortness of breath, chest heaviness, tightness, pain, a burning sensation, squeezing, or pressure either behind the breastbone or in the left arm, neck, or jaws. According to the American Heart Association, 64 percent of women and 50 percent of men who died suddenly of heart disease had no previous symptoms of the disease.

Diagnosis

Diagnosis begins with a doctor's review of the medical history, discussion of symptoms, listening to the heart, and performing basic screening tests. These tests measure blood lipid levels, blood pressure, fasting blood-glucose levels, weight, and other indicators. Other diagnostic tests include resting and exercise electrocardiograms,

echocardiography, radionuclide scans, and coronary **angiography**. The treadmill exercise (stress) test is an appropriate screening test for those with high risk factors even though they feel well.

Angiogram

Coronary angiography is considered the most accurate method for making a diagnosis of heart disease, but it is also the most invasive. This test involves taking x ray pictures of the coronary arteries and the vessels that supply blood to the heart. During coronary angiography the patient is awake but sedated. The cardiologist inserts a catheter into a blood vessel and guides it into the heart. A contrast dye (a radiopaque substance that is visible on x ray) is injected into the catheter and x rays are taken. This dye makes the blood vessels visible when an X-ray is taken of them. Angiography allows doctors to clearly see how blood flows into the heart. This helps them to pinpoint problems with the coronary arteries. Angiography may be recommended for patients with angina or those with suspected coronary artery disease. The test gives doctors valuable information on the condition of the coronary arteries, such as atherosclerosis, regurgitation (blood flowing backwards through the heart valves), or pooling of blood in a chamber because of a valve malfunction. Coronary angiography is performed in a **cardiac catheterization** laboratory in either an outpatient or an inpatient surgery unit.

Radionuclide angiography enables physicians to see the blood flow of the coronary arteries. Nuclear scans are performed by injecting a small amount of radiopharmaceutical, such as thallium, into the bloodstream. As the patient lies on a table, a camera that uses gamma rays to produce an image of the radioactive material passes over the patient and records pictures of the heart. Radionuclide angiography is usually performed in a hospital's nuclear medicine department. The radiation exposure is about the same as that in a **chest x ray**.

Echocardiogram

An echocardiogram uses sound waves (ultrasound) to create a picture of the heart. The recorded waves show the shape, texture, and movement of the heart valves, as well as the size of the heart chambers and how well they are working. A technician applies gel to a hand-held transducer and then presses it against the patient's chest. The heart's sound waves are converted into an image that can be displayed on a monitor. An echocardiogram may be done to determine whether a stroke was caused by a heart condition and can also help determine if there is a risk of blood clots forming in the heart. It may also be recommended if the patient is experiencing abnormal heart sounds, shortness of breath, palpitations, angina, or has a history of stroke. It is very useful in diagnosing heart valve problems. It does not reveal the coronary arteries themselves but can detect abnormalities in the heart wall caused by heart disease. Typically performed in a doctor's office or outpatient facility, the test takes 30 to 60 minutes.

Electrocardiogram

An electrocardiogram (ECG or EKG) is a test that checks how the heart is functioning by measuring the electrical activity of the heart. Electrodes are placed on the patient's chest, arms, and legs. They send impulses of the heart's activity through an oscilloscope (a monitor) to a recorder that traces them on paper. With each heart beat, an electrical impulse (wave) travels through the heart. This wave causes the muscle to squeeze and pump blood from the heart. By measuring how long the electrical wave takes to pass through the heart, a cardiologist can determine if the electrical activity is normal, fast, or irregular. The cardiologist may also be able to determine if the heart is enlarged or overworked. It may be recommended if the patient is experiencing arrhythmia, palpitations, dizziness, excessive fatigue, or angina. An ECG is used to:

- Detect abnormal heart rhythms that may have caused blood clots to form.
- Detect heart problems, including a recent or ongoing heart attack, abnormal heart rhythms (arrhythmias), coronary artery blockage, areas of damaged heart muscle (from a prior heart attack), enlargement of the heart, and inflammation of the sac surrounding the heart (pericarditis).
- Detect non-heart conditions such as electrolyte imbalances and lung diseases.
- Monitor recovery from a heart attack, progression of heart disease, or the effectiveness of certain heart medications or a pacemaker.
- Rule out hidden heart disease in patients about to undergo surgery.

Exercise stress test

This test measures how the heart and blood vessels respond to exertion when the patient is exercising on a treadmill or a stationary bike. It can be performed in a physician's office or outpatient facility.

Treatment

Heart disease can be treated many ways. The choice of treatment depends on the patient and the severity of the disease. Treatments include lifestyle changes, drug therapy, and coronary artery bypass surgery. (Recommendations for persons with coronary artery disease are available through the American Heart Association Web site at http://www.americanheart.org/presenter.jhtml?identifier=3039477.) These, however, are not a cure. Heart disease is a chronic disease requiring lifelong care.

There is no cure for heart disease, but there are many treatments, such as medications, surgery, and lifestyle changes, that can slow down its progression.

Medications

People with moderate heart disease may gain adequate control through lifestyle changes and drug therapy. Drugs such as nitrates, beta-blockers, and **calcium channel blockers** relieve chest pain and complications of heart disease, but they cannot clear blocked arteries. Nitrates improve blood flow to the heart, and beta-blockers reduce the amount of oxygen required by the heart during stress. Calcium channel blockers help keep the arteries open and reduce blood pressure. **Aspirin** helps prevent blood clots from forming on plaques, reducing the likelihood of a heart attack and stroke. Cholesterol-lowering medications are also indicated in many cases.

ANTIPLATELETS. Antiplatelets help prevent dangerous blood clots from forming. They may be used to reduce the risk of clot-induced heart attack or stroke, which is called preventive or prophylactic treatment. One of the most common antiplatelets is aspirin. Ticlopidine (Ticlid) may be prescribed to stroke survivors or those who are at high risk of stroke, particularly if they are not able to take aspirin. Clopidogrel (Plavix) is an antiplatelet drug that is effective in preventing strokes and heart attacks and is often prescribed for patients who receive a coronary stent. Dipyridmalole (Persantine) may also be given with other antiplatelet or anticoagulant medications. It can also be given by injection during tests on the heart.

ACE INHIBITORS. Angiotensin converting enzyme (ACE) inhibitors are usually given to people with high blood pressure, congestive heart failure, or people with a high likelihood of developing coronary artery disease. They may also be given after a heart attack to prevent more complications and to people living with congestive heart failure. They help control blood pressure to make it easier for the heart to pump. ACE inhibitors may also make people with CAD feel less tired and short of breath, reduce the time they spend in a hospital, and help them live longer. ACE inhibitors have been shown to reduce the risk of heart attack, stroke, and death in people with a history of coronary artery disease. Since ACE inhibitors are used to control and prevent conditions of the heart, they are usually prescribed for the long term.

BETA BLOCKERS. **Beta blockers** are used to treat high blood pressure, congestive heart failure, abnormal heart rhythms, and chest pain. They are sometimes used to prevent future heart attacks in someone who has had a heart attack and to treat **tremors** caused by an overactive thyroid, as well as anxiety or migraines. Beta blocker is short for beta-adrenergic blocking drugs. Beta blockers block the responses from the beta nerve receptors. This slows the heart rate and lowers blood pressure to reduce the workload on the heart.

CALCIUM CHANNEL BLOCKERS. Calcium channel blockers, sometimes called calcium channel antagonists, are used to control high blood pressure, chest pain caused by coronary artery disease, and irregular heartbeats. Calcium channel blockers are often taken in combination with beta blockers or **diuretics** to help reduce blood pressure. Calcium channel blockers are **vasodilators**, which means they widen (dilate) blood vessels, letting blood flow through more easily. By relaxing blood vessels, the blood pressure drops and the heart doesn't have to work as hard.

NITRATES. Nitrates are vasodilators and can be used to prevent chest pain, limit the number of angina attacks, relieve the pain of a current attack, or treat the symptoms of congestive heart failure. Nitroglycerin is a type of nitrate.

Medical procedures

ANGIOPLASTY WITH STENT. Percutaneous Coronary Intervention (PCI), commonly called **angioplasty** with a stent, is a non-surgical procedure that uses a catheter (a thin flexible tube) to place a small structure called a stent (a small tubular structure made of stainless steel or plastic) to open up blood vessels in the heart that have been narrowed by plaque buildup. PCI improves blood flow, thus decreasing heart-related chest pain, making the patient feel better and increasing his or her ability to be physically active. During the procedure, a catheter is inserted into the blood vessels either in the groin or in the arm. Using a special type of X-ray called fluoroscopy, the catheter is threaded through the blood vessels into the heart where the coronary artery is narrowed. When the tip is in place, a balloon tip covered with a stent is inflated. The balloon tip compresses the plaque and expands the stent. Once the plaque is compressed and the stent is in place, the balloon is deflated and withdrawn. The stent stays in the artery, holding it open. The doctor may use a coated stent or a bare metal stent. A coated stent has medicine on its outside that slows the regrowth of the artery wall and blocking the stent. If a coated stent is used, the patient will need to take Plavix for at least two years, perhaps for life.

CORONARY ARTERY BYPASS SURGERY. Coronary artery bypass surgery improves the blood flow to the heart muscle. It is commonly referred to as bypass surgery or Coronary Artery Bypass Graft (CABG, pronounced like cabbage) surgery. Bypass surgery is performed to improve blood flow problems to the heart muscle caused by the buildup of plaque in the coronary arteries. The surgery involves using a piece of blood vessel (artery, vein) taken from elsewhere in the body to create a detour or bypass around the blocked portion of the coronary artery. By improving blood flow, bypass surgery may decrease heart-related chest pain, making patients feel better and increasing their ability for physical activity.

In coronary artery bypass surgery, a piece of a healthy blood vessel from the patient's leg, arm, or chest will be removed to be used as the bypass. Unless a patient is undergoing one of the newer procedures (minimally-invasive bypass or off-pump or beating-heart surgery), the heart is stopped so the surgeons can work on it. A machine called the heart-lung machine will take over the work of the heart and lungs while the surgeon is operating on the heart. The section of healthy blood vessel is attached above and below the blocked artery. When the heart is restarted, blood flow is diverted through the bypass around the narrowed portion of the diseased artery. Depending upon the number of blockages, one to five bypasses may be created.

COUNTER PULSATION. Another medical procedure that can help with CAD is counter pulsation. In this procedure, inflatable cuffs are placed on the legs and lower abdomen. When the heart relaxes, the cuffs inflate and push blood into the blood vessels of the heart. This procedure is repeated over a few days and it stimulates improved blood flow to the heart. Counter pulsation can't be done in people with dilated aortas or who have severe **peripheral vascular disease**.

Heart attack (myocardial infarction)

When someone is experiencing a heart attack or believes they are, they should seek immediate emergency help. In the United States, call or have someone else call 911 and request paramedics or emergency medical technicians (EMTs). Most fire departments in the United States and Canada have paramedics and/or EMTs. Doctors also recommend that at the first sign of a heart attack, the patient chew and swallow an adult (325 mg) aspirin, which can help improve blood flow to the heart. Only aspirin can improve blood flow, no other pain medications, such as **acetaminophen** (Tylenol) or ibuprofen (Advil), will work. Until medical help arrives, the patient should sit or lie down. If the patient is on the drug nitroglycerine, they should take a normal dose. Following a heart attack, patients may be put on nitrates, ACE inhibitors, beta-blockers, and antiplatelets (all described under coronary artery disease medications). Other drugs used include thrombolytic drugs, used to dissolve blood clots that are blocking the coronary arteries, and anticoagulants, used to thin the blood and prevent clots from forming in the arteries. Surgical treatments include angioplasty and coronary bypass (both described under coronary artery disease medical procedures).

Congenital heart disease

The heart defects of congenital heart disease are treated with several medications, including ACE inhibitors, beta blockers, diuretics, and **digoxin**. Diuretics act on the kidneys to produce more urine and remove excess salt and water from the body. By decreasing water and salt, diuretics lower blood pressure and help reduce the workload on the heart. This may make it easier for the heart to pump, improve shortness of breath, reduce swelling and bloating, reduce the time spent in a hospital, and help patients live longer. Digoxin helps the heart pump stronger and slows down the heart rate to improve its pumping action.

In many cases, the strain to the heart requires procedures that either fix holes between the chambers, replace valves, or repair or reconnect major blood vessels. In severe cases, heart **transplant surgery** may be needed. Several other surgical procedures can be used to repair and correct congenital heart defects They include:

- Cardiac catheterization is often used to repair simple holes in the heart. A catheter (thin tube) is inserted into a blood vessel in the groin or arm and guided to the heart so that a surgeon can insert a plug inside the hole to repair it.
- Angioplasty is used to repair defective cardiac valves that can be either too narrow or leaky. A tiny balloon is guided to the heart inside a catheter (a thin tube). When the balloon is inflated, it can stretch the opening of a narrowed heart valve and restore normal blood flow. It is removed once blood flow returns.

Rheumatic heart disease

If heart damage from rheumatic fever is identified in childhood or young adulthood, daily antibiotics may be required until the age of 25 or 30 to help prevent recurrence of rheumatic fever and avoid the development of infective bacterial **endocarditis**, an infection of the heart valves or lining of the heart. Additional treatment will depend on the type of heart damage. Surgery may be required to repair or replace damaged heart valves. In rare cases, heart transplant surgery may be recommended.

Other treatment options

Herbal-medicine practitioners recommend a variety of remedies that may have a beneficial effect on heart disease. They may suggest garlic (*Allium sativum*), myrrh (*Commiphora molmol*), and oats (*Avena sativa*) to help reduce cholesterol, and hawthorn (*Crataegus* spp.), linden (*Tilia europaea*), and yarrow (*Achillea millefolium*) to control high blood pressure, a risk factor for heart disease. Tea, especially green tea (*Camellia sinensis*), is high in **antioxidants**, and studies have shown that it may have a preventive effect against atherosclerosis. Coenzyme Q10 has been shown to be beneficial for patients with congestive heart failure. Taurine, an amino acid found in meat and fish proteins, has also been suggested as a way to treat heart arrhythmia.

Some alternative-medicine practitioners believe that **yoga** and other bodywork, massage, relaxation, **aromatherapy**, and music therapies may also help prevent heart disease and stop, or even reverse, the progression of atherosclerosis. Vitamin and mineral supplements that are believed to reduce, reverse, or protect against heart disease include B-complex **vitamins**, calcium, chromium, magnesium, L-carnitine, zinc, and the antioxidant vitamins C and E. Notably, a study in 2004 showed a relationship between high doses of supplemental vitamin C and reduced coronary heart disease but found little risk reduction with supplemental vitamin E.

Traditional Chinese medicine (TCM) may recommend herbal remedies, massage, **acupuncture**, and dietary modification. A healthy diet (including cold water fish as a source of essential fatty acids) and exercise are important components of both alternative and conventional prevention and treatment strategies.

Nutrition and diet concerns

A healthy diet includes a variety of foods that are low in fat, especially saturated fat; low in cholesterol; and high in fiber. It includes plenty of fruits and vegetables and limits salt. According to the American Heart Association, fats should comprise no more than 25 to 35 percent of total daily calories and should total less than 7 percent saturated fats, less than 1 percent trans fats, and the remainder as monounsaturated and polyunsaturated fats from such sources as nuts, seeds, fish, and vegetable oils. Cholesterol intake should be limited to 300 mg per day for the average person. Those individuals who have coronary heart disease or who have an LDL cholesterol level of 100 mg/dL or more should lower their daily cholesterol intake to less than 200 mg per day. Eating cold-water fish or taking comparable omega-3 polyunsaturated fatty acid supplements can help prevent cardiac death. The American Heart Association advocates eating fish (particularly fatty fish) at least twice a week. It also recommends adding soybeans (including tofu), canola, walnut, and flaxseed, and their oils to the diet because these contain alpha-linolenic acid than can transform into omega-3 fatty acid in the body. The association also notes that individuals consult with their doctor before taking omega-3 fatty acid supplements in excess of 3 grams per day because of the potential for bleeding.

Cholesterol, a waxy substance containing fats, is found in foods such as meat, dairy, eggs, and other animal products. It is also produced in the liver. Soluble fiber can help lower cholesterol. Dietary cholesterol should be below 300 milligrams per day. Many popular lipid-lowering drugs can reduce LDL cholesterol by an average of 25 to 30 percent or more when used with a low-fat, low-cholesterol diet.

Antioxidants are chemical compounds in plant foods. When people eat antioxidant-rich foods, they may improve the function of the arteries and prevent arterial plaque formation and reduce their risk of **cancer**. Colorful vegetables and fruits are sources of antioxidants and are rich in fiber, vitamins, and **minerals**. They are low in calories and nearly fat-free. Vitamin C and beta-carotene, found in many fruits and vegetables, keep LDL-cholesterol from turning into a form that damages coronary arteries. Whole grains, especially whole oats and oat bran, reduce cholesterol.

Excess **sodium** can increase the risk of high blood pressure. Many processed foods contain large amounts of sodium. Daily intake should be limited to about 2,300 milligrams, about the amount in a teaspoon of salt.

New reports on diet and heart disease have answered some questions, but others remain unclear. While one study concludes that four servings per day of fruit and vegetables are associated with a slight drop in risk of heart disease, eight or more servings per day can produce a significant drop in risk. Another study showed that consuming legumes at least four times per week lowered risk of heart disease from 11 percent to 22 percent compared with consuming legumes less than once a week. Research on antioxidants continues to produce mixed findings, with some reports showing that vitamins E, C, and other antioxidants can help prevent heart disease and other studies showing they have no effect. Although scientists and medical professionals had not reached a consensus about the benefits of antioxidants as of 2008, the American Heart Association reported that up to 30 percent of Americans take antioxidant supplements. As of 2008, however, the association did not recommend supplements. Instead, it advised a diet containing a variety of nutrient-rich foods, including fruits, vegetables, whole grains, and nuts.

The Food Guide Pyramid developed by the Center for Nutrition Policy and Promotion, an organization of the U.S. Department of Agriculture, provides easy-to-follow guidelines for daily heart-healthy eating.

Exercising regularly

Regular aerobic exercise can lower blood pressure, help control weight, and increase HDL (good) cholesterol. It also may keep the blood vessels more flexible. The American Heart Association recommends moderate-to-vigorous intensity aerobic activity (50 to 85 percent of the maximum heart rate) for at least 30 minutes on most days of the week. Those 30 minutes can be divided into two 15-minute or three 10-minute sessions throughout the day. Aerobic exercise—activities such as walking, jogging, and cycling—uses the large muscle groups and forces the body to use oxygen more efficiently. It also can include everyday activities such as active gardening, climbing stairs, or brisk housework. People with heart disease or risk factors should consult a doctor before beginning an exercise program.

Maintaining a desirable body weight

People who are 20 percent or more above their ideal body weight have an increased risk of developing heart disease. Losing weight can help decrease total and LDL cholesterol, reduce **triglycerides**, and boost HDL cholesterol. It may also reduce blood pressure. Eating right and exercising are two essential components of losing weight.

Quitting smoking

Smoking has many adverse effects on the heart. It increases the heart rate, constricts major arteries, and can create irregular heartbeats. It also raises blood pressure, contributes to the development of plaque, increases the formation of blood clots, and causes blood platelets to cluster and impede blood flow. When smokers quit the habit, heart damage can be repaired. Several studies have shown that ex-smokers face the same risk of heart disease as non-smokers within 5 to 10 years after they quit.

Drinking in moderation

Modest consumption of alcohol may actually protect against heart disease because alcohol appears to raise levels of HDL cholesterol. The American Heart Association defines moderate consumption as one to two daily drinks for men and one daily drink for women, or one ounce of alcohol per day. The association defines one drink as 4 ounces of wine, 12 ounces of beer, 1.5 ounces of 80-proof spirits, or 1 ounce of 100-proof spirits.

Seeking diagnosis and treatment for hypertension

High blood pressure, one of the most common and serious risk factors for heart disease, can be completely controlled through lifestyle changes and medication. Seeking diagnosis and treatment is critical because **hypertension** often exhibits no symptoms, so many people do not know they have it. Moderate hypertension can be controlled by reducing dietary intake of sodium and fat, exercising regularly, managing stress, abstaining from smoking, and drinking alcohol in moderation.

Managing stress

Everyone experiences stress. Stress can sometimes be avoided and, when it is inevitable, it can be managed through relaxation techniques, exercise, and other methods.

Prevention

The only way to prevent rheumatic heart disease is to prevent rheumatic fever or successfully treat rheumatic fever before it can damage heart valves. There is no way to prevent congenital heart disease, since it is an inherited (genetic) disorder that develops in the womb.

People can lower their risk of coronary artery disease and heart attack by knowing and controlling their blood pressure, diabetes, and cholesterol. It is also important to lead a healthy lifestyle by not smoking and being physically active (exercising regularly), eating a healthy diet that is lower in fat, especially saturated and trans fat, achieving and maintaining a healthy weight, limiting alcohol use, and reducing stress. Seniors can reduce stress by regularly socializing with friends and family and with such activities as yoga and **meditation**. Many doctors also recommend taking a low-dose (81mg) of aspirin daily.

KEY TERMS

Angina—Chest pain.

Angiogram—An X-ray photograph of one or more blood vessels.

Angioplasty—A surgical operation to clear a narrowed or blocked artery.

Arrhythmia—An irregular heartbeat.

Atherosclerosis—A buildup of plaque in the arteries, also called hardening of the arteries.

Beta-blocker—A drug that blocks some of the effects of fight-or-flight hormone adrenaline (epinephrine and norepinephrine), slowing the heart rate and lowering the blood pressure.

Calcium channel blocker—A drug that blocks the entry of calcium into the muscle cells of small blood vessels (arterioles) and keeps them from narrowing.

Coronary arteries—The main arteries that provide blood to the heart. The coronary arteries surround the heart like a crown, coming out of the aorta, arching down over the top of the heart, and dividing into two branches. These are the arteries in which heart disease occurs.

Echocardiogram—An image of the heart created by ultrasound waves.

Electrocardiogram—A test that measures the electrical activity of the heart. Also called an ECG or EKG.

HDL cholesterol—High-density lipoprotein cholesterol is a component of cholesterol that helps protect against heart disease. HDL is nicknamed "good cholesterol."

LDL cholesterol—Low-density lipoprotein cholesterol is the primary cholesterol molecule. High levels of LDL increase the risk of coronary heart disease. LDL is nicknamed "bad cholesterol."

Plaque—A compound made up of fat, cholesterol, calcium, and other substances found in the blood. It can stick to the walls of arteries, partially or totally blocking blood flow.

Triglyceride—A fat that comes from food or is made from other energy sources in the body. Elevated triglyceride levels contribute to the development of atherosclerosis.

Ultrasound—A technique that uses high-frequency sound waves for medical diagnosis and treatment by creating images of internal organs.

Vasodilator—A class of drugs that widen the blood vessels, that in turn decreases resistance to blood flow and lowers blood pressure.

A healthy lifestyle can help prevent heart disease and slow its progress. A heart-healthy lifestyle includes maintaining a healthy diet and weight, performing regular exercise, refraining from smoking, engaging in moderate drinking, controlling hypertension, and managing stress. **Cardiac rehabilitation** programs are excellent ways to help prevent recurring coronary problems for people who are at risk and who have had coronary events and procedures.

Caregiver concerns

Patients with heart disease may have as many as five (or more) medications that need to be taken daily. Caregivers should have a system to make sure that the patient takes the medications when and how they are prescribed. Alarms or timers can be used to remind the patient when to take each pill. Also, weekly pill dispensers can help to insure patients only take the dose that is prescribed. Caregivers may want to keep a medicine calendar and note every time the patient takes a dose, or have the patient do it themselves. It is vital that the caregiver makes sure that prescriptions are refilled before they run out. Make sure that the patient is not taking anything that is contraindicated by their condition or that may interact with their medication. Examples include such things as herbal supplements, **antihistamines**, and **analgesics**. Check with the patient's doctor or pharmacist for possible **drug interactions**. Also, people who take nitrates (such as nitroglycerine) should not take medications for **erectile dysfunction** (ED), including sildenafil (Viagra), vardenafil (Levitra), and tadalafil (Cialis).

Helping a patient stick to their diet and exercise routine is critical to their overall health. One way to ensure adherence to a restricted diet is to prepare meals for the patient. If this is not feasible, the caregiver can try to limit the amount of forbidden foods that are present in the patient's home. The level of exercise required of a patient will depend on their overall health, but for most patients, frequent walks are beneficial. If the caregiver can accompany them on their walks it will make the experience more enjoyable and increase adherence. Perhaps the most important role of a caregiver is providing emotional support. Simply being there to listen to the patient's concerns and to provide encouragement can keep them on the path toward better health. In some cases, the patient may require at-home **oxygen therapy**. The caregiver should learn how the oxygen equipment is used and to make sure more oxygen is ordered well before the patient's current supply runs out.

Prognosis

Advances in medicine and the adoption of healthier lifestyles have caused a substantial decline in death rates from heart disease since the mid-1980s. New diagnostic techniques enable doctors to identify and treat heart disease in its earliest stages. New technologies and surgical procedures have extended the lives of many patients who would have otherwise died. Research continues, and valuable organizations continue to educate clinicians, patients, and healthy individuals alike, in the fight against heart disease

Resources

BOOKS

American Medical Association, Martin S. Lipsky, Marla Mendelson, and Stephen Havas. *American Medical Association Guide to Preventing and Treating Heart Disease: Essential Information You and Your Family Need to Know about Having a Healthy Heart*. Indianapolis, IN: Wiley, 2008.

Esselstyn, Caldwell B. *Prevent and Reverse Heart Disease: The Revolutionary, Scientifically Proven, Nutrition-Based Cure*. New York: Avery, 2008.

Katzenstein, Larry. *An AARP Guide: Living With Heart Disease: Everything You Need to Know to Safeguard Your Health and Take Control of Your Life*. New York: Sterling, 2007.

Lipsky, Martin S, et al. *American Medical Association Guide to Preventing and Treating Heart Disease: Essential Information You and Your Family Need to Know About Having a Healthy Heart*. Hoboken, NJ: Wiley, 2008.

Sinatra, Stephen T., et al. *Reverse Heart Disease Now: Stop Deadly Cardiovascular Plaque Before It's Too Late*. Hoboken, NJ: Wiley, 2008.

PERIODICALS

Grant, Ruth Ann. "Study: Elderly Lacking Heart Attack Care."*McKnight's Long-Term Care News* (September 2007): 6.

Guthrie, Catherine. "Damage Control: The 6 Best Natural Supplements to Protect Against Heart Disease, Choles terol, and High Blood Pressure." *Natural Health* (February 2008): 62(6).

Hanna, Ibrahim R., and Nanette K. Wenger. "Secondary Prevention of Coronary Heart Disease in Elderly Patients." *American Family Physician* (June 15, 2005): 2289.

Kuriyama, Shinichi, et al. "Green Tea Consumption and Mortality Due to Cardiovascular Disease, Cancer, and All Causes in Japan: The Ohsaki Study." *Journal of the American Medical Association*. 296, no. 10 (September 13, 2006): 1255–1265.

Lowry, Fran. "Gastric Bypass Also Cuts Cancer, Diabetes, Heart Disease Mortality."*Family Practice News* (February 1, 2008): 38.

Mast, Carlotta. "Go With the Flow: Support Your Circu latory System and Lower Your Risk of Stroke and Heart Disease With These Drug-Free Recommendations." *Delicious Living* (February 2008): 41(4).

Sherman, Carl. "Reducing the Risk of Heart Disease in Women: Incorporating New Research Findings, the American Heart Association's Updated Guidelines Make Several Changes in the Previous Recommendations."*Clinical Advisor* (January 2008): 49(3).

OTHER

"Hormone Therapy: Is It Right for You?" *MayoClinic.com* February 12, 2008. http://www.mayoclinic.com/health/hormone-therapy/WO00046.

ORGANIZATIONS

Adult Congenital Heart Association, 6757 Greene St., Suite 335, Philadelphia, PA, 19119-3508, (215) 849-1260, (888) 921-2242, (215) 849-1261, info@achaheart.org, http://www.achaheart.org.

American Heart Association, 7272 Greenville Ave., Dallas, TX, 75231, (301) 223-2307, (800) 242-8721, http://www.americanheart.org.

Association of Black Cardiologists, 5355 Hunter Road, Atlanta, GA, 30349, (404) 201-6600, (800) 753-9222, (404) 201-6601, abcardio@abcardio.org, http://www.abcardio.org.

European Society of Cardiology, The European Heart House, 2035 Route des Colles, B.P. 179-Les Templiers, Sophia-Antipolis, France, 06903, 33 4 9294 7600, 33 4 9294 7601, http://www.escardio.org.

Heart Foundation, 80 William St., Level 3, SydneyNSW, Australia, 2011, 02 9219 2444, 300 36 27 87, http://www.heartfoundation.org.au.

National Heart, Lung, and Blood Institute, P.O. Box 30105, Bethesda, MD, 20824-0105, (301) 592-8573, (204) 629-3246, nhlbiinfo@nhlbi.nih.gov, http://www.nhlbi.nih.gov.

Paula Ford-Martin
Ken R. Wells
Laura Jean Cataldo, RN, Ed.D.

Heart failure

Definition

Heart failure is a condition in which the heart has lost the ability to pump enough blood to the body's tissues. With too little blood being delivered, the organs and other tissues do not receive enough oxygen and nutrients to function properly.

Description

According to the American Heart Association, about 5 million Americans are living with congestive heart failure. Ten of every 1,000 people over age 65 have this condition. There are about 550,000 new cases each year.

Heart failure happens when a disease affects the heart's ability to deliver enough blood to the body's tissues. Often, a person with heart failure may have a buildup of fluid in the tissues, called **edema**. Heart failure with this kind of fluid buildup is called congestive heart failure. Where edema occurs in the body depends on the part of the heart that is affected by heart failure. Heart failure caused by abnormality of the lower left chamber of the heart (left ventricle) means that the left ventricle cannot pump blood out to the body as fast as it returns from the lungs. Because blood cannot get back to the heart, it begins to back up in the blood vessels of the lungs. Some of the fluid in the blood is forced into the breathing space of the lungs, causing **pulmonary edema**. A person with pulmonary edema has **shortness of breath**, which may be acute, severe and life threatening. A person with congestive heart failure feels tired because not enough blood circulates to supply the body's tissues with the oxygen and nutrients they need. Abnormalities of the heart structure and rhythm also can be responsible for left ventricular congestive heart failure.

In right-sided heart failure, the lower right chamber of the heart (right ventricle) cannot pump blood to the lungs as fast as it returns from the body through the veins. Blood then engorges the right side of the heart and the veins. Fluid backed up in the veins is forced out into the tissues, causing swelling (edema), usually in the feet and legs. Congestive heart failure of the right ventricle often is caused by abnormalities of the heart valves and lung disorders.

When the heart cannot pump enough blood, it tries to make up for this by becoming larger. By becoming enlarged (hypertrophic) the ventricle can contract more strongly and pump more blood. When this happens, the heart chamber becomes larger and the muscle in the heart wall becomes thicker. The heart also compensates by pumping more often to improve blood output and circulation. The kidneys try to compensate for a failing heart by retaining more salt and water to increase the volume of blood. This extra fluid also can cause edema. Eventually, as the condition worsens over time these measures are not enough to keep the heart pumping enough blood needed by the body. Kidneys often weaken under these circumstances, further aggravating the situation and making therapy more difficult.

For most people, heart failure is a chronic disease with no cure. However, it can be managed and treated with medicines and changes in diet, **exercise**, and lifestyle habits. **Heart transplantation** is considered in some cases.

Causes and symptoms

The most common causes of heart failure are:

- coronary artery disease and heart attack (which may be "silent")
- cardiomyopathy
- high blood pressure (hypertension)
- heart valve disease
- congenital heart disease
- alcoholism and drug abuse

The most common cause of heart failure is **coronary artery disease**. In coronary artery disease, the arteries supplying blood to the heart become narrowed or blocked. When blood flow to an area of the heart is completely blocked, the person has a **heart attack**. Some heart attacks go unrecognized. The heart muscle suffers damage when its blood supply is reduced or blocked. If the damage affects the heart's ability to pump blood, heart failure develops.

Cardiomyopathy is a general term for disease of the heart muscle. Cardiomyopathy may be caused by coronary artery disease and various other heart problems. Sometimes the cause of cardiomyopathy cannot be found. In these cases the heart muscle disease is called idiopathic cardiomyopathy. Whatever the cause, cardiomyopathy can weaken the heart, leading to heart failure.

High blood pressure is another common cause of heart failure. High blood pressure makes the heart work harder to pump blood. After a while, the heart cannot keep up and the symptoms of heart failure develop.

Defects of the heart valves, congenital heart diseases, **alcoholism**, and drug **abuse** cause damage to the heart that can all lead to heart failure.

A person with heart failure may experience the following:

- shortness of breath
- frequent coughing, especially when lying down
- swollen feet, ankles, and legs
- abdominal swelling and pain
- fatigue
- dizziness or fainting
- sudden death

A person with left-sided heart failure may have shortness of breath and coughing caused by the fluid buildup in the lungs. Pulmonary edema may cause the person to **cough** up bubbly phlegm that contains blood. With right-sided heart failure, fluid build-up in the veins and body tissues causes swelling in the feet, legs, and abdomen. When body tissues, such as organs and muscles, do not receive enough oxygen and nutrients they cannot function as well, leading to tiredness and **dizziness**.

Diagnosis

Diagnosis of heart failure is based on:

- symptoms
- medical history
- physical examination
- chest x ray
- electrocardiogram (ECG; also called EKG)
- other imaging tests
- cardiac catheterization

A person's symptoms can provide important clues to the presence of heart failure. Shortness of breath while engaging in activities and episodes of shortness of breath that wake a person from sleep are classic symptoms of heart failure. During the **physical examination**, the physician listens to the heart and lungs with a stethoscope for telltale signs of heart failure. Irregular heart sounds, "gallops," a rapid heart rate, and murmurs of the heart valves may be heard. If there is fluid in the lungs a crackling sound may be heard. Rapid breathing or other changes in breathing may also be present. Patients with heart failure also may have a rapid pulse.

By pressing on the abdomen, the physician can feel if the liver is enlarged. The skin of the fingers and toes may have a bluish tint and feel cool if not enough oxygen is reaching them.

A **chest x ray** can show if there is fluid in the lungs and if the heart is enlarged. Abnormalities of heart valves and other structures also may be seen on chest x ray.

An electrocardiogram gives information on the heart rhythm and the size of the heart. It can show if the heart chamber is enlarged and if there is damage to the heart muscle from blocked arteries.

Besides chest x ray, other imaging tests may help make a diagnosis. **Echocardiography** uses sound waves to make images of the heart. These images can show if the heart wall or chambers are enlarged and if there are any abnormalities of the heart valves. An echocardiogram also can be used to find out how much blood the heart is pumping. It determines the amount of blood in the ventricle (ventricular volume) and the amount of blood the ventricle pumps each time it beats (called the ejection fraction). A healthy heart pumps at least one-half the amount of blood in the left ventricle with each heartbeat. Radionuclide ventriculography also measures the ejection fraction by imaging with very low doses of an injected radioactive substance as it travels through the heart.

A new test that measures the level of a particular hormone in the blood was introduced in 2003 and researchers said the test may be useful for testing for heart failure in physicians' offices because it could provide results in 15 minutes.

Cardiac catheterization involves using a small tube (catheter) that is inserted through a blood vessel into the heart. It is used to measure pressure in the heart and the amount of blood pumped by the heart. This test can help find abnormalities of the coronary arteries, heart valves, and heart muscle, and other blood vessels. Combined with echocardiography and other tests, cardiac catheterization can help find the cause of heart failure. It is not always necessary, however.

Treatment

Heart failure usually is treated with lifestyle changes and medicines. Sometimes surgery is needed to correct abnormalities of the heart or heart valves. Heart transplantation is a last resort to be considered in certain cases.

Dietary changes to maintain proper weight and reduce salt intake may be needed. Reducing salt intake helps to lessen swelling in the legs, feet, and abdomen. Appropriate exercise also may be recommended, but it is important that heart failure patients only begin an exercise program with the advice of their doctors. Walking, bicycling, swimming, or low-impact aerobic exercises may be recommended. There are good heart **rehabilitation** programs at most large hospitals.

Other lifestyle changes that may reduce the symptoms of heart failure include stopping **smoking** or other tobacco use, eliminating or reducing alcohol consumption, and not using harmful drugs.

One or more of the following types of medicines may be prescribed for heart failure:

- diuretics
- digitalis
- vasodilators
- beta blockers
- angiotensin converting enzyme inhibitors (ACE inhibitors)
- angiotensin II receptor blockers (ARBs)

KEY TERMS

Angioplasty—A technique for treating blocked coronary arteries by inserting a catheter with a tiny balloon at the tip into the artery and inflating it.

Angiotensin-converting enzyme (ACE) inhibitor—A drug that relaxes blood vessel walls and lowers blood pressure.

Arrhythmias—Abnormal heartbeat.

Atherosclerosis—Buildup of a fatty substance called a plaque inside blood vessels.

Calcium channel blocker—A drug that relaxes blood vessels and lowers blood pressure.

Cardiac catheterization—A diagnostic test for evaluating heart disease; a catheter is inserted into an artery and passed into the heart.

Cardiomyopathy—Disease of the heart muscle.

Catheter—A thin, hollow tube.

Congenital heart defects—Abnormal formation of structures of the heart or of its major blood vessels present at birth.

Congestive heart failure—A condition in which the heart cannot pump enough blood to supply the body's tissues with sufficient oxygen and nutrients; back up of blood in vessels and the lungs causes buildup of fluid (congestion) in the tissues.

Coronary arteries—Arteries that supply blood to the heart muscle.

Coronary artery bypass—Surgical procedure to reroute blood around a blocked coronary artery.

Coronary artery disease—Narrowing or blockage of coronary arteries by atherosclerosis.

Digitalis—A drug that helps the heart muscle to have stronger pumping action.

Diuretic—A type of drug that helps the kidneys eliminate excess salt and water.

Edema—Swelling caused by fluid buildup in tissues.

Ejection fraction—A measure of the portion of blood that is pumped out of a filled ventricle.

Heart valves—Valves that regulate blood flow into and out of the heart chambers.

Hypertension—High blood pressure.

Hypertrophic—Enlarged.

Idiopathic cardiomyopathy—Cardiomyopathy without a known cause.

Pulmonary edema—Buildup of fluid in the tissue of the lungs.

Vasodilator—Any drug that relaxes blood vessel walls.

Ventricles—The two lower chambers of the heart.

- calcium channel blockers
- blood thinners
- potassium

Diuretics help eliminate excess salt and water from the kidneys by making patients urinate more often. This helps reduce the swelling caused by fluid buildup in the tissues. Digitalis helps the heart muscle to have stronger pumping action. **Vasodilators**, ACE inhibitors, ARBs, and **calcium channel blockers** lower blood pressure and expand the blood vessels so blood can move more easily through them. This action makes it easier for the heart to pump blood through the vessels. Cholesterol-lowering drugs called statins can help prevent **death** from heart failure. A 2003 study showed a 62% drop in the mortality rate among patients with severe heart failure who took statin therapy.

In 2005, the U.S. Food and Drug Administration (FDA) approved a new noninvasive procedure for patients with congestive heart failure. Called **enhanced external counterpulsation** (EECP), it consists of inflating three sets of pneumatic cuffs attached to the patient's legs. The therapy had positive effects on the blood pressure and reduced frequency of episodes of **angina (pain)** in a clinical trial by as much as 70%.

Surgery is used to correct certain heart conditions that cause heart failure. Congenital heart defects and abnormal heart valves can be repaired with surgery. Blocked coronary arteries usually can be treated with **angioplasty** or coronary artery bypass surgery.

With severe heart failure, the heart muscle may become so damaged that available treatments do not help. Patients with this stage of heart failure are said to have end-stage heart failure. Heart transplant usually is considered for patients with end-stage heart failure when all other treatments have stopped working.

Prognosis

Most patients with mild or moderate heart failure can be successfully treated with dietary and exercise programs and the right medications. In fact, in 2003, the American Heart Association said that even those awaiting heart transplants could benefit from exercise. Many people are able to participate in normal daily activities and lead relatively active lives.

Patients with severe heart failure may eventually have to consider heart transplantation. Approximately 50% of patients diagnosed with congestive heart failure live for five years with the condition. Women with heart failure usually live longer than men with heart failure.

Prevention

Heart failure usually is caused by the effects of some type of heart disease. The best way to try to prevent heart failure is to eat a healthy diet and get regular exercise, but many causes of heart failure cannot be prevented. People with risk factors for coronary disease (such as high blood pressure and high cholesterol levels) should work closely with their physician to reduce likelihood of heart attack and heart failure.

Heart failure sometimes can be avoided by identifying and treating any conditions that might lead to heart disease. These include high blood pressure, alcoholism, and coronary artery disease. Regular blood pressure checks and obtaining immediate medical care for symptoms of coronary artery disease, such as chest pain, will help to get these conditions diagnosed and treated early, before they can damage the heart muscle.

A 2003 initiative called OPTIMIZE H-F was aimed at preventing severe heart failure and deaths among patients discharge from hospitals. The project created a registry or database of patients with heart failure that could be shared among hospitals. Finally, diagnosing and treating heart failure before the heart becomes severely damaged can improve the prognosis. With proper treatment, many patients may continue to lead active lives for a number of years.

Resources

BOOKS

Roberts, Jillian, and Sheryl MacMath. *Starting a Conversation: School Children With Congenital Heart Disease.* Calgary, AB: Detselig Enterprises, 2006.

Swan, Lorna, et al. *Adult Congenital Heart Disease: A Practical Guide*. Oxford, UK: 2005.

Webb, Gary D. *Adult Congenital Heart Disease, An Issue of Cardiology Clinics*. Burlington, MA: 2006.

PERIODICALS

Frieden, Joyce. "Time to Rethink Adult Congenital Heart Disease."*Family Practice News* (March 1, 2006) 15.

MacNeil, Jane Salodof. "Improved Imaging Tracks Congenital Heart Disease: New Tools Allow Physicians to Image the Heart and Other Structures in Small Pediatric Patients."*Pediatric News* (May 2006): 52.

McGrath, Jacqueline M. "Early Detection and Immediate Management of Congenital Heart Disease is Important to Long-Term Outcomes." *Journal of Perinatal & Neonatal Nursing* (October-December 2006): 285–286.

Moons, P., et al. "Changes in Perceived Health of Children With Congenital Heart Disease After Attending a Special Sports Camp."*Pediatric Cardiology* (February 2006): 67–72.

Rhodes, Jonathan, et al. "Sustained Effects of Cardiac Rehabilitation in Children With Serious Congenital Heart Disease."*Pediatrics* (September 2006): 225–226.

Thompson, Lucy. "Care of the Patient With Adult Con genital Heart Disease." *Critical Care Nursing Quarterly* (January-March 2007): 3–11.

ORGANIZATIONS

Adult Congenital Heart Disease Association, 6757 Greene St., Suite 335, Philadelphia, PA, 19119-3508, (215) 849-1260, (215) 849-1261, (888) 921-ACHA, Info@acha heart.org, http://www.achaheart.org.

American Heart Association National Center, 7272 Greenville Avenue, Dallas, TX, 75231, (800) 242-8721, Review.personal.info@heart.org.

Heart and Stroke Foundation of Canada, 222 Queen Street, Suite 1402, Ottawa, CanadaON, K1P 5V9, (613) 569-4361, (613) 569-3278, http://www.heartandstroke.com.

Heart Association of Australia, Level 3, 80 William Street, Sydney, Australia, NSW 2011, (02) 02)9219 2444, reception.sydney@heartfoundation.org.au, http://www.heartfoundation.org.au.

National Heart Lung and Blood Institute Health Information Center, P.O. Box 30105, Bethesda, MD, 20824-0105, (301) 592-8573, (240) 629-3246, http://www.nhlbi.nih.gov.

Toni Rizzo
Ken R. Wells

Heart murmurs

Definition

A heart murmur is an abnormal extra sound during the heartbeat cycle made by blood moving through the heart and its valves. It is detected by the physician's examination using a stethoscope and may sound like a swishing or whooshing noise. Some heart murmurs are congenital (present at birth) while others develop later in life. In adults, most abnormal heart murmurs are caused by infections, other diseases, or **aging**.

Demographics

Innocent heart murmurs are quite common in the general population. Exact statistics are difficult to obtain; however, one Dutch study reported in the mid-1990s that 41% of schoolchildren between the ages of 5 and 14 years had grade 1 (barely audible) innocent heart murmurs, while 14% had grade 2 or grade 3 murmurs.

Description

A heart which is beating normally makes two sounds, "lubb," which is heard when the valves between the atria and ventricles close; and "dupp," which is heard when when the valves between the ventricles and the major arteries close. The first sound (lubb) is known as S1 in medical shorthand, and the second heart sound (dupp or dub) is known as S2. A heart murmur is a series of vibratory sounds made by turbulent blood flow. The sounds are longer than normal heart sounds and can be heard between the normal sounds of the heart.

Heart murmurs are common in children and can also result from heart or valve defects. Nearly two-thirds of heart murmurs in children are produced by normal hearts and are harmless. This type of heart murmur is usually called an "innocent" heart murmur. It can also be called "functional" or "physiologic." Innocent heart murmurs are usually very faint, intermittent, and occur in a small area of the chest. Pathologic heart murmurs may indicate the presence of a serious heart defect. They are louder, continual, and may be accompanied by a click or gallop.

Some heart murmurs are continually present; others occur only when the heart is working harder than usual, including during **exercise** or certain types of illness. Heart murmurs can be diastolic or systolic. Those that occur during relaxation of the heart between beats are called diastolic murmurs. Those that occur during contraction of the heart muscle are called systolic murmurs. Murmurs that can be heard throughout the heartbeat cycle are called continuous murmurs. The characteristics of the murmur may suggest specific alterations in the heart or its valves.

Heart murmurs are evaluated according to several characteristics:

- Timing. Timing refers to whether the murmur is systolic, diastolic, or continuous.
- Shape. Shape refers to the loudness of the murmur over time. Some grow louder (crescendo); some grow softer (decrescendo); and some grow louder and then softer (crescendo/decrescendo).
- Location. This characteristic refers to the place on the front of the chest where the doctor can best hear the murmur.
- Radiation. Radiation refers to the direction of the movement of the sound of the murmur. In general, heart murmurs radiate in the direction of the blood flow.
- Intensity. Intensity refers to the loudness of the murmur and is graded on a scale of 1 to 6. A grade 1 murmur is difficult to hear at all; grade 3 can be heard all over the portion of the chest over the heart; grade 5 can be heard with the stethoscope partly off the chest; and grade 6 is loud enough to be heard with the stethoscope completely off the chest.
- Pitch. The pitch of a murmur can be low, medium, or high.
- Quality. This characteristic refers to unusual aspects of the murmur's sound. Some murmurs can be described as harsh, rumbling, blowing, or even musical.

Risk factors

Risk factors for heart murmurs in an unborn child include:

- Family history of heart murmurs or heart defects-
- Illnesses during pregnancy, particularly poorly controlled diabetes and rubella (German measles)-
- Using alcohol or illegal drugs during pregnancy-

There are no known risk factors for innocent heart murmurs in the general population as of 2010.

Causes and symptoms

Heart murmurs in general are caused by the turbulence of blood flowing through the chambers and valves of the heart or the blood vessels near the heart strongly enough to produce audible sounds. Sometimes **anxiety**, **stress**, **fever**, anemia, an overactive thyroid gland, and **pregnancy** will cause innocent murmurs that can be heard by a physician using a stethoscope. Pathologic heart murmurs, however, are caused by structural abnormalities of the heart. These include defective heart valves or holes in the walls of the heart. Valve problems are more common. Valves that do not open completely cause blood to flow through a smaller opening than normal, while those that do not close properly may cause blood to go back through the valve. A hole in the wall between the left and right sides of the heart, called a septal defect, can cause heart murmurs. Some septal defects close on their own; others require surgery to prevent progressive damage to the heart.

The symptoms of heart murmurs differ depending on the cause of the heart murmur. Innocent heart murmurs and those which do not impair the function of the heart have no symptoms. Murmurs that are due to severe abnormalities of a heart valve may cause **shortness of breath**, **dizziness**, chest pains, faintness, a bluish discoloration of the skin of the fingertips and lips, swollen veins in the neck, heavy sweating with little exertion, **palpitations**, and lung congestion.

Diagnosis

The diagnosis of a heart murmur begins with taking a careful patient history. The doctor may ask about a family history of heart murmurs or heart disease. The doctor may also ask about symptoms that may be associated with heart disorders, such as **fainting**, chest **pain**, a bluish tinge to the complexion, shortness of breath, weight gain, and swelling. The doctor will also check the size of the patient's liver by feeling the abdomen, and look for swollen neck veins.

Examination

Heart murmurs can be heard during an office examination when a pediatrician or primary care physician listens to the heart through a stethoscope during a regular checkup. The doctor's listening to heart or other body sounds is called auscultation. After listening to the heart sounds, the doctor will also check for any unusual sounds in the lungs. Very loud heart murmurs and those with clicks or extra heart sounds should be evaluated further. The doctor may ask the patient to stand, squat, hold the breath while bearing down, or squeeze an object in the hand during auscultation. These maneuvers help the doctor to evaluate the location and possible cause of the murmur.

Infants with heart murmurs who do not thrive, eat, or breathe properly, and older children who lose consciousness suddenly or are intolerant of exercise should also be evaluated. If the murmur sounds suspicious, the physician may order a **chest x ray**, an electrocardiogram, and an echocardiogram. A primary care physician may refer the patient to a cardiologist, who is a doctor who specializes in diagnosing and treating heart disorders.

Tests

An electrocardiogram (ECG) displays the heart's activity and may reveal muscle thickening, damage, or a lack of oxygen. Electrodes covered with conducting jelly are placed on the patient's chest, arms, and legs. They send impulses of the heart's activity through a monitor (oscilloscope) to a recorder which traces them on paper. The test takes about 10 minutes and is commonly performed in a physician's office. An exercise ECG can reveal additional information.

An echocardiogram (cardiac ultrasound), may be ordered to identify a structural problem that is causing the heart murmur. An echocardiogram uses sound waves to create an image of the heart's chambers and valves. The technician applies gel to a hand-held transducer, then presses it against the patient's chest. The sound waves are converted into an image that can be displayed on a monitor. Performed in a cardiology outpatient diagnostic laboratory, the test takes 30 minutes to an hour.

In some cases the doctor may administer a drug to further evaluate a murmur. The two compounds used most often for such tests are amyl nitrite, which expands blood vessels and lowers blood pressure, and methoxamine, which has the opposite effect, namely constricting blood vessels and raising blood pressure.

Procedures

In some cases the doctor may recommend **cardiac catheterization** to evaluate the condition of the patient's heart. This procedure involves the use of x-ray and ultrasound imaging to guide a long thin tube called a catheter through a major blood vessel into the heart. The doctor can inject a dye visible on x ray through the catheter and trace its flow through the

KEY TERMS

Atria (singular, atrium)—The upper two chambers of the heart.

Auscultation—The medical term for listening to the sounds of the heart or other body organs.

Cardiologist—A doctor who specializes in diagnosing and treating disorders of the heart.

Congenital—Present at birth.

Echocardiogram—A non-invasive ultrasound test that shows an image of the inside of the heart. An echocardiogram can be performed to identify any structural problems which cause a heart murmur.

Electrocardiogram—A test that shows the electrical activity of the heart by placing electronic sensors on the patient. This test can be used to confirm the presence of a heart murmur.

Innocent—The medical term for a harmless heart murmur.

Pathologic—Characterized by disease or the structural and functional changes due to disease. Pathologic heart murmurs may indicate a heart defect.

Ventricles—The lower two chambers of the heart.

chambers of the heart in order to identify problems in the valves or other structures of the heart.

Treatment

Traditional

Innocent heart murmurs do not affect the patient's health and require no treatment. Treatment when needed is directed toward the cause of the heart murmur. Heart murmurs due to septal defects may require surgery. Those due to valvular defects may require **antibiotics** to prevent infection during certain surgical or dental procedures. Severely damaged or diseased valves can be repaired or replaced through surgery.

Drugs

Some heart murmurs can be managed with various medications. Depending on the specific cause of the murmur, the doctor might prescribe one or more of the following types of drugs:

- Diuretics. Diuretics, sometimes called water pills, are drugs that remove fluid from the blood by increasing urinary output. They can be used to lower blood pressure, as high blood pressure can worsen a heart murmur.
- Angiotensin-converting enzyme (ACE) inhibitors. These are another class of drugs often prescribed to lower high blood pressure.
- Statins. Statins are a group of drugs given to control blood cholesterol levels. High blood cholesterol is a risk factor for making some heart valve problems worse.
- Digoxin (Lanoxin). Also known as digitalis, digoxin is a drug that increases the strength of the heart muscle's contractions, making the heart pump blood more efficiently.
- Aspirin or other anticoagulants. Anticoagulants, sometimes called blood thinners, are drugs that prevent blood clots from forming in the heart, thus lowering the risk of a stroke or heart attack.

Alternative

There are no alternative treatments for heart murmurs that require surgical treatment, although there are alternative therapies that are helpful for pre- and post-surgical support of the patient. If the heart murmur is innocent, heart activity can be supported using the herb hawthorn (*Crataegus laevigata* or *C. oxyacantha*) or coenzyme Q10. These remedies improve heart contractility and the heart's ability to use oxygen. If the murmur is valvular in origin, herbs that act like antibiotics as well as options that build resistance to infection in the valve areas may be considered.

Prognosis

The prognosis of a heart murmur depends on its cause. Most children with innocent heart murmurs grow out of them by the time they reach adulthood. Severe causes of heart murmurs may progress to severe symptoms and **death**.

Prevention

Apart from keeping diabetes under control and avoiding drug or alcohol **abuse** during pregnancy, there is no known way to prevent heart murmurs as of 2010.

Resources

BOOKS

Auscultation Skills: Breath and Heart Sounds, 4th ed. Philadelphia:Wolters Kluwer/Lippincott Williams and Wilkins Health, 2010.

Driscoll, David J. *Fundamentals of Pediatric Cardiology*. Philadelphia: Lippincott Williams and Wilkins, 2006.

PERIODICALS

Conn, R.D., and J.H. O'Keefe. "Cardiac Physical Diagnosis in the Digital Age: An Important But Increasingly Neglected Skill (from Stethoscopes to Microchips)." *American Journal of Cardiology* 104, August 15, 2009: 590–95.

Dunn, F.G. "Physical Examination: Include Heart Murmurs." *BMJ* 340, January 19, 2010: c290.

Federspiel, M.G. "Cardiac Assessment in the Neonatal Population." *Neonatal Network* 29, May-June 2010: 135–42.

Guntheroth, W.G. "Innocent Murmurs: A Suspect Diagnosis in Non-pregnant Adults." *American Journal of Cardiology* 104, September 2009: 735–37.

Hanifin, C. "Cardiac Auscultation 101: A Basic Science Approach to Heart Murmurs." *Journal of the American Academy of Physician Assistants* 23, April 2010: 44–48.

Teixeira, O.H. "Distinguishing Innocent from Pathologic Murmurs in Neonates." *Journal of Pediatrics* 155, August 2009: 300.

OTHER

American Heart Association (AHA). *Innocent Heart Murmurs*. http://www.americanheart.org/presenter.jhtml?identifier=170.

Mayo Clinic. *Heart Murmurs*. http://www.mayoclinic.com/health/heart-murmurs/DS00727.

MedlinePlus Medical Encyclopedia. *Heart Murmurs and Other Sounds*. http://www.nlm.nih.gov/medlineplus/ency/article/003266.htm.

National Heart, Lung, and Blood Institute (NHLBI). *Heart Murmur*. http://www.nhlbi.nih.gov/health/dci/Diseases/heartmurmur/hmurmur_what.html

National Heart, Lung, and Blood Institute (NHLBI). *How the Heart Works: Heart Contraction and Blood Flow*. http://www.nhlbi.nih.gov/health/dci/Diseases/hhw/hhw_pumping.html.

Seattle Children's Hospital. *Heart Murmurs*. http://www.seattlechildrens.org/medical-conditions/heart-blood-conditions/heart-murmurs/.

ORGANIZATIONS

American College of Cardiology (ACC), Heart House, 2400 N Street NW, Washington, DC, 20037, 202-375-6000, 202-375-7000, http://www.acc.org/.

American Heart Association, 7272 Greenville Avenue, Dallas, TX, 75231, 301-592-8573, 800-242-8721, 301-592-8563, www.americanheart.org.

Center for Adults with Congenital Heart Disease, University of Chicago Medical Center, 5841 S. Maryland Avenue, Chicago, IL, 60637, 888-UCH-0200, http://www.uchospitals.edu/specialties/heart/services/adult-congenital-heart/.

National Heart, Lung, and Blood Institute (NHLBI), Health Information Center, P.O. Box 30105, Bethesda, MD, 20824-0105, 301-592-8573, 240-629-3246, nhlbiinfo@nhlbi.nih.gov, http://www.nhlbi.nih.gov/.

Lori De Milto
Rebecca J. Frey, PhD

Heart muscle infection *see* **Myocarditis**
Heart scan *see* **Echocardiography**
Heart septal defect *see* **Atrial septal defect**
Heart sonogram *see* **Echocardiography**

Heart surgery for congenital defects

Definition

A variety of surgical procedures that are performed to repair the many types of heart defects that may be present at birth.

Purpose

Heart surgery for congenital defects is performed to repair a defect as much as possible and improve the flow of blood and oxygen to the body. While congenital heart defects vary in their severity, most require surgery. Surgery is recommended for congenital heart defects that result in a lack of oxygen, a poor quality of life, or a patient who does not thrive. Some types of congenital heart defects that don't cause symptoms are treated surgically because they can lead to serious complications.

Precautions

There are many types of surgery for congenital heart defects and many considerations in the decision to operate. The patient's cardiologist or surgeon will discuss these issues on an individual basis.

Description

There are many types of congenital heart defects. Most obstruct the flow of blood in the heart, or the vessels near it, or cause an abnormal flow of blood through the heart. Rarer types include newborns born with one ventricle, one side of the heart that is not completely formed, or the pulmonary artery and the aorta coming out of the same ventricle. Most congenital heart defects require surgery during infancy or childhood. Recommended ages for surgery for the most common congenital heart defects are:

- atrial septal defects: during the preschool years
- patent ductus arteriosus: between ages one and two
- coarctation of the aorta: in infancy, if it's symptomatic, at age four otherwise
- Tetralogy of Fallot: age varies, depending on the patient's signs and symptoms
- transposition of the great arteries: often in the first weeks after birth, but before the patient is 12 months old

Surgical procedures seek to repair the defect as much as possible and restore circulation to as close to normal as possible. Sometimes, multiple, serial, surgical procedures are necessary. Smaller congenital heart defects can now be repaired in a **cardiac catheterization** lab instead of an operating room. Catheterization procedures include balloon atrial septostomy and **balloon valvuloplasty**. Surgical procedures include arterial switch, Damus-Kaye-Stansel procedure, Fontan procedure, Ross procedure, shunt procedure, and venous switch or intra-atrial baffle.

Catheterization procedures

Balloon atrial septostomy and balloon valvuloplasty are cardiac catheterization procedures. Cardiac catheterization procedures can save the lives of critically ill neonates and in some cases eliminate or delay more invasive surgical procedures. It is expected that catheterization procedures will continue to replace more types of surgery for congenital heart defects in the future. A thin tube called a catheter is inserted into

KEY TERMS

Atresia—A congenital defect in which the blood pumped through the body has too little oxygen. In tricuspid atresia, the baby lacks a triscupid valve. In pulmonary atresia, a pulmonary valve is missing.

Coarctation of the aorta—A congenital defect in which severe narrowing or constriction of the aorta obstructs the flow of blood.

Congenital heart defects—Congenital means conditions which are present at birth. Congenital heart disease includes a variety of defects that babies are born with.

Patent ductus arteriosus—A congenital defect in which the temporary blood vessel connecting the left pulmonary artery to the aorta in the fetus doesn't close in the newborn.

Septal defects—These are holes in the septum, the muscle wall separating the right and left sides of the heart. Atrial septal defects are openings between the two upper heart chambers and ventricular septal defects are openings between the two lower heart chambers.

Stenosis—A narrowing of the heart's valves. This congenital defect can occur in the pulmonary (lung) or aortic (the main heart artery) valve.

Tetralogy of Fallot—A cyanotic defect in which the blood pumped through the body has too little oxygen. Tetralogy of Fallot includes four defects: a large hole between the ventricles, narrowing at or beneath the pulmonary valve, an overly muscular right ventricle, and an aorta over the large hole.

Transposition of the great arteries—A cyanotic defect in which the blood pumped through the body has too little oxygen. The pulmonary artery and the aorta are reversed.

an artery or vein in the leg, groin, or arm and threaded into the area of the heart that needs repair. The patient receives a local anesthetic at the insertion site and is awake but sedated during the procedure.

BALLOON ATRIAL SEPTOSTOMY. Balloon atrial septostomy is the standard procedure for correcting **transposition of the great arteries**; it is sometimes used in patients with mitral, pulmonary, or tricupsid atresia (atresia is a defect that causes the blood to carry too little oxygen to the body). Balloon atrial septostomy enlarges the atrial opening. A special balloon-tipped catheter is inserted into the right atrium and inflated to create a large opening in the atrial septum.

BALLOON VALVULOPLASTY. Balloon valvuloplasty uses a balloon-tipped catheter to open a narrowed heart valve, improving the flow of blood. It is the procedure of choice in pulmonary stenosis and is sometimes used in aortic stenosis. Balloons made of plastic polymers are placed at the end of the catheter and inflated to relieve the obstruction in the heart valve. Long-terms results are excellent in most cases. The operative **death** rate is 2–4%.

Surgical procedures

These procedures are performed under **general anesthesia**. Some require the use of a heart-lung machine, which cools the body to reduce the need for oxygen and takes over for the heart and lungs during the procedure.

ARTERIAL SWITCH. Arterial switch is performed to correct transposition of the great arteries, where the position of the pulmonary artery and the aorta are reversed. The procedure involves connecting the aorta to the left ventricle and the pulmonary artery to the right ventricle.

DAMUS-KAYE-STANSEL PROCEDURE. Transposition of the great arteries can also be corrected by the Damus-Kaye-Stansel procedure, in which the pulmonary artery is cut in two and connected to the ascending aorta and right ventricle.

FONTAN PROCEDURE. For tricuspid atresia and pulmonary atresia, the Fontan procedure connects the right atrium to the pulmonary artery directly or with a conduit, and the atrial defect is closed. Survival is over 90%.

PULMONARY ARTERY BANDING. Pulmonary artery banding is narrowing the pulmonary artery with a band to reduce blood flow and pressure in the lungs. It is used for **ventricular septal defect**, atrioventricular canal defect, and tricuspid atresia. Later, the band can be removed and the defect corrected with open heart surgery.

ROSS PROCEDURE. To correct aortic stenosis, the Ross procedure grafts the pulmonary artery to the aorta.

SHUNT PROCEDURE. For **Tetralogy of Fallot**, tricuspid atresia, or pulmonary atresia, the shunt procedure creates a passage between blood vessels, sending blood into parts of the body that need it.

VENOUS SWITCH. For transposition of the great arteries, venous switch creates a tunnel inside the atria to re-direct oxygen-rich blood to the right ventricle and aorta and venous blood to the left ventricle and pulmonary artery.

OTHER TYPES OF SURGERY. These surgical procedures are also used to treat common congenital heart defects. A medium to large ventricular or **atrial septal defect** can be closed by suturing it or covering it with a Dacron patch. For **patent ductus arteriosus**, surgery consists of dividing the ductus into two and tying off the ends. If performed within the patient's first few years, there is practically no risk associated with this operation. Surgery for **coarctation of the aorta** involves opening the chest wall, removing the defect, and reconnecting the ends of the aorta. If the defect is too long to be reconnected, a Dacron graft is used to replace the missing piece. In uncomplicated cases, the risk of the operation is 1–2%.

Preparation

Before surgery for congenital heart defects, the patient will receive a complete evaluation, which includes a physical exam, a detailed family history, a **chest x ray**, an electrocardiogram, an echocardiogram, and usually cardiac catheterization. For six to eight hours before the surgery, the patient cannot eat or drink anything. An electrocardiogram shows the heart's activity and may reveal a lack of oxygen. Electrodes covered with conducting jelly are placed on the patient's chest, arms, and legs and the heart's impulses are traced on paper. An echocardiogram uses sound waves to create an image of the heart's chambers and valves. Gel is applied to a hand-held transducer and then pressed against the patient's chest. Cardiac catheterization is an invasive diagnostic technique used to evaluate the heart in which a long tube is inserted into a blood vessel and guided into the heart. A contrast solution is injected to make the heart visible on x rays.

Aftercare

After heart surgery for congenital defects, the patient goes to an intensive care ward where he or she is connected to a variety of tubes and monitors, including a ventilator. Patients are monitored every 15 minutes until vital signs are stable. Heart sounds, oxygenation, and the electrocardiogram are monitored. Chest tubes will be checked to ensure that they're draining properly and there is no hemorrhage. **Pain** medications will be administered. Complications such as **stroke**, lung **blood clots**, and reduced blood flow to the kidneys will be monitored. After the ventilator and breathing tube are removed, **chest physical therapy** and exercises to improve circulation will be started.

Risks

Complications from heart surgery for congenital defects can be severe. They include **shock**, congestive **heart failure**, lack of oxygen or too much carbon dioxide in the blood, irregular heartbeat, stroke, infection, kidney damage, lung blood clot, low blood pressure, hemorrhage, cardiac arrest, and death.

ORGANIZATIONS

American Heart Association National Center, 7272 Greenville Avenue, Dallas, TX, 75231, (800) 242-8721, Review.personal.info@heart.org.

Congenital Heart Information Network (C.H.I.N.), 101 N. Washington Ave., Suite 1A, Margate City, NJ, 08402-1195, (609) 882-1572, (609) 822-1574, mb@tchin.org, http://tchin.org/.

Texas Heart Institute. Heart Information Service, MC 3-116, PO Box 20345, Houston, TX, 77225, (832) 355-4011, (800) 292-2221, http://www.texasheart.org.

Lori De Milto

Heart transplantation

Definition

Heart transplantation, also called cardiac transplantation, is the replacement of a patient's diseased or injured heart with a healthy donor heart.

Purpose

Heart transplantation is performed on patients with end-stage **heart failure** or some other life-threatening heart disease. Before a doctor recommends heart transplantation for a patient, all other possible treatments for his or her disease must have been tried. The purpose of heart transplantation is to extend and improve the life of a person who would otherwise die from heart failure. Most patients who receive a new heart were so sick before transplantation that they could not live a normal life. Replacing a patient's diseased heart with a healthy, functioning donor heart often allows the recipient to return to normal daily activities.

Precautions

Because healthy donor hearts are in short supply, strict rules dictate who should or should not get a heart transplant. Patients who have conditions that might

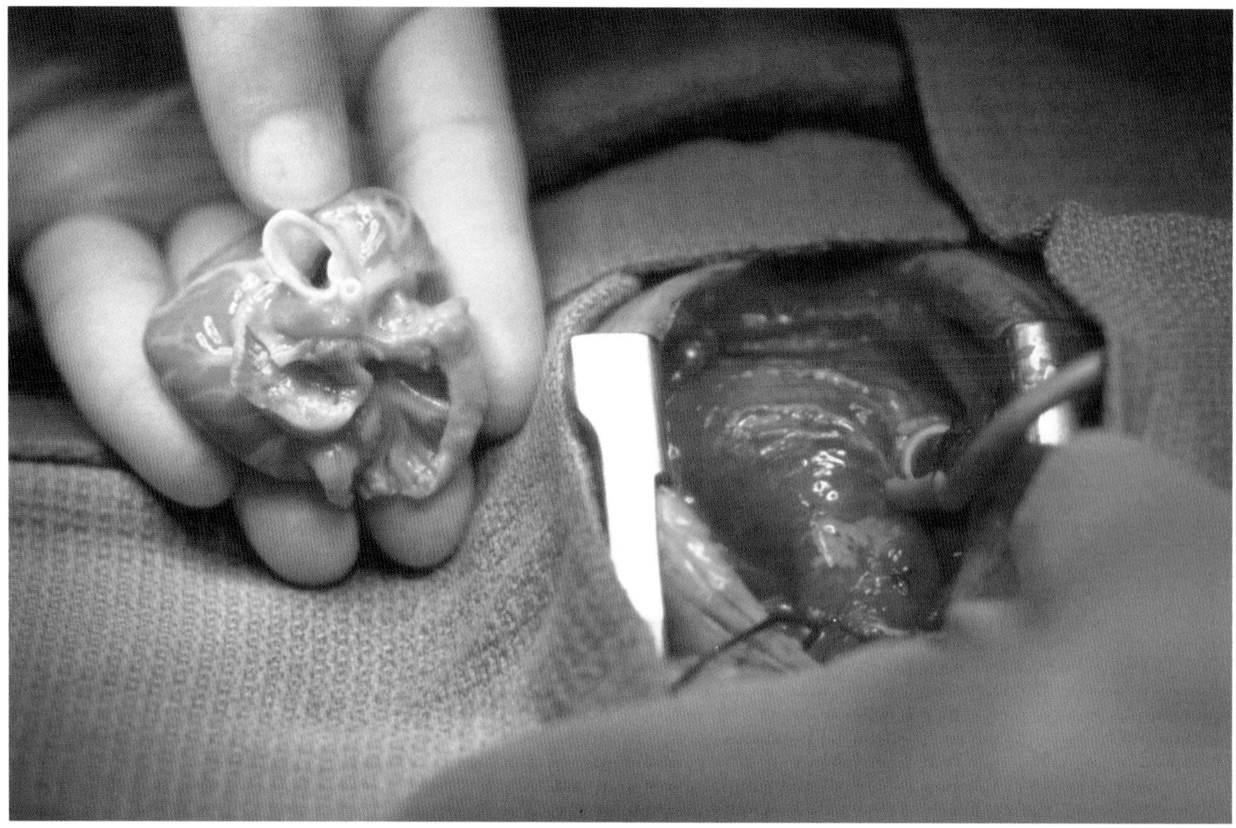

A comparison of the old and new hearts of Dylan Stork. At the time, he was the smallest heart transplant recipient in the world. Dylan was seven weeks old and weighed 5.5 pounds (2.5 kg) at the time of the operation. *(Alexander Tsiaras/Photo Researchers, Inc.)*

cause the new heart to fail should not have a heart transplant. Similarly, patients who may be too sick to survive the surgery or the side effects of the drugs they must take to keep their new heart working would not be good transplant candidates.

Patients who have any of the following conditions may not be eligible for heart transplantation:

- active infection
- pulmonary hypertension
- chronic lung disease with loss of more than 40% of lung function
- untreatable liver or kidney disease
- diabetes that has caused serious damage to vital organs
- disease of the blood vessels in the brain, such as a stroke
- serious disease of the arteries
- mental illness or any condition that would make a patient unable to take the necessary medicines on schedule
- continuing alcohol or drug abuse

Description

Patients with end-stage heart disease that threatens their life even after medical treatment may be considered for heart transplantation. Potential candidates must have a complete medical examination before they can be put on the transplant waiting list. Many types of tests are done, including blood tests, x rays, and tests of heart, lung, and other organ function. The results of these tests indicate to doctors how serious the heart disease is and whether or not a patient is healthy enough to survive the **transplant surgery**.

Organ waiting list

A person approved for heart transplantation is placed on the heart transplant waiting list of a heart transplant center. All patients on a waiting list are registered with the United Network for Organ Sharing (UNOS). UNOS has organ transplant specialists who run a national computer network that connects all the transplant centers and organ-donation organizations.

National transplant waiting list by organ type (June 2010)

Organ needed	Persons waiting
Kidney	85,296
Liver	16,031
Heart	3,141
Kidney/Pancreas	2,199
Lung	1,802
Pancreas	1,450
Intestine	242
Heart/Lung	79

SOURCE: U.S. Department of Health and Human Services, Organ Procurement and Transplantation Network. Available online at: http://optn.transplant.hrsa.gov/data/default.asp (accessed June 8, 2010).

(Table by PreMediaGlobal. Reproduced by permission of Gale, a part of Cengage Learning.)

When a donor heart becomes available, information about it is entered into the UNOS computer and compared to information from patients on the waiting list. The computer program produces a list of patients ranked according to blood type, size of the heart, and how urgently they need a heart. Because the heart must be transplanted as quickly as possible, the list of local patients is checked first for a good match. After that, a regional list and then a national list are checked. The patient's transplant team of heart and transplant specialists makes the final decision as to whether a donor heart is suitable for the patient.

The transplant procedure

When a heart becomes available and is approved for a patient, it is packed in a sterile cold solution and rushed to the hospital where the recipient is waiting.

Heart transplant surgery involves the following basic steps:

- A specialist in cardiovascular anesthesia gives the patient general anesthesia.
- Intravenous antibiotics are usually given to prevent bacterial wound infections.
- The patient is put on a heart/lung machine, which performs the functions of the heart and lungs and pumps the blood to the rest of the body during surgery. This procedure is called cardiopulmonary bypass.
- After adequate blood circulation is established, the patient's diseased heart is removed.
- The donor heart is attached to the patient's blood vessels.
- After the blood vessels are connected, the new heart is warmed up and begins beating. If the heart does not begin to beat immediately, the surgeon may start it with an electrical shock.
- The patient is taken off the heart/lung machine.
- The new heart is stimulated to maintain a regular beat with medications for two to five days after surgery, until the new heart functions normally on its own.

Heart transplant recipients are given immunosuppressive drugs to prevent the body from rejecting the new heart. These drugs are usually started before or during the heart transplant surgery. Immunosuppressive drugs keep the body's immune system from recognizing and attacking the new heart as foreign tissue. Normally, immune system cells recognize and attack foreign or abnormal cells, such as bacteria, **cancer** cells, and cells from a transplanted organ. The drugs suppress the immune cells and allow the new heart to function properly. However, they can also allow infections and other adverse effects to occur to the patient.

Because the chance of rejection is highest during the first few months after the transplantation, recipients are usually given a combination of three or four immunosuppressive drugs in high doses during this time. Afterwards, they must take maintenance doses of immunosuppressive drugs for the rest of their lives.

Cost and insurance coverage

The total cost for heart transplantation varies, depending on where it is performed, whether transportation and lodging are needed, and on whether there are any complications. The costs for the surgery and first year of care are estimated to be about $250,000. The medical tests and medications after the first year cost about $21,000 per year.

Insurance coverage for heart transplantation varies depending on the policy. Most commercial insurance companies pay a certain percentage of heart transplant costs. Medicare pays for heart transplants if the surgery is performed at Medicare-approved centers. Medicaid pays for heart transplants in 33 states and in the District of Columbia.

Preparation

Before patients are put on the transplant waiting list, their blood type is determined so a compatible donor heart can be found. The heart must come from a person with the same blood type as the patient, unless it is blood type O. A blood type O heart can be transplanted into a person with any type of blood.

A panel reactive antibodies (PRA) test is also done before heart transplantation. This test tells doctors whether or not the patient is at high risk for having a hyperacute reaction against a donor heart. A hyperacute reaction is a strong immune response against the new heart that happens within minutes to hours after the new heart is transplanted. If the PRA shows that a patient has a high risk for this kind of reaction, then a crossmatch is done between a patient and a donor heart before transplant surgery. A crossmatch checks how close the match is between the patient's tissue type and the tissue type of the donor heart.

Most people are not high risk, and a crossmatch usually is not done before the transplant because the surgery must be done as quickly as possible after a donor heart is found.

While waiting for heart transplantation, patients are given treatment to keep the heart as healthy as possible. They are regularly checked to make sure the heart is pumping enough blood. Intravenous medications may be used to improve cardiac output. If these drugs are not effective, a mechanical pump can help keep the heart functioning until a donor heart becomes available. Inserted through an artery into the aorta, the pump assists the heart in pumping blood.

Aftercare

Immediately following surgery, patients are monitored closely in the intensive care unit (ICU) of the hospital for 24–72 hours. Most patients need to receive oxygen for 4 to 24 hours following surgery. Blood pressure, heart function, and other organ functions are carefully monitored during this time.

Heart transplant patients start taking immunosuppressive drugs before or during surgery to prevent immune rejection of the heart. High doses of immunosuppressive drugs are given at this time, because rejection is most likely to happen within the first few months after the surgery. A few months after surgery, lower doses of immunosuppressive drugs usually are given and must be taken for the rest of the patient's life.

For six to eight weeks after the transplant surgery, patients usually come back to the transplant center twice a week for physical examinations and medical tests. These tests check for any signs of infection, rejection of the new heart, or other complications.

In addition to a **physical examination**, the following tests may be done during these visits:

- laboratory tests to check for infection
- chest x ray to check for early signs of lung infection
- electrocardiogram (ECG) to check heart function
- echocardiogram to check the function of the ventricles in the heart
- blood tests to check liver and kidney function
- complete blood counts (CBC) to check the numbers of blood cells
- taking of a small tissue sample from the donor heart (endomyocardial biopsy) to check for signs of rejection

During the physical examination, the blood pressure is checked and the heart sounds are listened to with a stethoscope to determine if the heart is beating properly and pumping enough blood. Kidney and liver function are checked because these organs may lose function if the heart is being rejected.

An endomyocardial biopsy is the removal of a small sample of the heart muscle. This is done with a very small instrument that is inserted through an artery or vein and into the heart. The heart muscle tissue is examined under a microscope for signs that the heart is being rejected. Endomyocardial biopsy is usually done weekly for the first four to eight weeks after transplant surgery and then at longer intervals after that.

Risks

The most common and dangerous complications of heart transplant surgery are organ rejection and infection. Immunosuppressive drugs are given to prevent rejection of the heart. Most heart transplant patients have a rejection episode soon after transplantation, but doctors usually diagnose it immediately when it will respond readily to treatment. Rejection is treated with combinations of immunosuppressive drugs given in higher doses than maintenance immunosuppression. Most of these rejection situations are successfully treated.

Infection can result from the surgery, but most infections are a side effect of the immunosuppressive drugs. Immunosuppressive drugs keep the immune system from attacking the foreign cells of the donor heart. However, the suppressed immune cells are also unable to adequately fight bacteria, viruses, and other microorganisms. Microorganisms that normally do not affect persons with healthy immune systems can cause dangerous infections in transplant patients taking immunosuppressive drugs.

Patients are given **antibiotics** during surgery to prevent bacterial infection. Patients may also be given an antiviral drug to prevent virus infections. Patients who develop infections may need to have their immunosuppressive drugs changed or the dose adjusted. Infections are treated with antibiotics or other drugs, depending on the type of infection.

KEY TERMS

Anesthesia—Loss of the ability to feel pain, caused by administration of an anesthetic drug.

Angina—Characteristic chest pain which occurs during exercise or stress in certain kinds of heart disease.

Cardiopulmonary bypass—Mechanically circulating the blood with a heart/lung machine that bypasses the heart and lungs.

Cardiovascular—Having to do with the heart and blood vessels.

Complete blood count (CBC)—A blood test to check the numbers of red blood cells, white blood cells, and platelets in the blood.

Coronary artery disease—Blockage of the arteries leading to the heart.

Crossmatch—A test to determine if patient and donor tissues are compatible.

Donor—A person who donates an organ for transplantation.

Echocardiogram—A test that visualizes and records the position and motion of the walls of the heart using ultrasound waves.

Electrocardiogram (ECG)—A test that measures electrical conduction of the heart.

End-stage heart failure—Severe heart disease that does not respond adequately to medical or surgical treatment.

Endomyocardial biopsy—Removal of a small sample of heart tissue to check it for signs of damage caused by organ rejection.

Fatigue—Loss of energy; tiredness.

Graft—A transplanted organ or other tissue.

Immunosuppressive drug—Medication used to suppress the immune system.

Inotropic drugs—Medications used to stimulate the heart beat.

Pulmonary hypertension—An increase in the pressure in the blood vessels of the lungs.

Recipient—A person who receives an organ transplant.

Other complications that can happen immediately after surgery are:

- bleeding
- pressure on the heart caused by fluid in the space surrounding the heart (pericardial tamponade)
- irregular heart beats
- reduced cardiac output
- increased amount of blood in the circulatory system
- decreased amount of blood in the circulatory system

About half of all heart transplant patients develop **coronary artery disease** 1–5 years after the transplant. The coronary arteries supply blood to the heart. Patients with this problem develop chest pains called **angina**. Other names for this complication are coronary allograft **vascular disease** and chronic rejection.

Outcomes

Heart transplantation is an appropriate treatment for many patients with end-stage heart failure. The outcomes of heart transplantation depend on the patient's age, health, and other factors. About 73% of heart transplant patients are alive four years after surgery.

After transplant, most patients regain normal heart function, meaning the heart pumps a normal amount of blood. A transplanted heart usually beats slightly faster than normal because the heart nerves are cut during surgery. The new heart also does not increase its rate as quickly during **exercise**. Even so, most patients feel much better and their capacity for exercise is dramatically improved from before they received the new heart. About 85% of patients return to work and other daily activities. Many are able to participate in sports.

Resources

OTHER

"What Every Patient Needs to Know." *United Network for Organ Sharing (UNOS)*. http://www.unos.org/docs/WEPNTK.pdf.

ORGANIZATIONS

American Society of Transplantation, 15000 Commerce Parkway, Suite C, Mt. Laurel, NJ, 08054, (856) 439-9986, (856) 439-9982, info@a-s-t.org, http://www.a-s-t.org/.

Health Services and Resources Administration, Division of Organ Transplantation, 5600 Fishers Lane, Rockville, MD, 20857, (888) 275-4772, ask@hrsa.gov, http://organdonor.gov.

United Network for Organ Sharing (UNOS), 700 N. 4th Street, PO Box 2484, Richmond, VA, 23218, (804) 782-4800, (804) 782-4817, (888) 894-6361, http://www. unos.org.

Toni Rizzo

Heart tumors *see* **Myxoma**

Heart valve repair

Definition

Heart valve repair is a surgical procedure used to correct a malfunctioning heart valve. Repair usually involves separating the valve leaflets (the one-way "doors" of the heart valve which open and close to pump blood through the heart) or forcing them open with a balloon catheter, a technique known as *balloon valvuloplasty*.

Purpose

To correct damage to the mitral, aortic, pulmonary, or tricuspid heart valves caused by a systemic infection, **endocarditis**, rheumatic heart disease, a congenital heart defect, or mitral and/or aortic valve disease. Damaged valves may not open properly (stenosis) or they may not close adequately (valve regurgitation, insufficiency, or incompetence).

KEY TERMS

Angiogram—An angiogram uses a radiopaque substance, or dye, to make the blood vessels or arteries visible under x ray.

Calcified—Hardened by calcium deposits.

Catheter—A long, thin, flexible tube used in valvuloplasty to widen the valve opening.

Echocardiogram—Ultrasound of the heart; generates a picture of the heart through the use of soundwaves.

Edema—Fluid accumulation in the body.

Scintigram—A nuclear angiogram; a scintigram involves injection of a radioactive substance into the patient's circulatory system. As the substance travels through the body, a special scanning camera takes pictures.

Stenosis—Narrowing of the heart valve opening.

Precautions

Patients who have a diseased heart valve that is badly scarred or calcified may be better candidates for valve replacement surgery.

Description

Heart valve repair is performed in a hospital setting by a cardiac surgeon. During valve repair surgery, the patient's heart is stopped, and his/her blood is circulated outside of the body through an *extracorporeal bypass circuit*, also called heart-lung machine or just "the pump." The extracorporeal circuit consists of tubing and medical devices that take over the function of the patient's heart and lungs during the procedure. As blood passes through the circuit, carbon dioxide is removed from the bloodstream and replaced with oxygen. The oxygenated blood is then returned to the body. Other components may also be added to the circuit to filter fluids from the blood or concentrate red blood cells.

In cases of valve disease where the leaflets have become fused together, a procedure known as a valvulotomy is performed. In valvulotomy, the leaflets of the valves are surgically separated, or partially resected, with an incision to increase the size of the valve opening. The surgeon may also make adjustments to the chordae, the cord-like tissue that connects the valve leaflets to the ventricle muscles, to improve valve function.

Another valve repair technique, **balloon valvuloplasty**, is used in patients with pulmonary, aortic, and **mitral valve stenosis** to force open the valve. Valvuloplasty is similar to a cardiac **angioplasty** procedure in that it involves the placement of a balloon-tipped catheter into the heart. Once inserted into the valve, the balloon is inflated and the valve dilates, or opens. Valvuloplasty does not require a bypass circuit.

Preparation

A number of diagnostic tests may be administered prior to valve repair surgery. **Magnetic resonance imaging** (MRI), echocardiogram, angiogram, and/or scintigram are used to help the surgeon get an accurate picture of the extent of damage to the heart valve and the status of the coronary arteries.

Aftercare

The patient's blood pressure and vital signs will be carefully monitored following a valve repair procedure, and he or she watched closely for signs of **edema** or congestive **heart failure**.

Echocardiography or other diagnostic tests are ordered for the patient at some point during or after surgery to evaluate valvular function. A **cardiac rehabilitation** program may also be recommended to assist the patient in improving **exercise** tolerance after the procedure.

Risks

As with any invasive surgical procedure, hemorrhage, infarction, **stroke**, **heart attack**, and infection are all possible complications of heart valve repair. The overall risks involved with the surgery depend largely on the complexity of the procedure and physical condition of the patient.

Normal results

Ideally, a successful heart valve repair procedure will return heart function to age-appropriate levels. If valvuloplasty is performed, a follow-up valve repair or replacement surgery may be necessary at a later date.

Resources

BOOKS

Surhone, Lambert M., Mariam T. Tennoe, and Susan F. Henssonow, eds. *Heart Valve Repair*. Beau Bassin, Mauritius: Betascript, 2010.

Paula Anne Ford-Martin

Heart valve replacement

Definition

Heart valve replacement is a surgical procedure during which surgeons remove a damaged valve from the heart and substitute a healthy one.

Purpose

Four valves direct blood to and from the body through the heart: the aortic valve, the pulmonic valve, the tricuspid valve, and the mitral valve. Any of these valves may malfunction because of a birth defect, infection, disease, or trauma. When the malfunction is so severe that it interferes with blood flow, an individual will have heart **palpitations**, **fainting** spells, and/or difficulty breathing. These symptoms will progressively worsen and cause **death** unless the damaged valve is replaced surgically.

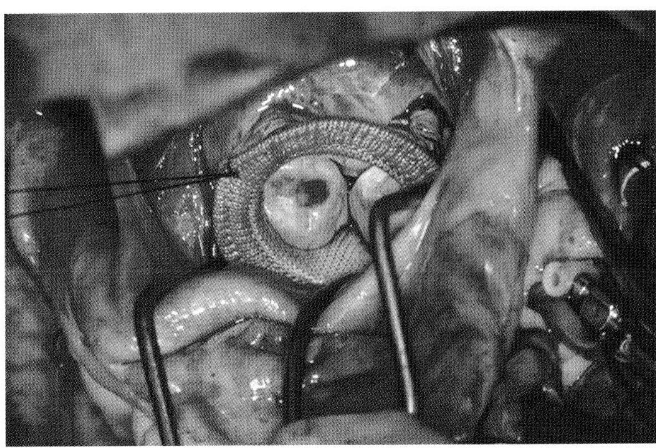

Open heart surgery showing replacement of a valve. *(David Leah/Photo Researchers, Inc.)*

Precautions

Abnormal tricuspid valves usually are not replaced because they do not cause serious symptoms. Mildly or even moderately diseased mitral valves may not need to be replaced because their symptoms are tolerable or they can be treated with such drugs as **beta blockers** or **calcium** antagonists, which slow the heart rate. However, a severely diseased mitral valve should be repaired or replaced unless the person is too ill to tolerate the operation because of another condition or illness.

Description

After cutting through and separating the breastbone and ribs, surgeons place the patient on a cardiopulmonary bypass machine, which will perform the functions of the heart and lungs during the operation. They then open the heart and locate the faulty valve. Slicing around the edges of the valve, they loosen it from the tendons that connect it to the rest of the heart and withdraw it. The new valve is inserted and sutured into place. The patient is then taken off the bypass machine and the chest is closed. The surgery takes three to five hours and is covered by most insurance plans.

There are three types of replacement valves. One class is made from animal tissue, usually a pig's aortic valve. Another is mechanical and is made of metal and plastic. The third, includes human valves that have been removed from an organ donor or that, rarely, are the patient's own pulmonic valve.

There is no single ideal replacement valve. The choice between an animal valve or a mechanical valve depends largely on the age of the patient. Because valves obtained from animals have a life expectancy of 7–15 years, they usually are given to older patients. Mechanical valves are used in younger patients because they are more durable. Because mechanical valves are made of foreign material, however, **blood clots** can form on their surface. Therefore, patients who receive these valves must take anticoagulants the rest of their lives.

Donor or pulmonic valves are given only to those patients who will deteriorate rapidly because of a narrowing of the passageway between the aorta and the

KEY TERMS

Anticoagulants—Drugs that prevent blood clots from forming.

Aortic valve—A fold in the channel leading from the aorta to the left ventricle of the heart. The aortic valve directs blood flow that has received oxygen from the lungs to the aorta which transmits blood to the rest of the body.

Cardiac catheterization—A thin tube called a catheter is inserted into an artery or vein in the leg, groin or arm. The catheter tube is carefully threaded into the area of the heart needing surgical repair. A local anaesthesia is used at the insertion sites.

Cardiopulmonary bypass machine—A mechanical instrument that takes over the circulation of the body while heart surgery is taking place.

Echocardiography—A diagnostic instrument that assesses the structure of the heart using sound waves.

Electrocardiography—A diagnostic instrument that evaluates the function of the heart by measuring the electrical activity generated by the beating of the heart.

Mitral valve—A fold in between the left atrium and the left ventricle of the heart that directs blood that has received oxygen from the lungs to the aortic valve and the aorta.

Pulmonic valve—A fold in the pulmonary artery that directs blood to the lungs. It may be transferred to replace a severely diseased aortic valve during heart valve replacement surgery for aortic stenosis.

Tricuspid valve—A fold in between the right atrium and the right ventricle of the heart that directs blood that needs oxygen to the lungs.

left ventrical (aortic stenosis). These valves are limited in their use because of the small supply available from donors and the strain that could be caused by removing and transferring a patient's own pulmonic valve.

Preparation

Before patients undergo heart valve replacement, they must be evaluated carefully for any signs that they may not tolerate the surgery.

Preoperative tests include:

- electrocardiography, which assesses the electrical activity of the heart
- echocardiography, which uses sound waves to show the extent of the obstruction of blood flow through the heart and determine the degree of loss of heart function due to the malfunctioning valve
- chest x ray, which provides an overall view of the anatomy of the heart and the lungs

Cardiac catheterization may also be performed to further asses the valve and to determine if coronary bypass surgery should also be done.

Aftercare

A patient usually spends one to three days in the hospital intensive care unit (ICU) after heart valve replacement so that the working of his or her heart and circulation can be monitored closely. When first brought to the ICU after surgery, the patient undergoes a neurological examination to be sure he or she has not suffered a **stroke**. The patient continues to breathe by means of a tube inserted in the trachea at the time of surgery. This mechanical ventilation is not withdrawn until the patient is fully awake from anesthesia, shows signs that he or she can breathe satisfactorily without mechanical support, and has steadfast circulation.

Once stablilized, the patient is transferred to a standard medical/surgical unit where he or she receives drugs that will prevent excess fluid from building up around the heart. As soon as possible, the patient begins walking and exercising to regain strength. He or she is also placed on a diet that is low in salt and cholesterol.

After being released from the hospital, the patient continues a daily **exercise** program that includes vigorous walking, and he or she may also join a recommended **cardiac rehabilitation** program. He or she usually can return to work or other normal activities within two months of the surgery.

Risks

Complications following heart valve replacement are not common, but can be serious. All valves made from animal tissue will develop calcium deposits over time. If these deposits hamper the function of the valve, it must be replaced. Valves may become dislodged. Blood clots may form on the surface of the substitute valve, break off into the general circulation, and become wedged in an artery supplying blood to the brain, kidneys, or legs. These blood clots may cause fainting spells, stroke, kidney failure, or loss of circulation to the legs. These blood clots can be treated with drugs or surgery.

Infection of heart muscle affects up to 2% of patients who have heart valve replacement. Such an infection is treated with intravenous **antibiotics**. If the infection persists, the new valve may have to be replaced.

Normal results

Few patients die as a result of the surgery. Approximately 3% of all patients die during or immediately after heart valve replacement, and less than 1% of patients below the age of 65 die because of the operation. The vast majority of patients who have heart valve replacement return to normal activity after the surgery. Depending on the type of valve they receive, these patients will have no symptoms of valve abnormality for at least seven years. Also, their quality of life will improve because they may no longer have difficulty breathing, fainting spells, or palpitations.

Resources

BOOKS

Pick, Adam. *The Patient's Guide To Heart Valve Surgery*. El Segundo, CA: Adam Pick, 2006.

ORGANIZATIONS

American College of Cardiology, Heart House, 2400 N Street NW, Washington, DC, 20037, (202) 375-6000, ext 5603, (202) 375-7000, (800) 223-4636, ext. 5603, resource@acc.org, http://www.acc.org.

American College of Surgeons, 633 North St. Clair St., Chicago, IL, 60611-3211, (212) 202-5000, (312) 202-5001, (800) 621-4111, postmaster@facs.org, http://www.facs.org.

American Heart Association National Center, 7272 Greenville Avenue, Dallas, TX, 75231, (800) 242-8721, Review.personal.info@heart.org.

Karen Marie Sandrick

Heartburn

Definition

Heartburn is a burning sensation in the chest that can extend to the neck, throat, and face; it is worsened by bending or lying down. It is the primary symptom of gastroesophageal reflux, which is the movement of stomach acid into the esophagus. On rare occasions, it is due to **gastritis** (stomach lining inflammation).

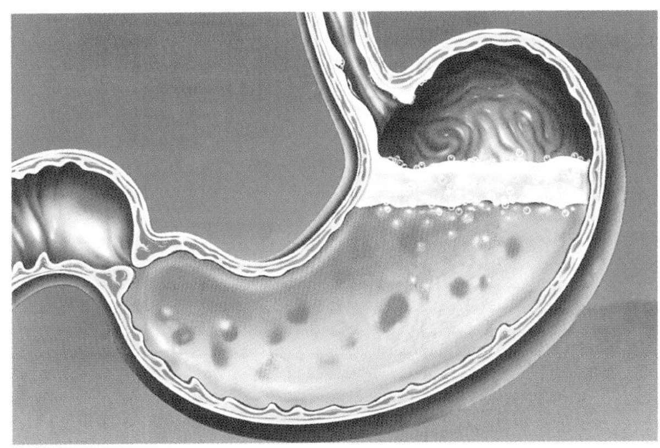

An illustration of foaming antacid on top of the contents of a human stomach. Heartburn is caused by a backflow of the stomach's acidic contents into the esophagus, causing inflammation and a sense of pain that can rise to the throat. *(Custom Medical Stock Photo, Inc. Reproduced by permission.)*

Demographics

Heartburn is extremely common. More than one-third of the population is afflicted by heartburn, with about one-tenth afflicted daily. Infrequent heartburn is usually without serious consequences, but chronic or frequent heartburn (recurring more than twice per week) can have severe consequences. Accordingly, early management is important.

Description

Understanding heartburn depends on understanding the structure and action of the esophagus. The esophagus is a tube connecting the throat to the stomach. It is about 10 in (25 cm) long in adults, lined with squamous (plate-like) epithelial cells, coated with mucus, and surrounded by muscles that push food to the stomach by sequential waves of contraction (peristalsis). The lower esophageal sphincter (LES) is a thick band of muscles that encircles the esophagus just above the uppermost part of the stomach. This sphincter is usually tightly closed and normally opens only when food passes from the esophagus into the stomach. Thus, the contents of the stomach are normally kept from moving back into the esophagus.

The stomach has a thick mucous coating that protects it from the strong acid it secretes into its interior when food is present, but the much thinner esophageal coating doesn't provide protection against acid. Thus, if the LES opens inappropriately or fails to close completely, and stomach contents leak into the esophagus, the esophagus can be burned by acid. The resulting burning sensation is called heartburn.

Occasional heartburn has no serious long-lasting effects, but repeated episodes of gastroesophageal reflux can ultimately lead to esophageal inflammation (esophagitis) and other damage. If episodes occur more frequently than twice a week, and the esophagus is repeatedly subjected to acid and digestive enzymes from the stomach, ulcerations, scarring, and thickening of the esophagus walls can result. This thickening of the esophagus wall causes a narrowing of the interior of the esophagus. Such narrowing affects swallowing and peristaltic movements. Repeated irritation can also result in changes in the types of cells that line the esophagus. The condition associated with these changes is termed Barrett's syndrome and can lead to **esophageal cancer**.

Causes and symptoms

Causes

A number of different factors may contribute to LES malfunction with its consequent gastroesophageal acid reflux:

- The eating of large meals that distend the stomach can cause the LES to open inappropriately.
- Lying down within two to three hours of eating can cause the LES to open.
- Obesity, pregnancy, and tight clothing can impair the ability of the LES to stay closed by putting pressure on the abdomen.
- Certain drugs, notably nicotine, alcohol, diazepam (Valium), meperidine (Demerol), theophylline, morphine, prostaglandins, calcium channel blockers, nitrate heart medications, anticholinergic and adrenergic drugs (drugs that limit nerve reactions), including dopamine, can relax the LES.
- Progesterone is thought to relax the LES.
- Greasy foods and some other foods such as chocolate, coffee, and peppermint can relax the LES.
- Paralysis and scleroderma can cause the LES to malfunction.
- Hiatus hernia may also cause heartburn according to some gastroenterologists. (Hiatus hernia is a protrusion of part of the stomach through the diaphragm to a position next to the esophagus.)

Symptoms

Heartburn itself is a symptom. Other symptoms also caused by gastroesophageal reflux can be associated with heartburn. Often heartburn sufferers salivate excessively or regurgitate stomach contents into their mouths, leaving a sour or bitter taste. Frequent gastroesophageal reflux leads to additional complications including difficult or painful swallowing, **sore throat**, hoarseness, coughing, **laryngitis**, **wheezing**, **asthma**, **pneumonia**, gingivitis, **bad breath**, and earache.

Diagnosis

Gastroenterologists and internists are best equipped to diagnose and treat gastroesophageal reflux. Diagnosis is usually based solely on patient histories that report heartburn and other related symptoms. Additional diagnostic procedures can confirm the diagnosis and assess damage to the esophagus, as well as monitor healing progress. The following diagnostic procedures are appropriate for anyone who has frequent, chronic, or difficult-to-treat heartburn or any of the complicating symptoms noted in the previous paragraph.

X rays taken after a patient swallows a barium suspension can reveal esophageal narrowing, ulcerations or a reflux episode as it occurs. However, this procedure cannot detect the structural changes associated with different degrees of esophagitis. This diagnostic procedure has traditionally been called the "upper GI series" or "barium swallow."

Esophagoscopy is a procedure that uses a thin flexible tube to view the inside of the esophagus directly. It should be done by a gastroenterologist or gastrointestinal endoscopist. It gives an accurate picture of any damage present and gives the physician the ability to distinguish between different degrees of esophagitis.

Other tests may also be used. They include pressure measurements of the LES; measurements of esophageal acidity (pH), usually throughout a 24-hour period; and microscopic examination of biopsied tissue from the esophageal wall (to inspect esophageal cell structure for Barrett's syndrome and malignancies).

Recent technology allows for continuous monitoring of pH levels to help determine the cause. A tiny wireless capsule can be delivered to the lining of the esophagus through a catheter and data recorder on a device the size of a pager that is clipped to the patient's belt or purse for 48 hours. The capsule eventually sloughs off and passes harmlessly through the gastrointestinal tract in 7 to 10 days.

Note: A burning sensation in the chest is usually heartburn and is not associated with the heart. However, chest **pain** that radiates into the arms and is not accompanied by regurgitation is a warning of a possible serious heart problem. Anyone with these symptoms should contact a doctor immediately.

KEY TERMS

Barrett's syndrome—Also called Barrett's esophagus or Barrett's epithelia, this is a condition where the squamous epithelial cells that normally line the esophagus are replaced by thicker columnar epithelial cells.

Digestive enzymes—Molecules that catalyze the breakdown of large molecules (usually food) into smaller molecules.

Esophagitis—Inflammation of the esophagus.

Fundoplication—A surgical procedure that increases pressure on the LES by stretching and wrapping the upper part of the stomach around the sphincter.

Gastroesophageal reflux—The flow of stomach contents into the esophagus.

Hiatus hernia—A protrusion of part of the stomach through the diaphragm to a position next to the esophagus.

Metabolic—Refers to the chemical reactions in living things.

Mucus—Thick, viscous, gel-like material that functions to moisten and protect inner body surfaces.

Peristalsis—A sequence of muscle contractions that progressively squeeze one small section of the digestive tract and then the next to push food along the tract, something like pushing toothpaste out of its tube.

Scleroderma—An autoimmune disease with many consequences, including esophageal wall thickening.

Squamous epithelial cells—Thin, flat cells found in layers or sheets covering surfaces such as skin and the linings of blood vessels and esophagus.

Ulceration—An open break in surface tissue.

Treatment

Drugs

Occasional heartburn is probably best treated with over-the-counter **antacids**. These products go straight to the esophagus and immediately begin to decrease acidity. However, they should not be used as the sole treatment for heartburn sufferers who either have two or more episodes per week or who suffer for periods of more than three weeks. There is a risk of kidney damage and other metabolic changes.

H2 blockers (histamine receptor blockers, such as Pepsid AC, Zantac, Tagamet) decrease stomach acid production and are effective against heartburn. H2 blocker treatment also allows healing of esophageal damage but is not very effective when there is a high degree of damage. It takes 30–45 minutes for these drugs to take effect, so they must be taken prior to an episode. Thus, they should be taken daily, usually two to four times per day for several weeks. Six to twelve weeks of standard-dose treatment relieves symptoms in about one-half the patients. Higher doses relieve symptoms in a greater fraction of the population, but at least 25% of heartburn sufferers are not helped by H2 blockers.

Proton-pump inhibitors also inhibit acid production by the stomach, but are much more effective than H2 blockers for some people. They are also more effective in aiding the healing process. Esophagitis is healed in about 90% of the patients undergoing proton-pump inhibitor treatment.

The long-term effects of inhibiting stomach acid production are unknown. Without the antiseptic effects of a consistently very acidic stomach environment, users of H2 blockers or proton-pump inhibitors may become more susceptible to bacterial and viral infection. Absorption of some drugs is also lowered by this less-acidic environment.

Prokinetic agents (also known as motility drugs) act on the LES, stimulating it to close more tightly, thereby keeping stomach contents out of the esophagus. It is not known how effectively these drugs promote healing. Some of the early motility drugs had serious neurological side effects, but a newer drug, cisapride, seems to act only on digestive system nerve connections.

Surgery

Fundoplication, a surgical procedure to increase pressure on the LES by stretching and wrapping the upper part of the stomach around the sphincter, is a treatment of last resort. About 10% of heartburn sufferers undergo this procedure. It is not always effective and its effectiveness may decrease over time, especially several years after surgery. Dr. Robert Marks and his colleagues at the University of Alabama reported in 1997 on the long-term outcome of this procedure. They found that 64% of the patients in their study who had fundoplication between 1992 and 1995 still suffered from heartburn and reported an impaired quality of life after the surgery.

However, **laparoscopy** (an examination of the interior of the abdomen by means of the laparoscope) now provides hope for better outcomes. Fundoplication performed with a laparoscope is less invasive. Five small incisions are required instead of one large incision. Patients recover faster, and it is likely that studies will show they suffer from fewer surgical complications.

Alternative treatment

Prevention, as outlined below, is a primary feature for heartburn management in alternative medicine and traditional medicine. Dietary adjustments can eliminate many causes of heartburn.

Herbal remedies include bananas, aloe vera gel, chamomile (*Matricaria recutita*), ginger (*Zingiber officinale*), and citrus juices, but there is little agreement here. For example, ginger, which seems to help some people, is claimed by other practitioners to *cause* heartburn and is thought to relax the LES. There are also many recommendations to *avoid* citrus juices, which are themselves acidic. Licorice (*Glycyrrhiza uralensis*) can help relieve the symptoms of heartburn by reestablishing balance in the acid output of the stomach.

Several homeopathic remedies are useful in treating heartburn symptoms. Among those most often recommended are *Nux vomica, Carbo vegetabilis*, and *Arsenicum album*. **Acupressure** and **acupuncture** may also be helpful in treating heartburn.

Sodium bicarbonate (baking soda) is an inexpensive alternative to use as an antacid. It reduces esophageal acidity immediately, but its effect is not long-lasting and should not be used by people on sodium-restricted **diets**.

Moderate **exercise** can also help relieve heartburn symptoms, but intense activity may exacerbate the condition.

Prognosis

The prognosis for people who get heartburn only occasionally or people without esophageal damage is excellent. The prognosis for people with esophageal damage who become involved in a treatment program that promotes healing is also excellent. The prognosis for anyone with esophageal **cancer** is very poor. There is a strong likelihood of a painful illness and a less than 5% chance of surviving more than five years.

Prevention

Given the lack of completely satisfactory treatments for heartburn or its consequences and the lack of a cure for esophageal cancer, prevention is of the utmost importance. Proponents of traditional *and* alternative medicine agree that people disposed to heartburn should:

- avoid eating large meals
- avoid alcohol, caffeine, fatty foods, fried foods, hot or spicy foods, chocolate, peppermint, and nicotine
- avoid drugs known to contribute to heartburn, such as nitrates (heart medications such as Isonate and Nitrocap), calcium channel blockers (e.g., Cardizem and Procardia), and anticholinergic drugs (e.g., Probanthine and Bentyl), and check with their doctors about any drugs they are taking
- avoid clothing that fits tightly around the abdomen
- control body weight
- wait about three hours after eating before going to bed or lying down
- elevate the head of the bed 6–9 inches to alleviate heartburn at night. This can be done with bricks under the bed or with a wedge designed for this purpose.

Preventing heartburn's switch to cancer begins with preventing heartburn in the first place. A study in Great Britain in 2004 also looked at using a combination of **aspirin** and an anti-ulcer drug to try to prevent Barrett's esophagus from forming in patients with long-term heartburn. Aspirin has been found in previous studies to reduce cases of esophageal cancer. However, since one of its side effects is an increased risk of stomach ulcers, the researchers were including an effective anti-ulcer drug for participants.

Resources

PERIODICALS

Ferri, F.F. Ferri's Clinical Advisor 2009: *Instant Diagnosis and Treatment*. Philadelphia, PA.: Mosby Elsevier, 2009:1232.

Kahrillas, P.J., et al. *American Gastrointestinal Association Medical Position Statement on the Management of Gastroesophageal Reflux Disease. Gastroenterology*. (2008), 135:1383-1391.

ORGANIZATIONS

The American College of Gastroenterology (ACG), PO Box 3099, Alexandria, VA, 22302, (800) HRT-BURN, https://www.healthtouch.com.

The American Gastroenterological Association (AGA), 7910 Woodmont Ave., 7th Floor, Bethesda, MD, 20814, (310) 654-2055, http://www.gastro.org/index.html.

American Society for Gastrointestinal Endoscopy, 13 Elm St, Manchester, MA, 01944, (508) 526-8330, http://www.asge.org.

National Digestive Diseases Information Clearinghouse, 2 Information Way, Bethesda, MD, 20892-3570, (800) 891-5389, www.niddk.nih.gov/health/digest/nddic.htm.

Lorraine Lica, PhD
Teresa G. Odle
Karl Finley

Heat cramps *see* **Heat disorders**

Heat disorders

Definition

Heat disorders are a group of physically related illnesses caused by prolonged exposure to hot temperatures, restricted fluid intake, or failure of the body's temperature regulation mechanisms. Disorders of heat exposure include heat cramps, heat exhaustion, and heat **stroke** (also called sunstroke). Hyperthermia is the general name given to heat-related illnesses. The two most common forms of hyperthermia are heat exhaustion and heat stroke, which is especially dangerous and requires immediate medical attention.

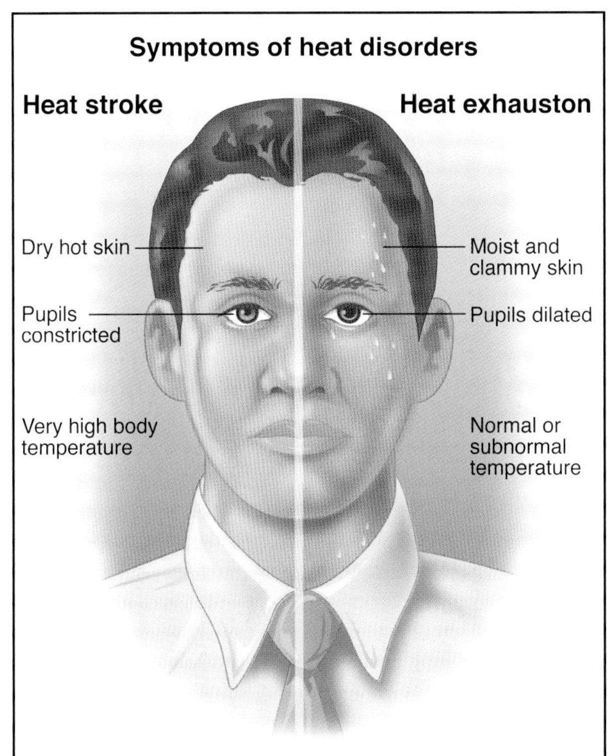

Symptoms of heat stroke and heat exhaustion. *(Illustration by Electronic Illustrators Group. Reproduced by permission of Gale, a part of Cengage Learning.)*

Demographics

Anyone can develop hyperthermia. However, seniors and young children are more likely to be affected than young or middle-aged adults. The United States Centers for Disease Control and Prevention (CDC) report that more than 330 individuals die of heat-related causes each year. More deaths occur in years that have significant heat waves, and more individuals die of heat-related illness during the summer months. More than 40% of the individuals who die of heat-related causes each year are over the age of 65.

Description

Heat disorders are harmful to people of all ages, but their severity is likely to increase as people age. Heat cramps in a 16-year-old may be heat exhaustion in a 45-year-old and heat stroke in a 65-year-old.

Regardless of extreme weather conditions, the healthy human body keeps a steady temperature of approximately 98.6°F (37°C). The body's temperature regulating mechanisms rely on the thermal regulating centers in the brain. Through these complex centers, the body tries to adapt to high temperatures by adjusting the amount of salt in the perspiration. Salt helps the cells in body tissues retain water. In hot weather, a healthy body will lose enough water to cool the body while creating the lowest level of chemical imbalance. In hot weather, or during vigorous activity, the body perspires. As perspiration evaporates from the skin, the body is cooled. If the body loses too much salt and fluids, the symptoms of **dehydration** can occur.

Risk factors

The very young, very old, obese individuals and those with cardiovascular problems are at increased risk of experiencing a heat disorder. Alcohol and diseases that impair the ability to sweat are associated with a higher risk of heat-related illness.

Individuals taking certain medications are more likely to be affected because the medications can interfere with the body's normal cooling mechanisms. Individuals taking some blood pressure and heart medications, allergy medications, diet pills, water pills, cold medicines, medicines to prevent seizures, **laxatives**, and thyroid pills are at increased risk for hyperthermia.

Heat cramps

Heat cramps are the least severe of the heat-related illnesses. This heat disorder is often the first signal that the body is having difficulty with increased temperature. Individuals exposed to excessive heat should think of heat cramps as a warning sign to a potential heat-related emergency.

Heat exhaustion

Heat exhaustion is a more serious and complex condition than heat cramps. Heat exhaustion can result from prolonged exposure to hot temperatures, restricted fluid intake, or failure of temperature regulation mechanisms of the body. It often affects athletes, firefighters, construction workers, factory workers, and anyone who wears heavy clothing in hot humid weather.

Heatstroke

Heat exhaustion can develop rapidly into heatstroke. Heatstroke can be life threatening. Because of its seriousness and its high potential for causing **death**, immediate medical attention is critical when problems first begin. Heat stroke, like heat exhaustion, is also a result of prolonged exposure to hot temperatures, restricted fluid intake, or failure of temperature regulation mechanisms of the body. However, the severity of impact on the body is much greater with heatstroke.

Causes and symptoms

Heat cramps

Heat cramps are painful **muscle spasms** caused by the excessive loss of salts (electrolytes) due to heavy perspiration. The muscle tissue becomes less flexible, causing **pain**, difficult movement, and involuntary tightness. Heavy exertion in extreme heat, restricted fluid intake, or failure of temperature regulation mechanisms of the body may lead to heat cramps. This disorder occurs more often in the legs and abdomen than in other areas of the body. Individuals at higher risk are those working in extreme heat, elderly people, young children, people with health problems, and those who are unable to naturally and properly cool their bodies. Individuals with poor circulation and who take medications to reduce excess body fluids (**diuretics**) can be at risk when conditions are hot and humid.

Heat exhaustion

Heat exhaustion is caused by exposure to high heat and humidity for many hours, resulting in excessive loss of fluids and salts through heavy perspiration. The skin may appear cool, moist, and pale. The individual may complain of **headache** and **nausea** with a feeling of overall weakness and exhaustion. **Dizziness**, faintness, and mental confusion are often present, as is rapid and weak pulse. Breathing becomes fast and shallow. Fluid loss reduces blood volume and lowers blood pressure. Yellow or orange urine often is a result of inadequate fluid intake, along with associated intense thirst. Insufficient water and salt intake or a deficiency in the production of sweat place an individual at high risk for heat exhaustion.

Heatstroke

Heatstroke is caused by overexposure to extreme heat, resulting in a breakdown in the body's heat regulating mechanisms. The body's temperature reaches a dangerous level, as high as 106°F (41.1°C). An individual with heat stroke has a body temperature higher than 104°F (40°C). Other symptoms include mental confusion with possible combativeness and bizarre behavior, staggering, and faintness.

The pulse becomes strong and rapid (160–180 beats per minute) with the skin taking on a dry and flushed appearance. There is often very little perspiration. The individual can quickly lose consciousness or have convulsions. Before heat stroke, an individual experiences heat exhaustion and the associated symptoms. When the body can no longer maintain a normal temperature, heat exhaustion becomes heatstroke. Heatstroke is a life-threatening medical emergency that requires immediate initiation of life-saving measures.

KEY TERMS

Convulsions—Also termed seizures; a sudden violent contraction of a group of muscles.

Electrolyte—Ions in the body that participate in metabolic reactions. The major human electrolytes are sodium (Na+), potassium (K+), calcium (Ca 2+), magnesium (Mg2+), chloride (Cl-), phosphate (HPO4 2-), bicarbonate (HCO3-), and sulfate (SO4 2-). Careful and regular monitoring of electrolytes and intravenous replacement of fluid and electrolytes are part of the acute care in many illnesses.

Intravenous (IV)—The process of giving a liquid through a vein.

Rehydration—The restoration of water or fluid to a body that has become dehydrated.

Diagnosis

The diagnosis of heat cramps usually involves observation of symptoms such as muscle cramping and thirst. Diagnosis of heat exhaustion or heatstroke, however, may require a physician to review the medical history, document symptoms, and obtain a blood pressure and temperature reading. The physician also may take blood and urine samples for further laboratory testing. A test to measure the body's electrolytes also can give valuable information about chemical imbalances caused by the heat-related illness.

Treatment

Heat cramps

The care of heat cramps includes placing the individual at rest in a cool environment, while giving cool water with one teaspoon of salt per quart of water or giving a commercial sports drink (e.g., Gatorade). Usually rest and liquids are all that is needed for the patient to recover. Mild stretching and massaging of the muscle area follows once the condition improves. The individual should not take salt tablets since this may actually worsen the condition. When the cramps stop, the person usually can start activity again if there are no other signs of illness. The individual needs to continue drinking fluids and should be watched carefully for further signs of heat-related illnesses.

Heat exhaustion

An individual who shows signs of heat exhaustion should stop all physical activity and immediately be moved to a cool place out of the sun, preferably a cool, air-conditioned location. She or he should then lay down with feet slightly elevated, remove or loosen clothing, and drink cold (but not iced), slightly salty water or a commercial sports drink. Rest and replacement of fluids and salt is usually all the treatment that is needed, and hospitalization is rarely required. Following rehydration, the person usually recovers rapidly.

Heatstroke

Simply moving the individual afflicted with heatstroke to a cooler place is not enough to reverse internal overheating. Emergency medical assistance should be called immediately. While waiting for help to arrive, quick action to lower body temperature must take place. Treatment involves getting the victim to a cool place, loosening clothes or undressing the heat stroke victim, and allowing air to circulate around the body. The next important step is wrapping the individual in wet towels or clothing, and placing ice packs in areas with the greatest blood supply. These areas include the neck, under the arm and knees, and in the groin. The individual can even be placed into a bathtub full of cool water to help speed cooling. A fan can be used to circulate air over dampened skin to simulate sweating and help the cooling process. Once the patient is under medical care, **cooling treatments** may continue as appropriate. The individual's body temperature will be monitored constantly to guard against overcooling. Breathing and heart rate will be monitored closely, and fluids and electrolytes will be replaced intravenously. **Anticonvulsant drugs** may be given to help reduce shivering, which warms the body up. After severe heat stroke, bed rest may be recommended for several days.

Prognosis

Prompt treatment for heat cramps is usually very effective with the individual returning to activity thereafter. Treatment of heat exhaustion usually brings full recovery in one to two days. Heatstroke is a very serious condition and its outcome depends upon general health and age. Due to the high internal temperature of heatstroke, permanent damage to internal organs is possible.

Prevention

Because heat cramps, heat exhaustion, and heatstroke are all essentially different levels of severity of the same disorder, the prevention of the onset of all heat disorders is similar. Strenuous **exercise** should be avoided when it is very hot or humid. Individuals exposed to extreme heat conditions should drink plenty of fluids. Wearing light and loose-fitting clothing in hot weather is important, regardless of the activity. It is important to consume water often and not to wait until thirst develops. If perspiration is excessive, fluid intake should be increased. When urine output decreases, fluid intake should also increase. Eating lightly salted foods can help replace salts lost through perspiration. Ventilation in any working areas in warm weather must be adequate. This can be achieved as simply as opening a window or using an electric fan. Proper ventilation will promote adequate sweat evaporation to cool the skin.

Resources

BOOKS

Barton, Bob. *Safety, Risk, and Adventure in Outdoor Activities*. Thousand Oaks, CA: Paul Chapman, 2007.

Spengler, Daniel P., Andrew Connaughton, and Andrew T. Pittman. *Risk Management in Sport and Recreation*. Champaign, IL: Human Kinetics, 2006.

PERIODICALS

Holcomb, Susan Simmons. "Pediatric Heatstroke." *Nursing* (September 2009) 39(9):64.

"What Can Be Done to Avoid Or At Least Recognize Heatstroke Before It's Too Late For Help?" *Mayo Clinic Health Letter* (July 2009) 27(7): 8.

"When Does Heat Stroke Occur, and What Are the Signs?" *Johns Hopkins Medical Letter* (August 2000) 21(6): 8.

OTHER

Medline Plus. Heat Illness. December 5, 2009. http://www.nlm.nih.gov/medlineplus/heatillness.html

University of Maryland Medical Center. Dehydration and Heat Stroke. January 25, 2008. http://www.umm.edu/non_trauma/dehyrat.htm

Jeffrey P. Larson, RPT
Tish Davidson, A.M.

Heat exhaustion *see* **Heat disorders**

Heat treatments

Definition

Heat treatments are applications of therapeutic thermal agents to specific body areas experiencing injury or dysfunction.

Purpose

The general purpose of a heat treatment is to increase the extensibility of soft tissues, remove toxins from cells, enhance blood flow, increase function of the tissue cells, encourage muscle relaxation, and help relieve **pain**. There are two types of heat treatments: superficial and deep. Superficial heat treatments apply heat to the outside of the body. Deep heat treatments direct heat toward specific inner tissues through ultrasound or by electric current. Heat treatments are beneficial prior to **exercise**, providing a warm-up effect to the soft tissues involved.

Precautions

Heat treatments should not be used on individuals with circulation problems, heat intolerance, or lack of sensation in the affected area. Low blood circulation may contribute to heat-related injuries. Heat treatments also should not be used on individuals afflicted with heart, lung, or kidney diseases. Deep heat treatments should not be used on areas above the eye, heart, or on a pregnant patient. Deep heat treatments over areas with metal surgical implants should be avoided in case of rapid temperature increase and subsequent injury.

Description

There are four different ways to convey heat:

- Conduction is the transfer of heat between two objects in direct contact with each other.
- Conversion is the transition of one form of energy to heat.
- Radiation involves the transmission and absorption of electromagnetic waves to produce a heating effect.
- Convection occurs when a liquid or gas moves past a body part creating heat.

Hot packs, water bottles, and heating pads

Hot packs are a very common form of heat treatment utilizing conduction as a form of heat transfer. Moist heat packs are readily available in most hospitals, **physical therapy** centers, and athletic training rooms. Treatment temperature should not exceed 131°F (55°C). The pack is used over multiple layers of toweling to achieve a comfortable warming effect for approximately 30 minutes. More recently, several manufacturers have developed packs that may be warmed in a microwave over a specified amount of time prior to use.

Hot-water bottles are another form of superficial heat treatment. The bottles are filled half way with hot water between 115–125°F (46.1–52°C). Covered by protective toweling, the hot-water bottle is placed on the treatment area and left until the water has cooled off.

Electrical heating pads continue to be used, however, because of the need for an electrical outlet, safety and convenience become an issue.

Paraffin

Paraffin, a conductive form of superficial heat, is often used for heating uneven surfaces of the body such as the hands. It consists of melted paraffin wax and mineral oil. Paraffin placed in a small bath unit becomes solid at room temperature and is used as a liquid heat treatment when heated at 126–127.4°F (52–53°C). The most common form of paraffin application is called the dip and wax method. In this technique, the patient will dip 8 to 12 times and then the extremity will be covered with a plastic bag and a towel for insulation. Most treatment sessions are about 20 minutes.

Hydrotherapy

Hydrotherapy is used in a form of heat treatment for many musculoskeletal disorders. The hydrotherapy tanks and pools are all generally set at warm temperatures, never exceeding 150°F (65.6°C). Because the patient often performs resistance exercises while in the water, higher water temperatures become a concern as the treatment becomes more physically draining. Because of this, many hydrotherapy baths are now being set at 95–110°F (35–43.3°C). There are also units available with moveable turbine jets, which provide a light massage effect. Hydrotherapy is helpful as a warm-up prior to exercise.

Fluidotherapy

Fluidotherapy is a form of heat treatment developed in the 1970s. It is a dry heat modality consisting of cellulose particles suspended in air. Units come in different sizes and some are restricted to only treating a hand or foot. The turbulence of the gas-solid mixture provides thermal contact with objects that are immersed in the medium. Temperatures of this treatment range from 110–123°F (43.3–50.5°C). Fluidotherapy allows the patient to exercise the limb during the treatment, and also massages the limb, increasing blood flow.

Ultrasound

Ultrasound heat treatments penetrate the body to provide relief to inner tissue. Ultrasound energy comes from the acoustic or sound spectrum and is undetectable to the human ear. By using conducting agents such as gel or mineral oil, the ultrasound transducer warms areas of the musculoskeletal system Some areas of the musculoskeletal system absorb ultrasound better that others. Muscle tissue and other connective tissue such as ligaments and tendons absorb this form of energy very well. However, fat absorbs to a much lesser degree. Ultrasound has a relatively long-lasting effect, continuing up to one hour.

Diathermy

Diathermy is another deep heat treatment. An electrode drum is used to apply heat to an affected area. It consists of a wire coil surrounded by dead space and other insulators such as a plastic housing. Plenty of toweling must be layered between the unit and the patient. This device is unique in that it utilizes the basis of a magnetic field on connective tissues. One advantage of diathermy over various other heat treatments is that fat does resist an electrical field, which is not the case with a magnetic field. It is found to be helpful with those experiencing chronic **low back pain** and **muscle spasms**. Prior to ultrasound technology, diathermy was a popular heat therapy of the 1940s–1960s.

Preparation

Before administering any form of heat treatment, heat sensitivity is accessed and the skin over the affected area is cleansed. When a patient is undergoing any form of heat treatment, supervision should always be present especially in the treatment of hydrotherapy.

Aftercare

Once the heat treatment has been completed, any symptoms of **dizziness** and **nausea** should be noted and documented along with any skin irritations or discoloring not present prior to the heat treatment. A one hour interval between treatments should be adhered to in order to avoid restriction of blood flow.

Risks

All heat treatments have the potential of tissue damage resulting from excessive temperatures. Proper insulation and treatment duration should be carefully administered for each method. Overexposure during a superficial heat treatment may result in redness, blisters, **burns**, or reduced blood circulation. During ultrasound therapy, excessive treatment over bony areas with little soft tissue (such as hand, feet, and elbow) can cause excessive heat resulting in pain and possible tissue damage. Exposure to the electrode drum during diathermy may produce hot spots.

ORGANIZATIONS

American Physical Therapy Association, 1111 North Fairfax St., Alexandria, VA, 22314-1488, (703) 684-2782, (703) 684-7343, (800) 999-2782, http://www.apta.org/.

Jeffrey P. Larson, RPT

Heatstroke *see* **Heat disorders**

Heavy menstruation *see* **Dysfunctional uterine bleeding**

Heavy metal poisoning

Definition

Heavy metal **poisoning** is the toxic accumulation of heavy metals in the soft tissues of the body.

Description

Heavy metals are chemical elements that have a specific gravity (a measure of density) at least five times that of water. The heavy metals most often implicated in accidental human poisoning are lead, mercury, arsenic, and cadmium. More recently, thallium has gained some attention in the media as the poison used in several murder cases in the 1990s. Some heavy metals, such as zinc, copper, chromium, iron, and manganese, are required by the body in small amounts, but these same elements can be toxic in larger quantities.

Heavy metals may enter the body in food, water, or air, or by absorption through the skin. Once in the body, they compete with and displace essential **minerals**, such as zinc, copper, magnesium, and **calcium**, and interfere with organ system function. People may come in contact with heavy metals in industrial work, pharmaceutical manufacturing, and agriculture. Children may be poisoned as a result of playing in contaminated soil. **Lead poisoning** in adults has been traced to the use of lead-based glazes on pottery vessels intended for use with food, and contamination of Ayurvedic and other imported herbal remedies. Arsenic and thallium have been mixed with food or beverages to attempt **suicide** or poison others.

Another form of **mercury poisoning** that is seen more and more frequently in the United States is self-injected mercury under the skin. Some boxers inject themselves with mercury in the belief that it adds muscle bulk. Metallic mercury is also used in folk medicine or religious rituals in various cultures. These practices increase the risk of mercury poisoning of children in these ethnic groups or subcultures.

Causes and symptoms

Symptoms will vary, depending on the nature and the quantity of the heavy metal ingested. Patients may complain of **nausea**, **vomiting**, **diarrhea**, stomach **pain**, **headache**, sweating, and a metallic taste in the mouth. Depending on the metal, there may be blue-black lines in the gum tissues. In severe cases, patients exhibit obvious impairment of cognitive, motor, and language skills. The expression "mad as a hatter" comes from the mercury poisoning prevalent in 17th-century France among hatmakers who soaked animal hides in a solution of mercuric nitrate to soften the hair.

Diagnosis

Heavy metal poisoning may be detected using blood and urine tests, hair and tissue analysis, or x ray. The diagnosis is often overlooked, however, because many of the early symptoms of heavy metal poisoning are nonspecific. The doctor should take a thorough patient history with particular emphasis on the patient's occupation.

In childhood, blood lead levels above 80 ug/dL generally indicate lead poisoning, however, significantly lower levels (>30 ug/dL) can cause **mental retardation** and other cognitive and behavioral problems in affected children. The Centers for Disease Control and Prevention considers a blood lead level of 10 ug/dL or higher in children a cause for concern. In adults, symptoms of lead poisoning are usually seen when blood lead levels exceed 80 ug/dL for a number of weeks.

Blood levels of mercury should not exceed 3.6 ug/dL, while urine levels should not exceed 15 ug/dL. Symptoms of mercury poisoning may be seen when mercury levels exceed 20 ug/dL in blood and 60 ug/dL in urine. Mercury levels in hair may be used to gauge the severity of chronic mercury exposure.

Since arsenic is rapidly cleared from the blood, blood arsenic levels may not be very useful in diagnosis. Arsenic in the urine (measured in a 24-hour collection following 48 hours without eating seafood) may exceed 50 ug/dL in people with arsenic poisoning. If acute arsenic or thallium poisoning is suspected, an x ray may reveal these substances in the abdomen (since both metals are opaque to x rays). Arsenic may also be detected in the hair and nails for months following exposure.

Cadmium toxicity is generally indicated when urine levels exceed 10 ug/dL of creatinine and blood levels exceed 5 ug/dL.

Thallium poisoning often causes hair loss (**alopecia**), **numbness**, and a burning sensation in the skin as well as nausea, **vomiting**, and **dizziness**. As little as 15–20 mg of thallium per kilogram of body weight is fatal in humans; however, smaller amounts can cause severe damage to the nervous system.

Treatment

When heavy metal poisoning is suspected, it is important to begin treatment as soon as possible to minimize long-term damage to the patient's nervous system and digestive tract. Heavy metal poisoning is considered a medical emergency, and the patient should be taken to a hospital emergency room.

The treatment for most heavy metal poisoning is **chelation therapy**. A chelating agent specific to the metal involved is given either orally, intramuscularly, or intravenously. The three most common chelating agents are calcium disodium edetate, dimercaprol (BAL), and penicillamine. The chelating agent encircles and binds to the metal in the body's tissues, forming a complex; that complex is then released from the tissue to travel in the bloodstream. The complex is filtered out of the blood by the kidneys and excreted in the urine. This process may be lengthy and painful, and typically requires hospitalization. Chelation therapy is effective in treating lead, mercury, and arsenic

KEY TERMS

Alopecia—Loss of hair.

Chelation—The process by which a molecule encircles and binds to a metal and removes it from tissue.

Heavy metal—One of 23 chemical elements that has a specific gravity (a measure of density) at least five times that of water.

Prussian blue—The common name of potassium ferric hexacyanoferrate, a compound approved in the United States for treatment of thallium poisoning. Prussian blue gets its name from the fact that it was first used by artists in 1704 as a dark blue pigment for oil paints. It has also been used in laundry bluing and fabric printing.

poisoning, but is not useful in treating cadmium poisoning. To date, no treatment has been proven effective for cadmium poisoning. Thallium poisoning is treated with a combination of Prussian blue (potassium ferric hexacyanoferrate) and a diuretic because about 35% of it is excreted in the urine; however, if treatment is not started within 72 hours of ingesting the poisoning, damage to the patient's nervous system may be permanent.

In cases of acute mercury, arsenic, or thallium ingestion, vomiting may be induced. **Activated charcoal** may be given in cases of thallium poisoning. Washing out the stomach (gastric lavage) may also be useful. The patient may also require treatment such as intravenous fluids for such complications of poisoning as **shock**, anemia, and kidney failure.

Patients who have taken arsenic, thallium, or mercury in a suicide attempt will be seen by a psychiatrist as part of emergency treatment.

Prognosis

The chelation process can only halt further effects of the poisoning; it cannot reverse neurological damage already sustained.

Prevention

Because arsenic and thallium were commonly used in rat and insect poisons at one time, many countries have tried to lower the rate of accidental poisonings by banning the use of heavy metals in pest control products. Thallium was banned in the United States as a rodent poison in 1984. As a result, almost all recent cases of arsenic and thallium poisoning in the United States were deliberate rather than accidental.

Because exposure to heavy metals is often an occupational hazard, protective clothing and respirators should be provided and worn on the job. Protective clothing should then be left at the work site and not worn home, where it could carry toxic dust to family members. Industries are urged to reduce or replace the heavy metals in their processes wherever possible. Exposure to environmental sources of lead, including lead-based paints, plumbing fixtures, vehicle exhaust, and contaminated soil, should be reduced or eliminated.

People who use Ayurvedic or traditional Chinese herbal preparations as alternative treatments for various illnesses should purchase them only from reliable manufacturers.

Resources

BOOKS

Beers, Mark H., Robert S. Porter, and Thomas V. Jones, eds. *The Merck Manual of Diagnosis and Therapy*. 18th ed. Whitehouse Station, NJ: Merck Research Laboratories, 2006.

Wilson, Billie Ann, Margaret T. Shannon, and Kelly Shields. *Pearson Nurse's Drug Guide 2010*. Upper Saddle River, NJ: Prentice Hall, 2009.

PERIODICALS

Boyarsky, Igor, DO, and Adrain D. Crisan, MD. "Toxicity, Thallium." *eMedicine* (August 3, 2004). <http://www.emedicine.com/emerg/topic926.htm.>

Centers for Disease Control and Prevention (CDC). "Adult Blood Lead Epidemiology and Surveillance—United States, 2002." *Morbidity and Mortality Weekly Report* 53 (July 9, 2004): 578–582.

Counter, S. A., and L. H. Buchanan. "Mercury Exposure in Children: A Review." *Toxicology and Applied Pharmacology* 198 (July 15, 2004): 209–230.

Prasad, V. L. "Subcutaneous Injection of Mercury: 'Warding Off Evil'." *Environmental Health Perspectives* 111 (September 2004): 1326–1328.

Schilling, U., R. Muck, and E. Heidemann. "Lead Poisoning After Ingestion of Ayurvedic Drugs." [in German] *Medizinische Klinik* 99 (August 15, 2004): 476–480.

Thompson, D. F., and E. D. Callen. "Soluble or Insoluble Prussian Blue for Radiocesium and Thallium Poison ing?" *Annals of Pharmacotherapy* 38 (September 2004): 1509–1514.

ORGANIZATIONS

American Society of Health-System Pharmacists (ASHP), 7272 Wisconsin Avenue, Bethesda, MD, 20814, (301) 657-3000, (866) 279-0681, http://www.ashp.org.

Centers for Disease Control and Prevention (CDC), 1600 Clifton Road, Atlanta, GA, 30333, (800) 232-4636, cdcinfo@cdc.gov, http://www.cdc.gov.

Food and Drug Administration. Consumer Information. , HFI-40, 5600 Fishers La.,-Rockville, MD, 20857, (888) 463-6332, ConsumerInfo@fda.hhs.gov, http://www.fda.gov.

National Center for Environmental Health, 1600 Clifton Road, Atlanta, GA, 30333, (800) 232-4636, cdcinfo@cdc.gov, http://www.cdc.gov/nceh.

Bethany Thivierge
Rebecca J. Frey, PhD

Heel spurs

Definition

A heel spur is a bony projection on the sole (plantar) region of the heel bone (also known as the calcaneous). This condition may accompany or result from severe cases of inflammation to the structure called plantar fascia. This associated plantar fascia is a fibrous band of connective tissue on the sole of the foot, extending from the heel to the toes.

Description

Heel spurs are a common foot problem resulting from excess bone growth on the heel bone. The bone growth is usually located on the underside of the heel bone, extending forward to the toes. One explanation for this excess production of bone is a painful tearing of the plantar fascia connected between the toes and heel. This can result in either a heel spur or an inflammation of the plantar fascia, medically termed plantar fascitis. Because this condition is often correlated to a decrease in the arch of the foot, it is more prevalent after the age of six to eight years, when the arch is fully developed.

Causes and symptoms

One frequent cause of heel spurs is an abnormal motion and mal-alignment of the foot called pronation. For the foot to function properly, a certain degree of pronation is required. This motion is defined as an inward action of the foot, with dropping of the inside arch as one plants the heel and advances the weight distribution to the toes during walking. When foot pronation becomes extreme from the foot turning in and dropping beyond the normal limit, a condition known as excessive pronation creates a mechanical problem in the foot. In some cases the sole or bottom of the foot flattens and becomes unstable because of this excess pronation, especially during critical times of walking and athletic activities. The portion of the plantar fascia attached into the heel bone or calcaneous begins to stretch and pull away from the heel bone.

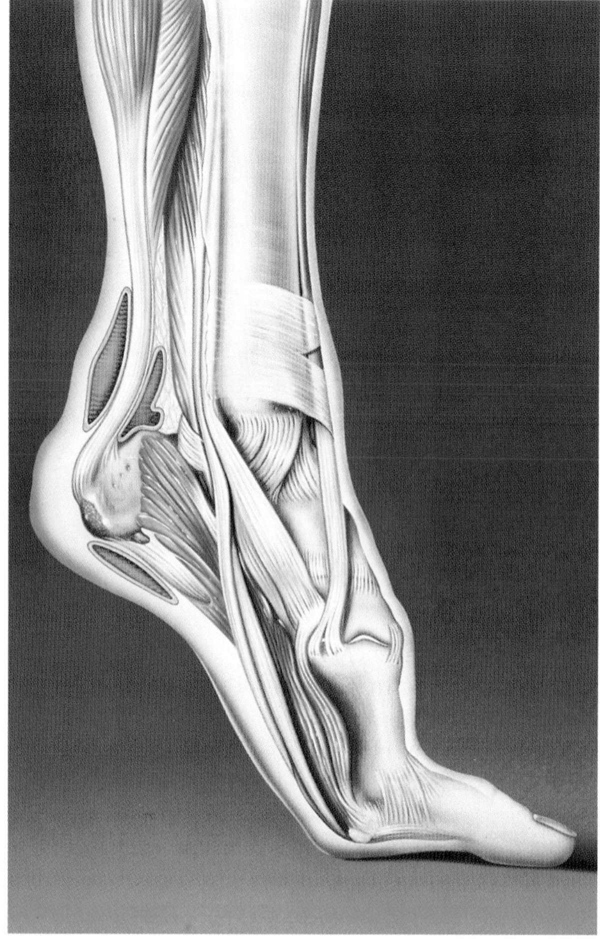

Illustration of a bony projection, a spur, which developed from chronic irritation. *(Photo Researchers, Inc.)*

At the onset of this condition, **pain** and swelling become present, with discomfort particularly noted as pushing off with the toes occurs during walking. This movement of the foot stretches the fascia that is already irritated and inflamed. If this condition is allowed to continue, pain is noticed around the heel region because of the newly formed bone, in response to the **stress**. This results in the development of the heel spur. It is common among athletes and others who run and jump a significant amount.

An individual with the lower legs angulating inward, a condition called genu valgum or "knock knees," can have a tendency toward excessive pronation. As a result, this too can lead to a fallen arch resulting in plantar fascitis and heel spurs. Women tend to have more genu valgum than men do. Heel spurs can also result from an abnormally high arch.

Other factors leading to heel spurs include a sudden increase in daily activities, an increase in weight, or a change of shoes. Dramatic increase in training intensity or duration may cause plantar fascitis. Shoes that are too flexible in the middle of the arch or shoes that bend before the toe joints will cause an increase in tension in the plantar fascia and possibly lead to heel spurs.

The pain this condition causes forces an individual to attempt walking on his or her toes or ball of the foot to avoid pressure on the heel spur. This can lead to other compensations during walking or running that in turn cause additional problems to the ankle, knee, hip, or back.

KEY TERMS

Calcaneous—The heel bone.

Genu valgum—Deformity in which the legs are curved inward so that the knees are close together, nearly or actually knocking as a person walks with ankles widely apart of each other.

Plantar fascia—A tough fibrous band of tissue surrounding the muscles of the sole of the foot. Also called plantar aponeurosis.

Pronation—The lowering or descending of the inner edge of the foot by turning the entire foot outwards.

Diagnosis

A thorough medical history and physical exam by a physician is always necessary for the proper diagnosis of heel spurs and other foot conditions. X rays of the heel area are helpful, as excess bone production will be visible.

Treatment

Conservative

Heel spurs and plantar fascitis are usually controlled with conservative treatment. Early intervention includes stretching the calf muscles while avoiding reinjuring the plantar fascia. Decreasing or changing activities, losing excess weight, and improving the proper fitting of shoes are all important measures to decrease this common source of foot pain. Modification of footwear includes shoes with a raised heel and better arch support. Shoe orthotics recommended by a healthcare professional are often very helpful in conjunction with exercises to increase strength of the foot muscles and arch. The orthotic prevents excess pronation and lengthening of the plantar fascia and continued tearing of this structure. To aid in this reduction of inflammation, applying ice for 10–15 minutes after activities and use of anti-inflammatory medication can be helpful. **Physical therapy** can be beneficial with the use of heat modalities, such as ultrasound that creates a deep heat and reduces inflammation. If the pain caused by inflammation is constant, keeping the foot raised above the heart and/or compressed by wrapping with an ace bandage will help.

Corticosteroid injections are also frequently used to reduce pain and inflammation. Taping can help speed the healing process by protecting the fascia from reinjury, especially during stretching and walking.

Heel surgery

When chronic heel pain fails to respond to conservative treatment, surgical treatment may be necessary. Heel surgery can provide relief of pain and restore mobility. The type of procedure used is based on examination and usually consists of releasing the excessive tightness of the plantar fascia, called a plantar fascia release. Depending on the presence of excess bony build up, the procedure may or may not include removal of heel spurs. Similar to other surgical interventions, there are various modifications and surgical enhancements regarding surgery of the heel.

Alternative treatment

Acupuncture and accupressure have been used to address the pain of heel spurs, in addition to using friction massage to help break up scar tissue and delay onset of bony formations.

Prognosis

Usually, heel spurs are curable with conservative treatment. If not, heel spurs are curable with surgery. About 10% of those that continue to see a physician for plantar fascitis have it for more than a year. If there is limited success after approximately one year of conservative treatment, patients are often advised to have surgery.

Prevention

To prevent this condition, wearing shoes with proper arches and support is very important. Proper stretching is always a necessity, especially when there is an increase in activities or a change in running technique. It is not recommended to attempt working through the pain, as this can change a mild case of heel spurs and plantar fascitis into a long lasting and painful episode of this condition.

ORGANIZATIONS

American Orthopaedic Foot and Ankle Society, 6300 N. River Road, Suite 510, Rosemont, IL, 60018, (847) 698-4654, (800) 235-4855.

American Podiatric Medical Association, 9312 Old Georgetown Road, Bethesda, MD, 20814-1621, (301) 581-9200, http://www.apma.org.

Jeffrey P. Larson, RPT

Heimlich maneuver

Definition

The Heimlich maneuver is an emergency procedure for removing a foreign object lodged in the airway that is preventing a person from breathing. It is also known as abdominal thrusts.

Purpose

Each year, between 2,800 and 4,000 adults die in the United States because they accidentally inhale rather than swallow food. The food gets stuck and blocks their trachea (windpipe), making breathing impossible. **Death** follows rapidly unless the food or other foreign material can be displaced from the airway. This condition is so common it has been nicknamed the "café coronary."

In 1974, Dr. Henry Heimlich first described an emergency technique for expelling foreign material blocking the trachea. This technique, now called the Heimlich maneuver or abdominal thrust, is simple enough that it can be performed immediately by anyone trained in the maneuver. The Heimlich maneuver is a standard part of all **first aid** courses.

The theory behind the Heimlich maneuver is that by compressing the abdomen below the level of the diaphragm, air is forced out of the lungs under pressure. This air dislodges the obstruction in the trachea and brings the foreign material back up into the mouth.

The Heimlich maneuver is used mainly when such solid materials as food, coins, vomit, or small toys are blocking the airway. There has been some controversy about whether the Heimlich maneuver is appropriate to use routinely on **near-drowning** victims. After several studies of the effectiveness of the Heimlich maneuver on reestablishing breathing in near-drowning victims, the American Red Cross and the American Heart Association both recommend that the Heimlich maneuver be used only as a last resort after traditional airway clearance techniques and **cardiopulmonary resuscitation** (CPR) have been tried repeatedly and failed; or if it is clear that a solid foreign object is blocking the airway.

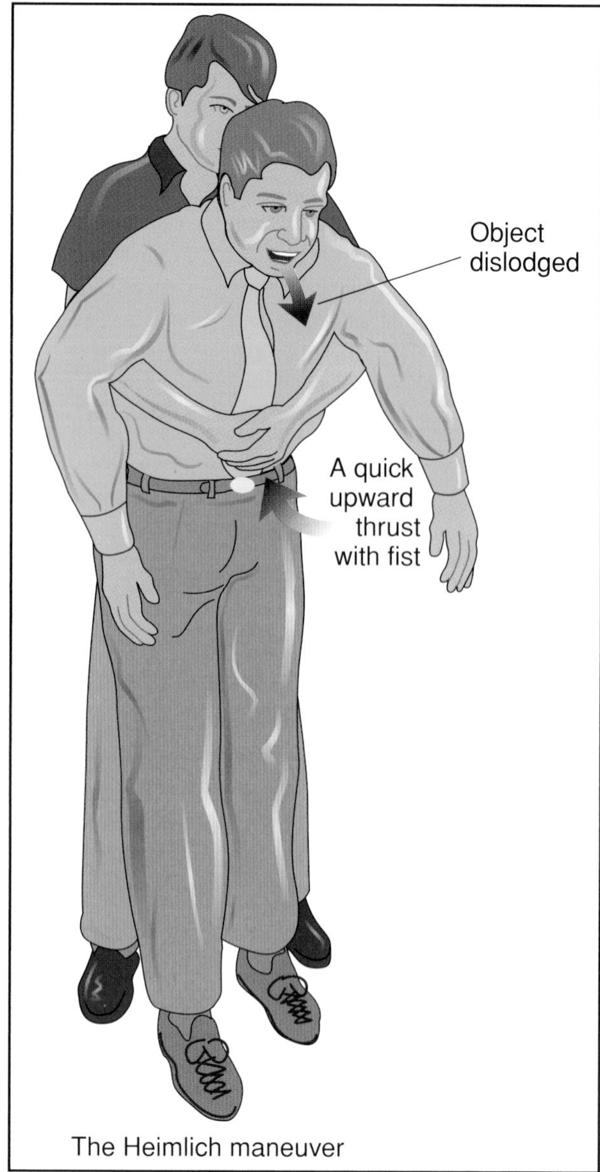

To perform the Heimlich maneuver on a conscious adult (as illustrated above), the rescuer stands behind the victim and encircles his waist. The rescuer makes a fist with one hand and places the other hand on top, positioned below the rib cage and above the waist. The rescuer then applies pressure by a series of upward and inward thrusts to force the foreign object back up the victim's trachea. *(Illustration by Electronic Illustrators Group. Reproduced by permission of Gale, a part of Cengage Learning.)*

Demographics

There are no exact statistics on the number of times the Heimlich maneuver is performed in an average year, or the circumstances or age groups of the persons treated, although one study done in California stated that 4% of 513 patients treated for a foreign body in the airway died and that the average age of patients treated was 65. The Heimlich maneuver was the most commonly used intervention, with an 86% success rate.

Description

The Heimlich maneuver can be performed on all people. Modifications are necessary if the person **choking** is very obese, pregnant, a child, or an infant. Indications that a person's airway is blocked include:

- inability to speak or cry out
- face turning blue from lack of oxygen
- desperate grabbing at the throat
- weak cough with labored breathing producing a high-pitched noise
- all of the above, followed by unconsciousness

Performing the Heimlich maneuver on adults

To perform the Heimlich maneuver on a conscious adult, the rescuer stands behind the affected person, who may be either sitting or standing. The rescuer makes a fist with one hand and places it, thumb toward the person choking, below the rib cage and above the waist. The rescuer encircles the other person's waist, placing the other hand on top of the fist.

In a series of 6 to 10 sharp and distinct thrusts upward and inward, the rescuer attempts to develop enough pressure to force the foreign object back up the trachea. If the maneuver fails, it is repeated. It is important not to give up if the first attempt fails. As the choking person is deprived of oxygen, the muscles of the trachea relax slightly. Because of this loosening, it is possible that a foreign object may be expelled on a second or third attempt.

If the individual choking is unconscious, the rescuer should place the person supine on the floor; bend the chin forward; make sure the tongue is not blocking the airway; and feel in the mouth for any **foreign objects**, being careful not to push them further into the airway. The rescuer kneels astride the choking person's thighs and places the fists between the bottom of the choking person's breastbone and navel. The rescuer then executes a series of 6 to 10 sharp compressions by pushing inward and upward.

After the abdominal thrusts, the rescuer repeats the process of lifting the chin, moving the tongue, feeling for and possibly removing any foreign material. If the airway is not clear, the rescuer repeats the abdominal thrusts as often as necessary. If the foreign object has been removed, but the victim is not breathing, the rescuer starts CPR.

Performing the Heimlich maneuver under special circumstances

OBVIOUSLY PREGNANT OR VERY OBESE PEOPLE. The main difference in performing the Heimlich maneuver on this group of people is in the placement of the fists. Instead of using abdominal thrusts, chest thrusts are used. The rescuer's fists are placed against the middle of the breastbone (sternum), and the motion of the chest thrust is in and downward, rather than upward. If the person choking is unconscious, the chest thrusts are similar to those used in CPR.

CHILDREN. The technique in children over one year of age is the same as in adults, except that the amount of force used is less than that used with adults, in order to avoid damaging a child's ribs, breastbone, and internal organs.

INFANTS UNDER ONE YEAR OLD. The rescuer sits down and positions the infant along the rescuer's forearm with the infant's face pointed toward the floor and at a lower level than the infant's chest. The rescuer's hand supports the infant's head. The forearm rests on the rescuer's own thigh for additional support. Using the heel of the other hand, the rescuer administers four or five rapid blows to the infant's back between the shoulder blades.

After administering the back blows, the rescuer sandwiches the infant between both arms. The infant is turned over so that it lies face up, supported by the rescuer's opposite arm. Using the free hand, the rescuer places the index and middle finger on the center of the breastbone and makes four sharp chest thrusts. This series of back blows and chest thrusts is alternated until the foreign object is expelled.

SELF-ADMINISTRATION OF THE HEIMLICH MANEUVER. To apply the Heimlich maneuver to oneself, a choking person should make a fist with one hand and place it in the middle of the body at a spot above the navel and below the breastbone, then grasp the fist with the other hand and push sharply inward and upward. If this fails, the choking person should press the upper abdomen over the back of a chair, edge of a table, porch railing or something similar, and thrust up and inward until the object is dislodged.

KEY TERMS

Aspiration—The entry of body secretions or foreign material into the trachea and lungs.

Diaphragm—The thin layer of muscle that separates the chest cavity, which contains the lungs and heart, from the abdominal cavity, which contains the intestines and digestive organs.

Sternum—The breastbone. The sternum is located over the heart, is the point of attachment for ribs at the front of the body and provides protection to the heart beneath it.

Trachea—The windpipe. A tube extending from below the voice box into the chest where it splits into two branches, the bronchi, that lead to each lung.

Benefits

The Heimlich maneuver usually results in the expulsion and removal of an obstruction in the throat; in many situations, the person's life is saved. The choking person suffers no permanent effects from the episode.

Precautions

If possible, have someone nearby call 911 while the rescuer performs the Heimlich maneuver.

It is important to have training and practice in the correct use of the maneuver. Incorrect application of the Heimlich maneuver can damage the chest, ribs, heart, or internal organs of the person on whom it is performed. People may also vomit after being treated with the Heimlich maneuver. It is important to prevent aspiration of the vomitus.

Preparation

Any adult, adolescent, or responsible older child can be trained to perform the Heimlich maneuver. Knowing how to perform it may save someone's life. Before doing the maneuver, it is important to determine whether the airway is completely blocked. If the choking person can talk or cry, the Heimlich maneuver is not appropriate. If the airway is not completely blocked, the choking person should be allowed to try to **cough** up the foreign object without assistance.

Aftercare

Once the obstruction is removed, most persons who experience an episode of choking recover without any further care. Persons who have an obstruction that cannot be dislodged but are able to breathe should be taken to an emergency room for treatment.

Risks

Many people vomit after being treated with the Heimlich maneuver. Depending on the length and severity of the choking episode, the person may need to be taken to a hospital emergency room. In addition, even when the maneuver is performed correctly, the person being treated often suffers **bruises** in the abdominal area. Occasionally, one or more ribs of the choking person may be broken during administration of the Heimlich maneuver. The elderly are more likely to suffer bruises or broken ribs during the maneuver than younger adults.

Applying the Heimlich maneuver too vigorously may result in an injury to the internal organs of the choking person. There may be some local **pain** and tenderness at the point where the rescuer's fist was placed. In infants, a rescuer should never attempt to sweep the baby's mouth without looking to remove foreign material. This is likely to push the material farther down the trachea. If the foreign material is not removed, the person choking will die from lack of oxygen.

Health care team roles

Anyone can be trained to successfully apply the Heimlich maneuver. Most of the applications each year are provided by trained volunteers. Health professionals may become involved. Paramedics may apply the Heimlich maneuver to a choking person. Physicians, physician assistants and nurses may provide additional treatment in a hospital emergency room. Nurses may provide some follow-up care.

Research and general acceptance

There is some debate as of 2010 over the benefit of slapping the person's upper back to help dislodge the material in the windpipe. Dr. Heimlich has long maintained that back slaps should not be done because they drive the material deeper into the windpipe. However, the American Red Cross and the American Heart Association presently recommend the use of hard blows with the heel of the rescuer's hand on the upper back of the victim. The number to be used varies by training organization, but is usually between 5 and 20. The back slap is designed to create pressure behind the blockage, assisting the patient in dislodging the article in the airway. The Mayo Clinic article listed in the Resources section of this article recommends five back slaps before beginning the abdominal thrusts of the Heimlich maneuver, and alternating between five back blows and five abdominal thrusts until the food or other object is dislodged.

Resources

BOOKS

American Academy of Orthopaedic Surgeons. *First Aid, CPR, and AED Standard*. Sudbury, MA: Jones and Bartlett Publishers, 2010.

Dvorchak, George E., Jr. *The Pocket First Aid Field Guide: Treatment of Outdoor Emergencies*. New York: Skyhorse Publishing, 2010.

National Safety Council. *Basic Pediatric First Aid, CPR, and AED*. Boston: McGraw-Hill Higher Education, 2008.

PERIODICALS

Chillag, S., et al. "The Heimlich Maneuver: Breaking Down the Complications." *Southern Medical Journal* 103 (February 2010): 147–150.

Drinka, P. "Broken Ribs Following CPR or the Heimlich Maneuver." *Journal of the American Medical Directors Association* 10 (May 2009): 283–84.

Lee, S.L., et al. "Complications as a Result of the Heimlich Maneuver." *Journal of Trauma* 66 (March 2009): E34–E35.

Soroudi, A., et al. "Adult Foreign Body Airway Obstruction in the Prehospital Setting." *Prehospital Emergency Care* 11 (January-March 2007): 25–29.

OTHER

American Heart Association. *Heimlich Maneuver*. http://www.americanheart.org/presenter.jhtml?identifier=4605.

Broomfield, James, MD. "Heimlich Maneuver on Self." *Discovery Health*, January 4, 2007. http://health.discovery.com/encyclopedias/illnesses.html?article=671.

Heimlich Institute. *How to Do the Heimlich Maneuver*. http://www.heimlichinstitute.org/page.php?id=34.

Howcast. *How to Perform the Heimlich Maneuver*. This is a video demonstration of the maneuver that takes about 2-1/2 minutes to watch. http://www.youtube.com/watch?v=tEIiEAn7b-U.

Mayo Clinic. *Choking: First Aid*. http://www.mayoclinic.com/health/first-aid-choking/FA00025.

MedlinePlus Medical Encyclopedia. *Heimlich Maneuver*. http://www.nlm.nih.gov/medlineplus/ency/article/000047.htm.

Nathan, Joan. "A Heimlich in Every Pot." *New York Times*, February 3, 2009. http://www.nytimes. com/2009/02/04/opinion/04nathan.html?ref=opinion.

ORGANIZATIONS

American Heart Association National Center, 7272 Greenville Avenue, Dallas, TX, 75231, 800-AHA-USA-1, http://www.americanheart.org/presenter.jhtml?identifier=1200000.

American Red Cross National Headquarters, 2025 E Street, NW, Washington, DC, 20006, 202-303-5000, http://www.redcross.org/.

Heimlich Institute, 311 Straight Street, Cincinnati, OH, 45219, 513-559-2100, http://www.heimlichinstitute.org/default.php.

L. Fleming Fallon, Jr., MD, PhD, DrPH
Rebecca J. Frey, PhD

Helicobacter pylori infection *see* **Helicobacteriosis**

Helicobacteriosis

Definition

Helicobacteriosis refers to infection of the gastrointestinal tract with the bacteria, *Helicobacter pylori* (*H. pylori*). While there are other, more rare strains of *Helicobacter* species that can infect humans, only *H. pylori* has been convincingly shown to be a cause of disease in humans. The organism was first documented to cause injury to the stomach in 1983 by two researchers in Australia, who ingested the organism to prove their theory. Since then, *H. pylori* has been

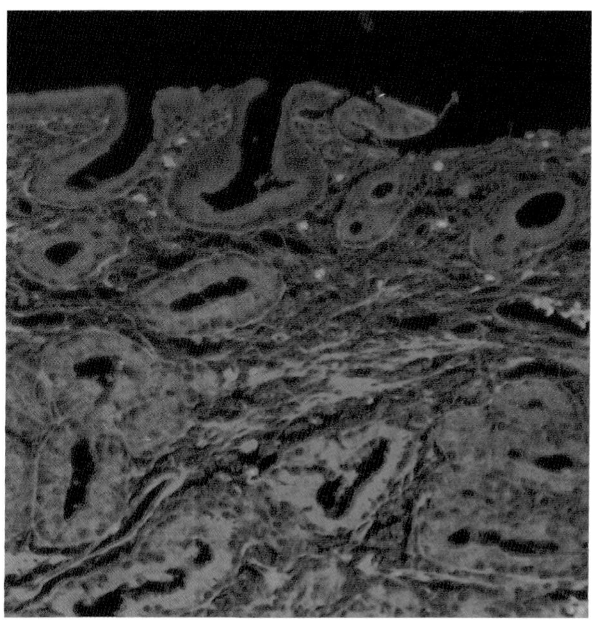

A light microscopic image of a stomach ulcer. Gastric and duodenal ulcers are usually caused by infection with the bacteria Helicobacter pylori. This bacterium is also believed to be a cause of various cancers of the stomach. *(Custom Medical Stock Photo, Inc. Reproduced by permission.)*

shown to be the main cause of ulcer disease, and has revolutionized the treatment of peptic ulcer disease. It also is believed to be linked to various cancers of the stomach.

Description

H. pylori is a gram-negative, spiral-shaped organism, that contains flagella (tail-like structures) and other properties. In addition to flagella, which help the organism to move around in the liquid mucous layer of the stomach, *H. pylori* also produces an enzyme called urease, that protects it from gastric acid present in the stomach. As the production of this enzyme is relatively unusual, new diagnostic tests have enabled rapid identification of the bacteria.

H. pylori also produces two other chemicals: a cytotoxin called vacA and a protein known as cagA. Patients with ulcer disease are more likely to produce the cytotoxin (vacA). The cagA protein not only occurs frequently in ulcer disease but also in **cancer**. It is still not known how these substances enable *H. pylori* to cause disease.

Causes and symptoms

Infection with *H. pylori* is largely dependent on two factors; age and income status. The bacteria is acquired mainly in childhood, especially in areas of poor hygiene or overcrowding. *H. pylori* is two to three times more prevalent in developing, non-industrialized countries. In the United States for example, the organism is believed to be present in about one-third of the population.

The exact way in which *H. pylori* gets passed from one individual to another is uncertain, but person to person transmission is most likely. In most cases, children are felt to be the source of spread. Reinfection of those who have been cured has been documented, especially in areas of overcrowding.

The bacteria is well adapted to survival within the stomach. Not only does it survive there for years, but once infection begins, a form of chronic inflammation (chronic **gastritis**) always develops. In most individuals, initial infection causes little or no symptoms; however, some individuals, such as the original researchers who ingested the bacteria, wind up with abdominal **pain** and **nausea**.

In about 15% of infected persons, ulcer disease develops either in the stomach or duodenum. Why some develop ulcer disease and others do not remains unclear. Ulcer symptoms are characterized by upper abdominal pain that is typically of a burning or "gnawing" type and usually is rapidly relieved by **antacids** or food.

Acid secretion increases in most patients with duodenal ulcers. This increase returns to normal once *H. pylori* is eliminated. It is now known that elimination of the bacteria will substantially decrease the risk of recurrent bouts of ulcer disease in the vast majority of patients. In fact, a 2003 report showed that by eradicating H. pylori, ulcer bleeding rarely recurs.

In the last decade it has been shown that *H. pylori* is not only the prime cause of ulcer disease of the stomach and duodenum, but is also strongly associated with various tumors of the stomach. Bacterial infection is nine times more common in patients with cancer of the stomach, and seven times more common in those with lymphoma of the stomach (tumor of the lymphatic tissue), called a MALT tumor. It is believed that the prolonged inflammation leads to changes in cell growth and tumors. Eliminating *H. pylori* can lead to regression of some tumors.

In addition to the above damage caused by *H. pylori*, some individuals lose normal gastric function, such as the ability to absorb vitamin B_{12}.

Diagnosis

There are basically two types of tests to identify infection: one group is "invasive" in that it involves the use of an **endoscopy** to obtain biopsy specimens for evaluation, while the other "noninvasive" methods depend on blood or breath samples. Invasive tests can be less accurate because of technical limitations: the biopsy may miss the area where the bacteria hides.

Invasive studies make use of tissue obtained by endoscopic biopsy to identify the organism. The bacteria can be searched for in pieces of biopsy tissue or grown (cultured) from the specimen. However, *H. pylori* is not easy to culture. Another method uses the bacteria's production of the enzyme urease. Biopsy specimens are placed on a card that changes color if urease is present. Results often are available within a few minutes, but can take up to 24 hours.

Noninvasive tests are of two types: blood tests and breath test. Blood tests measure antibodies to make a diagnosis accurately within minutes. This can be done immediately in the doctor's office. In addition, antibody levels can be measured several months after treatment, to see if *H. pylori* has been eradicated.

The breath test uses radioactive or non-radioactive forms of a compound called urea, which the patient drinks. The method that uses a radioactive form of urea is easier to perform, as the equipment is commonly

KEY TERMS

Antibiotic—A medication that is designed to kill or weaken bacteria.

Endoscope, Endoscopy—An endoscope as used in the field of gastroenterology is a thin flexible tube that uses a lens or miniature camera to view various areas of the gastrointestinal tract. When the procedure is performed to examine certain organs, such as the bile ducts or pancreas, the organs are not viewed directly, but indirectly through the injection of x ray. The performance of an exam using an endoscope is referred by the general term endoscopy. Diagnosis through biopsies or other means and therapeutic procedures can be done with these instruments.

Gram-negative—Refers to the property of many bacteria in which they do not take or color with Gram's stain, a method which is used to identify bacteria. Gram-positive bacteria that take up the stain turn purple, while Gram-negative bacteria which do not take up the stain turn red.

available in x ray departments. Radiation exposure is less than that of a **chest x ray**. The test that uses non-radioactive urea is safer for children. A 2003 study in Brazil showed that the urea breath test and H. pylori stool antigen test also worked well to detect the bacteria in children. The breath test is the best way to be sure of elimination of *H. pylori*. The test can be used within 30 days after treatment. This is an advantage over following antibody levels that take six months or longer to diminish.

Treatment

H. pylori peptic ulcers are treated with drugs to kill the bacteria, drugs to reduce stomach acid, and drugs to protect the lining of the stomach. The **antibiotics** most commonly used to kill the bacteria are amoxicillin, clarithromycin, metronidazole, and tetracycline. Drugs used to reduce stomach acid may be histamine blockers or **proton pump inhibitors**. The most commonly used histamine blockers are cimetidine, famotidine, nizatidine, and ranitidine. The most commonly used proton pump inhibitors are lansoprazole and omeprazole. The drug bismuth subsalicylate (a component of Pepto-Bismol) is used to protect the stomach lining.

The most common drug treatment is a two-week course of treatment called triple therapy. This treatment regimen involves taking two antibiotics to kill the bacteria and either an acid reducer or a stomach-lining shield. This therapy has been shown to kill the bacteria, reduce ulcer symptoms, and prevent ulcer recurrence in over 90% of patients.

The main drawback of triple therapy is that some patients find it difficult to follow because it often requires taking as many as 20 pills a day. The antibiotics also may cause unpleasant side effects that may make certain patients less likely to follow the treatment protocol. These side effects include dark stools, **diarrhea**, **dizziness**, **headache**, a metallic taste in the mouth, nausea, **vomiting**, and yeast infections in women.

Prognosis

The elimination of *H. pylori* and cure of ulcer disease is now possible in more than 90% of those infected. The finding that most ulcers are due to an infectious agent has brought a dramatic change in treatment and outlook for those suffering from the disease. Some patients will wind up with repeated infection, but this is most common in overcrowded areas.

Prevention

Attempts to develop a vaccine to protect against infection may be worthwhile in areas where the *H. pylori* infection rate and occurrence of cancer of the stomach is high. Research has shown such a vaccine would likely be safe in humans, but a vaccine has yet to be fully identified and developed as of mid-2003.

Resources

PERIODICALS

"Urea Breath, Stool Antigen Tests Work Well to Detect H. Pylori in Children." *Health & Medicine Week*. September 22, 2003: 315.

"Vaccination Against H. Pylori Is an Achievable Goal." *Drug Week*. July 18, 2003: 153.

Worcester, Sharon. "Eradicating H. Pylori May Prevent Bleeding Ulcers: No [Histamine. Sub2] Blockers Needed." *Internal Medicine News*. September 15, 2003: 33.

OTHER

"H. Pylori and Peptic Ulcer." National Institutes of Health. http://www.niddk.nih.gov/health/digest/pubs/hpylori/hpylori.htm.

"Management Strategies for Helicobacter pylori Seropositive Patients with Dyspepsia." http://www.acponline.org/journals/annals/15feb97/treatcounsel.htm.

"Treating Stomach Ulcers and H. pylori Infection." http://www.aafp.org/patientinfo/ulcers.html.

"What Is Helicobacter pylori Infection?" Centers for Disease Control. http://www.cdc.gov/ncidod/aip/research/hp.html#what_is_hp.

Paul A. Johnson, Ed.M.
Teresa G. Odle

Hellerwork

Definition

Hellerwork is a system of bodywork that combines deep tissue massage, body movement education, and verbal dialogue. It is designed to realign the body's structure for overall health, improvement of posture, and reduction of physical and mental **stress**.

Purpose

Hellerwork improves posture and brings the body's natural structure into proper balance and alignment. This realignment can bring relief from general aches and pains, improve breathing, and relieve physical and mental stress. Hellerwork has been used to treat such specific physical problems as chronic back, neck, shoulder, and joint **pain** as well as repetitive stress injuries, including **carpal tunnel syndrome**. Hellerwork is also used to treat and prevent athletic injuries.

Description

Origins

Joseph Heller (1940–) developed Hellerwork, a system of structural integration patterned after **Rolfing**. Heller received a degree in engineering and worked for NASA's Jet Propulsion Laboratory in Pasadena, California, before he became interested in humanistic psychology in the 1970s. He spent two years studying bioenergetics and **Gestalt therapy** as well as studying under architect and futurist Buckminster Fuller (1895–1983), flotation tank therapy developer John Lilly, family therapist Virginia Satir, and body movement pioneer Judith Aston.

During this period, he trained for six years with Dr. Ida P. Rolf (1896-1979), the founder of Rolfing, and became a certified Rolfer in 1972. After Heller developed his own system of bodywork, he founded Hellerwork in 1979 and established a training facility in Mt. Shasta, California, where he continues his work.

Hellerwork is based largely on the principles of Rolfing, in which the body's connective tissue is manipulated or massaged to realign and balance the body's structure. Because Heller believes that physical realignment is insufficient, he expanded his system to include movement education and verbal dialogue as well as deep tissue massage.

Connective tissue massage

The **massage therapy** aspect of Hellerwork is designed to release the tension that exists in the deep connective tissue, called fascia, and return it to a normal alignment. The fascia is plastic and highly adaptable. It can tighten and harden in response to the general effects of gravity on the body, other ongoing physical stresses, negative attitudes and emotions, and periodic physical traumas. One example of ongoing physical stress is carrying a briefcase, which pulls down the shoulder on one side of the body. Over time, the connective tissue becomes hard and stiff; the body becomes adapted to that position even when the person is not carrying a briefcase. In trying to adjust to the uneven weight distribution, the rest of the body becomes unbalanced and out of proper alignment.

Heller believes that as people age, more of these stress and trauma patterns become ingrained in the connective tissue, further throwing the body out of alignment. As stress accumulates, the body shortens and stiffens, a process commonly attributed to **aging**. Hellerwork seeks to recondition the body and make the connective tissue less rigid.

Movement education

The second component of Hellerwork, movement education, trains patients in the proper physical movements needed to keep the body balanced and correctly aligned. Movement education focuses on common actions, such as sitting, standing, and walking. Hellerwork practitioners also teach better patterns of movement for activities that are specific to each individual, such as their job and favorite sports or social activities.

Verbal dialogue

Verbal dialogue is the third aspect of Hellerwork. It is designed to teach awareness of the relationships among emotions, life attitudes, and the body. Hellerwork practitioners believe that as patients become responsible for their attitudes, their body movements and patterns of self-expression improve. Dialogue focuses on the theme of each session and the area of the body that is worked on during that session.

JOSEPH HELLER (1940–)

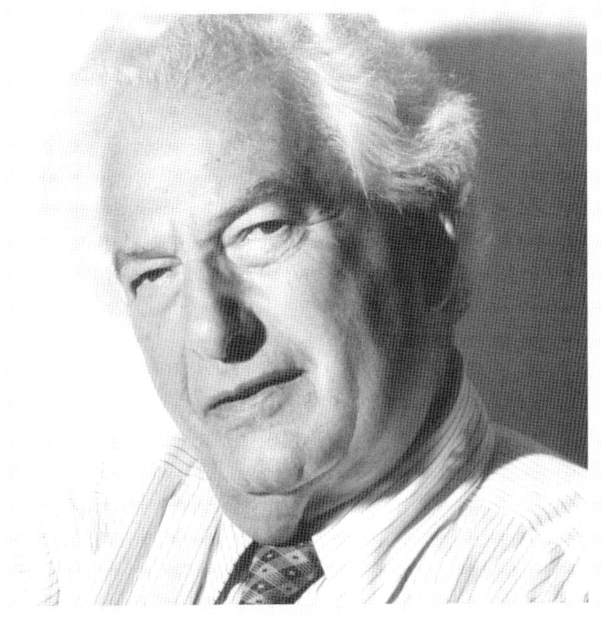

(AP Images.)

Born in Poland, Joseph Heller attended school in Europe until age 16, when he immigrated to the United States. Living in Los Angeles, he attended the California Institute of Technology in Pasadena and graduated in 1962 with a degree in engineering. He worked for 10 years at the National Aeronautics and Space Administration's Jet Propulsion Laboratory (JPL) in Pasadena as an aerospace engineer. During his service at JPL, Heller became interested in humanistic psychology. After leaving JPL in 1972, he became director of Kairos, a center for human development in Los Angeles. He spent two years studying bioenergetics and gestalt. He also trained under Buckminster Fuller, flotation tank therapy developer John Lilly, self-esteem trainer Virginia Satir, and body movement pioneer Judith Aston.

He became a certified Rolfer in 1972 and spent the next six years studying structural integration under Rolfing founder Ida P. Rolf. He became the first president of the Rolf Institute in 1975. During his training with Rolf, Heller began developing his own system of bodywork. He left the institute in 1978 and moved to Northern California where he founded Hellerwork, which he continues to operate today. According to Hellerwork's website (http://www.hellerwork.com/), his program is a unique and powerful combination of deep-tissue structural integration bodywork, movement education and dialogue. The 11 section series is designed to transform a person's relationship with his body and with the experience of being alive.

Hellerwork consists of 11 90-minute sessions costing about $90–100 each. The first three sessions focus on the surface layers of the fascia and on developmental issues of infancy and childhood. The next four sessions are the core sessions and work on the deep layers and on adolescent developmental issues. The final four treatments are the integrative sessions, and build upon all the previous ones, while also looking at questions of maturity.

Preparations

No advance preparations are required to begin Hellerwork treatment. The treatment is usually done on a massage table with the patient wearing only undergarments.

Precautions

Since Hellerwork involves vigorous deep tissue massage, it is often described as uncomfortable and sometimes painful, especially during the first several sessions. As it requires the use of hands, it may be a problem for people who do not like or are afraid of being touched. It is not recommended as a treatment for any disease or a chronic inflammatory condition such as arthritis, and can worsen such a condition. Anyone with a serious medical condition, including heart disease, diabetes, or respiratory problems, should consult a medical practitioner before undergoing Hellerwork.

Side effects

There are no reported serious side effects associated with Hellerwork when delivered by a certified practitioner to adults and juveniles.

Research and general acceptance

As with many alternative or holistic treatments, there is little mainstream scientific research documenting the effectiveness of Hellerwork therapy. Since the deep tissue massage aspect of Hellerwork is similar to Rolfing, scientific studies of Rolfing may be useful in evaluating Hellerwork. A 1988 study published in the *Journal of the American Physical Therapy Association* indicated that Rolfing stimulates the parasympathetic

KEY TERMS

Bioenergetics—A system of therapy that combines breathing and body exercises, psychological therapy, and the free expression of emotions to release blocked physical and psychic energy.

Bodywork—A term that covers a variety of therapies that include massage, realignment of the body, and similar techniques to treat deeply ingrained stresses and traumas carried in the tissues of the body.

Chronic—A disease or condition that progresses slowly but persists or reoccurs over time.

Fascia—The sheet of connective tissue that covers the body under the skin and envelops the muscles and various organs.

Gestalt therapy—A form of therapy that focuses on helping patients reconnect with their bodies and their feelings directly, as contrasted with verbal intellectual analysis.

Kinesiology—The study of the anatomy and physiology of body movement, particularly in relation to therapy.

Rolfing—A deep-tissue therapy that involves manipulating the body's fascia to realign and balance the body's structure.

nervous system, which can help speed the recovery of damaged tissue. An article in *The Journal of Orthopaedic and Sports Physical Therapy* reported that Rolfing can provide effective and sustained pain relief from lower back problems.

Resources

BOOKS

Benjamin, Patricia J. *Tappan's Handbook of Healing Massage Techniques*. 5th ed. Upper Saddle River, NJ: Prentice Hall, 2009.

Schenkman, Steven. *Massage Therapy: What It Is and How It Works*. Florence, KY; Cengage Learning, 2009.

Stewart, Nicola. *The Complete Body Massage Course: An Introduction to the Most Popular Massage Therapies*. London: Collins & Brown, 2010.

Weintraub, Michael I., Ravinder Mamtani, and Marc S. Micozzi, eds. *Complementary and Integrative Medicine in Pain Management*. New York: Springer, 2008.

ORGANIZATIONS

American Massage Therapy Association, 500 Davis St., Evanston, IL, 60201, (877) 905-2700, http://www.amtamassage.org.

Hellerwork, 406 Berry St., Mt. Shasta, CA, 96067, (530) 926-2500, http://www.hellerwork.com.

The Center for Mindfulness in Medicine, Health Care and Society. University of Massachusetts Medical School., 55 Lake Avenue North, Worcester, MA, 01655, (508) 856-2656, (508) 856-1977, mindfulness@umassmed.edu, http://www.umassmed.edu/cfm/.

Ken R. Wells
Laura Jean Cataldo, RN, EdD

HELLP syndrome *see* **Preeclampsia and eclampsia**

Hemangiomas *see* **Birthmarks**

Hematocrit

Definition

The hematocrit measures how much space in the blood is occupied by red blood cells. It is useful when evaluating a person for anemia.

Purpose

Blood is made up of red and white blood cells, and plasma. A decrease in the number or size of red cells also decreases the amount of space they occupy, resulting in a lower hematocrit. An increase in the number or size of red cells increases the amount of space they occupy, resulting in a higher hematocrit. **Thalassemia** is a condition which can cause an increased number of red blood cells but a decreased size and hematocrit.

The hematocrit is usually done on a person with symptoms of anemia. An anemic person has fewer or smaller than normal red cells. A low hematocrit, combined with other abnormal blood tests, confirms the diagnosis.

Some conditions, such as polycythemia, cause an overproduction of red blood cells, resulting in an increased hematocrit.

Transfusion decisions are based on the results of laboratory tests, including hematocrit. Transfusion is not considered if the hematocrit level is reasonable. The level differs for each person, depending on his or her clinical condition.

Description

Blood drawn from a fingerstick is often used for hematocrit testing. The blood fills a small tube, which is

KEY TERMS

Anemia—A condition where a person has fewer or smaller than normal red blood cells.

Hemoglobin—The percentage of space in blood occupied by red blood cells.

then spun in a small centrifuge. As the tube spins, the red blood cells go to the bottom of the tube, the white blood cells cover the red in a thin layer called the buffy coat, and the liquid plasma rises to the top. The spun tube is examined for the line that divides the red cells from the buffy coat and plasma. The height of the red cell column is measured as a percent of the total blood column. The higher the column of red cells, the higher the hematocrit.

The hematocrit test can also be done on an automated instrument as part of a **complete blood count**. It is also called Packed Red Cell Volume or Packed Cell Volume, or abbreviated as Hct or Crit. The test is covered by insurance when medically necessary. Results are usually available the same or following day.

Preparation

To collect the blood by fingerstick, a healthcare worker punctures a finger with a lancet and allows the blood to fill a small tube held to the puncture site.

Tests done on an automated instrument require 5–7 mL of blood. A healthcare worker ties a tourniquet on the person's upper arm, locates a vein in the inner elbow region, and inserts a needle into that vein. Vacuum action draws the blood through the needle into an attached tube. Collection of the sample takes only a few minutes.

Aftercare

Discomfort or bruising may occur at the puncture site or the person may feel dizzy or faint. Pressure to the puncture site until the bleeding stops reduces bruising. Warm packs to the puncture site relieve discomfort.

Normal results

Normal values vary with age and sex. Adult male range is 42–52%, adult female 36–48%.

Abnormal results

Hematocrit values decrease when the size or number of red cells decrease. This is most common in anemia, but other conditions have similar effects: excessive bleeding, damaged cells due to a mechanical heart valve, **liver disease**, and cancers affecting the bone marrow. Additional tests and the person's symptoms and medical history help distinguish these conditions or diagnose a specific type of anemia. Hematocrit values increase when the size or number of red cells increase, such as in polycythemia.

Fluid volume in the blood affects the hematocrit. Pregnant women have extra fluid, which dilutes the blood, decreasing the hematocrit. **Dehydration** concentrates the blood, increasing the hematocrit.

Resources

OTHER

"Hemocrit." *Medline Plus*. http://www.nlm.nih.gov/medlineplus/ency/article/003646.htm.

Nancy J. Nordenson

Hemiplegia *see* **Paralysis**

Hemochromatosis

Definition

Hemochromatosis is an inherited blood disorder that causes the body to retain excessive amounts of iron. This iron overload can lead to serious health consequences, most notably **cirrhosis** of the liver.

Description

Hemochromatosis is also known as iron overload, bronze diabetes, hereditary hemochromatosis and familial hemochromatosis. The inherited disorder causes increased absorption of intestinal iron, well beyond that needed to replace the body's loss of iron. Iron overload diseases afflict as many as 1.5 million persons in the United States. The most common of these, as well as one of the most common genetic disorders in the United States, is hereditary hemochromatosis. Men and women are equally affected by hemochromatosis, but women are diagnosed later in life because of blood loss from menstruation and **childbirth**. It most commonly appears in patients between the ages of 40–60 years, since it takes many years for the body to accumulate excessive iron. Symptoms appear later in females than in males—usually after **menopause**.

Hemochromatosis causes excess iron storage in several organs of the body including the liver, pancreas, endocrine glands, heart, skin, joints, and intestinal lining. The buildup of iron in these organs can lead to serious complications, including **heart failure**, **liver cancer**, and cirrhosis of the liver. It is estimated that about 5% of cirrhosis cases are caused by hereditary hemochromatosis.

Idiopathic pulmonary hemosiderosis, a disorder afflicting children and young adults, is a similar overload disorder characterized by abnormal accumulation of hemosiderin. Hemosiderin is a protein found in most tissues, especially the liver. It is produced by digestion of hematin, an iron-related substance.

Hemochromatosis is one of the most common genetic disorders in the United States. Approximately one in nine individuals have one abnormal hemochromatosis gene (11% of the population). Since everyone has two copies of each gene, these individuals have an abnormal *HFE* gene and a normal gene. They are called carriers. Between 1/200 and 1/400 individuals have two abnormal genes for hemochromatosis and no normal gene.

With most autosomal recessive conditions, an affected person's parents are carriers. If more than one family member has the condition, they are siblings. Hemochromatosis is so common, however, that families are seen in which both parents are affected, or one parent is affected and the other parent is a carrier. More than one generation may be affected, which is not usually seen in rare autosomal recessive conditions.

Causes and symptoms

Hereditary hemochromatosis is an autosomal recessive condition. This means that individuals with hemochromatosis have inherited an altered (mutated) gene from both of their parents. Affected individuals have two abnormal hemochromatosis genes and no normal hemochromatosis gene.

The gene that causes hemochromatosis has been identified, and the most common abnormalities of the gene have been described. The gene is on chromosome 6; it is called *HFE*. Scientists have not confirmed the function of the normal gene product; they do know that it interacts with the cell receptor for transferrin. Transferrin binds and transports iron in the blood.

Because it is an autosomal recessive condition, siblings of individuals who have hemochromatosis are at a 25% risk to also be affected. However, the likelihood that an individual will develop symptoms depends on which gene mutation he or she has as well as environmental factors. The two most common changes in the *HFE* gene are *C282Y* and *H63D*. The age at which symptoms begin is variable, even within the same family.

The symptoms of hemochromatosis include **fatigue**, weight loss, weakness, **shortness of breath**, heart **palpitations**, chronic abdominal **pain**, and impaired sexual performance. The patient may also show symptoms commonly connected with heart failure, diabetes, or cirrhosis of the liver. Changes in the pigment of the skin may appear, such as grayness in certain areas or a tanned or yellow (**jaundice**) appearance. The age of onset and initial symptoms vary.

Idiopathic pulmonary hemosiderosis may first, and only, appear as paleness of the skin. Sometimes the patient will experience spitting of blood from the lungs or bronchial tubes.

Diagnosis

The most common diagnostic methods for hemochromatosis are blood studies of iron, genetic blood studies, **magnetic resonance imaging** (MRI), and **liver biopsy**. Blood studies of transferrin–iron saturation and ferritin concentration are often used to screen for iron overload. Ferritin is a protein that transports iron and liver enzymes. Additional studies are performed to confirm the diagnosis.

Blood studies used to confirm the diagnosis include additional iron studies and/or genetic blood studies. Genetic blood studies became available in the late 1990s. **Genetic testing** is a reliable method of diagnosis. However, in the year 2001 scientists and physicians began to study how accurately having a hemochromatosis mutation predicts whether a person will develop symptoms. Most individuals affected with hemochromatosis (87%) have two identifiable gene mutations; that is, genetic testing will confirm the diagnosis in most individuals. Genetic studies are also be used to determine whether the affected person's family members are at risk for hemochromatosis. The results of genetic testing are the same whether or not a person has developed symptoms.

MRI scans and/or liver biopsy may be necessary to confirm the diagnosis. MRI studies of the liver (or other iron absorbing organs), with quantitative assessment of iron concentration, may reveal abnormal iron deposits. For the liver biopsy, a thin needle is inserted into the liver while the patient is under **local anesthesia**. The needle will extract a small amount of liver tissue, which can be analyzed microscopically to measure its iron content and other signs of hemochromatosis. Diagnosis of idiopathic pulmonary hemosiderosis begins with blood tests and x ray studies of the chest.

Treatment

Patients who show signs of iron overload will often be treated with **phlebotomy**. Phlebotomy is a procedure that involves drawing blood from the patient, just like **blood donation**. Its purpose as a treatment is to rid the

KEY TERMS

Autosomal—Relating to any chromosome besides the X and Y sex chromosomes. Human cells contain 22 pairs of autosomes and one pair of sex chromosomes.

Cirrhosis—A chronic degenerative disease of the liver, in which normal cells are replaced by fibrous tissue. Cirrhosis is a major risk factor for the later development of liver cancer.

Diabetes mellitus—The clinical name for common diabetes. It is a chronic disease characterized by inadequate production or use of insulin.

Phlebotomy—The taking of blood from the body through an incision in the vein, usually in the treatment of disease.

body of excess iron storage. Patients may need these procedures one or two times a week for a year or more. Less frequent phlebotomy may be continued in subsequent years to keep excess iron from accumulating. Patients who cannot tolerate phlebotomy due to other medical problems can be treated with Desferal (desferrioxamine). Diet restrictions may also be prescribed to limit the amount of iron ingested. Complications from hemochromatosis, such as cirrhosis or diabetes, may also require treatment. Treatment for idiopathic pulmonary hemosiderosis is based on symptoms.

Diet restrictions may help lower the amount of iron in the body, but do not prevent or treat hemochromatosis. Individuals who are affected or who know they have two *C282Y* and/or *H63D* genes may reduce iron intake by avoiding iron and mineral supplements, excess vitamin C, and uncooked seafood. If a patient is symptomatic, he/she may be advised to abstain from drinking alcohol.

Prognosis

With early detection and treatment, the prognosis is usually good. All potential symptoms are prevented if iron levels are kept within the normal range, which is possible if the diagnosis is made before an individual is symptomatic. If a patient is symptomatic but treated successfully before he/she develops liver cirrhosis, the patient's life expectancy is near normal. However, if left untreated, complications may arise which can be fatal. These include liver **cancer**, liver cirrhosis, **diabetes mellitus**, congestive heart failure, and difficulty depleting iron overload through phlebotomy. Liver biopsy can be helpful in determining prognosis of more severely affected individuals. Genetic testing may also be helpful, as variable severity has been noted in patients who have two *C282Y* genes compared to patients with two *H63D* genes or one of each. Men are two times more likely than women to develop severe complications. The prognosis for patients with idiopathic pulmonary hemosiderosis is fair, depending on detection and complications.

Prevention

Screening for hemochromatosis is cost effective, particularly for certain groups of people. Relatives of patients with hemochromatosis—including children, siblings, and parents—should be tested by the most appropriate method. The best screening method may be iron and ferritin studies or genetic testing. If the affected person's diagnosis has been confirmed by genetic testing, relatives may have genetic testing to determine whether or not they have the genetic changes present in the affected individual. Many medical groups oppose genetic testing of children. Relatives who are affected but do not have symptoms can reduce iron intake and/or begin phlebotomy prior to the onset of symptoms, possibly preventing ever becoming symptomatic.

In the winter of 2000, population screening for hereditary hemochromatosis was widely debated. Many doctors and scientists wanted population screening because hemochromatosis is easily and cheaply treated, and quite common. Arguments against treatment include the range of symptoms seen (and not seen) with certain gene mutations, and the risk of discrimination in health and life insurance. Whether or not population screening becomes favored by a majority, the publicity is beneficial. Hemochromatisis is a common, easily and effectively treated condition. However, diagnosis may be difficult because the presenting symptoms are the same as those seen with many other medical problems. The screening debate has the positive effect of increasing awareness and suspicion of hemochromatisis. Increased knowledge leads to earlier diagnosis and treatment of symptomatic individuals, and increased testing of their asymptomatic at-risk relatives.

Resources

BOOKS

Garrison, Cheryl D. *The Iron Disorders Institute Guide to Hemochromatosis*. Naperville, IL: Cumberland House.

OTHER

Hemochromatosis Information Sheet. National Institute of Diabetes & Digestive & Kidney Diseases (NIDDK).

http://www.niddk.nih.gov/health/digest/pubs/hemochrom/hemochromatosis.htm.

Hereditary Hemochromatosis. Lecture by Richard Fass, MD, hematologist, Advanced Oncology Associates, given April 25, 1999. http://www.advancedoncology.org/listen.htm.

MacFarlane, Julie, George Papanikalaou, and Y. Paul Goldberg. "Hemochromatosis." *GeneReviews*. http://www.ncbi.nlm.nih.gov/bookshelf/br.fcgi?book=gene&part=jh.

ORGANIZATIONS

American Liver Foundation, 75 Maiden Lane, Suite 603, New York, NY, 10038, (212) 668-1000, (212) 483-8179, http://www.liverfoundation.org/.

Hemochromatosis Foundation, PO Box 675, Taylor, SC, 29687, (864) 292-1878, (888) 565-4766 , patientservices@irondisorders.org, http://www.hemochromatosis.org.

Iron Disorders Institute, P.O. Box 675, Taylors, SC, 29687, (864) 292-1175, (864) 292-1878, (888) 565-IRON (4766), http://www.irondisorders.org.

Iron Overload Diseases Association, Inc., West Palm Beach, FL, 33405, (561) 586-8246, iod@ironoverload.org, http://www.ironoverload.org/.

The Hemochromatosis Information Center, P.O. Box 675, Taylors, SC, 29687, (864) 292-1175, (864) 292-1878, (888) 565-4766, patientservices@irondisorders.org, http://www.hemochromatosis.org/.

Michelle Q. Bosworth, MS, CGC

Hemodialysis *see* **Dialysis, kidney**

Hemoglobin electrophoresis

Definition

Hemoglobin electrophoresis (also called Hgb electrophoresis), is a test that measures the different types of hemoglobin in the blood. The method used is called electrophoresis, a process that causes movement of particles in an electric field, resulting in formation of "bands" that separate toward one end or the other in the field.

Purpose

Hgb electrophoresis is performed when a disorder associated with abnormal hemoglobin (hemoglobinopathy) is suspected. The test is used primarily to diagnose diseases involving these abnormal forms of hemoglobin, such as sickle cell anemia and **thalassemia**.

Precautions

Blood transfusions within the previous 12 weeks may alter test results.

Description

Hemoglobin (Hgb) is comprised of many different types, the most common being A_1, A_2, F, S, and C.

Hgb A_1 is the major component of hemoglobin in the normal red blood cell. Hgb A_2 is a minor component of normal hemoglobin, comprising approximately 2–3% of the total.

Hgb F is the major hemoglobin component in the fetus, but usually exists only in minimal quantities in the normal adult. Levels of Hgb F greater than 2% in patients over three years of age are considered abnormal.

Hgb S is an abnormal form of hemoglobin associated with the disease of sickle cell anemia, which occurs predominantly in African Americans. A distinguishing characteristic of **sickle cell disease** is the crescent-shaped red blood cell. Because the survival rate of this type of cell is limited, patients with sickle cell disease also have anemia.

Hgb C is another hemoglobin variant found in African Americans. Red blood cells containing Hgb C have a decreased life span and are more readily destroyed than normal red blood cells, resulting in mild to severe **hemolytic anemia**.

Each of the major hemoglobin types has an electrical charge of a different degree, so the most useful method for separating and measuring normal and abnormal hemoglobins is electrophoresis. This process involves subjecting hemoglobin components from dissolved red blood cells to an electric field. The components then move away from each other at different rates, and when separated form a series of distinctly pigmented bands. The bands are then compared with those of a normal sample. Each band can be further assessed as a percentage of the total hemoglobin, thus indicating the severity of any abnormality.

Preparation

This test requires a blood sample. No special preparation is needed before the test.

Risks

Risks for this test are minimal, but may include slight bleeding from the blood-drawing site, **fainting** or feeling lightheaded after venipuncture, or hematoma (blood accumulating under the puncture site).

KEY TERMS

Hemoglobin C disease—A disease of abnormal hemoglobin, occurring in 2–3% of African Americans. Only those who have two genes for the disease develop anemia, which varies in severity. Symptoms include episodes of abdominal and joint pain, an enlarged spleen and mild jaundice.

Hemoglobin H disease—A thalassemia-like syndrome causing moderate anemia and red blood cell abnormalities.

Heterozygous—Two different genes controlling a specified inherited trait.

Homozygous—Identical genes controlling a specified inherited trait.

Thalassemias—The name for a group of inherited disorders resulting from an imbalance in the production of one of the four chains of amino acids that make up hemoglobin. Thalassemias are categorized according to the amino acid chain affected. The two main types are alpha-thalassemia and beta-thalassemia. The disorders are further characterized by the presence of one defective gene (thalassemia minor) or two defective genes (thalassemia major). Symptoms vary, but include anemia, jaundice, skin ulcers, gallstones, and an enlarged spleen.

Normal results

Normal reference values can vary by laboratory, but are generally within the following ranges.

Adults:

- Hgb A_1: 95–98%
- Hgb A_2: 2–3%
- Hgb F: 0.8–2%
- Hgb S: 0%
- Hgb C: 0%.

Child (Hgb F):

- 6 months: 8%
- greater than 6 months: 1–2%
- newborn (Hgb F): 50–80%

Abnormal results

Abnormal reference values can vary by laboratory, but when they appear within these ranges, results are usually associated with the conditions that follow in parentheses.

Hgb A_2:

- 4–5.8% (β-thalassemia minor)
- under 2% (Hgb H disease)

Hgb F:

- 2–5% (β-thalassemia minor)
- 10–90% (β-thalassemia major)
- 5–35% (Heterozygous hereditary persistence of fetal hemoglobin, or HPFH)
- 100% (Homozygous HPFH)
- 15% (Homozygous Hgb S)

Homozygous Hgb S:

- 70–98% (Sickle cell disease).

Homozygous Hgb C:

- 90–98% (Hgb C disease)

Resources

BOOKS

Barton, James C., et al. *Handbook of Iron Overload Disorders.* Cambridge, UK; New York: Cambridge University Press, 2010.

Pagana, Kathleen Deska, and Timothy J. Pagana. *Mosby's Manual of Diagnostic and Laboratory Tests.* 4th ed. St. Louis: Mosby, 2009.

Janis O. Flores

Hemoglobin F test *see* **Fetal hemoglobin test**

Hemoglobin test

Definition

Hemoglobin is a protein inside red blood cells that carries oxygen throughout the body. A hemoglobin test reveals how much hemoglobin is in a person's blood, helping to diagnose and monitor anemia and **polycythemia vera**.

Purpose

A hemoglobin test is done when a person is ill or during a general **physical examination**. Good health requires an adequate amount of hemoglobin. The amount of oxygen in the body tissues depends on how much hemoglobin is in the red cells. Without enough hemoglobin, the tissues lack oxygen and the heart and lungs must work harder to try to compensate.

If the test indicates a "less than" or "greater than" normal amount of hemoglobin, the cause of the decrease or increase must be discovered. A low hemoglobin usually means the person has anemia. Anemia results from conditions that decrease the number or size of red cells, such as excessive bleeding, a dietary deficiency, destruction of cells because of a **transfusion** reaction or mechanical heart valve, or an abnormally formed hemoglobin.

A high hemoglobin may be caused by polycythemia vera, a disease in which too many red blood cells are made.

Hemoglobin levels also help determine if a person needs a blood transfusion. Usually a person's hemoglobin must be below 8 gm/dL before a transfusion is considered.

Description

Hemoglobin is made of heme, an iron compound, and globin, a protein. The iron gives blood its red color. Hemoglobin tests make use of this red color. A chemical is added to a sample of blood to make the red blood cells burst. When they burst, the red cells release hemoglobin into the surrounding fluid, coloring it clear red. By measuring the color using an instrument called a spectrophotometer, the amount of hemoglobin is determined.

Hemoglobin is often ordered as part of a **complete blood count** (CBC), a test that includes other blood cell measurements.

Some people inherit hemoglobin with an abnormal structure. These abnormal hemoglobins cause diseases, such as sickle cell or Hemoglobin C disease. Special tests, using a process called **hemoglobin electrophoresis**, identify abnormal hemoglobins.

Preparation

This test requires 5 mL of blood. A healthcare worker ties a tourniquet on the person's upper arm, locates a vein in the inner elbow region, and inserts a needle into that vein. Vacuum action draws the blood through the needle into an attached tube. Collection of the sample takes only a few minutes.

The person should avoid **smoking** before this test as smoking can increase hemoglobin levels.

Aftercare

Discomfort or bruising may occur at the puncture site or the person may feel dizzy or faint. Pressure to the puncture site until the bleeding stops reduces bruising. Warm packs to the puncture site relieve discomfort.

KEY TERMS

Anemia—A condition characterized by a decrease in the size or number of red blood cells.

Hemoglobin—A protein inside red blood cells that carries oxygen to body tissues.

Polycythemia vera—A disease in which the bone marrow makes too many red blood cells.

Normal results

Normal values vary with age and sex. Women generally have lower hemoglobin values than men. Men have 14.0–18.0 g/dL, while women have levels of 12.0–16.0 g/dL.

Abnormal results

A low hemoglobin usually indicates the person has anemia. Further tests are done to discover the cause and type of anemia. Dangerously low hemoglobin levels put a person at risk of a **heart attack**, congestive **heart failure**, or **stroke**.

A high hemoglobin indicates the body is making too many red cells. Further tests are done to see if this is caused by polycythemia vera or as a reaction to illness, high altitudes, heart failure, or lung disease.

Fluid volume in the blood affects hemoglobin values. Pregnant women and people with **cirrhosis** have extra fluid, which dilutes the blood, decreasing the hemoglobin. **Dehydration** concentrates the blood, increasing the hemoglobin.

Resources

PERIODICALS

Hsia, Connie C. W. "Respiratory Function of Hemoglobin. "*New England Journal of Medicine* 338 (January 1998): 239-247.

Nancy J. Nordenson

Hemoglobinopathies

Definition

Hemoglobinopathies are genetic (inherited) disorders of hemoglobin, the oxygen-carrying protein of the red blood cells.

Description

The hemoglobin molecule is composed of four separate polypeptide chains of amino acids, two alpha chains, and two beta chains, as well as four iron-bearing heme groups that bind oxygen. The alpha chains are coded for by two similar genes on chromosome 16; the beta chains by a single gene on chromosome 11. Mutations and deletions in these genes cause one of the many hemoglobinopathies.

In general, hemoglobinopathies are divided into those in which the gene abnormality results in a qualitative change in the hemoglobin molecule and those in which the change is quantitative. Sickle cell anemia (**sickle cell disease**) is the prime example of the former, and the group of disorders known as the **thalassemias** constitute the latter. It has been estimated that one-third of a million people worldwide are seriously affected by one of these genetic disorders.

Causes and symptoms

Sickle cell anemia (SSA), an autosomal recessive disorder more common in the Black population, is caused by a single mutation in the gene that codes for the beta polypeptide. Approximately 1/400 to 1/600 African Americans are born with the disorder, and, one in 10 is a carrier of one copy of the mutation. In certain parts of the African continent, the prevalence of the disease reaches 1 in 50 individuals.

The sickle cell mutation results in the substitution of the amino acid valine for glutamic acid in the sixth position of the beta polypeptide. In turn, this alters the conformation of the hemoglobin molecule and causes the red blood cells to assume a characteristic sickle shape under certain conditions. These sickle-shaped cells, no longer able to pass smoothly through small capillaries, can block the flow of blood. This obstruction results in symptoms including growth retardation, severe **pain** crises, tissue and organ damage, splenomegaly, and strokes. Individuals with SSA are anemic and prone to infections, particularly **pneumonia**, a significant cause of **death** in this group. Some or all of these symptoms are found in individuals who have the sickle mutation in both copies of their beta-globin gene. Persons with one abnormal gene and one normal gene are said to be carriers of the sickle cell trait. Carriers are unaffected because of the remaining normal copy of the gene.

The thalassemias are a diverse group of disorders characterized by the fact that the causative mutations result in a decrease in the amount of normal hemoglobin. Thalassemias are common in Mediterranean populations as well as in Africa, India, the Mideast, and Southeast Asia. The two main types of thalassemias are alpha-thalassemia due to mutations in the alpha polypeptide and beta-thalassemia resulting from beta chain mutations.

Since individuals possess a total of four genes for the alpha polypeptide (two genes on each of their two chromosomes 16), disease severity depends on how many of the four genes are abnormal. A defect in one or two of the genes has no clinical effect. Abnormalities of three results in a mild to moderately severe anemia (hemoglobin H disease) and splenomegaly. Loss of function of all four genes usually causes such severe oxygen deprivation that the affected fetus does not survive. A massive accumulation of fluid in the fetus (hydrops fetalis) results in **stillbirth** or neonatal death.

Beta thalassemias can range from mild and clinically insignificant (beta **thalassemia** minor) to severe and life-threatening (beta thalassemia major, also known as Cooley's anemia), depending on the exact nature of the gene mutation and whether one or both copies of the beta gene are affected. While the milder forms may only cause slight anemia, the more severe types result in growth retardation, skeletal changes, splenomegaly, vulnerability to infections, and death as early as the first decade of life.

Diagnosis

Many countries, including the United States, have made concerted efforts to screen for sickle cell anemia at birth because of the potential for beginning early treatment and counseling parents about their carrier status. Diagnosis is traditionally made by blood tests, including **hemoglobin electrophoresis**. Similar tests are used to determine whether an individual is a sickle cell or thalassemia carrier. In certain populations with a high prevalence of one of the mutations, carrier testing is common. If both members of a couple are carriers of one of these conditions, it is possible through prenatal **genetic testing** to determine if the fetus will be affected, although the severity of the disease cannot always be predicted.

Treatment

Treatment of SSA has improved greatly in recent years with a resulting increase in life expectancy. The use of prophylactic (preventative) antibiotic therapy has been particularly successful. Other treatments include fluid therapy to prevent **dehydration**, oxygen supplementation, pain relievers, blood transfusions,

KEY TERMS

Amino acids—Organic compounds that form the building blocks of protein. There are 20 different amino acids.

Autosomal recessive—A pattern of inheritance in which both copies of an autosomal gene must be abnormal for a genetic condition or disease to occur. An autosomal gene is a gene that is located on one of the autosomes or non-sex chromosomes. When both parents have one abnormal copy of the same gene, they have a 25% chance with each pregnancy that their offspring will have the disorder.

Hemoglobin—Protein-iron compound in the blood that carries oxygen to the cells and carries carbon dioxide away from the cells.

Hydroxyurea—A drug that has been shown to induce production of fetal hemoglobin. Fetal hemoglobin has a pair of gamma-globin molecules in place of the typical beta-globins of adult hemoglobin. Higher-than-normal levels of fetal hemoglobin can prevent sickling from occurring.

Phlebotomy—Drawing blood from a vein for diagnosis or treatment. Phlebotomy is sometimes used in the treatment of hemoglobinopathies to lower the iron concentration of the blood.

Sickle cell—A red blood cell that has assumed an elongated shape due to the presence of hemoglobin S.

Splenomegaly—Enlargement of the spleen.

and several different types of medications. Recent interest has focused on **bone marrow transplantation**, which has been successful in selected patients.

Since the clinically important thalassemias are characterized by severe anemia, the traditional treatment has been blood **transfusion**, but the multiple transfusions needed to sustain life lead to an iron overload throughout the tissues of the body and eventual destruction of the heart and other organs. For this reason, transfusion therapy must also include infusions of medications such as deferoxamine (desferroxamine) to rid the body of excess iron. **Phlebotomy** is another technique that has been used with some success to lower the concentration of iron in the patient's blood. As with sickle cell anemia, bone marrow therapy has been successful in some cases.

Until very recently, patients being treated with bone marrow transplants had to find a sibling or other closely related donor in order to avoid rejection of the transplant. Advances in the preparation of the transplanted cells, however, have made the use of bone marrow from unrelated donors (URD) an option for patients with hemoglobinopathies. The National Marrow Donor Program reports that about 40% of bone marrow transplants involve a patient in the United States receiving marrow from an international donor or an international patient receiving marrow from a donor in the United States.

Emphasis is also being placed on developing drugs that treat sickle cell anemia directly. The most promising of these drugs in the late 1990s was hydroxyurea, a drug that was originally designed for anticancer treatment. Hydroxyurea has been shown to reduce the frequency of painful crises and acute chest syndrome in adults, and to lessen the need for blood transfusions. Hydroxyurea seems to work by inducing a higher production of fetal hemoglobin. The major side effects of the drug include decreased production of platelets, red blood cells, and certain white blood cells. The effects of long-term hydroxyurea treatment are unknown; however, a nine-year follow-up study of 299 adults with frequent painful crises reported in 2003 that taking hydroxyurea was associated with a 40% reduction in mortality.

Another promising development for the treatment of hemoglobinopathies is **gene therapy**, which has interested researchers since the early 1990s. In late 2001, genetic scientists reported that they had designed a gene that might lead to a future treatment of sickle cell anemia. Although the gene had not been tested in humans, early results showed that the injected gene protected cells from sickling. Experiments in gene therapy for sickle cell disease have been carried out in mice, using lentiviral vectors to transfer the corrective gene into the mouse's stem cells. This technique, however, has not yet been attempted in human subjects.

Prognosis

Hemoglobinopathies are life-long disorders. The prognosis depends upon the exact nature of the mutation and the availability of effective treatment, as well as the individual's compliance with therapies. Hemoglobinopathies significantly complicate **pregnancy** and increase the risk of infant mortality.

Prevention

Because the hemoglobinopathies are inherited diseases, primary prevention involves carriers making reproductive decisions to prevent passage of the abnormal gene to their offspring. At present, most prevention is targeted toward the symptoms using treatments such as those described above.

Resources

BOOKS

Beers, Mark H., Robert S. Porter, and Thomas V. Jones, eds. *The Merck Manual of Diagnosis and Therapy*. 18th ed. Whitehouse Station, NJ: Merck Research Laboratories, 2006.

Kliegman, Robert M., and Waldo Emerson Nelson. *Nelson Textbook of Pediatrics*. 18th ed. Philadelphia: Saunders, Elsevier, 2007.

PERIODICALS

Davies, S. C., and A. Gilmore. "The Role of Hydroxyurea in the Management of Sickle Cell Disease." *Blood Reviews* 17 (June 2003): 99–109.

Koduri, P. R. "Iron in Sickle Cell Disease: A Review Why Less Is Better." *American Journal of Hematology* 73 (May 2003): 59–63.

Krishnamurti, L., S. Abel, M. Maiers, and S. Flesch. "Availability of Unrelated Donors for Hematopoietic Stem Cell Transplantation for Hemoglobinopathies." *Bone Marrow Transplantation* 31 (April 2003): 547–550.

Markham, M. J., R. Lottenberg, and M. Zumberg. "Role of Phlebotomy in the Management of Hemoglobin SC Disease: Case Report and Review of the Literature." *American Journal of Hematology* 73 (June 2003): 121–125.

Nienhuis, A. W., H. Hanawa, N. Sawai, et al. "Development of Gene Therapy for Hemoglobin Disorders." *Annals of the New York Academy of Science* 996 (May 2003): 101–111.

Steinberg, M. H., F. Barton, O. Castro, et al. "Effect of Hydroxyurea on Mortality and Morbidity in Adult Sickle Cell Anemia: Risks and Benefits up to 9 Years of Treatment." *Journal of the American Medical Association* 289 (April 2, 2003): 1645–1651.

ORGANIZATIONS

American Sickle Cell Anemia Association, Cleavand Clinic, 10681 Carnegie Avenue, Cleveland, OH, 44106, (216) 229-8600, (216) 229-4500, http://www.ascaa.org/.

National Marrow Donor Program, 3001 Broadway Street Northeast, Suite 100, Minneapolis, MN, 55413-1753, (800) 627-7692, patientinfo@nmdp.org, https://www.marrow-donor.org.

Sickle Cell Disease Association of America, Inc., 231 East Baltimore Street, STE 800, Baltimore, MD, 21202, (800)421-8453, scdaa@sicklecelldisease.org, http://sicklecelldisease.org.

Sallie Boineau Freeman, PhD
Rebecca J. Frey, PhD

Hemolytic-uremic syndrome

Definition

Hemolytic-uremic syndrome (HUS) is a rare condition that affects mostly children under the age of 10, but also may affect the elderly as well as persons with other illnesses. HUS, which most commonly develops after a severe bowel infection with certain toxic strains of a bacteria, is characterized by destruction of red blood cells, damage to the lining of blood vessel walls, and in severe cases, kidney failure.

Description

Most cases of HUS occur after an infection in the digestive system that has been caused by toxin-producing strains of the bacterium ***Escherichia coli***. About 75% of HUS cases in the United States are caused by the strain referred to as *E. coli* O157:H7, which is found in the intestinal tract of cattle, while the remaining cases are caused by non-O157 strains. Some children infected with *E. coli* O157:H7 will develop HUS. HUS also can follow respiratory infection episodes in young children. In the United States, there are about 20,000 infections and 250 deaths annually that are caused by *E. coli* O157:H7. HUS has also been known to occur in persons using drugs such as **oral contraceptives**, immunosuppressors, and antineoplastics and in women during the postpartum period.

E. coli. O157:H7, first identified in 1982 and isolated with increasing frequency since then, is found in contaminated foods such as meat, dairy products, and juices. Infection with *E. coli*. O157:H7 causes severe **gastroenteritis**, which can include abdominal **pain**, **vomiting**, and bloody **diarrhea**. For most children, the vomiting and diarrhea stop within two to three days. However, about 5 to 10% of the children will develop HUS and will become pale, tired, and irritable. Toxins produced by the bacteria enter the blood stream, where they destroy red blood cells and platelets, which contribute to the clotting of blood. The damaged red blood cells and platelets clog tiny blood vessels in the kidneys, or form lesions in the kidneys, making it difficult for the kidneys to remove wastes and extra fluid from the body, resulting in **hypertension**, fluid accumulation, and reduced production of urine.

Causes and symptoms

The most common way an *E. coli* O157:H7 infection is contracted is through the consumption of undercooked ground beef (e.g., eating hamburgers that are still pink inside). Healthy cattle carry *E. coli* within their intestines. During the slaughtering process, the meat can become contaminated with the *E. coli* from the intestines. When contaminated beef is ground up, the *E. coli* bacteria are spread throughout the meat. Additional ways to contract an *E. coli* infection include drinking contaminated water and unpasteurized milk and juices, eating contaminated fruits and vegetables, and working with cattle. The infection is also easily transmitted from an infected person to others in settings such as day care centers and nursing homes when improper sanitary practices are used.

Symptoms of an *E. coli* O157:H7 infection start about seven days after infection with the bacteria. The first symptom is sudden onset of severe abdominal cramps. After a few hours, watery diarrhea starts, causing loss of fluids and electrolytes (**dehydration**), which causes the person to feel tired and ill. The watery diarrhea lasts for about a day, and then changes to bright red bloody stools, as the infection causes sores to form in the intestines. The bloody diarrhea lasts for two to five days, with as many as 10 bowel movements a day. Additional symptoms may include **nausea** and vomiting, without a **fever**, or with only a mild fever. After about 5 to 10 days, HUS can develop, which is characterized by paleness, irritability, and **fatigue**, as well as reduced urine production.

Diagnosis

The diagnosis of an *E. coli* infection is made through a **stool culture**. The culture must be taken within the first 48 hours after the start of the bloody diarrhea. If a positive culture is obtained, the patient should be monitored for the development of HUS, with treatment initiated as required.

Children should not go to day care until they have had two negative stool cultures. Older people in nursing homes should stay in bed until two stool cultures are negative.

Treatment

Treatment of HUS is supportive, with particular attention to management of fluids and electrolytes. Treatment generally is provided in a hospital setting. Blood transfusions may be required. In about 50% of the cases, short term replacement of kidney function is required in the form of dialysis. Most patients will recover kidney function and be able to discontinue dialysis.

Some studies have shown that the use of **antibiotics** and antimotility agents during an *E. coli* infection may worsen the course of the infection and should be avoided. However, other studies have been less definitive. Physicians should stay informed so that clinical practices matches medical advances on this aspect of treatment.

KEY TERMS

Antineoplastics—Agents that inhibit or prevent the development, maturation, and proliferation of malignant cells.

Gastroenteritis—An acute inflammation of the lining of the stomach and intestines, characterized by nausea, diarrhea, abdominal pain and weakness, which has various causes, including food poisoning due to infection with such organisms as *Escherichia coli*, *Staphylococcus aureus*, and *Salmonella* species, consumption of irritating food or drink, or psychological factors, such as anger, stress and fear.

Alternative treatment

Persons with HUS must be under the care of health care professionals skilled in the treatment of HUS.

Prognosis

Ninety percent of children with HUS who receive careful supportive care survive the initial acute stages of the condition, with most having no long-term effects. However, between 10 and 30% of survivors will have kidney damage that will lead to kidney failure immediately or within several years. The children with kidney failure require on-going dialysis to remove waste and extra fluids from their bodies, or may require a kidney transplant.

Prevention

Prevention of HUS caused by ingestion of foods contaminated with *E. coli* O157:H7 and other toxin-producing bacteria is accomplished through practicing hygienic food preparation techniques, including adequate handwashing, cooking of meat thoroughly, defrosting meats safely, vigorous washing of fruits and vegetables, and handling leftovers properly. Irradiation of meat has been approved by the United States Food and Drug Administration and the United States Department of Agriculture in order to decrease bacterial contamination of consumer meat supplies.

Resources

OTHER

National Kidney and Urologic Diseases Information Clearinghouse. Fact Sheet: Hemolytic Uremic Syndrome. NIH Publication No. 99-4570. March 2000. http://www.niddk.nih.gov/health/kidney/summary/hus/.

Judith Sims

Hemolytic anemia

Definition

Red blood cells have a normal life span of approximately 90–120 days, at which time the old cells are destroyed and replaced by the body's natural processes. Hemolytic anemia is a disorder in which the red blood cells are destroyed prematurely. The cells are broken down at a faster rate than the bone marrow can produce new cells. Hemoglobin, the component of red blood cells that carries oxygen, is released when these cells are destroyed.

Description

As a group, **anemias** (conditions in which the number of red blood cells or the amount of hemoglobin in them is below normal) are the most common blood disorders. Hemolytic anemias, which result from the increased destruction of red blood cells, are less common than anemias caused by excessive blood loss or by decreased hemoglobin or red cell production.

Since a number of factors can increase red blood cell destruction, hemolytic anemias are generally identified by the disorder that brings about the premature destruction. Those disorders are classified as either inherited or acquired. Inherited hemolytic anemias are caused by inborn defects in components of the red blood cells—the cell membrane, the enzymes, or the hemoglobin. Acquired hemolytic anemias are those that result from various other causes. With this type, red cells are produced normally, but are prematurely destroyed because of damage that occurs to them in the circulation.

Causes and symptoms

Inherited hemolytic anemias involve conditions that interfere with normal red blood cell production. Disorders that affect the red blood cell membrane include hereditary spherocytosis, in which the normally disk-shaped red cells become spherical, and hereditary elliptocytosis, in which the cells are oval, rather than disk-shaped. Other hereditary conditions that cause hemolytic anemia include disorders of the hemoglobin, such as sickle cell anemia and **thalassemia**, and red blood cell enzyme deficiencies, such as G6PD deficiency.

The causes of acquired hemolytic anemias vary, but the most common are responses to certain medications and infections. Medications may cause the body to develop antibodies that bind to the red blood cells and cause their destruction in the spleen. Immune hemolytic anemia most commonly involves antibodies that react against the red blood cells at body temperature (warm-antibody hemolytic anemia), which can cause premature destruction of the cells. About 20% of hemolytic anemias caused by warm antibodies come from diseases such as lymphocytic leukemia, 10% from an autoimmune disease, and others are drug-induced. Cold-antibody hemolytic anemia is a condition in which the antibodies react with the red blood cells at a temperature below that of normal body temperature. Red blood cells can also receive mechanical damage as they circulate through the blood vessels. Aneurysms, artificial heart valves, or very high blood pressure can cause the red cells to break up and release their contents. In addition, hemolytic anemia may be caused by a condition called **hypersplenism**, in which a large, overactive spleen rapidly destroys red blood cells.

Major symptoms of hemolytic anemias are similar to those for all anemias, including **shortness of breath**; noticeable increase in heart rate, especially with exertion; **fatigue**; pale appearance; and dark urine. A yellow tint, or **jaundice**, may be seen in the skin or eyes of hemolytic anemia patients. Examination may also show an enlarged spleen. A more emergent symptom of hemolytic anemia is **pain** in the upper abdomen. Severe anemia is indicated if there are signs of **heart failure** or an enlarged liver.

Diagnosis

In order to differentiate hemolytic anemia from others, physicians will examine the blood for the number of young red blood cells, since the number of young cells is increased in hemolytic anemia. The physician will also examine the abdominal area to check for spleen or liver enlargement. If the physician knows the duration of hemolysis, it may also help differentiate between types of anemia. There are a number of other indications that can be obtained from blood samples

KEY TERMS

Antibody—Antibodies are parts of the immune system which counteract or eliminate foreign substances or antigens.

Erythrocyte—The name for red blood cells or red blood corpuscles. These components of the blood are responsible for carrying oxygen to tissues and removing carbon dioxide from tissues.

Hemolysis—The process of breaking down red blood cells. As the cells are destroyed, hemoglobin, the component of red blood cells which carries the oxygen, is liberated.

Thalassemia—One of a group of inherited blood disorders characterized by a defect in the metabolism of hemoglobin, or the portion of the red blood cells that transports oxygen throughout the blood stream.

that will help a physician screen for hemolytic anemia. An antiglobulin (Coomb's) test may be performed as the initial screening exam after determining hemolysis. In the case of immune hemolytic anemia, a direct Coomb's test is almost always positive.

Treatment

Treatment will depend on the cause of the anemia and may involve treatment of the underlying cause. If the hemolytic anemia was brought on by hereditary spherocytosis, the spleen may be removed. Corticosteroid medications, or adrenal **steroids**, may be effective, especially in hemolytic anemia due to antibodies. If the cause of the disorder is a medication, the medication should be stopped. When anemia is severe in conditions such as sickle cell anemia and thalassemia, blood transfusions may be indicated.

Prognosis

Hemolytic anemias are seldom fatal. However, if left untreated, hemolytic anemia can lead to heart failure or liver complications.

Prevention

Hemolytic anemia due to inherited disorders can not be prevented. Acquired hemolytic anemia may be prevented if the underlying disorder is managed properly.

ORGANIZATIONS

American Autoimmune Related Diseases Association, Inc., 22100 Gratiot Avenue, Eastpointe, MI, 48021, (586) 776-3900, (586) 776-3903, http://www.aarda.org.

American Society of Hematology, 2021 L St. NW, Suite 900, Washington, DC, 20036, (202) 776-0544, (202) 776-0545, http://www.hematology.org.

National Heart Lung and Blood Institute Health Information Center, P.O. Box 30105, Bethesda, MD, 20824-0105, (301) 592-8573, (240) 629-3246, http://www.nhlbi.nih.gov.

Teresa Odle

Hemophilia

Definition

Hemophilia is a coagulation disorder arising from a genetic defect of the X chromosome; the defect can either be inherited or result from spontaneous gene mutation. In each type of hemophilia (hemophilias A, B, and C), a critical coagulation protein is missing, causing individuals to bleed for long periods of time before clotting occurs. Depending on the degree of the disorder in the affected individual, uncontrolled bleeding may occur spontaneously with no known initiating event or occur after specific events, such as surgery, dental procedures, immunizations, or injury.

Demographics

According to the National Heart, Lung, and Blood Institute (NHLBI), hemophilia affects about 18,000 people in the United States, and each year about 400 babies are born with the disorder, which usually occurs only in males with very rare exceptions. Worldwide, hemophilia A is the most common type of the disorder with about 1 in 4,000 males born with the disorder. As for hemophilia B, it occurs approximately in 1 of 20,000 newborn males. In 2008, an Orphanet report estimated the European prevalence of hemophilia at 7.7 per 100,000 persons. The mortality rate for patients with hemophilia is twice that of the healthy male population. For severe hemophilia, the rate is increased 4–6 times.

Hemophilia A and B are observed in all ethnic and racial groups, with some prevalence reported in Chinese populations.

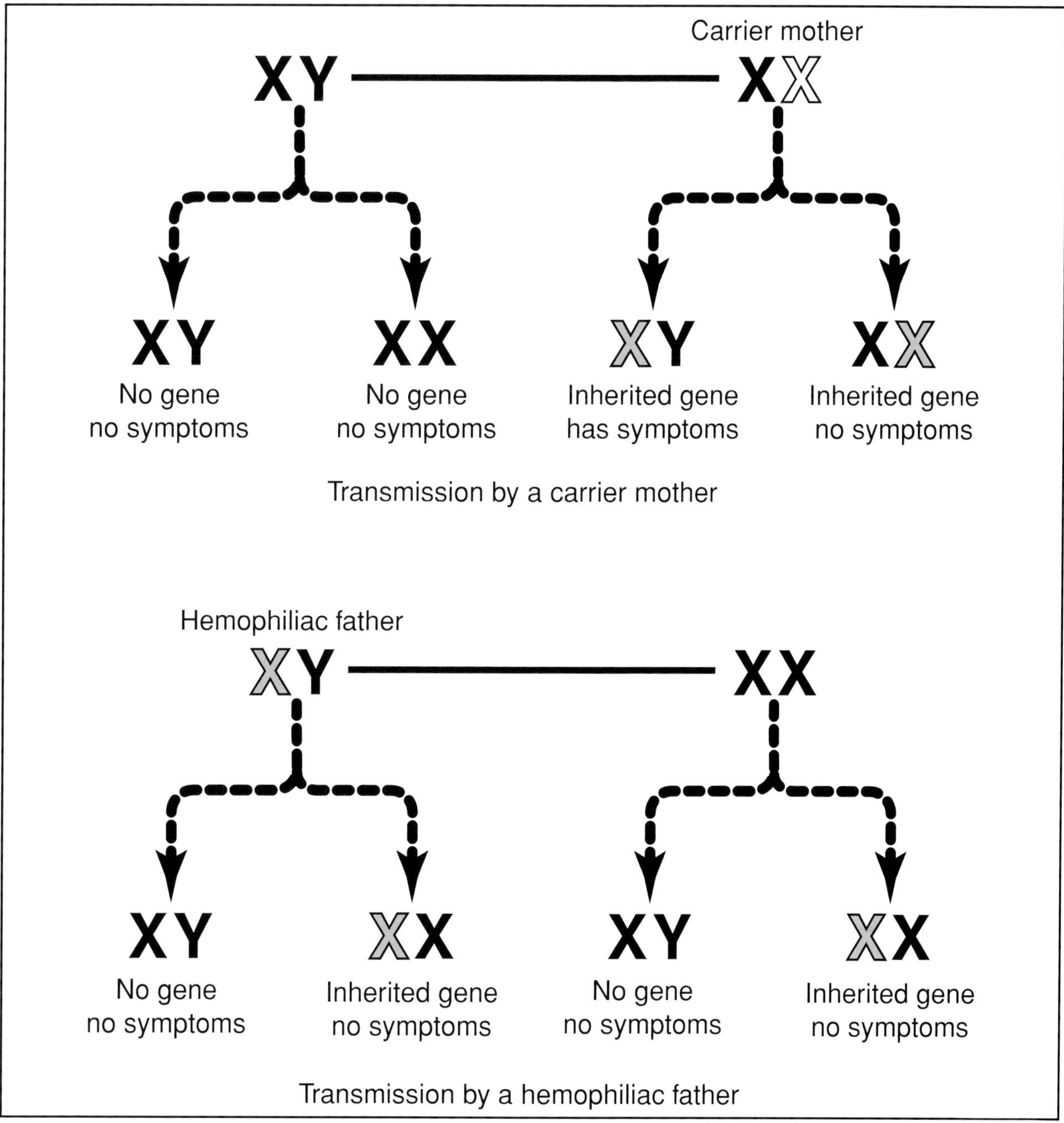

Hemophilia A and B are both caused by a genetic defect present on the X chromosome. Approximately 70% of people with hemophilia A or B inherited the disease, while the remaining 30% have hemophilia due to a spontaneous genetic mutation. *(Illustration by Electronic Illustrators Group. Reproduced by permission of Gale, a part of Cengage Learning.)*

Description

The normal mechanism for blood clotting is a complex series of events (coagulation cascade) involving interaction between the injured blood vessel, blood cells called platelets, 13 specific coagulation factors (designated by Roman numerals I through XIII), and other substances that circulate in the blood.

When a blood vessel is injured in a way that causes bleeding, platelets collect over the injured area, and form a temporary plug to prevent further bleeding. This temporary plug, however, is too disorganized to serve as a long–term solution, so a series of chemical events occur, resulting in the formation of a more reliable plug. The final plug involves tightly woven fibers of a material called fibrin. The production of fibrin requires the interaction of several chemicals, in particular a series of proteins called clotting factors. At least 13 different clotting factors have been identified.

The clotting cascade, as it is usually called, is the series of events required to form the final fibrin clot. The cascade uses a technique called amplification to rapidly produce the proper sized fibrin clot from the small number of molecules initially activated by the injury.

In hemophilia, certain clotting factors are either decreased in quantity, absent, or improperly formed. Because the clotting cascade uses amplification to rapidly plug up a bleeding area, absence or inactivity of just one clotting factor can greatly increase **bleeding time**.

Hemophilia A is the most common type of bleeding disorder and involves decreased activity of factor VIII. There are three levels of factor VIII deficiency: severe, moderate, and mild. This classification is based on the percentage of normal factor VIII activity present:

- Individuals with less than 1% of normal factor VIII activity level have severe hemophilia. Half of all people with hemophilia A fall into this category. Such individuals frequently experience spontaneous bleeding, most frequently into their joints, skin, and muscles. Surgery or trauma can result in life–threatening hemorrhage and must be carefully managed.
- Individuals with 1–5% of normal factor VIII activity level have moderate hemophilia and are at risk for heavy bleeding after seemingly minor traumatic injury.
- Individuals with 5–40% of normal factor VIII activity level have mild hemophilia, and must prepare carefully for any surgery or dental procedures.

Individuals with hemophilia B have symptoms very similar to those of hemophilia A, but the deficient factor is factor IX. This type of hemophilia is also known as Christmas disease.

Hemophilia C is very rare and is much more mild than hemophilia A or B; it involves factor XI.

Risk factors

Hemophilia is a genetic disorder, which is usually inherited. The hemophilia gene is passed down from a parent to a child. Individuals with a family history of the condition are accordingly at higher risk for hemophilia.

Causes and symptoms

Hemophilia A and B are both caused by a genetic defect present on the X chromosome. (Hemophilia C is inherited in a different fashion.) About 70% of all people with hemophilia A or B inherited the disease. The other 30% develop from a spontaneous genetic mutation.

The following concepts are important to understanding the inheritance of these diseases. All humans have two chromosomes determining their gender: females have XX, males have XY. Because the trait is carried only on the X chromosome, it is called "sex–linked." The chromosome's flawed unit is referred to as the gene.

Both factors VIII and IX are produced by a genetic defect of the X chromosome, so hemophilia A and B are both sex–linked diseases. Because a female child always receives two X chromosomes, she nearly always will receive at least one normal X chromosome. Therefore, even if she receives one flawed X chromosome, she will still be capable of producing a sufficient quantity of factors VIII and IX to avoid the symptoms of hemophilia. Such a person who has one flawed chromosome, but does not actually suffer from the disease, is called a carrier. She carries the flaw that causes hemophilia and can pass it on to her offspring. If, however, she has a son who receives her flawed X chromosome, he will be unable to produce the right quantity of factors VIII or IX, and he will suffer some degree of hemophilia. (Males inherit one X and one Y chromosome, and therefore have only one X chromosome.)

In rare cases, a hemophiliac father and a carrier mother can pass on the right combination of parental chromosomes to result in a hemophiliac female child. This situation, however, is rare. The vast majority of people with either hemophilia A or B are male.

About 30% of all people with hemophilia A or B are the first member of their family to ever have the disease. These individuals have had the unfortunate occurrence of a spontaneous mutation, meaning that in their early development, some random genetic accident befell their X chromosome, resulting in the defect causing hemophilia A or B. Once such a spontaneous genetic mutation takes place, offspring of the affected person can inherit the newly–created, flawed chromosome.

In the case of severe hemophilia, the first bleeding event usually occurs prior to 18 months of age. In some babies, hemophilia is suspected immediately, when a routine **circumcision** (removal of the foreskin of the penis) results in unusually heavy bleeding. Toddlers are at particular risk, because they fall frequently and may bleed into the soft tissue of their arms and legs. These small bleeds result in bruising and noticeable lumps, but don't usually need treatment. As a child becomes more active, bleeding may occur

KEY TERMS

Amplification—A process by which something is made larger. In clotting, only a very few chemicals are released by the initial injury; they result in a cascade of chemical reactions which produces increasingly larger quantities of different chemicals, resulting in an appropriately–sized, strong fibrin clot.

Coagulation—Blood clotting.

Coagulation factors—Specific coagulation proteins in the blood required for clotting. Coagulation proteins are designated with roman numerals I through XIII.

Factors—Coagulation factors are substances in the blood, such as proteins and minerals, that are necessary for clotting. Each clotting substance is designated with roman numerals I through XIII.

Fibrin—The final substance created through the clotting cascade, which provides a strong, reliable plug to prevent further bleeding from the initial injury.

Hemorrhage—Very severe, massive bleeding that is difficult to control. Hemorrhage can occur in hemophiliacs after what would be a relatively minor injury to a person with normal clotting factors.

Mutation—A permanent change in the genetic material that may alter a trait or characteristic of an individual, or manifest as disease, and can be transmitted to offspring.

Platelets—Small disc–shaped structures that circulate in the blood stream and participate in blood clotting.

Trauma—Injury.

into the muscles, which is a much more painful and debilitating problem. These muscle bleeds result in **pain** and pressure on the nerves in the area of the bleed. Damage to nerves can cause **numbness** and decreased ability to use the injured limb.

Some of the most problematic and frequent bleeds occur into the joints, particularly into the knees and elbows. Repeated bleeding into joints can result in scarring within the joints and permanent deformities. Individuals may develop arthritis in joints that have suffered continued irritation from the presence of blood. Mouth injuries can result in compression of the airway, and, therefore, can be life–threatening. A blow to the head, which might be totally insignificant in a normal individual, can result in bleeding into the skull and brain. Because the skull has no room for expansion, the hemophiliac is at risk for brain damage due to blood taking up space and exerting pressure on the delicate brain tissue.

People with hemophilia are at very high risk of hemorrhage (severe, heavy, uncontrollable bleeding) from injuries, such as motor vehicle accidents, and also from surgery.

Some other rare clotting disorders such as **Von Willebrand disease** present similar symptoms but are not usually called hemophilia.

Diagnosis

Examination

If hemophilia is suspected, or if a person has a bleeding problem, a physician typically takes personal and family medical histories to establish whether the family has a history of frequent or heavy bleeding and bruising.

Tests

Various tests are available to measure, under very carefully controlled conditions, the length of time it takes to produce certain components of the final fibrin clot. The activated **partial thromboplastin time** (APTT) is performed and will typically be prolonged while a **prothrombin time** (PT) will likely be normal. Factor assays, which are measurement methods performed by the clinical laboratory, can determine the percentage of factors VIII and IX present compared to normal percentages. This information helps to confirm a diagnosis of hemophilia and identifies the type and severity of hemophilia present.

Hemophilia A and B are classified as mild, moderate, or severe, depending on the amount of clotting factor VIII or IX in the blood. Mild hemophilia is diagnosed if 5–30% of the normal clotting factors are present. With 1–5% of the normal clotting factors present, the haemophilia is diagnosed as moderate, and as severe when less than 1% of the normal clotting factors are present.

Procedures

Individuals with a family history of hemophilia may benefit from **genetic counseling** before deciding to have a baby. Families with a positive history of hemophilia can also have tests done during a

pregnancy to determine whether the fetus is a hemophiliac. A test called chorionic villius sampling examines proteins for the defects that lead to hemophilia. This test, which is associated with a 1% risk of **miscarriage**, can be performed at 10–12 weeks. A test called **amniocentesis** examines the DNA of fetal cells shed into the amniotic fluid for genetic mutations. Amniocentesis, which is associated with a 1 in 200 risk of miscarriage, is performed at 16–18 weeks gestation.

Treatment

Traditional

The most important thing that individuals with hemophilia can do to prevent complications of his disease is to avoid injury. This is accomplished with replacement therapy to replace the clotting factor that is missing or present in low amounts. Hemophiliacs are also typically vaccinated against hepatitis.

In replacement therapy, various types of factors VIII and IX are available to replace a patient's missing factors. These are administered intravenously (directly into the patient's veins by needle). Cryoprecipitate, for example, is a single– or multiple–donor human plasma preparation rich in coagulation factors; it is available as a frozen concentrate. Fresh frozen plasma is a single–donor preparation of factor–rich plasma; it is used primarily for replacing factor XI in individuals with hemophilia C. Concentrated factor preparations may be obtained from a single donor by pooling the donations of as many as thousands of donors or by laboratory creation through highly advanced genetic techniques. These preparations are administered directly into the individual's veins (intravenous administration). In 2008, the United States Food and Drug Administration (FDA) approved a new formulation of the genetically engineered version of Factor VIIa that can be stored at room temperature for up to two years.

The frequency of treatment with factors depends on the severity of the individual patient's disease. Patients with relatively mild disease will only require treatment in the event of injury, or to prepare for scheduled surgical or dental procedures. Patients with more severe disease will require regular treatment to avoid spontaneous bleeding.

While appropriate treatment of hemophilia can both decrease suffering and be life–saving, complications associated with treatment can also be quite serious. About 20% of all patients with hemophilia A begin to produce chemicals in their bodies which rapidly destroy infused factor VIII. The presence of such a chemical may greatly hamper efforts to prevent or stop a major hemorrhage.

Individuals who receive factor prepared from pooled donor blood are at risk for serious infections that may be passed through blood. Hepatitis, a severe and potentially fatal viral liver infection, may be contracted from pooled factor preparations. Recently, a good deal of concern has been raised about the possibility of hemophiliacs contracting a fatal slow virus infection of the brain (Creutzfeldt–Jakob disease) from blood products. Unfortunately, pooled factor preparations in the early 1980s were contaminated with human **immunodeficiency** virus (HIV), the virus which causes **AIDS**. A large number of hemophiliacs were infected with HIV and some statistics show that HIV is still the leading cause of **death** among hemophiliacs. Currently, careful methods of donor testing, as well as methods of inactivating viruses present in donated blood, have greatly lowered this risk.

Drugs

Desmopressin (DDAVP) is a synthetic hormone used in the treatment of mild to moderate hemophilia A. DDAVP is not used to treat hemophilia B or severe hemophilia A. DDAVP usually is given by injection or as nasal spray. Since it wears off when used often, DDAVP is given only in specific situations. For example, before dental work or before certain physical activities to prevent or reduce bleeding. Antifibrinolytic medicines, such as tranexamic acid and aminocaproic acid, may also be used with replacement therapy. These medications are typically used before dental work or to treat bleeding from the mouth or nose or mild intestinal bleeding.

Medications or drugs that promote bleeding, such as **aspirin**, should be avoided.

Alternative

The most exciting new treatments currently being researched involve efforts to transfer new genes to hemophiliacs. These new genes would have the ability to produce the missing factors. As yet, these techniques are not being performed on humans, but there is great hope that eventually this type of **gene therapy** will be available.

Clinical trials for the treatment of hemophilia are currently sponsored by the National Institutes of Health (NIH) and other agencies. In 2009, NIH reported 196 on–going or recently completed studies. Some examples include the following:

- The evaluation of the safety of gene transfer for the treatment of severe hemophilia B. (NCT00076557)

- The study of musculoskeletal function in people with hemophilia in developing countries. (NCT00324493)
- The study of allergic reactions to factor IX in patients with hemophilia B. (NCT00195221)
- A study evaluating inhibitor specificity in hemophilia A. (NCT00151385)

Clinical trial information is constantly updated by NIH and the most recent information on hemophilia trials can be found at: http://clinicaltrials.gov/ct2/results?term = hemophilia

Home remedies

At home, certain steps can help avoid excessive bleeding. They include regular **exercise** to build up muscles and protect joints, avoiding aspirin and non-steroidal anti–inflammatory drugs (Advil, Motrin, others) that can aggravate bleeding, practising good dental hygiene to avoid having teeth pulled out, and using protective equipment in sports and physical activities to minimize injuries.

Prognosis

Prognosis is very difficult to generalize. Because there are so many variations in the severity of hemophilia and because much of what befalls a hemophiliac patient will depend on issues such as physical activity level and accidental injuries, statistics on prognosis are not generally available.

Prevention

Because of its genetic origins, hemophilia cannot be prevented in those born with the inherited defects or factor deficiencies. However, individuals who have a family history of hemophilia may benefit from **genetic testing** and counseling before deciding to have a baby. The most important way for individuals with hemophilia to prevent complications of the disease is to avoid activities that may lead to injury. Those individuals who require dental work or any type of surgery may need to be pre–treated with an infusion of factor VIII to avoid hemorrhage. Hemophiliacs should also avoid medications or drugs that promote bleeding; aspirin is one such medication, and many prescription drugs have anticoagulant properties.

Resources

BOOKS

Freedman, Jeri. *Hemophilia (Genetic Diseases)*. New York, NY: Rosen Publishing Group, 2006.

Gray, Laura, and Christine Chamberlain. *The Gift of Experience: Conversations About Hemophilia*. Brunswick, ME: Camden Writers, 2008.

Lee, Christine A., et al., eds. *Textbook of Hemophilia*. Boston, MA: Blackwell Publishing, 2010.

Parker, Philip M. *Hemophilia — A Bibliography and Dictionary for Physicians, Patients, and Genome Researchers*. San Diego, CA: Icon Health Publications, 2007.

Raabe, Michelle. *Hemophilia (Genes and Disease)*. New York, NY: Chelsea House Publishers, 2008.

PERIODICALS

Douma–van Riet, D. C., et al. "Physical fitness in children with haemophilia and the effect of overweight." *Haemophilia* 15, no. 2 (March 2009): 519–527.

Ghosh, K., and S. Shetty. "Immune response to FVIII in hemophilia A: an overview of risk factors." *Clinical Reviews in Allergy & Immunology* 37, no. 2 (October 2009): 58–66.

Kessler, C. M. "Advances in the treatment of hemophilia." *Clinical Advances in Hematology & Oncology* 6, no. 3 (March 2008): 184–187.

Oldenburg, J., et al. "Haemophilia care then, now and in the future." *Haemophilia* 15, suppl. 1 (January 2009): 2–7.

Petrini, P., and A. Seuser. "Haemophilia care in adolescents —compliance and lifestyle issues." *British Journal of Haematology* 15, suppl. 1 (January 2009): 15–19.

Rodriguez, N. I., and W. K. Hoots. "Advances in hemophilia: experimental aspects and therapy." *Pediatric Clinics of North America* 55, no. 2 (April 2008): 357–376.

Sherry, D. D. "Avoiding the impact of musculoskeletal pain on quality of life in children with hemophilia." *Orthopaedic Nursing* 27, no. 2 (March–April 2008): 103–108.

Stine, K. C., and D. L. Becton. "Bleeding disorders: when is normal bleeding not normal?" *Journal of the Arkansas Medical Society* 106, no. 2 (August 2009): 40–42.

Viiala, N. O., et al. "Gene therapy for hemophilia: clinical trials and technical tribulations." *Seminars in Thrombosis and Hemostasis* 35, no. 1 (February 2009): 81–92.

Zhang, B. "Recent developments in the understanding of the combined deficiency of FV and FVIII." *British Journal of Haematology* 145, no. 1 (April 2009): 15–23.

OTHER

"Frequently Asked Questions About Hemophilia." *World Federation of Hemophilia*. Information Page. http://www.wfh.org/index.asp?lang = EN&url = 2/1/1_1_1_FAQ.htm (accessed December 17, 2009).

"Hemophilia." *Medline Plus*. Health Topic. http://www.nlm.nih.gov/medlineplus/hemophilia.html (accessed December 17, 2009).

"Hemophilia." *Genetics Home Reference*. Information Page. http://ghr.nlm.nih.gov/condition = hemophilia (accessed December 17, 2009).

"Hemophilia." *NHLBI*. Information Page. http://www.nhlbi.nih.gov/health/dci/Diseases/hemophilia/hemophilia_what.html (accessed December 17, 2009).

ORGANIZATIONS

American Society of Pediatric Hematology and Oncology (ASPHO), 4700 W. Lake Ave., Glenview, IL, 60025, (847) 375-4716, info@aspho.org, http://www.aspho.org.

National Heart, Lung, and Blood Institute (NHLBI), P.O. Box 30105, Bethesda, MD, 20824-0105, (301) 592-8573, (240) 629-3246, nhlbiinfo@nhlbi.nih.gov, http://www.nhlbi.nih.gov.

National Hemophilia Foundation, 116 West 32nd St., 11th Floor, New York, NY, 10001, (212) 328-3700, (212) 328-3777, handi@hemophilia.org, http://www.hemophilia.org.

World Federation of Hemophilia, 1425 René Lévesque Blvd. W., Suite 1010, MontréalQC, Canada, H3G 1T7, (514) 875-7944, (514) 875-8916, wfh@wfh.org, http://www.wfh.org.

Jennifer F. Wilson, MS
Culvert L. Lee, MS
Monique Laberge, PhD

Hemophilus ducreyi infection *see* **Chancroid**

Hemophilus infections

Definition

Hemophilus infections, most of which are due to *Haemophilus influenzae* infections, are a group of contagious diseases that are caused by a gram-negative bacterium and affect only humans. Some hemophilus infections are potentially fatal.

Description

H. influenzae is a common organism worldwide; it has been found in the nasal secretions of as many as 90% of healthy individuals in the general population. Hemophilus infections are characterized by acute inflammation with a discharge (exudate). They may affect almost any organ system, but are most common in the respiratory tract. The organism can be transmitted by person-to-person contact or by contact with nasal discharges and other body fluids. Hemophilus infections in the United States are most likely to spread in the late winter or early spring.

The primary factor influencing the rate of infection is age; children between the ages of six months and four years are most vulnerable to *H. influenzae*. In previous years, about 50% of children would acquire a hemophilus infection before reaching one year of age; almost all children would develop one before age three. These figures are declining, however, as a result of the increasing use of hemophilus vaccines for children.

Adults are also susceptible to hemophilus diseases. *H. influenzae*pneumonia is a common nosocomial infection (illnesses contracted in hospitals). The rate of hemophilus infections in the adult population has increased over the past 40 years. The reasons for this change are unclear, but some researchers speculate that the overuse of **antibiotics** has led to the development of drug-resistant strains of *H. influenzae*. The risk factors for hemophilus infections among adults include:

- smoking
- alcoholism
- chronic lung disease
- old age
- living in a city or institutional housing with a large group of people
- poor nutrition and hygiene
- hIV infection or other immune system disorder

Causes and symptoms

Hemophilus infections are primarily caused by *Haemophilus influenzae*, a gram-negative bacterium that is capable of spreading from the nasal tissues and upper airway, where it is usually found, to the chest, throat, or middle ear. The organism sometimes invades localized areas of tissue, producing **meningitis**, **infectious arthritis**, **conjunctivitis**, **cellulitis**, **epiglottitis**, or inflammation of the membrane surrounding the heart. The most serious infections are caused by a strain called *H. influenzae* b (Hib). Before routine **vaccination**, Hib was the most common cause of bacterial meningitis and was responsible for most of the cases of acquired **mental retardation** in the United States.

Hemophilus infections in children

BACTERIAL SEPSIS IN THE NEWBORN. Bacterial **sepsis** (the presence of illness-causing microorganisms, or their poisons, in the blood) is a potentially fatal illness in newborn infants. The child may acquire the disease organism as it passes through the mother's birth canal or from the hospital environment. *H. influenzae* can also produce inflammations of the eye (conjunctivitis) in newborn children. The signs of sepsis may include **fever**, crankiness, feeding problems, breathing difficulties, pale or mottled skin, or drowsiness. Premature birth is the most significant risk factor for hemophilus infections in newborns.

EPIGLOTTITIS. Epiglottitis is a potentially fatal hemophilus infection. Although children are more likely to develop epiglottitis, it can occur in adults as well. When the epiglottis (a piece of cartilage behind the tongue which protects the opening to the windpipe by opening and closing) is infected, it can swell to the point where it blocks the windpipe. The symptoms of epiglottitis include a sudden high fever, drooling, the feeling of an object stuck in the throat, and **stridor**. The epiglottis will look swollen and bright red if the doctor examines the patient's throat with a laryngoscope (a viewing device).

MENINGITIS. Meningitis caused by Hib is most common in children between nine months and four years of age. The child usually develops upper respiratory symptoms followed by fever, loss of appetite, **vomiting**, **headache**, and a stiff or sore neck or back. In severe cases, the child may have convulsions or go into **shock** or **coma**.

OTHER INFECTIONS. Hib is the second most common cause of middle ear infection and **sinusitis** in children. The symptoms of sinusitis include fever, **pain**, **bad breath**, and coughing. Children may also develop infectious arthritis from Hib. The joints most frequently affected are the large weight-bearing joints.

Hemophilus infections in adults

PNEUMONIA. Hib **pneumonia** is the most common hemophilus infection in adults. The symptoms include **empyema** (sputum containing pus) and fever. The hemophilus organism can usually be identified from sputum samples. Hib pneumonia is increasingly common in the elderly.

MENINGITIS. Meningitis caused by Hib can develop in adults as a complication of an ear infection or sinusitis. The symptoms are similar to those in children but are usually less severe in adults.

Diagnosis

The diagnosis is usually based on a combination of the patient's symptoms and the results of blood counts, cultures, or antigen detection tests.

Laboratory tests

Laboratory tests can be used to confirm the diagnosis of hemophilus infections. The bacterium can be grown on chocolate agar or identified by blood cultures or Gram stain of body fluids. Antigen detection tests can be used to identify hemophilus infections in children. These tests include latex agglutination and electrophoresis.

Other laboratory findings that are associated with hemophilus infections include anemia (low red blood cell count) and a drop in the number of white blood cells in children with severe infections. Adults often show an abnormally high level of white blood cells; cell counts of 15,000–30,000/mm^3 are not unusual.

Treatment

Because some hemophilus infections are potentially fatal, treatment is started without waiting for the results of laboratory tests.

Medications

Hemophilus infections are treated with antibiotics. Patients who are severely ill are given ampicillin or a third-generation cephalosporin, such as cefotaxime or ceftriaxone, intravenously. Patients with milder infections are given oral antibiotics, including amoxicillin, cefaclor, erythromycin, or trimethoprim-sulfamethoxazole. Patients who are allergic to penicillin are usually given cefaclor or trimethoprim-sulfamethoxazole.

Patients with Hib strains that are resistant to ampicillin may be given chloramphenicol. Chloramphenicol is not a first-choice drug because of its side effects, including interference with bone marrow production of blood cells.

The duration of antibiotic treatment depends on the location and severity of the hemophilus infection. Adults with respiratory tract infections, or Hib pneumonia, are usually given a 10–14 day course of antibiotics. Meningitis is usually treated for 10–14 days, but a seven-day course of treatment with ceftriaxone appears to be sufficient for infants and children. Ear infections are treated for 7 to 10 days.

Supportive care

Patients with serious hemophilus infections require bed rest and a humidified environment (such as a **croup** tent) if the respiratory tract is affected. Patients with epiglottitis frequently require intubation (insertion of a breathing tube) or a **tracheotomy** to keep the airway open. Patients with inflammation of the heart membrane, pneumonia, or arthritis may need surgical treatment to drain infected fluid from the chest cavity or inflamed joints.

Supportive care also includes monitoring of blood cell counts for patients using chloramphenicol, ampicillin, or other drugs that may affect production of blood cells by the bone marrow.

Prognosis

The most important factors in the prognosis are the severity of the infection and promptness of treatment. Untreated hemophilus infections—particularly meningitis, sepsis, and epiglottitis—have a high mortality rate. Bacterial sepsis of the newborn has a mortality rate between 13 and 50%. The prognosis is usually good for patients with mild infections who are treated

KEY TERMS

Bacterium—A microscopic one-celled organism. *Haemophilus influenzae* is a specific bacterium.

Epiglottitis—Inflammation of the epiglottis. The epiglottis is a piece of cartilage behind the tongue that closes the opening to the windpipe when a person swallows. An inflamed epiglottis can swell and close off the windpipe, thus causing the patient to suffocate.

Exudate—A discharge produced by the body. Some exudates are caused by infections.

Gram-negative—A term that means that a bacterium will not retain the violet color when stained with Gram's dye. *Haemophilus influenzae* is a gram-negative bacterium.

Intubation—The insertion of a tube into the patient's airway to protect the airway from collapsing. Intubation is sometimes done as an emergency procedure for patients with epiglottitis.

Nosocomial—Contracted in a hospital. Pneumonia caused by *H. influenzae* is an example of a nosocomial infection.

Sepsis—Invasion of body tissues by disease organisms or their toxins. Sepsis may be either localized or generalized. *Haemophilus influenzae* can cause bacterial sepsis in newborns.

Stridor—A harsh or crowing breath sound caused by partial blockage of the patient's upper airway.

Tracheotomy—An emergency procedure in which the surgeon cuts directly through the patient's neck into the windpipe in order to keep the airway open.

without delay. Children who develop Hib arthritis sometimes have lasting problems with joint function.

Prevention

Hemophilus vaccines

There are three different vaccines for hemophilus infections used to immunize children in the United States: PRP-D, HBOC, and PRP-OMP. PRP-D is used only in children older than 15 months. HBOC is administered to infants at two, four, and six months after birth, with a booster dose at 15–18 months. PRP-OMP is administered to infants at two and four months, with the third dose at the child's first birthday. All three vaccines are given by intramuscular injection. About 5% of children may develop a fever or soreness in the area of the injection.

Other measures

Other preventive measures include isolating patients with respiratory hemophilus infections; treating appropriate contacts of infected patients with rifampin; maintaining careful standards of cleanliness in hospitals, including proper disposal of soiled tissues; and washing hands properly.

Resources

BOOKS

McPhee, Stephen, and Maxine Papadakis. *Current Medical Diagnosis and Treatment, 2010*, 49th ed. New York: McGraw–Hill Medical, 2009.

Rebecca J. Frey, PhD

Hemophilus influenzae infections *see* **Hemophilus infections**

Hemoptysis

Definition

Hemoptysis is the coughing up of blood or bloody sputum from the lungs or airway. It may be either self-limiting or recurrent. Massive hemoptysis is defined as 200–600 mL of blood coughed up within a period of 24 hours or less.

Description

Hemoptysis can range from small quantities of bloody sputum to life-threatening amounts of blood. The patient may or may not have chest **pain**.

Causes and symptoms

Hemoptysis can be caused by a range of disorders:

- Infections. These include pneumonia; tuberculosis; aspergillosis; and parasitic diseases, including ascariasis, amebiasis, and paragonimiasis.
- Tumors that erode blood vessel walls.
- Drug abuse. Cocaine can cause massive hemoptysis.
- Trauma. Chest injuries can cause bleeding into the lungs.
- Vascular disorders, including aneurysms, pulmonary embolism, and malformations of the blood vessels.
- Bronchitis. Its most common cause is long-term smoking.
- Foreign object(s) in the airway.
- Blood clotting disorders.

- Bleeding following such surgical procedures as bronchial biopsies and heart catheterization.

Diagnosis

The diagnosis of hemoptysis is complicated by the number of possible causes.

Patient history

It is important for the doctor to distinguish between blood from the lungs and blood coming from the nose, mouth, or digestive tract. Patients may aspirate, or breathe, blood from the nose or stomach into their lungs and **cough** it up. They may also swallow blood from the chest area and then vomit. The doctor will ask about stomach ulcers, repeated **vomiting**, **liver disease**, **alcoholism**, **smoking**, **tuberculosis**, mitral valve disease, or treatment with anticoagulant medications.

Physical examination

The doctor will examine the patient's nose, throat, mouth, and chest for bleeding from these areas and for signs of chest trauma. The doctor also listens to the patient's breathing and heartbeat for indications of heart abnormalities or lung disease.

Laboratory tests

Laboratory tests include blood tests to rule out clotting disorders, and to look for food particles or other evidence of blood from the stomach. Sputum can be tested for fungi, bacteria, or parasites.

X ray and bronchoscopy

Chest x rays and **bronchoscopy** are the most important studies for evaluating hemoptysis. They are used to evaluate the cause, location, and extent of the bleeding. The bronchoscope is a long, flexible tube used to identify tumors or remove **foreign objects**.

Imaging and other tests

Computed tomography scans (CT scans) are used to detect aneurysms and to confirm x-ray results. Ventilation-perfusion scanning is used to rule out **pulmonary embolism**. The doctor may also order an angiogram to rule out pulmonary **embolism**, or to locate a source of bleeding that could not be seen with the bronchoscope.

In spite of the number of diagnostic tests, the cause of hemoptysis cannot be determined in 20–30% of cases.

KEY TERMS

Aneurysm—A sac formed by the dilation of the wall of an artery, vein, or heart; it is filled with clotted blood or fluid.

Angiography—A technique for imaging the blood vessels by injecting a substance that is opaque to x rays.

Aspergillosis—A lung infection caused by the mold *Aspergillus fumigatus*.

Intubation—The insertion of a tube into a body canal or hollow organ, as into the trachea or stomach.

Pulmonary embolism—The blocking of an artery in the lung by a blood clot.

Treatment

Massive hemoptysis is a life-threatening emergency that requires treatment in an intensive care unit. The patient will be intubated (the insertion of a tube to help breathing) to protect the airway, and to allow evaluation of the source of the bleeding. Patients with lung **cancer**, bleeding from an aneurysm (blood clot), or persistent traumatic bleeding require chest surgery.

Patients with tuberculosis, **aspergillosis**, or bacterial **pneumonia** are given **antibiotics**.

Foreign objects are removed with a bronchoscope.

If the cause cannot be determined, the patient is monitored for further developments.

Prognosis

The prognosis depends on the underlying cause. In cases of massive hemoptysis, the mortality rate is about 15%. The rate of bleeding, however, is not a useful predictor of the patient's chances for recovery.

Resources

BOOKS

McPhee, Stephen, and Maxine Papadakis. *Current Medical Diagnosis and Treatment, 2010*, 49th ed. New York: McGraw–Hill Medical, 2009.

Rebecca J. Frey, PhD

Hemorrhagic colitis *see* *Escherichia* **coli**

Hemorrhagic fever with renal syndrome *see* **Hantavirus infections**

Hemorrhagic fevers

Definition

Hemorrhagic fevers are caused by viruses that exist throughout the world. However, they are most common in tropical areas. Early symptoms, such as muscle aches and **fever**, can progress to a mild illness or to a more debilitating, potentially fatal disease. In severe cases, a prominent symptom is bleeding, or hemorrhaging, from orifices and internal organs.

Description

Although hemorrhagic fevers are regarded as emerging diseases, they probably have existed for many years. This designation isn't meant to imply that they are newly developing, but rather that human exposure to the causative viruses is increasing to the point of concern.

These viruses are maintained in nature in arthropod (insects, spiders and other invertebrates with external hard skeletons) or animal populations—so-called disease reservoirs. Individuals within these populations become infected with a virus but do not die from it. In many cases, they don't even develop symptoms. Then the viruses are transmitted from a reservoir population to humans by vectors—either members of the reservoir population or an intervening species, such as mosquitoes.

Hemorrhagic fevers are generally either endemic or linked to specific locations. If many people reside in an endemic area, the number of cases may soar. For example, **dengue fever**, a type of hemorrhagic fever, affects approximately 100 million people annually. A large percentage of those infected live in densely populated Southeast Asia, an area in which the disease vector, a mosquito, thrives. Some hemorrhagic fevers are exceedingly rare because people very infrequently encounter the virus. Marburg hemorrhagic fever, which has affected fewer than 40 people since its discovery in 1967, provides one such example. Fatality rates are also variable. In cases of dengue hemorrhagic fever–dengue **shock** syndrome, 1–5% of the victims perish. On the other end of the spectrum is Ebola, an African hemorrhagic fever, that kills 30–90% of those infected.

The onset of hemorrhagic fevers may be sudden or gradual, but all of them are linked by the potential for hemorrhaging. However, not all cases progress to this very serious symptom. Hemorrhaging may be attributable to the destruction of blood coagulating factors or to increased permeability of body tissues. The severity of bleeding ranges from petechiae, which are pinpoint hemorrhages under the skin surface, to distinct bleeding from such body orifices as the nose or vagina.

Causes and symptoms

The viruses that cause hemorrhagic fevers are found most commonly in tropical locations; however, some are found in cooler climates. Typical disease vectors include rodents, ticks, or mosquitoes, but person-to-person transmission in health care settings or through sexual contact can also occur.

Filoviruses

Ebola is the most famous of the Filoviridae, a virus family that also includes the Marburg virus. Ebola is endemic to Africa, particularly the Republic of the Congo and Sudan; the Marburg virus is found in sub-Saharan Africa. The natural reservoir of filoviruses is unknown. The incubation period, or time between infection and appearance of symptoms, is thought to last three to eight days, possibly longer.

Symptoms appear suddenly, and include severe **headache**, fever, chills, muscle aches, malaise, and appetite loss. These symptoms may be accompanied by **nausea**, **vomiting**, **diarrhea**, and abdominal **pain**. Victims become apathetic and disoriented. Severe bleeding commonly occurs from the gastrointestinal tract, nose and throat, and vagina. Other bleeding symptoms include petechiae and oozing from injection sites. Ebola is fatal in 30–90% of cases.

Arenaviruses

Viruses of the Arenaviridae family cause Argentinian, Brazilian, Bolivian, and Venezuelan hemorrhagic fevers. Lassa fever, which occurs in west Africa, also arises from an arenavirus. Infected rodents, the natural reservoir, shed virus particles in their urine and saliva, which humans may inhale or otherwise come in contact with.

Fever, muscle aches, malaise, and appetite loss gradually appear one to two weeks after infection with the South American viruses. Initial symptoms are followed by headache, back pain, **dizziness**, and gastrointestinal upset. The face and chest appear flushed and the gums begin to bleed. In about 30% of cases, the disease progresses to bleeding under the skin and from the mucous membranes and/or to effects on the nervous system, such as **delirium**, **coma**, and convulsions. Untreated, South American hemorrhagic fevers have a 10–30% fatality rate.

Lassa fever also begins gradually, following an 8–14 day incubation. Initial symptoms resemble those of the South American hemorrhagic fevers, followed by a **sore throat**, muscle and joint pain, severe headache, pain above the stomach, and a dry **cough**. The face and neck become swollen, and fluid may accumulate in the lungs. Bleeding occurs in 15–20% of infected individuals, mostly from the gums and nose. Overall, the fatality rate is lower than 2%, but hospitals may encounter 20% fatality rates, treating typically the most serious of cases.

Flaviviruses

The Flaviviridae family includes the viruses that cause yellow and dengue fevers.

Yellow fever occurs in tropical areas of the Americas and Africa and is transmitted from monkeys to humans by mosquitoes. The virus may produce a mild, possibly unnoticed illness, but some individuals are suddenly stricken with a fever, weakness, **low back pain**, muscle pain, nausea, and **vomiting**. This phase lasts one to seven days, after which the symptoms recede for one to two days. Symptoms then return with greater intensity, along with **jaundice**, delirium, seizures, stupor, and coma. Bleeding occurs from the mucous membranes and under the skin surface, and dark blood appears in stools and vomit.

Mosquitoes also transmit the dengue virus. Dengue fever is endemic in Southeast Asia and areas of the Americas. Cases have also been reported in the Caribbean, Saudi Arabia, and northern Australia. In 2004 several cases were reported along the border between Texas and Mexico in the southwestern United States. This virus causes either the mild dengue fever or the more serious dengue hemorrhagic fever–dengue shock syndrome (DHF-DSS).

In children, dengue fever is characterized by a sore throat, runny nose, slight cough, and a fever lasting for a week or less. Older children and adults experience more severe symptoms: fever, headache, muscle and joint pain, loss of appetite, and a rash. The skin appears flushed, and intense pain occurs in the bones and limbs. After nearly a week, the fever subsides for one to two days before returning. Minor hemorrhaging, such as from the gums, or more serious gastrointestinal bleeding may occur.

DHF-DSS primarily affects children younger than 15 years. The symptoms initially resemble those of dengue fever in adults, without the bone and limb pain. As the fever begins to abate, the individual's condition worsens and hemorrhaging occurs from the nose, gums, and injection sites. Bleeding is also seen from the gastrointestinal, genitourinary, and respiratory tracts.

Bunyaviruses

The Bunyaviridae family includes several hundred viruses but only a few are responsible for hemorrhagic fevers in humans.

Rift Valley fever is caused by the phlebovirus, found in sub-Saharan Africa and the Nile Delta. Natural reservoirs are wild and domestic animals, and transmission occurs through contact with infected animals or through mosquito **bites**. The incubation period lasts 3–12 days. Most cases of Rift Valley fever are mild and may be symptomless. If symptoms develop, they include fever, backache, muscle and joint pain, and headache. Hemorrhagic symptoms occur rarely, while **death**, which occurs in fewer than 3% of cases, is attributable to massive liver damage.

Crimean-Congo hemorrhagic fever is caused by nairovirus and occurs in central and southern Africa, Asia, Eurasia, and the Middle East. The virus is found in hares, birds, ticks, and domestic animals and may be transmitted by ticks or by contact with infected animals. The nairovirus incubation period is 3 to 12 days, after which an individual experiences fever, chills, headache, severe muscle pain, pain above the stomach, nausea, vomiting, and appetite loss. Bleeding under the skin and gastrointestinal and vaginal bleeding may develop in the most severe cases. Death rates range from 10% in southern Russia to 50% in parts of Asia.

Hemorrhagic fever with renal (kidney) syndrome is caused by the hantaviruses: Hantaan, Seoul, Puumala, and Dobrava. Hantaan virus occurs in northern Asia, the Far East, and the Balkans; Seoul virus is found worldwide; Puumala virus is found in Scandinavia and northern Europe; while Dobrava virus occurs in the Balkans. Wild rodents are the natural reservoirs and transmit the virus via their excrement or body fluids or through direct contact. Initial symptoms develop within 10–40 days and include fever, headache, muscle pain, and dizziness. Other symptoms are blurry vision, abdominal and back pain, nausea, and vomiting. High levels of protein in the urine signal kidney damage; hemorrhaging may also occur. Death rates range from 0–10%.

Diagnosis

Since the hemorrhagic fevers share symptoms with many other diseases, positive identification of the disease relies on evidence of the viruses in the bloodstream—such as detection of antigens and antibodies—or **isolation** of the virus from the body. Disruptions in the normal levels of bloodstream components may be helpful in determining some, but not all, hemorrhagic fevers.

Treatment

Lassa fever, and possibly other hemorrhagic fevers, respond to ribavirin, an antiviral medication. However, most of the hemorrhagic fever viruses can only be treated with supportive care. Interferon is not useful and may in fact complicate management. Such care centers around maintaining correct fluid and electrolyte balances in the body and protecting the patient against secondary infections. Heparin and vitamin K administration, coagulation factor replacement, and blood transfusions may be effective in lessening or stopping hemorrhage in some cases.

Some researchers are investigating the possibility of targeting tissue factor (TF) as a way of treating viral hemorrhagic fevers. TF is a protein that activates the coagulation process in these illnesses, and experimental models suggest that a blockade of tissue factor assists the body's immune response to hemorrhagic fever viruses.

Prognosis

Recovery from some hemorrhagic fevers is more certain than from others. The filoviruses are among the most lethal; fatality rates for Ebola range from 30–90%, while DHF-DSS cases result in a 1–5% fatality rate. Whether a case occurs during an epidemic or as an isolated case also has a bearing on the outcome. For example, isolated cases of yellow fever have a 5% mortality rate, but 20–50% of epidemic cases may be fatal.

Permanent disability can occur with some types of hemorrhagic fever. About 10% of severely ill Rift Valley fever victims suffer retina damage and may be permanently blind, and 25% of South American hemorrhagic fever victims suffer potentially permanent deafness.

Proper treatment is vital. In cases of DHF-DSS, fatality can be reduced from 40–50% to less than 2% with adequate medical care. For individuals who survive hemorrhagic fevers, prolonged convalescence is usually inevitable. However, survivors seem to gain lifelong immunity against the virus that made them ill.

Prevention

Hemorrhagic fevers can be prevented through vector control and personal protection measures. Attempts have been made in urban and settled areas to destroy mosquito and rodent populations. In areas where such measures are impossible, individuals can use insect repellents, mosquito netting, and other methods to minimize exposure.

Vaccines have been developed against yellow fever, Argentinian hemorrhagic fever, and Crimean-Congo hemorrhagic fever. Vaccines against other hemorrhagic fevers are being researched. Another possible preventive measure is increasing the number of natural killer (NK) cells in the body. These cells appear to be an important innate source of protection against Ebola and other filoviruses.

Prevention of epidemics of hemorrhagic fevers has acquired a new importance in the early 2000s from concern that the causative viruses might be used as weapons of bioterrorism. These viruses can be

KEY TERMS

Antibody—A molecule created by the body's immune system to combat a specific infectious agent, such as a virus or bacteria.

Antigen—A specific feature, such as a protein, on an infectious agent. Antibodies use this feature as a means of identifying infectious intruders.

Coagulating factors—Components within the blood that help form clots.

Endemic—Referring to a specific geographic area in which a disease may occur.

Hemorrhage—As a noun, this refers to the point at which blood is released. As a verb, this refers to bleeding.

Incubation—The time period between exposure to an infectious agent, such as a virus or bacteria, and the appearance of symptoms of illness.

Petechiae—Pinpoint hemorrhages that appear as reddish dots beneath the surface of the skin.

Reservoir—A population in which a virus is maintained without causing serious illness to the infected individuals.

Ribavirin—A drug that is used to combat viral infections.

Tissue factor—A glycoprotein involved in blood coagulation.

Vector—A member of the reservoir population or an intervening species that can transmit a virus to a susceptible victim. Mosquitoes are common vectors, as are ticks and rodents.

transmitted in aerosol form as well as having a high mortality rate.

Resources

BOOKS

Beers, Mark H., Robert S. Porter, and Thomas V. Jones, eds. *The Merck Manual of Diagnosis and Therapy*. 18th ed. Whitehouse Station, NJ: Merck Research Laboratories, 2006.

Professional Guide to Diseases. 9th ed. Philadelphia; London: Wolters Kluwer Health, 2008.

PERIODICALS

Izadi, S., K. H. Naieni, S. R. Madjdzadeh, and A. Nadim. "Crimean-Congo Hemorrhagic Fever in Sistan and Baluchestan Province of Iran, A Case-Control Study on Epidemiological Characteristics." *International Journal of Infectious Diseases* 8 (September 2004): 299–306.

Mahanty, S., and M. Bray. "Pathogenesis of Filoviral Haemorrhagic Fevers." *Lancet Infectious Diseases* 4 (August 2004): 487–498.

Ruf, W. "Emerging Roles of Tissue Factor in Viral Hemor rhagic Fever." *Trends in Immunology* 25 (September 2004): 461–464.

Salvaggio, M. R., and J. W. Baddley. "Other Viral Biowea pons: Ebola and Marburg Hemorrhagic Fever." *Dermatologic Clinics* 22 (July 2004): 291–302.

Setlick, R. F., D. Ouellette, J. Morgan, et al. "Pulmonary Hemorrhage Syndrome Associated with an Autochthonous Case of Dengue Hemorrhagic Fever." *Southern Medical Journal* 97 (July 2004): 688–691.

Warfield, K. L., J. G. Perkins, D. L. Swenson, et al. "Role of Natural Killer Cells in Innate Protection against Lethal Ebola Virus Infection." *Journal of Experimental Medicine* 200 (July 19, 2004): 169–179.

OTHER

Centers for Disease Control and Prevention, Special Pathogens Branch. "Ebola Hemorrhagic Fever," August 23, 2004. http://www.cdc.gov/ncidod/dvrd/spb/mnpages/dispages/ebola.htm.

Centers for Disease Control and Prevention, Special Pathogens Branch. "Marburg Hemorrhagic Fever," August 23, 2004. http://www.cdc.gov/ncidod/dvrd/spb/mnpages/dispages/marburg.htm.

ORGANIZATIONS

Centers for Disease Control and Prevention (CDC), 1600 Clifton Road, Atlanta, GA, 30333, (800) 232-4636, cdcinfo@cdc.gov, http://www.cdc.gov.

Infectious Diseases Society of America (IDSA), 1300 Wilson Blvd., Suite 300, Arlington, VA, 22209, (703) 299-0200, (703) 299-0204, http://www.idsociety.org/.

World Health Organization (WHO), Avenue Appia 201211, Geneva, Switzerland, 27, 4122791-2111, info@who.int, http://www.who.int.

Julia Barrett
Rebecca J. Frey, PhD

Hemorrhoids

Definition

Hemorrhoids are enlarged veins in the anus or lower rectum. They often go unnoticed and usually clear up after a few days, but can cause long-lasting discomfort, bleeding and excruciatingly pain. Effective medical treatments are available, however.

Demographics

Hemorrhoids are a very common medical complaint. More than 75% of Americans have hemorrhoids at some point in their lives, typically after age 30. Pregnant women often develop hemorrhoids, but the condition usually clears up after **childbirth**. Men are more likely than women to suffer from hemorrhoids that require professional medical treatment.

Description

Hemorrhoids (also called piles) can be divided into two kinds, internal and external. Internal hemorrhoids lie inside the anus or lower rectum, beneath the anal or rectal lining. External hemorrhoids lie outside the anal opening. Both kinds can be present at the same time.

Causes and symptoms

Precisely why hemorrhoids develop is unknown. Researchers have identified a number of reasons to explain hemorrhoidal swelling, including the simple fact that people's upright posture places a lot of pressure on the anal and rectal veins. **Aging**, **obesity**, **pregnancy**, chronic **constipation** or **diarrhea**, excessive use of **enemas** or **laxatives**, straining during bowel

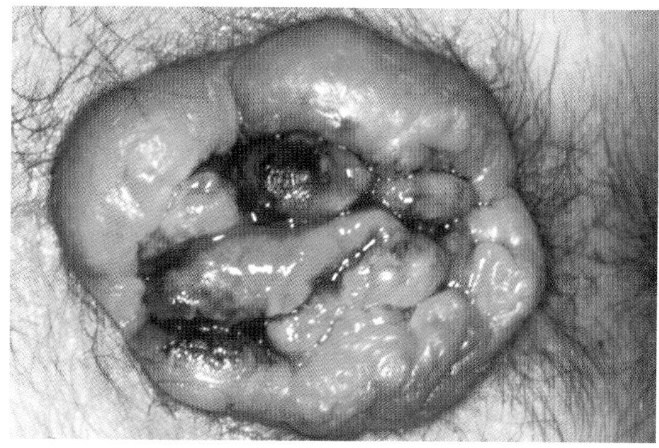

Clinical photo of a thrombosed external hemorrhoid. *(Custom Medical Stock Photo, Inc. Reproduced by permission.)*

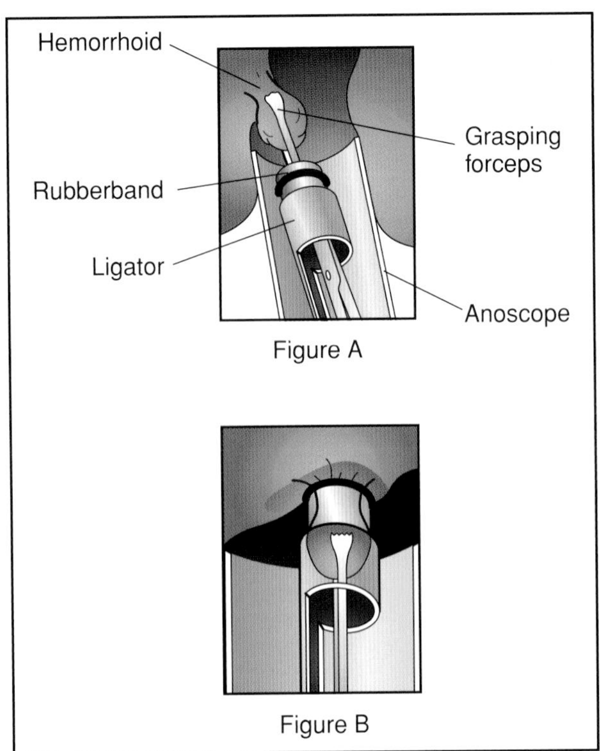

Rubber band ligation is probably the most widely used treatment for internal hemorrhoids. An applicator is used to place one or two small rubber bands around the base of the hemorrhoid, cutting off its blood supply (figures A and B). After 3-10 days, the rubber bands and the hemorrhoid fall off, leaving a scab which disappears within a week or two. *(Illustration by Electronic Illustrators Group. Reproduced by permission of Gale, a part of Cengage Learning.)*

movements, and spending too much time on the toilet are considered contributing factors. Heredity may also play a part in some cases. There is no reason to believe that hemorrhoids are caused by jobs requiring, for instance, heavy lifting or long hours of sitting, although activities of that kind may make existing hemorrhoids worse.

The most common symptom of internal hemorrhoids is bright red blood in the toilet bowl or on one's feces or toilet paper. When hemorrhoids remain inside the anus they are almost never painful, but they can prolapse (protrude outside the anus) and become irritated and sore. Sometimes, prolapsed hemorrhoids move back into the anal canal on their own or can be pushed back in, but at other times they remain permanently outside the anus until treated by a doctor.

Small external hemorrhoids usually do not produce symptoms. Larger ones, however, can be painful and interfere with cleaning the anal area after a bowel movement. When, as sometimes happens, a blood clot forms in an external hemorrhoid (creating what is called a thrombosed hemorrhoid), the skin around the anus becomes inflamed and a very painful lump develops. On rare occasions the clot will begin to bleed after a few days and leave blood on the underwear. A thrombosed hemorrhoid will not cause an **embolism**.

Diagnosis

Diagnosis begins with a visual examination of the anus, followed by an internal examination during which the doctor carefully inserts a gloved and lubricated finger into the anus. The doctor may also use an anoscope, a small tube that allows him or her to see into the anal canal. Under some circumstances the doctor may wish to check for other problems by using a sigmoidoscope or colonoscope, a flexible instrument that allows inspection of the lower colon (in the case of the sigmoidoscope) or the entire colon (in the case of the colonoscope).

Treatment

Hemorrhoids can often be effectively dealt with by dietary and lifestyle changes. Softening the feces and avoiding constipation by adding fiber to one's diet is important because hard feces lead to straining during defecation. Fruit, leafy vegetables, and whole-grain breads and cereals are good sources of fiber, as are bulk laxatives and fiber supplements, such as Metamucil or Citrucel. Exercising, losing excess weight, and drinking six to eight glasses a day of water or another liquid (not alcohol) also helps. Soap or toilet paper that is perfumed may irritate the anal area and should be avoided, as should excessive cleaning, rubbing, or wiping of that area. Reading in the bathroom is also considered a bad idea, because it adds to the time one spends on the toilet and may increase the strain placed on the anal and rectal veins. After each bowel movement, wiping with a moistened tissue or pad sold for that purpose helps lessen irritation. Hemorrhoid **pain** is often eased by sitting in a tub of warm water for about 10 or 15 minutes two to four times a day (**sitz bath**). A cool compress or ice pack to reduce swelling is also recommended (the ice pack should be wrapped in a cloth or towel to prevent direct contact with the skin). Many people find that over-the-counter hemorrhoid creams and foams bring relief, but these medications do not make hemorrhoids disappear.

When painful hemorrhoids do not respond to home-based remedies, professional medical treatment is necessary. The choice of treatment depends on the type of hemorrhoid, what medical equipment is available, and other considerations.

KEY TERMS

Anus—The opening at the lower end of the rectum. The anus and rectum are both part of the large intestine, a digestive system organ.

Colon—The major part of the large intestine, a digestive system organ.

Defecation—Passage of feces through the anus.

Embolism—Obstruction of blood flow in an artery by a blood clot or other substance arising from another site. An untreated embolism can endanger health and even cause death.

Enema—The introduction of water or another liquid into the bowels through a tube inserted into the anus. Enemas are used to treat constipation and for other purposes.

Feces—Undigested food and other waste that is eliminated through the anus; also called stools.

Rectum—The lower section of the large intestine, a digestive system organ. After food has passed through the stomach and intestines and been digested, the leftover material, in the form of feces, enters the rectum, where it stays until defecation.

Suppository—A medicinal substance that slowly dissolves after being inserted into the rectum (or other body cavity).

Rubber band ligation is probably the most widely used of the many treatments for internal hemorrhoids (and the least costly for the patient). This procedure is performed in the office of a family doctor or specialist or in a hospital on an outpatient basis. An applicator is used to place one or two small rubber bands around the base of the hemorrhoid, cutting off its blood supply. After 3 to 10 days in the bands, the hemorrhoid falls off, leaving a sore that heals in a week or two. Because internal hemorrhoids are located in a part of the anus that does not sense pain, anesthetic is unnecessary and the procedure is painless in most cases. Although there can be minor discomfort and bleeding for a few days after the bands are applied, complications are rare and most people are soon able to return to work and other activities. If more than one hemorrhoid exists or if banding is not entirely effective the first time (as occasionally happens), the procedure may need to be repeated a few weeks later. After five years, 15–20% of patients experience a recurrence of internal hemorrhoids, but in most cases all that is needed is another banding.

External hemorrhoids, and some prolapsed internal hemorrhoids, are removed by conventional surgery in a hospital. Depending on the circumstances, this requires a local, regional, or general anesthetic. Surgery does cause a fair amount of discomfort, but an overnight hospital stay is usually not necessary. Full healing takes two to four weeks, but most people are able to resume normal activities at the end of a week. Hemorrhoids rarely return after surgery.

Alternative treatment

Like mainstream practitioners, alternative practitioners stress the importance of a high-fiber diet. To prevent hemorrhoids by strengthening the veins of the anus, rectum, and colon, they recommend blackberries, blueberries, cherries, vitamin C, butcher's broom (*Ruscus aculeatus*), and flavonoids (plant pigments found in fruit and fruit products, tea, and soy). Herbal teas, ointments, and suppositories, and other kinds of herbal preparations, are suggested for reducing discomfort and eliminating hemorrhoids. In particular, pilewort (*Ranunculusficaria*), applied in an ointment or taken as a tea, can reduce the pain of external hemorrhoids. **Acupuncture**, **acupressure**, **aromatherapy**, and homeopathy are also used to treat hemorrhoids.

Prognosis

Hemorrhoids do not cause **cancer** and are rarely dangerous or life threatening. Most clear up after a few days without professional medical treatment. However, because colorectal cancer and other digestive system diseases can cause anal bleeding and other hemorrhoid-like symptoms, people should always consult a doctor when those symptoms occur.

Prevention

A high-fiber diet and the other lifestyle changes recommended for coping with existing hemorrhoids also help to prevent hemorrhoids. Not straining during bowel movements is essential.

Resources

PERIODICALS

Grucela A, Salinas H, Khaitov S, et al. "Prospective Analysis of Clinician Accuracy in the Diagnosis of Benign Anal Pathology: Comparison Across

Specialties and Years of Experience. *Dis Colon Rectum*, Jan 2010, 53(1):47-52.
Kaidar-Person O., et al. "Hemorrhoidal disease: A comprehensive review." *Journal of the American College of Surgeons*. (2007) 204:102.

ORGANIZATIONS

National Digestive Diseases Information Clearinghouse, 2 Information Way, Bethesda, MD, 20892-3570, (800) 891-5389, http://www.niddk.nih.gov/health/digest/nddic.htm.

Howard Baker
Karl Finley

Henoch-Schönlein purpura *see* **Allergic purpura**

Hepatic carcinoma *see* **Liver cancer, primary**

Hepatic encephalopathy *see* **Liver encephalopathy**

Hepatitis-associated antigen (HAA) test *see* **Hepatitis virus tests**

Hepatitis A

Definition

Hepatitis A is an **infectious disease** of the liver caused by the HAV virus. The disease is usually transmitted by food or water contaminated by human wastes containing the virus or by close human contact. As far as is known, only humans can get hepatitis A; it is not carried by other animals.

Hepatitis A was previously known as infectious hepatitis because it spread relatively easily from those infected to close household contacts.

Demographics

Hepatitis A is much more common in Africa, Asia, and South America than in the United States. The rates of hepatitis A in North America have been steadily dropping since the 1980s due to improvements in public health policies and sanitation; on the other hand, the rates of hepatitis A among frequent travelers have been rising during the same time period.

In 1988 the Centers for Disease Control and Prevention (CDC) reported 32,000 cases in the United States; in 2003, 7653 cases were reported. The CDC estimates that nearly 25,000 people contracted hepatitis A in the United States in 2007, although the number of reported cases is much lower because many people do not show symptoms of the disease. In developing countries, children below the age of 2 account for most new cases of hepatitis A; in the United States, the age group most often affected is children between the ages of 5 and 14.

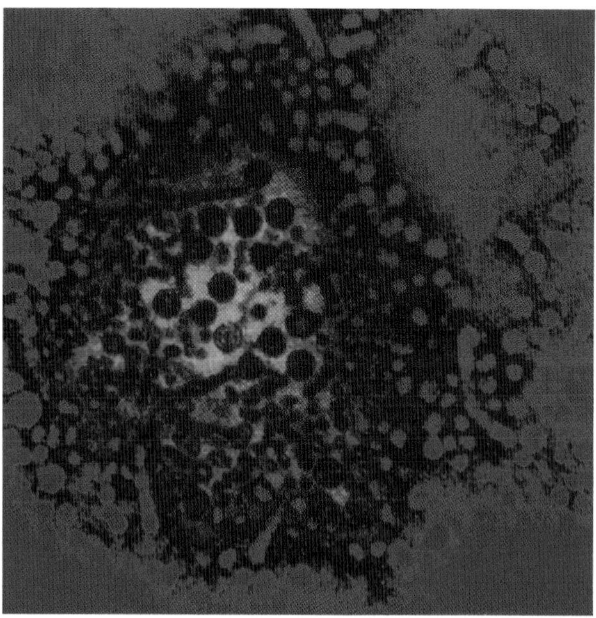

Hepatitis A virus magnified 225,000 times. *(Custom Medical Stock Photo, Inc. Reproduced by permission.)*

The states with the highest incidence of hepatitis A account for 50 percent of the reported cases. According to the American Academy of Pediatrics, 11 states have a rate of HAV infection that is at least twice the national average, or 20 cases per every 100,000 people. The states are Arizona, Alaska, California, Idaho, Nevada, New Mexico, Oklahoma, Oregon, South Dakota, Utah, and Washington.

Males and females are equally likely to get hepatitis A, as are people from all races and ethnic groups in the United States.

Description

Hepatitis A is an inflammation of the liver caused by the HAV virus, also called enterovirus 72, which was first identified in 1973. It differs from **hepatitis B** and **hepatitis C** in that it does not cause long-term liver damage. Even though people can take several weeks or months to recover completely from hepatitis A, they have lifelong immunity afterward. Complications from hepatitis A are rare and usually limited to people with chronic **liver disease** or those who have received a liver transplant.

Hepatitis A varies in severity, running an acute course, generally starting within two to six weeks after contact with the virus, and lasting no longer than two or three months. Children and younger adults may have no symptoms at all, although they can still spread the disease. In general, adults are more likely to have noticeable symptoms than children or teenagers. The most common symptom is loss of energy and overall tiredness.

Some people develop a mild flu-like illness with **diarrhea**, low-grade **fever**, **nausea**, **vomiting**, and **muscle cramps**. People with more severe symptoms may have **pain** in the abdomen in the area of the liver (below the rib cage on the right side of the body); they may notice that their urine has turned dark brown or that they have jaundice—yellowing of the skin and the whites of the eyes. Some have an itchy skin rash.

HAV may occur in single cases after contact with an infected relative or sex partner. Alternately, epidemics may develop when food or drinking water is contaminated by the feces of an infected person. In the public's mind, outbreaks of hepatitis A usually are linked with the eating of contaminated food at a restaurant. It is true that food-handlers, who may themselves have no symptoms, can start an alarming, widespread epidemic. Many types of food can be infected by sewage containing HAV, but such shellfish as clams and oysters are common culprits.

Most people diagnosed with hepatitis A feel better within four to six weeks after the symptoms begin, although about 15 percent of patients may take up to 9 months to regain their energy and feel normal again.

Risk factors

Some people are at increased risk of hepatitis A, including:

- People who travel to parts of the world with high rates of the disease and poor sanitation, including the Middle East, South America, Eastern Europe, Mexico and Central America, Africa, Southeast Asia, and the Caribbean.
- Male homosexuals.
- People who use illicit drugs, whether injected or taken by mouth.
- Medical researchers and laboratory workers who may be exposed to HAV.
- Child care workers and children in day care centers. Children at day care centers make up an estimated 14–40% of all cases of HAV infection in the United States. Changing diapers transmits infection through fecal-oral contact. Toys and other objects may remain contaminated for some time. Often a child without symptoms brings the infection home to siblings and parents.
- Troops living under crowded conditions at military camps or in the field.
- Homeless people.

Causes and symptoms

Causes

Hepatitis A is caused by a virus that is transmitted by close personal contact with an infected person, by needle sharing, and by eating food or drinking water contaminated by fecal matter. After the virus enters the body, it multiplies in the cells of the liver, causing inflammation of the liver and a general response from the immune system that leads to most of the symptoms of the illness.

The HAV virus is shed from the liver into the bile (a digestive fluid secreted by the liver) and then into the person's stools between 15 and 45 days before symptoms appear. That means that people can spread the virus through their feces before they know that they are sick. In the United States, hepatitis A is most commonly spread by food handlers who do not wash their hands properly after using the bathroom; by childcare workers who do not wash their hands after changing a baby's diaper; by anal sex; and by eating raw shellfish harvested from sewage-polluted waters. In very rare cases the virus can be transmitted through blood transfusions.

Symptoms

Often the first symptoms to appear are **fatigue** and general achiness. Those who like to drink coffee or smoke cigarettes may lose their taste for them. The liver often enlarges, causing pain or tenderness in the right upper part of the abdomen. As many as three out of four children have no symptoms of HAV infection, but about 85% of adults will have symptoms.

In addition to fatigue, the most common symptoms of hepatitis A include:

- Low-grade fever (101°F)
- Nausea, vomiting, and diarrhea
- Loss of appetite and weight loss
- Swelling of the liver and pain in the area of the abdomen over the liver
- Tea- or coffee-colored urine
- Jaundice
- An itchy rash or a generalized sensation of itching
- Pale or clay-colored stools
- Muscle pains

KEY TERMS

Antibody—A substance made by the body in response to a foreign body, such as a virus, which is able to attack and destroy the invading virus.

Antiemetic—A type of drug given to control nausea and vomiting.

Bile—A yellow-green fluid secreted by the liver that aids in the digestion of fats.

Contamination—The process by which an object or body part becomes exposed to an infectious agent such as a virus.

Epidemic—A situation where a large number of infections by a particular agent, such as a virus, develops in a short time. The agent is rapidly transmitted to many individuals.

Hepatitis—The medical term for inflammation of the liver. It can be caused by toxic substances or alcohol as well as infections.

Immune globulin—A preparation of antibodies that can be given before exposure for short-term protection against hepatitis A and for persons who have already been exposed to hepatitis A virus. Immune globulin must be given within two weeks after exposure to hepatitis A virus for maximum protection.

Incubation period—The interval from initial exposure to an infectious agent, such as a virus, and the first symptoms of illness.

Jaundice—A yellowish discoloration of the skin and whites of the eyes caused by increased levels of bile pigments from the liver in the patient's blood.

Relapse—A temporary recurrence of the symptoms of a disease.

Vaccine—A substance prepared from a weakened or killed microorganism which, when injected, helps the body to form antibodies that will prevent infection by the natural microorganism.

Diagnosis

Diagnosis of hepatitis A is made on the basis of the patient's history, findings during an office examination, and a blood test for HAV.

Examination

The doctor may suspect that a patient has hepatitis A during a **physical examination** in the office by feeling the area over the liver for signs of swelling and pain; taking the patient's temperature; and checking the skin and eyes for signs of **jaundice**.

Tests

A definite diagnosis is provided by a blood test for antibodies to the HAV virus. There is a specific antibody called hepatitis A IgM antibody that develops when HAV is present in the body. This test always registers positive when a patient has symptoms and should continue to register positive for four to six months. However, hepatitis A IgM antibody will persist lifelong in the blood and is protective against reinfection.

In some cases the doctor may also have the sample of blood checked for abnormally high levels of liver enzymes.

Treatment

Traditional

There is no specific drug treatment for hepatitis A, as **antibiotics** cannot be used to treat virus infections. Most people can care for themselves at home by making sure they get plenty of fluids and adequate **nutrition**. People whose appetite has been affected may benefit from eating small snacks throughout the day rather than three main meals and by eating soft and easily digested foods.

Patients with hepatitis A should avoid drinking alcohol, which makes it harder for the liver to recover from inflammation. Patients should also tell their doctor about any over-the-counter or prescription drugs they are taking because the drugs may need to be stopped temporarily or have the dosages changed.

Drugs

Patients with hepatitis A may take **acetaminophen** to reduce fever and relieve pain. Patients with mild **vomiting** may be prescribed antiemetics (drugs to control nausea); the drug most commonly prescribed for hepatitis patients is metoclopramide (Reglan). Those with severe vomiting may need to be hospitalized in order to receive intravenous fluids.

Prognosis

Most people recover fully from hepatitis A within a few weeks or months. Between 3 and 20% have relapses (temporary recurrences of symptoms) for as long as six to nine months after infection. In the United States, serious complications are infrequent and deaths are very rare. As many as 75% of adults over 50 years of age in North America will have blood test evidence of previous hepatitis A.

About 1 percent of patients develop liver failure following HAV infection, mostly those over 60 or those with chronic liver disease. In these cases **liver transplantation** may be necessary for the patient's survival. There are about 100 deaths from hepatitis A reported each year in the United States.

Prevention

Hepatitis A can be prevented by a vaccine called Havrix that is given before exposure to the HAV virus. The vaccine is given in two shots, the second given between 6 and 18 months after the first. It confers immunity against hepatitis A for at least 20 years. Those who should receive the vaccine include people in the military and those who travel abroad frequently; men who have sex with other men; people who use intravenous drugs; people with **hemophilia** who must receive human blood products; and people who have chronic hepatitis B or C infection.

People who have been exposed to the HAV virus should be given immune globulin to protect them against getting sick, because Havrix is not effective in people who have already been exposed to HAV. Children under the age of 2 should be given immune globulin or a vaccine called Epaxal that was introduced in 2007 rather than Havrix to protect them against HAV.

A vaccine against hepatitis A introduced in 2007 is called Epaxal; there is a version for children called Epaxal Junior that appears to be a good choice for mass **vaccination** programs. Unlike Havrix, Epaxal Junior can be given to children above the age of one year.

Everyone can reduce their risk of hepatitis A by observing the following precautions:

- Practice good personal hygiene; wash hands frequently, especially after using the toilet or changing a child's diaper.
- When traveling, drink only bottled water; avoid raw or undercooked meat or shellfish; and avoid eating fresh fruits or vegetables unless you have washed and peeled them yourself.
- Avoid sharing drinking glasses and eating utensils. If someone in the family has hepatitis A, wash their glasses and utensils separately in hot, soapy water.
- Avoid sexual contact with anyone who has hepatitis A.

Resources

BOOKS

Dworkin, Mark S. *Outbreak Investigations around the World: Case Studies in Infectious Disease Field Epidemiology*. Sudbury, MA: Jones and Bartlett, Publishers, 2010.

Feigin, Ralph D., et al, eds. *Feigin and Cherry's Textbook of Pediatric Infectious Diseases*, 6th ed. Philadelphia, PA : Saunders/Elsevier, 2009.

Richman, Douglas D., Richard J. Whitley, and Frederick G. Hayden, eds. *Clinical Virology*, 3rd ed. Washington, DC: ASM Press, 2009.

Younossi, Zobair M., ed. *Practical Management of Liver Diseases*. New York: Cambridge University Press, 2008.

PERIODICALS

Ackerman, L.K. "Update on Immunizations in Children and Adolescents." *American Family Physician* 77 (June 1, 2008): 1561–68.

Bovier, P.A. "Epaxal: A Virosomal Vaccine to Prevent Hepatitis A Infection." *Expert Review of Vaccines* 7 (October 2008): 1141–1150.

Costas, L., et al. "Vaccination Strategies against Hepatitis A in Travelers Older Than 40 Years: An Economic Evaluation." *Journal of Travel Medicine* 16 (September-October 2009): 344–48.

Degertekin, B., and A.S. Lok. "Update on Viral Hepatitis: 2008." *Current Opinion in Gastroenterology* 25 (May 2009): 180–85.

Dentinger, C.M. "Emerging Infections: Hepatitis A." *American Journal of Nursing* 109 (August 2009): 29–33.

Gitto, S., et al. "Alcohol and Viral Hepatitis: A Mini-Review." *Digestive and Liver Disease* 41 (January 2009): 67–70.

Lugoboni, F., et al. "Bloodborne Viral Hepatitis Infections among Drug Users: The Role of Vaccination." *International Journal of Environmental Research and Public Health* 6 (January 2009): 400–413.

Todd, E.C., et al. "Outbreaks Where Food Workers Have Been Implicated in the Spread of Foodborne Disease. Part 4. Infective Doses and Pathogen Carriage." *Journal of Food Protection* 71 (November 2008): 2339–2373.

OTHER

American Liver Foundation. *Hepatitis A*. http://www.liverfoundation.org/education/info/hepatitisa/

Centers for Disease Control and Prevention (CDC). *Hepatitis A Vaccination*. http://www.cdc.gov/vaccines/vpd-vac/hepa/default.htm

Gilroy, Richard A., and Sandeep Mukherjee. "Hepatitis A." *eMedicine*, August 26, 2008. http://emedicine.medscape.com/article/177484-overview

Mayo Clinic. *Hepatitis A*. http://www.mayoclinic.com/health/hepatitis-a/DS00397

National Institute of Allergy and Infectious Diseases (NIAID). *Hepatitis A*. http://www3.niaid.nih.gov/topics/hepatitis/hepatitisA/

ORGANIZATIONS

American College of Gastroenterology (ACG), P.O. Box 342260, Bethesda, MD, 20827-2260, (301)263-9000, http://www.acg.gi.org/.

American Liver Foundation (ALF), 75 Maiden Lane, Suite 603, New York, NY, 10038, (212)668-1000, (212)483-8179, http://www.liverfoundation.org/.

Centers for Disease Control and Prevention (CDC), 1600 Clifton Road, Atlanta, GA, 30333, (800)232-4636, cdcinfo@cdc.gov, http://www.cdc.gov.

National Institute of Allergy and Infectious Diseases (NIAID), 6610 Rockledge Drive, MSC 6612, Bethesda, MD, 20892-6612, (301)496-5717, (866)284-4107, (301)402-3573, http://www3.niaid.nih.gov.

World Health Organization (WHO), Avenue Appia 20, 1211 Geneva 27, Switzerland, + 41 22 791 21 11, + 41 22 791 31 11, info@who.int, http://www.who.int/en/.

Larry I. Lutwick, MD
Monique Laberge, PhD
Rebecca J. Frey, PhD

Hepatitis, alcoholic

Definition

Alcoholic hepatitis is an inflammation of the liver caused by alcohol.

Description

Irritation, whether from toxins or infections, causes a similar response in body organs. The response is known as inflammation and consists of:

- an increase in the blood to the affected organ
- redness and swelling of the organ
- influx of immune agents like white blood cells and their arsenal of chemical weapons
- pain

As the acute process subsides, there is either healing or lingering activity. Lingering activity—chronic disease—has a milder presentation with similar ingredients. Healing often takes the form of scarring, wherein normal functioning tissue is replaced by tough, fibrous, and non-productive scar. Both chronic disease and healing can happen simultaneously, so that scar tissue progressively replaces normal tissue. This leads to **cirrhosis**, a liver so scarred it is unable to do its job adequately.

KEY TERMS

Cirrhosis—Disruption of normal liver structure and function caused by any type of chronic disease such as hepatitis and alcohol abuse.

Fatty liver—An abnormal amount of fat tissue in the liver caused by alcohol abuse.

Hemolysis—Disintegration of red blood cells.

Protozoa—One-celled microscopic organisms like amoeba.

Alcohol can cause either an acute or a chronic disease in the liver. The acute disease can be severe, even fatal, and can bring with it hemolysis–blood cell destruction. Alcohol can also cause a third type of **liver disease**, **fatty liver**, in which the continuous action of alcohol turns the liver to useless fat. This condition eventually progresses to cirrhosis if the poisoningcontinues.

Causes and symptoms

Inflammation of the liver can be caused by a great variety of agents—poisons, drugs, viruses, bacteria, protozoa, and even larger organisms like worms. Alcohol is a poison if taken in more than modest amounts. It favors destroying stomach lining, liver, heart muscle, and brain tissue. The liver is a primary target because alcohol travels to the liver after leaving the intestines. Those who drink enough to get alcohol **poisoning** have a tendency to be undernourished, since alcohol provides ample calories but little **nutrition**. It is suspected that both the alcohol and the poor nutrition produce alcoholic hepatitis.

Diagnosis

Hepatitis of all kinds causes notable discomfort, loss of appetite, **nausea**, **pain** in the liver, and usually **jaundice** (turning yellow). Blood test abnormalities are unmistakably those of hepatitis, but selecting from so many the precise cause may take additional diagnostic work.

Treatment

As with all poisonings, removal of the offending agent is primary. There is no specific treatment for alcohol poisoning. General supportive measures must see the patient through until the liver has healed by itself. In the case of fulminant (sudden and severe) disease, the liver may be completely destroyed and have to be replaced by a transplant.

Prognosis

The liver is robust. It can heal without scarring after one or a few episodes of hepatitis that resolve without lingering. It can, moreover, regrow from a fragment of its former self, provided there is not disease or poison still inhibiting it.

Prevention

Alcohol is lethal in many ways when ingested in excess. Research suggests that the maximum healthy dose of alcohol per day is roughly one pure ounce—the amount in two cocktails, two glasses of wine, or two beers.

ORGANIZATIONS

Alcoholics Anonymous, World Services, P.O. Box 459, New York, NY, 10163, (212) 870-3400, http://www. aa.org.

American Liver Foundation, 75 Maiden Lane, Suite 603, New York, NY, 10038, (212) 668-1000, (212) 483-8179, http://www.liverfoundation.org/.

J. Ricker Polsdorfer, MD

Hepatitis, autoimmune

Definition

A form of liver inflammation in which the body's immune system attacks liver cells.

Description

Autoimmunity causes the body's defense mechanisms to turn against itself. Many of the tissues in the body can be the target of such an attack. While one tissue type predominates, others may be involved in a general misdirection of immune activity, perhaps because the specific target antigen is present in differing quantities in each of the affected tissues. There seem to be hereditary causes for autoimmunity, since these diseases tend to run in families and have genetic markers. Among the more common diseases believed to fall within this category are **rheumatoid arthritis**, **systemic lupus erythematosus**, **multiple sclerosis**, and **psoriasis**.

The process of autoimmune disease is very similar to **infectious disease** and allergy, so that great caution is observed in placing a disorder in this class. Germs were found to cause several diseases originally thought to be autoimmune. Allergens cause others. Many more may be uncovered. Autoimmunity is often believed to originate with a virus infection. A chemical in the virus resembles a body chemical so closely that the immune system attacks both.

Autoimmune hepatitis is similiar to viral hepatitis, a disease of the liver. It can be an acute disease that kills over a third of its victims within six months, can persist for years, or can return periodically. Some patients develop **cirrhosis** of the liver which, over time, causes the liver to cease functioning.

KEY TERMS

Allergen—Any chemical that causes an immune reaction only in people sensitive to it.

Antigen—Any chemical that can be the target of an immune response.

Biopsy—Surgical removal of a piece of tissue for examination.

Jaundice—A yellow color to the skin from bile that backs up into the circulation.

Causes and symptoms

Symptoms of autoimmune hepatitis resemble those of other types of hepatitis. Patients who develop autoimmune hepatitis experience **pain** under the right ribs, **fatigue** and general discomfort, loss of appetite, **nausea**, and sometimes **vomiting** and **jaundice**. In addition, other parts of the body may be involved and contribute their own symptoms.

Diagnosis

Extensive laboratory testing may be required to differentiate this disease from viral hepatitis. The distinction may not even be made during the initial episode. There are certain markers of autoimmune disease in the blood that can lead to the correct diagnosis if they are sought. In advanced or chronic cases a **liver biopsy** may be necessary.

Treatment

Autoimmune hepatitis is among the few types of hepatitis that can be treated effectively. Since treatment itself introduces problems in at least 20% of patients, it is reserved for the more severe cases. Up to 80% of patients improve with cortisone treatment, although a cure is unlikely. Another drug—azathioprine—is sometimes used concurrently. Treatment continues for over a year and may be restarted during a relapse. At least half the patients relapse at some point, and most will still continue to have progressive liver scarring.

If the liver fails, transplant is the only recourse.

Prognosis

In spite of treatment, autoimmune hepatitis can re-erupt at any time and may continue to damage and scar the liver. The rate of progression varies considerably from patient to patient.

ORGANIZATIONS

American Liver Foundation, 75 Maiden Lane, Suite 603, New York, NY, 10038, (212) 668-1000, (212) 483-8179, http://www.liverfoundation.org/.

J. Ricker Polsdorfer, MD

Hepatitis B

Definition

Hepatitis B is a viral infection of the liver transmitted through the blood or body fluids of someone who is infected. It is also called serum hepatitis because it can be transmitted through blood serum, the liquid portion of blood.

Hepatitis B is the most common serious liver infection worldwide. The disease has two forms: an acute form that lasts a few weeks, and a chronic form that can last for years, leading to **cirrhosis**, liver failure, **liver cancer**, and even **death**. Acute hepatitis B has a 5 percent chance of leading to the chronic form of the infection in adults. However, infants infected during the mother's **pregnancy** have a 90 percent chance of developing chronic hepatitis B, and children have a 25–50 percent chance.

Demographics

There are about 100,000 new cases of hepatitis B in the United States each year; it is estimated that 1–1.4 million people carry the disease and that 12 million Americans (1 in 20) have been infected by the disease. Hepatitis B causes about 5100 deaths in the United States each year; on average, one American health care worker dies each day from hepatitis B. In the rest of the world, as many as a third of the population (2 billion people) are chronic carriers of the disease. Chronic hepatitis B affects approximately 400 million people around the world as of 2009 and contributes to an estimated 1 million deaths worldwide each year.

The age group most commonly affected by hepatitis B in the United States is adults between the ages of 20 and 50. The routine immunization of children

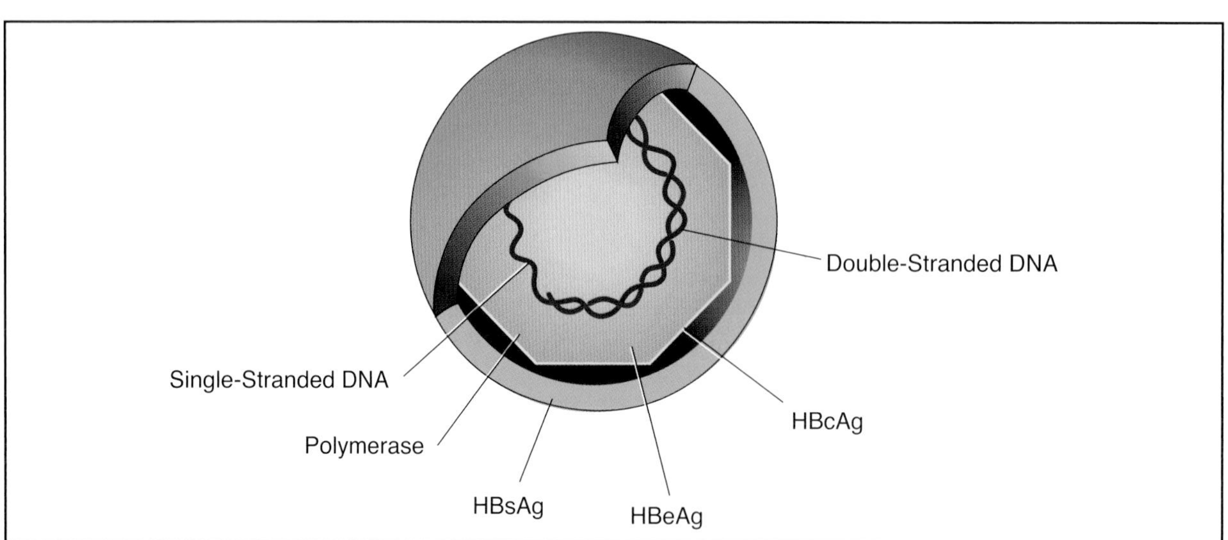

Hepatitis B virus (HBV) is composed of an inner protein core and an outer protein capsule. The outer capsule contains the hepatitis B surface antigen (HBsAg). The inner core contains HBV core antigen (HBcAg) and hepatitis B e-antigen (HBeAg). This cell also contains polymerase, which catalyzes the formation of the cell's DNA. HBV is the only hepatitis-causing virus that has DNA, instead of RNA. *(Illustration by Electronic Illustrators Group. Reproduced by permission of Gale, a part of Cengage Learning.)*

against the disease since 1990 has led to a decline in the rate of acute hepatitis in North America for the past two decades. African Americans are more likely to be infected than either Hispanics or Caucasians; however, Alaskan Eskimos and Pacific Islanders have higher rates of carrier status than members of other racial groups. Asian Americans are at increased risk of severe liver damage from hepatitis B compared to members of other racial groups. More males than females are infected with hepatitis B in all races and age groups.

Description

Hepatitis B has an incubation period of 1–6 months. About 50 percent of people with the acute form of the disease have no symptoms at all; the others experience loss of appetite, **nausea** and **vomiting**, and **jaundice** around 12 weeks after getting infected. Some patients may also have joint **pain**, itchy skin, or abdominal pain. Many of these patients assume that they have **influenza**.

Patients with chronic hepatitis may have no symptoms at all. The one-third who do eventually fall ill have the same symptoms as patients with the acute form of the disease. About two-thirds of people with chronic HBV are carriers of the virus. They may never get sick themselves but they can transmit the infection to others. The remaining one-third of people with chronic hepatitis B develop **liver disease** that can lead to permanent scarring of the liver. Between 15 and 25 percent of people with chronic hepatitis B eventually die of liver disease.

Although there are many ways of passing on HBV, the virus is not very easily transmitted by indirect contact because it is a bloodborne pathogen. There is no need to worry that such casual contact as shaking hands will expose one to hepatitis B, and there is no reason not to share a workplace or even a restroom with an infected person. On the other hand, hepatitis B virus is a durable virus that can survive outside the body for at least seven days. During that time, the virus can still cause disease if it enters the body of a person who is not infected. For that reason it is necessary to clean any surface contaminated by blood spills (including those that have dried) carefully with a mixture of chlorine bleach and water. Medical or dental instruments must be sterilized with particular care.

People who have been infected by HBV and have recovered from the infection are protected against hepatitis B for the rest of their lives. People can also be protected by receiving a vaccine against the disease but must have a repeat **vaccination** every 5–10 years.

Risk factors

Risk factors for hepatitis B include:

- Having unprotected sex with a partner regardless of sexual orientation.
- Having a large number of sexual partners.
- Being infected with another sexually transmitted disease (STD), particularly gonorrhea or chlamydia.
- Sharing needles with other intravenous drug users.
- Having a family member with chronic HBV infection.
- Having had a blood transfusion or use of blood products before 1972.
- Needing hemodialysis for kidney disease.
- Frequent travels to parts of the world with high rates of hepatitis B. These include the Middle East, southern Africa, China, Southeast Asia, Brazil, and the Pacific Islands.
- Emigrating from or adopting a child from any of the countries listed above.
- Working in a hospital, clinic, or other facility requiring frequent exposure to blood, open wounds, or other body secretions. Health care workers at risk include dentists and dental hygienists as well as physicians, nurses, and laboratory technicians.
- Working as a police officer, firefighter, or other emergency first responder.
- Being a prison inmate.
- Living or working in a facility for the developmentally disabled.

Causes and symptoms

Causes

Hepatitis B is caused by a virus known as HBV. With the exception of HBV, all the common viruses that cause hepatitis are known as RNA viruses because they contain ribonucleic acid or RNA as their genetic material. HBV is the only deoxyribonucleic acid or DNA virus that is a major cause of hepatitis. HBV is made up of several fragments called antigens that stimulate the body's immune system to produce the antibodies that can neutralize or even destroy the infecting virus. It is in fact the immune reaction, not the virus, that seems to cause the liver inflammation associated with hepatitis B.

Hepatitis B is primarily a bloodborne infection but can also be transmitted through contact with the semen, vaginal secretions, or saliva of an infected person. The virus enters the body through injection, a

KEY TERMS

Antibody—A substance formed in the body in response to a foreign body, such as a virus, which can then attack and destroy the invading virus.

Antigen—Part of an invading microorganism, such as a virus, that causes tissue damage (in hepatitis, to the liver), and that also stimulates the body's immune system to produce antibodies.

Carrier—A person who is infected with a virus or other disease organism but does not develop the symptoms of the disease.

Chronic—Long-term or recurrent.

Cirrhosis—Disruption of normal liver function by the formation of scar tissue and nodules in the liver.

Fulminant—Referring to a disease that comes on suddenly with great severity.

Hepatitis—A general term for inflammation of the liver. It can be caused by toxic substances or alcohol as well as infections.

Jaundice—A yellowish discoloration of the skin and whites of the eyes caused by increased levels of bile pigments from the liver in the patient's blood.

Pathogen—Any biological agent that causes illness or disease in its host. A pathogen may be a virus, bacterium, fungus, or prion.

Vaccine—A substance prepared from a weakened or killed virus which, when injected, helps the body to form antibodies that will attack an invading virus and may prevent infection altogether.

break in the skin, or contact with the mucous membranes that line the mouth, genitals, and rectum. People cannot get hepatitis B from food or from shaking hands, sneezing or coughing, **breastfeeding**, or casual contact with an infected person.

Symptoms

ACUTE HEPATITIS B. In the United States, a majority of acute HBV infections occur in teenagers and young adults. Half of these youth never develop symptoms, and only about 20%—or one in five infected patients—develop severe symptoms and yellowing of the skin (jaundice). Jaundice occurs when the infected liver is unable to get rid of certain colored substances, or pigments, as it normally does. The remaining 30% of patients have only "flu-like" symptoms and will probably not even be diagnosed as having hepatitis unless certain blood tests are performed.

The most commom symptoms of acute hepatitis B are loss of appetite, **nausea**, generally feeling poorly, and pain or tenderness in the right upper part of the abdomen (where the liver is located). Compared to patients with **hepatitis A** or C, those with HBV infection are less able to continue their usual activities and require more time resting in bed.

Occasionally patients with HBV infection will develop joint swelling and pain (arthritis), as well as **hives** or a skin rash before jaundice appears. The joint symptoms usually last no longer than three to seven days.

Typically the symptoms of acute hepatitis B do not persist longer than two or three months. If they continue for four months, the patient has an abnormally long-lasting acute infection. In a small number of patients—probably fewer than 3%—the infection keeps getting worse as the liver cells die off. Jaundice deepens, and patients may bleed easily when the levels of coagulation factors (normally made by the liver) decrease. Large amounts of fluid collect in the abdomen and beneath the skin (**edema**).

A few people (less than 1% of patients) develop a severe form of hepatitis B known as fulminant hepatitis. This form of the disease appears rapidly and can cause death if not treated at once. Its symptoms include:

- Sudden collapse
- Mental confusion, hallucinations, or extreme sleepiness
- Jaundice
- Noticeable swelling of the abdomen

CHRONIC HEPATITIS B. HBV infection lasting longer than six months is said to be chronic. After this time it is much less likely that the infection will disappear. Most infants infected with HBV at birth and many children infected between 1 and 5 years of age become chronically infected. Not all carriers of the virus develop chronic liver disease; in fact, a majority of carriers have no symptoms. About one in every four HBV carriers, however, develops liver disease that gets worse over time as the liver becomes more and more scarred and less able to carry out its normal functions. The hepatitis B virus accounts for 5–10% of cases of chronic end-stage liver disease in the United States. A badly scarred liver is called cirrhosis. Patients are likely to have an enlarged liver and spleen, as well as tiny clusters of abnormal blood vessels in the skin that resemble spiders.

The most serious complication of chronic HBV infection is liver **cancer**. Worldwide this is the most common cancer to occur in men. Nevertheless, the overall chance that liver cancer will develop at any time in a patient's life is probably much lower than 10%. Patients with chronic hepatitis B who drink or smoke are more likely to develop liver cancer. It is not unusual for a person to simultaneously have HBV infection and infection by HIV (human **immunodeficiency** virus, the cause of **AIDS**). One study reported that men infected with both HIV and HBV were more likely to die from liver disease than people infected with just one of the diseases.

Diagnosis

Hepatitis B is diagnosed by one or more blood tests, since patients may not have any apparent symptoms. In a number of cases, the person is diagnosed following a routine blood test given as part of an annual health checkup. The most common clue is abnormal liver function results.

Examination

Many patients infected with hepatitis B will not have any visible symptoms during a routine office examination. In some cases, however, the doctor may observe swelling or tenderness in the right upper quadrant of the patient's abdomen; enlargement of the spleen; a low-grade **fever**; reddening of the palms of the hands; and signs of jaundice. If the disease has progressed to cirrhosis, the doctor may be able to detect the presence of fluid in the abdomen.

Tests

To confirm the diagnosis of hepatitis B, the doctor will take one or more blood samples for testing:

- A test of the patient's liver function, if this has not already been done.
- Tests for antibodies to the hepatitis B virus. A positive result means that the person has either been effectively vaccinated against HBV or has been infected at some point in the past and has recovered.
- Tests for the surface antigen of the hepatitis B virus (HBsAg). The surface antigen is the outer coating of the virus. A positive HBsAg test means that the patient is currently infected and can pass on the virus to others.
- Hepatitis B DNA test. This blood test measures the levels of virus in the patient's blood.

Procedures

Patients with chronic active hepatitis B may be given a computed tomography (CT) scan or ultrasound imaging of the liver to see whether the liver has been damaged by the infection. The doctor may also perform a **liver biopsy**. This test involves inserting a long hollow needle into the patient's liver through the abdomen and withdrawing a small amount of tissue for examination under a microscope.

Treatment

Traditional

There are few treatment options for chronic hepatitis B. If the patient has no symptoms and little sign of liver damage, the doctor may suggest monitoring the levels of HBV in the patient's blood periodically rather than starting drug treatment right away.

If the patient develops fulminant hepatitis B or their liver is otherwise severely damaged by HBV, the only option is a liver transplant. This is a serious operation with a lengthy recovery period; its success also depends on finding a suitable donor liver.

Drugs

Patients who know that they have been exposed to the hepatitis B virus can be treated by administering three shots of the HBV vaccine to prevent them from developing an active infection. Those who have already developed symptoms of the acute form of the disease may be given intravenous fluids to prevent **dehydration** or antinausea medications to stop **vomiting**. There is no medication as of late 2009 that can prevent acute hepatitis B from becoming chronic once the symptoms begin.

There are seven different drugs approved in the United States to treat chronic hepatitis B in adults as of 2009, but they do not work in all patients and may produce severe side effects. These drugs include adefovir dipivoxil (Hepsera), alpha interferon (Intron A), pegylated interferon (Pegasys), entecavir (Baraclude), telbivudine (Telzeka), tenofovir (Viread), and lamivudine (Zeffix or Epivir-HBV). The two interferons are given by injection; the other five drugs are taken by mouth in pill form once a day. Most doctors will wait until the patient's liver function begins to worsen before administering these drugs. The drugs do not cure the infection; what they do is lower the patient's risk of severe liver damage by slowing or preventing the hepatitis B virus from reproducing further.

The only drugs approved as of 2009 for treating chronic hepatitis B in children are alpha interferon (Intron A) and lamivudine (Zeffix or Epivir-HBV).

Alternative

There are no alternative or complementary therapies that are definitely known to be useful in treating or preventing hepatitis B. One herbal remedy, milk thistle (*Silybum marianum*), has been recommended by some alternative practitioners as beneficial to liver function and as a treatment for cirrhosis and viral hepatitis. The seeds of the plant are used to make capsules, extracts, and herbal teas to be taken by mouth.

Several studies have been done on the benefits of milk thistle; however, the studies are of uneven quality and the findings inconclusive as of 2009. The only major side effects of milk thistle are headaches and mild gastrointestinal upset (**diarrhea**, laxative effect, and nausea). While milk thistle is not known to be harmful, patients diagnosed with hepatitis B who wish to try this herb should consult their doctor first.

Prognosis

Each year an estimated 150,000 persons in the United States get hepatitis B. More than 10,000 will require hospital care, and as many as 5,000 will eventually die from complications of the infection. About 90% of all those infected will have acute disease only. It is the remaining 10% with chronic infection who account for most serious complications and deaths from HBV infection. Even when no symptoms of liver disease develop, chronic carriers remain a threat to others by serving as a source of infection.

Patients with acute hepatitis B usually recover; the symptoms go away in 2–3 weeks, and the liver itself returns to normal in about 4 months. Other patients have a longer period of illness with very slow improvement. The course of chronic HBV infection in any particular patient is unpredictable. Some patients who do well at first may later develop serious complications. Chronic hepatitis leads to an increased risk of cirrhosis and liver cancer, and eventual death in about 1 percent of cases.

Prevention

Hepatitis B can be prevented by vaccination with a vaccine called Engerix-B. An adult patient is given the first two doses of the vaccine a month apart and the third dose 6 months later. The vaccine is recommended for all persons under the age of 20; it can be given to newborns and infants as part of their regular vaccination series. Children usually receive the first vaccine between birth and two months of age, the second shot at one to four months, and the third at 6 to 18 months. The vaccine is generally required for all children born on or after January 1, 1992, before they enter school. The vaccine is available for older children who may have not been immunized before 1992 and is recommended to be given before age 11 or 12.

Others who should be vaccinated include health care workers, military personnel, firefighters and police, people who travel frequently to countries with high rates of hepatitis B, people with **hemophilia**, people who must be treated for **kidney disease**, people who inject illegal drugs, and men who have sex with men. A study published in 2009 reported that the immunity conferred by the vaccine lasts for at least 22 years.

Other preventive measures include:

- Practicing safe sex
- Not sharing needles, razors, toothbrushes, or any other personal item that might have blood on it
- Avoiding getting a tattoo or body piercing, as some people who perform these procedures do not sterilize their needles and other equipment properly
- Getting tested for HBV infection if pregnant, as the virus can be transmitted from a mother to her unborn baby
- Consulting a doctor before taking an extended trip to any country with high rates of hepatitis B.
- Carefully disinfecting any bloodstained surface or material with a mixture of chlorine bleach and water

Resources

BOOKS

Feigin, Ralph D., et al, eds. *Feigin and Cherry's Textbook of Pediatric Infectious Diseases*, 6th ed. Philadelphia, PA : Saunders/Elsevier, 2009.

Freedman, Jeri. *Hepatitis B*. New York: Rosen Publishing, 2009.

Mathet, Veronica B. *Genetic Diversity and Variability of Hepatitis B virus (HBV)*. New York: Nova Science Publishers, 2009.

Richman, Douglas D., Richard J. Whitley, and Frederick G. Hayden, eds. *Clinical Virology*, 3rd ed. Washington, DC: ASM Press, 2009.

Wilt, Timothy J., et al. *Management of Chronic Hepatitis B*. Rockville, MD: U.S. Department of Health and Human Services, Agency for Healthcare Research and Quality, 2008.

Younossi, Zobair M., ed. *Practical Management of Liver Diseases*. New York: Cambridge University Press, 2008.

PERIODICALS

Bertoletti, A., and A. Gehring. "Therapeutic Vaccination and Novel Strategies to Treat Chronic HBV Infection." *Expert Review of Gastroenterology and Hepatology* 3 (October 2009): 561–69.

Carey, I., and P.M. Harrison. "Monotherapy Versus Combination Therapy for the Treatment of Chronic Hepa titis B." *Expert Opinion on Investigational Drugs* 18 (November 2009): 1655–66.

Degertekin, B., and A.S. Lok. "Update on Viral Hepatitis: 2008." *Current Opinion in Gastroenterology* 25 (May 2009): 180–85.

Jones, J., et al. "Adefovir Dipivoxil and Pegylated Interferon-alpha for the Treatment of Chronic Hepatitis B: An Updated Systematic Review and Economic Evalu ation." *Health Technology Assessment* 13 (July 2009): 1–172.

Kim, H.N., et al. "Hepatitis B Vaccination in HIV-infected Adults: Current evidence, Recommendations and Practical Considerations." *International Journal of STD and AIDS* 20 (September 2009): 595–600.

Lim, S.G., et al. "Prevention of Hepatocellular Carcinoma in Hepatitis B Virus Infection." *Journal of Gastroenterology and Hepatology* 24 (August 2009): 1352–57.

Lugoboni, F., et al. "Bloodborne Viral Hepatitis Infections among Drug Users: The Role of Vaccination." *International Journal of Environmental Research and Public Health* 6 (January 2009): 400–413.

McMahon, B.J., et al. "Antibody Levels and Protection after Hepatitis B Vaccine: Results of a 22-year Follow-up Study and Response to a Booster Dose." *Journal of Infectious Diseases* 200 (November 1, 2009): 1390–96.

Poynard, T., et al. "Impact of Interferon-alpha Treatment on Liver Fibrosis in Patients with Chronic Hepatitis B: An Overview of Published Trials." *Gastroentérologie clinique et biologique* 33 (October-November 2009): 916–22.

Wong, V.W., and H.L. Chan. "Severe Acute Exacerbation of Chronic Hepatitis B: A Unique Presentation of a Common Disease." *Journal of Gastroenterology and Hepatology* 24 (July 2009): 1179–86.

OTHER

American Liver Foundation. Hepatitis B. http://www.liverfoundation.org/education/info/hepatitisb/.

Centers for Disease Control and Prevention (CDC). Hepatitis B. http://www.cdc.gov/hepatitis/HepatitisB.htm.

Mayo Clinic. Hepatitis B. http://www.mayoclinic.com/health/hepatitis-b/DS00398.

National Center for Complementary and Alternative Med icine (NCCAM). Herbs at a Glance: Milk Thistle. http://nccam.nih.gov/health/milkthistle/ataglance.htm.

National Library of Medicine (NLM). *Hepatitis B.* http://www.nlm. nih.gov/medlineplus/tutorials/hepatitisb/htm/index.htm.

Pyrsopoulos, Nikolaos T., and K. Rajender Reddy. "Hepatitis B." *eMedicine*, June 19, 2009. http://emedicine.medscape.com/article/177632-overview.

ORGANIZATIONS

American College of Gastroenterology (ACG), P.O. Box 342260, Bethesda, MD, 20827-2260, (301) 263-9000, http://www.acg.gi.org/.

American Liver Foundation (ALF), 75 Maiden Lane, Suite 603, New York, NY, 10038, (212) 668-1000, (212) 483-8179, http://www.liverfoundation.org/.

Centers for Disease Control and Prevention (CDC), 1600 Clifton Road, Atlanta, GA, 30333, (800) 232-4636, cdcinfo@cdc.gov, http://www.cdc.gov.

Hepatitis B Foundation, 3805 Old Easton Road, Doylestown, PA, 18902, (215) 489-4900, (215) 489-4313, info@hepb.org, http://www.hepb.org/.

National Institute of Allergy and Infectious Diseases (NIAID), 6610 Rockledge Drive, MSC 6612, Bethesda, MD, 20892-6612, (301) 496-5717, (866) 284-4107, (301) 402-3573, http://www3.niaid.nih.gov.

World Health Organization (WHO), Avenue Appia 20, 1211 Geneva 27, Switzerland, + 41 22 791 21 11, + 41 22 791 31 11, info@who.int, http://www.who.int/en/.

David A. Cramer, MD
Monique Laberge, PhD
Rebecca J. Frey, PhD

Hepatitis C

Definition

Hepatitis C infection is an inflammatory disease of the liver caused by the hepatitis C virus or HCV. The virus is most commonly transmitted from person to person through contaminated blood. It is sometimes called non-A non-B hepatitis.

Demographics

Hepatitis C is the major source of chronic liver infection in North America; it accounts for about 15 percent of cases of acute viral hepatitis, 60 to 70 percent of cases of chronic hepatitis, and up to 50 percent of cases of **cirrhosis**, end-stage **liver disease**, and **liver cancer**. There are approximately 20,000–30,000 new infections and 8,000–10,000 deaths from hepatitis C each year in the United States. It is estimated that 4 million persons in the United States have been infected by the virus and 3.2 million of these have the chronic form of the infection as of 2009. HCV infection presently accounts for 40 percent of referrals to liver clinics. The cost of treating hepatitis C in the United States is estimated to be more than $600 million a year.

Hepatitis C is more common among Hispanics and African Americans than among Caucasians, Asian Americans, or Native Americans. In terms of age groups, 65 percent of persons with HCV infection are between the ages of 30 and 49 years. According to the Centers for Disease Control and Prevention (CDC), the rates of hepatitis C infection are highest among people born between 1945 and 1965. Most of these persons were likely infected during the 1970s and 1980s, when rates of hepatitis C in North America were at their peak.

The World Health Organization (WHO) estimates that 170 million individuals worldwide are infected with the hepatitis C virus. The rates vary considerably from country to country, however, from 0.02% of the population in the United Kingdom to 6.5% in Africa to 22% in Egypt.

Description

Hepatitis C is an infection that often goes undetected until it has done significant damage to a patient's liver. The infection is divided into two phases, an acute phase (the first six months) and a chronic phase (after the first six months). A minority of patients clear the virus from their bodies during the acute phase, but 60–85 percent have a chronic HCV infection.

People may have no symptoms of illness at all during the acute phase of HCV infection and possibly only a mild flu-like syndrome later. Such symptoms of severe liver damage as **nausea**, **vomiting**, collection of fluid in the abdomen, and mental changes or severe psychiatric disturbances may not develop for 10 or 20 years after the initial infection with the virus.

Risk factors

People who are at increased risk of hepatitis C include:

- Those who abuse intravenous drugs (60 percent of new cases)
- People who use any form of cocaine, including non-injected (smoked or snorted) cocaine
- People who have unprotected sex with a large number of partners
- People who require hemodialysis for kidney disorders
- People who need frequent blood transfusions
- People who received clotting factor concentrates made before 1987
- Children born to mothers with hepatitis C
- People who are HIV-positive (about 25% of HIV-positive patients in North America are also infected with hepatitis C)
- Health care workers who may get needlestick injuries

There have been several notorious cases of hepatitis C transmission in healthcare settings when syringes, other injectable medications, or intravenous solutions were mishandled and became contaminated. In 2000–2001, there was an outbreak of HCV infection in Nebraska that affected almost a hundred patients at a **cancer** clinic. A physician's wife who began treatment for **breast cancer** at the clinic in 2001 was surprised to find out in 2002 that she was infected with hepatitis C. Her husband discovered on checking his records that several of his patients were also infected; what they had in common was undergoing cancer therapy at the same clinic.

An investigation of the clinic found that the HCV virus had been transmitted to patients through contamination of the saline solution used to cleanse **chemotherapy** equipment. In March 2000, a patient known to have hepatitis C began treatment at the cancer clinic. The clinic nurse used a syringe to rinse the patient's chemotherapy port with saline solution and then used the same syringe to draw more saline from a large common container. In the process, HCV virus was transferred from the infected patient's chemotherapy port to the large container of saline. From there the virus was transmitted to other patients via the saline solution and repeated use of other contaminated syringes.

Causes and symptoms

Causes

Hepatitis C is caused by the HCV virus, which is a spherical, single-stranded RNA virus belonging to the family Flaviviridae. HCV is most often transmitted from one person to another through infected blood or blood products, but it can also be transmitted from mother to child during **childbirth** or through sexual intercourse. Before 1992, the virus was sometimes transmitted through blood transfusions, hemodialysis, or transplanted organs from infected donors, but these are now rare events. In 1992, researchers invented a new test for checking blood products for HCV; as a result, new infections per year in the United States declined from 240,000 in the 1980s to about 20,000–30,000 per year as of 2009. The most common cause of HCV transmission at present is intravenous drug use; transfusion-related cases of hepatitis C now occur only once in every 2 million transfused units of blood.

Hepatitis C infection is sometimes divided into an early phase called the acute stage and a later phase called the chronic stage. The acute stage begins when the virus enters the body; it lasts for about six months. Antibodies to the virus can usually be detected between 3 and 12 weeks after infection. About 15–25 percent of people who are infected clear the virus from their bodies during this phase, while the other 75–85 percent go on to develop chronic hepatitis C infection. Doctors do not yet know why some patients clear the virus without treatment and others do not. It is this second

KEY TERMS

Antibody—A substance made by the body in response to a foreign body, such as a virus, which is able to attack and destroy the invading virus.

Ascites—Accumulation of fluid in the abdomen.

Chronic—Recurrent or long-term. Chronic hepatitis C refers to an infection that has lasted longer than 6 months and has not been cleared by the patient's body.

Cirrhosis—Disruption of normal liver function by the formation of scar tissue and nodules in the liver. It is most commonly caused by alcoholism or hepatitis C.

Contamination—The process by which an object or body part becomes exposed to an infectious agent such as a virus.

Genotype—The genetic makeup of a cell or organism. There are six genotypes of the virus that causes hepatitis C.

Hepatitis—Inflammation of the liver. It can be caused by toxic substances or alcohol as well as infections.

Jaundice—A yellowish discoloration of the skin and whites of the eyes caused by increased levels of bile pigments from the liver in the patient's blood.

Relapse—A temporary recurrence of the symptoms of a disease.

group of patients who run the risk of suffering cirrhosis or other forms of liver or kidney damage years later.

Symptoms

Eighty percent of patients infected by the hepatitis C virus in its early stage do not have any symptoms, or have mild and nonspecific symptoms like **fatigue**. In patients who do develop symptoms, the average time period from exposure to symptom onset is 4–12 weeks, although some feel sick in as little as two weeks after exposure. Others have a flu-like syndrome marked by poor appetite or nausea, soreness in the area of the abdomen over the liver, or pains in the joints and muscles. Some may notice that their urine is darker than normal and looks like tea or cola.

If chronic HCV infection leads to liver disease 10–20 years later, the patient may have the following symptoms:

- Severe loss of appetite
- Nausea and vomiting, with blood in the vomit
- Low-grade fever
- Itchy skin
- Jaundice. This is a yellowish discoloration of the whites of the eyes and the skin caused by an increase in the amount of bile pigments from the liver in the patient's blood.
- Sleep disturbances
- Swelling of the abdomen caused by fluid retention
- Diarrhea
- Clay-colored stools
- Difficulty urinating
- Confusion, hallucinations, difficulty concentrating, or other mental disturbances

Diagnosis

The diagnosis of hepatitis C infection is often delayed for years because many patients with chronic HCV infection do not have noticeable or troublesome symptoms until damage to the liver has already occurred. In some cases a person with chronic hepatitis C is detected through routine blood testing for abnormal liver function or because they have a history of intravenous drug **abuse**, organ transplantation, hemodialysis treatment, or HIV infection. The diagnosis is based on a combination of the patient's history and the results of blood tests.

Examination

Many patients infected with hepatitis C will not have any visible symptoms during a routine office examination. In some cases, however, the doctor may observe swelling or tenderness in the right upper quadrant of the patient's abdomen; enlargement of the spleen; signs of **jaundice**; scratches or abrasions on the skin; swollen ankles; and evidence of muscle wasting. The doctor may also be able to detect the presence of fluid in the patient's abdomen (**ascites**).

Tests

Testing for chronic HCV infection begins with blood tests that indicate the presence of antibodies to the hepatitis C virus. Since antibody tests cannot tell whether the person is currently infected, however, a second blood test that looks for the virus's characteristic RNA is performed.

If the results are positive for both tests, the doctor will order a third blood test that determines the virus's specific genotype or genetic makeup. There are six known genotypes of the HCV virus as of 2009, and more than 50 subtypes have been identified. Knowing which type is involved helps to guide the patient's treatment. The most common HCV genotype in patients in North America is genotype 1, found in 75% of patients diagnosed with chronic hepatitis C. Unfortunately, this genotype is less responsive to therapy than the others. Genotype 1 also may be associated with more severe liver disease and a higher risk of liver cancer.

Genotypes 1 and 2 are found worldwide whereas the others are limited to specific geographical regions. Genotype 3 is found in Australia, India, and Thailand. Genotype 4 is the most common HCV genotype in Egypt and the Middle East. Genotype 5 is found in South Africa, while genotype 6 is more common in Southeast Asia, particularly in Hong Kong, Macao, and Vietnam.

Other tests that are performed to guide treatment and monitor the effects of the drugs used to treat hepatitis C include a **complete blood count** (CBC); **liver function tests**; screening for co-infection with HIV or **hepatitis B**; and screening for alcohol and drug abuse.

Procedures

To determine the extent of damage to the patient's liver, the doctor may order a **liver biopsy**. In this procedure, a needle is inserted into the patient's liver through the abdomen in order to remove a small sample of tissue for analysis.

The doctor may also order an ultrasound of the liver. Other imaging studies are not particularly useful in diagnosing hepatitis C.

Treatment

Traditional

The goals of treatment for hepatitis C are 1) to achieve persistent absence of HCV RNA in the patient's blood six months and longer after the end of drug therapy; and 2) prevent the disease from progressing to cirrhosis and liver cancer.

Drugs

The first line of treatment in hepatitis C is two medications known as Intron A, a drug that resembles the antibodies that the body makes naturally to fight viruses; and Virazole, which is an antiviral drug. The combination of these drugs works better than Intron A alone. Intron A is given as a shot once a week and Virazole is taken as a pill twice a day. The length of treatment depends on the genotype of the HCV virus; patients with genotype 2 and 3 are treated for 24 weeks whereas patients with genotypes 1 or 4 must undergo 48 weeks of treatment. The cure rates for genotypes 1 and 3 are between 60 and 75 percent; the cure rate for genotype 1 is 50 percent and for genotype 4, 65 percent. Unfortunately, Intron A and Virazole produce unpleasant side effects for patients that range from depression and irritability to weight loss, nausea, and muscle pains. In addition to side effects in adult patients, Virazole cannot be given at all to pregnant women because it can harm the unborn child. In rare cases, patients treated with Intron A for hepatitis C have had psychotic episodes.

Combination therapy with these drugs is not recommended for patients who have already developed cirrhosis due to hepatitis C, or for patients who have received kidney, liver, or heart transplants. Other patients who should not be given these drugs include those with lupus or other autoimmune diseases; severe psychiatric disorders; **coronary artery disease**; inability to practice birth control; and active alcohol or **substance abuse**.

Patients treated for hepatitis C are monitored for levels of HCV RNA in their blood during treatment, usually at the 12-week mark; at the completion of therapy; and six months after the completion of therapy. If the patient has a detectable level of HCV RNA at this point, they are considered to have a relapse. There are few treatment options for patients who do not respond to drug therapy or have a relapse as of 2009.

Surgery

The only treatment for cirrhosis or severe liver disease as of 2009 is **liver transplantation**. Chronic HCV infection, in fact, is the leading indication for liver transplants in the United States. The problem, however, is that there are many more patients waiting for donated livers than there are suitable organs available. In addition, liver transplantation does not cure HCV infection; most people who receive transplanted livers will develop a recurrence of the virus. About 30% of recipients die, develop cirrhosis, or have the transplanted liver fail within five years of surgery, with the rate of failure increasing with each year of follow-up. The effectiveness of medication treatment of hepatitis C following a liver transplant is unclear as of 2009.

Patients with chronic hepatitis C should stop drinking alcohol, as even small amounts can speed up the rate of liver damage. They should also be vaccinated against **hepatitis A** and hepatitis B.

Prognosis

The prognosis of hepatitis C is guarded for most patients. The **antiviral drugs** presently used to treat the infection cure only about 60% of patients. According to the CDC, between 75 and 85 percent of people infected with HCV will develop chronic HCV infection, and 60–70 percent will develop some form of chronic liver disease. Twenty percent of these chronically infected persons will develop cirrhosis of the liver within 20 years of infection; 1–5 percent of chronically infected people will eventually die of liver disease.

Women with chronic hepatitis C have better outcomes than men, and patients infected at younger ages have better outcomes than those infected in middle age. The reason for these differences is not clear as of 2009.

A small percentage of patients with hepatitis C develop medical conditions that are not related to the liver. It is thought that these conditions result from the body's immune response to the HCV virus. These conditions include **diabetes mellitus**; skin **rashes**; inflammation of the kidney (**glomerulonephritis**); non-Hodgkin lymphoma; and essential mixed cryoglobulinemia, a condition marked by the presence of abnormal proteins in the blood.

Prevention

There is no vaccine that can prevent hepatitis C infection as of 2009, and there is no treatment that can prevent someone who recovered from one genotype of the virus from contracting a different genotype. Prevention depends on careful observation of good health practices in hospitals and clinics, and on individual lifestyle changes. The CDC recommends the following ways that individuals can lower their risk of getting hepatitis C:

- Do not use intravenous drugs. People who cannot quit should never share their needles, syringes, water, or other materials used to inject drugs. They should also get vaccinated against hepatitis A and hepatitis B.
- Do not share personal items (razors, toothbrushes, nail clippers, etc.) that might have blood on them.
- Avoid getting tattoos or body piercing. People who do get a tattoo, however, should at least make sure that the operator who performs the tattoo is using proper sterile procedure.
- Use latex condoms when having sex. Although it is rare for hepatitis C to be transmitted through sexual intercourse, it can happen.
- People who discover that they are infected with hepatitis C should not donate blood, organs, or tissues.
- Health care personnel must take special precautions when performing or assisting with surgical or dental procedures on patients with hepatitis C.

Resources

BOOKS

Everson, Gregory T., and Hedy Weinberg. *Living with Hepatitis C: A Survivor's Guide*, 5th ed. New York: Hatherleigh, 2009.

Fabry, Stephen, and R. Anand Narasimhan. *100 Questions and Answers about Hepatitis C: A Lahey Clinic Guide*. Sudbury, MA: Jones and Bartlett Publishers, 2006.

Lawford, Christopher K., and Diana Sylvestre. *Healing Hepatitis C*. New York: Harper, 2009.

McKnight, Evelyn V. *A Never Event: The Story of the Largest American Outbreak of Hepatitis C in History*. New York: Arbor Books, 2008.

Tang, Hengli, ed. *Hepatitis C: Methods and Protocols*, 2nd ed. Totowa, NJ: Humana Press, 2009.

Younossi, Zobair M., ed. *Practical Management of Liver Diseases*. New York: Cambridge University Press, 2008.

PERIODICALS

Asthana, S., and N. Kneteman. "Operating on a Patient with Hepatitis C." *Canadian Journal of Surgery* 52 (August 2009): 337–342.

Cheng, Y., et al. "Prolonged Psychosis Associated with Interferon Therapy in a Patient with Hepatitis C: Case Study and Literature Review." *Psychosomatics* 50 (September-October 2009): 538–42.

Degertekin, B., and A.S. Lok. "Update on Viral Hepatitis: 2008." *Current Opinion in Gastroenterology* 25 (May 2009): 180–85.

Foster, G. R. "Quality of Life Considerations for Patients with Chronic Hepatitis C." *Journal of Viral Hepatitis* 16 (September 2009): 605–11.

Garg, G., and P. Kar. "Management of HCV Infection: Current Issues and Future Options." *Tropical Gastroenterology* 30 (January-March 2009): 11–18.

Houghton, M. "The Long and Winding Road Leading to the Identification of the Hepatitis C Virus." *Journal of Hepatology* 51 (November 2009): 939–48.

Singal, A.K., and B.S. Anand. "Management of Hepatitis C Virus Infection in HIV/HCV Co-infected Patients: Clinical Review." *World Journal of Gastroenterology* 15 (August 14, 2009): 3713–3724.

Sockalingam, S., and S.E. Abbey. "Managing Depression during Hepatitis C Treatment." *Canadian Journal of Psychiatry* 54 (September 2009): 614–25.

Vogel, M., et al. " Treatment of Acute Hepatitis C in HIV-Positive Individuals: What Are the Challenges?" *Journal of HIV Therapy* 14 (March 2009): 8–12.

Watt, K., et al. "A Practical Guide to the Management of HCV Infection following Liver Transplantation." *American Journal of Transplantation* 9 (August 2009): 1707–13.

OTHER

American Association for the Study of Liver Diseases (AASLD). *AASLD Practice Guideline: Diagnosis, Management and Treatment of Hepatitis C*. http://www.aasld.org/practiceguidelines/Practice%20Guideline%

20Archive/Diagnosis,%20Management%20and%20 Treatment% 20of%20Hepatitis%20C.pdf

American Liver Foundation (ALF). *Hepatitis C.* http://www.liverfoundation.org/education/info/ hepatitisc/.

Centers for Disease Control and Prevention (CDC). *Hepatitis C.* http://www.cdc.gov/hepatitis/ ChooseC.htm.

Mayo Clinic. *Hepatitis C.* http://www.mayoclinic.com/ health/hepatitis-c/DS00097.

Mukherjee, Sandeep, and Vinod K. Dhawan. "Hepatitis C." *eMedicine*, June 18, 2009. http://emedicine.medscape. com/article/177792-overview.

National Institute of Diabetes and Digestive and Kidney Diseases (NIDDK). *Chronic Hepatitis C: Current Disease Management.* http://digestive.niddk.nih.gov/ddiseases/pubs/chronichepc/.

ORGANIZATIONS

American Association for the Study of Liver Diseases (AASLD), 1001 North Fairfax, Suite 400, Alexandria, VA, 22314, (703) 299-9766, (703) 299-9622, aasld@ aasld.org, http://www.aasld.org/Pages/ Default.aspx.

American Liver Foundation (ALF), 75 Maiden Lane, Suite 603, New York, NY, 10038, (212) 668-1000, (212) 483-8179, http://www.liverfoundation.org/.

Centers for Disease Control and Prevention (CDC), 1600 Clifton Road, Atlanta, GA, 30333, (800) 232-4636, cdcinfo@cdc.gov, http://www.cdc.gov.

National Institute of Allergy and Infectious Diseases (NIAID), 6610 Rockledge Drive, MSC 6612, Bethesda, MD, 20892-6612, (301) 496-5717, (866) 284-4107, (301) 402-3573, http://www3.niaid.nih.gov.

National Institute of Diabetes and Digestive and Kidney Diseases (NIDDK), Building 31. Rm 9A06, 31 Center Drive, MSC 2560, Bethesda, MD, 20892-2560, (301) 496-3583, http://www2.niddk.nih.gov/Footer/Contact NIDDK.htm, http://www2.niddk.nih.gov/.

World Health Organization (WHO), Avenue Appia 20, 1211 Geneva 27, Switzerland, + 41 22 791 21 11, + 41 22 791 31 11, info@who.int, http://www.who.int/en/.

Rebecca J. Frey, PhD

Hepatitis D

Definition

Hepatitis D (or delta, the Greek letter "D"), is a form of liver inflammation that occurs only in patients who also are infected by the **hepatitis B** virus. Infection by the hepatitis delta virus (HDV) either occurs at the same time as hepatitis B develops or develops later when infection by hepatitis B virus (HBV) has entered the chronic (long-lasting) stage.

Description

Delta hepatitis can be quite severe, but it is seen only in patients already infected by HBV. In the late 1970s, Italian physicians discovered that some patients with hepatitis B had another type of infectious agent in their liver cells. Later the new virus—HDV—was confirmed by experimentally infecting chimpanzees. When both viruses are present, acute infection tends to be more severe. Furthermore, patients with both infections are more likely than those with HBV alone to develop chronic **liver disease**, and, when it occurs, it is more severe.

About 300 million persons worldwide carry HBV. Of them, at least 5% probably also have delta hepatitis. In North America HDV infection appears to be less frequent: 4% of all patients with acute hepatitis B have HDV infection. The delta virus causes an estimated 2% of all cases of acute viral hepatitis in the United States. The rate of HDV infection varies widely in different parts of the world; it is a very serious infection in some countries and quite mild in others. Chronic delta hepatitis is a more serious disease than either chronic hepatitis B alone or **hepatitis C**.

Certain individuals—the same ones who are at increased risk of developing hepatitis B—are the prime candidates to be infected by HDV. For example:

- Not infrequently, HDV infection occurs in patients with chronic HBV infection who also have hemophilia, a bleeding disease. These patients are at risk because they require large amounts of transfused blood and blood products that may contain HDV.
- In some areas, one-fourth to one-half of patients with chronic HBV infection who inject themselves with illicit drugs become infected by HDV as well. Drug abusers who share contaminated needles are likely to infect one another.
- Patients who get HBV infection by sexual contact may also be infected by HDV, although the delta virus is less often spread in this way than is HBV itself. Between 10–25% of homosexual men with chronic HBV infection harbor the delta virus.
- Like hepatitis B, HDV infection may develop in health-care workers who are victims of a needle stick, and it also can be spread within households when personal items such as a razor or toothbrush are shared.

Causes and symptoms

The delta virus is a small and incomplete viral particle. Perhaps this is why it cannot cause infection

KEY TERMS

Alpha-interferon—A natural body substance that now can be made in large quantities and is an effective treatment for some types of viral inflammatory disease, including hepatitis C.

Antibody—A substance formed in the body in response to an invading microorganism, such as a virus, which can attack and destroy the invading virus.

Coinfection—Invasion of the body by two viruses at about the same time.

Hemophilia—A bleeding disease that may call for the transfusion of large amounts of blood and blood products.

Superinfection—Infection by a second virus after a previous infection by a different virus has become well established.

on its own. Its companion virus, HBV, actually forms a covering over the HDV particle. In chronically ill patients (those whose virus persists longer than six months), the combined viruses cause inflammation throughout the liver and eventually destroy the liver cells, which are then replaced by scar tissue. This scarring is called **cirrhosis**.

When HBV and HDV infections develop at the same time, a condition called coinfection, recovery is the rule. Only 2–5% of patients become chronic carriers (have the virus remain in their blood more than six months after infection). It may be that HDV actually keeps HBV from reproducing as rapidly as it would if it were alone, so chronic infection is less likely.

When HBV infection occurs first and is followed by HDV infection, the condition is called superinfection. This is a more serious situation. Between half and two-thirds of patients with superinfection develop severe acute hepatitis. Once the liver cells contain large numbers of HBV viruses, HDV tends to reproduce more actively. Massive infection and liver failure are more common in superinfection. The risk of **liver cancer**, however, is no greater than from hepatitis B alone.

As with other forms of hepatitis, the earliest symptoms are **nausea**, loss of appetite, joint pains, and tiredness. There may be **fever** (not marked), and an enlarged liver may cause discomfort or actual **pain** in the right upper part of the abdomen. Later, **jaundice** (a yellowing of the skin and whites of the eyes that occurs when the liver is no longer able to eliminate certain pigmented substances) may develop.

Diagnosis

HDV infection may be diagnosed by detecting the antibody against the virus. Unfortunately this test cannot detect acute coinfection or superinfection as early as when symptoms first develop. Antibody against HDV usually is found no sooner than 30 days after symptoms appear. Until recently, the virus itself could only be identified by testing a small sample of liver tissue. Scientists now are developing a blood test for HDV that should make diagnosis faster and easier. When HDV is present, liver enzymes (proteins made by the liver) are present in abnormally high amounts. In some patients with coinfection, the enzyme levels peak twice, once when HBV infection starts and again at the time of HDV infection.

Treatment

As in any form of hepatitis, patients in the acute stage should rest in bed as needed, eat a balanced diet, and avoid alcohol. Alpha-interferon, the natural body substance which helps control hepatitis C, has generally not been found helpful in treating hepatitis D. If the liver is largely destroyed and has stopped functioning, **liver transplantation** is an option. Even when the procedure is successful, the disease often recurs and cirrhosis may actually develop more rapidly than before.

Prognosis

A large majority of patients with coinfection of HBV and HDV recover from an episode of acute hepatitis. However, about two-thirds of patients chronically infected by HDV go on to develop cirrhosis of the liver. In one long-term study, just over half of patients who became carriers of HDV had moderate or severe liver disease, and one-fourth of them died. If very severe liver failure develops, the chance of a patient surviving is no better than 50%. A liver transplant may improve this figure to 70%. When transplantation is done for cirrhosis, rather than for liver failure, nearly 90% of patients live five years or longer. The major concern with transplantation is infection of the transplanted liver; this may occur in as many as 40% of transplant patients.

When a child with viral hepatitis develops cirrhosis, HDV infection is commonly responsible. A woman who develops delta hepatitis while pregnant will do as well as if she were not pregnant, and there is no increased risk that the newborn will be malformed in any way.

Prevention

The vaccine against hepatitis B also prevents delta hepatitis, since it cannot occur unless HBV infection is present. Hopefully, a vaccine can be developed that will keep delta infection from developing in chronic HBV carriers. However, if a person already has HBV infection, any exposure to blood should be strictly avoided. A high level of sexual activity with multiple partners is also a risk factor for delta hepatitis.

ORGANIZATIONS

American Liver Foundation, 75 Maiden Lane, Suite 603, New York, NY, 10038, (212) 668-1000, (212) 483-8179, http://www.liverfoundation.org/.

David A. Cramer, MD

Hepatitis, drug-induced

Definition

Inflammation of the liver due to an adverse reaction with a drug.

Description

The liver is a very important organ to the body. It is a large internal organ weighing more than three pounds in the average adult. It performs over 100 functions including formation of bile; **detoxification** of harmful substances; vitamin storage; and metabolism of carbohydrates, fats, and proteins. Serious complications could arise when the liver becomes inflamed due to hepatitis when it is not able to perform these tasks. A virus most often causes hepatitis but certain drugs can also induce it.

Drug-induced hepatitis (also called toxic hepatitis) occurs in eight in every 10,000 people because the liver reacts abnormally during drug exposure, leading to liver damage. This pathology causes the liver not to function properly and the symptoms can begin to be seen. Women tend to be affected almost twice as often as men. Older people are more prone to this type of hepatitis because their bodies aren't able to repair themselves as fast as younger people. Drugs that can be associated with drug-induced hepatitis include **acetaminophen**, vitamin A, and PTU (a drug treatment for **tuberculosis**).

Causes and symptoms

There are three general types of drug-induced hepatitis: toxic, metabolic idiosyncrasy, and immunologic idiosyncrasy. With toxic hepatitis liver damage as the result of a drug complication with hepatotoxins happens to everyone who takes that particular drug. On the other hand, hepatitis resulting from a metabolic or immunologic idiosyncrasy only happens to certain people, those predisposed to particular idiosyncrasy.

In patients with a metabolic idiosyncrasy the person metabolizes the drug differently than most people causing a harmful by-product that damages the liver. A metabolic idiosyncrasy is seen in 0.1-2% of people and it is complicated by use of alcohol.

With an immunologic idiosyncrasy the patient's body recognizes the metabolized drug by-products as foreign. This leads to the destruction of liver cells containing the by-product via the immune system resulting in hepatitis. An immunologic idiosyncrasy is seen in less than one person per 10,000 (0.01%) people and is more than twice as common in women.

The symptoms of drug-induced hepatitis are similar to viral hepatitis. Drug induced hepatitis tends to be acute. If it is not caught soon enough the damage could be permanent resulting in chronic hepatitis. Some of the common symptoms are:

- nausea
- vomiting
- headache
- anorexia
- jaundice
- clay color stools
- dark urine
- hepatomegaly

Diagnosis

Diagnosis is typically made through a physical exam along with a patient history to identify any possible hepatotoxins. Blood tests are usually done as well. An increased **white blood cell count** is typical.

Treatment

There isn't any specific treatment other than immediate discontinuance of the causative agent. Rest

KEY TERMS

Hepatitis—General inflammation of the liver.

Hepatomegaly—General swelling of the liver.

Hepatotoxin—A substance that is toxic to the liver.

Idiosyncrasy—A defect in that particular pathway resulting in an abnormality.

during the acute phase of the disease is vital along with the intake of fluids to maintain hydration.

Prognosis

Usually the symptoms will go away after the drug has been eliminated due to the liver repairing itself. A full recovery is typically expected unless it wasn't treated quickly resulting in more liver damage being done than normal.

Prevention

If there is a history of liver damage certain medications should not be taken. Doctors will be familiar with these.

Resources

BOOKS

Sleisenger, Marvin H., et al. *Sleisenger & Fordtran's Gastrointestinal and Liver Disease: Pathophysiology, Diagnosis, Management*. St. Louis, MO: MD Consult, 2009.

Thomas Scott Eagan
Ronald Watson, PhD

Hepatitis E

Definition

The hepatitis E virus (HEV) is a common cause of hepatitis that is transmitted via the intestinal tract, and is not caused by the **hepatitis A** virus. Spread most often by contaminated drinking water, HEV infection occurs mainly in developing countries.

Description

Hepatitis E is also known as epidemic non-A, non-B hepatitis. Like hepatitis A, it is an acute and short-lived illness that can sometimes cause liver failure. HEV, discovered in 1987, is spread by the fecal-oral route. It is constantly present (endemic) in countries where human waste is allowed to get into drinking water without first being purified. Large outbreaks (epidemics) have occurred in Asian and South American countries where there is poor sanitation. In the United States and Canada no outbreaks have been reported, but persons traveling to an endemic region may return with HEV.

Causes and symptoms

There are at least two strains of HEV, one found in Asia and another in Mexico. The virus may start dividing in the gastrointestinal tract, but it grows mostly in the liver. After an incubation period (the time from when a person is first infected by a virus until the appearance of the earliest symptoms) of two to eight weeks, infected persons develop a **fever**, may feel nauseous, lose their appetite, and often have discomfort or actual **pain** in the right upper part of the abdomen where the liver is located. Some develop yellowing of the skin and the whites of the eyes (**jaundice**). Most often the illness is mild and disappears within a few weeks with no lasting effects. Children younger than 14 years and persons over age 50 seldom have jaundice or show other clinical signs of hepatitis.

Hepatitis E never becomes a chronic (long-lasting) illness, but on rare occasions the acute illness damages and destroys so many liver cells that the liver can no longer function. This is called fulminant liver failure and may cause **death**. Pregnant women are at much higher risk of dying from fulminant liver failure; this increased risk is not true of any other type of viral hepatitis. The great majority of patients who recover from acute infection do not continue to carry HEV and cannot pass on the infection to others.

Diagnosis

HEV can be found by microscopically examining a stool sample, but this is not a reliable test, as the virus often dies when stored for a short time. Like other hepatitis viruses, HEV stimulates the body's immune system to produce a substance called an antibody, which can swallow up and destroy the virus. Blood tests can determine elevated antibody levels, which indicate the presence of HEV virus in the body. Unfortunately, such antibody blood tests are not widely available.

Treatment

There is no way of effectively treating the symptoms of any acute hepatitis, including hepatitis E.

KEY TERMS

Antibody—A substance made by the body's immune system in response to an invading virus, the antibodies then attack and destroy the virus.

Incubation period—The time from when a person is first infected by a virus until the appearance of the earliest symptoms.

Jaundice—Yellowing of the skin that occurs when pigments normally eliminated by the liver collect in high amounts in the blood.

Sanitation—The process of keeping drinking water, foods, or any anything else with which people come into contact free of microorganisms such as viruses.

Vaccine—A substance prepared from a weakened or killed virus which, when injected, stimulates the immune system to produce antibodies that can prevent infection by the natural virus.

During acute infection, a patient should eat a balanced diet and rest in bed as needed.

Prognosis

In the United States hepatitis E is not a fatal illness, but elsewhere about 1–2% of those infected die of advanced liver failure. In pregnant women the death rate is as high as 20%. It is not clear whether having hepatitis E once guarantees against future HEV infection.

Prevention

Most attempts to use blood serum containing HEV antibody to prevent hepatitis in those exposed to HEV have failed. Hopefully, this approach can be made to work so that pregnant women living in endemic areas can be protected. No vaccine is available, though several are being tested. It also is possible that effective anti-viral drugs will be found. The best ways to prevent hepatitis E are to provide safe drinking water and take precautions to use sterilized water and beverages when traveling.

ORGANIZATIONS

American Liver Foundation, 75 Maiden Lane, Suite 603, New York, NY, 10038, (212) 668-1000, (212) 483-8179, http://www.liverfoundation.org/.

David A. Cramer, MD

Hepatitis G

Definition

Hepatitis G is a newly discovered form of liver inflammation caused by hepatitis G virus (HGV), a distant relative of the **hepatitis C** virus.

Description

HGV, also called hepatitis GB virus, was first described early in 1996. Little is known about the frequency of HGV infection, the nature of the illness, or how to prevent it. What is known is that transfused blood containing HGV has caused some cases of hepatitis. For this reason, patients with **hemophilia** and other bleeding conditions who require large amounts of blood or blood products are at risk of hepatitis G. HGV has been identified in between 1–2% of blood donors in the United States. Also at risk are patients with **kidney disease** who have blood exchange by hemodialysis and those who inject drugs into their veins. It is possible that an infected mother can pass on the virus to her newborn infant. Sexual transmission also is a possibility.

Often patients with hepatitis G are infected at the same time by the **hepatitis B** or C virus, or both. In about three of every thousand patients with acute viral hepatitis, HGV is the only virus present. There is some indication that patients with hepatitis G may continue to carry the virus in their blood for many years, and so might be a source of infection in others.

Causes and symptoms

Some researchers believe that there may be a group of GB viruses, rather than just one. Others remain doubtful that HGV actually causes illness. If it does, the type of acute or chronic (long-lasting) illness that results is not clear. When diagnosed, acute HGV infection has usually been mild and brief. There is no evidence of serious complications, but it is possible that, like other hepatitis viruses, HGV can cause severe liver damage resulting in liver failure. The virus has been identified in as many as 20% of patients with long-lasting viral hepatitis, some of whom also have hepatitis C.

Diagnosis

The only method of detecting HGV is a complex and costly DNA test that is not widely available. Efforts are under way, however, to develop a test for the HGV antibody, which is formed in response to invasion by the virus. Once antibody is present,

KEY TERMS

Antibody—A substance made by the body's immune system in response to an invading virus; antibodies then attack and destroy the virus.

Hemophilia—A bleeding disorder that often makes it necessary to give patients dozens or even hundreds of units of blood and blood products over time.

however, the virus itself generally has disappeared, making the test too late to be of use.

Treatment

There is no specific treatment for any form of acute hepatitis. Patients should rest in bed as needed, avoid alcohol, and be sure to eat a balanced diet.

Prognosis

What little is known about the course of hepatitis G suggests that illness is mild and does not last long. When more patients have been followed up after the acute phase, it will become clear whether HGV can cause severe liver damage.

Prevention

Since hepatitis G is a blood-borne infection, prevention relies on avoiding any possible contact with contaminated blood. Drug users should not share needles, syringes, or other equipment.

ORGANIZATIONS

American Liver Foundation, 75 Maiden Lane, Suite 603, New York, NY, 10038, (212) 668-1000, (212) 483-8179, http://www.liverfoundation.org/.

David A. Cramer, MD

Hepatitis virus studies *see* **Hepatitis virus tests**

Hepatitis virus tests

Definition

Viral hepatitis is any type of liver inflammation caused by a viral infection. The three most common viruses now recognized to cause **liver disease** are **hepatitis A**, **hepatitis B**, and hepatitis non-A, non-B (also called **hepatitis C**). Several other types have been recognized: **hepatitis D**, **hepatitis E**, and the recently identified **hepatitis G**. A seventh type (hepatitis F) is suspected but not yet confirmed.

Purpose

The different types of viral hepatitis produce similar symptoms, but they differ in terms of transmission, course of treatment, prognosis, and carrier status. When the clinical history of a patient is insufficient for differentiation, hepatitis virus tests are used as an aid in diagnosis and in monitoring the course of the disease. These tests are based primarily on antigen-antibody reactions—an antigen being a protein foreign to the body, and an antibody another type of protein manufactured by lymphocytes (a type of white blood cell) to neutralize the antigen.

Description

There are five major types of viral hepatitis. The diseases, along with the antigen-antibody tests available to aid in diagnosis, are

Hepatitis A

Commonly called infectious hepatitis, this is caused by the hepatitis A virus (HAV). It is usually a mild disease, most often spread by food and water contamination, but sometimes through sexual contact. Immunologic tests are not commercially available for the HAV antigen, but two types of antibodies to HAV can be detected. IgM antibody (anti-HAV/IgM), appears approximately three to four weeks after exposure and returns to normal within several months. IgG (anti-HAV/IgG) appears approximately two weeks after the IgM begins to increase and remains positive. Acute hepatitis is suspected if IgM is elevated; conversely, if IgG is elevated without IgM, a convalescent stage of HAV is presumed. IgG antibody can remain detectable for decades after infection.

Hepatitis B

Commonly known as serum hepatitis, this is caused by the hepatitis B virus (HBV). The disease can be mild or severe, and it can be acute (of limited duration) or chronic (ongoing). It is usually spread by sexual contact with another infected person, through contact with infected blood, by intravenous drug use, or from mother to child at birth.

HBV, also called the Dane particle, is composed of an inner protein core surrounded by an outer protein capsule. The outer capsule contains the hepatitis B surface antigen (HBsAg), formerly called the Australia antigen. The inner core contains HBV core antigen (HBcAg), and the hepatitis B e-antigen (HBeAg). Antibodies to these antigens are called anti-HBs, anti-HBc, and anti-HBe. Testing for these antigens and antibodies is as follows:

- Hepatitis B surface antigen (HBsAg). This is the first test for hepatitis B to become abnormal. HBsAg begins to elevate before the onset of clinical symptoms, peaks during the first week of symptoms, and usually disappears by the time the accompanying jaundice (yellowing of the skin and other tissues) begins to subside. HBsAg indicates an active HBV infection. A person is considered to be a carrier if this antigen persists in the blood for six or more months.
- Hepatitis B surface antibody (anti-HBs). This appears approximately one month after the disappearance of the HBsAg, signaling the end of the acute infection period. Anti-HBs is the antibody that demonstrates immunity after administration of the hepatitis B vaccine. Its presence also indicates immunity to subsequent infection.
- Hepatitis B core antigen (HBcAg). No tests are commercially available to detect this antigen.
- Hepatitis B core antibody (anti-HBc). This appears just before acute hepatitis develops and remains elevated (although it slowly declines) for years. It is also present in chronic hepatitis. The hepatitis B core antibody is elevated during the time lag between the disappearance of the hepatitis B surface antigen and the appearance of the hepatitis B surface antibody in an interval called the "window." During this time, the hepatitis B core antibody is the only detectable marker of a recent hepatitis B infection.
- Hepatitis B e-antigen (HBeAg). This is more useful as an index of infection than for diagnostic purposes. The presence of this antigen correlates with early and active disease, as well as with high infectivity in patients with acute HBV infection. When HBeAg levels persist in the blood, the development of chronic HBV infection is suspected.
- Hepatitis B e-antibody (anti-HBe). In the bloodstream, this indicates a reduced risk of infectivity in patients who have previously been HBeAg positive. Chronic hepatitis B surface antigen carriers can be positive for either HBeAg or anti-HBe, but are less infectious when anti-HBe is present. Antibody to e antigen can persist for years, but usually disappears earlier than anti-HBs or anti-HBc.

Hepatitis C

Previously known as non-A non-B hepatitis, this disease is primarily caused by the hepatitis C virus (HCV). It is generally mild, but more likely than hepatitis B to lead to chronic liver disease, possible liver failure, and the eventual need for transplant. Chronic carrier states develop in more than 80% of patients, and chronic liver disease is a major problem. As many as 20% of patients with chronic hepatitis C will develop liver failure or **liver cancer**. HCV is spread through sexual contact, as well as through sharing drug needles, although nearly half of infections can't be traced as to origin.

Hepatitis C is detected by HCV serology (tests on blood sera). A specific type of assay called enzyme-linked immunosorbent assay (ELISA) was developed to detect antibody to hepatitis C for diagnostic purposes, as well as for screening blood donors. Most cases of post-transfusion non-A, non-B hepatitis are caused by HCV, but application of this test has virtually eliminated post-transfusion hepatitis. An HCV viral titer to detect HCV RNA in the blood is now available, and recently, IgM anti-HCV core is proving to be a useful acute marker for HCV infection.

Hepatitis D

Also called delta hepatitis, this is caused by the hepatitis D virus (HDV). The disease occurs only in those who have HBV in the blood from a past or simultaneously occurring infection. Experts believe transmission may occur through sexual contact, but further research is needed to confirm that. Most cases occur among those who are frequently exposed to blood and blood products. Many cases also occur among drug users who share contaminated needles. Hepatitis D virus (HDV) antigen can be detected by radioimmunoassay within a few days after infection, together with IgM and total antibodies to HDV.

Hepatitis E

Caused by the hepatitis E virus (HEV), this is actually another type of non-A non-B hepatitis. The virus is most often spread through fecally contaminated water, but the role of person-to-person transmission is unclear. This form of hepatitis is quite rare in the United States. There are currently no antigen or antibody tests widely available to accurately detect HEV.

Preparation

Hepatitis virus tests require a blood sample. It is not necessary for the patient to withhold food or fluids before any of these tests, unless requested to do so by the physician.

Risks

Risks for these tests are minimal for the patient, but may include slight bleeding from the blood-drawing site, **fainting** or feeling lightheaded after venipuncture, or hematoma (blood accumulating under the puncture site).

Normal results

Reference ranges for the antigen/antibody tests are as follows:

- hepatitis A antibody, IgM: Negative
- hepatitis B core antibody: Negative
- hepatitis B e antibody: Negative
- hepatitis B e-antigen: Negative
- hepatitis B surface antibody: Varies with clinical circumstance (Note: As the presence of anti-HBs indicates past infection with resolution of previous hepatitis B infection, or vaccination against hepatitis B, additional patient history may be necessary for diagnosis.)
- hepatitis B surface antigen: Negative
- hepatitis C serology: Negative
- hepatitis D serology: Negative.

Abnormal results

Hepatitis A: A single positive anti-HAV test may indicate previous exposure to the virus, but due to the antibody persisting so long in the bloodstream, only evidence of a rising anti-HAV titer confirms hepatitis A. Determining recent infection rests on identifying the antibody as IgM (associated with recent infection). A negative anti-HAV test rules out hepatitis A.

Hepatitis B: High levels of HBsAg that continue for three or more months after onset of acute infection suggest development of chronic hepatitis or carrier status. Detection of anti-HBs signals late convalescence or recovery from infection. This antibody remains in the blood to provide immunity to reinfection.

Hepatitis C (non-A non-B hepatitis): Anti-HBc develops after exposure to hepatitis B. As an early indicator of acute infection, antibody (IgM) to core antigen (anti-HBc IgM) is rarely detected in chronic infection, so it is useful in distinguishing acute from chronic infection, and hepatitis B from non-A, non-B.

Resources

BOOKS

Pagana, Kathleen Deska, and Timothy J. Pagana. *Mosby's Manual of Diagnostic and Laboratory Tests*. 4th ed. St. Louis: Mosby, 2009.

Janis O. Flores

Hepatobiliary scan *see* **Gallbladder nuclear medicine scan**

Hepatocellular carcinoma *see* **Liver cancer, primary**

Hepatolenticular degeneration *see* **Wilson's disease**

Hepatoma *see* **Liver cancer, primary**

Herbal medicine *see* **Herbalism, western**

Herbalism, traditional Chinese

Definition

Chinese herbalism is one of the major components of **traditional Chinese medicine** (TCM), or Oriental medicine (OM). In TCM, herbs are often used in conjunction with other techniques, such as **acupuncture** or massage. Chinese herbalism is a holistic medical system, meaning that it looks at treating a patient as a whole person, looking at the mental and spiritual health, as well as the physical health, of the individual. Illness is seen as a disharmony or imbalance among these aspects of the individual. Chinese herbalism has been practiced for over 4,000 years.

One of the earliest and certainly the most important Chinese herbal text is the *Huang Ti Nei Ching*, or *Yellow Emperor's Classic of Internal Medicine*. It is believed to be authored by Huang Ti during his reign over China, which started about 2697 B.C. Since that time, herbal practices have been more extensively documented and refined. In modern China, traditional Chinese

Five popular Chinese herbs used in the United States

Herb	Purpose
Astragalus (huang qi)	Builds immune system; offsets side effects of chemotherapy and radiation treatments
Dong quai (dang gui)	Stimulates the production of red blood cells and bone marrow; increases cardiovascular endurance; regulates menstrual disorders
Ginseng (ren shen)	Increases physical stamina; general tonic
Reishi mushroom (ling zhi)	Eliminates toxins; increases physical stamina
Schisandra (wu wei zu)	Prevents fluid loss (e.g., excessive sweating, runny nose, incontinence)

(Table by PreMediaGlobal. Reproduced by permission of Gale, a part of Cengage Learning.)

herbalism is taught alongside conventional Western pharmacology. Chinese herbal remedies have been used in the West only relatively recently, over the past two decades. These remedies are more gentle and natural that conventional medicines. In addition, they have fewer unpleasant side effects. Individuals with chronic disorders in particular are increasingly drawn to the holistic aspect of Chinese herbalism and TCM in general.

Purpose

Because it is a safe, inexpensive solution to health problems of all kinds, Chinese herbalism is very popular in China. In recent years, herbalism has been modernized with the introduction of quality control. For example, herbs are subjected to absorption spectrometry to determine levels of heavy metals found in some. Because they are standardized, Chinese herbs are safer for self-treatment. This puts the individual, not the physician, in charge of the individual's health; that is a basic goal of Chinese herbalism.

Chinese herbalism offers unique advice regarding what foods can help and what can hinder, and an herbalist can help an individual discover foods that might cause an allergic reaction. In addition, Chinese herbs stimulate the immune system and provide beneficial nutrients, aside from their role in curing illness.

At M.D. Anderson Hospital in Texas, medical research has confirmed that patients undergoing **chemotherapy** were shown to have an improved degree of immune function when they took the tonic herb astragulus (*huang qi*). (It is well known that chemotherapy suppresses the immune system.) Research also showed that T-cell and macrophage activity and interferon production was increased in patients using the Chinese herbs ganoderma, lentinus, and polyporous, helping the body fight **cancer** cells. Agents also found in ganoderma were found to inhibit platelet aggregation and thrombocyte formation, which would be helpful to counter circulation and heart problems.

An ingredient of **ginseng** was found to promote adrenal function, which would give the herb properties of enhancing many hormone functions in the body.

Description

Origins

HISTORICAL BACKGROUND. Traditional Chinese medicine originated in the region of eastern Asia that today includes China, Tibet, Vietnam, Korea, and Japan. Tribal shamans and holy men who lived as hermits in the mountains of China as early as 3500 B.C. practiced what was called the "Way of Long Life." This regimen included a diet based on herbs and other plants; kung-fu exercises; and special breathing techniques that were thought to improve vitality and life expectancy.

After the Han dynasty, the next great age of Chinese medicine was under the Tang emperors, who ruled from A.D. 608 to 906. The first Tang emperor established China's first medical school in A.D. 629 Under the Song (A.D. 960–1279) and Ming (A.D. 1368–1644) dynasties, new medical schools were established, their curricula and qualifying examinations were standardized, and the traditional herbal prescriptions were written down and collected in encyclopedias. One important difference between the development of medicine in China and in the West is the greater interest in the West in surgical procedures and techniques.

PHILOSOPHICAL BACKGROUND: THE COSMIC AND NATURAL ORDER. In Taoist thought, the Tao, or universal first principle, generated a duality of opposing principles that underlie all the patterns of nature. These principles, yin and yang, are mutually dependent as well as polar opposites. They are basic concepts in traditional Chinese medicine. Yin represents everything that is cold, moist, dim, passive, slow, heavy, and moving downward or inward; while yang represents heat, dryness, brightness, activity, rapidity, lightness, and upward or outward motion. Both forces are equally necessary in nature and in human well-being, and neither force can exist without the other. The dynamic interaction of these two principles is reflected in the cycles of the seasons, the human life cycle, and other natural phenomena. One objective of traditional Chinese medicine is to keep yin and yang in harmonious balance within a person.

In addition to yin and yang, Taoist teachers also believed that the Tao produced a third force, primordial energy or qi (also spelled chi or ki). The interplay between yin, yang, and qi gave rise to the Five Elements of water, metal, earth, wood, and fire. These entities are all reflected in the structure and functioning of the human body.

THE HUMAN BEING. Traditional Chinese physicians did not learn about the structures of the human body from dissection because they thought that cutting open a body insulted the person's ancestors. Instead they built up an understanding of the location and functions of the major organs over centuries of observation, and then correlated them with the principles of yin, yang, qi, and the Five Elements. Thus wood is related to the liver (yin) and the gall bladder (yang); fire to the heart (yin) and the small intestine (yang); earth to the spleen (yin) and the stomach (yang); metal to the lungs (yin) and the large intestine (yang); and water to the kidneys (yin) and the bladder (yang). The Chinese also believed that the body contains Five Essential Substances, which include blood, spirit, vital essence (a principle of growth and development produced by the body from qi and blood), fluids (all body fluids other than blood, such as saliva, spinal fluid, sweat, etc.), and qi.

Chinese herbal treatment differs from **Western herbalism** in several respects. In Chinese practice, several different herbs may be used, according to each plant's effect on the individual's Qi and the Five Elements. There are many formulas used within traditional Chinese medicine to treat certain common imbalance patterns. These formulas can be modified to fit specific individuals more closely.

A traditional Chinese herbal formula typically contains four classes of ingredients, arranged in a hierarchical order: a chief (the principal ingredient, chosen for the patient's specific illness); a deputy (to reinforce the chief's action or treat a coexisting condition); an assistant (to counteract side effects of the first two ingredients); and an envoy (to harmonize all the other ingredients and convey them to the parts of the body that they are to treat).

Methods of diagnosis

A Chinese herbalist will not prescribe a particular herb on the strength of symptoms only, but will take into consideration the physical condition, emotional health, and mental state of the patient. He or she may look at the condition of the patient's hair, skin, and tongue, as well as the appearance of the eyes, lips, and general complexion. The practitioner then listens to the sounds the body makes when breathing. He or she may smell the breath, body odor, or sputum in diagnosis.

TCM practitioners take an extensive medical history of a patient. He or she may ask about dietary habits, lifestyle, and sleep patterns. The patient will be questioned about chief medical complaints, as well as on his or her particular emotional state and sexual practices.

Chinese herbalists employ touch as a diagnostic tool. They may palpate the body or use light massage to assess the patient's physical health. Another chief component of Chinese medical diagnosis is pulse diagnosis, or sphygmology. This is a very refined art that takes practitioners years to master. Some practitioners can detect 12 different pulse points that correspond to the 12 major organs in Chinese medicine. There are over 30 pulse qualities that practitioners are able to detect on each point. The strength, speed, quality, and rhythm of the pulse, to name a few, will be determined before a diagnosis is given.

Herbs

Chinese herbs may be used alone or in combination. Relatively few are used alone for medicinal purposes. Practitioners believe that illness can be effectively treated by combining herbs based on their various characteristics and the patient's overall health. Every herb has four basic healing properties: nature, taste, affinity, and effect.

An herb's nature is described according to its yin or yang characteristics. Yang, or warming, herbs treat cold deficiencies. They are frequently used in the treatment of the upper respiratory tract, skin, or extremities. Yin, or cooling, herbs, treat hot excess conditions. They are most often used to treat internal conditions and problems with organs. Herbs can also be neutral in nature.

An herb's taste does not refer to its flavor, but to its effect on qi, blood, fluids, and phlegm. Sour herbs have a concentrating action. They are prescribed to treat bodily excess conditions, such as **diarrhea**, and concentrate qi. Bitter herbs have an eliminating or moving downward action. They are used to treat coughs, **constipation**, and heart problems. Sweet or bland herbs have a harmonizing action. They are used as restorative herbs and to treat **pain**. Spicy herbs have a stimulating action. They are prescribed to improve blood and qi circulation. Salty herbs have a softening action. They are used to treat constipation and other digestion problems.

An herb's affinity describes its action on a specific bodily Organ. (Note that Chinese medicine does not have the anatomical correlation for organ names. They correspond more closely to the organ's function.) Sour herbs have an affinity for the Liver and Gallbladder. Bitter herbs act on the Heart and Small Intestine. Sweet and bland herbs affect the Stomach and Spleen. Spicy herbs have an affinity for Lungs and Large Intestine, whereas salty herbs act on the Kidneys and Bladder.

Chinese herbs are lastly classified according to their specific actions, which are divided into four effects. Herbs that dispel are used to treat an accumulation, sluggishness, or spasm by relaxing or redistributing. Herbs with an astringent action are used to consolidate or restrain a condition characterized by discharge or excessive elimination. Herbs that purge treat an obstruction or "poison" by encouraging elimination and **detoxification**. Tonifying herbs nourish, support, and calm where there is a deficiency.

Treatment of diabetes

The incidence of diabetes has increased quite dramatically in recent years, especially in the United States, where in general people take less **exercise**, and food is

KEY TERMS

Absorption spectrometry—A scientific procedure to determine chemical makeup of samples.

Interferon—A substance proved to be necessary in the body to help fight cancer cells.

Immune function—The body's defense system against bacteria, viruses and fungi, and any malfunction of the organism.

Pharmaco-dynamics—The study of the relationships and interactions of herbs.

Platelet aggregation—The clumping together of blood cells, possibly forming a clot.

Thrombocyte—Another name for platelet.

taken in greater quantity with a general reduction in quality. This has lead to a scramble to find new solutions to the problem, and many researchers have focused their interest on Chinese herbal remedies. In the search for more effective and more convenient treatments, the alkaloid berberine has come under close scrutiny for its many uses, including the treatment of diabetes. In trials, rats given a mixture of berberine and alloxan showed less likelihood of incurring a rise in blood sugar. Patients suffering from type II diabetes who were given between 300 and 600 mg of berberine daily for between one and three months, showed a reduction in blood sugar levels, when taken in conjunction with a controlled diet.

Treatment of AIDS and cancer

Independent researchers are investigating indications that Chinese herbalism can reduce the toxicity of chemotherapy and other medications, in addition to stimulating immune responses.

Preparations

Those who are unfamiliar with Chinese herbs and their uses should consult a practitioner before starting any treatment. Once a remedy is prescribed, it may be found at Oriental markets or health food stores. The remedies used in Chinese herbalism are standardized and sold prepared for use, with instructions for dosage. A Chinese herbalist may prescribe herbs to be made into tea, or taken as capsules.

Precautions

When treating a patient, the herbalist will aim to gently "nudge" the system into shape, rather than producing any immediate reaction. A return to health, therefore, may take time, and it is important that the patient realizes the principle of the treatment. Some practitioners estimate that treatment will take a month for every year that a chronic condition has existed. The advantage of the slow pace is that if there is a bad reaction to any herb, which is rare, it will be mild because the treatment itself is gentle.

As with most naturopathic therapies, Chinese herbal remedies work best when taken in conjunction with a healthy lifestyle and program of exercise.

Side effects

Some Chinese herbs are incompatible with certain prescription drugs, certain foods, or should not be taken during **pregnancy**. To be certain, a Chinese herbalist should be consulted.

Research and general acceptance

At present, there is renewed interest in the West in traditional Chinese medicine and Chinese herbalism. Of the 700 herbal remedies used by traditional Chinese practitioners, over 100 have been tested and found effective by the standards of Western science. Several United States agencies, including the National Institutes of Health, the Office of Alternative Medicine, and the Food and Drug Administration are currently investigating Chinese herbal medicine as well as acupuncture and *Tui na* massage. In general, however, Western studies of Chinese medicine focus on the effects of traditional treatments and the reasons for those effects, thus attempting to fit traditional Chinese medicine within the Western framework of precise physical measurements and scientific hypotheses.

ORGANIZATIONS

California State Oriental Medial Association, 703 Market Street, Suite 250, San Francisco, CA, 94103-2100, (800) 477-4564, info@csomaonline.org, http://www.csomaonline.org.

Crane Herb Company, 745 Falmouth Road, Mashpee, MA, 02649, (508) 539-1700, (508) 539-2369, info@craneherb.com, https://www.craneherb.com.

National Center for Complementary and Alternative Medicine (NCCAM), P.O. Box 7923, Gaitherburg, MD, 20898, (866) 464-3616, (888) 644-6226, info@nccam.nih.gov, http://nccam.nih.gov/.

Traditional Chinese Medicine Association and Alumni, Inc. (TCMAA), 108-A East 38th Street, New York, NY, 10016, (212) 889-4802, (643) 309-7633, peng8@verizon.net, http://www.tcmaa.org/.

Patricia Skinner

Herbalism, Western

Definition

Western herbalism is a form of the healing arts that draws from herbal traditions of Europe and the Americas and that emphasizes the study and use of European and Native American herbs in the treatment and prevention of illness. Western herbalism is based on physicians' and herbalists' clinical experience and traditional knowledge of medicinal plant remedies preserved by oral tradition and in written records over thousands of years. Western herbalism, like the much older system of **traditional Chinese medicine**, relies on the synergistic and curative properties of the plant to treat symptoms and disease and maintain health.

Western herbalism is based upon pharmocognosy, the study of natural products. Pharmocognosy includes the identification, extraction methods, and applications of specific plant constituents responsible for specific therapeutic actions, such as the use of **digoxin** from Digitalis leaf for **heart failure**. These constituents are extracted, purified and studied in vitro, in vivo, and in clinical research. They may be concentrated to deliver standardized, set doses. Sometimes, the natural constituent can be synthesized in the lab, or changed and patented. Practitioners may choose to use fresh medicinal plants, simple extracts, or standardized extracts.

In standardized extracts, a specific quantity of a constituent is called a marker compound, and it may or may not be the active constituent(s) in the plant medicine. There are preparations with standardized active constituent quantities and preparations with greater emphasis on quality of crude plant material and traditional preparation methodology than on finalized total quantity of marker compounds. The preference between the two for precision dosing is philosophical, practical and variable. When using plant extracts in which the active constituents and their cofactors are well established, or the therapeutic and lethal dose are close, standardized products are often preferred. When using plant extracts whose active constituents remain obscure, or the active constituents when purified produce weaker therapeutic results or more undesirable side effects, the products produced under good manufacturing processes and according to the traditional *National Formulary U. S. Dispensatory* or *U. S. Pharmacopeia* are preferred.

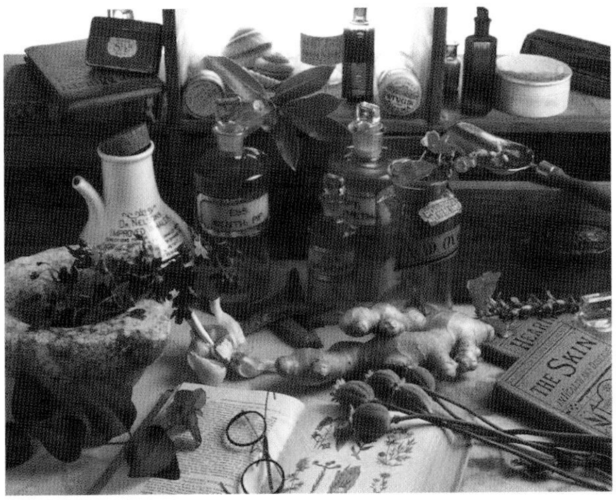

A selection of Western herbal medical equipment and traditional herbs, including foxglove (upper right), ginger (center right), and periwinkle (lower left). *(Photo Researchers, Inc.)*

Purpose

The benefits of botanical medicine may be subtle or dramatic, depending on the remedy used and the symptom or problem being addressed. Herbal remedies usually have a much slower effect than pharmaceutical drugs. Some herbal remedies have a cumulative effect and work slowly over time to restore balance, and others are indicated for short-term treatment of acute symptoms. When compared to the pharmaceutical drugs, herbal remedies prepared from the whole plant have relatively few side effects. This is due to the complex chemistry and synergistic action of the full range of phytochemicals present in the whole plant and the relatively lower concentrations. They are generally safe when used in properly designated therapeutic dosages and less costly than the isolated chemicals or synthetic prescription drugs available from western pharmaceutical corporations.

Description

Origins

More than 2,500 years ago Hippocrates wrote, "In medicine one must pay attention not to plausible theorizing but to experience and reason together." This Greek physician and herbalist from the fourth century B.C. is considered the father of Western medicine. He stressed the importance of diet, water quality, climate, and social environment in the development of disease. Hippocrates believed in treating the whole person, rather than merely isolating and treating symptoms. He recognized the innate capacity of the body to heal itself, and emphasized the importance of keen observation in the medical practice. He recommended simple herbal remedies to assist the body in restoring health.

Ancient Greek medicine around the fifth century B.C. was a fertile ground for contrasting philosophies and religions. Greek physicians were influenced by the accumulated medical knowledge from Egypt, Persia, and Babylon. Medical advances flourished and practitioners and scholars were free to study and practice without religious and secular constraints. In the fourth century B.C., Theophrastus wrote the *Historia Plantarum*, considered to be the founding text in the science of botany.

During the first century A.D. Dioscorides, a Greek physician who traveled with the Roman legions, produced five medical texts. His herbal text, known as the *De Materia Medica* is considered to be among the most influential of all western herbal texts. It became a standard reference for practitioners for the next 1,500 years. This influential book also included information on medicinal herbs and treatments that had been used for centuries in Indian **Ayurvedic medicine**. Galen of Pergamon, who also lived in the first century A.D., was a Roman physician and student of anatomy and physiology. He authored a recipe book containing 130 antidotes and medicinal preparations. These elaborate mixtures, known as galenicals, sometimes included up to one hundred herbs and other substances. This complex approach to herbal medicine was a dramatic change from the simple remedies recommended by Hippocrates and employed by traditional folk healers. Galen developed a rigid system of medicine in which the physician, with his specialized knowledge of complex medical formulas, was considered the ultimate authority in matters of health care. The Galenic system, relying on theory and scholarship rather than observation, persisted throughout the Middle Ages. The Galenical compounds, along with bloodletting and purging, were among the drastic techniques practiced by the medical professionals during those times; however, traditional herbal healers persisted outside the mainstream medical system.

During the eighth century a medical school was established in Salerno, Italy, where the herbal knowledge accumulated by Arab physicians was preserved. The Arabian Muslims conducted extensive research on medicinal herbs found in Europe, Persia, India, and the Far East. Arab businessmen opened the first herbal pharmacies early in the ninth century. The *Leech Book of Bald*, the work of a Christian monk, was compiled in the tenth century. It preserved important medical writings that had survived from the work of physicians in ancient Greece and Rome.

The Middle Ages in Europe was a time of widespread **death** from plagues and pestilence. The Black **Plague** of 1348, particularly, and other health catastrophes in later years, claimed so many lives that survivors began to lose faith in the dominant Galenic medical system. Fortunately, the knowledge of traditional herbal medicine had not been lost. Medieval monks who cultivated extensive medicinal gardens on the monastery grounds, also patiently copied the ancient herbal and medical texts. Folk medicine as practiced in Europe by traditional healers persisted, even though many women herbalists were persecuted as witches and enemies of the Catholic church and their herbal arts were suppressed.

The growing spice trade and explorations to the New World introduced exotic plants, and a whole new realm of botanical medicines became available to Europeans. Following the invention of the printing press in the fifteenth century, a large number of herbal texts, also simply called herbals, became available for popular use. Among them were the beautifully illustrated works of the German botanists Otto Brunfels and Leonhard Fuchs published in 1530 and the Dutch herbal of Belgian physician Rembert Dodoens, a popular work that was later reproduced in English. In 1597, the physician and gardener John Gerard published one of the most famous of the English herbal, still in print today. Gerard's herbal, known as *The Herball or General Historie of Plantes* was not an original work. Much of the content was taken from the translated text of his Belgian predecessor Dodoens. Gerard did, however, include descriptions of some of the more than 1,000 species of rare and exotic plants and English flora from his own garden.

The correspondence of astrology with herbs was taught by Arab physicians who regarded astrology as a science helpful in the selection of medicines and in the treatment of diseases. This approach to western herbalism was particularly evident in the herbal texts published in the sixteenth and seventeenth centuries. One of the most popular and controversial English herbals is *The English Physician Enlarged* published in 1653. The author, Nicholas Culpeper, was an apothecary by trade. He also published a translation of the Latin language *London Pharmacopoeia* into English. Culpeper was a nonconformist in loyalist England, and was determined to make medical knowledge more accessible to the apothecaries, the tradesmen who prescribed most of the herbal remedies. Culpeper's herbal was criticized by the medical establishment for its mix of magic and astrology with botanical medicine, but it became one of the most popular compendiums of botanical medicine of its day. Culpeper also accepted the so-called "Doctrine of Signatures," practiced by medieval monks in their medicinal gardens. This theory teaches that the appearance of plants is the clue to their curative powers. Plants were chosen for treatment of particular medical conditions based on their associations with the four natural elements and with a planet or sign. The place where the plant grows, its dominant physical feature, and the smell and taste of an herb determined the plant's signature. Culpeper's herbal is still in print in facsimile copies, and some pharmocognosists and herbalists in the twenty-first century voice the same criticisms that Culpeper's early critics did.

European colonists brought their herbal knowledge and plant specimens to settlements in North America where they learned from the indigenous Americans how to make use of numerous nutritive and medicinal plants, native to the New World. Many European medicinal plants escaped cultivation from the early settlements and have become naturalized throughout North America. The first record of Native American herbalism is found in the manuscript of the native Mexican Indian physician, Juan Badianus published in 1552. The American Folk tradition of herbalism developed as a blend of traditional European medicine and Native American herbalism. The pioneer necessity for self-reliance contributed to the perseverance of folk medicine well into the twentieth century.

In Europe in the seventeenth century, the alchemist Paracelsus changed the direction of western medicine with the introduction of chemical and mineral medicines. He was the son of a Swiss chemist and physician. Paracelsus began to apply chemicals, such as arsenic, mercury, sulfur, iron, and copper sulfate to treat disease. His chemical approach to the treatment of disease was a forerunner to the reliance in the twentieth century on chemical medicine as the orthodox treatment prescribed in mainstream medical practice.

The nineteenth and twentieth centuries brought a renewed interest in the practice of Western herbalism and the development of natural therapies and health care systems that ran counter to the mainstream methods of combating disease symptoms with synthetic pharmaceuticals.

In the late eighteenth century, the German physician Samuel Hahnemann developed a system of medicine known as homeopathy. This approach to healing embraces the philosophy of "like cures like." Homeopathy uses extremely diluted solutions of herbs, animal products, and chemicals that are believed to hold a "trace memory" or energetic imprint of the substance used. Homeopathic remedies are used to amplify the patient's symptoms with remedies that would act to produce the same symptom in a healthy person. Homeopathy holds that the symptoms of illness are evidence of the body's natural process of healing and eliminating the cause of the disease.

In 1895, the European medical system known as Naturopathy was introduced to the North America. Like homeopathy, this medical approach is based on the Hippocratic idea of eliminating disease by assisting the body's natural healing abilities. The naturopath uses nontoxic methods to assist the body's natural healing processes, including **nutritional supplements**, herbal remedies, proper diet, and **exercise** to restore health.

Western herbalism is regaining popularity at a time when the world is assaulted by the **stress** of overpopulation and development that threatens the natural biodiversity necessary for these valuable medicinal plants to survive. The American herb market is growing rapidly and increasing numbers of individuals are choosing alternative therapies over the mainstream allopathic Western medicine. Consumers spend more than $7 billion a year on herbal products. An estimated 2,400 acres of native plant habitat are lost to development every day. As much as 29% of all plant life in North America is in danger of extinction, including some of the most important native medicinal plants, according to the 1997 World Conservation Union Red List of Threatened Plants.

Though research into the efficacy and safety of traditional herbal remedies is increasing, it has been limited by the high costs of clinical studies and laboratory research, and by the fact that whole plants and their constituents are not generally patentable (therefore, there is no drug profit after market introduction). Outside the United States, herbalism has successfully combined with conventional medicine and in some countries is fully integrated into the nation's health care systems. At the beginning of the twenty-first century, 80% of the world's population continues to rely on herbal treatments. The World Health Organization, an agency of the United Nations, promotes traditional herbal medicine for treatment of many local health problems, particularly in the third world where it is affordable and already well-integrated into the cultural fabric.

In the United States, the re-emergence of interest in holistic approaches to health care is evident. Citizens are demanding access to effective, safe, low-cost, natural medicine. Legislative and societal change is needed, however, before natural therapies can be fully integrated into the orthodox allopathic health care system and provide citizens with a wide range of choices for treatment. If the current trend continues, U. S. citizens will benefit from a choice among a variety of safe and effective medical treatments.

Herbs are generally defined as any plant or plant part that may be used for medicinal, nutritional, culinary, or other beneficial purposes. The active constituents of plants (if known) may be found in varying amounts in the root, stem, leaf, flower, and fruit, etc. of the plant. Herbs may be classified into many different categories. Some western herbalists categorize herbal remedies according to their strength, action, and characteristics. Categories may include sedatives, stimulants, **laxatives**, febrifuges (to reduce **fever**), and many others. One system of classification is based on a principle in traditional Chinese medicine that categorizes herbs into four classes: tonics, specifics, heroics, and cleansers and protectors. Within these broad classifications are the numerous medicinal actions of the whole herb which may be due to a specific chemical or combination of chemicals in the plant.

- Tonics. Herbs in this classification are also known as alteratives in western herbalism. They are generally mild in their action and act slowly in the body, providing gentle stimulation and nutrition to specific organs and systems. Tonic herbs act over time to strengthen and nourish the whole body. These herbs are generally safe and may be used regularly, even in large quantities. These tonic herbs are known as "superior" remedies in traditional Chinese medicine. The therapeutic dose of tonic remedies is far removed from the possible toxic dose. American ginseng is an example of a tonic herb.
- Specifics. Herbs in this classification are strong and specific in their therapeutic action. They are generally used for short periods of time in smaller dosages to treat acute conditions. Herbs classified as specifics are not used beyond the therapeutic treatment period. Echinacea is a specific herb.
- Heroic. These herbs offer high potency but are potentially toxic and should not be used in self-treatment. Because the therapeutic dosage may be close to the lethal dosage, these herbs are presented cautiously and closely monitored or avoided by trained clinicians. They should not be used continuously or without expert supervision. Poke (*Phytolacca americana*) is an example of a heroic remedy.
- Cleansers and protectors. These herbs, plants, and plant tissues remove wastes and pollutants, while minimally affecting regular body processes. An example of a cleanser is pectin. Pectins are the water soluble substances that bind cell walls in plant tissues, and some believe that they help remove heavy metals and environmental toxins from the body.

Preparations

Herbal preparations are commercially available in a variety of forms, including tablets or capsules, tinctures, teas, fluid extracts, douches, washes, suppositories, dried herbs, and many other forms. The medicinal properties of herbs are extracted from the fresh or dried plant parts by the use of solvents appropriate to the particular herb. Alcohol, oil, water, vinegar, glycerin, and propylene glycol are some of the solvents used to extract and concentrate the medicinal properties. Steam distillation and cold-pressing techniques are used to extract the essential oils. The quality of any herbal remedy and the potency of the phytochemicals found in the herb depends greatly on the conditions of weather and soil where the herb was grown, the timing and care in harvesting, and the manner of preparation and storage.

KEY TERMS

In vitro—A biological reaction occurring in a laboratory apparatus.

In vivo—Occurring in a living organism.

Phyto-, as in phytochemical, phytomedicinal, and phytotherapy—Meaning, or pertaining to, a plant or plants.

Wildcrafting—Gathering of herbs or other natural materials.

Precautions

Herbal remedies prepared by infusion, decoction, or alcohol tincture from the appropriate plant part, such as the leaf, root, or flower, are generally safe when ingested in properly designated therapeutic dosages. However, many herbs have specific contraindications for use when certain medical conditions are present. Not all herbal remedies may be safely administered to infants or small children. Many herbs are not safe for use by pregnant or lactating women. Some herbs are toxic, even deadly, in large amounts, and there is little research on the chronic toxicity that may result from prolonged use. Herbal remedies are sold in the United States as dietary supplements and are not regulated for content or efficacy. Self-diagnosis and treatment with botanical medicinals may be risky. A consultation with a clinical herbalist, Naturopathic physician, or certified clinical herbalist is prudent before undertaking a course of treatment.

Essential oils are highly concentrated and should not be ingested as a general rule. They should also be diluted in water or in a non-toxic carrier oil before application to the skin to prevent **contact dermatitis** or photo-sensitization. The toxicity of the concentrated essential oil varies depending on the chemical constituents of the herb.

The American Professor of Pharmacognosy, Varro E. Tyler, believes that "herbal chaos" prevails in the United States with regard to herbs and phytomedicinals. In part he blames the herb producers and marketers of crude herbs and remedies for what he terms unproven hyperbolic, poor quality control, deceptive labeling, resistance to standardization of dosage forms, and continued sale of herbs determined to be harmful.

Side effects

Herbs have a variety of complex phytochemicals that act on the body as a whole or on specific organs and systems. Some of these chemical constituents are mild and safe, even in large doses. Other herbs contain chemicals that act more strongly and may be toxic in large doses or when taken continuously. **Drug interactions** are possible with certain herbs when combined with certain pharmaceutical drugs. Some herbs are tonic in a small amount and toxic in larger dosages.

Research and general acceptance

Western herbalism is experiencing a revival of popular and professional interest. The number of training schools and qualified herbal practitioners is growing to meet the demand. Western herbalism is incorporated into the medical practice of licensed Naturopathic doctors, who receive special training in clinical herbalism. Folk herbalists, heir to the continuing oral traditions passed from generation to generation in many rural areas, as well as amateur, self-taught herbalists, keep the practice of botanical medicine alive at the grassroots level. Traditional western herbalism relies on traditional use and *materia medica*, folk wisdom, and recent clinical research and advances in the extraction processes. These advances provide increased quality control on the concentration and potency of the active ingredients. Western physicians, educated in allopathic medicine, typically receive no training in the use of herbs. These doctors rely on pharmaceutical drugs for their patients, and some cite the following reasons for continuing to do so: lack of standardized dosages, lack of quality control in the preparation of herbal medicinals, and the dearth of clinical research verifying the safety and effectiveness of many traditional herbal remedies.

Herbalism is widely practiced throughout Europe, particularly in England, France, Italy, and Germany, where phytomedicinals are available in prescription form and as over-the-counter remedies. In Germany, plant medicines are regulated by a special government body known as the Commission E. In the United States, however, despite increasing popularity, traditional herbalism is not integrated into the allopathic medical system. Phytomedicinals are sold as dietary supplements rather than being adequately researched and recognized as safe and effective drugs. The Dietary Supplement Health and Education Act of 1994 circumvented a U. S. Food and Drug Administration (FDA) effort to effectively remove botanicals from the marketplace and implement regulations restricting sale. Massive popular outcry against the proposed regulations on the sale of herbs and phytomedicinals resulted in this Congressional action. In 2000, U.S. President Bill Clinton, by executive order, created the White House Commission on Alternative Medicine in an effort to hold alternative medicine therapies "to the same standard of scientific rigor as more traditional health care interventions." That Commission is charged with recommending federal guidelines and legislation regarding the use of alternative medical therapies in the twenty-first century.

Resources

OTHER

Hobbs, Christopher. "Specific and Tonic Immune Herbs: Exploring a Practical System of Western Herbalism." Health World. http://www.healthy.net.

Oracle Tree New Age Mall. "Western Medical Astrology: A Brief History." http://ww.oracletree.com/avalonphysics/wesmedas.html.

Wicke, Roger, Ph.D. "A World History of Herbology and Herbalism: Oppressed Arts." Rocky Mountain Herbal Institute. http://www.rmhiherbal.org/a/f.ahr1.hist.html.

ORGANIZATIONS

American Herbalists Guild, PO Box 230741, Boston, MA, 02123, (857) 350-3128, ahgoffice@earthlink.net, http://americanherbalistsguild.com.

Clare Hanrahan

Herbs *see* **Echinacea; Ginkgo biloba; Ginseng; Saw palmetto; St. John's wort**

Hereditary cerebral hemorrhage with amyloidosis *see* **Cerebral amyloid angiopathy**

Hereditary chorea *see* **Huntington's disease**

Hereditary fructose intolerance

Definition

Hereditary fructose intolerance is an inherited condition where the body does not produce the chemical needed to break down fructose (fruit sugar).

KEY TERMS

Aldolase B—Also called fructose 1-phosphate aldolase, this chemical is produced in the liver, kidneys, and brain. It is needed for the breakdown of fructose, a sugar found in fruits, vegetables, honey, and other sweeteners.

Hyperbilirubinemia—A condition where there is a high level of bilirubin in the blood. Bilirubin is a natural by-product of the breakdown of red blood cells, however, a high level of bilirubin may indicate a problem with the liver.

Liver biopsy—A surgical procedure where a small piece of the liver is cut out for examination. A needle or narrow tube may be inserted either directly through the skin and muscle or through a small incision and passed into the liver for collection of a sample of liver tissue.

Description

Fructose is a sugar found naturally in fruits, vegetables, honey, and table sugar. Fructose intolerance is a disorder caused by the body's inability to produce an enzyme called aldolase B (also called fructose 1-phosphate aldolase) that is necessary for absorption of fructose. The undigested fructose collects in the liver and kidneys, eventually causing liver and kidney failure. One person in about 20,000 is born with this disorder. It is reported more frequently in the United States and Northern European countries than in other parts of the world. It occurs with equal frequency in males and females.

Causes and symptoms

Fructose intolerance is an inherited disorder passed on to children through their parents' genes. Both the mother and father have the gene that causes the condition, but may not have symptoms of fructose intolerance themselves. (This is called an autosomal recessive pattern of inheritance.) The disorder will not be apparent until the infant is fed formula, juice, fruits, or baby foods that contain fructose. Initial symptoms include **vomiting**, **dehydration**, and unexplained **fever**. Other symptoms include extreme thirst and excessive urination and sweating. There will also be a loss of appetite and a failure to grow. **Tremors** and seizures caused by low blood sugar can occur. The liver becomes swollen and the patient becomes jaundiced with yellowing of the eyes and skin. Left untreated, this condition can lead to **coma** and **death**.

Diagnosis

Urine tests can be used to detect fructose sugar in the urine. Blood tests can also be used to detect *hyperbilirubinemia* and high levels of liver enzymes in the blood. A **liver biopsy** may be performed to test for levels of enzymes present and to evaluate the extent of damage to the liver. A fructose-loading test where a dose of fructose is given to the patient in a well-controlled hospital or clinical setting may also be used to confirm fructose intolerance. Both the biopsy and the loading test can be very risky, particularly in infants that are already sick.

Treatment

Once diagnosed, fructose intolerance can be successfully treated by eliminating fructose from the diet. Patients usually respond within three to four weeks and can make a complete recovery if fructose-containing foods are avoided. Early recognition and treatment of the disease is important to avoid damage to the liver, kidneys, and small intestine.

Prognosis

If the condition is not recognized and the diet is not well controlled, death can occur in infants or young children. With a well-controlled diet, the child can develop normally.

Prevention

Carriers of the gene for hereditary fructose intolerance can be identified through DNA analysis. Anyone who is known to carry the disease or who has the disease in his or her family can benefit from **genetic counseling**. Since this is a hereditary disorder, there is currently no known way to prevent it other than assisting at-risk individuals with family planning and reproductive decisions.

Resources

OTHER

"What Is Hereditary Fructose Intolerance?" Hereditary Fructose Intolerance & Aldolase Homepage. http://www.bu.edu/aldolase.

ORGANIZATIONS

National Institute of Diabetes and Digestive and Kidney Diseases, NIDDK, NIH Bldg 31, Rm 9A06 31 Center Drive, MSC 2560, Bethesda, MD, 20892-2560, (301) 496.3583, http://www2.niddk.nih.gov.

Altha Roberts Edgren

KEY TERMS

Autosomal dominant—A pattern of inheritance in which the dominant gene on any non-sex chromosome carries the defect.

Chromosome—A threadlike structure in the cell which transmits genetic information.

Hereditary hemorrhagic telangiectasia

Definition

Hereditary hemorrhagic telangiectasia is an inherited condition characterized by abnormal blood vessels which are delicate and prone to bleeding. Hereditary hemorrhagic telangiectasia is also known as Rendu-Osler-Weber disease.

Description

The term telangiectasia refers to a spot formed, usually on the skin, by a dilated capillary or terminal artery. In hereditary hemorrhagic telangiectasia these spots occur because the blood vessel is fragile and bleeds easily. The bleeding may appear as small, red or reddish-violet spots on the face, lips, inside the mouth and nose or the tips of the fingers and toes. Other small telangiectasias may occur in the digestive tract.

Unlike **hemophilia**, where bleeding is caused by an ineffective clotting mechanism in the blood, bleeding in hereditary hemorrhagic telangiectasia is caused by fragile blood vessels. However, like hemophilia, bleeding may be extensive and can occur without warning.

Causes and symptoms

Hereditary hemorrhagic telangiectasia, an autosomal dominant inherited disorder, occurs in one in 50,000 people.

Recurrent nosebleeds are a nearly universal symptom of this condition. Usually the nosebleeds begin in childhood and become worse with age. The skin changes begin at **puberty**, and the condition becomes progressively worse until about 40 years of age, when it stabilizes.

Diagnosis

The physician will look for red spots on all areas of the skin, but especially on the upper half of the body, and in the mouth and nose and under the tongue.

Treatment

There is no specific treatment for hereditary hemorrhagic telangiectasia. The bleeding resulting from the condition can be stopped by applying compresses or direct pressure to the area. If necessary, a laser can be used to destroy the vessel. In severe cases, the leaking artery can be plugged or covered with a graft from normal tissue.

Prognosis

In most people, recurrent bleeding results in an iron deficiency. It is usually necessary to take iron supplements.

Prevention

Hereditary hemorrhagic telangiectasia is an inherited disorder and cannot be prevented.

ORGANIZATIONS

American Medical Association, 515 N. State St., Chicago, IL, 60654, (800) 621-8335, http://www.ama-assn.org/.

Association of Birth Defect Children, 3526 Emerywood Lane, Orlando, FL, 32806, (305) 859-2821.

Dorothy Elinor Stonely

Hereditary hyperuricemia *see* **Lesch-Nyhan syndrome**

Hereditary spinocerebellar ataxia *see* **Friedreich's ataxia**

Hermaphroditism *see* **Intersex states**

Hernia

Definition

Hernia is a general term used to describe a bulge or protrusion of an organ through the structure or muscle that normally contains it.

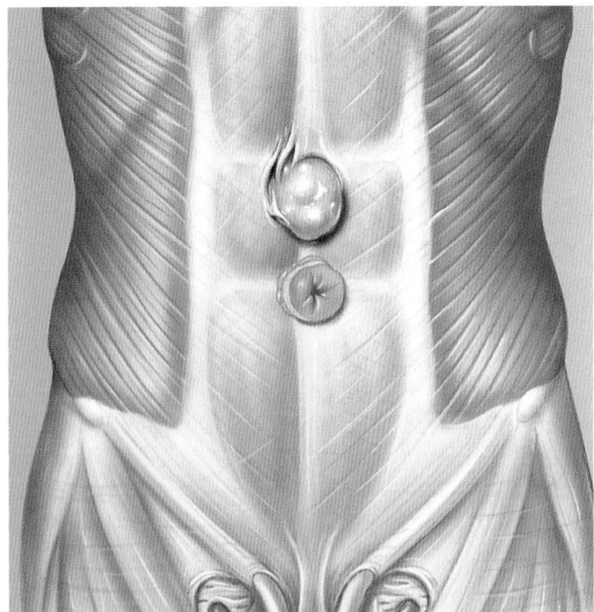

An illustration of an epigastric (abdominal) hernia in an adult male. The torso is shown with its skin removed. Epigastric hernia is caused commonly by a congenital weakness in muscles of the central upper abdomen; the intestine bulges out through the muscle at a point between the navel and breastbone. *(John Bavosi/Photo Researchers, Inc.)*

Demographics

The frequency of hernias varies greatly depending on the type of hernia. Hernias tend to be more common in the elderly than in younger individuals. Hernias also are more common in infants and children, often caused by the abdominal wall not closing completely after birth.

Hiatal hernias are very common, although most do not produce serious symptoms and many individuals never even know they have one. About 10% of individuals under the age of 40 have hiatal hernias. This number increases with age, with about 70% of individuals over age 70 having this type of hernia.

Abdominal hernias are more common in males than in females. About 25% of men have an inguinal hernia at some time in their lives, and only about 2% of women ever have one. Over 1 million surgeries are performed each year to repair abdominal hernias.

Description

There are many different types of hernias. The most familiar type is that which occur in the abdomen when part of the intestine protrudes through the abdominal wall. This may occur in different areas and, depending on the location, the hernia is given a different name.

An inguinal hernia appears as a bulge in the groin and may come and go depending on the position of the person or their level of physical activity. It can occur with or without **pain**. In men, the protrusion may descend into the scrotum. Inguinal hernias account for 80% of all hernias and are more common in men.

Femoral hernias are similar to inguinal hernias but appear as a bulge slightly lower. They are more common in women and are often caused by the strain that **pregnancy** puts on the abdominal area.

A ventral hernia is also called an incision hernia because it generally occurs as a bulge in the abdomen at the site of an old surgical scar. It is caused by thinning or stretching of scar tissue It occurs more frequently in people who are obese or pregnant.

An umbilical hernia appears as a soft bulge at the navel (umbilicus). It is caused by a weakening of the area or an imperfect closure of the area in infants. This type of hernia is more common in women due to pregnancy and in Chinese and African American infants. Some umbilical hernias in infants disappear without treatment within the first year.

A hiatal or diaphragmatic hernia is different from abdominal hernias in that it is not visible on the outside of the body. With a **hiatal hernia**, the stomach bulges upward through the muscle that separates the chest from the abdomen (the diaphragm). This type of hernia occurs more often in women than in men, and it is treated differently from other types of hernias.

Causes and symptoms

Most hernias result from a weakness in the abdominal wall. In many cases an infant is born with this weakness (congenital), and in other cases weakness can develop later in life. Any increase in pressure in the abdomen, such as recurring coughing, straining, heavy lifting, or pregnancy, can be a considered a causative factor in developing an abdominal hernia. **Obesity** or recent excessive weight loss, as well as **aging** and previous surgery, are also risk factors.

Most abdominal hernias appear suddenly when the abdominal muscles are strained. The individual may feel tenderness, a slight burning sensation, or a feeling of heaviness in the bulge. It may be possible for the individual to push the hernia back into place with gentle pressure, or the hernia may disappear by itself when the person reclines. Being able to push the hernia back is called reducing it. On the other hand, some hernias cannot be pushed back into place and are termed incarcerated or irreducible.

KEY TERMS

Endoscopy—A diagnostic procedure in which a tube is inserted through the mouth, into the esophagus and stomach. It is used to visualize various digestive disorders, including hiatal hernias.

Herniorrhaphy—Surgical repair of a hernia.

Incarcerated hernia—A hernia that cannot be reduced, or pushed back into place inside the abdominal wall.

Laparoscopic surgery—A minimally invasive surgery in which a camera and surgical instruments are inserted through a small incision.

Reducible hernia—A hernia that can be gently pushed back into place or that disappears when the person lies down.

Strangulated hernia—A hernia that is so tightly incarcerated outside the abdominal wall that the intestine is blocked and the blood supply to that part of the intestine is cut off.

A hiatal hernia may also be caused by obesity, pregnancy, aging, or previous surgery. About 50% of all people with hiatal hernias do not have any symptoms. If symptoms exist they usually include **heartburn**, usually 30–60 minutes following a meal. There may be some mid chest pain due to gastric acid from the stomach being pushed up into the esophagus (gastric reflux). The pain and heartburn usually are worse when lying down. Frequent belching and feelings of abdominal fullness may also be present.

Diagnosis

Generally, abdominal hernias need to be seen and felt to be diagnosed. Usually the hernia will increase in size with an increase in abdominal pressure, so the doctor may ask the person to **cough** while he or she feels the area. Once a diagnosis of an abdominal hernia is made, the doctor usually will refer the individual to a surgeon for a consultation. Surgery provides the only cure for a hernia through the abdominal wall.

With a hiatal hernia, the preliminary diagnosis is based on the symptoms reported by the person. The doctor may then order tests to confirm the diagnosis. One possible test is called a barium swallow test. During this procedure, the individual drinks a chalky white barium solution and then undergoes an abdominal x ray. The barium causes any protrusion through the diaphragm show up more clearly on the x ray. Hiatal hernias often are diagnosed using **endoscopy**. This procedure is done by a gastroenterologist (a specialist in digestive diseases). During an endoscopy the person is given an intravenous sedative and a small tube is inserted through the mouth, then into the esophagus and stomach where the doctor can look at the hernia using a small tube or camera. The procedure takes about 30 minutes and usually causes no discomfort. It is done on an outpatient basis.

Treatment

Once an abdominal hernia occurs it tends to increase in size. Some patients with abdominal hernias take a watch and wait approach before deciding on surgery. In these cases, they must avoid strenuous physical activity such as heavy lifting or straining with **constipation**. They may also wear a truss, which is a support worn like a belt to keep a small hernia from protruding. People can tell if their hernia is getting worse if they develop severe constant pain, **nausea and vomiting**, or if the bulge does not return to normal when lying down or when they try to gently push it back in place. In these cases they, should consult their doctor immediately. In most cases, surgery is eventually required to correct the hernia.

Surgery

There are risks to not surgically repairing a hernia. Left untreated, a hernia may become incarcerated, which means it can no longer be reduced or pushed back into place. With an incarcerated hernia, the intestine become trapped, or strangulated, outside the abdomen. This can lead to a blockage in the intestine. If strangulation is severe, it may cut off the blood supply to the intestine and part of the intestine will die. Because of the risk of tissue **death** (necrosis) and **gangrene**, and because the hernia can block food from moving through the bowel, a strangulated hernia is a medical emergency requiring immediate surgery. Repairing a hernia before it becomes incarcerated or strangulated is much safer than waiting until complications develop.

Surgical repair of a hernia is called a herniorrhaphy. The surgeon will push the bulging part of the intestine back into place and sew the overlying muscle back together. When the muscle is not strong enough, the surgeon may reinforce it with a synthetic mesh.

Surgery can be done on an outpatient basis. It usually takes 30 minutes in children and 60 minutes in adults. It can be done under either local or **general anesthesia** and is frequently done laparoscopically. In this type of surgery, a tube that allows visualization of the abdominal cavity is inserted through a small puncture wound. Several small punctures are made to allow surgical instruments to be inserted. This type of surgery avoids a larger incision and significantly reduces the time required for recovery.

Hiatal hernias normally are treated without surgery. The focus of the treatment is to reduce the symptoms associated with **gastroesophageal reflux disease** (GERD) associated with the hernia. Treatments include:

- avoiding reclining after meals
- avoiding spicy foods, acidic foods, alcohol, and tobacco
- eating small, frequent, bland meals
- eating a high-fiber diet

Several types of medications can help manage the symptoms of gastric reflux and heartburn a hiatal hernia. **Antacids** are used to neutralize gastric acid and decrease heartburn. Drugs that reduce the amount of acid produced in the stomach (H2 blockers) are also used. This class of drugs includes famotidine (Pepcid), cimetidine (Tagamet), and ranitidine (Zantac). Omeprazole (Prilosec) is a proton pump inhibitor (PPI) drug, which is another class of drugs that suppress gastric acid secretion and are used for symptoms associated with hiatal hernias. Another option may be metoclopramide (Reglan), a drug that increases the tone of the muscle around the esophagus and causes the stomach to empty more quickly. This drug, however, can have serious side effects.

Alternative treatment

Visceral manipulation, done by a trained therapist, can help replace the stomach to its proper positioning. An alternative to H2 blocker and PPI drugs is deglycyrrhizinated licorice (DGL). This helps balance stomach acid by improving the protective substances that line the stomach and intestines and by improving blood supply to these tissues. DGL does not interrupt the normal function of stomach acid.

As with traditional therapy, dietary modifications are important. Small, frequent meals will keep pressure down on the esophageal sphincter. Also, raising the head of the bed several inches with blocks or books can help with both the quality and quantity of sleep.

Prognosis

Abdominal hernias generally do not recur in children but can recur in up to 10% of adult patients. Surgery is considered the only cure, and the prognosis is excellent if the hernia is corrected before it becomes strangulated.

Hiatal hernias are treated successfully with medication and diet modifications 85% of the time.

Prevention

Some hernias can be prevented by maintaining a reasonable weight, not **smoking**, avoiding heavy lifting, preventing constipation, and following a moderate **exercise** program to maintain good abdominal muscle tone.

Resources

PERIODICALS

Goran, Augustin, et al. "Abdominal Hernias in Pregnancy." *Journal of Obstetrics and Gynecology Research* (April 2009) 35(2): 203–211.

Kingsnorth, Andrew N. "Hernia Surgery: From Guidelines to Clinical Practice." *Annals of the Royal College of Surgeons of England* (May 2009) 91(4): 273–279.

OTHER

Hernia Resource Center. All About Hernias. 2007. http://www.herniainfo.com/content/about.aspx.

Medline Plus. Hernia. February 8, 2010. http://www.nlm.nih.gov/medlineplus/hernia.html.

ORGANIZATIONS

The British Hernia Centre, 87 Watford Way, London, England, United Kingdom, NW4 4RS, + 44-20 8201 7000, + 44 20 8202 6714, experts@hernia.org, http://www.hernia.org/.

Joyce S. Siok, RN
Tish Davidson, A.M.

Hernia repair

Definition

Hernia repair is a surgical procedure to return an organ that protrudes through a weak area of muscle to its original position.

Purpose

Hernias occur when a weakness in the wall of the abdomen allows an organ, usually the intestines, to bulge out of place. Hernias may result from a genetic predisposition toward this weakness. They can also be the result of weakening the muscle through improper **exercise** or poor lifting techniques. Both children and adults get hernias. Some are painful, while others are not.

There are three levels of hernias. An uncomplicated hernia is one where the intestines bulge into the peritoneum (the membrane lining the abdomen), but they can still be manipulated back into the body (although they

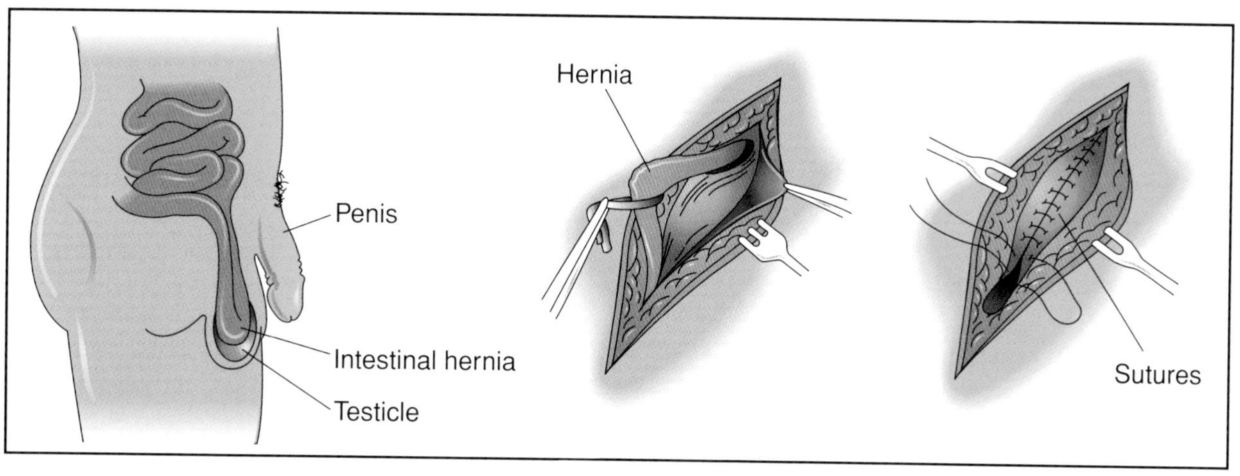

In this inguinal hernia repair, an incision is made in the abdomen. The hernia is located, and the intestines are returned to the abdomen. The abdominal wall is then sutured together to close any space and reinforce the weak area. *(Illustration by Electronic Illustrators Group. Reproduced by permission of Gale, a part of Cengage Learning.)*

don't stay in place without corrective surgery). This is termed a reducible hernia.

If the intestines bulge through the hernia defect and become trapped, this is called an incarcerated hernia. If the blood supply to an incarcerated hernia is shut off, the hernia is called a strangulated hernia. Strangulated hernias can result in **gangrene**.

Both incarcerated and strangulated hernias are medical emergencies and require emergency surgery to correct. For this reason, doctors generally recommend the repair of an uncomplicated hernia, even if it causes no discomfort to the patient.

Precautions

Hernia repair can be performed under local, regional, or **general anesthesia**. The choice depends on the age and health of the patient and the type of hernia. Generally hernia repair is very safe surgery, but—as with any surgery—the risk of complications increases if the patient smokes, is obese, is very young or very old, uses alcohol heavily, or uses illicit drugs.

Description

Hernia repairs are performed in a hospital or outpatient surgical facility by a general surgeon. Depending on the patient's age, health, and the type of hernia, he or she may be able to go home the same day or may remain hospitalized for up to three to five days.

There are two types of hernia repair. A herniorrhaphy is used for simpler hernias. The intestines are returned to their proper place and the defect in the abdominal wall is mended. A hernioplasty is used for larger hernias. In this procedure, plastic or steel mesh is added to the abdominal wall to repair and reinforce the weak spot.

There are five kinds of common hernia repairs. They are named for the part of the body closest to the hernia, or bulge.

Femoral hernia repair

This procedure repairs a hernia that occurs in the groin where the thigh meets the abdomen. It is called a femoral hernia repair because it is near the spot where the femoral artery and vein pass from the leg into the trunk of the body. Sometimes this type of hernia creates a noticeable bulge.

An incision is made in the groin area. The tissues are separated from the hernia sac, and the intestines are returned to the abdomen. The area is often reinforced with webbing before it is sewn shut. The skin is closed with sutures or metal clips that can be removed in about one week.

Inguinal hernia repair

Inguinal hernia repair closes a weakness in the abdominal wall that is near the inguinal canal, the spot where the testes descend from the body into the scrotum. This type of hernia occurs in about 2 percent of adult males.

An incision is made in the abdomen, then the hernia is located and repaired. The surgeon must be alert not to injure the spermatic cord, the testes, or the blood supply to the testes. If the hernia is small, it is simply repaired. If it is large, the area is reinforced with mesh to prevent a recurrence. External skin sutures can be removed in about a week. Patients should not resume sexual activity until being cleared by their doctor.

Umbilical hernia repair

This procedure repairs a hernia that occurs when the intestines bulge through the abdomen wall near the navel. Umbilical hernias are most common in infants.

An incision is made near the navel. The hernia is located and the intestines are returned to the abdomen. The peritoneum is closed, then the large abdominal muscle is pulled over the weak spot in such a way as to reinforce the area. External sutures or skin clips can be removed in about 10 days.

Incisional hernia repair

Incisional hernias occur most frequently at the site of a scar from earlier abdominal surgery. Once again, the abdomen is opened and the intestines returned to their proper place. The area is reinforced with mesh, and the abdominal wall is reconstructed to prevent another hernia from developing. External sutures can be removed in about a week.

Hiatal hernia

A **hiatal hernia** repair is slightly different from the other hernias described here, because it corrects a weakness or opening in the diaphragm, the muscle that separates the chest cavity from the abdominal cavity. This surgery is done to prevent the stomach from shifting up into the chest cavity and to prevent the stomach from spilling gastric juices into the esophagus, causing **pain** and scarring.

An incision is made in the abdomen or chest, and the hole or weakness in the diaphragm is located and repaired. The top of the stomach is wrapped around the bottom of the esophagus, and they are sutured together to hold the stomach in place. Sometimes the vagus nerve is cut in order to decrease the amount of acid the stomach produces. External sutures can be removed in about one week. This type of hernia repair often requires a longer hospital stay than the other types, although techniques are being improved that reduce invasiveness of the surgery and the length of the hospital stay.

Preparation

Before the operation, the patient will have blood and urine collected for testing. X rays are taken of the affected area. In a hiatal hernia, an **endoscopy** (a visual inspection of the organs) is done.

KEY TERMS

Endoscopy—A procedure in which an instrument containing a camera is inserted into the gastrointestinal tract so that the doctor can visually inspect the gastrointestinal system.

Gangrene—Death and decay of body tissue because the blood supply is cut off. Tissues that have died in this way must be surgically removed.

Peritoneum—The transparent membrane lining the abdominal cavity that holds organs such as the intestines in place.

Patients should meet with the anesthesiologist before the operation to discuss any medications or conditions that might affect the administration of anesthesia. Patients may be asked to temporarily discontinue certain medications. The day of the operation, patients should not eat or drink anything. They may be given an enema to clear the bowels.

Aftercare

Patients should eat a clear liquid diet until the gastrointestinal tract begins functioning again. Normally this is a short period of time. After that, they are free to eat a healthy, well-balanced diet of their choice. They may bathe normally, using a gentle, unscented soap. An antibiotic ointment may be prescribed for the incision. After the operation, a hard ridge will form along the incision line. With time, this ridge softens and becomes less noticeable. Patients who remain in the hospital will have blood drawn for follow-up studies.

Patients should begin easy activities, such as walking, as soon as they are comfortable, but should avoid strenuous exercise for four to six weeks, and especially avoid heavy lifting. Learning and practicing proper lifting techniques is an important part of patient education after the operation. Patients may be given a laxative or stool softener so that they will not strain to have bowel movements. They should discuss with their doctor when to resume driving and sexual activity.

Risks

As with any surgery, there exists the possibility of excessive bleeding and infection after the surgery. In inguinal and femoral hernia repair, a slight risk of damage to the testicles or their blood supply exists for male patients. Accidental damage may be caused to the intestinal tract, but generally complications are few.

Normal results

The outcome of surgery depends on the age and health of the patient and on the type of hernia. Although most hernias can be repaired without complications, hernias recur in 10–20% of people who have had hernia surgery.

Resources

OTHER

"Hernia Repair." *ThriveOnline*. http://thriveonline.oxygen.com.

Tish Davidson, A.M.

Herniated disk

Definition

Disk herniation is a rupture of fibrocartilagenous material (annulus fibrosis) that surrounds the intervertebral disk. This rupture involves the release of the disk's center portion containing a gelatinous substance called the nucleus pulposus. Pressure from the vertebrae above and below may cause the nucleus pulposus to be forced outward, placing pressure on a spinal nerve and causing considerable **pain** and damage to the nerve. This condition most frequently occurs in the lumbar region and is also commonly called herniated nucleus pulposus, prolapsed disk, ruptured intervertebral disk, or slipped disk.

Description

The spinal column is made up of 26 vertebrae that are joined together and permit forward and backward bending, side bending, and rotation of the spine. Five distinct regions comprise the spinal column, including the cervical (neck) region, thoracic (chest) region, lumbar (low back) region, sacral, and coccygeal (tailbone) region. The cervical region consists of seven vertebrae, the thoracic region includes 12 vertebrae, and the lumbar region contains five vertebrae. The sacrum is

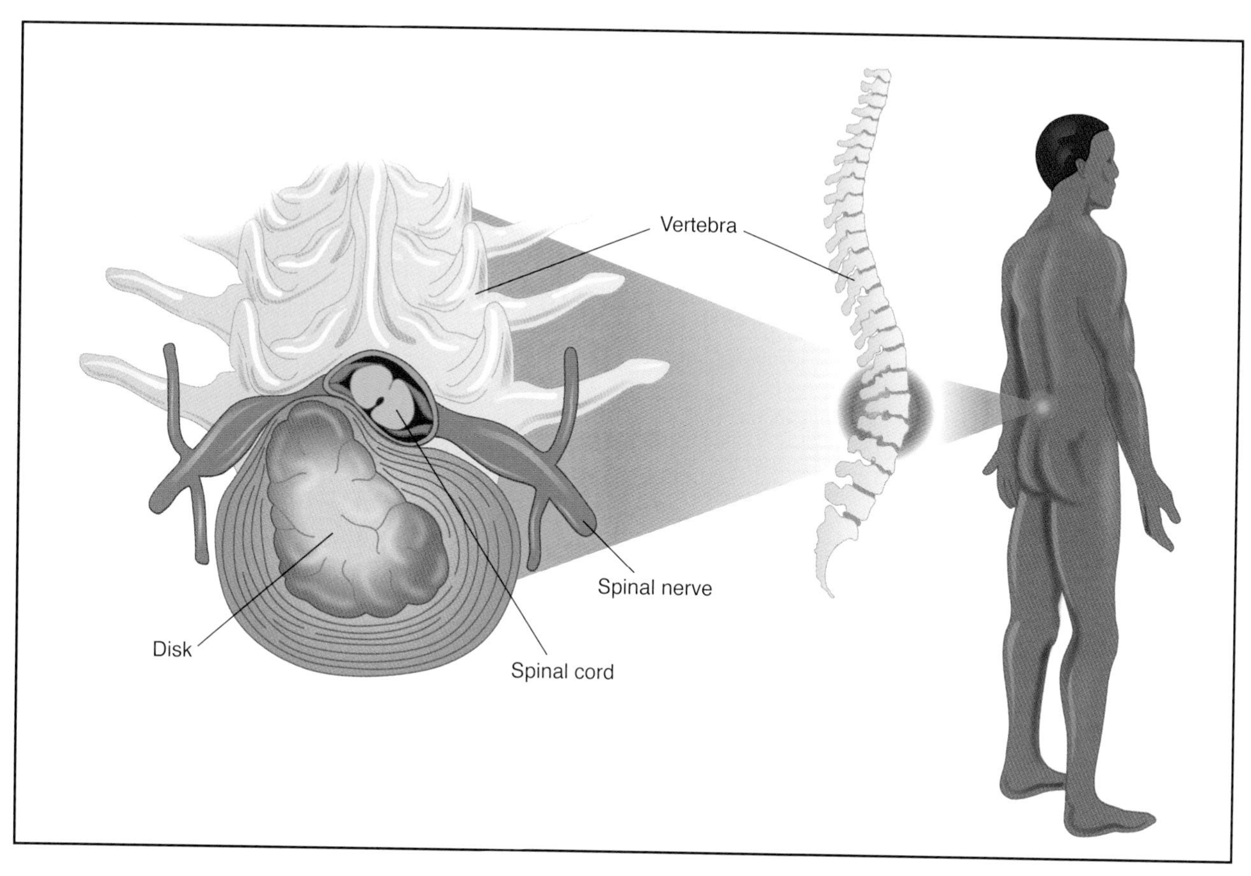

A herniated disk refers to the rupture of fibrocartilagenous material, called the annulus fibrosis, that surrounds the intervertebral disk. When this occurs, pressure from the vertebrae above and below may force the disk's center portion, a gel-like substance, outward, placing additional pressure on the spinal nerve and causing pain and damage to the nerve. *(Illustration by Electronic Illustrators Group. Reproduced by permission of Gale, a part of Cengage Learning.)*

composed of five fused vertebrae, which are connected to four fused vertebrae forming the coccyx. Intervertebral disks lie between each adjacent vertebra.

Each disk is composed of a gelatinous material in the center, called the nucleus pulposus, surrounded by rings of a fiberous tissue (annulus fibrosus). In disk herniation, an intervertebral disk's central portion herniates or slips through the surrounding annulus fibrosus into the spinal canal, putting pressure on a nerve root. Disk herniation most commonly affects the lumbar region between the fifth lumbar vertebra and the first sacral vertebra. However, disk herniation can also occur in the cervical spine. The incidence of cervical disk herniation is most common between the fifth and sixth cervical vertebrae. The second most common area for cervical disk herniation occurs between the sixth and seventh cervical vertebrae. Disk herniation is less common in the thoracic region.

Predisposing factors associated with disk herniation include age, gender, and work environment. The peak age for occurrence of disk herniation is between 20–45 years of age. Studies have shown that males are more commonly affected than females in lumbar disk herniation by a 3:2 ratio. Prolonged exposure to a bent-forward work posture is correlated with an increased incidence of disk herniation.

There are four classifications of disk pathology:

- A protrusion may occur where a disk bulges without rupturing the annulus fibrosis.
- The disk may prolapse where the nucleus pulposus migrates to the outermost fibers of the annulus fibrosis.
- There may be a disk extrusion, which is the case if the annulus fibrosis perforates and material of the nucleus moves into the epidural space.
- The sequestrated disk may occur as fragments from the annulus fibrosis and nucleus pulposus are outside the disk proper.

Causes and symptoms

Any direct, forceful, and vertical pressure on the lumbar disks can cause the disk to push its fluid contents into the vertebral body. Herniated nucleus pulposus may occur suddenly from lifting, twisting, or direct injury, or it can occur gradually from degenerative changes with episodes of intensifying symptoms. The annulus may also become weakened over time, allowing stretching or tearing and leading to a disk herniation. Depending on the location of the herniation, the herniated material can also press directly on nerve roots or on the spinal cord, causing a shock-like pain (**sciatica**) down the legs, weakness, **numbness**, or problems with bowels, bladder, or sexual function.

Diagnosis

Several radiographic tests are useful for confirming a diagnosis of disk herniation and locating the source of pain. These tests also help the surgeon indicate the extent of the surgery needed to fully decompress the nerve. X rays show structural changes of the lumbar spine. **Myelography** is a special x ray of the spine in which a dye or air is injected into the patient's spinal canal. The patient lies strapped to a table as the table tilts in various directions and spot x rays are taken. X rays showing a narrowed dye column in the intervertebral disk area indicate possible disk herniation.

A computed tomography scan (CT or CAT scan) exhibits the details of pathology necessary to obtain consistently good surgical results. **Magnetic resonance imaging** (MRI) analysis of the disks can accurately detect the early stages of disk **aging** and degeneration. Electomyograms (EMGs) measure the electrical activity of the muscle contractions and possibly show evidence of nerve damage. An EMG is a powerful tool for assessing muscle **fatigue** associated with muscle impairment with **low back pain**.

Treatment

Drugs

Unless serious neurologic symptoms occur, herniated disks can initially be treated with pain medication and up to 48 hours of bed rest. There is no proven benefit from resting more than 48 hours. Patients are then encouraged to gradually increase their activity. Pain medications, including antiinflammatories, muscle relaxers, or in severe cases, **narcotics**, may be continued if needed.

Epidural steroid injections have been used to decrease pain by injecting an antiinflammatory drug, usually a corticosteroid, around the nerve root to reduce inflammation and **edema** (swelling). This partly relieves the pressure on the nerve root as well as resolves the inflammation.

Physical therapy

Physical therapists are skilled in treating acute back pain caused by the disk herniation. The physical therapist can provide noninvasive therapies, such as ultrasound or diathermy to project heat deep into the tissues of the back or administer manual therapy, if mobility of the spine is impaired. They may help improve posture and develop an **exercise** program for recovery and long-term protection. Appropriate exercise can help take pressure off inflamed nerve structures, while improving overall posture and flexibility. **Traction** can be used to try to decrease pressure on the disk. A lumbar support can be helpful for a herniated disk at this level as a temporary measure to reduce pain and improve posture.

Surgery

Surgery is often appropriate for conditions that do not improve with the usual treatment. In this event, a strong, flexible spine is important for a quick recovery after surgery. There are several surgical approaches to treating a herniated disk, including the classic discectomy, microdiscectomy, or percutanteous discectomy. The basic differences among these procedures are the size of the incision, how the disk is reached surgically, and how much of the disk is removed.

Discectomy is the surgical removal of the portion of the disk that is putting pressure on a nerve causing the back pain. In the classic disectomy, the surgeon first enters through the skin and then removes a bony portion of the vertebra called the lamina, hence the term **laminectomy**. The surgeon removes the disk material that is pressing on a nerve. Rarely is the entire lamina or disk entirely removed. Often, only one side is removed and the surgical procedure is termed hemilaminectomy.

In microdiscectomy, through the use of an operating microscope, the surgeon removes the offending bone or disk tissue until the nerve is free from compression or stretch. This procedure is possible using **local anesthesia**. Microsurgery techniques vary and have several advantages over the standard discectomy, such as a smaller incision, less trauma to the musculature and nerves, and easier identification of structures by viewing into the disk space through microscope magnification.

Percutaneous disk excision is performed on an outpatient basis, is less expensive than other surgical procedures, and does not require a **general anesthesia**. The purpose of percutaneous disk excision is to reduce the volume of the affected disk indirectly by partial removal of the nucleus pulposus, leaving all the structures important to stability practically unaffected. In this procedure, large incisions are avoided by inserting devices that have cutting and suction capability. Suction is applied and the disk is sliced and aspirated.

Arthroscopic microdiscectomy is similar to percutaneous discectomy, however it incorporates modified arthroscopic instruments, including scopes and suction devices. A suction irrigation of saline solution is established through two entry sites. A video discoscope is introduced from one site and the deflecting instruments from the opposite side. In this way, the surgeon is able to search and extract the nuclear fragments under direct visualization.

Laser disk decompression is performed using similar means as percutaneous excision and arthroscopic microdiscectomy, but laser energy is used to remove the disk tissue. Here, laser energy is percutanteously introduced through a needle to vaporize a small volume of nucleus pulposus, thereby dropping the pressure of the disk and decompressing the involved neural tissues. One disadvantage of this procedure is the high initial cost of the laser equipment. It is important to realize that only a very small percentage of people with herniated lumbar disks go on to require surgery. Further, surgery should be followed by appropriate **rehabilitation** to decrease the chance of reinjury.

Chemonucleolysis

Chemonucleolysis is an alternative to surgical excision. Chymopapain, a purified enzyme derived from the papaya plant, is injected percutaneously into the disk space to reduce the size of the herniated disks. It hydrolyses proteins, thereby decreasing water-binding capacity, when injected into the nucleus pulposus inner disk material. The reduction in size of the disk relieves pressure on the nerve root.

Spinal fusion

Spinal fusion is the process by which bone grafts harvested from the iliac crest (thick border of the ilium located on the pelvis) are placed between the intervertebral bodies after the disk material is removed. This approach is used when there is a need to reestablish the normal bony relationship between the vertebrae. A total discectomy may be needed in some cases because lumbar spinal fusion can help prevent recurrent lumbar disk herniation at a particular level.

Alternative treatment

Acupuncture involves the use of fine needles inserted along the pathway of the pain to move energy locally and relieve the pain. An acupuncturist determines the location of the nerves affected by the herniated disk and positions the needles appropriately. Massage therapists may also provide short-term relief from a herniated disk. Following manual examination and x-ray diagnosis, **chiropractic** treatment usually includes manipulation to correct muscle and joint malfunctions, while care is taken not to place an additional strain on the injured disk. If a full trial of conservative therapy fails, or if neurologic problems (weakness, bowel or bladder problems, and sensory loss) develop, the next step is usually evaluation by an orthopedic surgeon.

Prognosis

Only 5–10% of patients with unrelenting sciatica and neurological involvement, leading to chronic pain of the lumbar spine, need to have a surgical procedure performed. This strongly suggests that many patients with herniated disks at the lumbar level respond well to conservative treatment. For those patients who do require surgery for lumbar disk herniation, the reviewed procedures of nerve root decompression caused by disk herniation is favorable. Results of studies varied from 60–90% success rates. Disk surgery has progressively evolved in the direction of decreasing invasiveness. Each surgical procedure is not without possible complications, which can lead to chronic low back pain and restricted lifestyle.

Prevention

Proper exercises to strengthen the lower back and abdominal muscles are key in preventing excess **stress** and compressive forces on lumbar disks. Good posture will help prevent problems on cervical, thoracic, and lumbar disks. A good flexibility program is critical for prevention of muscle and spasm that can cause an increase in compressive forces on disks at any level. Proper lifting of heavy objects is important for all muscles and levels of the individual disks. Good posture in sitting, standing, and lying down is helpful for the spine. Losing weight, if needed, can prevent weakness and unnecessary stress on the disks caused by **obesity**. Choosing proper footwear may also be helpful to reduce the impact forces to the lumbar disks while walking on hard surfaces. Wearing special back support devices may be helpful if heavy lifting is required with combinations of twisting.

Resources

OTHER

"Back Pain." Healthtouch Online Page. http://www.healthtouch.com.

Jeffrey P. Larson, RPT

Hernioplasty *see* **Hernia repair**

Herniorrhaphy *see* **Hernia repair**

Herpes *see* **Cold sore**

Herpes encephalitis *see* **Encephalitis**

Herpes genitalis *see* **Genital herpes**

Herpes simplex *see* **Cold sore**

Herpes simplex type 2 *see* **Genital herpes**

Herpes type 2 *see* **Genital herpes**

Herpes zoster infection *see* **Shingles**

Heterotopic transplant *see* **Liver transplantation**

Heterotropia *see* **Strabismus**

HFRS *see* **Hantavirus infections**

Hiatal hernia

Definition

A hiatal hernia is a condition in which a weakness or actual gap or tear in the large muscle of the diaphragm serves as an opening through which the stomach can enter the chest. Hiatal hernias can exist at birth (congenital hiatal hernia) or can develop later in life.

The diaphragm is a large dome-shaped sheet of muscle tissue that spans from the left to the right ribcage. It divides the chest area (thoracic cavity) from the abdominal cavity. The esophageal hiatus is the area of the diagphragm where the esophagus penetrates, joining the stomach below.

Along with other muscles of the abdomen and thoracic cavity, the diaphragm plays an important role in the process of respiration (breathing). During inspiration (breathing in), the muscle of the diaphragm contracts. This increases the volume of the thoracic cavity, and suction allows air to enter the lungs. During expiration, the diaphragm relaxes, and air is expelled from the lungs. The esophagus passes through an area of the diaphragm (the hiatus) on the way to the stomach, which helps prevent the backflow of stomach acid up the esophagus. The diaphragm plays a role in other functions, by virtue of its ability to increase pressure within the abdomen (intra-abdominal pressure)—in this capacity, it is crucial to the acts of **vomiting**, defecation, and urination.

Demographics

A hiatal hernia can occur due to an injury, or can develop over time due to some inherent weakness in the muscle fibers. Greatly increased intra-abdominal pressure, as may occur during **pregnancy**, can also induce a hiatal hernia. The following factors may contribute to the development of a hiatal hernia:

- Obesity
- Family history of hiatal hernia

- Repeated straining due to constipation
- Smoking
- Heavy lifting
- Chronic cough
- Extreme bouts of violent vomiting
- Age (about 60% of people develop some degree of hiatal hernia by the time they reach the age of 60)

Description

A hiatal hernia occurs when the stomach enters the chest cavity through a weakness or tear in the area of the diaphragm where the esophagus passes through. The most common form of hiatal hernia occurs when the gastroesophageal junction (the area where the esophagus enters the stomach) slides upward through the hernia opening. This is referred to as a sliding hiatal hernia. A rolling or paraesophageal hiatal hernia is much more rare. In this instance, the gastroesophageal junction doesn't protrude up into the thoracic cavity; instead, a portion of the stomach slides up alongside the esophagus, and protrudes into the chest cavity through the hiatal opening. This type of hiatal hernia is more dangerous, since there is a risk that the narrow confines through which the stomach protrudes will prevent proper blood circulation into this area of the stomach, causing its tissue to become oxygen deprived (strangulated).

While some people can have a hiatal hernia without any recognizable symptoms, other people have clear-cut discomfort related to the condition. Symptoms of a hiatal hernia are very similar to symptoms of gastric acid reflux, and include

- heartburn
- chest pain
- nausea
- frequent belching

Symptoms often get worse based on position (lying down, leaning forward) and activity (lifting heavy objects, straining for any reason). Over time, symptoms can worsen and cause coughing and asthma-like symptoms, **sore throat**, and swallowing problems (dysphagia). Anemia can develop when chronic acid reflux causes esophagitis with erosions of the esophagus or upper stomach.

Diagnosis/Preparations

Hiatal hernia is sometimes diagnosed when a **chest x ray** is performed for some other reason. In other instances, tests such as a barium swallow (upper GI series) or upper **endoscopy** may be performed specifically to look for the presence of a hiatal hernia.

Treatment

Treatment of a hiatal hernia often starts with treatment of the symptoms of gastroesophageal reflux that it induces, including medications such as **antacids**, **H-2 blockers**, and **proton pump inhibitors**. Practical recommendations include weight loss, stopping **smoking**, elevating the head of the bed at night, so that gravity discourages acid reflux, adjusting the diet to avoid **constipation** (and therefore straining at stool), and avoiding activities that cause straining (such as heavy lifting).

In some cases, surgical interventions will be required, particularly with very large hiatal hernias or with the rolling or paraesophageal form of hiatal hernia. Several surgical approaches may be utilized, all with the purpose of pulling the stomach back down into the abdomen, and decreasing the size of the hiatal opening. The surgery may be performed through an incision in the chest (thoracic access), abdomen (abdominal access), or using minimally invasive, laparoscopic techniques. Some of the surgeries used include Nissen fundoplication, Belsey (Mark IV) fundoplication, and Hill repair.

Resources

BOOKS

Feldman, M., et al. *Sleisenger & Fordtran's Gastrointestinal and Liver Disease*. 8th ed. St. Louis: Mosby, 2005.

Khatri, V. P., and J. A. Asensio. *Operative Surgery Manual*. 1st ed. Philadelphia: Saunders, 2003.

Townsend, C. M., et al. *Sabiston Textbook of Surgery*. 17th ed. Philadelphia: Saunders, 2004.

Rosalyn Carson-DeWitt, MD

Hiccups

Definition

Hiccups are the result of an involuntary, spasmodic contraction of the diaphragm followed by the closing of the throat.

Demographics

A hiccup bout is an episode lasting more than a few minutes. If hiccups last longer than 48 hours, they are considered persistent or protracted. Hiccups lasting longer than one month are termed intractable. The longest recorded attack is six decades.

Hiccups can occur at any age and in utero. Preterm infants spend up to 2.5% of their time hiccupping.

Although hiccups occur less frequently with age, intractable hiccups are more common in adult life. Females develop hiccups more frequently during early adulthood than males of the same age.

Hiccups are one of the most common, but thankfully mildest, disorders to which humans are prey. Virtually everyone experiences them at some point, but they rarely last long or require a doctor's care. Occasionally, a bout of hiccups will last longer than two days, earning it the name "persistent hiccups." Very few people will experience intractable hiccups, in which hiccups last longer than one month.

Description

A hiccup involves the coordinated action of the diaphragm and the muscles that close off the windpipe (trachea). The diaphragm is a dome-shaped muscle separating the chest and abdomen, normally responsible for expanding the chest cavity for inhalation. Sensation from the diaphragm travels to the spinal cord through the phrenic nerve and the vagus nerve, which pass through the chest cavity and the neck. Within the spinal cord, nerve fibers from the brain monitor sensory information and adjust the outgoing messages that control contraction. These messages travel along the phrenic nerve.

Irritation of any of the nerves involved in this loop can cause the diaphragm to undergo involuntary contraction, or spasm, pulling air into the lungs. When this occurs, it triggers a reflex in the throat muscles. Less than a tenth of a second afterward, the trachea is closed off, making the characteristic "hic" sound.

Causes and symptoms

Hiccups can be caused by central nervous system disorders, injury or irritation to the phrenic and vagus nerves, and toxic or metabolic disorders affecting the central or peripheral nervous systems. They may be of unknown cause or may be a symptom of psychological **stress**. Hiccups often occur after drinking carbonated beverages or alcohol. They may also follow overeating or rapid temperature changes. Persistent or intractable hiccups may be caused by any condition which irritates or damages the relevant nerves, including:

- overstretching of the neck
- laryngitis
- heartburn (gastroesophageal reflux)
- irritation of the eardrum (which is innervated by the vagus nerve)
- general anesthesia
- surgery
- bloating
- tumor
- infection
- diabetes

Diagnosis

Hiccups are diagnosed by observation, and by hearing the characteristic sound. Diagnosing the cause of intractable hiccups may require imaging studies, blood tests, pH monitoring in the esophagus, and other tests.

Treatment

Most cases of hiccups will disappear on their own. Home remedies that interrupt or override the spasmodic nerve circuitry are often effective. Such remedies include:

- holding one's breath for as long as possible
- breathing into a paper bag
- swallowing a spoonful of sugar
- bending forward from the waist and drinking water from the wrong side of a glass

Treating any underlying disorder will usually cure the associated hiccups. Chlorpromazine (Thorazine) relieves intractable hiccups in 80% of cases. Metoclopramide (Reglan), carbamazepam, valproic acid (Depakene), and phenobarbital are also used. As a last resort, surgery to block the phrenic nerve may be performed, although it may lead to significant impairment of respiration.

Prognosis

Most cases of hiccups last no longer than several hours, with or without treatment.

Prevention

Some cases of hiccups can be avoided by drinking in moderation, avoiding very hot or very cold food, and avoiding cold showers. Carbonated beverages when drunk through a straw deliver more gas to the stomach than when sipped from a container; therefore, avoid using straws.

Resources

PERIODICALS

Krysiak W. et al. "Hiccups as a Myocardial Ischemia Symptom." *Pol Arch Med Wewn.* March 2008, 118(3):148-51.

Suh W. M., and S. C. Krishnan. "Violent hiccups: An Infrequent Cause of Bradyarrhythmias." *West J Emerg Med.* August 2009, 10(3):176-7.

Richard Robinson
Karl Finley

High-altitude sickness *see* **Altitude sickness**

High-risk pregnancy

Definition

A **pregnancy** that has maternal or fetal complications requiring special medical attention or bed rest is considered high-risk. Complications, as used here, mean that the risk of illness or **death** before or after delivery is greater than normal for the mother or baby.

Demographics

According to the U.S. Centers for Disease Control and Prevention (CDC) there were 13.1 maternal deaths for every 100,000 live births in the United States in 2004. There was a large racial disparity in maternal deaths, with African American women experiencing 36.1 deaths per 100,00 live births in 2004 and white women experiencing 9.8 deaths per 100,000 live births the same year. The rate for Hispanic women was 8.5 per 100,000 live births. Over the past 100 years deaths due to pregnancy and **childbirth** have declined hugely. In the early 1900s, giving birth was one of the most dangerous things a woman could do, with more than 600 women dying for every 100,000 live births in the year 1915.

Other statistics provide maternal mortality information by total female population, instead of per number of live births. In 2006, there were 115 deaths per 100,000 population due to pregnancy and childbirth among African American women, 70 deaths per 100,000 population among Hispanic and Latino women, 113 deaths per 100,000 population among white women, and 20 deaths per 100,000 population among Asian women. Common causes of death in women of childbearing age are problems related to pregnancy and delivery, including **blood clots** that travel to the lungs, anesthesia complications, bleeding, infection, and high blood pressure complications (preeclampsia and **eclampsia**).

A baby dies before, during, or shortly after birth in 16 out of 1,000 deliveries in the United States. Almost 50% of these deaths are stillbirths, which are sometimes unexplained. In 2005 there were 4.54 deaths in newborns before age 28 days per 1,000 live births, a total of 18,782 neonatal deaths. Risk factors for **stillbirth** and neonatal can be present before pregnancy occurs or develop during the course of the pregnancy.

Description

Risk factors in pregnancy are those findings discovered during prenatal assessment that are known to have a potentially negative effect on the outcome of the pregnancy, either for the woman or the fetus. This evaluation determines whether the mother has characteristics or conditions that make her or her baby more likely to become sick or die during the pregnancy.

The pregnant woman's interview at her first visit to the health care provider is conducted by the nurse, who obtains the data necessary to begin the high-risk screening. The physician or midwife caring for the pregnant woman will review the prenatal assessment sheet, order lab data, and obtain ultrasounds to determine if any risk factors are present. If it is determined that a woman has a high-risk pregnancy, she should be referred to a perinatologist for advanced care. This is the specialist who establishes and implements the medical regimen needed for the particular maternal/fetal complications likely to occur and the interdisciplinary team associated with the perinatal center works in its management. The perinatal team usually comprises a nutritionist, social worker, nurse educators, geneticists, ultrasonographers, and additional nursing staff who are responsible for the monitoring and supervising of ongoing team care of the patient.

Causes and symptoms

All risk factors do not threaten pregnancy to the same extent. The risk of complications is increased by **smoking**, poor nutritional habits, drug and alcohol **abuse**, domestic violence, prepregnancy maternal health status, psychosocial factors, prior health care, the presence of chronic medical problems in the mother, past history of repeated preterm delivery, multiple gestation, and abnormalities of the fetus or placenta. A woman with a high-risk pregnancy may have an earlier labor and delivery depending upon the fetal or maternal complication present and, likewise, present with symptoms dependent on the condition. Since the placenta supplies the baby with its nutrients and oxygen, any condition that threatens the blood supply to it threatens fetal development.

The threat of a preterm delivery is the most common reason for a referral to a perinatal center, which is linked to obstetric and newborn services that provide

KEY TERMS

Amniocentesis—A procedure that uses ultrasound to guide a needle into the amniotic sac (bag of waters) surrounding the baby and obtain fluid to analyze for genetic abnormalities.

Antepartum—This refers to the time period of the woman's pregnancy from conception and onset of labor.

Down syndrome—The most prevalent of a class of genetic defects known as trisomies, in which cells contain three copies of certain chromosomes rather than the usual two. Down syndrome, or trisomy 21, usually results from three copies of chromosome 21.

Perinatal—Refers to the period shortly before and after birth, generally from around the 20th week of pregnancy to one to four weeks after birth.

Perinatologist—A specialist in the branch of obstetrics that deals with the high-risk pregnant woman and her fetus.

Preconceptional—This refers to the time period before pregnancy, i.e., conception, occurs.

Ultrasonographer—The person who performs the radiologic technique of ultrasound in which deep structures of the body are visualized.

the highest level of care for a pregnant woman and her baby. A preterm delivery may occur because of a **premature rupture of membranes** (the bag of water surrounding the baby breaks) or preterm labor. There is a strong correlation of vaginal or uterine infection with the pregnant woman's water breaking, and there are laboratory tests that are predictive of a woman's risk of experiencing preterm labor.

Diagnosis

A risk-scoring sheet is used by many health care agencies during the prenatal assessment to establish if a woman may be at risk for complications during her pregnancy. This score sheet is implemented at the first prenatal visit, becomes a part of the woman's record, and is updated throughout the pregnancy as necessary. A woman's age affects pregnancy risk, as girls 15 years old and under are more likely to develop high blood pressure, protein in the urine and fluid accumulation, or seizures. They also are more likely to have underweight or undernourished babies. A woman 35 or older has a greater risk of developing high blood pressure or diabetes, as well as a much higher risk of having a chromosomal abnormality such as **Down syndrome**. A woman shorter than five feet or a woman weighing less than 100 pounds before pregnancy has a greater risk of having a small or preterm baby.

Laboratory data and ultrasound also are used to determine high-risk pregnancies by specific blood tests and imaging of the baby. A pregnancy may begin classified as low risk but be changed to a classification of high risk secondary to complications determined from the ongoing assessment of the pregnant woman. Since many of these complications can be managed with proper treatment, it is essential that a pregnant woman make and keep regular obstetric appointments.

Treatment

Treatment will vary, depending upon the maternal or fetal complication present. Generally, a woman with severe high-risk factors in pregnancy should be referred to a perinatal center to obtain the highest level of care for herself and her baby. Interventions to improve health status might include nutritional assessment; **physical examination**; teaching modalities for smoking cessation, drug and alcohol programs; prescribing medications related to the condition or changing pre-pregnancy medications (known to cause problems in the fetus); serial ultrasounds to learn fetal status; **amniocentesis**; fetal transfusions; fetal surgery; **antepartum testing**; bed rest; home health care; hospitalization; and early delivery. In a post-term pregnancy (greater than 42 weeks), the death of a baby is three times more likely than that of a normal term pregnancy (37–40 weeks). The treatment in this case would be to induce labor or perform a **cesarean section** before problems start to occur.

Prognosis

Advances in the management of complications in high-risk pregnancies have provided women with a means of controlling their risks, which substantially increases the potential for a successful outcome. Since it is impossible to guarantee a good outcome in a normal pregnancy, it is even more difficult to ensure that a high-risk pregnancy will result in a healthy infant and mother. A woman who strictly adheres to the medical regimen established for her, however, will greatly increase her chances of a positive result.

Prevention

The early weeks of pregnancy are the most crucial ones for the fetus. Many women do not know they are pregnant until several weeks after conception, so education about the need for preconceptional care is essential. Preconception counseling guides a woman in planning a healthy pregnancy. These are some of the factors to which attention must be paid:

- family history
- medical history
- past pregnancies
- current medications
- lifestyle
- environment
- infections

The number one preventable cause of **mental retardation** in infants is the alcohol use during pregnancy. Alcohol can cause problems ranging from **miscarriage** to severe behavioral problems in the baby or developing child even if no obvious physical **birth defects** are apparent. **Fetal alcohol syndrome** is seen in about 2 out of 1,000 live births.

Cigarette smoking is the most common **addiction** among pregnant women in the United States, and despite the health hazards of smoking being well known, only about 20% of these women actually quit during pregnancy. One risk of smoking during pregnancy is having a baby who may die from **sudden infant death syndrome** (SIDS).

Drugs known to cause birth defects when taken during pregnancy include: alcohol, dilantin (phenytoin), any drug that interferes with the actions of **folic acid**, lithium, streptomycin, tetracycline, thalidomide, warfarin (Coumadin), and isotretinoin (Accutane), which is prescribed for **acne**.

Infections that may cause birth defects include: herpes simplex, viral hepatitis, the flu, **mumps**, German **measles (rubella)**, **chickenpox** (varicella), **syphilis**, **toxoplasmosis** (occurs from eating undercooked meat and handling kitty litter), **listeriosis**, and infections from the coxsackievirus or cytomegalovirus (CMV). Many adults have been exposed to coxsackievirus and CMV when they were younger, but many have not. Those who have not been exposed should pay careful attention to any illnesses they have early in their pregnancy, noting the onset, presence of **fever**, muscle aches and pains, and duration of illness to report to their physician.

Hemolytic disease of the newborn (destruction of the red blood cells) can occur when Rh incompatibility exists between child and mother. The most common cause of incompatible blood types is Rh incompatibility, such as when the mother has Rh-negative blood and the father has Rh-positive blood. The baby may have Rh-positive blood, in which case the mother's body produces antibodies against the baby's blood. Fortunately, the mother can be treated with Rhogham [Rh0(D)immune globulin], which can be given to the mother in the first 72 hours after delivery and at the twenty-eighth week of pregnancy; it will destroy any antibodies produced by her blood and significantly decrease the risk associated with pregnancies with Rh-factor incompatibilities.

There are, however, other incompatible blood factors during the prenatal assessment period that can cause anemia in the fetus and require ongoing monitoring. The greatest gift a woman can give to herself and her baby is to plan her pregnancy with preconceptional counseling. Many women are frequently deficient in folic acid, a B vitamin used in the synthesis of ribonucleic acid (RNA) and essential, in large quantities, for optimal protein synthesis in the fetus. This is especially true in the early weeks of pregnancy, when all cell division and organ development is occurring. Thus, the best prevention for a high risk pregnancy is good planning.

Resources

BOOKS

Gilbert, Elizabeth S. *Manual of High Risk Pregnancy and Delivery*, 5th ed. Maryland Heights, MO: Mosby Elsevier, 2011.

James, David K., ed. *High Risk Pregnancy: Management Options*, 5th ed. Philadelphia, PA: Saunders/Elsevier, 2011.

Platt, Elizabeth S. *100 Questions and Answers about Your High-Risk Pregnancy*. Sudbury, MA: Jones & Bartlett Publishers, 2008.

Raab, Diana, with Errol Norwitz. *Your High-Risk Pregnancy: A Practical and Supportive Guide*. Alameda, CA: Hunter House, 2009.

PERIODICALS

Holland, Marium G., et al. "Late Preterm Birth: How Often is it Avoidable?" *American Journal of Obstetrics and Gynecology* (October 2009), 104(4), 404.e1-4.

Vidaeff, Alex C., and Susan M. Ramin. "Management Strategies for the Prevention of Preterm Birth." *Current Opinion in Obstetrics and Gynecology* (December 2009), 21(6), 480-484.

ORGANIZATIONS

American Academy of Pediatrics, 141 Northwest Point Boulevard, Elk Grove Village, IL, 60007-1098, (847) 434-4000, (847) 434-8000, http://www.aap.org.

American College of Obstetricians and Gynecologists, P.O. Box 96920, Washington, DC, 20090-6920, (202)638-5577, http://www.acog.org.

American Pregnancy Association, 431 Greenway Drive, Suite 800, Irving, TX, 75038, (972) 550-0140, (972) 550-0800, Questions@AmericanPregnancy.org, http://www.americanpregnancy.org.

Linda K. Bennington, R.N.C., M.S.N., C.N.S.
Tish Davidson, A.M.

High blood phosphate level *see* **Phosphorus imbalance**

High blood pressure *see* **Pulmonary hypertension**

High calcium blood level *see* **Hypercalcemia**

High cholesterol *see* **Cholesterol, high**

High potassium blood level *see* **Hyperkalemia**

High sodium blood level *see* **Hypernatremia**

Hindu medicine *see* **Ayurvedic medicine**

Hip bath *see* **Sitz bath**

Hip replacement *see* **Joint replacement**

Hirschsprung's disease

Definition

Hirschsprung's disease, also known as congenital megacolon or aganglionic megacolon, is an abnormality in which certain nerve fibers are absent in segments of the bowel, resulting in severe bowel obstruction. It was first identified in 1886 by a physician named Harold Hirschsprung.

Description

Hirschsprung's disease is caused when certain nerve cells (called parasympathetic **ganglion** cells) in the wall of the large intestine (colon) do not develop before birth. Without these nerves, the affected segment of the colon lacks the ability to relax and move bowel contents along. This causes a constriction and as a result, the bowel above the constricted area dilates due to stool becoming trapped, producing megacolon (dilation of the colon). The disease can affect varying lengths of bowel segment, most often involving the region around the rectum. In up to 10% of children, however, the entire colon and part of the small intestine are involved. This condition is known as total colonic aganglionosis, or TCA.

Hirschsprung's disease occurs once in every 5,000 live births, and it is about four times more common in males than females. Between 4% and 50% of siblings are also afflicted. The wide range for recurrence is due to the fact that the recurrence risk depends on the gender of the affected individual in the family (i.e., if a female is affected, the recurrence risk is higher) and the length of the aganglionic segment of the colon (i.e., the longer the segment that is affected, the higher the recurrence risk).

Causes and symptoms

Hirschsprung's disease occurs early in fetal development when, for unknown reasons, there is either failure of nerve cell development, failure of nerve cell migration, or arrest in nerve cell development in a segment of the bowel. The absence of these nerve fibers, which help control the movement of bowel contents, is what results in intestinal obstruction accompanied by other symptoms.

There is a genetic basis to Hirschsprung's disease, and it is believed that it may be caused by different genetic factors in different subsets of families. Proof that genetic factors contribute to Hirschprung's disease is that it is known to run in families, and it has been seen in association with some chromosome abnormalities. For example, about 10% of children with the disease have **Down syndrome** (the most common chromosomal abnormality). Molecular diagnostic techniques have identified many genes that cause susceptibility to Hirschprung's disease. As of the early 2000s, a total of six genes have been identified: the RET gene, the glial cell line-derived neurotrophic factor gene, the endothelin-B receptor gene, endothelin converting enzyme, the endothelin-3 gene, and the Sry-related transcription factor SOX10. Mutations that inactivate the RET gene are the most frequent, occurring in 50% of familial cases (cases which run in families) and 15–20% of sporadic (non-familial) cases. Mutations in these genes do not cause the disease, but they make the chance of developing it more likely. Mutations in other genes or environmental factors are required to develop the disease, and these other factors are not understood. At least three chromosomes are known to be involved: 13q22, 21q22, and 10q. Hirschsprung's disease has also been reported in association with abnormal forms of chromosome 18.

For persons with a ganglion growth beyond the sigmoid segment of the colon, the inheritance pattern is autosomal dominant with reduced penetrance (risk closer to 50%). For persons with smaller segments involved, the inheritance pattern is multifactorial (caused by an interaction of more than one gene and environmental factors, risk lower than 50%) or autosomal recessive (one disease gene inherited from each parent, risk closer to 25%) with low penetrance.

The initial symptom is usually severe, continuous **constipation**. A newborn may fail to pass meconium (the first stool) within 24 hours of birth, may repeatedly vomit yellow- or green-colored bile and may have a distended (swollen, uncomfortable) abdomen. Occasionally, infants may have only mild or intermittent constipation, often with **diarrhea**.

While two-thirds of cases are diagnosed in the first three months of life, Hirschsprung's disease may also be diagnosed later in infancy or childhood. Occasionally, even adults are diagnosed with a variation of the disease. In older infants, symptoms and signs may include anorexia (lack of appetite or inability to eat), lack of the urge to move the bowels or empty the rectum on **physical examination**, distended abdomen, and a mass in the colon that can be felt by the physician during examination. It should be suspected in older children with abnormal bowel habits, especially a history of constipation dating back to infancy and ribbon-like stools.

Occasionally, the presenting symptom may be a severe intestinal infection called enterocolitis, which is life-threatening. The symptoms are usually explosive, watery stools and **fever** in a very ill-appearing infant. It is important to diagnose the condition before the intestinal obstruction causes an overgrowth of bacteria that evolves into a medical emergency. Enterocolitis can lead to severe diarrhea and massive fluid loss, which can cause **death** from **dehydration** unless surgery is done immediately to relieve the obstruction.

Hirschsprung's disease sometimes occurs in children with other disorders of the autonomic nervous system, such as congenital central hypoventilation syndrome, a breathing disorder. Other syndromes associated with Hirschsprung disease include congenital deafness and Waardenburg syndrome, a genetic disorder characterized by facial abnormalities and the loss of normal pigmentation in the hair, skin, and the iris of the eye.

Diagnosis

Hirschsprung's disease in the newborn must be distinguished from other causes of intestinal obstruction. The diagnosis is suspected by the child's medical history and physical examination, especially the rectal exam. The diagnosis is confirmed by a **barium enema** x ray, which shows a picture of the bowel. The x ray will indicate if a segment of bowel is constricted, causing dilation and obstruction. A biopsy of rectal tissue will reveal the absence of the nerve fibers. Adults may also undergo manometry, a balloon study (device used to enlarge the anus for the procedure) of internal anal sphincter pressure and relaxation.

Treatment

Hirschsprung's disease is treated surgically. The goal is to remove the diseased, nonfunctioning segment of the bowel and restore bowel function. This is often done in two stages. The first stage relieves the intestinal obstruction by performing a **colostomy**. This is the creation of an opening in the abdomen (stoma) through which bowel contents can be discharged into a waste bag. When the child's weight, age, or condition is deemed appropriate, surgeons close the stoma, remove the diseased portion of bowel, and perform a "pull-through" procedure, which repairs the colon by connecting functional bowel to the anus. The pull-through operation usually establishes fairly normal bowel function.

Children with total colonic aganglionosis occasionally fail to benefit from a pull-through procedure. One option in treating these patients is the construction of an ileoanal S-pouch.

The surgeon may recommend a permanent **ostomy** if the child has Down syndrome in addition to Hirschsprung disease, as these children usually have more difficulty with bowel control.

Prognosis

Overall, prognosis is very good. Most infants with Hirschsprung's disease achieve good bowel control after surgery, but a small percentage of children may have lingering problems with soilage or constipation. These infants are also at higher risk for an overgrowth of bacteria in the intestines, including subsequent episodes of enterocolitis, and should be closely followed by a physician. Mortality from enterocolitis or surgical complications in infancy is 25–30%.

Prevention

Hirschsprung's disease is a congenital abnormality that has no known means of prevention. It is important to diagnose the condition early in order to prevent the development of enterocolitis. **Genetic counseling** can be offered to a couple with a previous child with the disease or to an affected individual considering **pregnancy** to discuss recurrence risks and treatment options. Prenatal diagnosis is not available as of the early 2000s.

Resources

BOOKS

Beers, Mark H., Robert S. Porter, and Thomas V. Jones, eds. *The Merck Manual of Diagnosis and Therapy*. 18th ed. Whitehouse Station, NJ: Merck Research Laboratories, 2006.

PERIODICALS

Chen, M. L., and T. G. Keens. "Congenital Central Hypoventilation Syndrome: Not Just Another Rare Disorder." *Paediatric Respiratory Reviews* 5 (September 2004): 182–189.

Lal, D. R., P. F. Nichol, B. A. Harms, et al. "Ileo-Anal S-Pouch Reconstruction in Patients with Total Colonic Aganglionosis after Failed Pull-Through Procedure." *Journal of Pediatric Surgery* 39 (July 2004): e7–e9.

Prabhakara, K., H. E. Wyandt, X. L. Huang, et al. "Recurrent Proximal 18p Monosomy and 18q Trisomy in a Family with a Maternal Pericentric Inversion of Chromosome 18." *Annales de génétique* 47 (July-September 2004): 297–303.

ORGANIZATIONS

American Pseudo-Obstruction & Hirschsprung's Society, 158 Pleasant St., North Andover, MA, 01845-2797, (978) 685-4477, (978) 685-4488, aphs@tiac.net.

National Organization for Rare Disorders, P.O. Box 8923, New Fairfield, CT, 06812-8923, (800) 999-6673, http://www.rarediseases.org.

Pull-thru Network, 2312 Savoy Street, Hoover, AL, 35226-1528, (205) 978-2930, PTNmail@charter.net, http://www.pullthrunetwork.org.

Amy Vance, MS, CGC
Rebecca J. Frey, PhD

Hirsutism

Definition

Excessive growth of facial or body hair in women is called hirsutism.

Description

Hirsutism is not a disease. The condition usually develops during **puberty** and becomes more pronounced as the years go by. However, an inherited tendency, overproduction of male hormones (androgens), medication, or disease, can cause it to appear at any age.

Women who have hirsutism usually have irregular menstrual cycles. They sometimes have small breasts and deep voices, and their muscles and genitals may become larger than women without the condition.

Types of hirsutism

Idiopathic hirsutism is probably hereditary, because there is usually a family history of the disorder. Women with idiopathic hirsutism have normal menstrual cycles and no evidence of any of the conditions associated with secondary hirsutism.

Secondary hirsutism is most often associated with **polycystic ovary syndrome** (an inherited hormonal disorder characterized by menstrual irregularities, biochemical abnormalities, and **obesity**). This type of hirsutism may also be caused by:

- malfunctions of the pituitary or adrenal glands
- use of male hormones or minoxidil (Loniten), a drug used to widen blood vessels
- adrenal or ovarian tumors.

Causes and symptoms

Hirsutism is rarely caused by a serious underlying disorder. **Pregnancy** occasionally stimulates its development. Hirsutism triggered by tumors is very unusual.

Hair follicles usually become enlarged, and the hairs themselves become larger and darker. A woman whose hirsutism is caused by an increase in male hormones has a pattern of hair growth similar to that of a man. A woman whose hirsutism is not hormone-related has long, fine hairs on her face, arms, chest, and back.

Diagnosis

Diagnosis is based on a family history of hirsutism, a personal history of menstrual irregularities, and masculine traits. Laboratory tests are not needed to assess the status of patients whose menstrual cycles are normal and who have mild, gradually progressing hirsutism.

A family physician or endocrinologist may order blood tests to measure hormone levels in women with long-standing menstrual problems or more severe hirsutism. **Computed tomography scans** (CT scans) are sometimes performed to evaluate diseases of the adrenal glands. Additional diagnostic procedures may be used to confirm or rule out underlying diseases or disorders.

Treatment

Primary hirsutism can be treated mechanically. Mechanical treatment involves bleaching or physically removing unwanted hair by:

- cutting
- electrolysis
- shaving
- tweezing
- waxing
- using hair-removing creams (depilatories)

Low-dose dexamethasone (a synthetic adrenocortical steroid), birth-control pills, or medications that suppress male hormones (for example, spironolactone) may be prescribed for patients whose condition stems from high androgen levels.

Treatment of secondary hirsutism is determined by the underlying cause of the condition.

Prognosis

Birth-control pills alone cause this condition to stabilize in one of every two patients and to improve in 1 of every 10.

When spironolactone (Aldactone) is prescribed to suppress hair growth, 70% of patients experience improvement within six months. When women also take birth-control pills, menstrual cycles become regular and hair growth is suppressed even more.

ORGANIZATIONS

American Society for Reproductive Medicine, 1209 Montgomery Highway, Birmingham, AL, 35216-2809, (205) 978-5000, (205) 978-5005, asrm@asrm.org, http://www.asrm.org.

Maureen Haggerty

Hispanic American health *see* **Minority health**
Histamine *see* **Antiulcer drugs**
Histamine headache *see* **Cluster headache**

Histiocytosis X

Definition

Histiocytosis X is a generic term that refers to an increase in the number of histiocytes, a type of white blood cell, that act as scavengers to remove foreign material from the blood and tissues. Since recent research demonstrated Langerhan cell involvement as well as histiocytes, this led to a proposal that the term Langerhans Cell Histiocytosis (LCH) be used in place of histiocytosis X. Either term refers to three separate illnesses (listed in order of increasing severity): eosinophilic granuloma, Hand-Schuller-Christian disease, and Letterer-Siwe disease.

Description

Epidermal (skin) Langerhans cells (a form of dendritic cell) accumulate with other immune cells in various parts of the body and cause damage by the release of chemicals. Normally, Langerhans cells recognize foreign material, including bacteria, and stimulate the immune system to react to them. Langerhans cells are usually found in skin, lymph nodes, lungs, and the gastrointestinal tract. Under abnormal conditions these cells affect skin, bone, and the pituitary gland as well as the lungs, intestines, liver, spleen, bone marrow, and brain. Therefore, the disease is not confined to areas where Langerhans cells are normally found. The disease is more common in children than adults and tends to be most severe in very young children.

Histiocytosis X or LCH is a family of related conditions characterized by a distinct inflammatory and proliferative process but differs from each other in which parts of the body are involved. The least severe of the histiocytosis X/LCH family is eosinophilic granuloma. Approximately 60–80% of all diagnosed cases are in this classification, which usually occurs in children aged 5–10 years. The bones are involved 50–75% of the time, which includes the skull or mandible, and the long bones. If the bone marrow is involved, anemia can result. With skull involvement, growths can occur behind the eyes, bulging them forward. One case study involved swelling of the eyes caused by histiocytosis in a three-year-old girl. The lungs are involved less than 10% of the time, and this involvement signals the worst prognosis.

Next in severity is Hand-Schuller-Christian disease, a chronic, scattered form of histiocytosis. It occurs most commonly from the age of one to three years and is a slowly progressive disease that affects the softened areas of the skull, other flat bones, the eyes, and skin. Letterer-Siwe disease is the acute form of this series of diseases. It is generally found from the time of birth to one year of age. It causes an enlarged liver, bruising and **skin lesions**, anemia, enlarged lymph glands, other organ involvement, and extensive skull lesions.

Causes and symptoms

This is a rare disorder affecting approximately 1 in 200,000 children or adults each year. The International Histiocyte Society formed a registry in 2000 that has registered a total of about 300 adults from 13 countries. Because histiocytic disorders are so rare, little research has been done to determine their cause. Over time, histiocytosis may lessen in its assault on the body but there are still problems from damage to the tissues. There are no apparent inheritance patterns in these diseases with the exception of a form involving the lymphatic system; of the 274 adults in the international registry, only one came from a family with a history of the disease.

The symptoms of histiocytosis are caused by substances called cytokines and prostaglandins, which are normally produced by histiocytes and act as messengers between cells. When these chemicals are produced in excess amounts and in the wrong places, they cause tissue swelling and abnormal growth. Thus, symptoms may include painful lumps in the skull and limbs as well as **rashes** on the skin. General symptoms may include: poor appetite, failure to gain weight, recurrent **fever**, and irritability. Symptoms from other possible sites of involvement include:

- gums: swelling, usually without significant discomfort
- ear: chronic discharge
- liver or spleen: abdominal discomfort or swelling
- pituitary: This gland at the base of the brain is affected at some stage in approximately 20%–30% of children causing a disturbance in water balance to produce thirst and frequent urination.
- eyes: Due to the bony disease, behind-the-eye bulging may occur (exophthalmos).
- lungs: breathing problems

Diagnosis

The diagnosis can be made only by performing a biopsy, that is, taking a tissue sample under anesthesia from a site in the patient thought to be involved. Blood and urine tests, chest and other x rays, **magnetic resonance imaging** (MRI) and **computed tomography scans** (CT scans) (to check the extent of involvement), and possibly bone marrow or breathing tests may be required to confirm the diagnosis.

Treatment

Although this disease is not **cancer**, most patients diagnosed with it are treated in cancer clinics. There are two reasons for this:

- Historically, cancer specialists treated it before the cause was known.
- The treatment requires the use of drugs typically required to treat cancer.

Any cancer drugs utilized are usually given in smaller doses, which diminishes the severity of their side effects. **Radiation therapy** is rarely used, and special drugs may be prescribed for skin symptoms. If there is only one organ affected, **steroids** may be injected locally, or a drug called indomethacin may be used. Indomethacin is an anti-inflammatory medication that may achieve a similar response with less severe side effects.

Prognosis

The disease fluctuates markedly. If only one system is involved, the disease often resolves by itself. Multisystem disease usually needs treatment although it may disappear spontaneously. The disease is not normally fatal unless organs vital to life are damaged. In general, the younger the child at diagnosis and the more organs involved, the poorer the outlook. If the condition resolves, there could still be long-term complications because of the damage done while the disease was active.

Resources

BOOKS

Beers, Mark H., Robert S. Porter, and Thomas V. Jones, eds. *The Merck Manual of Diagnosis and Therapy*. 18th ed. Whitehouse Station, NJ: Merck Research Laboratories, 2006.

Kliegman, Robert M., and Waldo Emerson Nelson. *Nelson Textbook of Pediatrics*. 18th ed. Philadelphia: Saunders, Elsevier, 2007.

PERIODICALS

Arico, M., M. Girschikofsky, T. Genereau, et al. "Langer hans Cell Histiocytosis in Adults. Report from the International Registry of the Histiocyte Society." *European Journal of Cancer* 39 (November 2003): 2341–2348.

Eckhardt, A., and A. Schulze. "Maxillofacial Manifestations of Langerhans Cell Histiocytosis: A Clinical and Therapeutic Analysis of 10 Patients." *Oral Oncology* 39 (October 2003): 687–694.

Levy, J., T. Monos, J.Kapelushnik, et al. "Langerhans Cell Histiocytosis with Periorbital Cellulitis." *American Journal of Ophthalmology* 136 (November 2003): 939–942.

ORGANIZATIONS

Histiocytosis Association of America, 332 North Broadway, Pittman, NJ, 08071, (856) 589-6614, (800) 548-2758, Association@histio.org, http://www.histio.org.

Linda K. Bennington, CNS
Rebecca J. Frey, PhD

Histoplasmosis

Definition

Histoplasmosis is an **infectious disease** caused by inhaling the microscopic spores of the fungus *Histoplasma capsulatum*. The disease exists in three forms. Acute or primary histoplasmosis causes flu-like symptoms. Most people who are infected recover without medical intervention. Chronic histoplasmosis affects the lungs and can be fatal. Disseminated histoplasmosis affects many organ systems in the body and is often fatal, especially to people with acquired **immunodeficiency** syndrome (**AIDS**).

Description

Histoplasmosis is an airborne infection. The spores that cause this disease are found in soil that has been contaminated with bird or bat droppings. In the United States, the disease is most common in eastern and midwestern states and is widespread in the upper Mississippi, Ohio, Missouri, and St. Lawrence river valleys. Sometimes histoplasmosis is called Ohio Valley disease, Central Mississippi River Valley disease, Appalachian Mountain disease, Darling's disease, or *Histoplasma capsulatum* infection.

Anyone can get histoplasmosis, but people who come in contact with bird and bat excrement are more likely to be infected. This includes farmers, gardeners, bridge inspectors and painters, roofers, chimney cleaners, demolition and construction workers, people installing or servicing heating and air conditioning units, people restoring old or abandoned buildings, and people who explore caves.

The very young and the elderly, especially if they have a pre-existing lung disease or are heavy smokers, are more likely to develop symptoms that are more severe. People who have a weakened immune system, either from diseases, such as AIDS or leukemia, or as the result of medications they take (**corticosteroids**, **chemotherapy** drugs), are more likely to develop chronic or disseminated histoplasmosis.

Causes and symptoms

When the spores of *H. capsulatum* are inhaled, they lodge in the lungs where they divide and cause lesions. This is known as acute or primary histoplasmosis. It is not contagious.

Many otherwise healthy people show no symptoms of infection at all. When symptoms do occur, they appear 3–17 days after exposure (average time is 10 days). The symptoms are usually mild and resemble those of a cold or flu: **fever**, dry **cough**, enlarged lymph glands, tiredness, and a general feeling of ill health. A small number of people develop bronchopneumonia. About 95% of people who are infected either experience no symptoms or have symptoms that clear up spontaneously. These people then have partial immunity to re-infection.

In some people, the spores that cause the disease continue to live in the lungs. In about 5% of people who are infected, usually those with chronic lung disease, diabetes mellitis, or weakened immune systems, the disease progresses to chronic histoplasmosis. This can take months or years. Symptoms of chronic histoplasmosis resemble those of **tuberculosis**. Cavities form in the lung tissue, parts of the lung may collapse, and the lungs fill with fluid. Chronic histoplasmosis is a serious disease that can result in **death**.

The most rare form of histoplasmosis is disseminated histoplasmosis. Disseminated histoplasmosis is seen almost exclusively in patients with AIDS or other immune defects. In disseminated histoplasmosis the infection may move to the spleen, liver, bone marrow, or adrenal glands. Symptoms include a worsening of those found in chronic histoplasmosis, as well as weight loss, **diarrhea**, the development of open sores in the mouth and nose, and enlargement of the spleen, liver, and adrenal gland.

Diagnosis

A simple skin test similar to that given for tuberculosis will tell if a person has previously been infected by the fungus *H. capsulatum*. Chest x rays often show lung damage caused by the fungus, but do not lead to a definitive diagnosis because the damage caused by other diseases has a similar appearance on the x ray. Diagnosis of chronic or disseminated histoplasmosis can be made by culturing a sample of sputum or other body fluids in the laboratory to isolate the fungus. The urine, blood serum, washings from the lungs, or cerebrospinal fluid can all be tested for the presence of an antigen produced in response to the infection. Most cases of primary histoplasmosis go undiagnosed.

Treatment

Acute primary histoplasmosis generally requires no treatment other than rest. Non-prescription drugs such as **acetaminophen** (Tylenol) may be used to treat **pain** and relieve fever. Avoiding smoke and using a cool air humidifier may ease chest pain.

Patients with an intact immune system who develop chronic histoplasmosis are treated with the drug ketoconazole (Nizoral) or amphotericin B (Fungizone). Patients with suppressed immune systems are treated with amphotericin B, which is given intravenously. Because of its potentially toxic side effects, hospitalization is often required. The patient may also receive other drugs to minimize the side effects of the amphotericin B.

Patients with AIDS must continue to take the drug itraconazole (Sporonox) orally for the rest of their lives in order to prevent a relapse. If the patient can not tolerate itraconazole, the drug fluconazole (Diflucan) can be substituted.

Alternative treatment

In non-immunocompromised patients, alternative therapies can be very successful. Alternative treatment for fungal infections focuses on creating an environment where the fungus cannot survive. This is accomplished by maintaining good health and eating a diet low in dairy products; sugars, including honey and fruit juice; and foods like beer that contain yeast. This is complemented by a diet high in raw food. Supplements of antioxidant **vitamins** C, E, and A, along with B complex, may also be added to the diet. *Lactobacillus acidophilus* and *Bifodobacteria* will replenish the good bacteria in the intestines. Antifungal herbs, like garlic, can be consumed in relatively large doses and for an extended period of time in order to be most effective.

Prognosis

Most people recover from primary histoplasmosis in a few weeks without medical intervention. Patients with chronic histoplasmosis who are treated with antifungal drugs generally recover rapidly if they do not have an underlying serious disease. When left untreated, or if serious disease is present, histoplasmosis can be fatal.

AIDS patients with disseminated histoplasmosis vary in their response to amphotericin B, depending on their general health and how well they tolerate the side effects of the drug. Treatment often suppresses the infection temporarily, but patients with AIDS are always in danger of a relapse and must continue to take medication for the rest of their lives to keep the infection at bay. New combinations of therapies and new drugs are constantly being evaluated, making hard statistics on prognosis difficult to ascertain. AIDS patients have problems with multiple opportunistic infections, making it difficult to isolate death rates due to any one particular fungal infection.

Prevention

Since the spores of *H. capsulatum* are so widespread, it is almost impossible to prevent exposure in endemic areas. Dust suppression measures when working with contaminated soil may help limit exposure. Individuals who are at risk of developing the more severe forms of the disease should avoid situations where they will be exposed to bat and bird droppings.

Resources

OTHER

Histoplasmosis: Protecting Workers at Risk. Centers for Disease Control and Prevention. http://www.cdc.gov/niosh/97146eng.html.

ORGANIZATIONS

American Lung Association, 1301 Pennsylvania Ave. NW, Suite 800, Washington, DC, 20001, (202) 758-3355, (202) 452-1805, (800) 548-8252, info@lungusa.org, http://www.lungusa.org/.

National Center for Preparedness, Detection, and Control of Infectious Diseases, 1600 Clifton Road, Atlanta, GA, 30333, (888) 232-4636, cdcinfo@cdc.gov, http://www.cdc.gov/ncpdcid.

National Institute for Occupational Safety and Health, 1600 Clifton Road, Atlanta, GA, 30333, (800) 232-4636, cdcinfo@cdc.gov, http://www.cdc.gov/niosh.

Tish Davidson, A.M.

HIV infection *see* **AIDS**

Hives

Definition

Hives are due to an allergic skin reaction and cause localized redness, swelling, and **itching**.

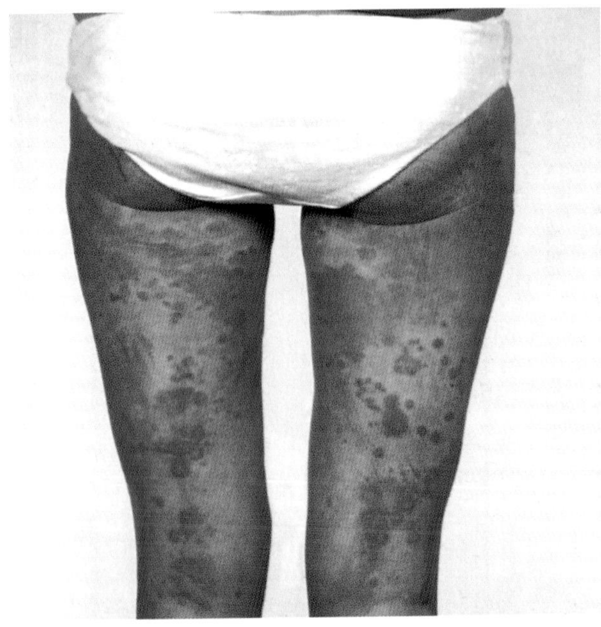

Hives on the back of a young woman's legs. The accompanying inflammation develops as an allergic reaction which ranges in size from small spots to patches measuring several inches across. *(Custom Medical Stock Photo, Inc. Reproduced by permission.)*

Description

Hives are a reaction of the body's immune system that causes areas of the skin to swell, itch, and become reddened (wheals). When the reaction is limited to small areas of the skin, it is called "urticaria." Involvement of larger areas, such as whole sections of a limb, is called "angioedema." Hives can be round or they can form rings or large patches. Hives can also form wheals or welts, which are red lesions with a red flare at the borders.

Demographics

It is estimated that 5 percent of all people will develop urticaria at some point in their lives. Hives are more common in women than in men. Of those with chronic hives, lasting six weeks or more, about 80% are idiopathic, meaning no cause, allergic or otherwise, can be found.

Causes and symptoms

Causes

Hives occur due to an allergic reaction. The body's immune system is normally responsible for protection from foreign invaders. When it becomes sensitized to normally harmless substances, the resulting reaction is called an allergy. An attack of hives is set off when such a substance, called an allergen, is ingested, inhaled, or otherwise contacted. The allergen interacts with immune cells called mast cells, which reside in the skin, airways, and digestive system. When mast cells encounter an allergen, they release histamine and otherchemicals, both locally and into the bloodstream. These chemicals cause blood vessels to become more porous, allowing fluid to accumulate in tissue and leading to the swollen and reddish appearance of hives. Some of the chemicals released sensitize **pain** nerve endings, causing the affected area to become itchy and sensitive.

A wide variety of substances may cause hives in sensitive people, including foods, drugs, and insect **bites** or **stings**. Common culprits include:

- nuts, especially peanuts, walnuts, and Brazil nuts
- fish, mollusks, and shellfish
- eggs
- wheat
- milk
- strawberries
- food additives and preservatives
- penicillin or other antibiotics
- flu vaccines
- tetanus toxoid vaccine
- gamma globulin
- bee, wasp, and hornet stings
- bites of mosquitoes, fleas, and scabies

Symptoms

Urticaria is characterized by redness, swelling, and itching of small areas of the skin. These patches usually grow and recede in less than a day, but may be replaced by hives in other locations. Angioedema is characterized by more diffuse swelling. Swelling of the airways may cause **wheezing** and respiratory distress. In severe cases, airway obstruction may occur.

Diagnosis

Hives are easily diagnosed by visual inspection. The cause of hives is usually apparent, but may require a careful medical history in some cases.

Treatment

Mild cases of hives are treated with **antihistamines**, such asdiphenhydramine (Benadryl) or desloratadine (Clarinex). Clarinex is non-sedating, meaning it will not make patients drowsy. More severe cases may require oral **corticosteroids**, such as prednisone. Topical corticosteroids are not effective. Airway swelling may require emergency injection of epinephrine (adrenaline).

Alternative treatment

An alternative practitioner will try to determine what allergic substance is causing the reaction and help the patient eliminate or minimize its effects.To deal with the symptoms of hives, an oatmeal bath may help to relieve itching. Chickweed (*Stellaria media*), applied as a poultice (crushed or chopped herbs applied directly to the skin) or added to bath water, may also help relieve itching. Several homeopathic remedies, including *Urtica urens* and *Apis* (*Apis mellifica*), may help relieve the itch, redness, or swelling associated with hives.

Prognosis

Most cases of hives clear up within one to seven days without treatment, providing the cause (allergen) is found and avoided.

Prevention

Preventing hives depends on avoiding the allergen causing them. Analysis of new items in the diet or new drugs taken may reveal the likely source of their action. Chronic hives may be aggravated by **stress**, **caffeine**, alcohol, or tobacco; avoiding these may reduce the frequency of reactions.

Resources

PERIODICALS

Kirn, F. Timothy. "Desloratadine Improves Urticaria in Clinical Setting." *Skin & Allergy News*. September 2004:41.

ORGANIZATIONS

American Academy of Dermatology (AAD), 930 E. Wood field Rd., Schaumburg, IL, 60173, http://www.aad.org.

American Podiatric Medical Association (APMA), 9312 Old Georgetown Rd., Bethesda, MD, 20814–1698, (301) 571–9200, http://www.apma.org.

Richard Robinson
Teresa G. Odle
Karl Finley

HLA-B27 antigen test *see* **Tissue typing**

HLA test *see* **Human leukocyte antigen test**

HMG-CoA reductase inhibitors *see* **Cholesterol-reducing drugs**

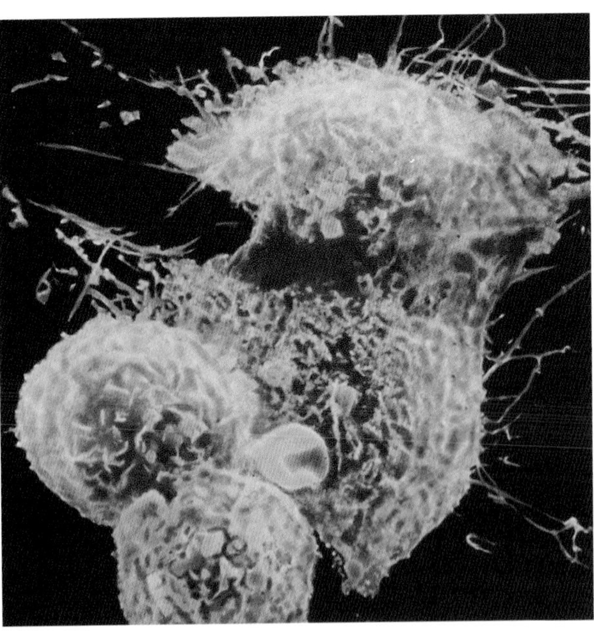

A scanning electron micrograph (SEM) image of dividing Hodgkin's cells from the pleural effusions (abnormal accumulations of fluid in the lungs) of a 55-year-old male patient. *(Dr. Andrejs Liepins/Photo Researchers, Inc.)*

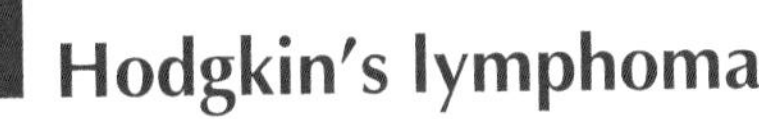

Hodgkin's lymphoma

Definition

Hodgkin's lymphoma is a rare lymphoma, a **cancer** of the lymphatic system.

Demographics

The American Cancer Society estimated there were 8,510 new cases of Hodgkin's lymphoma in the United States in 2009—3,870 in females and 4,640 in males. It is estimated that 800 men and 490 women in the United States died of the disease in 2009.

Hodgkin's lymphoma can occur at any age. However, the majority of cases develop in early adulthood (ages 15–40) and late adulthood (after age 55). Approximately 10–15% of cases are in children under age 17. It is more common in boys than in girls under the age of 10. The disease is very rare in children under age five.

Description

Hodgkin's lymphoma, or Hodgkin's disease, was first described in 1832 by British physician Thomas Hodgkin's. Hodgkin's clearly differentiated between this disease and the much more common non-Hodgkin's lymphomas. Prior to 1970, few individuals survived Hodgkin's lymphoma. Due to significant treatment advancements, the majority of individuals with this cancer can be cured.

The lymphatic system is part of the body's immune system, for fighting disease, and a part of the blood-producing system. It includes the lymph vessels and nodes, the spleen, bone marrow, and thymus. The narrow lymphatic vessels carry lymphatic fluid throughout the body. The lymph nodes are small organs that filter the lymphatic fluid and trap foreign substances, including viruses, bacteria, and cancer cells. The spleen, in the upper left abdomen, removes old cells and debris from the blood. The bone marrow, the tissue inside the bones, produces new red and white blood cells.

Lymphocytes are white blood cells that recognize and destroy disease-causing organisms. Lymphocytes are produced in the lymph nodes, spleen, and bone marrow. They circulate throughout the body in the blood and lymphatic fluid. Clusters of immune cells also exist in major organs.

Hodgkin's lymphoma is a type of lymphoma in which antibody-producing cells of the lymphatic system begin to grow abnormally. It usually begins in a lymph node and progresses slowly, in a fairly predictable way, spreading via the lymphatic vessels from one group of lymph nodes to the next. Sometimes it invades organs that are adjacent to the lymph nodes. If the cancer cells spread to the blood, the disease can reach almost any site in the body. Advanced cases of Hodgkin's lymphoma may involve the spleen, liver, bone marrow, and lungs.

There are different subtypes of Hodgkin's lymphoma:

- nodular sclerosis (60–80% of cases); most common subtype affecting younger patients
- mixed cellularity (15–30% of cases) most common subtypes in patients diagnosed after age 55
- lymphocyte predominant or lymphocyte rich (5% of cases)
- lymphocyte depleted (less than 1% of cases)

These four subtypes are referred to as classic Hodgkin's lymphoma. A fifth subtype, nodular lymphocyte predominant Hodgkin's lymphoma (NLPHD), which accounts for about 5% of cases, is a subtype that is clinically unique from the other subtypes and is treated differently.

Risk factors

Although the exact cause of Hodgkin's lymphoma is not yet known, several risk factors related to the disease have been identified including:

- Previous infection with the Epstein Barr virus/infectious mononucleosis (mono). The overall risk of developing Hodgkin's lymphoma after this infection is small. According to a study conducted in Denmark and Sweden, the average time between illness with infectious mononucleosis and diagnosis of Hodgkin's lymphoma was about three years.
- Age—Individuals in their twenties and adults over the age of 55 are more likely to be diagnosed with Hodgkin's lymphoma.
- Gender—Males are more likely to be diagnosed with this type of lymphoma. In children, up to 85% of cases are diagnosed in boys.
- Family history—Siblings of patients who have been diagnosed with Hodgkin's lymphoma are at higher risk than the general population. An identical twin of an individual who has been diagnosed with Hodgkin's is at even higher risk. However, less than 5% of cases are diagnosed in family members.
- Patients with human immunodeficiency virus (HIV) infection are more likely to develop Hodgkin's lymphoma than those not diagnosed with HIV.

Causes and symptoms

The cause of Hodgkin's lymphoma is not known. It is suspected that some interaction between an individual's genetic makeup, environmental exposures, and infectious agents may be responsible. Immune system deficiencies may be involved.

Early symptoms of Hodgkin's lymphoma are similar to those of the flu:

- fevers, night sweats, chills
- fatigue
- itching
- swelling of one or more lymph nodes
- loss of appetite
- weight loss
- pain after drinking alcoholic beverages (occurs in less than 10% of patients)

Sudden or emergency symptoms of Hodgkin's lymphoma include:

- sudden high fever
- loss of bladder and/or bowel control
- numbness in the arms and legs and a loss of strength

As lymph nodes swell, they may push on other structures, causing a variety of symptoms:

- pain due to pressure on nerve roots
- loss of function in muscle groups served by compressed nerves
- coughing or shortness of breath due to compression of the windpipe and/or airways by swollen lymph nodes in the chest
- kidney failure from compression of the ureters, the tubes that carry urine from the kidneys to the bladder
- swelling in the face, neck, or legs, due to pressure on veins
- paralysis in the legs due to pressure on the spinal cord

As Hodgkin's lymphoma progresses, the immune system becomes less effective at fighting infection. Thus, patients with Hodgkin's lymphoma become more susceptible to both common infections caused by bacteria and opportunistic infections.

As many as 75% of individuals with Hodgkin's lymphoma do not have any typical symptoms.

Diagnosis

As with many forms of cancer, diagnosis of Hodgkin's lymphoma has two major components.

- Identification of Hodgkin's lymphoma as the cause of the patient's disease.
- Staging of the disease to determine how far the cancer has spread.

KEY TERMS

Excisional biopsy—Removal of an entire lymph node; often the most suspicious-looking node is removed for testing.

Incisional biopsy—Removal of a part of a lymph node for diagnostic purposes.

Lymph node—Small, round-shaped organs of the lymph system found throughout the body that are connected by lymph vessels.

Lymphatic system—A system of the body that includes lymph vessels and nodes, the spleen, bone marrow, and the thymus.

Lymphoma—Cancer originating in a lymph node or in the lymph system.

Reed-Sternberg cells—Cancerous cells that, when present in the body, are indicative of Hodgkin's lymphoma

Examination

The initial diagnosis of Hodgkin's lymphoma often results from abnormalities in a chest x-ray that was performed because of nonspecific symptoms. The physician then takes a medical history to check for the presence of symptoms and conducts a complete **physical examination**.

The size, tenderness, firmness, and location of swollen lymph nodes are determined and correlated with any signs of infection. In particular, lymph nodes that do not shrink after treatment with **antibiotics** may be a cause for concern. The lymph nodes that are most often affected by Hodgkin's lymphoma include those of the neck, above the collarbone, under the arms, and in the chest above the diaphragm.

Tests

Laboratory tests that may be ordered as part of the diagnostic workup for Hodgkin's lymphoma include:

- Lactate dehydrogenase (LDH) level—High levels of LDH may be indicative of more extensive disease.
- Complete blood count (CBC)—Anemia may be present if there is disease in the bone marrow. The platelet count may be increased or decreased.
- Alkaline phosphatase (ALP) levels—ALP may be increased if there is disease in the liver and/or bone.
- An HIV test should be done if HIV infection is suspected. Antiviral therapies to treat HIV should be initiated because they have a positive impact in HIV-positive patients diagnosed with Hodgkin's lymphoma

Procedures

Diagnosis of Hodgkin's lymphoma requires either the removal of an entire enlarged lymph node (an excisional biopsy) or an incisional biopsy (the recommended procedure), in which only a small part of a large tumor is removed. If the node is near the skin, the biopsy is performed with a local anesthetic. If it is inside the chest or abdomen, **general anesthesia** is required.

The sample of biopsied tissue is examined under a microscope. Giant cells called Reed-Sternberg cells must be present to confirm a diagnosis of Hodgkin's lymphoma. These cells, which usually contain two or more nuclei, are named for the two pathologists who discovered them. Normal cells have only one nucleus (the organelle within the cell that contains the genetic material). Affected lymph nodes may contain only a few Reed-Sternberg cells and they may be difficult to recognize. Characteristics of other types of cells in the biopsied tissue help to diagnose the subtype of Hodgkin's lymphoma.

A fine needle aspiration (FNA) biopsy, in which a thin needle and syringe are used to remove a small amount of fluid and bits of tissue from a tumor, has the advantage of not requiring surgery. An FNA may be performed prior to an excisional or incisional biopsy, to check for infection or for the spread of cancer from another organ. However, an FNA biopsy does not provide enough tissue to diagnose Hodgkin's lymphoma. FNA is generally indicated only when a **head and neck cancer** is suspected.

Occasionally, additional biopsies are required to diagnose Hodgkin's lymphoma. In rare instances, other tests that detect certain substances on the surfaces of cancer cells or changes in the DNA of cells are used to distinguish Hodgkin's lymphoma from non-Hodgkin's's lymphoma.

Staging is very important in Hodgkin's lymphoma. This is because the cancer usually spreads in a predictable pattern, without skipping sets of lymph nodes until late in the progression of the disease.

Tests

Imaging of the abdomen, chest, and pelvis is used to identify areas of enlarged lymph nodes and abnormalities

DOROTHY MENDENHALL (1874–1964)

Dorothy Reed Mendenhall, the last of three children, was born September 22, 1874, in Columbus, Ohio, to William Pratt Reed, a shoe manufacturer, and Grace Kimball Reed, both of whom had descended from English settlers who came to America in the seventeenth century. Mendenhall attended Smith College and obtained a baccalaureate degree. Although she initially contemplated a career in journalism, Mendenhall's interest in medicine was inspired by a biology course she attended.

Dorothy Reed Mendenhall was a well-respected researcher, obstetrician, and pioneer in methods of childbirth. She was the first to discover that Hodgkin's lymphoma was not a form of tuberculosis, as had been thought. This finding received international acclaim. As a result of her work, the cell type characteristic of Hodgkin's lymphoma bears her name. The loss of her first child due to poor obstetrics changed her research career to a lifelong effort to reduce infant mortality rates. Mendenhall's efforts paid off with standards being set for weight and height for children ages birth to six and also in programs that stressed the health of both the mother and child in the birthing process.

in the spleen or other organs. Computerized axial tomography (CT or CAT) scans use a rotating x ray beam to obtain pictures. Chest x rays also may be taken. These images reveal rounded lumps called nodules in the affected lymph nodes and other organs.

Positron emission tomography (PET) scan, considered to be an essential diagnostic tool in Hodgkin's lymphoma, is an extremely accurate method for staging Hodgkin's lymphoma. A very low dose of radioactive glucose, a sugar, is injected into the body. The glucose travels to metabolically active sites, including cancerous regions that require large amounts of glucose. The **PET** scan detects the radioactivity and produces images of the entire body that distinguish between cancerous and non-cancerous tissues.

Anemia (a low red-blood-cell count), fevers, or night sweats are indications that Hodgkin's lymphoma may be in the bone marrow. In these cases, a bone-marrow biopsy, in which a large needle is used to remove a narrow, cylindrical piece of bone, may be necessary to determine the spread of the cancer. Alternatively, an aspiration, in which a needle is used to remove small bits of bone marrow, may be used. The marrow usually is removed from the back of the hip or other large bone.

Rarely, further staging, called pathological staging or a staging laparotomy, is used for Hodgkin's lymphoma. In this operation, a surgeon checks the abdominal lymph nodes and other organs for cancer and removes small pieces of tissue. A pathologist examines the tissue samples for Hodgkin's lymphoma cells. Usually the spleen is removed (a **splenectomy**) during the laparotomy. The splenectomy helps with staging Hodgkin's lymphoma, as well as removing a disease site. The staging laparotomy is infrequently used.

Treatment

All of the available treatments for Hodgkin's lymphoma have serious side effects, both short and long-term. Goals of treatment include minimizing treatment for patients who have been diagnosed with low-risk disease in early stages. With accurate staging, physicians and patients often can choose the minimum treatment that will cure the disease. The staging system used most often to stage Hodgkin's lymphoma is the Ann Arbor Staging Classification System.

Hodgkin's lymphoma is divided into four stages, with additional substages:

- Stage I: The disease is confined to one lymph node area or to one site outside of a lymph node.
- Stage II: The disease is in two or more lymph node areas on one side of the diaphragm (the muscle below the lungs).
- Stage III: The disease is in lymph node areas on both sides of the diaphragm.
- Stage IV: The disease has spread from the lymphatic system to one or more other organs, such as the bone marrow or liver.

Treatment for Hodgkin's lymphoma depends both on the stage of the disease and whether or not symptoms are present. Stages are labeled with an A if no symptoms are present. If symptoms are present, the stage is labeled with a B. These symptoms include:

- unexplained or unintended loss of more than 10% of body weight over the previous six months
- fevers above 100°F (37.7°C)
- drenching night sweats

Drugs

Combined modality treatment incorporating **radiation therapy** and/or **chemotherapy** (drug therapy) are the standard treatments for Hodgkin's lymphoma. If the disease is confined to one area of the body, radiotherapy is usually used. This treatment, with x rays or other high-energy rays, is used when the disease is in bulky areas such as the chest, where chemotherapeutic drugs cannot reach all of the cancer. External-beam radiation, a focused beam from an external machine, is used to irradiate only the affected lymph nodes. This procedure is called involved field radiation. Chemotherapy is also used to treat early stage disease to enhance the effects of the radiation therapy; this is called a synergistic effect.

Involved field radiation may also be used in patients with advanced disease who have disease remaining after treatment with chemotherapy.

Since external-beam radiation damages healthy tissue near the cancer cells, the temporary side effects of radiotherapy can include sunburn-like skin damage, **fatigue**, **nausea**, and **diarrhea**. Other temporary side effects may include a **sore throat** and difficulty swallowing. Long-term side effects depend on the dose and the location of the radiation and the age of the patient. Since radiation of the ovaries causes permanent sterility (the inability to have offspring), the ovaries of girls and young women are protected during radiotherapy. Sometimes the ovaries are surgically moved from the region to be irradiated. The testes should also be shielded if they are in a radiation field.

Chemotherapy utilizes a combination of drugs, each of which kills cancer cells in a different way. The most common chemotherapy regimens for Hodgkin's lymphoma are MOPP (either mechlorethamine or methotrexate with oncovin, procarbazine, and prednisone) and ABVD (adriamycin or doxorubicin, bleomycin, vincristine, dacarbazine). Each of these consists of four different drugs. ABVD, now considered the standard regimen to treat Hodgkin's lymphoma, is used more frequently than MOPP because it has fewer severe side effects such as sterility and because ABVD has been proven to be superior in terms of outcomes. Use of ABVD also reduces the risk of development of a secondary leukemia. MOPP may be used for individuals who are at risk for **heart failure**. The chemotherapeutic drugs may be injected into a vein or taken orally (prednisone).

Children who are sexually mature when they develop Hodgkin's lymphoma, and whose muscle and bone mass are almost completely developed, usually receive the same treatment as adults. Younger children usually are treated with chemotherapy, since radiation will adversely affect bone and muscle growth. However, radiation may be used in low dosages in combination with chemotherapy. Chemotherapy for children with Hodgkin's lymphoma usually includes more drugs than ABVD and MOPP.

The side effects of chemotherapy for Hodgkin's lymphoma depend on the dose of drugs and the length of time they are taken. Since these drugs target rapidly dividing cancer cells, they also affect normal cells that grow rapidly. These include the cells of the bone marrow, the linings of the mouth and intestines, and hair follicles. Damage to bone marrow leads to lower white blood cell counts and lower resistance to infection. It also leads to lower red blood cell counts, which can result in fatigue and easy bleeding and bruising. Damage to intestinal cells leads to a loss of appetite, nausea, and **vomiting**. Mouth sores and hair loss also are common side effects of chemotherapy. These side effects disappear when the chemotherapy is discontinued. Some drugs can reduce or prevent the **nausea and vomiting**.

Chemotherapy for Hodgkin's lymphoma may lead to long-term complications. The drugs may damage the heart, lungs, kidneys, and liver. In children, growth may be impeded. Some chemotherapy can cause sterility, so men may choose to have their sperm frozen prior to treatment. Women may stop ovulating and menstruating during chemotherapy. This may or may not be permanent.

The development of a second type of cancer is the most serious risk from radiation and chemotherapy treatment for Hodgkin's lymphoma. In particular, there is a risk of developing leukemia, **breast cancer**, bone cancer, or **thyroid cancer**. Chemotherapy, particularly MOPP, or chemotherapy in conjunction with radiotherapy, significantly increases the risk for leukemia.

Following treatment, the original diagnostic tests for Hodgkin's lymphoma are repeated, to determine whether all traces of the cancer have been eliminated and to check for long-term side effects of treatment. In resistant Hodgkin's lymphoma, some cancer cells remain following treatment. If the cancer continues to spread during treatment, it is called progressive Hodgkin's lymphoma. If the disease returns after treatment, it is known as recurrent Hodgkin's lymphoma. It may recur in the area where it first started or elsewhere in the body. It may recur immediately after treatment or many years later.

Additional treatment is necessary with these types of Hodgkin's lymphoma. Salvage therapy for refractory or recurrent Hodgkin's lymphoma includes the chemotherapy regimens ICE (ifosfamide, mesna, carboplatin, and etoposide), the DHAP regimen (cisplatin, cytarabine, and dexamethasone), and the EPOCH regimen (etoposide, vincristine, doxorubicin, cyclophosphamide, and prednisone).

An autologous bone marrow and/or a peripheral blood **stem cell transplantation** (PBSCT) often is recommended for treating resistant or recurrent Hodgkin's lymphoma, particularly if the disease recurs within a few months of a chemotherapy-induced remission. These transplants are autologous because they utilize the individual's own cells. The patient's bone marrow cells or peripheral blood stem cells (immature bone marrow cells found in the blood) are collected and frozen prior to high-dosage chemotherapy, which destroys bone marrow cells. A procedure called leukapheresis is used to collect the stem cells. Following the high-dosage chemotherapy, and possibly radiation, the bone marrow cells or stem cells are reinjected into the individual.

Most complementary therapies for Hodgkin's lymphoma are designed to stimulate the immune system to destroy cancer cells and repair normal cells that have been damaged by treatment. These therapies are used in conjunction with standard treatment.

Targeted **immunologic therapies**, also known as immunotherapies, biological therapies, or biological response modifier therapies, utilize substances that are produced by the immune system. These include interferon (an immune system protein), monoclonal antibodies (specially engineered antibodies), colony-stimulating (growth) factors (such as filgrastim), and vaccines. Many immunotherapies for Hodgkin's lymphoma are being evaluated and most are available only through clinical trials. As of 2010, targeted immunotherapy agents have shown modest effects when used to treat refractory or recurrent Hodgkin's lymphoma.

Prognosis

Hodgkin's lymphoma, particularly in children, is one of the most curable forms of cancer. Approximately 90% of individuals are cured of the disease with chemotherapy and/or radiation.

The one-year relative survival rate following treatment for Hodgkin's lymphoma is 93%. Relative survival rates do not include individuals who die of causes other than Hodgkin's lymphoma. The percentage of individuals who have not died of Hodgkin's lymphoma within five years of diagnosis is 90–95% for those with stage I or stage II disease. The figure is 85–90% for those diagnosed with stage III Hodgkin's and approximately 65% for those diagnosed with stage IV disease. The 15-year relative survival rate is 63%. Approximately 75% of children are alive and cancer free 20 years after the original diagnosis of Hodgkin's's.

Acute myelocytic leukemia, a very serious cancer, may develop in as many as 2–6% of individuals receiving certain types of treatment for Hodgkin's lymphoma. Women under the age of 30 who are treated with radiation to the chest have a much higher risk for developing breast cancer. Both men and women are at higher risk for developing lung or thyroid cancers as a result of chest irradiation.

Individuals with the type of Hodgkin's lymphoma known as nodular lymphocytic predominance have a 2% chance of developing non-Hodgkin's lymphoma. This appears to be a result of the Hodgkin's lymphoma itself and not the treatment.

Prevention

As it is not known exactly what causes Hodgkin's lymphoma, it is not possible to prevent the occurrence of this type of cancer.

Most relapses of disease after treatment with Hodgkin's lymphoma occur within the first three years after treatment has been completed. Therefore, compliance with scheduled follow-up visits is extremely important. A typical schedule for follow-up after completion of treatment of Hodgkin's lymphoma is as follows:

- every two to four months during the first two years
- every three to six months during the next three to five years

Resources

PERIODICALS

Ferme, C., et al. "Chemotherapy Plus Involved-Field Radiation in Early-Stage Hodgkin's lymphoma." *New England Journal of Medicine* 357, no. 19 (November 8, 2007): 1916–27.

Hjalgrim, H., et al. "Infectious Mononucleosis, Childhood Social Environment, and Risk of Hodgkin's Lymphoma." *Cancer Research* 67, no. 5 (March 1, 2007): 2382–8.

Hoppe, R.T., Advani, R.H., et al. "Hodgkin's lymphoma/Lymphoma." *Journal of National Comprehensive Cancer Network* 6, no. 6 (July 2008): 594–622.

Mani, H., and E.S. Jaffe. "Hodgkin's Lymphoma: An Update on its Biology with New Insights into Classification." *Clinical Lymphoma, Myeloma, and Leukemia* 9, no. 3 (June 2009): 206–16.

OTHER

Dessain, Scott, James L. Spears, and Athanassios Argiris. "Hodgkin's lymphoma." *eMedicine*. August 20, 2010. http://emedicine.medscape.com/article/201886-overview (accessed October 6, 2010).

"Hodgkin's lymphoma." American Cancer Society. August 29, 2010. http://www.cancer.org/cancer/Hodgkin'sDisease/DetailedGuide/Hodgkin's-disease-what-is-Hodgkin's-disease (accessed October 6, 2010).

ORGANIZATIONS

American Cancer Society, (800) 227-2345, http://www.cancer.org.

The Leukemia and Lymphoma Society, 1311 Mamaroneck Ave., White Plains, NY, 10605, (800) 955-4572, http://www.leukemia-lymphoma.org.

Rosalyn Carson-DeWitt, MD
Margaret Alic, PhD
Melinda Granger Oberleitner
RN, DNS, APRN, CNS

Holistic medicine

Definition

Holistic medicine is a term used to describe therapies that attempt to treat the patient as a whole person. That is, instead of treating an illness, as in orthodox allopathy, holistic medicine looks at an individual's overall physical, mental, spiritual, and emotional well-being before recommending treatment. A practitioner with a holistic approach treats the symptoms of illness as well as looking for the underlying cause of the illness. Holistic medicine also attempts to prevent illness by placing a greater emphasis on optimizing health. The body's systems are seen as interdependent parts of the person's whole being. Its natural state is one of health, and an illness or disease is an imbalance in the body's systems. Holistic therapies tend to emphasize proper **nutrition** and avoidance of substances—such as chemicals—that pollute the body. Their techniques are non-invasive.

Some of the world's health systems that are holistic in nature include **naturopathic medicine**, homeopathy, and **traditional Chinese medicine**. Many alternative or natural therapies have a holistic approach, although that is not always the case. The term complementary medicine is used to refer to the use of both allopathic and holistic treatments. It is more often used in Great Britain, but is gaining acceptance in the United States.

There are no limits to the range of diseases and disorders that can be treated in a holistic way, as the principle of holistic healing is to balance the body, mind, spirit, and emotions so that the person's whole being functions smoothly. When an individual seeks holistic treatment for a particular illness or condition, other health problems improve without direct treatment, due to improvement in the performance of the immune system, which is one of the goals of holistic medicine.

Origins

The concept of holistic medicine is not new. In the 4th century B.C., Socrates warned that treating one part of the body only would not have good results. Hippocrates considered that many factors contribute to the health of a human being, including weather, nutrition, emotional factors, and in our time, a host of different sources of pollution can interfere with health. Of course, holistic medicine existed even before ancient Greece in some ancient healing traditions, such as those from India and China, which date back over 5,000 years. However, the term "holistic" only became part of everyday language in the 1970s, when Westerners began seeking an alternative to allopathic medicine.

Interestingly, it was only at the beginning of the twentieth century that the principles of holistic medicine fell out of favor in Western societies, with the advent of major advances in what we now call allopathic medicine. Paradoxically, many discoveries of the twentieth century have only served to confirm many natural medicine theories. In many cases, researchers have set out to debunk holistic medicine, only to find that their research confirms it, as has been the case, for example, with many herbal remedies.

Purpose

Many people are now turning to holistic medicine, often when suffering from chronic ailments that have not been successfully treated by allopathic means. Although many wonderful advances and discoveries have been made in modern medicine, surgery and drugs alone have a very poor record for producing optimal health because they are designed to attack illness. Holistic medicine is particularly helpful in treating chronic illnesses and maintaining health through proper nutrition and **stress** management.

Description

There are a number of therapies that come under the umbrella of "holistic medicine." They all use basically the same principles, promoting not only physical health, but also mental, emotional, and spiritual health. Most emphasize quality nutrition. Refined foods typically eaten in the twenty-first century United States contain chemical additives and preservatives, are high in fat, cholesterol, and sugars, and promote disease. Alternative nutritionists counter that by recommending whole foods whenever possible and minimizing the amount of meat—especially red meat—that is consumed. Many alternative therapies promote **vegetarianism** as a method of **detoxification**.

The aim of holistic medicine is to bring all areas of an individual's life, and most particularly the energy flowing through the body, back into harmony. Ultimately, of course, only the patient can be responsible for this, for no practitioner can make the necessary adjustments to diet and lifestyle to achieve health. The practice of holistic medicine does not rule out the practice of allopathic medicine; the two can complement each other.

A properly balanced holistic health regimen, which takes into consideration all aspects of human health and includes noninvasive and nonpharmaceutical healing

ANDREW WEIL (1942–)

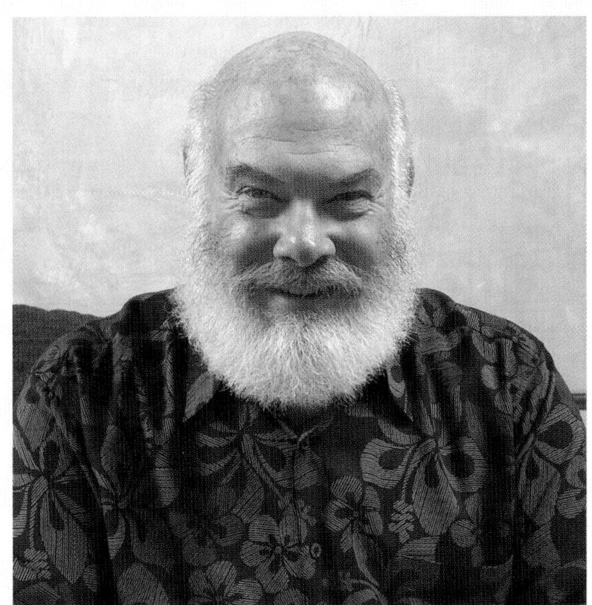

(AP Images.)

Dr. Andrew Weil, a Harvard-educated physician, adds credibility and expertise to the natural healing methods he espouses in his best-selling books, on his website, in his talk show appearances, and in his popular audio CD of music and meditation. Weil's *Spontaneous Healing* spent more than a year on the best-seller list, and his 1997 book, *Eight Weeks to Optimum Health*, also was a runaway best-seller. Perhaps the best-known proponent of naturalistic healing methods, Weil established a field he calls integrative medicine. He is director of Tucson's Center for Integrative Medicine (http://integrativemedicine.arizona.edu/), which he founded in 1993. In 1997, he began training doctors in the discipline at the University of Arizona, where he teaches.

After getting his bachelor's degree in botany from Harvard University, Weil applied for admission to Harvard Medical School in 1964. During his second year, he led a group of students who argued they could succeed better studying on their own than going to classes; in fact, the group got higher scores on their final exams than their classmates. After graduating from Harvard Medical School, he volunteered at the notorious counter-cultural Haight-Asbury Free Clinic in San Francisco, CA. Later in 1969, Weil got a job in Washington, DC, with the National Institute of Mental Health's Drug Studies Division. From 1971 to 1975, he traveled extensively in South America and Africa, soaking up information about medicinal plants, shamanism, and natural healing techniques. He never returned to the practice of conventional medicine.

His approach to alternative medicine is eclectic, mingling traditional medicine with herbal therapy, acupuncture, homeopathy, chiropractic, hypnotism, cranial manipulation, and other alternative healing methods. Though his books discuss the benefits of everything from healing touch to herbal cures, Weil doesn't dismiss the benefits of standard Western medicine when appropriate.

Today, Weil continues to teach and practice alternative medicine, news about which can be found on http://www.drweil.com. He also started the Weil Foundation, a nonprofit organization dedicated to supporting integrative medicine through training, education, and research.

methods, can often completely eradicate even acute health conditions safely. If a patient is being treated with allopathic medicine, holistic therapies may at least support the body during treatment, and alleviate the symptoms that often come with drug treatments and surgery. In addition, holistic therapies aim at the underlying source of the illness, to prevent recurrence.

Here are some of the major holistic therapies:

- herbal medicine
- homeopathy
- naturopathic medicine
- traditional Chinese medicine
- Ayurvedic medicine
- nutritional therapies
- chiropractic
- stress reduction
- psychotherapy
- massage

Because holistic medicine aims to treat the whole person, holistic practitioners sometimes may advise treatment from more than one type of practitioner. This is to ensure that all aspects of health are addressed. Some practitioners also specialize in more than one therapy, and so may be able to offer more comprehensive assistance.

Preparations

How to choose a holistic practitioner:

- How did you hear of this therapist? A personal referral can sometimes be more reliable than a professional one. What do other professionals say about this therapist? What qualifications, board certification, or affiliations does this practitioner have?

- How do you feel personally about this practitioner? Do you feel comfortable in his/her office and with his/her staff? Is your sense of well being increased? Are you kept waiting for appointments?
- Do you have confidence in this practitioner, does he/she respect you as a person? Does he/she show an interest in your family, lifestyle, and diet? Are various treatment options explained to you?
- Is your personal dignity respected?
- Do you feel that this practitioner is sensitive to your feelings and fears regarding treatment?
- Is this practitioner a good advertisement for his/her profession? Signs of stress or ill health may mean that you would be better off choosing another practitioner.
- Do you feel that you are rushed into decisions, or do you feel that you are allowed time to make an informed choice regarding treatment?
- Are future health goals outlined for you? And do you feel that the practitioner is taking your progress seriously?
- Do you feel unconditionally accepted by this practitioner?
- Would you send your loved ones to this practitioner?

If you answered yes to all the above, then you have found a suitable practitioner. The cost of treatment by a holistic therapist varies widely, depending on the level of qualification and the discipline, so it is best to discuss how much treatment can be expected to cost with a practitioner before beginning a course. Some forms of holistic treatment may be covered by health insurance.

Precautions

Many people who try holistic therapies focus on one area of their health only, often detoxification and nutrition. However, practitioners stress that it is only when all areas of a person's potential well being are tackled that total health and happiness can be achieved. They stress that the spiritual and emotional health contribute just as much as physical and mental health to a person's overall state of well-being.

When seeking treatment from a holistic practitioner, it is important to ensure that they are properly qualified. Credentials and reputation should always be checked. In addition, it is important that allopathic physicians and alternative physicians communicate about a patient's care.

Side effects

One of the main advantages of holistic therapies is that they have few side effects when used correctly. If a reputable practitioner is chosen and guidelines are adhered to, the worst that typically happens is that when lifestyle is changed and fresh nutrients are provided, the body begins to eliminate toxins that may have accumulated in the cells over a lifetime.

Often this results in what is known in alternative medicine circles as a "healing crisis." This comes about when the cells eliminate poisons into the blood stream all at the same time, throwing the system into a state of toxic overload until it can clear the "backlog." Symptoms such as **nausea**, headaches, or sensitivities to noise and other stimulations may be experienced.

The answer to most otherwise healthy patients is often just to lie quietly in a darkened room and take herbal teas. However, in the case of someone who has a serious illness, such as arthritis, **colitis**, diabetes, or **cancer**, (the list is much longer than this), it is strongly advised that they seek the help of a qualified practitioner. Therapists can help patients achieve detoxification in a way that causes the least stress to their bodies.

Research and general acceptance

Traditionally, holistic medicine, in all its different forms, has been regarded with mistrust and skepticism on the part of the allopathic medical profession. This situation is gradually changing. As of the year 2000, many insurance companies will provide for some form of alternative, or complementary, treatment.

In addition, many allopathic physicians, recognizing the role alternative medicine can play in overall health and well being, are actually referring patients to reputable practitioners, particularly **chiropractic** and relaxation therapists, for help with a varied range of complaints.

Training and certification

Holistic or alternative medicine practitioners are usually affiliated with an organization in their field. Training varies tremendously with the category, and ranges from no qualifications at all—experience only—to holding a Ph.D. from an accredited university. Again, credentials and memberships should be checked by prospective patients.

An excellent source for qualified practitioners is the American Board of Holistic Medicine, (AHBM), which was incorporated in 1996. Also, the American Holistic Medicine Association has a comprehensive list of practitioners in all types of therapies across the United States, which they call "the holistic doctor finder." However, they stress that it is the responsibility of the patient to check each practitioner's credentials prior to treatment.

The ABHM has established the core curriculum upon which board certification for holistic medicine will be based. It includes the following 12 categories:

Body

Physical and environmental health

- nutritional medicine
- exercise medicine
- environmental medicine

Mind

Mental and emotional health

- behavioral medicine

Spirit

Spiritual health

- spiritual attunement
- social health

The six specialized areas:

- biomolecular diagnosis and therapy
- botanical medicine
- energy medicine
- ethno-medicine—including traditional Chinese medicine, Ayurveda, and Native American medicine
- homeopathy
- manual medicine

Founded in 1978 for the purpose of uniting practitioners of holistic medicine, membership of the AHMA is open to licensed medical doctors (MDs) and doctors of osteopathic medicine (DOs) from every specialty and to medical students studying for those degrees. Associate membership is open to health care practitioners who are certified, registered or licensed in the state in which they practice. The mission of the AHMA is to support practitioners in their personal and professional development as healers, and to educate physicians about holistic medicine.

ORGANIZATIONS

American Holistic Medical Association, 23366 Commerce Park, Suite 101B, Beachwood, OH, 44122, (216) 292-6644, (216) 292-6688, info@holisticmedicine.org, http://www.holisticmedicine.org.

Holistic Medicine, http://www.holisticmed.com/whatis. html.

Patricia Skinner

Holter monitoring

Definition

Holter monitoring is continuous monitoring of the electrical activity of a patient's heart muscle (**electrocardiography**) for 24 hours, using a special portable device called a Holter monitor. Patients wear the Holter monitor while carrying out their usual daily activities.

Purpose

Holter monitoring is used to help determine whether someone has an otherwise undetected heart disease, such as abnormal heart rhythm (cardiac arrhythmia), or inadequate blood flow through the heart. Specifically, it can detect abnormal electrical activity in the heart that may occur randomly or only under certain circumstances, such as during sleep or periods of physical activity or **stress**,

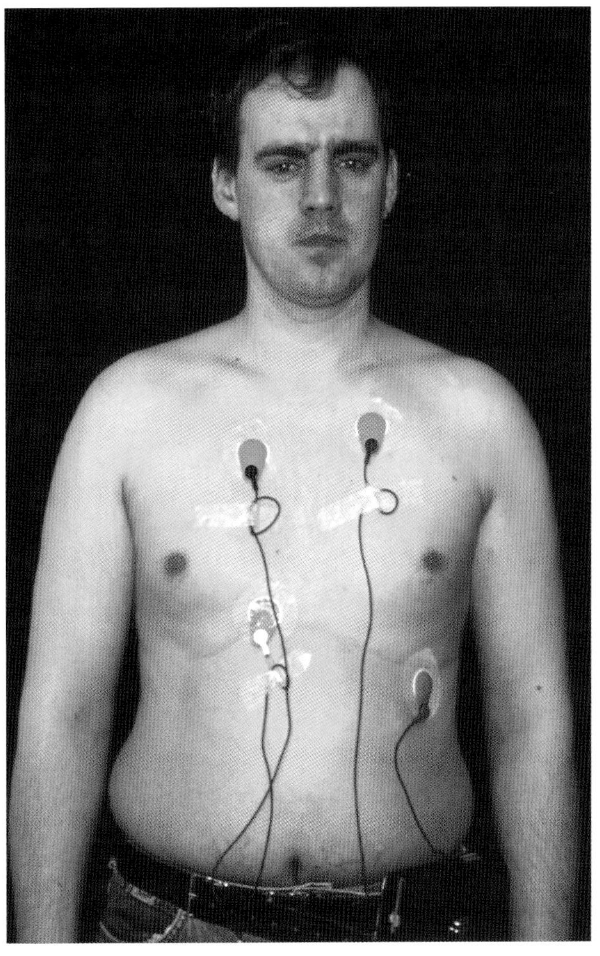

A male patient wears electrodes attached to his chest, which is connected to a Holter monitor at his waist. *(Dr. P. Marazzi/ Photo Researchers, Inc.)*

which may or may not be picked up by standard, short-term electrocardiography performed in a doctor's office.

Traditionally, an exercise **stress test** has been used to screen people for "silent" heart disease (heart disease with none of the usual symptoms). However, an exercise stress test is not completely foolproof, often producing false negative results (indicating no heart disease when heart disease is actually present) and false positives (indicating heart disease when there is none). Furthermore, some people cannot undergo exercise stress testing because of other medical conditions, such as arthritis.

Holter monitoring, also known as ambulatory or 24-hour electrocardiography, offers an alternate means of testing people for heart disease. By monitoring electrocardiographic activity throughout the day, Holter monitoring can uncover heart problems that occur during the patient's everyday activities. It can also help to recognize any activities that may be causing the heart problems. And it can define and correlate symptoms that may be caused by irregularities of the heart.

Precautions

Holter monitoring is an extremely safe procedure and no special precautions are required.

Description

The technician affixes electrodes on the surface of the skin at specific areas of the patient's chest, using adhesive patches with special gel that conducts electrical impulses. Typically, electrodes are placed under each collarbone and each bottom rib, and several electrodes are placed across the chest in a rough outline of the heart. The electrodes are attached to a portable electrocardiographic device called a Holter monitor, which records the electrical activity of the heart over 24–48 hours. The device is worn over the patient's shoulder or attached to a belt around the waist.

The Holter monitor records the continuous electrical activity throughout the course of the day, while the patient carries out his or her daily activities. During this time, the patient also keeps a detailed log or diary, recording his or her various activities, such as exercise, eating, sleeping, straining, breathing too hard (hyperventilating), and any stressful situations. The patient also notes the time and circumstances of any symptoms–especially chest **pain**, **dizziness**, **shortness of breath**, heart **palpitations**, and any other signs of heart trouble. Some Holter monitors allow patients to record their symptoms electronically, highlighting the portion of the electrocardiogram recorded while the symptoms are occurring.

After 24–48 hours, the Holter monitor is removed. A computer-assisted analysis is performed on the electrocardiographic recording, and the doctor compares the recording against the patient's log to see if there is any correlation between electrocardiographic abnormalities and any of the patient's activities or symptoms. The physician makes a final interpretation.

Preparation

In the doctor's office, electrodes are attached to the patient's chest. In some cases, the patient's chest hair may have to be shaved to facilitate attaching the electrodes. The patient then begins carrying the monitor on a shoulder harness, in a pocket, or on the belt while carrying out his or her usual daily routine. The patient should inform the doctor of any drugs he or she may be taking, because certain drugs can alter heart rhythms and may affect the results of the test.

Aftercare

The patient returns to the doctor's office to have the monitor and electrodes removed. No special measures need to be taken following Holter monitoring. The test results are usually available within a few days after the monitor is removed.

Risks

There are no known risks associated with Holter monitoring. The main complaint that people have with Holter monitoring is that the monitor may be cumbersome and interfere with certain activities, especially sleeping. Bathing and showering are not allowed during the study.

Normal results

A normal Holter monitoring test shows relatively normal electrical activity in the heart around the clock and no evidence of silent **ischemia** (deprivation of oxygen-rich blood).

Abnormal results

An abnormal result on Holter monitoring may indicate ischemia to the heart muscle or heart rhythm disturbances. Abnormalities are especially likely to show up during periods of stress or heavy activity, but sometimes serious abnormalities are recorded while the patient is sleeping.

ORGANIZATIONS

American Heart Association National Center, 7272 Greenville Avenue, Dallas, TX, 75231, (800) 242-8721, Review.personal.info@heart.org.

National Heart Lung and Blood Institute Health Informa tion Center, P.O. Box 30105, Bethesda, MD, 20824-0105, (301) 592-8573, (240) 629-3246, http://www.nhlbi. nih.gov.

Robert Scott Dinsmoor

Holtzman ink blot test

Definition

The Holtzman Inkblot Technique (HIT) is a projective personality assessment test for persons ages five and up.

Purpose

The HIT is used to assess the personality structure of a test subject. It is sometimes used as a diagnostic tool in assessing **schizophrenia**, depression, **addiction**, and character disorders.

Precautions

Psychometric testing requires a clinically trained examiner. The HIT should be administered and interpreted by a trained psychologist, psychiatrist, or appropriately trained mental health professional.

Some consider projective tests to be less reliable than objective personality tests. If the examiner is not well-trained in psychometric evaluation, subjective interpretations may affect the outcome of the test.

Description

The HIT, developed by psychologist Wayne Holtzman and colleagues, was introduced in 1961. The test was designed to overcome some of the deficiencies of its famous predecessor, the Rorschach Inkblot Test.

Unlike the Rorschach, the Holtzman is a standardized measurement with clearly defined objective scoring criteria. The HIT consists of 45 inkblots. The test administrator, or examiner, has a stack of 47 cards with inkblots (45 test cards and 2 practice cards) face down in front of him or her. The examiner hands each card to the subject and asks the test subject what he or she sees in the inkblot. Only one response per inkblot is requested. Occasionally, the examiner may ask the test subject to clarify or elaborate on a response. The administration of the HIT typically takes 50–80 minutes. The HIT is then scored against 22 personality-related characteristics.

The HIT can also be administered in a group setting. In group testing, 30–45 inkblots are projected onto a screen and test subjects provide written responses to each inkblot.

Medicare reimbursement rates for psychological and neuropsychological testing is $58.35 an hour. Billing time typically includes test administration, scoring and interpretation, and reporting. Many insurance plans cover all or a portion of diagnostic psychological testing.

Normal results

Because of the complexity of the scoring process and the projective nature of the test, results for the HIT should only be interpreted by a clinically trained psychologist, psychiatrist, or appropriately trained mental health professional.

ORGANIZATIONS

American Psychological Association (APA), 750 First St. NE, Washington, DC, 20002-4242, (202) 336-5500, (800) 374-2721, http://www.apa.org/.

Paula Anne Ford-Martin

Homeopathic medicine

Definition

Homeopathy, or homeopathic medicine, is a holistic system of treatment that originated in the late eighteenth century. The name homeopathy is derived from two Greek words that mean "like disease." The system is based on the idea that substances that produce symptoms of sickness in healthy people will have a curative effect when given in very diluted quantities to sick people who exhibit those same symptoms. Homeopathic remedies are believed to stimulate the body's own healing processes. Homeopaths use the term "allopathy," or "different than disease," to describe the use of drugs used in conventional medicine to oppose or counteract the symptom being treated.

Purpose

Homeopathic physicians seek to cure their patients on the physical, mental and emotional levels, and each treatment is tailored to a patient's individual needs. Homeopathy is generally a safe treatment, as it uses medicines in extremely diluted quantities, and there are usually minimal side effects. Its non-toxicity makes it a

Examples of popular homeopathic remedies

Aconite	Commonly known as monkshood, aconite is highly toxic. A nontoxic, diluted extract is used in homeopathy to treat symptoms similar to that of poison.
Allium cepa	Commonly known as red onion, homeopathic physicians use a diluted extract of red onion to treat symptoms similar to that of red onion—watery eyes, burning, etc.
Apis	Commonly known as the honey bee, apis as a homeopathic remedy is made from the body of the bee. It is used to treat symptoms similar to that of a bee sting—redness, swelling, etc.
Arnica	Commonly known as the mountain daisy, arnica is used by homeopaths to treat bruises, sprains, and strains.
Arsenicum album	Also known as ars alb, arsenicum album is a diluted form of arsenic, a metallic poison. It is used by homeopathic physicians to treat symptoms similar to the effects of arsenic poisoning—dehydration, burning pain, etc.
Belladonna	Commonly known as deadly nightshade, belladonna is used in homeopathy to treat symptoms of dry mouth, nausea, delirium, etc.
Bryonia	Commonly known as wild hops, bryonia is used in homeopathy to treat vomiting, diarrhea, inflammation, etc.
Calcarea carbonica	Also known as calcium carbonate or calc carb, calcarea carbonica is used in homeopathy to treat symptoms of exhaustion, depression, and anxiety.
Cantharis	Commonly known as Spanish fly, cantharis is used in homeopathy to treat conditions with symptoms of abdominal cramps, vomiting, diarrhea, convulsions, etc.
Chamomilla	Derived from German chamomile, chamomilla is used in homeopathy to treat irritability, impatience, etc. It is most often prescribed to children.
Ferrum phosphoricum	Also known as ferrum phos or iron phosphate, it is used to treat symptoms of low energy and anemia.
Gelsemium	Also known as yellow jasmine, gelsemium is used to treat conditions that affect vision, balance, thought, and locomotion.
Hepar sulphuris	Derived from the inner layer of oyster shells, hepar sulphuris is used to treat infection.
Hypericum perforatum	Commonly known as St. John's wort, hypericum is used to treated nerve damage.
Ignatia	Derived from the bean of a small tree, this homeopathic remedy is prescribed to treat conditions with symptoms such as headache, cramping, and tremors.
Ipecac	Ipecac induces vomiting and causes gastrointestinal distress. Homeopaths prescribe it to treat similar symptoms.
Kali bichromicum	Commonly known as potassium bichromate, kali bichromicum is a poison used also in textile dyes, wood stain, etc. Homeopaths use it to treat localized pain.
Lachesis	Derived from the venom of the bushmaster snake, this homeopathic remedy is used to treat conditions that cause the same symptoms as the venom.
Ledum	Also known as marsh tea, ledum is used to treat infections, most often from animal bites, stings, cuts, etc.
Lycopodium	Commonly known as club moss, lycopodium is used to treat diarrhea, stomach upset, etc.
Mercurius vivus	Also known as quicksilver, it is used to treat symptoms of sweats, shaking, nausea, etc.
Natrum muriaticum	Commonly known as salt, it is used to treat conditions that cause excessive thirst and salt cravings.
Phosphorus	Phosphorus is used to treat symptoms of excessive thirst, fatigue, and nervousness.
Pulsatilla	Pulsatilla is used to treat conditions that are accompanied by discharge, such as bedwetting, sinusitis, etc.
Rhus toxicodendron	Commonly known as poison ivy, homeopaths use it to treat conditions with symptoms of fever, swollen glands, and restlessness.
Ruta	Ruta, or rue, is used to treat conditions associated with pain and strain, such as tennis elbow, sciatica, etc.
Sepia	Sepia is the discharge used by the cuttlefish to disappear from a predator. Homeopaths use sepia to treat symptoms of apathy and weakness.
Silica	Also called flint, silica is used by homeopaths to treat conditions that cause weakness, sweating, and sensitivity to cold.
Sulphur	Sulphur is used to treat conditions with symptoms of itching, burning pains, and odor.

(Table by PreMediaGlobal. Reproduced by permission of Gale, a part of Cengage Learning.)

good choice for the treatment of children. Another benefit of homeopathy is the cost of treatments; homeopathic remedies are inexpensive, often a fraction of the cost of conventional drugs.

Homeopathic treatment has been shown effective in treating many conditions. Colds and flu may be effectively treated with aconite and bryonia. **Influenza** suffers in a double-blind study found that they were twice as likely to recover in 48 hours when they took homeopathic remedies. Studies have been published in British medical journals confirming the efficacy of homeopathic treatment for **rheumatoid arthritis**. Homeopathic remedies are effective in treating infections, circulatory problems, respiratory problems, heart disease, depression and nervous disorders, migraine headaches, **allergies**, arthritis, and diabetes. Homeopathy is a good treatment to explore for acute and chronic illnesses, particularly if these are found in the early stages and where there is not severe damage. Homeopathy can be used to assist the healing process after surgery or **chemotherapy**.

Description

Origins

Homeopathy was founded by German physician Samuel Hahnemann (1755–1843), who was much disturbed by the medical system of his time, believing that its cures were crude and some of its strong drugs and treatments did more harm than good to patients. Hahnemann performed experiments on himself using Peruvian bark, which contains quinine, a **malaria** remedy. He concluded that in a healthy person, quinine creates the same symptoms as malaria, including fevers and chills, which is the reason why it is effective as a remedy. He then began to analyze the remedies available in nature by what he called provings. Provings of homeopathic remedies are still compiled by dosing healthy adults with various substances and documenting the results, in terms of the dose needed to produce the symptoms and the length of the dose's effectiveness. The provings are collected in large homeopathic references called *materia medica* or materials of medicine.

Hahnemann formulated these principles of homeopathy:

- Law of Similars (like cures like)
- Law of the Infinitesimal Dose (The more diluted a remedy is, the more potent it is.)
- illness is specific to the individual

Hahnemann's Law of Similars was based on thinking that dated back to Hippocrates in the fourth century B.C. It is the same thinking that provided the basis for vaccines created by Edward Jenner (1749–1823) and Louis Pasteur (1822–1895). These vaccines provoke a reaction in the individual that protects against the actual disease. Allergy treatments work the same way. By exposing a person to minute quantities of the allergen, the person's tolerance levels are elevated.

The Law of the Infinitesimal Dose has always caused controversy among those outside the field of homeopathy. Hahnemann contended that as he diluted his remedies with water and alcohol and succussed, or shook, them, the remedies actually worked more effectively. In fact, diluted homeopathic remedies may have no chemical trace of the original substance. Practitioners believe that the electromagnetic energy of the original substance is retained in the dilution, but toxic side effects of the remedy are not. It is this electrochemical "message" that stimulates the body to heal itself, although there is no scientific proof of this.

Homeopathic practitioners believe that illness is specific to an individual. In other words, two people with severe headaches may not receive the same remedies. The practitioner will ask the patient questions about lifestyle, dietary habits, and personality traits, as well as specific questions about the nature of the **headache** and when it occurs. This information gathering is called profiling or case-taking.

In the early 1900s, homeopathy was popular in the United States, with over 15% of all doctors being homeopathic. There were 22 major homeopathic medical schools, including Boston University and the University of Michigan. However, with the formation of the American Medical Association, which restricted and closed down alternative practices, homeopathy declined for half a century. When the 1960s invigorated back-to-nature trends and distrust of artificial drugs and treatments, homeopathy began to grow again dramatically through the next decades. In 1993, *The New England Journal of Medicine* reported that 2.5 million Americans used homeopathic remedies and 800,000 patients visited homeopaths in 1990, and it has continued to grow. Homeopathy is much more popular in Europe than in the United States. French pharmacies are required to make homeopathic remedies available along with conventional medications. Homeopathic hospitals and clinics are part of the national health system in Britain. It is also practiced in India and Israel, among other countries.

A visit to a homeopath can be a different experience than a visit to a regular physician. The initial visit often includes a long questionnaire about a patient's medical and family history, and then a long interview with the practitioner, who prompts the patient with many questions. Sometimes a homeopathic practitioner will use lab tests to establish a patient's general level of health. The initial interview usually lasts between one and two hours.

The purpose of homeopathy is the restoration of the body to homeostasis, or healthy balance, which is its natural state. The symptoms of a disease are regarded as the body's own defensive attempt to correct its imbalance, rather than as enemies to be defeated. Because a homeopath regards symptoms as positive evidence of the body's inner intelligence, he or she will prescribe a remedy designed to stimulate this internal curative process, rather than suppress the symptoms.

In homeopathy, the curative process extends beyond the relief of immediate symptoms of illness. Healing may come in stages, as the practitioner treats layers of symptoms that are remnants of traumas or chronic disease in the patient's past. This is part of Hering's Laws of Cure, named for Constantine Hering, the father of homeopathy in the United States. Hering believed that healing starts from the deepest parts of the body to the extremities, and from the upper parts of the body to the lower parts. Hering's Laws also state that homeopaths should treat disease symptoms in reverse chronological order, from the most recent to the oldest, restoring health in stages. Sometimes, the patient may feel worse before feeling better. This is called a healing crisis.

SAMUEL HAHNEMANN (1755–1843)

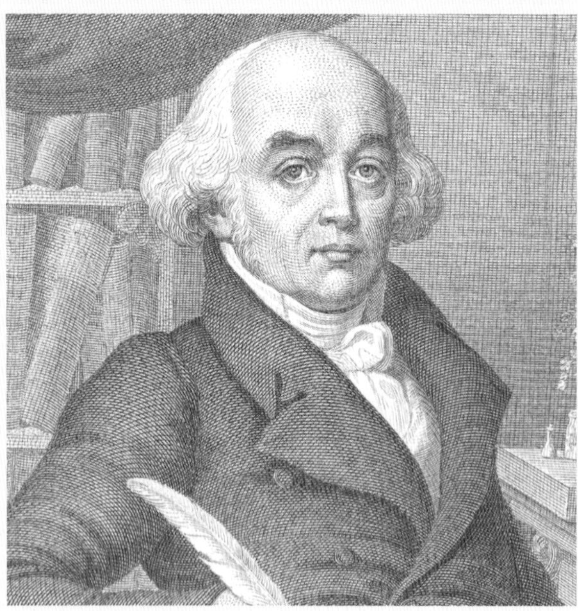

(© Bettmann/Corbis.)

Samuel Christian Hahnemann created and developed the system called homeopathy. It is also known as *similia similibus curentor* or like cures like. Although his new methods initially met with ridicule and criticism, by the time of his death they were accepted the world over as a result of the great success he had with his new cure.

Hahnemann was born in Meissen, Saxony (now part of Germany) into a financially challenged middle class family. His parents initially educated him at home, where his father taught him never to accept anything he learned without first questioning it. He graduated as a physician at Erlangen in 1779 after studying at Leipzig and Vienna. He was also fluent in English, German, Italian, French, Greek, Arabic, Latin, and Hebrew.

At age 27 he married his first wife, Johanna Henriette Kuchler, the daughter of an apothecary, with whom he had 11 children.

Living in poverty, Hahnemann began practicing medicine in 1781 and translating scientific texts to supplement his income. However, disillusioned with medicine, he eventually gave it up entirely.

He discovered the concept of homeopathy when considering the effect of quinine on malaria, and went on to cure soldiers and then sufferers of a typhus epidemic with astounding success. He documented his discoveries in the *Organon,* a treatise on his work. Homeopathy also proved its worth in 1831 when there was an outbreak of cholera. Hahnemann used homeopathic treatment with a 96% success rate, compared to the 41% of allopathic medicine. He also wrote his *Materia Medica Pura.*

In 1834, Hahnemann met his second wife, Marie Melanie d'Hervilly. Despite a great difference in age, they were happily married until his death in Paris on July 2, 1843, at the age of 88.

When prescribing a remedy, homeopaths will match a patient's symptoms with the proper remedy in a repertory or *materia medica* that has been compiled throughout the history of homeopathy. Classical homeopaths prescribe only one remedy at a time. However, it is becoming more common, especially in Europe, to use combination formulas of several remedies for the treatment of some combinations of symptoms.

The cost of homeopathic care can vary. The cost of visits will be comparable to conventional medicine, with initial visits ranging from $50 to $300. Non-M.D. homeopaths can charge from $50 to $250. Follow-up visits are less, at about $35 to $100. Homeopathic medicine is significantly cheaper than pharmaceuticals, and most remedies cost between $2 and $10. Homeopaths rarely use lab tests, which reduces the cost of treatment further. In general, homeopathy is much more economical than conventional medicine. In 1991, the French government did a study on the cost of homeopathic medicine, and found that it costs half as much to treat patients, considering all costs involved. The study did not look at the effectiveness of homeopathy treatment versus conventional treatment.

When homeopaths are licensed professionals, most insurance companies will pay for their fees. Consumers should consult their insurance policies to determine individual regulations. Insurance usually will not cover visits to homeopathic practitioners or homeopathic medicine.

Precautions

Although homeopathic remedies sometimes use substances that are toxic, they are diluted and prescribed in non-toxic doses. Remedies should be prescribed by a homeopathic practitioner. Those preparing to take homeopathic remedies should also avoid taking *antidotes*, substances which homeopathic doctors believe cancel the effects of their remedies. These substances include alcohol, coffee, peppermint (in toothpaste and mouthwash), camphor (in salves and lotions), and very spicy foods. Homeopathic medicine should also be

KEY TERMS

Acute prescribing—Homeopathic treatment for self-limiting illnesses with abrupt onset.

Allopathy—Conventional medical treatment of disease symptoms that uses substances or techniques to oppose or suppress the symptoms.

Law of similars—The basic principle of homeopathic medicine that governs the selection of a specific remedy. It holds that a substance of natural origin that produces certain symptoms in a healthy person will cure those same symptoms in a sick person.

Modalities—The factors and circumstances that cause a patient's symptoms to improve or worsen.

Mother tincture—The first stage in the preparation of a homeopathic remedy, made by soaking a plant, animal, or mineral product in a solution of alcohol.

Potentization—The process of increasing the power of homeopathic preparations by successive dilutions and succussions of a mother tincture.

Succussion—The act of shaking diluted homeopathic remedies as part of the process of potentization.

Trituration—The process of diluting a nonsoluble substance for homeopathic use by grinding it to a fine powder and mixing it with lactose powder.

handled with care, and should not be touched with the hands or fingers, which can contaminate it.

Side effects

A homeopathic *aggravation* sometimes occurs during initial treatment with homeopathic remedies. This means that symptoms can temporarily worsen during the process of healing. Although this is usually mild, the aggravation can sometimes be severe. Homeopaths see aggravation as a positive sign that the remedy is a good match for the patient's symptoms. The healing crisis, which happens when the patient is undergoing treatment for layers of symptoms, may also cause the patient to feel worse before feeling better. Some patients can experience emotional disturbances like weeping or depression, if suppressed emotional problems led to the illness in the first place.

Research and general acceptance

Since the early 1900s, when the American Medical Association and pharmacists waged a battle against it, homeopaths believe that homeopathy has been neglected and sometimes ridiculed by mainstream medicine. Much of this is because there are few controlled scientific studies of homeopathy that would meet the criteria for approval by the U.S. Food and Drug Administration (FDA), or for acceptance for publication in the major reputable medical journals in the United States. Aside from politics, part of the reason for this skepticism is that there are some aspects of homeopathy which have not been completely explained scientifically. For instance, homeopaths have found that the more they dilute and succuss a remedy, the greater effect it seems to have on the body. Some homeopathic remedies are so diluted that not even a single molecule of the active agent remains in a solution. Also, homeopathy puts an emphasis on analyzing symptoms and then applying remedies to these symptoms, rather than working by classifying diseases. Thus, some people with the same disease may require different homeopathic medicines and treatments. Furthermore, conventional medicine strives to find out how medicines work in the body before they use them; homeopathy is less concerned with the intricate biochemistry involved than with whether a remedy ultimately works and heals holistically. For all these reasons, conventional medicine claims that homeopathy is not scientific.

There continue to be many studies that homeopaths believe affirm the effectiveness of homeopathic treatments. Among the most celebrated, the *British Medical Journal* in 1991 published a large analysis of homeopathic treatments that were given over the course of 25 years. This project involved over 100 studies of patients with problems ranging from vascular diseases, respiratory problems, infections, stomach problems, allergies, recovery from surgeries, arthritis, trauma, psychological problems, diabetes, and others. The study found improvement with homeopathic treatment in most categories of problems, and concluded that the evidence was "sufficient for establishing homeopathy as a regular treatment for certain indications."

Resources

BOOKS

Schmukler, Alan. *Homeopathy: An A to Z Home Hand book*Woodbury, MN: Llewellyn Publications, 2006.

Wauters, Ambika. *The Homeopathy Bible: The Definitive Guide to Remedies*. New York: Sterling Publishing, 2007.

PERIODICALS

Brewitt, Barbara. "Natural Laws Put Homeopaths and Medical Scientists in Harm's Way in the Political Arena: American's Access to Health Care Innovations

Blocked." *Townsend Letter: The Examiner of Alterna tive Medicine* (December 2007): 13(3).

Khuda-Bukhsh, Anisur R. "Laboratory Research in Homeopathy: Pro." *Integrative Cancer Therapies* (December 2006): 320(13).

Moffett, John R., et al. "Laboratory Research in Homeo pathy: Con." *Integrative Cancer Therapies* (December 2006): 333(10).

Solan, Matthew. "Beyond the M.D.: What Can a Homeo-path, Naturopath, or TCM Doctor Do for You? Plenty, if You Know What to Look For."

ORGANIZATIONS

American Institute of Homeopathy, 801 N. Fairfax St., Suite 306, Alexandria, VA, 22314, (888) 445-9988, http://www.homeopathyusa.org.

Council for Homeopathic Certification, PMB 187, 16915 SE 272nd St., Suite 100, Covington, WA, 98042, (866) 242-3399, http://www.homeopathicdirectory.com.

Homeopathic Medical Council of Canada, 3910 Bathurst St., Suite 202, Toronto, ON, Canada, M3H 3N8, (416) 638-4622, http://www.hmcc.ca.

Ken R. Wells

Homeopathic medicine, acute prescribing

Definition

Acute homeopathic prescribing is that part of homeopathy that treats illness which has an abrupt onset and needs immediate attention. In **homeopathic medicine**, acute refers primarily to the speed of onset and self-limiting character of the disorder rather than its seriousness. Colds, **influenza**, sore throats, insect **stings**, cuts, **bruises**, **vomiting**, **diarrhea**, **fever**, muscle aches, and short-term **insomnia** are all examples of conditions that are treated by acute prescribing. The remedies given in acute homeopathic prescribing are intended to stimulate the body's internal ability to heal itself; they do not kill germs or suppress symptoms. Acute prescribing can be done—within limits—by patients at home, as well as by homeopathic practitioners. Study courses, self-treatment guides, and homeopathic home medicine kits are now available by mail order from homeopathic pharmacies and educational services.

Purpose

Homeopathic physicians seek to cure their patients on physical, mental, and emotional levels, and each treatment is tailored to a patient's individual needs. Homeopathy is generally a safe treatment, as it uses medicines in extremely diluted quantities, and there are usually minimal side effects. Its non-toxicity makes it a choice for the treatment of children. Another benefit of homeopathy is the cost of treatments; homeopathic remedies are inexpensive, often a fraction of the cost of conventional drugs.

Acute homeopathic prescribing is thought to benefit a wide range of ailments. These include **altitude sickness**, Bell's palsy, the **common cold**, **allergies**, coughing, **dengue fever**, **dysentery**, earaches, migraine headaches, fever, **food poisoning**, grief, influenza, **motion sickness**, **shock**, **sore throat**, surgical complications, and reactions to vaccinations and drug therapy. Acute remedies may also be prescribed to treat insect stings, animal **bites**, and problems related to **poison oak** and **poison ivy**. It may be further employed in treating injuries including black eyes, **burns**, bruises, concussions, cuts, damaged tendons and ligaments, **dislocations**, **fractures**, herniated discs, nosebleeds, puncture **wounds**, sprains, and strains.

Description

Origins

Homeopathy is a gentle, painless, holistic system of healing developed during the 1790s by Samuel Hahnemann, a German physician. Experimenting on himself with the anti-malarial drug quinine, Hahnemann noticed that large doses of the medicine actually caused malaria-like symptoms, while smaller doses cured the symptoms. From this, he advanced his concept of *Similia similibus curentur*, or "let like be cured with like." Hahnemann then developed an extensive system of medicine based on this concept. He named it homeopathy, from the Greek words *homoios* (the same) and *pathos* (suffering).

Homeopathic remedies are almost always made from natural materials—plant, animal, or mineral substances—that have been treated to form base tinctures or nonsoluble powders. Liquid extracts are then potentized, or increased in power, by a series of dilutions and succussions, or shakings. It is thought that succussion is necessary to transfer the energy of the natural substance to the solution. In addition, the potency of the remedy is regarded as increasing with each dilution. After the tincture has been diluted to the prescribed potency, the resulting solution is added to a bottle of sucrose/lactose tablets, which are stored in a cool, dark place. If the remedy is not soluble in water, it is ground to a fine powder and triturated with powdered lactose to achieve the desired potency.

Proponents of homeopathy over the years have included Louisa May Alcott, Charles Dickens, Benjamin

Disraeli, Johann Wolfgang Goethe, Nathaniel Hawthorne, William James, Henry Wadsworth Longfellow, Pope Pius X, John D. Rockefeller, Harriet Beecher Stowe, William Thackeray, Daniel Webster, and W. B. Yeats. England's Royal Family has employed homeopathic practitioners since the 1830s.

Homeopathic prescribing differs in general from allopathic medicine in its tailoring of remedies to the patient's overall personality type and totality of symptoms, rather than to the disease. Whereas a conventional physician would prescribe the same medication or treatment regimen to all patients with the common cold, for example, a homeopathic practitioner would ask detailed questions about each patient's symptoms and the modalities, or factors, that make them better or worse. As a result, the homeopath might prescribe six different remedies for six different patients with the same illness. In acute prescribing homeopathy, consultations are more brief compared to constitutional homeopathic prescribing. A typical patient might spend just 10–15 minutes with the practitioner, compared to more than an hour for constitutional prescribing.

Homeopathic classification of symptoms

Homeopathic practitioners use the word symptom in a more inclusive fashion than traditional medicine. In homeopathy, symptoms include any change that the patient experiences during the illness, including changes in emotional or mental patterns.

Homeopaths classify symptoms according to a hierarchy of four categories for purposes of acute prescribing:

- Peculiar symptoms. These are symptoms unique to the individual that do not occur in most persons with the acute disease. Homeopaths make note of peculiar symptoms because they often help to determine the remedy.
- Mental and emotional symptoms. These are important general symptoms that inform the homeopath about the patient's total experience of the disorder.
- Other general symptoms. These are physical symptoms felt throughout the patient's body, such as tiredness, changes in appetite, or restlessness.
- Particular symptoms. Particular symptoms are localized in the body; they include such symptoms as nausea, skin rashes, headache, etc.

During homeopathic case-taking, the practitioner will evaluate the intensity of the patient's symptoms, assess their depth within the patient's body, note any peculiar symptoms, evaluate the modalities of each symptom, and make a list of key symptoms to guide the selection of the proper medicine.

Homeopathic remedies

There are several hundred homeopathic remedies. Homeopathic medicines are usually formulated from diluted or triturated natural substances, including plants, **minerals**, or even venom from snakes or stinging insects. Some remedies may be given in a spray, ointment, or cream, but the most common forms of administration are liquid dilutions and two sizes of pellets, or cylindrical tablets (for triturated remedies). A dose consists of one drop of liquid; 10–20 small pellets; or 1–3 large pellets. Since the remedies are so dilute, the exact size of the dose is not of primary importance. The frequency of dosing is considered critical, however; patients are advised not to take further doses until the first has completed its effect.

Homeopathic remedies can be kept indefinitely with proper handling. Proper handling includes storing the remedies in the original bottles and discarding them if they become contaminated by sunlight or other intense light; temperatures over 100°F (37.8°C); vapors from camphor, mothballs, or perfume; or from other homeopathic remedies being opened in the same room at the same time.

Preparations

Case-taking

The first step in acute prescribing is a lengthy interview with the patient, known as case-taking. In addition to noting the character, location, and severity of the patient's symptoms, the homeopath will ask about their modalities. The modalities are the circumstances or factors (e.g., weather, time of day, body position, behavior or activity, etc.) that make the symptoms either better or worse. Case-taking can be done by the patient or a family member as well as by a homeopath.

Selection and administration of a remedy

The choice of a specific remedy is guided by the patient's total symptom profile rather than by the illness. Homeopathic remedies are prescribed according to the law of similars, which holds that a substance that produces specific symptoms in healthy people cures those symptoms in sick people when given in highly diluted forms. For example, a patient with influenza who is irritable, headachy, and suffering from joint or muscle pains is likely to be given *bryonia* (wild hops), because this plant extract would cause this symptom cluster in a healthy individual.

Patients are instructed to avoid touching homeopathic medicines with their fingers. The dose can be poured onto a piece of white paper or the bottle's cap and tipped directly into the mouth. Homeopathic remedies are not taken with water; patients should not eat or drink anything for 15–20 minutes before or after taking the dose.

Precautions

Homeopathic acute prescribing is not recommended for the treatment of chronic conditions requiring constitutional prescribing, for severe infections requiring antibiotic treatment, or for conditions requiring major surgery. It is also not recommended for the treatment of mental health problems.

Persons who are treating themselves with homeopathic remedies should follow professional guidelines regarding the limitations of home treatment. Most homeopathic home treatment guides include necessary information regarding symptoms and disorders that require professional attention.

Homeopathic remedies may lose their potency if used at the same time as other products. Some homeopathic practitioners recommend the avoidance of mint and mentholated products (toothpastes, candies, chewing gum, mouth rinses), as well as camphor and camphorated products (including eucalyptus and Tiger Balm), patchouli and other essential oils, moth balls, strong perfumes, aftershaves, scented soaps, **stress**, x rays, coffee, nicotine, recreational drugs (**marijuana**), and certain therapeutic drugs (most notably cortisone and prednisone) during treatment. Patients are also advised to avoid electric blankets and dental work, as these are thought to adversely affect homeopathic therapy. Homeopathic remedies should never be placed near magnets.

Practitioners caution that high-potency preparations should be used only under the supervision of a homeopathic practitioner.

Side effects

Homeopathic medicines are so diluted that sometimes no trace of the original substance can be detected. These medicines are therefore considered non-toxic and generally free of harmful side effects. There may, however, be individual reactions to homeopathic medicine.

An intensified healing response may occur as treatment begins, which causes symptoms to worsen, but the phenomenon is usually temporary. In some patients, old symptoms may re-appear from past conditions from which recovery was not complete. Such phenomena are taken as positive indications that the healing process has started.

Research and general acceptance

As Samuel Hahnemann's healing system grew in popularity during the 1800s, it quickly attracted vehement opposition from the medical and apothecary professions. Since the early 1900s, when the American Medical Association and pharmacists waged a battle against it, homeopaths believe that homeopathy has been neglected and sometimes ridiculed by mainstream medicine. Much of this skepticism is because there are few controlled scientific studies of homeopathy that would meet the criteria of the U.S. Food and Drug Administration (FDA), or for acceptance for publication in the major reputable medical journals in the United States. Aside from politics, part of the reason for this skepticism is that there are some aspects of homeopathy which have not been completely explained scientifically. For instance, homeopaths have found that the more they dilute and succuss a remedy, the greater effect it seems to have on the body. Some homeopathic remedies are so diluted that not even a single molecule of the active agent remains in a solution, yet homeopaths maintain it still works; some studies have demonstrated this paradox, yet cannot explain it. Also, homeopathy puts an emphasis on analyzing symptoms and then applying remedies to these symptoms, rather than working by classifying diseases. Thus, some people with the same disease may require different homeopathic medicines and treatments. Furthermore, conventional medicine strives to find out how medicines work in the body before they use them; homeopathy is less concerned with the intricate biochemistry involved than with whether a remedy ultimately works and heals holistically. For all these reasons, conventional medicine claims that homeopathy is not scientific, but homeopaths reply that homeopathy has been developed and studied for centuries, with much documentation and success.

There continue to be many studies that homeopaths believe affirm the effectiveness of homeopathic treatments. Among the most celebrated, the *British Medical Journal* in 1991 published a large analysis of homeopathic treatments that were given over the course of 25 years. This project involved over 100 studies of patients with problems ranging from vascular diseases, respiratory problems, infections, stomach problems, allergies, recovery from surgeries, arthritis, trauma, psychological problems, diabetes, and others. The study found improvement with homeopathic treatment in most categories of problems, and concluded that the evidence was "sufficient for establishing homeopathy as a regular treatment for certain indications."

In the United Kingdom and other countries where homeopathy is especially popular, some medical doctors incorporate aspects of acute prescribing homeopathy into their practices. Countries in which homeopathy is popular include France, India, Pakistan, Sri Lanka, Brazil, and Argentina. Large homeopathic hospitals exist in London and Glasgow, and homeopathic medical centers can be found in India and South America.

Resources

BOOKS

Schmukler, Alan. *Homeopathy: An A to Z Home Handbook*. Woodbury, MN: Llewellyn Publications, 2006.

Wauters, Ambika. *The Homeopathy Bible: The Definitive Guide to Remedies*. New York: Sterling Publishing, 2007.

PERIODICALS

Brewitt, Barbara. "Natural Laws Put Homeopaths and Medical Scientists in Harm's Way in the Political Arena: American's Access to Health Care Innovations Blocked." *Townsend Letter: The Examiner of Alternative Medicine* (December 2007): 13(3).

Khuda-Bukhsh, Anisur R. "Laboratory Research in Homeopathy: Pro." *Integrative Cancer Therapies* (December 2006): 320(13).

Medhurst, Robert. "Homeopathy for Hypertension." *Journal of the Australian Traditional-Medicine Society* (March 2007): 29(2).

Moffett, John R., et al. "Laboratory Research in Homeopathy: Con." *Integrative Cancer Therapies* (December 2006): 333(10).

Reichenberg-Ullman, Judyth, and Robert Ullman. "The Best of Naturopathic Medicine: Homeopathy." *Townsend Letter: The Examiner of Alternative Medicine* (February-March 2007): 52(3).

ORGANIZATIONS

American Institute of Homeopathy, 101 South Whiting Street, Suite 16, Alexandria, VA, 22304, (888) 445-9988, admin@homeopathyusa.org, http://www.homeopathyusa.org.

Australian Homeopathic Association, PO Box7108, Toowoomba, Australia, (07) 4646 4380, (07) 4646 4393, admin@homeopathyoz.org, http://www.homeopathyoz.org.

Council for Homeopathic Certification, PMB 187, 16915 SE 272nd St., Suite 100, Covington, WA, 98042, (815) 366-7622, (866) 242-3399, http://www.homeopathicdirectory.com.

Homeopathic Medical Council of Canada, 31 Adelaide Street East, Box 605, Toronto, CanadaOntario, M5C 2J8, (416) 788-4622, Ontario@HMCC.ca, http://www.hmcc.ca.

Ken R. Wells

Homeopathic medicine, constitutional prescribing

Definition

Constitutional homeopathic prescribing, also called classical prescribing, is a holistic system of medicine that has been practiced for more than 200 years. Unlike acute homeopathic prescribing, constitutional prescribing refers to the selection and administration of homeopathic preparations over a period of time for treatment related to what practitioners call miasmic disorders, those caused by an inherited predisposition to a disease. The term miasm comes from a Greek word meaning stain or pollution. As in acute prescribing, constitutional prescribing is holistic in that it is intended to treat the patient on the emotional and spiritual levels of his or her being as well as the physical. Constitutional prescribing is also aimed at eventual cure of the patient, not just suppression or relief of immediate symptoms.

Purpose

Homeopathic physicians seek to treat their patients on physical, mental, and emotional levels, and each treatment is tailored to a patient's individual needs. Homeopathy is generally a safe treatment, as it uses medicines in extremely diluted quantities, and there are usually minimal side effects. Its non-toxicity makes it a choice for treating children. Another benefit of homeopathy is the cost of treatments; homeopathic remedies are inexpensive, often a fraction of the cost of conventional drugs.

Classical homeopathy has been used to treat a wide range of diseases and conditions, most of which tend to be long-term. These include: **alcoholism**, **allergies**, **anxiety**, arthritis, **asthma**, bladder conditions, **chronic fatigue syndrome**, depression, drug dependencies, gastrointestinal problems, Gulf War sickness, **headache**, hearing problems, herpes, hypersensitivity, immune disorders, **insomnia**, joint problems, kidney conditions, liver problems, **Lyme disease**, lower back problems, **malaria**, **menopause**, menstrual problems, migraine, **multiple sclerosis**, **paralysis**, **phobias**, **shingles**, sinus problems, skin disorders, repetitive stress injury, rheumatism, vertigo, vision problems, and yeast infections.

Description

Origins

Homeopathy was developed during the 1790s by Samuel Hahnemann, a German physician. Experimenting on himself with the anti-malarial drug quinine, Hahnemann noticed that large doses of the medicine actually caused malaria-like symptoms, while smaller doses cured the symptoms. From this, he advanced his concept of *Similia similibus curentur*, or "let like be cured with like." Hahnemann then developed an extensive system of medicine based on this concept. He named it homeopathy, from the Greek words *homoios* (the same) and *pathos* (suffering).

There are several hundred homeopathic remedies. They are almost always made from natural materials—plant, animal, or mineral substances—that have been treated to form base tinctures or nonsoluble powders. Liquid extracts are then potentized, or increased in power, by a series of dilutions and succussions, or shakings. It is thought that succussion is necessary to transfer the energy of the natural substance to the solution. In addition, the potency of the remedy is regarded as increasing with each dilution. After the tincture has been diluted to the prescribed potency, the resulting solution is added to a bottle of sucrose/lactose tablets, which are stored in a cool, dark place. If the remedy is not soluble in water, it is ground to a fine powder and triturated with powdered lactose to achieve the desired potency.

Proponents of homeopathy over the years have included Louisa May Alcott, Charles Dickens, Benjamin Disraeli, Johann Wolfgang Goethe, Nathaniel Hawthorne, William James, Henry Wadsworth Longfellow, Pope Pius X, John D. Rockefeller, Harriet Beecher Stowe, William Thackeray, Daniel Webster, and W. B. Yeats. England's Royal Family has employed homeopathic practitioners since the 1830s.

Constitutional prescribing is based on the patient's symptom profile and specific aspects of homeopathic theory.

Homeopathic classification of symptoms

Homeopathic practitioners use the word symptom in a more inclusive fashion than traditional medicine. In homeopathy, symptoms include any change that the patient experiences during the illness, including changes in emotional or mental patterns.

Homeopaths classify symptoms according to a hierarchy of four categories:

- Peculiar symptoms. These are symptoms unique to the individual that do not occur in most persons. Homeopaths make note of peculiar symptoms because they often help to determine the remedy.
- Mental and emotional symptoms. These are important general symptoms that inform the homeopath about the patient's total experience of the disorder.
- Other general symptoms. These are physical symptoms felt throughout the patient's body, such as tiredness, changes in appetite, or restlessness.
- Particular symptoms. Particular symptoms are localized in the body; they include such symptoms as nausea, skin rashes, or headaches.

Miasms

Homeopaths regard the patient's symptom profile as a systemic manifestation of an underlying chronic disorder called a miasm. Miasms are serious disturbances of what homeopaths call the patient's vital force that are inherited from parents at the time of conception. Hahnemann believed that the parents' basic lifestyle, their emotional condition, and habitual diet, and even the atmospheric conditions at the time of conception would affect the number and severity of miasms passed on to the child. Hahnemann himself distinguished three miasms: the psoric, which he considered the most universal source of chronic disease in humans; the syphilitic; and the sycotic, which he attributed to **gonorrhea**. Later homeopaths identified two additional miasms, the cancernic and the tuberculinic. The remaining major source of miasms is allopathic medicine. It is thought that specific allopathic treatments—particularly **smallpox** vaccinations, cortisone preparations, major tranquilizers, and antibiotics—can produce additional layers of miasms in the patient's constitution. There are no credible, mainstream scientific studies that support this. Constitutional prescribing evaluates the person's current state or miasmic picture, and selects a remedy intended to correct or balance that state. The homeopath may prescribe a different remedy for each miasmic layer over time, but gives only one remedy at a time directed at the person's current state. The basic principle governing the prescription of each successive remedy is the law of similars, or "like cures like."

Hering's laws of cure

The homeopathic laws of cure were outlined by Constantine Hering, a student of Hahnemann who came to the United States in the 1830s. Hering enunciated three laws or principles of the patterns of healing that are used by homeopaths to evaluate the effectiveness of specific remedies and the overall progress of constitutional prescribing:

- Healing progresses from the deepest parts of the organism to the external parts. Homeopaths consider the person's mental and emotional dimensions, together with the brain, heart, and other vital organs, as a person's deepest parts. The skin, hands, and feet are considered the external parts.
- Symptoms appear or disappear in the reverse of their chronological order of appearance. In terms of

constitutional treatment, this law means that miasms acquired later in life will resolve before earlier ones.

- Healing proceeds from the upper to the lower parts of the body.

Healing crises

Homeopaths use Hering's laws to explain the appearance of so-called healing crises, or aggravations, in the course of homeopathic treatment. It is not unusual for patients to experience temporary worsening of certain symptoms after taking their first doses of homeopathic treatment. For example, a person might notice that arthritic pains in the shoulders are better but that the hands feel worse. Hering's third law would indicate that the remedy is working because the symptoms are moving downward in the body. In constitutional prescribing, a remedy that removes one of the patient's miasmic layers will then allow the symptoms of an older miasm to emerge. Thus the patient may find that a physical disease is followed by a different set of physical problems or by emotional symptoms.

Preparations

The most important aspects of preparation for constitutional prescribing are the taking of a complete patient history and careful patient education.

Case-taking

Homeopathic case-taking for constitutional prescribing is similar to that for acute prescribing, but more in-depth. The initial interview generally takes one to two hours. The practitioner is concerned with recording the totality of the patient's symptoms and the modalities that influence their severity. Also included are general characteristics about the patient and his or her lifestyle choices. For example, a practitioner might ask the patient if he or she likes being outside or is generally hot or cold. There is also an emphasis on the patient's lifetime medical history, particularly records of allopathic treatments.

Patient education

Homeopaths regard patients as equal partners in the process of recovery. They will take the time to explain the theories underlying constitutional prescribing to the patient as well as taking the history. Patient education is especially important in constitutional prescribing in order to emphasize the need for patience with the slowness of results and length of treatment, and to minimize the possibility of self-treatment with allopathic drugs if the patient has a healing crisis.

Homeopathic remedies

In constitutional prescribing, one dose of the selected remedy is given. Patients then wait two to six weeks before following up with the homeopath, while the body begins the healing process. At the follow-up visit, the remedy may be repeated, or a different remedy prescribed. The preparation, selection, administration, and storage of remedies for constitutional prescribing are the same as for acute prescribing. These procedures are described more fully in the article on acute prescribing.

Precautions

Constitutional homeopathic prescribing is not appropriate for diseases or health crises requiring emergency treatment, whether medical, surgical, or psychiatric. In addition, constitutional prescribing should not be self-administered. Although home treatment kits of homeopathic remedies are available for acute self-limited disorders, the knowledge of homeopathic theory and practice required for constitutional evaluation is beyond the scope of most patients. Patients who are also seeing an allopathic doctor should make sure the physician is aware of the homeopathic treatment.

Patients are instructed to avoid touching homeopathic medicines with their fingers. The dose can be poured onto a piece of white paper or the bottle's cap and tipped directly into the mouth. Homeopathic remedies are not taken with water; patients should not eat or drink anything for 15–20 minutes before or after taking the dose.

Homeopathic remedies may lose their potency if used at the same time as other products. Some homeopathic practitioners recommend the avoidance of mint and mentholated products (toothpastes, candies, chewing gum, mouth rinses), as well as camphor and camphorated products (including eucalyptus and Tiger Balm), patchouli and other essential oils, moth balls, strong perfumes, aftershaves, scented soaps, stress, x rays, coffee, nicotine, recreational drugs (**marijuana**), and certain therapeutic drugs (most notably cortisone and prednisone) during treatment. Patients are also advised to avoid electric blankets and dental work, as these are thought to adversely affect homeopathic therapy. Homeopathic remedies should never be placed near magnets.

Side effects

Homeopathic medicines are so diluted that sometimes no trace of the original substance can be detected. These medicines are therefore considered by homeopathic practitioners as non-toxic and generally free of harmful side effects. The primary risks to the patient from constitutional homeopathic treatment are the symptoms of the healing crisis and individual reactions to **homeopathic medicine**. The complexity of constitutional prescribing requires homeopaths to have detailed knowledge of the *materia medica* and the repertories, and to take careful and extensive case notes.

An intensified healing response may occur as treatment begins, which causes symptoms to worsen, but the phenomenon is temporary. In some patients, old symptoms may re-appear from past conditions from which recovery was not complete. Such phenomena are taken as positive indications that the healing process has commenced.

Research and general acceptance

As Samuel Hahnemann's healing system grew in popularity during the 1800s, it quickly attracted vehement opposition from the medical and apothecary professions. Since the early 1900s, when the American Medical Association and pharmacists waged a battle against it, homeopathy has been neglected and sometimes ridiculed by mainstream medicine. Much of this is because there are few controlled scientific studies of homeopathy that would meet criteria of the U.S. Food and Drug Administration, or would be accepted for publication in the major reputable medical journals in the United States. Aside from politics, part of the reason for this is that there are some aspects of homeopathy which have not been completely explained scientifically. For instance, homeopaths have found that the more they dilute and succuss a remedy, the greater effect it seems to have on the body. Some homeopathic remedies are so diluted that not even a single molecule of the active agent remains in a solution, yet homeopaths maintain it still works; some studies have demonstrated this paradox, yet cannot explain it. Also, homeopathy puts an emphasis on analyzing symptoms and then applying remedies to these symptoms, rather than working by classifying diseases. Thus, some people with the same disease may require different homeopathic medicines and treatments. Furthermore, conventional medicine strives to find out how medicines work in the body before they use them; homeopathy is less concerned with the intricate biochemistry involved than with whether a remedy ultimately works and heals holistically. For all these reasons, conventional medicine claims that homeopathy is not scientific, but homeopaths reply that homeopathy has been developed and studied for centuries, with much documentation and success.

There continue to be many studies that affirm the effectiveness of homeopathic treatments. Among the most celebrated, the *British Medical Journal* in 1991 published a large analysis of homeopathic treatments that were given over the course of 25 years. This project involved over 100 studies of patients with problems ranging from vascular diseases, respiratory problems, infections, stomach problems, allergies, recovery from surgeries, arthritis, trauma, psychological problems, diabetes, and others. The study found improvement with homeopathic treatment in most categories of problems, and concluded that the evidence was "sufficient for establishing homeopathy as a regular treatment for certain indications."

In the United Kingdom and other countries where homeopathy is especially popular, some medical doctors incorporate aspects of acute prescribing homeopathy into their practices. Countries in which homeopathy is popular include France, India, Pakistan, Sri Lanka, Brazil, and Argentina. Large homeopathic hospitals exist in London and Glasgow, and homeopathic medical centers can be found in India and South America.

Resources

BOOKS

Schmukler, Alan. *Homeopathy: An A to Z Home Handbook*. Woodbury, MN: Llewellyn Publications, 2006.

Wauters, Ambika. *The Homeopathy Bible: The Definitive Guide to Remedies*. New York: Sterling Publishing, 2007.

PERIODICALS

Brewitt, Barbara. "Natural Laws Put Homeopaths and Medical Scientists in Harm's Way in the Political Arena: American's Access to Health Care Innovations Blocked." *Townsend Letter: The Examiner of Alternative Medicine* (December 2007): 13(3).

Khuda-Bukhsh, Anisur R. "Laboratory Research in Homeopathy: Pro." *Integrative Cancer Therapies* (December 2006): 320(13).

Moffett, John R., et al. "Laboratory Research in Homeopathy: Con." *Integrative Cancer Therapies* (December 2006): 333(10).

Monks, Richard. "Mass Consumers Become Homeopathic Consumers." *Chain Drug Review* (March 5, 2007): 41.

Ullman, Robert, and Judyth Reichenberg-Ullman. "Using Liquid Remedies for Greater Flexibility in Homeopathic Prescribing and Case Management." *Townsend Letter for Doctors and Patients*(May 2005): 104(2).

ORGANIZATIONS

American Institute of Homeopathy, 101 South Whiting Street, Suite 16, Alexandria, VA, 22304, (888) 445-9988, admin@homeopathyusa.org, http://www.homeopathyusa.org.

Australian Homeopathic Association, PO Box7108, Toowoomba, Australia, (07) 4646 4380, (07) 4646 4393, admin@homeopathyoz.org, http://www.homeopathyoz.org.

Council for Homeopathic Certification, PMB 187, 16915 SE 272nd St., Suite 100, Covington, WA, 98042, (815) 366-7622, (866) 242-3399, http://www.homeopathicdirectory.com.

Homeopathic Medical Council of Canada, 31 Adelaide Street East, Box 605, Toronto, Ontario, M5C 2J8, Canada, (416) 788-4622, Ontario@HMCC.ca, http://www.hmcc.ca.

Ken R. Wells

Homocysteine

Definition

Homocysteine is a naturally occurring amino acid found in blood plasma. High levels of homocysteine in the blood are believed to increase the chance of heart disease, **stroke**, **Alzheimer's disease**, and **osteoporosis**.

Description

Homocysteine is a sulfur-containing amino acid that occurs naturally in all humans. It is broken down in the body through two metabolic pathways. The chemical changes that must occur to break down homocysteine require the presence of **folic acid** (also called folate) and **vitamins** B^6 and B^{12}. The level of homocysteine in the blood is influenced by the presence of these substances.

Homocystinuria is a rare genetic disorder that occurs in about one in every 200,000 individuals. This congenital metabolic disorder causes large amounts of homocysteine to be excreted in the urine. Homocystinuria is associated **mental retardation** and the development of heart disease before age 30.

In the late 1960s, doctors documented that individuals with homocystinuria developed narrowing of the arteries at a very early age, sometimes even in childhood. Although homocystinuria is rare, this finding stimulated research on whether people who did not have homocystinuria but who did have unusually high levels of homocysteine in their blood were at greater risk of developing heart disease or stroke.

Many risk factors, including family history of heart disease, **smoking**, **obesity**, lack of **exercise**, diabetes, high levels of low-density lipoprotein cholesterol (LDL or "bad" cholesterol), low levels of high-density lipoprotein cholesterol (HDL or "good" cholesterol), and high blood pressure have been documented to increase the risk of stroke and heart disease. With so many other risk factors, it has been difficult to determine whether high levels of homocysteine are an independent risk factor for the development these diseases. However, a substantial number of controlled, well-designed, and well-documented studies have shown that individuals who have high levels of homocysteine in the blood are at increased risk of developing blocked blood vessels, a condition known as occlusive arterial disease or at risk to worsen **atherosclerosis** ("hardening of the arteries").

In the 2000s, studies also suggested that high levels of homocysteine were associated with poorer mental functioning, leading to ongoing investigations into the role of homocysteine in Alzheimer's disease. Additional studies have also suggested that high levels of homocysteine can lead to osteoporosis and an increased risk of broken bones in the elderly. Homocysteine was being tested in half a dozen clinical trials to determine its role in these and several other conditions. Information on clinical trials that are enrolling patients can be found online at www.clinicaltrials.gov.

Causes and symptoms

Homocysteine is thought to irritate the lining of the blood vessels, causing them to become scarred, hardened, and narrowed. This increases the work the heart must do, leading to heart disease. High levels of homocysteine also cause increased blood clotting. **Blood clots** can decrease or block the flow of blood through blood vessels, resulting in strokes and heart attacks. If and how homocysteine directly plays a role in osteoporosis and Alzheimer's disease is not clear.

The level of homocysteine in the blood naturally varies with age, gender, diet, hereditary factors, and general health, but it is estimated that 5–10% of the population has homocysteine levels that are considered high. With the exception of rare individuals who have congenital homocystinuria, people with high blood levels of homocysteine do not have any obvious signs or symptoms.

Diagnosis

The American Heart Association and the American College of Cardiology do not recommend routine screening of homocysteine levels, but they do recommend screening as part of a cardiac risk assessment for individuals who have a family history of **coronary artery disease** but no obvious symptoms of heart disease. The level of homocysteine in the blood can be measured with a simple blood test that is often, but not always, done after **fasting**. Homocysteine levels of 12 mmol/L are considered normal and levels below 10 mmol/L are considered desirable.

Treatment

Lowering homocysteine blood levels is linked to increasing the intake of folic acid and vitamins B_6 and B_{12}. The healthiest way to increase intake is by eating more foods that are high in these substances. Good sources of folic acid, vitamin B_6, and vitamin B_{12} include green leafy vegetables, fortified breakfast cereals, lentils, chickpeas, asparagus, spinach, and most beans. Taking a daily multivitamin is also a way to increase the levels of these substances. However, megadoses of folic acid, vitamin B_6, and vitamin B_{12} are not recommended. Individuals should discuss dosage with their doctor before beginning any supplements. It is important to note that a direct link between increased intake of folic acid, vitamin B_6, and vitamin B_{12} and decreased incidence stroke and **heart attack** has not been proven. However, one study published in the *Journal of the American Medical Association* found that women whose folic acid levels were in the lowest 25% were 69% more likely to die of coronary problems than women whose folic acid levels were in the top 25%.

Individuals with homocystinuria are treated with the drug betaine (Cystadane). This is a powder dissolved in water, juice, or milk and drunk usually twice a day with meals. This drug is not normally used simply to lower high levels of homocysteine in the absence of congenital disease.

Prognosis

Individuals who increase the folic acid, vitamin B_6, and vitamin B_{12} in their diet are expected to see a decrease in blood levels of homocysteine and as a result decrease their risk of heart disease and stroke.

Prevention

Certain drugs are suspected of increasing the level of homocysteine in the blood. People using these drugs should discuss with their doctor the advisability of increasing their intake of folic acid, vitamin B_6, and vitamin B_{12}. These drugs include:

- lipid-lowering drugs such as fenofibrate (Tricor) and bezafibrate (Bezalip)
- metformin (Glucophage), a drug to modify insulin resistance
- anti-epileptic drugs such as phenobarbital, phenytoin (Dilantin), primidone (Mysoline) and carbamazepine (Tegretol)
- levadopa (Sinemet) for treatment of Parkinson's disease
- methotrexate (Rheumatrex, Trexall) for treatment of cancer, psoriasis, rheumatoid arthritis, and systemic lupus erythematosus
- androgen treatment
- nitrous oxide ("laughing gas"), a mild anesthetic

Resources

BOOKS

Robinson, Killian C. *Homocysteine and Vascular Disease*, New York: Springer, 2010.

OTHER

Homocysteine.net, May 10, 2004. [cited March 23, 2005]. http://www.homocysteine.net

ORGANIZATIONS

American Heart Association National Center, 7272 Greenville Avenue, Dallas, TX, 75231, (800) 242-8721, Review.personal.info@heart.org, http://www.heart.org.

Tish Davidson, A.M.

Hong Kong flu *see* **Influenza**

Hookworm disease

Definition

Hookworm disease is an illness caused by one of two types of S-shaped worms that infect the intestine of humans (the worm's host).

Description

Two types of hookworm are responsible for hookworm disease in humans. *Necator americanus* and *Ancylostoma duodenale* have similar life cycles and similar methods of causing illness. The adult worm of both *Necator americanus* and *Ancylostoma duodenale* is about 10 mm long, pinkish-white in color and curved into an S-shape or double hook.

Both types of hookworm have similar life cycles. The females produce about 10,000–20,000 eggs per day. These eggs are passed out of the host's body in feces. The eggs enter the soil, where they incubate. After about 48 hours, the immature larval form hatches out of the eggs. These larvae take about six weeks to develop into the mature larval form that is capable of causing human infection. If exposed to human skin at this point (usually bare feet walking in the dirt or bare hands digging in the dirt), the larvae will bore through the skin and ride through the lymph circulation to the right side of the heart. The larvae are then pumped into the lungs. There

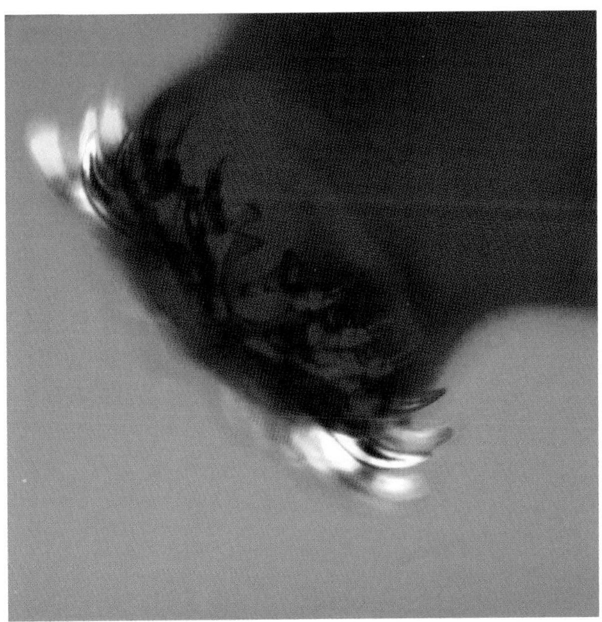

A micrograph image of the head of the hookworm *Ancylostoma spp.* *(Photo Researchers, Inc.)*

they bore into the tiny air sacs (alveoli) of the lungs. Their presence within the lungs usually causes enough irritation to produce coughing. The larvae are coughed up into the throat and mouth, and are then swallowed and passed into the small intestine. It is within the intestine that they develop into the adult worm, producing illness in their human host.

Ancylostoma duodenale is found primarily in the Mediterranean, the Middle East, and throughout Asia. *Necator americanus* is common in tropical areas including Asia, parts of the Americas, and throughout Africa. Research suggests that at least 25% of all people in the world have hookworm disease. In the United States, 700,000 people are believed to be infected with hookworms at any given time.

Causes and symptoms

Hookworms cause trouble for their human host when the worms attach their mouths to the lining of the small intestine and suck the person's blood.

An itchy, slightly raised rash called "ground itch" may appear around the area where the larvae first bored through the skin. The skin in this area may become red and swollen. This lasts for several days and commonly occurs between the toes.

When the larvae are in the lungs, the patient may have a **fever**, **cough**, and some **wheezing**. Some people, however, have none of these symptoms.

Once established within the intestine, the adult worms can cause abdominal **pain**, decreased appetite, **diarrhea**, and weight loss. Most importantly, the worms suck between 0.03–0.2 mL of blood per day. When a worm moves from one area of the intestine to another, it detaches its mouth from the intestinal lining, leaving an irritated area that may continue to bleed for some time. This results in even further blood loss. A single adult worm can live for up to 14 years in a patient's intestine. Over time, the patient's blood loss may be very significant. Anemia is the most serious complication of hookworm disease, progressing over months or years. Children are particularly harmed by such anemia, and can suffer from heart problems, **mental retardation**, slowed growth, and delayed sexual development. In infants, hookworm disease can be deadly.

Diagnosis

Diagnosis of hookworm disease involves collecting a stool sample for examination under a microscope. Hookworm eggs have a characteristic appearance. Counting the eggs in a specific amount of feces allows the healthcare provider to estimate the severity of the infection.

Treatment

Minor infections are often left untreated, especially in areas where hookworm is very common. If treatment is required, the doctor will prescribe a three-day dose of medication. One to two weeks later, another stool sample will be taken to see if the infection is still present.

Anemia is treated with iron supplements. In severe cases, blood **transfusion** may be necessary. Two medications, pyrantel pamoate and mebendazole, are frequently used with good results.

Prognosis

The prognosis for patients with hookworm disease is generally good. However, reinfection rates are extremely high in countries with poor sanitation.

Prevention

Prevention of hookworm disease involves improving sanitation and avoiding contact with soil in areas with high rates of hookworm infection. Children should be required to wear shoes when playing outside in such areas, and people who are gardening should wear gloves.

ORGANIZATIONS

Centers for Disease Control and Prevention (CDC), 1600 Clifton Road, Atlanta, GA, 30333, (800) 232-4636, cdcinfo@cdc.gov, http://www.cdc.gov.

Rosalyn Carson-DeWitt, MD

Hormone replacement therapy

Definition

Hormone replacement therapy (HRT)—now more commonly called menopausal hormone therapy (MRT)—is the use of synthetic or natural females hormones to compensate for the decline in the body's hormone production that occurs when a woman enters **menopause**.

Purpose

HRT is used relieve physical symptoms associated with menopause—the stage of midlife development when a woman's menstrual periods become irregular and eventually cease. Women usually begin the earliest stages of menopause—known as perimenopause—in their mid-30s. Over time the ovaries decrease their production of the sex hormones estrogen and progesterone. Women undergo natural menopause when they have their last menstrual period. Menopause is considered to be complete one year after the last menstruation. This most often occurs between the ages of 45 and 55. Women who have their ovaries removed undergo immediate surgical menopause.

In the years before and during menopause the levels of estrogen and progesterone fluctuate irregularly. Following menopause, estrogen levels are about one-tenth of premenopausal levels and progesterone is almost completely absent. Menopausal symptoms resulting from low estrogen that may be treated with HRT include:

- hot flashes
- vaginal dryness
- night sweats
- sleep disturbances
- mood swings
- frequent urination
- loss of sexual interest

HRT is also used to help prevent osteoporosis—a decrease in bone mass and density that causes the bones to become more fragile and can lead to **fractures**.

Demographics

At the turn of the twenty-first century, about 6 million American women were taking estrogen and

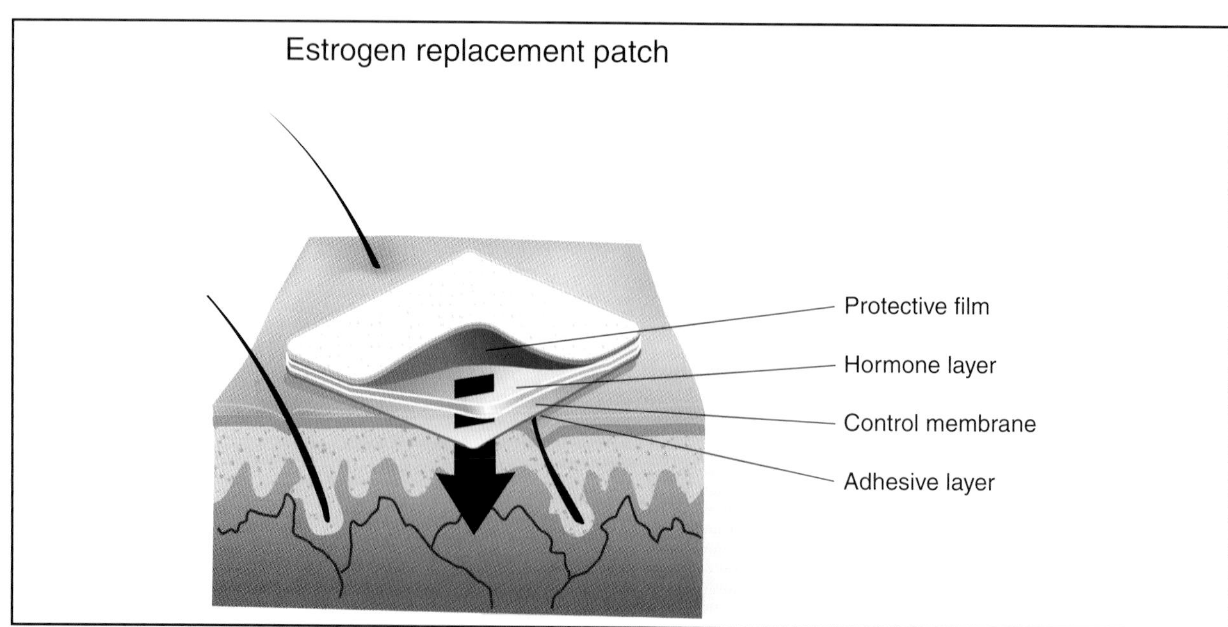

Estrogen replacement patches adhere to a patient's skin and slowly administer estrogen to the body. *(Illustration by Argosy, Inc. Reproduced by permission of Gale, a part of Cengage Learning.)*

progestin (a synthetic progesterone) as HRT. Although many women used HRT for only a couple of years to treat menopausal symptoms, some women used HRT indefinitely. Then, in 2002 and 2004, early results from the **Women's Health** Initiative (WHI) Hormone Program—a very large clinical study of HRT by the U.S. National Institutes of Health—indicated that postmenopausal women on HRT were at increased risk for **heart attack**, **stroke**, **blood clots**, and **breast cancer**. Since then millions of women have stopped taking the hormones. Recent decreases in the incidence of breast **cancer** in the United States have been attributed, in part, to this reduction in HRT.

Description

Estrogen relieves menopausal symptoms and may help prevent **osteoporosis**. Women who have had their uterus removed can use estrogen alone for HRT. Otherwise women must take progesterone or progestin along with the estrogen to reduce the risk of thickening of the lining of the uterus and uterine cancer.

Estrogen for HRT is available in many forms including:

- oral pills
- transdermal skin patches
- implants
- injections
- vaginal ring inserts
- vaginal tablets
- vaginal creams
- gels
- emulsions
- sprays

Estrogen patches and pills can relieve hot flashes, night sweats, and vaginal dryness. Vaginal rings, tablets, and creams are used to treat vaginal dryness, although vaginal ring inserts may help relieve some urinary tract symptoms.

There are different types of estrogens. Estradiol is the most important type in premenopausal women. If synthetic estradiol is injected or applied to the skin—rather than taken by mouth—it appears to work in the same way as estradiol made in the body. Estrone is the form of estrogen that is produced by the body in postmenopausal women. Conjugated estrogen is a mixture of estrone and other estrogens. Estriol is a weaker form of estrogen produced by the breakdown of other estrogens in the body and is the type most commonly used in Europe for HRT. Estrogen taken as a pill is chemically changed in the liver. Some studies have suggested that estrogen that enters through the skin, bypassing the liver, may present less risk for serious blood clots, stroke, and possibly gallbladder disease. Non-oral forms of estrogen also may relieve symptoms at a lower dosage than oral estrogen.

Progesterone or progestin is available in various forms including:

- pills
- combined with estrogen in pills
- combined with estrogen in skin patches
- injections
- as an intrauterine device (IUD)
- gels
- vaginal suppositories

HRT doses and timing of the doses vary. Sometimes estrogen and progesterone are taken daily. Sometimes estrogen is taken daily, whereas progesterone or progestin is taken for 10–14 days every four weeks to mimic premenopausal hormone production. This approach can cause some spotting or bleeding. Various other dosing regimes are also used.

Common types of HRT include:

- generic estradiol pills
- Gynodiol (estradiol pill)
- Menest (esterified estrogen pill)
- generic estropipate pills
- generic estradiol skin patches
- Estraderm (estradiol skin patch)
- FemRing (estradiol vaginal ring)
- Estring (estradiol vaginal ring)
- Premarin vaginal cream (conjugated equine estrogen)
- generic medroxyprogesterone pills
- Prempro (estrogen-progestin combination pill)
- Prefest (estrogen-progestin combination pill)
- Climara Pro (estrogen-progestin skin patch)
- Combipatch (estrogen-progestin skin patch)

Some women prefer natural progesterone because they find that it lacks the side effects of synthetic progestin. Natural progesterone is also available as an over-the-counter vitamin E oil suspension that is absorbed through the skin.

"Natural" or bio-identical estrogens and progesterones are made from plants such as soy or yams. Some of these hormones are chemically identical to those made by the female body. Sometimes these hormones are formulated by a physician according to the requirements of individual women and are put together or compounded by a compounding pharmacist.

Women's ovaries secrete small amounts of the male sex hormone testosterone throughout their lives. Women who have had both ovaries surgically removed are sometimes given testosterone along with estrogen for HRT. Women also sometimes use 1% testosterone cream to relieve vaginal soreness.

Origins

Physicians began prescribing estrogen to menopausal women during the 1960s, when it was referred to as estrogen replacement therapy (ERT). The use of HRT grew rapidly, in part because—until the results of the WHI—it was widely believed that HRT reduced the risk of heart disease, stroke, and cancer in postmenopausal women.

Benefits

HRT can significantly improve quality of life for some women. The WHI and other studies have found that 70–90% of menopausal women who take estrogen have an average reduction of 75% in the frequency of hot flashes and night sweats. Estrogen supplementation also reduces vaginal dryness and urinary symptoms associated with menopause. Estrogen appears to improve cholesterol levels, lowering LDL ("bad" cholesterol) and raising HDL ("good" cholesterol), although estrogen in pill form can cause increased triglycerides—fats in the blood. The estrogen patch does not seem to have this effect, but it also does not improve cholesterol levels to the same degree as the pill.

The WHI found that both estrogen-alone and estrogen-plus-progestin HRT lowered the risk of bone fractures. Estrogen-plus-progestin HRT also lowered the risk of colorectal cancer.

Precautions

Women aged 50–59 who have become menopausal within the past five years and are at low risk for heart disease can use HRT without increasing their risk for heart disease. However they will have an increased risk of breast cancer, blood clots, and stroke:

- Women should take the lowest dose of HRT that relieves symptoms and for the shortest possible time.
- HRT should be re-evaluated every six months.
- Women should not use HRT if their symptoms are mild and can be managed with lifestyle and habit changes, such as quitting smoking, sleeping in a cooler room, reducing stress, exercising regularly, and limiting caffeine and alcohol.
- Women should not use HRT after the first five to 10 years post-menopause.
- HRT is ineffective for—and can even worsen—conditions such as mood swings, irritability, depression, anxiety, cognitive difficulties, reduced libido, urinary incontinence, back or joint pain, chronic pain, stiffness, or fatigue.
- Bio-identical hormones compounded in pharmacies are not regulated by the U.S. Food and Drug Administration (FDA) and have not been shown to be more effective or safer than other HRTs.

Common side effects of HRT include:

- fluid retention
- bloating
- weight gain
- breast tenderness or soreness
- spotting or a return of monthly periods
- cramping
- leg cramps
- vaginal discharge
- severe headaches
- hair loss
- nausea and vomiting
- acne
- moodiness
- depression
- shortness of breath
- dizziness

Potentially serious side effects of HRT include:

- tissues growth in the uterus (fibroids)
- abnormal growth (hyperplasia) of uterine tissue
- gallstones
- thrombophlebitis
- hypoglycemia
- thyroid disorders
- high blood pressure

HRT can interact with other medications, including:

- corticosteroids
- anticoagulants
- rifampin

Drugs that can cause liver damage when combined with estrogens include:

- acetaminophen (Tylenol), when used in high doses over long periods
- anabolic steroids such as nandrolone (Anabolin) or oxymetholone (Anadrol)
- medicine for infections

KEY TERMS

Estrodiol—The most physiologically active form of estrogen.

Estrogen—Any of several naturally occurring or synthetic steroid hormones that promote the growth and maintenance of the female reproductive system.

Menopause—The female developmental stage at which menstruation ceases.

Osteoporosis—A disease characterized by low bone mass and structural deterioration of bone tissue, leading to bone fragility.

Progesterone—A female steroid sex hormone that is secreted after ovulation to prepare the lining of the uterus for implantation with a fertilized egg and secreted by the placenta to maintain pregnancy.

Progestin—Any natural or synthetic hormone that causes the effects of progesterone.

Testosterone—The primary male sex hormone.

Women's Health Initiative (WHI)—A very large clinical study supported by the National Heart, Lung, and Blood Institute and the National Cancer Institute of the U.S. National Institutes of Health that is examining a wide range of women's health issues including HRT.

- antiseizure medicines such as divalproex (Depakote), valproic acid (Depakene), or phenytoin (Dilantin)
- antianxiety drugs, including chlorpromazine (Thorazine), prochlorperazine (Compazine), and thioridazine (Mellaril)

Estrogens can interfere with the effects of bromocriptine (Parlodel) used to treat Parkinson's disease and other conditions. Estrogens can increase the chance of toxic side effects from cyclosporine (Sandimmune).

Other conditions and allergies

HRT should not be used by women with:

- heart disease
- diabetes, high cholesterol, high blood pressure, family history of heart disease, or other risk factors for heart disease
- breast cancer
- cancer of the ovaries or uterus
- history of stroke
- abnormal undiagnosed vaginal bleeding
- liver disease
- gallstones or gallbladder disease

Preparation

Women who are considering HRT should carefully discuss the benefits and risks with their doctor. They should have a variety of tests including:

- a Pap smear
- breast examination and mammogram
- urinalysis
- bone density
- red blood cell count
- blood sugar levels
- cholesterol levels
- liver and thyroid function

Before prescribing HRT many doctors administer a progesterone challenge test to determine whether a woman is still producing estrogen. Bleeding after taking progesterone for 10 days indicates that a woman's ovaries are still making estrogen.

Aftercare

Women on HRT should have their blood pressure tested and breasts examined at least twice a year. They should have a complete physical on a yearly basis. Any abnormal bleeding may require a tissue biopsy or dilatation and curettage to rule out uterine cancer.

The HRT dosage should be tapered off over a period of several months rather than discontinued abruptly. The gradual reduction minimizes the possibility of hot flashes and other side effects.

Risks

The WHI Estrogen-plus-Progestin Study was halted prematurely in July of 2002, when early results showed that the overall risks of Prempro outweighed the benefits, increasing the risk of breast cancer, heart disease, heart attack, stroke, serious blood clots in the legs and lungs, and **urinary incontinence**. Furthermore, the WHI Memory Study found that, in postmenopausal women aged 65 and older, estrogen-plus-progestin HRT doubled the risk for developing all types of **dementia**, including **Alzheimer's disease**.

The WHI Estrogen-Alone Study was halted prematurely in 2004, when researchers found an increased risk of stroke, blood clots, and urinary incontinence. It was also found that estrogen alone did not reduce the risk of heart disease.

It is unclear whether the results of the WHI Hormone Therapy Study apply to all forms of HRT. The study used only oral HRT, rather than patches or other forms of delivery, and only specific forms of estrogen and progestin at specific doses. Furthermore, the increased risk for heart disease and dementia applied only to women over age 60.

Resources

BOOKS

Kimes, Joanne, Elaine Ambrose, and Carolyn Chambers Clark. *Menopause Sucks: What To Do When Hot Flashes Make You and Everyone Else Miserable*. Avon, MA: Adams Media, 2008.

Parker-Pope, Tara. *The Hormone Decision*. New York: Pocket Books. 2008.

Seaman, Barbara. *The Greatest Experiment Ever Performed on Women: Exploding the Estrogen Myth*. New York: Seven Stories Press, 2009.

Seaman, Barbara, and Laura Eldridge. *The No-Nonsense Guide to Menopause*. New York: Simon & Schuster, 2008.

PERIODICALS

Hannon, Kerry. "Dealing with the Hormone Dilemma: Younger Women Tormented by Hot Flashes Are Coming Back for an Ultralow Dose." *U.S. News & World Report* 147, no. 2 (February 1, 2010): 51.

Holcomb, Susan Simmons. "Hormone Therapy for Menopausal Women." *Nurse Practitioner* 34, no. 12 (December 2009): 9.

International Menopause Society. "Menopause-Cardiology Consensus Statement on Cardiovascular Disease and on HRT." *Heart Disease Weekly* (December 13, 2009): 6.

Marchione, Marilynn. "Experts Warn Against 'Bioidentical' Hormones." *Los Angeles Times* (December 27, 2009): A39.

Potera, Carol. "Hormone Replacement Therapy: Is the Risk Overestimated?" *American Journal of Nursing* 109, no. 12 (December 2009): 20.

Singer, Natasha, and Duff Wilson. "Menopause, as Brought To You by Big Pharma." *New York Times* (December 13, 2009): BU1.

OTHER

"Hormone Replacement Therapy." *MedlinePlus*. http://www.nlm.nih.gov/medlineplus/hormonereplacementtherapy.html.

"Hormones and Menopause." *Tips from the National Institute on Aging*. http://www.nia.nih.gov/HealthInformation/Publications/hormones.htm.

"Menopausal Hormone Replacement Therapy Use and Cancer." *National Cancer Institute FactSheet*. http://www.cancer.gov/cancertopics/factsheet/Risk/menopausal-hormones.

"Menopausal Therapy Information." *National Institutes of Health*. http://www.nih.gov/PHTindex.htm.

"Menopause Drugs." *Consumer Reports Health*. http://www.consumerreports.org/health/best-buy-drugs/meno pause.htm.

ORGANIZATIONS

American College of Obstetricians and Gynecologists, PO Box 96920, Washington, DC, 20090-6920, (202) 638-5577, (800) 673-8444, resources@acog.org, http://www.acog.org.

National Cancer Institute, NCI Public Inquiries Office, 6116 Executive Boulevard, Room 3036A, Bethesda, MD, 20006, (800) 4-CANCER, http://www.cancer.gov.

National Heart, Lung and Blood Institute, NHLBI Health Information Center, PO Box 30105, Bethesda, MD, 20824-0105, (301) 592-8573, (240) 629-3246, nhlbiinfo@nhlbi.nih.gov, http://www.nhlbi.nih.gov.

National Institute on Aging, Information Center, P.O. Box 8057, Gaithersburg, MD, 20898-8057, (301) 496-1752, (301) 496-1072, http://www.nia.nih.gov.

North American Menopause Society, 5900 Landerbrook Drive, Suite 390, Mayfield Heights, OH, 44124, (440) 442-7550, (800) 774-5342, (440) 442-2660, info@menopause.org, http://www.menopause.org/.

Laith Farid Gulli, MD
Teresa G. Odle
Margaret Alic, PhD
Brenda W. Lerner

Hospital–acquired infections

Definition

A hospital–acquired infection, also called a nosocomial infection, is one that is unrelated to the patient's original condition and first appears after the patient is admitted to a hospital, nursing home, or other health care facility. Hospital–acquired infections can be bacterial, viral, or fungal.

Description

In the United States, the National Nosocomial Infections Surveillance (NNIS) System of the Centers for Disease Control and Prevention (CDC) tracks hospital–acquired infections. The CDC has estimated that about 10% of patients admitted to hospitals develop a nosocomial infection. In 2006, this amounted to close to 1.7 million patients and accounted for about 90,000 deaths.

Bacteria, viruses, fungi, or parasites can cause hospital–acquired infections. These microorganisms may already be present in the patient's body or may come from the environment, contaminated hospital equipment, health care workers, or other patients. Depending on the causal agents involved, an infection may start in any part of the body. A localized infection is limited to a specific part of the body and has local symptoms. For example, if a surgical wound in the abdomen becomes infected, the area of the wound becomes red, hot, and painful. A generalized infection is one that enters the bloodstream and causes general systemic symptoms such as **fever**, chills, low blood pressure, or mental confusion.

Hospital–acquired infections may develop from surgical procedures, catheters placed in the urinary tract or blood vessels, or from material from the nose or mouth that is inhaled into the lungs. The most common types of hospital–acquired infections are urinary tract infections (UTIs), pneumonia, and surgical wound infections.

Causes and symptoms

All hospitalized patients are susceptible to contracting a nosocomial infection. Some patients are at greater risk than others. Newborns, the elderly, and persons with compromised immune systems are more likely to get an infection. Other risk factors for getting a hospital–acquired infection are a long hospital stay, the use of indwelling catheters, failure of health care workers to wash their hands, and overuse of **antibiotics**.

Any type of invasive procedure can expose a patient to the possibility of infection. Common causes of hospital–acquired infections include:

- urinary bladder catheterization
- respiratory procedures
- surgery and wounds
- intravenous (IV) procedures

Urinary tract infection (UTI) is the most common type of hospital–acquired infection accounting for 32% of reported cases. Most hospital–acquired UTIs happen after urinary catheterization. Catheterization is the placement of a catheter through the urethra into the urinary bladder. This procedure is done to empty urine from the bladder, relieve pressure in the bladder, measure urine in the bladder, put medicine into the bladder, or for other medical reasons.

The healthy urinary bladder is sterile, which means it does not have any harmful bacteria or other microorganisms in it. There may be bacteria in or around the urethra but they normally cannot enter the bladder. A catheter can pick up bacteria from the urethra and allow them into the bladder, causing an infection to start.

Bacteria from the intestinal tract are the most common type to cause UTIs. Patients with poorly functioning immune systems, such as those with **AIDS** or who are taking antibiotics, are also at risk for infection by a fungus called *Candida*.

Pneumonia accounts for about 15% of hospital–acquired infections. Bacteria and other microorganisms are easily brought into the throat by respiratory procedures commonly done in the hospital. The microorganisms come from contaminated equipment or the hands of health care workers. Some of these procedures are respiratory intubation, suctioning of material from the throat and mouth, and mechanical ventilation. The introduced microorganisms quickly colonize the throat area. This means that they grow and form a colony, but do not yet cause an infection. Once the throat is colonized, it is easy for a patient to inhale the microorganisms into the lungs.

Patients who cannot **cough** or gag very well are most likely to inhale colonized microorganisms into their lungs. Some respiratory procedures can keep patients from gagging or coughing. Patients who are sedated or who lose consciousness may also be unable to cough or gag. The inhaled microorganisms grow in the lungs and cause an infection that can lead to pneumonia.

Surgical procedures increase a patient's risk of getting an infection in the hospital and account for about 22% of nosocomial infections. Surgery directly invades the patient's body, giving bacteria a way into normally sterile parts of the body. An infection can be acquired from contaminated surgical equipment or from health care workers. Following surgery, the surgical wound can become infected. Other **wounds** from trauma, **burns**, and ulcers may also become infected.

Many hospitalized patients need a steady supply of medications or nutrients delivered to their bloodstream. An intravenous (IV) catheter is placed in a vein and the medication or other substance is infused into the vein. Bacteria transmitted from the surroundings, contaminated equipment, or health care workers' hands can invade the site where the catheter is inserted. A local infection may develop in the skin around the catheter. Bacteria also can enter the blood through the vein and cause a generalized infection. Infections of the bloodstream account for about 14% of hospital–acquired infections. The longer a catheter is in place, the greater the risk of infection.

Other hospital procedures that put patients at risk for nosocomial infection are gastrointestinal procedures, obstetric procedures, and kidney dialysis.

In the 2000s, hospitals have had increasingly to contend with the development of antibiotic–resistant strains of bacteria. In fact, some organisms may be resistant to *multiple* antimicrobial agents (MDROs). Years of overprescribing and misuse of antibiotics and

KEY TERMS

Abscess—Localized collection of pus in any part of the body that is surrounded by swelling.

Antibiotic—A drug used to treat infections caused by bacteria and other microorganisms.

Antibiotic-resistant—Microorganisms that continue to multiply although exposed to antibiotics.

Antimicrobial agent—A substance that kills microorganisms such as bacteria or mold, or stops them from growing and causing disease.

Bacterium—A single-celled microorganism that can be seen only through a microscope. Many bacteria cause disease.

Immune system—The integrated body system of organs, tissues, cells, and cell products such as antibodies that protects the body from foreign organisms or substances.

Multidrug-resistant organisms (MDROs)—Bacteria that are resistant to one or more classes of antimicrobial agents and usually are resistant to all but one or two commercially available antimicrobial agents.

Pus—A generally viscous, yellowish-white fluid formed in infected tissue, consisting of white blood cells, cellular debris, and dead tissue.

the increased use of antibiotics in the production of meat and milk have resulted in the emergence of strains of bacteria that are resistant to many antibiotics. A bacterium is considered resistant when it can no longer be treated effectively using antibiotics that are commonly prescribed for that type of infection.

Methicillin-resistant *S. aureus.* is a strain of staph bacteria that is resistant to the antibiotic methicillin and other common antibiotics that normally control staph infections. Although this strain of staph has existed in hospitals for years, in the 1990s, MRSA began appearing in places other than hospitals. By 2007, two forms of MRSA were recognized, hospital-acquired MRSA (HA-MRSA) and community-acquired MRSA (CA-MRSA). Symptoms of a MRSA infection are similar to other staph infection symptoms, only MRSA is much more dangerous and has a much higher mortality rate because treatment with common antibiotics does not kill the bacterium.

Risk factors for acquiring HA-MRSA include hospitalization, especially in patients who need intravenous lines, feeding tubes, and catheters, residence in a nursing home, and recent treatment with certain antibiotics including the fluoroquinolone antibiotics ciprofloxacin (Cipro), ofloxacin (Floxin, Tarivid), levofloxacin (Levaquin, Elequine), and cephalosporin (Keflex). The Association of Professionals in **Infection Control** and Epidemiology estimates that in 2007 1.2 million hospital patients were infected with MRSA and about 423,000 were healthy carriers (i.e., they showed no symptoms) of the bacteria.

Fever is often the first sign of infection. Other symptoms and signs of infection are rapid breathing, mental confusion, low blood pressure, reduced urine output, and a high **white blood cell count**.

Patients with a UTI may have **pain** when urinating and blood in the urine. Symptoms of pneumonia may include difficulty breathing and coughing. A localized infection causes swelling, redness, and tenderness at the site of infection.

Diagnosis

An infection is suspected any time a hospitalized patient develops a fever that cannot be explained by a known illness. Some patients, especially the elderly, may not develop a fever. In these patients, the first signs of infection may be rapid breathing or mental confusion.

Diagnosis of a hospital-acquired infection is based on:

- symptoms and signs of infection
- examination of wounds and catheter entry sites
- review of procedures that might have led to infection
- laboratory test results

A complete **physical examination** is conducted in order to locate symptoms and signs of infection. Wounds and the skin where catheters have been placed are examined for redness, swelling, or the presence of pus or an **abscess**. The physician reviews the patient's record of procedures performed in the hospital to determine if any posed a risk for infection.

Laboratory tests are done to look for signs of infection. A complete blood count can reveal if the white blood cell count is high. White blood cells are immune system cells that increase in numbers in response to an infection. White blood cells or blood may be present in the urine when there is a UTI.

Cultures of blood, urine, sputum, other body fluids, or tissue are done to look for infectious microorganisms. If an infection is present, it is necessary to identify the microorganism so the patient can be treated with the correct medication. A sample of the fluid or tissue is placed in a special medium that bacteria grow in. Other tests can also be done on blood and body fluids to look for and identify bacteria, fungi, viruses, or other microorganisms responsible for an infection.

If a patient has symptoms suggestive of pneumonia, a **chest x ray** is done to look for infiltrates of white blood cells and other inflammatory substances in the lung tissue. Samples of sputum can be studied with a microscope or cultured to look for bacteria or fungi.

Treatment

Once the source of infection is identified, the patient is treated with antibiotics or other medication that kills the responsible microorganism. Many different antibiotics are available that are effective against different bacteria. Some common antibiotics are penicillin, **cephalosporins**, tetracyclines, and erythromycin. More and more commonly, some types of bacteria are becoming resistant to the standard antibiotic treatments. When this happens, a different, more powerful antibiotic must be used. Two strong antibiotics that have been effective against resistant bacteria are vancomycin and imipenem, although some bacteria are developing resistance to these antibiotics as well.

Fungal infections are treated with antifungal medications. Examples of these medications are amphotericin B, nystatin, ketoconazole, itraconazole, and fluconazole.

A number of **antiviral drugs** have been developed that slow the growth or reproduction of viruses. Acyclovir, ganciclovir, foscarnet, and amantadine are examples of antiviral medications.

Prognosis

Hospital–acquired infections are serious illnesses that cause death in about 1% of cases. Rapid diagnosis and identification of the responsible microorganism is necessary, so treatment can be started as soon as possible.

Prevention

Hospitals and other health care facilities have developed extensive infection control programs to prevent nosocomial infections. These programs focus on identifying high–risk procedures and other possible sources of infection. High–risk procedures such as **urinary catheterization** should be performed only when necessary and catheters should be left in for as little time as possible. Medical instruments and equipment must be properly sterilized to ensure they are not contaminated. Frequent hand washing by health care workers and visitors is necessary to avoid passing infectious microorganisms to hospitalized patients. In 2003, the Joint Commission on Accreditation of Health care Organizations (JCAHO) announced it would make prevention of nosocomial infections a major goal future years. JCAHO, the body that inspects hospitals for quality and accredits them accordingly, issued an alert stating that hospital–acquired infections are seriously underreported. In 2005, Pennsylvania and Florida became the first states to require hospitals to report data on hospital–acquired infections. Since then, many other states have passed similar legislation. Increasingly, lawsuits have been brought against hospitals by families of patients that have died from nosocomial infections. The problem of nosocomial infections has become more serious for hospitals to address as many bacteria are becoming resistant to antibiotics.

Antibiotics should be used only when necessary. Use of antibiotics creates favorable conditions for infection with the fungal organism *Candida.* Overuse of antibiotics is also responsible for the development of bacteria that are resistant to antibiotics.

Resources

BOOKS

Rokavec, Kathleen A. *The Hospital Book.* Raleigh, NC: lulu.com., 2009.

Wallach, Jacques. *Interpretation of Diagnostic Tests,* 8th ed. Philadelphia, PA: Lippincott Williams & Wilkins, 2006.

Zimring, Michael P. *Healthy Travel: Don't Travel Without It!* Laguna Beach, CA: Basic Health Publications, Inc., 2009.

OTHER

"Hospital–acquired Infections." eMedicine.com. (August 21, 2007) http://www.emedicine.com/ PED/topic 1619.htm (accessed September 11, 2010).

"Healthcare–associated Infections." Centers for Disease Control. http://www.cdc.gov/nci dod/dhqp/healthDis. html. (accessed September 11, 2010).

ORGANIZATIONS

Centers for Disease Control and Prevention (CDC), 1600 Clifton Rd., Atlanta, GA, 30333, (404) 498–1515, (800)311–3435, http://www.cdc.gov.

Hospital Infection Society, 162 Kings Cross Rd., London, England, WC1X 9DH, 020 7713 0273, http://www. his.org.uk.

National Heart, Lung, and Blood Institute, PO Box 30105, Bethesda, MD, 20824–0105, (301) 592–8573, (204) 629–3246, nhlbiinfo@nhlbi.nih.gov, http://www.nhlbi. nih.gov.

National Institute of Allergy and Infectious Diseases (NIAID), 6610 Rockledge Dr., MSC 6612, Bethesda, MD, 20892–6612, (301) 496–5717, (866) 284–4107, http://www3.niaid.nih.gov.

National Institutes of Health (NIH), 9000 Rockville Pike, Bethesda, MD, 20892, 301-496-4000, http://www.nih.gov/index.html.

World Health Organization (WHO), Avenue Appia 20, CH – 1211 Geneva 27, Switzerland, +41 22 791 2111, http://www.who.int/en.

Tish Davidson, A.M.
Teresa G. Odle
Laura Jean Cataldo, RN, Ed.D.

Hot-spot imaging *see* **Technetium heart scan**

HPV vaccination

Definition

HPV **vaccination** refers to the administration of a vaccine to protect against human papillovirus (HPV) infection.

Purpose

Human papillomavirus (HPV) is the most common sexually transmitted virus in the United States. Most HPV infections do not cause any symptoms and disappear on their own, but it is now known that HPV can cause **cervical cancer** in women. Every year in the United States, approximately 11,000 women are diagnosed with cervical **cancer** and 4,000 die from it. Cervical cancer is the second leading cause of cancer deaths among women around the world. It is estimated that as much as two-thirds of the cervical cancer deaths around the world could be eliminated if all women were immunized with the HPV vaccine prior to infection with HPV.

There are approximately 40 types of genital HPV. In the United States, about 20 million people are infected, with about 6.2 million new cases of genital HPV infection reported each year. Some HPV types can cause cervical cancer in women and can also cause other kinds of cancer in both men and women. HPV infection has been linked to oropharyngeal cancer and cancers of the anus, vulva, vagina, and penis. Other types of HPV can cause **genital warts** in both males and females or **warts** in the upper respiratory tract. The HPV vaccines work by preventing the most common types of HPV that cause cervical cancer and genital warts.

Description

In June 2006, the Advisory Committee on Immunization Practices (ACIP) voted to recommend the first vaccine developed to prevent cervical cancer and other diseases in females caused by certain types of genital human papillomavirus (HPV). This vaccine, Gardasil®, manufactured by the pharmaceutical company Merck, is a quadrivalent vaccine that protects against four HPV types (types 6, 11, 16, and 18), which together cause 70% of cervical cancers and 90% of genital warts. The Food and Drug Administration (FDA) licensed this vaccine for use in girls and women, between the ages of 9–26 years. Gardasil has also been approved by the FDA for use in males ages 9 to 26 years to prevent genital warts caused by HPV types 6 and 11.

In 2009, drug manufacturer GlaxoSmithKline released a second HPV vaccine, Cervarix. Cervarix is a bivalent vaccine, meaning it protects against HPV infection from two HPV types (types 16 and 18) that can cause precancerous and cancerous tumors of the cervix. Cervarix does not protect against genital warts (caused by HPV types 6 and 11). Cervarix has been approved by the FDA for use in females ages 10 to 25 years for the prevention of cervical cancer caused by HPV types 16 and 18.

Recommended dosage

The HPV vaccine is routinely administered to girls 11 and 12 years of age and is given in a series of three injections over a six–month period. The second and third doses are given one and six months after the first dose. Each dose of quadrivalent HPV vaccine is 0.5 mL, administered intramuscularly. It is important for girls to get vaccinated before their first sexual contact, i.e., before they can be exposed to HPV. For immunized girls, the vaccine can prevent almost 100% of the diseases caused by the types of HPVs targeted by the vaccine. Girls as young as 9 years old can receive the vaccine. The vaccine is also recommended for girls and women 13 through 26 years of age who did not receive it when they were younger. Additional (booster) doses are not recommended at this time. Studies are underway to determine whether booster vaccinations are necessary. HPV vaccine may be given at the same time as other vaccines.

Precautions

Vaccines can cause severe allergic reactions, like all medications. The risk of a vaccine causing serious harm, or **death**, is extremely small. Overwhelmingly, health practitioners recommend vaccination over the risk of suffering the disease against which it protects.

KEY TERMS

Cervical cancer—Cancer of the entrance to the womb (uterus). The cervix is the lower, narrow part of the uterus (womb).

Cervical cancer screening—Use of the Papanicolaou (Pap) smear test to detect cervical cancer in the early curable stage.

Intramuscularly—A medication given by needle into a muscle.

Pathogen—A disease-causing microorganism.

Quadrivalent vaccine—A vaccine that protects against four pathogens.

Virus—A microorganism smaller than a bacteria, which cannot grow or reproduce apart from a living cell. Viruses cause many common human infections, and are also responsible for many rare diseases.

Wart—A raised growth on the surface of the skin or other organ.

However, some girls should not get the HPV vaccine. They include:

- Any girl who has ever had a life–threatening allergic reaction to yeast, to any other component of HPV vaccine, or to a previous dose of HPV vaccine.
- Pregnant women should not get vaccinated since no data is yet available on its safety in mothers and the unborn baby. Women who are breast feeding may safely get the vaccine.
- Girls with moderate or severe illnesses should wait until they recover.

Protection from HPV vaccine is expected to be long–lasting. However, vaccinated women still need cervical cancer screening because the vaccine does not protect against all HPV types that cause cervical cancer.

Side effects

According to the CDC, the following problems may follow HPV vaccination:

- Pain at the injection site (8 people in 10)
- Redness or swelling at the injection site (1 person in 4)
- Mild fever (100°F/37.8°C) (1 person in 10)
- Itching at the injection site (1 person in 30)
- Moderate fever (102°F/38.9°C) (1 person in 65)

A small number of patients receiving the HPV vaccine have experienced syncope (**fainting**) or seizures. Patients receiving the vaccine should be observed for 15 minutes after receiving each dose.

Interactions

The FDA has licensed the HPV vaccine as safe and effective. This vaccine has been tested in thousands of females (9 to 26 years of age) around the world no serious interactions or side effects.

Some medicines may interact with HPV vaccine. Alkylating agents (eg, cyclophosphamide), antimetabolites (eg, fluorouracil, methotrexate), cytotoxics (eg, cisplatin), or **corticosteroids** (eg, prednisone) may decrease the HPV vaccine's effectiveness.

Resources

BOOKS

Campbell, Kenneth. *Infectious Causes of Cancer: A Guide for Nurses and Healthcare Professionals*. New York: Wiley, 2011.

Nardo, Don. *Human Papillomavirus (HPV)*. Farmington Hills, MI: Lucent Books (Gale), 2007.

PERIODICALS

Ault, K. A. "Long–term efficacy of human papillomavirus vaccination." *Gynecologic Oncology* 107, no. 2 (November 2007): S27–S30.

Brisson, M., Van de Velde, N., De Wals, P., Boily, M. C. "Estimating the number needed to vaccinate to prevent diseases and death related to human papillomavirus infection." *Canadian Medical Association Journal* 177, no. 5 (August 2007): 464–468.

Bryan, J. T. "Developing an HPV vaccine to prevent cervical cancer and genital warts." *Vaccine* 25, no. 16 (2007): 3001–3006.

Garcia, F. A., and D. Saslow. "Prophylactic human papillomavirus vaccination: a breakthrough in primary cervical cancer prevention." *Obstetrics and Gynecology Clinics of North America* 34, no. 4 (December 2007): 761–781.

Giuliano, A. R. "Human papillomavirus vaccination in males." *Gynecology and Oncolgy* 107, suppl. 2 (November 2007): S24–S26.

Hairon, N. "HPV vaccination of girls to help prevent cervical cancer." *Nursing Times* 103, no. 45 (2007): 23–24.

OTHER

HPV Vaccination. Webpage, CDC (June 1, 2007). http://www.cdc.gov/vaccines/vpd-vac/hpv/default.htm.

HPV Vaccine Questions and Answers. Webpage, CDC (August 2006). http://www.cdc.gov/std/hpv/STDFact-HPV-vaccine.htm.

Human Papillomavirus (HPV) Prevention and HPV Vaccine: Questions and Answers Webpage. Public Health Agency of Canada (June 18, 2006). http://www.phac-aspc.gc.ca/std-mts/hpv-vph/hpv-vph-vaccine_e.html.

Human Papillomavirus (HPV) Vaccines: Questions and Answers Webpage. National Cancer Institute (December 9, 2007). http://www.cancer.gov/cancertopics/factsheet/risk/HPV-vaccine.

Vaccine Information: Human papillomavirus (HPV) Webpage. National Network for Immunization Information (December 21, 2007). http://www.immunizationinfo.org/vaccineInfo/vaccine_detail.cfv?id=53.

ORGANIZATIONS

Centers for Disease Control and Prevention (CDC), 1600 Clifton Road, Atlanta, GA, 30333, (800) 232-4636, cdcinfo@cdc.gov, http://www.cdc.gov.

National Institute of Allergies and Infectious Diseases, 6610 Rockledge Drive, MSC 6612, Bethesda, MD, 20892-6612, (301) 496-5717, (301) 402-3573, (866) 284-4107, ocpostoffice@niaid.nih.gov, http://www.niaid.nih.gov.

National Network for Immunization Information, 301 University Blvd, Galveston, TX, 77555-0350, (409) 772-0199, (409) 772-5208, nnii@i4ph.org, http://www.immunizationinfo.org.

National Vaccine Program Office. U.S. Department of Health & Human Services, Room 715-H 200 Independence Avenue, SW, Washington, DC, 20201, (202) 690-5566, nvpo@hhs.gov, http://www.hhs.gov/nvpo.

Monique Laberge, PhD
Melinda Granger Oberleitner
RN, DNS, APRN, CNS

HRT *see* **Hormone replacement therapy**

HTLV-1 associated myelopathy *see* **Tropical spastic paraparesis**

HTLV-1 infection *see* **Tropical spastic paraparesis**

Huffing *see* **Inhalants and related disorders**

Human-potential movement

Definition

The human-potential movement is a term used for humanistic psychotherapies that first became popular in the 1960s and early 1970s. The movement emphasized the development of individuals through such techniques as encounter groups, sensitivity training, and primal therapy. Although the human-potential movement and humanistic therapy are sometimes used as synonyms, in reality, humanistic therapy preceded the human-potential movement and provided the movement's theoretical base. Humanistic therapy flourished in the 1940s and 1950s. Its theorists were mostly psychologists rather than medical doctors. They included Gordon Allport, Abraham Maslow, Everett Shostrom, Carl Rogers, and Fritz Perls.

The human-potential movement and humanistic therapy is distinguished by the following emphases:

- A concern for what is uniquely human rather than what humans share with other animals.
- A focus on each person's open-ended growth rather than reshaping individuals to fit society's demands.
- An interest in the here-and-now rather than in a person's childhood history or supposed unconscious conflicts.
- A holistic approach concerned with all levels of human being and functioning—not just the intellectual—including creative and spiritual functioning.
- A focus on psychological health rather than disturbance.

Purpose

The purpose of humanistic therapy is to allow a person to make full use of his or her personal capacities leading to self-actualization. Self-actualization requires the integration of all the components of one's unique personality. These elements or components of personality include the physical, emotional, intellectual, behavioral, and spiritual. The marks of a self-actualized person are maturity, self-awareness, and authenticity. Humanistic therapists think that most people—not only those with obvious problems—can benefit from opportunities for self-development. Humanistic therapy uses both individual and group approaches.

Precautions

Psychotic patients, substance abusers, and persons with severe **personality disorders** or disorders of impulse control may not be appropriate for treatment with humanistic methods.

Description

Humanistic approaches to individual treatment usually follow the same format as other forms of outpatient counseling. Therapists may be medical doctors, nurses, psychologists, social workers, or clergy. Humanistic group treatment formats are flexible, and a wide range of treatment methods are used, ranging from encounter groups and therapy groups to assertiveness training and consciousness-raising groups. In addition, the humanistic tradition has fostered the publication of self-help books for people interested in psychological self-improvement.

Risks

The chief risks include the reinforcement of self-centered tendencies in some patients and the dangers resulting from encounter groups led by persons without adequate training. Poorly led encounter groups can be traumatic to persons with low tolerance for confrontation or "uncovering" of private issues.

Normal results

The anticipated outcome of humanistic therapy is a greater degree of personal wholeness, self-acceptance, and exploration of one's potential. In group treatment, participants are expected to grow in interpersonal empathy and relationship skills. However, there have been few controlled studies to determine the reasonableness of these expectations.

Resources

BOOKS

Surhone, Lambert M., Miriam T. Timpledon, and Susan F. Marseken, eds. *Human Potential Movement.* Beau Bassin, Mauritius: Betascript, 2010.

Rebecca J. Frey, PhD

Human bite infections

Definition

Human bite infections are potentially serious infections caused by rapid growth of bacteria in broken skin.

Description

Bites—animal and human—are responsible for about 1% of visits to emergency rooms. Bite injuries are more common during the summer months.

Closed–fist injury

In adults, the most common form of human bite is the closed–fist injury, sometimes called the "fight bite." These injuries result from the breaking of the skin over the knuckle joint when a person's fist strikes someone's teeth during a fight.

Causes and symptoms

In children, bite infections result either from accidents during play or from fighting. Most infected bites in adults result from fighting.

KEY TERMS

Antibiotic—A drug used to treat infections caused by bacteria and other microorganisms.

Bacteria—Single–celled microorganisms that can be seen only through a microscope. Many bacteria cause disease.

The infection itself can be caused by a number of bacteria that live in the human mouth. These include streptococci, staphylococci, anaerobic organisms, and *Eikenella corrodens.* Infections that begin less than 24 hours after the injury are usually produced by a mixture of organisms and can cause a necrotizing infection (causing the **death** of a specific area of tissue), in which tissue is rapidly destroyed. If a bite is infected, the skin will be sore, red, swollen, and warm to the touch.

Diagnosis

In most cases the diagnosis is made by an emergency room physician on the basis of the patient's history.

Because the human mouth contains a variety of bacteria, the physician will order a laboratory culture to choose the most effective antibiotic.

Treatment

Treatment involves surgical attention as well as medications. Because bites cause puncturing and tearing of skin rather than clean-edged cuts, they must be carefully cleansed. The doctor will wash the wound with water under high pressure and debride it. **Debridement** is the removal of dead tissue and **foreign objects** from a wound to prevent infection. If the bite is a closed–fist injury, the doctor will look for torn tendons or damage to the spaces between the joints. Examination includes x rays to check for bone **fractures** or foreign objects in the wound.

Doctors do not usually suture a bite wound because the connective tissues and other structures in the hand form many small closed spaces that make it easy for infection to spread. Emergency room doctors often consult surgical specialists if a patient has a deep closed–fist injury or one that appears already infected.

The doctor will make sure that the patient is immunized against **tetanus**, which is routine procedure for any open wound. A study released in June 2004 showed that routine use of **antibiotics** for human bites may not be necessary, as physicians try to minimize overuse of antibiotics. Superficial **wounds** in low-risk areas may no longer need antibiotic treatment, but more serious human bites to high-risk areas such as the hands should be treated with antibiotics to prevent serious infection. Patients with closed–fist injuries may need inpatient treatment in addition to an intravenous antibiotic.

Prognosis

The prognosis depends on the location of the bite and whether it was caused by a child or an adult. Bites caused by children rarely become infected because they are usually shallow. Between 15–30% of bites caused by adults become infected, with a higher rate for closed–fist injuries.

Prevention

Prevention of human bite infections depends upon prompt treatment of any bite caused by a human being, particularly a closed–fist injury.

Resources

PERIODICALS

"Do All Human Bite Wounds Need Antibiotics?" *Emergency Medicine Alert*. June 2004: 3.

ORGANIZATIONS

Centers for Disease Control and Prevention (CDC), 1600 Clifton Rd., Atlanta, GA, 30333, 800-311-3435, http://www.cdc.gov.

National Institutes of Health (NIH), 9000 Rockville Pike, Bethesda, MD, 20892, 301-496-4000, http://www.nih.gov/index.html.

Rebecca J. Frey, Ph.D.
Teresa G. Odle
Laura Jean Cataldo, RN, Ed.D.

Human chorionic gonadotropin *see* **Infertility drugs**

Human chorionic gonadotropin pregnancy test

Definition

The most common test of **pregnancy** involves the detection of a hormone known as human chorionic gonadotropin (hCG) in a sample of blood or urine.

Purpose

To determine whether or not a woman is pregnant.

Description

Shortly after a woman's egg is fertilized by her male partner's sperm and is implanted in the lining or the womb (uterus), a placenta begins to form. This organ will help nourish the developing new life. The placenta produces hCG, whose presence, along with other hormones, helps maintain the early stages of pregnancy. Because hCG is produced only by placental tissue and the hormone can be found in the blood or urine of a pregnant woman, it has become a convenient chemical test of pregnancy.

After implantation, the level of detectable hCG rises very rapidly, approximately doubling in quantity every two days until a peak is reached between the sixth and eighth week. Over the next 10 or more weeks, the quantity of hCG slowly decreases. After this point, a much lower level is sustained for the duration of the pregnancy. Detectable levels of this hormone may even persist for a month or two after delivery.

Blood tests for hCG are the most sensitive and can detect a pregnancy earlier than urine tests. Blood tests for hCG can also distinguish normal pregnancies from impending miscarriages or pregnancies that occur outside of the uterus (ectopic pregnancies).

If a woman misses her menstrual period and wants to know if she may be pregnant, she can purchase one of many home pregnancy test kits that are available. Although each of these products may look slightly different and provide a different set of directions for use, each one detects the presence of hCG. This indicator contains chemical components called antibodies that are sensitive to a certain quantity of this hormone.

Precautions

Although home pregnancy tests may be advertised as having an accuracy of 97% or better, studies indicate that, in practice, pregnancy tests performed in the home may incorrectly indicate that a woman is not pregnant (a false positive result) between 25–50% of the time. Studies also indicate that the false negative results usually result from failing to follow the package directions or testing too soon after a missed menstrual period. Waiting a few days after the missed period was expected can increase the accuracy of the test. Blood and urine tests performed by a laboratory are from 97–100% accurate in detecting pregnancy.

Preparation

Generally, no preparation is required for a pregnancy test given in a doctor's office.

Home pregnancy test kits can be divided into two basic types. One type involves the use of a wand-like device that a woman must place into her urine stream for a brief period of time. The other type of kit involves the use of a cup, a dropper, and a wand or stick with a small well. The cup is used to collect the urine, and the dropper is used to transfer a specific number of drops into the well. Results are displayed by a color change. It's important to follow the package directions very carefully (the techniques vary from brand to brand) and to read the results in the time specified.

Aftercare

No special care is required after a urine test for hCG. Women who feel faint or who continue to bleed after a blood test should be observed until the condition goes away.

Risks

Tests for hCG levels pose no direct risk to a woman's health. The main risk with a home pregnancy test is a false negative result, which may be lessened by following the manufacturer's instructions carefully and waiting at least several days after the expected menstrual period to test. A false negative result can cause a delay in seeking prenatal care, which can pose a risk to both the woman and the baby.

Abnormal results

In most cases, a positive result is an indication of pregnancy. However, false positive results may also occur. If a pregnancy test is performed within a month or two of a recent birth or **miscarriage**, it is possible to test positive for pregnancy since hCG may still be detected in a woman's urine. Sometimes positive pregnancy tests provide clues of an early miscarriage that might have otherwise gone unrecognized because it occurred before or just after a missed period. An **ectopic pregnancy** (one in which an embryo implants outside the uterus), certain types of masses (such as an ovarian tumor or a **hydatidiform mole**), and the use of some fertility drugs that contain hCG are among other possibilities behind false positive results.

Normal results

A woman should notify her physician immediately if her home pregnancy test is positive. Pregnancy can then be confirmed with hCG urine or blood tests taken in the doctor's office and evaluated by laboratory personnel. If performed accurately, home pregnancy tests have been found to be highly reliable. However, the versions of these tests performed by qualified laboratory technologists are considered to be definitive. Often, such a test will produce positive results before a woman experiences symptoms or before a doctor's exam reveals signs of pregnancy.

Resources

PERIODICALS

Bastian, L. A., et al. "Is This Patient Pregnant?" *The Journal of the American Medical Association* 278, no. 7: 586–591.

Betty Mishkin

Human herpes *see* **Roseola**

Human leukocyte antigen test

Definition

The human leukocyte antigen test, also known as HLA, is a test that detects antigens (genetic markers) on white blood cells. There are four types of human leukocyte antigens: HLA-A, HLA-B, HLA-C, and HLA-D.

Purpose

The HLA test is used to provide evidence of tissue compatibility typing of tissue recipients and donors. It is also an aid in **genetic counseling** and in paternity testing.

Precautions

This test may have to be postponed if the patient has recently undergone a **transfusion**.

Description

Human leukocyte antigen (leukocyte is the name for white blood cell, while antigen refers to a genetic marker) is a substance that is located on the surface of white blood cells. This substance plays an important role in the body's immune response.

Because the HLA antigens are essential to immunity, identification aids in determination of the degree of tissue compatibility between transplant recipients and donors. Testing is done to diminish the likelihood of rejection after transplant, and to avoid graft-versus-host disease (GVHD) following major organ or **bone marrow transplantation**. It should be noted that risk of GVHD exists even when the donor and recipient share major antigens. As an example, it was recently discovered that a mismatch of HA-1 (a minor antigen) was a cause of GVHD in bone marrow grafts from otherwise HLA-identical donors.

HLA can aid in paternity exclusion testing, a highly specialized area of forensic medicine. To resolve cases of disputed paternity, a man who demonstrates a phenotype (two haplotypes: one from the father and one from the mother) with no haplotype or antigen pair identical to one of the child's is excluded as the father. Conversely, a man who has one haplotype identical to one of the child's may be the father (the probability varies with the appearance of that particular haplotype in the population). Because of the issues involved, this type of testing is referred to experts.

Certain HLA types have been linked to diseases, such as **rheumatoid arthritis**, **multiple sclerosis**, serum lupus erythematosus, and other **autoimmune disorders**. By themselves, however, none of the HLA types are considered definitive. Because the clinical significance of many of the marker antigens has not yet been well defined, definitive diagnosis of disease is obtained by the use of more specific tests.

Preparation

The HLA test requires a blood sample. There is no need for the patient to be **fasting** (having nothing to eat or drink) before the test.

Risks

Risks for this test are minimal, but may include slight bleeding from the blood-drawing site, **fainting** or feeling lightheaded after venipuncture, or hematoma (blood accumulating under the puncture site).

Normal results

Identification of specific leukocyte antigens, HLA-A, HLA-B, HLA-C and HLA-D.

Abnormal results

Incompatible groups between organ donors and recipients may cause unsuccessful tissue transplantation.

Certain diseases have a strong association with certain types of HLAs, which may aid in genetic counseling. For example, Hashimoto's **thyroiditis** (an autoimmune disorder involving underproduction by the thyroid gland) is associated with HLA-DR5, while B8 and Dw3 are allied with Graves' disease (another autoimmune disorder, but with overproduction by the thyroid gland). Hereditary **hemochromatosis** (too much iron in the blood) is associated with HLA-A3, B7, and B14. HLA-A3 is found in approximately 70% of patients with hemochromatosis, but as is the case with other HLA-associated disorders, the expense of HLA typing favors use of other tests. In cases of suspected hemochromatosis, for example, diagnosis is better aided by two tests called transferrin saturation and serum ferritin.

Resources

BOOKS

Pagana, Kathleen Deska, and Timothy J. Pagana. *Mosby's Manual of Diagnostic and Laboratory Tests*. 4th ed. St. Louis: Mosby, 2009.

Janis O. Flores

Human papilloma virus

Definition

HPV infection is a sexually transmitted disease (STD) caused by 30–40 of the 130 or so known strains of human papillomavirus, the name of a group of viruses that infect the skin and mucous membranes of humans and some animals. In humans these sexually transmitted strains can cause **genital warts**, precancerous changes in the tissues of the female vagina, or **cervical cancer**. Other strains of HPV are responsible for **warts** on the soles of the feet (plantar warts), common warts on the hands, and flat warts on the face or legs.

Demographics

In recent years HPV infection has become the most common STD in the United States. Approximately 20 million Americans are infected with HPV as of 2009, and another 6.2 million people become newly infected each year. According to one study, 27 percent of women between the ages of 14 and 59 are infected with one or more types of HPV, and 35% of homosexual men. The Centers for Disease Control and Prevention (CDC) estimates that more than 80 percent of American women will contract at least one strain of genital HPV by age 50. About 75–80 percent of sexually active Americans of either sex will be infected with HPV at some point in their lifetime.

Prevalence of HPV and related diseases

Human papillomavirus (HPV): Approximately 20 million Americans are currently infected with HPV and another 6 million become infected each year. HPV is so prevalent that half of all sexually active men and women contract it at some point in their lives.

Genital warts: About 1% of sexually active adults in the United States have genital warts.

Cervical cancer: On average, 12,000 women in the United States are diagnosed with cervical cancer each year.

Other cancers that can be caused by HPV:

- Vulvar cancer (3,700 women per year)
- Vaginal cancer (1,000 women per year)
- Penile cancer (1,000 men per year)
- Anal cancer (2,700 women and 1,700 men per year)

SOURCE: Centers for Disease Control and Prevention, "Genital HPV Infection Fact Sheet." Available online at: http://www.cdc.gov/std/hpv/stdfact-hpv.htm (accessed August 17, 2010).

(Table by PreMediaGlobal. Reproduced by permission of Gale, a part of Cengage Learning.)

As far as is known, men and women are at equal risk of being infected with HPV, as are members of all races and ethnic groups.

In terms of specific illnesses associated with HPV, 11,000 women are diagnosed with cervical **cancer** each year in the United States and 3,900 women die of the disease. Another 5,800 women are diagnosed with cancers of the vagina and the external female genitals, while 3,300 men are diagnosed with cancer of the penis or the anal area. The risk of **anal cancer** is 17 to 31 times higher among gay and bisexual men than among heterosexual men.

Description

The family of human papilloma viruses includes a large number of genetically related viruses. Many of these cause warts, including the warts commonly found on the skin. Another group of HPV preferentially infect the mucosal surfaces of the genitals, including the penis, vagina, vulva, and cervix. These are spread among adults by sexual contact. One group of HPV that infect the genitals causes soft warts, often designated condylomata acuminata. These genital warts are quite common and rarely if ever become cancerous. The most common of these low-risk HPV types are designated HPV 6 and 11.

The second group of viruses, termed high-risk HPV types, is associated with the development of cervical cancer. Individuals infected with these viruses are at higher risk for the development of precancerous lesions. Typically, infection with these viruses is common in adolescents and women in their twenties and usually do not result in cancerous growth. The most common high-risk HPV is type 16. The appearance of abnormal cells containing high-risk HPV types is seen most frequently in women over the age of 30 who have abnormal Pap smears.

It is possible that other viruses work together with human papilloma viruses to produce precancerous changes in tissue. Cases of tongue cancer have been reported in which HPV was found together with **Epstein-Barr virus**, or EBV. **Smoking**, the use of **oral contraceptives** for birth control for longer than five years, and suppression of the immune system are also thought to be factors that combine with HPV infection to lead to precancerous lesions in tissue.

Risk factors

Some people are at greater risk of sexually transmitted HPV than others:

- Gay and bisexual men.
- People with HIV or other diseases that weaken the immune system.
- Males or females below age 25. Younger people appear to be more biologically vulnerable to the HPV virus.
- People who have large numbers of sexual partners.
- People in relationships with partners who have sex with many other people.
- People who must take drugs that suppress the immune system.

Causes and symptoms

Causes

The cause of sexually transmitted HPV infection is one or more strains of the human papillomavirus. The virus enters the body through small breaks in the skin surface or in the mucous membranes lining the genitals. In most cases the body fights off the virus within a few weeks. In some people, however, HPV remains dormant for a period ranging from a few weeks to three years in one of the lower layers of skin cells. The virus then begins to replicate (copy itself) when these cells mature and move upward to the surface of the skin. The virus affects the shape of the cells, leading to the formation of noticeable warts, precancerous changes in skin cells, or cervical cancer. About 1 percent of sexually active adults in the United States have genital warts at any one time; about 10 percent of women with high-risk HPV in the tissues of their cervix will develop long-lasting HPV infections that put them at risk for cervical cancer.

The percentages of cancers caused by high-risk types of HPV are as follows:

- Cervical cancer: 100%
- Anal cancer: 90%
- Cancer of the vulva: 40%
- Vaginal cancer: 40%
- Oropharyngeal cancer: 12%
- Oral cancer: 3%

Symptoms in adults

Symptoms of sexually transmitted HPV infection may include:

- Genital warts. These appear as bumps or clusters of fleshy outgrowths around the anus or on the genitals. Some may grow into large cauliflower-shaped masses. Genital warts usually appear within weeks or months after sexual contact with an infected person. If left untreated, genital warts may go away, remain unchanged, or increase in size or number but will not turn into cancers. It is possible, however, for a person to be infected with a high-risk strain of HPV as well as one of the strains that cause genital warts; therefore the appearance of genital warts does not necessarily mean that the person is not at risk of cancer.
- Precancerous changes in the tissues of the female cervix. These are flat growths on the cervix that cannot be seen or felt by the infected woman.
- Cancer. High-risk strains of HPV can cause cancers of the mouth and throat as well as cancers of the anal area and the male and female genitals. These typically take years to develop after infection. In men, symptoms of anal cancer may include bleeding, pain, or a discharge from the anus, or changes in bowel habits. Early signs of cancer of the penis may include thickening of the skin, tissue growths, or sores.

It was not fully understood as of 2009 why most infections with high-risk HPV are of short duration, while a small percentage persist and eventually transform cervical cells to a state of cancerous growth.

Symptoms in children

In addition to producing precancerous lesions in some patients, HPV infections in women are a health concern because they can be transmitted to the respiratory tract of a baby during **childbirth**. This type of HPV infection may lead to a rare disorder known as juvenile-onset recurrent respiratory papillomatosis (JO-RRP) or laryngeal papillomatosis, in which papillomas or warts form in the child's airway, producing hoarseness or partial blockage of the windpipe. Although laryngeal papillomatosis can occur in HPV-infected adults, 60–80% of cases occur in children, most of them younger than three years.

Laryngeal papillomatosis is usually diagnosed by **laryngoscopy**. Surgery, whether traditional or **laser surgery**, is the usual treatment for JO-RRP, but the warts often recur and require additional surgery to remove them. In extreme cases, the patient may be given a **tracheotomy**, a procedure in which a hole is cut through the throat into the windpipe and a tube is inserted to keep the breathing hole open. A new treatment for the disorder is **photodynamic therapy** or PDT. In PDT, a special light-sensitive dye is injected into the patient's blood. The dye collects in the tumors rather than in healthy tissue. When bright light of a specific wavelength is shined on the throat, it destroys the tumors containing the dye.

Cidofovir and interferon are often given as adjuvant treatments for this disease as of the early 2000s. JO-RRP is a serious illness, leading to **death** in a significant number of affected children. In a very few cases, respiratory papillomatosis can lead to cancer as well as breathing difficulties.

Diagnosis

There is no general blood, urine, or imaging test for HPV infection. The diagnosis of genital warts is obvious based on their location and appearance. The doctor may, however, use a vinegar solution to identify HPV-infected areas on the skin of the genitals. The vinegar solution will turn white if HPV is present. Since genital warts are caused by low-risk strains of HPV, the doctor does not need to identify the specific strain of the virus that is present.

Sexually active women should be screened periodically for the presence of changes in the tissues of the cervix. The most common test is the Papanikolaou test or Pap smear, invented by a Greek physician in the 1940s. To perform a Pap smear, the doctor takes a small spatula to obtain cells from the outer surface of the cervix and smears the collected cells on a slide that is then examined in a laboratory for signs of any abnormal cells. If abnormal or questionable cells are found, the doctor may order an HPV DNA test, which can identify the DNA of 13 high-risk types of HPV in cells taken from the cervix.

There were no HPV screening tests for men as of 2009; however, some doctors suggested that anal Pap smears for men who have sex with men would be useful in early detection of anal cancer.

Tests

The relationship among HPV, precancerous cellular changes, and cervical cancer have led to the suggestion

KEY TERMS

Ablative—Also known as "ablation" and referring to the surgical removal of lesions associated with HPV.

Biopsy—The removal of a small bit of tissue for diagnostic examination.

Cervical intra-epithelial neoplasia (CIN)—A precancerous condition in which a group of cells grow abnormally on the cervix but do not extend into the deeper layers of this tissue.

Cervix—The narrow neck or outlet of a woman's uterus.

Colposcopy—Procedure in which the cervix is examined using a special microscope.

Condylomata acuminata (singular, condyloma acuminatum)—The medical term for infectious warts on the genitals caused by HPV.

Cryotherapy—The use of liquid nitrogen or other forms of extreme cold to destroy tissue.

Epithelial—Referring to the epithelium, the layer of cells forming the epidermis of the skin and the surface layer of mucous membranes.

High-risk HPV type—A member of the HPV family of viruses that is associated with the development of cervical cancer and precancerous growths.

Pap test—A screening test for cervical cancer devised by Giorgios Papanikolaou (1883–1962) in the 1940s.

Photodynamic therapy (PDT)—A treatment for tumors in which a light-sensitive dye is injected into the blood (or skin) to be taken up selectively by the tumors. Light of a specific wavelength is then applied to the affected area to kill the tumors.

Topical—Referring to a type of medication applied directly to the skin or outside of the body.

Tracheotomy—A surgical procedure in which a hole is cut through the neck to open a direct airway through an incision in the trachea (windpipe).

that testing for the presence of HPV can be a useful addition to Pap smears. Pap smears involve microscopic analysis of cells removed from the cervix. The results of these tests are generally reported as either normal or consistent with the presence of cancer or a precancerous condition. Patients receiving the latter diagnosis usually are treated either by excisional or ablative therapy surgery or some other means in order to remove the tumor or precancerous lesion.

In some cases the cytologist or pathologist examining a Pap smear reports a "borderline" result when abnormal cells are observed, but it is not possible to distinguish whether the changes seen are due to early precancerous changes or to inflammation caused by some infectious agent or irritant. In these cases, some physicians and scientists believe that testing for the presence of HPV can help to identify those women who should be closely followed for the development of early cancerous lesions, or who should undergo **colposcopy**, a procedure to examine the cervix for precancerous lesions. These cancer precursors, termed cervical intraepithelial neoplasia (CIN) when identified early, before they have become invasive, can almost always be completely removed by minor surgery, essentially curing the patient before the cancer has had a chance to develop. The cervical tissue removed, which includes the precancerous tissue, is examined as part of a biopsy to confirm the diagnosis, and if requested by a doctor, can be tested for the presence of high-risk HPV types.

Treatment

Traditional

Patients with genital warts should *never* use over-the counter-preparations designed to remove common or flat warts from the hands or face. Doctors can treat genital warts with various medical or surgical techniques:

- Cryotherapy. Cryotherapy uses liquid nitrogen to freeze the warts. The dead tissue in the wart falls away from the skin beneath in about a week.
- Imiquimod. Imiquimod (Aldara) is a topical cream that gets rid of genital warts by stimulating the body's immune system to fight the virus that causes the warts.
- Podofilox. Podofilox (Condylox) is a topical medication available in liquid or gel form that destroys the wart tissue.
- Surgery. The doctor can remove the wart by drying it out with an electric needle and then scraping the tissue with a sharp instrument called a curette. Lasers can also be used to remove genital warts.

Low-grade precancerous changes in the tissue of the female cervix are not usually treated directly because most of them will eventually go away on their own without developing into cancer. The patient should, however, see the doctor for follow-up Pap smears to make sure that the tissues are returning to normal. High-risk precancerous lesions are removed, usually by surgery, **cryotherapy**, electrocauterization, or laser surgery.

Since the incidence of latent and recurrent infections is high, the eradication of HPV is not always 100% effective. It is essential to be aware that HPV is a sexually transmitted disease and women must engage in safe sex practices to decrease the risk of spreading the virus or becoming reinfected. A vaccine effective against four of the HPV types most likely to cause genital warts or cervical cancer was approved for use in 2006; it is described more fully in the Prevention section of this article. As of 2009, researchers were working on developing vaccines to protect against additional types of the HPV virus.

Prognosis

The prognosis of sexually transmitted HPV infections depends on the patient's age, number of sexual partners, gender, and the condition of his or her immune system. Women are significantly more likely than men to develop cancers following HPV infection. However, most people of either sex with normally functioning immune systems who are infected with HPV will clear the infection from their bodies within two years.

Prevention

Preventive measures that people can take to lower their risk of HPV infection include:

- Abstaining from sex or having sex only with an uninfected partner who is faithful.
- Reducing the number of sexual partners.
- Using condoms regularly during sexual intercourse.
- For women, using a vaccine called Gardasil. Approved by the Food and Drug Administration (FDA) in 2006, Gardasil is protects against the four types of HPV that cause most cervical cancers and genital warts. The vaccine is recommended for 11- and 12-year-old girls. It is also recommended for girls and women age 13 through 26 who have not yet been vaccinated or completed the vaccine series. Gardasil works best in girls who have not yet been sexually active. It is given as a series of three shots over a six-month period.

A second human papillomavirus vaccine, Cervarix, was approved in Europe, Australia, and the Philippines in 2007. It received FDA approval for use in the United States in October 2009.

In addition to giving the available preventive vaccines to women, some doctors think it might be a useful preventive measure to vaccinate men as well to protect their female partners against infection. As of 2009, however, male **vaccination** for HPV is still under discussion rather than being put into clinical practice.

Resources

BOOKS

Gonzales, Lissette. *Frequently Asked Questions about Human Papillomavirus*. New York: Rosen, 2009.

Krueger, Hans, et al. *HPV and Other Infectious Agents in Cancer: Opportunities for Prevention and Public Health*. New York: Oxford University Press, 2010.

Marr, Lisa. *Sexually Transmitted Diseases: A Physician Tells You What You Need to Know*, 2nd ed. Baltimore, MD: Johns Hopkins University Press, 2007.

Nardo, Don. *Human Papillomavirus (HPV)*. Detroit, MI: Lucent Books, 2007.

Rosenblatt, Alberto. *Human Papillomavirus*. New York: Springer, 2009.

PERIODICALS

Burki, T. "Should Males Be Vaccinated against HPV?" *Lancet Oncology* 10 (September 2009): 845.

Haug, C. "The Risks and Benefits of HPV Vaccination." *Journal of the American Medical Association* 302 (August 19, 2009): 795–95.

Hershey, J.H., and L.F. Velez. "Public Health Issues Related to HPV Vaccination." *Journal of Public Health Manage ment and Practice* 15 (September-October 2009): 384–92.

Lindsey, K., et al. "Anal Pap Smears: Should We Be Doing Them?" *Journal of the American Academy of Nurse Practitioners* 21 (August 2009): 437–43.

O'Connor, M. B., and C. O'Connor. "The HPV Vaccine for Men." *International Journal of STD and AIDS* 20 (April 2009): 290–91.

Printz, C. "HPV Status Predicts Survival of Oropharyngeal Cancer Patients." *Cancer* 115 (September 15, 2009): 4045.

Samara, R. N., and S. N. Khleif. "HPV as a Model for the Development of Prophylactic and Therapeutic Cancer Vaccines." *Current Molecular Medicine* 9 (August 2009): 766–73.

Wang, Z., et al. " Detection of Human Papilloma Virus Subtypes 16 and P16(ink4a) in Invasive Squamous Cell Carcinoma of the Fallopian Tube and Concomitant Squamous Cell Carcinoma in Situ of the Cervix." *Journal of Obstetrics and Gynaecology Research* 35 (April 2009): 385–89.

OTHER

Centers for Disease Control and Prevention (CDC). *Human Papillomavirus (HPV) Infection*. http://www.cdc.gov/std/hpv/default.htm.

Centers for Disease Control and Prevention (CDC) Fact Sheet. *HPV and Men*. http://www.cdc.gov/std/hpv/STDFact-HPV-and-men.htm.

Gearhart, Peter A., and Thomas C. Randall. "Human Papillomavirus." *eMedicine*, August 4, 2009. http://emedicine.medscape.com/article/219110-overview.

Mayo Clinic. *HPV Infection*. http://www.mayoclinic.com/health/hpv-infection/DS00906.

National Cancer Institute (NCI). http://www.cancer.gov/cancertopics/factsheet/Risk/HPV.

National Institute of Allergy and Infectious Diseases (NIAID). *Human Papillomavirus and Genital Warts*. http://www3.niaid.nih.gov/topics/genitalWarts.

National Institute on Deafness and Other Communication Disorders (NIDCD). *Laryngeal Papillomatosis*. http://www.nidcd.nih.gov/health/voice/laryngeal.htm.

ORGANIZATIONS

American College of Obstetricians and Gynecologists (ACOG), 409 12th St., S.W., P.O. Box 96920, Washington, DC, 20090-6920, 202-638-5577, resources@acog.org, http://www.acog.org/.

American Social Health Association (ASHA), P.O. Box 13827, Research Triangle Park, NC, 27709, 919-361-8400, 800-227-8922, 919-361-8425, http://www.ashastd.org/index.cfm.

Centers for Disease Control and Prevention (CDC), 1600 Clifton Road, Atlanta, GA, 30333, 800-232-4636, cdcinfo@cdc.gov, http://www.cdc.gov.

National Cancer Institute, 6116 Executive Blvd., Room 3036A, Bethesda, MD, 20892-8322, 800-422-6237, cancergovstaff@mail.nih.gov, http://www.cancer.gov.

National Institute of Allergy and Infectious Diseases (NIAID), 6610 Rockledge Drive, MSC 6612, Bethesda, MD, 20892-6612, 301-496-5717, 866-284-4107, 301-402-3573, http://www3.niaid.nih.gov.

National Institute on Deafness and Other Communication Disorders (NIDCD), 31 Center Drive, MSC 2320, Bethesda, MD, 20892-2320, 800 241-1044, 301 770-8977, nidcdinfo@nidcd.nih.gov, http://www.nidcd.nih.gov/index.asp.

Warren Maltzman, PhD
Rebecca J. Frey, PhD

Humanistic therapy *see* **Gestalt therapy; Human-potential movement**

Humpback *see* **Kyphosis**

Hunchback *see* **Kyphosis**

Hunter's syndrome *see* **Mucopolysaccharidoses**

Huntington's disease

Definition

Huntington's disease (HD) is an inherited, progressive, neurodegenerative disease causing uncontrolled physical movements and mental deterioration. The disease was discovered by George Huntington of Pomeroy, Ohio, who first described a hereditary movement disorder.

Demographics

HD is estimated to occur in the United States at a rate of 4.1–8.4 cases per 100,000 people. In most European countries, prevalence ranges from 1.63–9.95 per 100,000 people. It is lower in Finland and Japan (less than 1 case per 100,000 people). Pockets of isolated populations with western European ancestors exist where the prevalence is higher. For example, these include the region of lake Maracaibo in Venezuela (700 per 100,000 people), the island of Mauritius (46 per 100,000 people), and Tasmania (17.4 per 100,000 people). HD is a disease that affects males and females equally.

The mean age at HD onset ranges from 35–44 years. HD onset in patients younger than 10 years and older than 70 years is rare. Modifying genes and environmental factors are thought to influence the age of onset. Fpr example, the Venezuelan age of onset (34.35 y) is on average higher than that of Americans (37.47 y) and Canadians (40.36 y).

Description

Huntington's disease is also called Huntington chorea, from the Greek word for "dance," referring to the involuntary movements that develop as the disease progresses. It is occasionally referred to as "Woody Guthrie disease" for the U.S. folk singer who died from it. Huntington's disease causes progressive loss of cells in areas of the brain responsible for some aspects of movement control and mental abilities. A person with HD gradually develops abnormal movements and changes in cognition (thinking), behavior and personality.

Risk factors

Children of a parent who carries the gene responsible for HD have a 50% chance of inheriting the abnormal gene.

Causes and symptoms

Mutations in the HTT gene cause Huntington's disease. This gene provides instructions for making a protein called huntingtin, a protein that is believed to play an important role in the development of brain neurons. The HTT mutation involves lengthening a DNA segment known as a CAG trinucleotide repeat. The extra building blocks in the huntingtin gene cause the protein that is made from it to contain an extra section. It is currently thought that this extra protein section interacts with

KEY TERMS

Chorea—Involuntary writhing movements.

Cognition—The mental activities associated with thinking, learning, and memory.

Computed tomography (CT) scan—An imaging procedure that produces a three–dimensional picture of organs or structures inside the body, such as the brain.

Deoxyribonucleic acid (DNA)—The genetic material in cells that holds the inherited instructions for growth, development, and cellular functioning.

Heimlich maneuver—An action designed to expel an obstructing piece of food from the throat. It is performed by placing the fist on the abdomen, underneath the breastbone, grasping the fist with the other hand (from behind), and thrusting it inward and upward.

Neurodegenerative—Relating to degeneration of nerve tissues.

Neuron—A cell that is specialized to conduct nerve impulses.

other proteins in brain cells where it occurs, and that this interaction ultimately leads to cell **death**.

The HD gene is a dominant gene, meaning that only one copy of it is needed to develop the disease. HD affects both males and females. The gene may be inherited from either parent, who will also be affected by the disease. A parent with the HD gene has a 50% chance of passing it on to each offspring. The chances of passing on the HD gene are not affected by the results of previous pregnancies.

The symptoms of HD fall into three categories: motor or movement symptoms, personality and behavioral changes, and cognitive decline. The severity and rate of progression of each type of symptom can vary from person to person.

Early motor symptoms include restlessness, twitching and a desire to move about. Handwriting may become less controlled, and coordination may decline. Later symptoms include:

- Dystonia, or sustained abnormal postures, including facial grimaces, a twisted neck, or an arched back.
- Chorea, in which involuntary jerking, twisting or writhing motions become pronounced.
- Slowness of voluntary movements, inability to regulate the speed or force of movements, inability to initiate movement, and slowed reactions.
- Difficulty speaking and swallowing due to involvement of the throat muscles.
- Localized or generalized weakness and impaired balance ability.
- Rigidity, especially in late–stage disease.

Personality and behavioral changes include depression, irritability, **anxiety**, and apathy. The person with HD may become impulsive, aggressive, or socially withdrawn.

Cognitive changes include loss of ability to plan and execute routine tasks, slowed thought, and impaired or inappropriate judgment. Short–term **memory loss** usually occurs, although long–term memory is usually not affected. The person with late–stage HD usually retains knowledge of his environment and recognizes family members or other loved ones, despite severe cognitive decline.

Diagnosis

Examination

Diagnosis of HD begins with a detailed medical history, and a thorough physical and **neurological exam**. Family medical history is very important as HD is inherited.

Tests

Magnetic resonance imaging (MRI) or computed tomography scan (CT scan) imaging may be performed to look for degeneration in the basal ganglia and cortex, the brain regions most affected in HD.

A genetic test is available for confirmation of the clinical diagnosis. In this test, a small blood sample is taken, and DNA from it is analyzed to determine the CAG repeat number. A person with a repeat number of 30 or below will not develop HD. A person with a repeat number between 35 and 40 may not develop the disease within their normal life span. A person with a very high number of repeats (70 or above) is likely to develop the juvenile–onset form. An important component of **genetic testing** is extensive **genetic counseling**

Prenatal testing is also available. A person at risk for HD may obtain fetal testing without determining whether she herself carries the gene. This test, also called a linkage test, examines the pattern of DNA near the gene in both parent and fetus, but does not analyze for the triple nucleotide repeat (CAG). If the DNA patterns do not match, the fetus can be assumed not to have inherited the HD gene, even if present in the parent. A pattern match indicates the fetus probably has the same genetic makeup of the at–risk parent.

Treatment

Traditional

There is no cure for HD, nor any treatment that can slow the rate of progression. Treatment is aimed at reducing the disability caused by the motor impairments, and treating behavioral and emotional symptoms.

Physical therapy is used to maintain strength and compensate for lost strength and balance. Stretching and range of motion exercises help minimize contracture, or muscle shortening, a result of weakness and disuse. The physical therapist also advises on the use of mobility aids such as walkers or wheelchairs.

Occupational therapy is used to design compensatory strategies for lost abilities in the activities of daily living, such as eating, dressing, and grooming. The occupational therapist advises on modifications to the home that improve safety, accessibility, and comfort.

Difficulty swallowing may be lessened by preparation of softer foods, blending food in an electric blender, and taking care to eat slowly and carefully. Use of a straw for all liquids can help. The potential for **choking** on food is a concern, especially late in the disease progression. Caregivers should learn the use of the **Heimlich maneuver**. In addition, passage of food into the airways increases the risk for **pneumonia**. A gastric feeding tube may be needed, if swallowing becomes too difficult or dangerous.

Speech difficulties may be partially compensated by using picture boards or other augmentative communication devices. Loss of cognitive ability affects both speech production and understanding. A speech–language pathologist can work with the family to develop simplified and more directed communication strategies, including speaking slowly, using simple words, and repeating sentences exactly.

Drugs

Motor symptoms may be treated with drugs, although some studies suggest that anti–chorea treatment rarely improves function. Chorea (movements caused by abnormal muscle contractions) can be suppressed with drugs that deplete dopamine, an important brain chemical regulating movement. As HD progresses, natural dopamine levels fall, leading to loss of chorea and an increase in rigidity and movement slowness. Treatment with L–dopa (which resupplies dopamine) may be of some value. Frequent reassessment of the effectiveness and appropriateness of any drug therapy is necessary. In August 2008 the Food and Drug Administration (FDA) approved tetrabenazine to treat Huntington's chorea, making it the first drug approved for use in the United States to treat HD.

Early behavioral changes, including depression and anxiety, may respond to drug therapy. Maintaining a calm, familiar, and secure environment is useful as the disease progresses. Support groups for both patients and caregivers form an important part of treatment.

Alternative

As of 2009, 548 clinical trials for the treatment of Huntington's disease were being sponsored by the National Institutes of Health (NIH)and other agencies. A few examples include:

- The study of early brain and behavioral changes in people who have the gene expansion for HD, but are currently healthy and have no symptoms. (NCT00051324)
- The evaluation of the effect of atomoxetine on daily activities such as attention and focus, thinking ability and muscle movements in subjects with early HD. (NCT00368849)
- The collection of prospective data from individuals who are part of HD family to learn more about HD, develop potential treatments for HD, and to plan for future research studies of experimental drugs aimed at slowing or postponing the onset and progression of HD. (NCT00313495)
- The evaluation of the safety of the drug ursodiol in people with HD and the study of how the compound is processed by the body. (NCT00514774)
- The evaluation of the safety and tolerability of dimebon in people with HD. (NCT00387270)
- The effectiveness of a music therapy program to improve holistically the psychological, somatic, and social symptoms of patients with HD. (NCT00178360)
- The assessment of the impact of minocycline on the progression of symptoms of HD. (NCT00277355)

Clinical trial information is constantly updated by NIH and the most recent information on Huntington's disease trials can be found at http://clinicaltrials.gov/search/term = Huntington%27s%20Disease

Prognosis

The person with Huntington's disease may be able to maintain a job for several years after diagnosis, despite the increase in disability. Loss of cognitive functions and increase in motor and behavioral symptoms eventually prevent the person with HD from continuing employment. Ultimately, severe motor symptoms prevent mobility. Death usually occurs 15–20 years after disease onset. Progressive weakness of respiratory and swallowing muscles leads to increased risk of respiratory infection and choking, the most common causes of death. Future research in this area is focusing on nerve cell transplantation.

Prevention

Genetic testing is available for HD and should be considered if there is a family history of the disease. The Huntington's Disease Society of America has reputable pre–test and post–test counseling information.

Resources

BOOKS

Knowles, Johanna. *Huntington's Disease*. New York, NY: Rosen Publishing Group, 2006.

Lawrence, David, M. *Huntington's Disease*. New York, NY: Chelsea House Publications, 2009.

Lo, Donald C., and Robert E. Hughes. *The Neurobiology of Huntington's Disease*. Boca Raton, FL: CRC Press, 2009.

Quarrell, Oliver W. J. *Huntington's Disease (The Facts)*. Oxford, UK: Oxford University Press, 2008.

Sulaiman, Sandy. *Learning to Live With Huntington's Disease: One Family's Story*. London, UK: Jessica Kingsley Publishers, 2007.

Wexler, Alice. *The Woman Who Walked into the Sea: Huntington's and the Making of a Genetic Disease*. Ann Harbor, MI: Sheridan Books, 2008.

PERIODICALS

Aubeeluck, A., and E. Wilson. "Huntington's disease. Part 1: essential background and management." *British Journal of Nursing* 17, no. 3 (February 2008): 146–151.

Blekher, T., et al. "Visual scanning and cognitive performance in prediagnostic and early–stage Huntington's disease. Part 2: treatment and management issues in juvenile HD." *Movement Disorders* 24, no. 4 (March 2009): 533–540.

Busse, M. E., et al. " Mobility and falls in people with Huntington's disease." *Journal of Neurology, Neurosurgery, and Psychiatry* 80, no. 1 (January 2009): 88–90.

Harper, S. Q. " Progress and challenges in RNA interference therapy for Huntington disease." *Archives of Neurology* 66, no. 8, (August 2009): 933–938.

Kim, M., et al. "Stem cell–based cell therapy for Huntington disease: a review." *Neuropathology* 28, no. 1 (February 2008): 1–9.

Lahiri, N., and S. J. Tabrizi. "Huntington's disease: a tale of two genes." *Neurology* 73, no. 16 (October 2009): 1254–1255.

Videnovic, A., et al. "Daytime somnolence and nocturnal sleep disturbances in Huntington disease." *Parkinsonism & related disorders* 15, no. 6 (July 2009): 471–474.

Williams, J. K., et al. "Caregiving by teens for family members with Huntington disease." *Journal of Family Nursing* 15, no. 3 (August 2009): 273–294.

OTHER

"Genetic Testing for Huntington's Disease." *HDSA*. Referral List. http://www.hdsa.org/living-with-huntingtons/family-care/living-at-risk/genetic-testing-centers.html (accessed December 12, 2009).

"Huntington's Disease." Genetics Home Reference. Information Page. http://ghr.nlm.nih.gov/condition=huntingtondisease (accessed December 12, 2009).

"Huntington's Disease." Madisons Foundation. Information Page. http://www.madisonsfoundation.org/index.php/component/option,com_mpower/diseaseID,190 (accessed December 12, 2009).

"Huntington's Disease." Medline Plus. Health Topic. http://www.nlm.nih.gov/medlineplus/huntingtonsdisease.html (accessed December 12, 2009).

"Huntington's Disease." NINDS. Information Page. http://www.ninds.nih.gov/disorders/huntington/huntington.htm (accessed December 12, 2009).

ORGANIZATIONS

Hereditary Disease Foundation., 3960 Broadway, 6th Floor, New York, NY, 10032, (212) 928-2121, (212) 928-2172, cures@hdfoundation.org, http://www.hdfoundation.org.

Huntington's Disease Society of America (HDSA), 505 Eighth Avenue, Suite 902, New York, NY, 10018, (212) 242-1968, (800) 345-4372, (212) 239-3430, hdsainfo@hdsa.org, http://www.hdsa.org.

Huntington Society of Canada, 151 Frederick Street, Suite 400, Kitchener, Ontario, NH2 2M2, Canada, (519) 749-7063, (800) 998-7398, (519) 749-8965, info@huntingtonsociety.ca, http://www.huntingtonsociety.ca.

International Huntington Association (IHA), Callunahof 8, St Harfsen, The Netherlands, 7217, + 31-573-431595, + 31-573-431719, iha@huntington-assoc.com, http://www.huntington-assoc.com.

National Institute of Neurological Disorders and Stroke (NINDS), PO Box 5801, Bethesda, MD, 20824, (301) 496-5751, (800) 352-9424, http://www.ninds.nih.gov.

Laith Gulli, MD
Monique Laberge, PhD

Hurler's syndrome *see* **Mucopolysaccharidoses**

HUS *see* **Hemolytic-uremic syndrome**

Hyaline *see* **Respiratory distress syndrome**

Hydatid *see* **Echinococcosis**

Hydatidiform mole

Definition

A hydatidiform mole is a relatively rare condition in which tissue around a fertilized egg that normally would have developed into the placenta instead develops as an abnormal cluster of cells. (This is also called a molar pregnancy.) This grapelike mass forms inside of the uterus after fertilization instead of a normal embryo. A hydatidiform mole triggers a positive **pregnancy** test and in some cases can become cancerous.

Description

A hydatidiform mole ("hydatid" means "drop of water" and "mole" means "spot") occurs in about 1 out of every 1,500 (1/1,500) pregnancies in the United States. In some parts of Asia, however, the incidence may be as high as 1 in 200 (1/200). Molar pregnancies are most likely to occur in younger and older women (especially over age 45) than in those between ages 20–40. About 1–2% of the time a woman who has had a molar pregnancy will have a second one.

A molar pregnancy occurs when cells of the chorionic villi (tiny projections that attach the placenta to the lining of the uterus) don't develop correctly. Instead, they turn into watery clusters that can't support a growing baby. A partial molar pregnancy includes an abnormal embryo (a fertilized egg that has begun to grow) that does not survive. In a complete molar pregnancy there is a small cluster of clear blisters or pouches that don't contain an embryo.

If not removed, about 15% of **moles** can become cancerous. They burrow into the wall of the uterus and cause serious bleeding. Another 5% will develop into fast-growing cancers called choriocarcinomas. Some of these tumors spread very quickly outside the uterus in other parts of the body. Fortunately, **cancer** developing from these moles is rare and highly curable.

Causes and symptoms

The cause of hydatidiform mole is unclear; some experts believe it is caused by problems with the chromosomes (the structures inside cells that contain genetic information) in either the egg or sperm, or both. It may be associated with poor **nutrition** or a problem with the ovaries or the uterus. A mole sometimes can develop from placental tissue that is left behind in the uterus after a **miscarriage** or **childbirth**.

Women with a hydatidiform mole will have a positive pregnancy test and often believe they have a normal pregnancy for the first three or four months. However, in these cases the uterus will grow abnormally fast. By the end of the third month, if not earlier, the woman will experience vaginal bleeding ranging from scant spotting to excessive bleeding. She may have **hyperthyroidism** (overproduction of **thyroid hormones** causing symptoms such as weight loss, increased appetite, and intolerance to heat). Sometimes, the grapelike cluster of cells itself will be shed with the blood during this time. Other symptoms may include severe **nausea and vomiting** and high blood pressure. As the pregnancy progresses, the fetus will not move and there will be no fetal heartbeat.

Diagnosis

The physician may not suspect a molar pregnancy until after the third month or later, when the absence of a fetal heartbeat together with bleeding and severe nausea and vomiting indicates something is amiss.

First, the physician will examine the woman's abdomen, feeling for any strange lumps or abnormalities in the uterus. A tubal pregnancy, which can be life threatening if not treated, will be ruled out. Then the physician will check the levels of human chorionic gonadotropin (hCG), a hormone that is normally produced by a placenta or a mole. Abnormally high levels of hCG together with the symptoms of vaginal bleeding, lack of fetal heartbeat, and an unusually large uterus all indicate a molar pregnancy. An ultrasound of the uterus to make sure there is no living fetus will confirm the diagnosis.

Treatment

It is extremely important to make sure that all of the mole is removed from the uterus, since it is possible that the tissue is potentially cancerous. Often, the tissue is naturally expelled by the fourth month of pregnancy. In some instances, the physician will give the woman a drug called oxytocin to trigger the release of the mole that is not spontaneously aborted.

If this does not happen, however, a vacuum aspiration can be performed to remove the mole. In a procedure similar to a **dilatation and curettage** (D & C), a woman is given an anesthetic (to deaden feeling during the procedure), her cervix (the structure at the bottom of the uterus) is dilated and the contents of the uterus is gently suctioned out. After the mole has been mostly removed, gentle scraping of the uterus lining is usually performed.

If the woman is older and does not want any more children, the uterus can be surgically removed (**hysterectomy**) instead of a vacuum aspiration because of the higher risk of cancerous moles in this age group.

Because of the cancer risk, the physician will continue to monitor the patient for at least two months after the end of a molar pregnancy. Since invasive disease is usually signaled by high levels of hCG that don't go down after the pregnancy has ended, the woman's hCG levels will be checked every two weeks. If the levels don't return to normal by that time, the mole may have become cancerous.

If the hCG level is normal, the woman's hCG will be tested each month for six months, and then every two months for a year.

If the mole has become cancerous, treatment includes removal of the cancerous issue and **chemotherapy**. If the cancer has spread to other parts of the body, radiation will be added. Specific treatment depends on how advanced the cancer is.

Women should make sure not to become pregnant within a year after hCG levels have returned to normal. If a woman were to become pregnant sooner than that, it would be difficult to tell whether the resulting high levels of hCG were caused by the pregnancy or a cancer from the mole.

Prognosis

A woman with a molar pregnancy often goes through the same emotions and sense of loss as does a woman who has a miscarriage. Most of the time, she truly believed she was pregnant and now has suffered a loss of the baby she thought she was carrying. In addition, there is the added worry that the tissue left behind could become cancerous.

In the unlikely case that the mole is cancerous the cure rate is almost 100%. As long as the uterus was not removed, it would still be possible to have a child at a later time.

Resources

BOOKS

Carlson, Karen J., Stephanie A. Eisenstat, and Terra Ziporyn. "Abortion." In *The New Harvard Guide to Women's Health*. Cambridge, MA: Harvard University Press, 2004.

Carol A. Turkington

Hydrocelectomy

Definition

Hydrocelectomy, also called hydrocele repair, is the surgical removal of a hydrocele. A hydrocele is a fluid-filled sac along the spermatic cord within a testicle. It forms from a backup of peritoneal (abdominal) fluid in a membrane called the tunica vaginalis, which covers the front and sides of the male testes.

Purpose

A hydrocelectomy is performed to remove a hydrocele and prevent its recurrence. In babies a hydrocelectomy is used to remove a congenital (present at birth) hydrocele that has not resolved on its own by the age of two. In adults hydrocelectomies are used to repair hydroceles that:

- are large, painful, or embarrassing
- cause swelling of the scrotum
- reoccur following aspiration of the hydrocele
- interfere with the blood supply in the testicle
- are associated with an inguinal hernia

Demographics

Hydroceles occur in at least 80% of male infants, but almost always disappear on their own by the age of two. They also can occur in older boys and men. About 1% of adult males over age 40 develop hydroceles.

Description

During development of the male fetus the testicles descend down a tube from the abdomen into the scrotum. Congenital hydroceles are most often caused by a failure of a portion of the testicular membrane—the processus vaginalis that descends with the testicles—to close normally. This failure to close allows peritoneal fluid to flow into the scrotum and becomes trapped. However the processus vaginalis usually closes spontaneously within the first year of life and the hydrocele disappears. The processus does not usually close spontaneously after the age of 18 months.

In adults hydroceles develop slowly and increase and decrease in size over time. They are usually a result either of a defect in the tunica vaginalis that causes overproduction of fluid or a blocked lymphatic flow that may be related to an obstruction in the spermatic cord. The latter type of hydrocele is more common in older men. Hydroceles can also develop from inflammation, injury, or infection of the epididymis or testicle, trauma to the scrotal area, or in association with an inguinal **hernia** or cancerous tumors in the groin.

Hydroceles usually appear as a soft swelling in the membrane surrounding the testes. Hydroceles typically occur in one testis—only 7–10% occur on both sides of the scrotum. They are not usually painful and do not damage the testes; however as the hydrocele fills with fluid some men may experience discomfort or **pain** from the increased size of the scrotum. If a hydrocele occurs in conjunction with **epididymitis** (inflammation of the epididymis), the testis may become painful and inflamed.

KEY TERMS

Aspiration—The process of removing fluids or gases from the body by suction.

Epididymis—A coiled segment of spermatic duct within the scrotum, attached to the back of the testis.

Epididymitis—Inflammation of the epididymis.

Hydrocele—An accumulation of fluid in the membrane that surrounds the testis.

Inguinal hernia—An opening, weakness, or bulge in the lining of the abdominal wall in the groin area, with protrusion of the large intestine.

Peritoneal fluid—Fluid from the abdominal cavity.

Processus vaginalis—A pouch of the peritoneum (lining of the abdominal cavity) that is carried into the scrotum with the descent of the testicles to become the tunica vaginalis.

Scrotum—The pouch of skin containing the testes, epididymis, and portions of the spermatic cords.

Testis (plural: testes)—The male sex gland, held within the scrotum.

Transillumination—A technique by which a strong light is shone through body tissues to examine an organ or structure.

Tunica vaginalis—A sac-like membrane covering the outer surface of the testis.

Hydroceles can sometimes be diagnosed in a doctor's office by visual examination and palpation (touch). Hydroceles are distinguished from other testicular problems by transillumination (shining a light source through the hydrocele so that the tissue lights up) and ultrasound examinations of the area around the groin and scrotum.

Although the fluid from a hydrocele can be removed through a needle by aspiration, this is usually a temporary measure because the hydrocele often recurs. Aspiration may have longer-term success when certain medications are injected during the procedure (sclerotherapy). However there also is a higher risk of infection with aspiration than with hydrocelectomy.

A hydrocelectomy is performed by a general surgeon or a urologist on an outpatient basis in a clinic, one-day surgery center, or hospital operating room, with no special precautions. Patients are given **general anesthesia**. The extent of the surgery depends on the presence of other problems:

- For a hydrocelectomy in a child, a small incision is made in the fold of the groin, the fluid is drained, and the hydrocele sac is removed. The muscle wall is then strengthened with stitches.
- For an uncomplicated hydrocele in an adult, an incision is made directly into the scrotum. The canal between the abdominal cavity and the scrotum is repaired, the hydrocele sac is removed, the fluid is drained from the scrotum, and the incision is closed with sutures.
- For more complicated hydrocelectomies, such as those associated with an inguinal hernia, the incision is made in the groin area and the hernia or other complicating factor is repaired along with hydrocele removal.
- Sometimes a hydrocelectomy is performed by minimally invasive laparoscopic surgery. A lighted, camera-tipped, tube-like instrument called a laparoscope is inserted through a tiny incision. Instruments can be passed through the laparoscope or inserted through other small incisions. The repair completed by visualizing images on a monitor in the operating room.

Benefits

Hydrocelectomy usually eliminates the hydrocele and completely corrects any underlying defect. Recurrence of hydroceles are rare and the long-term prognosis is excellent.

Precautions

Children can resume normal activities in four to seven days following a hydrocelectomy. Adults can resume most activities within 7 to 10 days, although heavy lifting and sexual activities may be delayed for up to six weeks. There may be swelling of the scrotum for a month or more after the procedure; however prolonged swelling, **fever**, or redness in the incision area should be reported to the surgeon immediately. There have been no reports of **death** following a hydrocele repair.

Preparation

Prior to the hydrocelectomy standard pre-operative blood and urine tests will be performed. Several days before the surgery adults may be asked to stop taking any drugs that affect blood clotting. These include **aspirin**, ibuprofen (Motrin, Advil), naproxen (Naprosyn, Aleve), and some herbal supplements. The patient may be asked to not eat or drink for at least six hours before the surgery. An anesthesiologist will discuss the patient's medical history to select the correct type and amount of anesthesia. The physician or nurse will explain the surgical procedure, the type of anesthesia, and, in some cases, the need to insert a temporary drain during surgery to reduce the risk of postoperative infection and fluid accumulation.

Aftercare

Immediately following the hydrocelectomy the patient will be moved to a recovery area and checked for any undue bleeding from the incision. Body temperature and blood pressure will be monitored. Patients usually return home within a few hours. A follow-up visit is usually required several weeks after the surgery to examine the incision for proper healing and any signs infection.

Risks

Hydrocelectomy is considered a very safe surgery, with only a 2% risk of infection or complications. It is possible for a hydrocelectomy to cause injury to spermatic vessels that can affect fertility. Most surgical procedures carry some risk of problems related to anesthesia, including allergic reactions or breathing difficulties. Most surgeries also carry some risk of bleeding from the incision, internal bleeding, **blood clots**, or infection.

Resources

BOOKS

Sandlow, J. I., H. N. Winfield, and M. Goldstein. "Surgery of the Scrotum and Seminal Vesicles." In: Wein, A. J., ed. *Campbell-Walsh Urology*, 9th ed. Philadelphia: Saunders Elsevier, 2007.

Schneck, F. X., and M. F. Bellinger. "Abnormalities of the Testes and Scrotum and Their Surgical Management." In: Wein, A. J., ed. *Campbell-Walsh Urology*, 9th ed. Philadelphia: Saunders Elsevier, 2007.

OTHER

"Hydrocele." *MedlinePlus*. http://www.nlm.nih.gov/medlineplus/ency/article/000518.htm.

"Hydrocele Repair—All Information." *Kernan Orthopaedics and Rehabilitation*. http://health.kernan.org/ency/article/002999all.htm.

ORGANIZATIONS

National Kidney and Urologic Diseases Information Clearinghouse, 3 Information Way, Bethesda, MD, 20892-3580, (703) 738-4929, (800) 891-5390, (703) 738–4929, nkudic@info.niddk.nih.gov, http://kidney.niddk.nih.gov.

L. Lee Culvert
Margaret Alic, PhD

Hydrocephalus

Definition

Hydrocephalus is an abnormal expansion of cavities (ventricles) within the brain that is caused by the accumulation of cerebrospinal fluid. Hydrocephalus comes from two Greek words: *hydros* means water and *cephalus* means head.

There are two main varieties of hydrocephalus: congenital and acquired. An obstruction of the cerebral aqueduct (aqueductal stenosis) is the most frequent cause of congenital hydrocephalus. Acquired hydrocephalus may result from **spina bifida**, intraventricular hemorrhage, **meningitis**, head trauma, tumors, and cysts.

Description

Hydrocephalus is the result of an imbalance between the formation and drainage of cerebrospinal fluid (CSF). Approximately 500 milliliters (about a pint) of CSF is formed within the brain each day, by epidermal cells in structures collectively called the choroid plexus. These cells line chambers called ventricles that are located within the brain. There are four ventricles in a human brain. Once formed, CSF usually circulates among all the ventricles before it is absorbed and returned to the circulatory system. The normal adult volume of circulating CSF is 150 mL. The CSF turn-over rate is more than three times per day. Because production is independent of absorption, reduced absorption causes CSF to accumulate within the ventricles.

There are three different types of hydrocephalus. In the most common variety, reduced absorption occurs when one or more passages connecting the ventricles become blocked. This prevents the movement of CSF to its drainage sites in the subarachnoid space just inside the skull. This type of hydrocephalus is called "noncommunicating." In a second type, a reduction in the absorption rate is caused by damage to the absorptive tissue. This variety is called "communicating hydrocephalus."

Both of these types lead to an elevation of the CSF pressure within the brain. This increased pressure pushes aside the soft tissues of the brain. This squeezes and distorts them. This process also results in damage to these tissues. In infants whose skull bones have not yet fused, the intracranial pressure is partly relieved by expansion of the skull, so that symptoms may not be as dramatic. Both types of elevated-pressure hydrocephalus may occur from infancy to adulthood.

A third type of hydrocephalus, called "normal pressure hydrocephalus," is marked by ventricle enlargement without an apparent increase in CSF pressure. This type affects mainly the elderly.

Hydrocephalus has a variety of causes including:

- congenital brain defects
- hemorrhage, either into the ventricles or the subarachnoid space
- infection of the central nervous system (syphilis, herpes, meningitis, encephalitis, or mumps)
- tumor

Hydrocephalus is believed to occur in approximately one to two of every 1,000 live births. The incidence of adult onset hydrocephalus is not known. There is no known way to prevent hydrocephalus.

Causes and symptoms

Hydrocephalus that is congenital (present at birth) is thought to be caused by a complex interaction of genetic and environmental factors. Aqueductal stenosis, an obstruction of the cerebral aqueduct, is the most frequent cause of congenital hydrocephalus. The genetic factors are not well understood. According to the British Association for Spina Bifida and Hydrocephalus, in very rare circumstances, hydrocephalus is due to hereditary factors, which might affect future generations.

Signs and symptoms of elevated-pressure hydrocephalus include:

- headache
- nausea and vomiting, especially in the morning
- lethargy
- disturbances in walking (gait)
- double vision
- subtle difficulties in learning and memory
- delay in children achieving developmental milestones

Irritability is the most common sign of hydrocephalus in infants. If this is not treated, it may lead to lethargy. Bulging of the fontanelles, or the soft spots between the skull bones, may also be an early sign. When hydrocephalus occurs in infants, fusion of the skull bones is prevented. This leads to abnormal expansion of the skull.

Symptoms of normal pressure hydrocephalus include **dementia**, gait abnormalities, and incontinence (involuntary urination or bowel movements).

Diagnosis

Imaging studies—x ray, computed tomography scan (CT scan), ultrasound, and especially **magnetic resonance imaging** (MRI)—are used to assess the presence and location of obstructions, as well as changes in brain tissue that have occurred as a result of the hydrocephalus. **Lumbar puncture** (spinal tap) may be performed to aid in determining the cause when infection is suspected.

Treatment

The primary method of treatment for both elevated and normal pressure hydrocephalus is surgical installation of a shunt. A shunt is a tube connecting the ventricles of the brain to an alternative drainage site, usually the abdominal cavity. A shunt contains a one-way valve to prevent reverse flow of fluid. In some cases of non-communicating hydrocephalus, a direct connection can be made between one of the ventricles and the subarachnoid space, allowing drainage without a shunt.

Installation of a shunt requires lifelong monitoring by the recipient or family members for signs of recurring hydrocephalus due to obstruction or failure of the shunt. Other than monitoring, no other management activity is usually required.

Some drugs may postpone the need for surgery by inhibiting the production of CSF. These include acetazolamide and furosemide. Other drugs that are used to delay surgery include glycerol, **digoxin**, and isosorbide.

Some cases of elevated pressure hydrocephalus may be avoided by preventing or treating the infectious diseases which precede them. Prenatal diagnosis of congenital brain malformation is often possible, offering the option of family planning.

Prognosis

The prognosis for elevated-pressure hydrocephalus depends on a wide variety of factors, including the cause, age of onset, and the timing of surgery. Studies indicate that about half of all children who receive appropriate treatment and follow-up will develop IQs greater than 85. Those with hydrocephalus at birth do better than those with later onset due to meningitis. For individuals with normal pressure hydrocephalus, approximately half will benefit by the installation of a shunt.

Resources

BOOKS

Cinalli, G., W. J. Maixner, and Christian Sainte–Rose. *Pediatric Hydrocephalus*. Milan; New York: Springer, 2004.

OTHER

"Hydrocephalus." *American Association of Neurological Surgeons*. http://www.aans.org/Patient%20Information/Conditions%20and%20Treatments/Hydrocephalus.aspx.

"Hydrocephalus." National Library of Medicine. MedlinePlus. http://www.nlm.nih.gov/medlineplus/hydrocephalus.html.

ORGANIZATIONS

Association for Spina Bifida and Hydrocephalus, 42 Park Rd, Peterborough, UK, PE1 2UQ, 44(0173) 355 5988, 44(017) 3355 5985, helpline@asbah.org, http://www.asbah.org.

The Hydrocephalus Foundation, Inc., (HyFI), 910 Rear Broadway, Saugus, MA, 01906, (781) 942-1161, HyFII@netscape.net, http://www.hydrocephalus.org/.

L. Fleming Fallon, MD, PhD, DrPH

Hydrochlorothiazide *see* **Diuretics**
Hydrocodone *see* **Analgesics, opioid**
Hydrogen peroxide *see* **Antiseptics**

Hydronephrosis

Definition

Hydronephrosis is the swelling of the kidneys when urine flow is obstructed in any of part of the urinary tract. Swelling of the ureter, which always accompanies hydronephrosis, is called hydroureter. Hydronephrosis implies that a ureter and the renal pelvis (the connection of the ureter to the kidney) are overfilled with urine.

Description

The kidneys filter urine out of the blood as a waste product. It collects in the renal pelvis and flows down the ureters into the bladder. The ureters are not simple tubes, but muscular passages that actively propel urine into the bladder. At their lower end is a valve (the ureterovesical junction) that prevents urine from flowing backward into the ureter. The bladder stores urine. The prostate gland surrounds the bladder outlet in males. Urine then flows through the urethra and out of the body as a waste product.

Because the urinary tract is closed save for the one opening at the bottom, urine cannot escape. Instead, the parts distend. Rupture is rare unless there is violent trauma like an automobile accident.

Obstructed flow anywhere along the drainage route can cause swelling of the upper urinary tract, but if the obstruction is below the bladder, the ureterovesical valve will protect the upper tract to a certain extent. Even then, with no place to go, the urine will back up all the way to its source. Eventually, the back pressure causes kidney function to deteriorate.

Obstruction need not be complete for problems to arise. Intermittent or partial obstruction is far more common than complete blockage, allowing time for the parts to enlarge gradually. Furthermore, if a ureterovesical valve is absent or incompetent, the pressure generated by bladder emptying will force urine backward into the ureter and kidney, causing dilation even without mechanical obstruction.

Causes and symptoms

Causes are numerous. Various congenital deformities of the ureter may sooner or later produce back pressure. **Kidney stones** are a common cause. They form in the renal pelvis and become lodged in the kidney, usually at the ureterovesical junction. In older men, the continued growth of the prostate gland leads commonly to restricted urine flow out of the bladder. **Prostate cancer**, and **cancer** anywhere else along the urine pathways, can obstruct flow. **Pregnancy** normally causes ureteral obstruction from the pressure of the enlarged uterus (womb) on the ureters.

Symptoms relate to the passage of urine. Sometimes, urine may be difficult to pass, irregular, or uncontrolled. **Pain** from distension of the structures is present. Blood in the urine may be visible, but it is usually microscopic.

In all cases where bodily fluids cannot flow freely, infection is inevitable. Symptoms of urinary infection may include:

- painful, burning urine
- cloudy urine
- pain in the back, flank, or groin
- fever, sweats, chills, and generalized discomfort

Patients often mistake a serious urinary infection for the flu.

Diagnosis

If the bladder is significantly distended, it can be felt through the abdomen. An analysis of the urine may reveal blood (if there is a stone), infection, or chemical changes suggesting kidney damage. Blood tests may also detect a decrease in kidney function.

All urinary obstructions will undergo imaging of some sort. Beginning with standard x rays to look for stones, radiologists, physicians specializing in the use of radiant energy for diagnostic purposes, will select from a wide array of tests. Ultrasound is simple, inexpensive, and very useful for these conditions. Standard x rays can be enhanced with contrast agents in several ways. If the kidneys are functioning, they will filter an x ray dye out of the blood and concentrate it in the urine, giving excellent pictures and also an assessment of kidney function. For better images of the lower urinary tract, contrast agents can be instilled from below. This is usually done with a cystoscope placed in the bladder. Through the cystoscope, a small tube can be threaded into the ureter through the ureterovesical valve, allowing dye to be injected all the way up to the kidney. CT and MRI scanning provide miraculous detail, more than is often needed for this condition.

Treatment

The obstruction must be relieved, even if it is partial or functional, as in the case of reflux from the bladder. If not, the kidney will ultimately be damaged, infection will appear, or both. The task may be as simple as placing a catheter through a restricting prostate or as complicated as removing a cancerous bladder and rebuilding a new one with a piece of bowel. In some cases, a badly damaged kidney may have to be removed.

Alternative treatment

Catheters or other urinary diversions may be better for weak or ill patients who cannot tolerate more extensive procedures. There is support using botanical medicine that can help the patient using a catheter avoid infections. Consultation with a trained health care practitioner is necessary.

Prognosis

After relief of the obstruction, a kidney may react with a brief flood of urine, but if the obstruction has been of short duration, normal kidney function will return. If one kidney is destroyed, the other will compensate for the lost organ.

Prevention

Kidney stones can be prevented by dietary changes and medication. Prompt evaluation of infections and urinary complaints will usually detect problems early enough to prevent long-term complications.

ORGANIZATIONS

American Association of Kidney Patients, 3505 E. Frontage Road, Suite 315, Tampa, FL, 33607, (813) 636-8122, (800) 749-2257, info@aakp.org, http://www.aakp.org.

American Kidney Fund (AKF), 6110 Executive Boulevard, Suite 1010, Rockville, MD, 20852, (800) 638-8299, http://www.kidneyfund.org.

National Kidney Foundation, Inc. , 30 East 33rd Street, New York, NY, 10016, (212) 889-2210, (212) 689-9261, (800) 622-9010, http://www.kidney.org/.

J. Ricker Polsdorfer, MD

Hydrotherapy

Definition

Hydrotherapy, or water therapy, is the use of water (hot, cold, steam, or ice) to relieve discomfort and promote physical well-being.

Purpose

Hydrotherapy can soothe sore or inflamed muscles and joints, rehabilitate injured limbs, lower fevers, soothe headaches, promote relaxation, treat **burns** and **frostbite**, ease labor pains, and clear up skin problems. The temperature of water used affects the therapeutic properties of the treatment. Hot water is chosen for its relaxing properties. It is also thought to stimulate the immune system. Tepid water can also be used for **stress reduction**, and may be particularly relaxing in hot weather. Cold water is selected to reduce inflammation. Alternating hot and cold water can stimulate the circulatory system and improve the immune system. Adding herbs and essential oils to water can enhance its therapeutic value. Steam is frequently used as a carrier for essential oils that are inhaled to treat respiratory problems.

Since the late 1990s, hydrotherapy has been used in critical care units to treat a variety of serious conditions, including such disorders of the nervous system as **Guillain-Barré syndrome**.

Description

Origins

The therapeutic use of water has a long history. Ruins of an ancient bath were unearthed in Pakistan and date as far back as 4500 B.C. Bathhouses were an essential part of ancient Roman culture. The use of steam, baths, and aromatic massage to promote well being is documented since the first century. Roman physicians Galen and Celsus wrote of treating patients with warm and cold baths in order to prevent disease.

By the seventeenth and eighteenth centuries, bathhouses were extremely popular with the public throughout Europe. Public bathhouses made their first American appearance in the mid 1700s.

In the early nineteenth century, Sebastien Kneipp, a Bavarian priest and proponent of water healing, began treating his parishioners with cold water applications after he himself was cured of **tuberculosis** through the same methods. Kneipp wrote extensively on the subject, and opened a series of hydrotherapy clinics known as the Kneipp clinics, which are still in operation today.

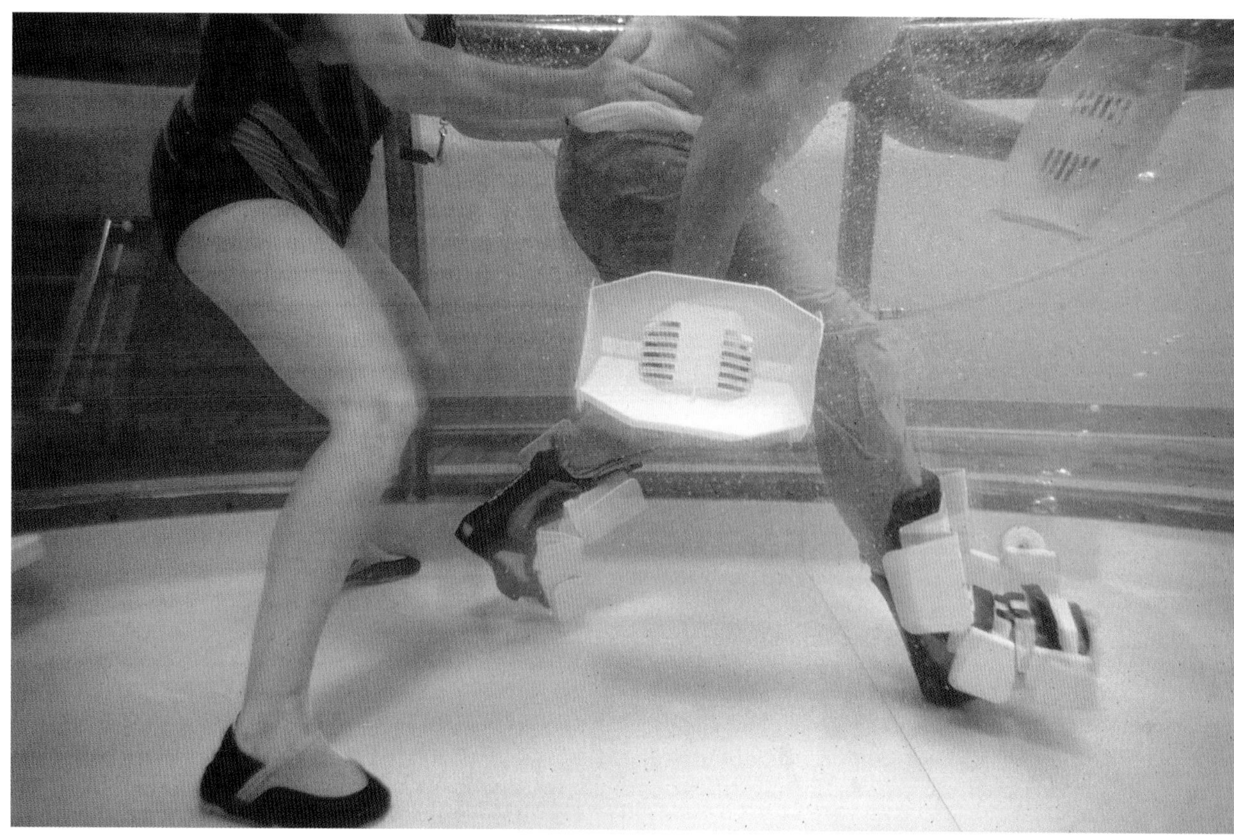

A patient (holding paddles) is undergoing a hydrotherapy treatment. *(Will & Deni McIntyre/Photo Researchers, Inc.)*

Around the same time in Austria, Vincenz Priessnitz was treating patients with baths, packs, and showers of cold spring water. Priessnitz also opened a spa that treated over 1,500 patients in its first year of operation, and became a model for physicians and other specialists to learn the techniques of hydrotherapy.

Water can be used therapeutically in a number of ways. Common forms of hydrotherapy include:

- Whirlpools, jacuzzis, and hot tubs. These soaking tubs use jet streams to massage the body. They are frequently used by physical therapists to help injured patients regain muscle strength and to soothe joint and muscle pain. Some midwives and obstetricians also approve of the use of hot tubs to soothe the pain of labor.
- Pools and Hubbard tanks. Physical therapists and rehabilitation specialists may prescribe underwater pool exercises as a low-impact method of rebuilding muscle strength in injured patients. The buoyancy experienced during pool immersion also helps ease pain in conditions such as arthritis.
- Baths. Tepid baths are prescribed to reduce a fever. Baths are also one of the oldest forms of relaxation therapy. Aromatherapists often recommend adding essential oils of lavender (*Lavandula angustifolia*) to a warm to hot bath to promote relaxation and stress reduction. Adding Epsom salts (magnesium sulfate) or Dead Sea salts to a bath can also promote relaxation and soothe rheumatism and arthritis.
- Showers. Showers are often prescribed to stimulate the circulation. Water jets from a shower head are also used to massage sore muscles. In addition, showering hydrotherapy has been shown to be preferable to immersion hydrotherapy for treating burn patients.
- Moist compresses. Cold, moist compresses can reduce swelling and inflammation of an injury. They can also be used to cool a fever and treat a headache. Hot or warm compresses are useful for soothing muscle aches and treating abscesses.
- Steam treatments and saunas. Steam rooms and saunas are recommended to open the skin pores and cleanse the body of toxins. Steam inhalation is prescribed to treat respiratory infections. Adding botanicals to the steam bath can increase its therapeutic value.
- Internal hydrotherapy. Colonic irrigation is an enema that is designed to cleanse the entire bowel. Proponents of the therapy say it can cure a number of

VINZENZ PRIESSNITZ (1799–1851)

Hydrotherapy inventor Vinzenz Priessnitz was the son of a Silesian farmer from a remote Austrian territory in the Jeseniky Mountains. From the age of 12, Priessnitz dutifully provided for his blind father, his elderly mother, and his sister. His formal education was sporadic at best. However, Priessnitz possessed a level head and a high degree of intelligence along with a keen and active mind. As he matured he became extremely aware of his surroundings in nature.

At age 16, Priessnitz fell from a horse and was seriously hoofed by the animal. He received the morbid prognosis that he might be crippled at best, or might die at worst. He set to treating his own chest wound with cold packs, in emulation of a doe that he had once observed bathing a wound in a cool mountain stream. The hydrotherapy regimen proved highly effective and drew considerable attention to his small hometown of Gräfenberg. In 1822 he rebuilt the family home, renovating its wooden frame into a solid brick spa structure. The spa, known as the castle, housed as many as 1,500 guests each year by 1939. Among the guests were medical professionals who were intent upon exposing the therapy as a sham.

Detractors notwithstanding, word of the simple and effective treatment spread to Vienna, where Priessnitz traveled on occasion to provide counsel at the emperor's court. Priessnitz, for his remarkable discovery, received the Austrian Gold Civil Merit Medal First Class, the highest civilian honor of the Austrian government.

Priessnitz died on November 28, 1851. He was survived by a wife, Zofie Priessnitz, and a young son, Vinzenz Pavel. Joseph Schindler took over the operation of the spa at Gräfenberg following the death of its founder.

digestive problems. Douching, another form of internal hydrotherapy, directs a stream of water into the vagina for cleansing purposes. The water may or may not contain medications or other substances. Douches can be self-administered with kits available at most drug stores.

Preparations

Because of the expense of the equipment and the expertise required to administer effective treatment, hydrotherapy with pools, whirlpools, Hubbard tanks, and saunas is best taken in a professional healthcare facility, and/or under the supervision of a healthcare professional. However, baths, steam inhalation treatments, and compresses can be easily administered at home.

Bath preparations

Warm to hot bath water should be used for relaxation purposes, and a tepid bath is recommended for reducing fevers. Herbs can greatly enhance the therapeutic value of the bath for a variety of illnesses and minor discomforts.

Herbs for the bath can be added to the bath in two ways—as essential oils or whole herbs and flowers. Whole herbs and flowers can be placed in a muslin or cheesecloth bag that is tied at the top to make an herbal bath bag. The herbal bath bag is then soaked in the warm tub, and can remain there throughout the bath. When using essential oils, add five to 10 drops of oil to a full tub. Oils can be combined to enhance their therapeutic value. Marjoram (*Origanum marjorana*) is good for relieving sore muscles; juniper (*Juniperus communis*) is recommended as a detoxifying agent for the treatment of arthritis; lavender, ylang ylang (*Conanga odorata*), and chamomile (*Chamaemelum nobilis*) are recommended for **stress** relief; cypress (*Cupressus sempervirens*), yarrow (*Achillea millefolium*), geranium (*Pelargonium graveolens*), clary sage (*Savlia sclaria*), and myrtle (*Myrtus communis*) can promote healing of **hemorrhoids**; and spike lavender and juniper (*Juniperus communis*) are recommended for rheumatism.

To prepare salts for the bath, add one or two handfuls of epsom salts or Dead Sea salts to boiling water until they are dissolved, and then add them to the tub.

A **sitz bath**, or hip bath, can also be taken at home to treat hemorrhoids and promote healing of an **episiotomy**. There is special apparatus available for taking a seated sitz bath, but it can also be taken in a regular tub partially filled with warm water.

Steam inhalation

Steam inhalation treatments can be easily administered with a bowl of steaming water and a large towel. For colds and other conditions with nasal congestion, aromatherapists recommend adding five drops of an essential oil that has decongestant properties, such as peppermint (*Mentha piperita*) and eucalyptus blue gum (*Eucalyptus globulus*). Oils that act as **expectorants**, such as myrtle (*Myrtus communis*) or rosemary (*Rosmarinus officinalis*), can also be used. After the oil is added, the individual should lean over the bowl of water and place the towel over head to trap the steam. After approximately three minutes of inhaling the steam, with eyes closed, the towel can be removed.

Other herbs and essential oils that can be beneficial in steam inhalation include:

- tea tree oil (*Melaleuca alternaifolia*) for bronchitis and sinus infections
- sandalwood (*Santalum album*), virginian cedarwood (*Juniperus virginiana*), and frankincense (*Boswellia carteri*) for sore throat
- lavender (*Lavandula angustifolia*) and thyme (*Thymus vulgaris*) for cough

Compresses

A cold compress is prepared by soaking a cloth or cotton pad in cold water and then applying it to the area of injury or distress. When the cloth reaches room temperature, it should be resoaked and reapplied. Applying gentle pressure to the compress with the hand may be useful. Cold compresses are generally used to reduce swelling, minimize bruising, and to treat headaches and sprains.

Warm or hot compresses are used to treat abscesses and muscle aches. A warm compress is prepared in the same manner as a cold compress, except steaming water is used to wet the cloth instead of cold water. Warm compresses should be refreshed and reapplied after they cool to room temperature.

Essential oils may be added to moist compresses to increase the therapeutic value of the treatment. Peppermint, a cooling oil, is especially effective when added to cold compresses. To add oils to compresses, place five drops of the oil into the bowl of water the compress is to be soaked in. Never apply essential oils directly to a cloth, as they may irritate the skin in undiluted form.

Precautions

Individuals with **paralysis**, frostbite, or other conditions that impair the nerve endings and cause reduced sensation should only take hydrotherapy treatments under the guidance of a trained hydrotherapist, physical therapist, or other appropriate healthcare professional. Because these individuals cannot accurately sense temperature changes in the water, they run the risk of being seriously burned without proper supervision. Diabetics and people with **hypertension** should also consult their healthcare professional before using hot tubs or other heat hydrotherapies.

Hot tubs, jacuzzis, and pools can become breeding grounds for bacteria and other infectious organisms if they are not cleaned regularly, maintained properly, kept at the appropriate temperatures, and treated with the proper chemicals. Individuals should check with their healthcare provider to ensure that the hydrotherapy equipment they are using is sanitary. Those who are using hot tubs and other hydrotherapy equipment in their homes should follow the directions for use and maintenance provided by the original equipment manufacturer.

Certain essential oils should not be used by pregnant or nursing women or by people with specific illnesses or physical conditions. Individuals suffering from any chronic or acute health condition should inform their healthcare provider before starting treatment with any essential oil.

Essential oils such as cinnamon leaf, juniper, lemon, eucalyptus blue gum, peppermint, and thyme can be extremely irritating to the skin if applied in full concentration. Oils used in hydrotherapy should always be diluted in water before they are applied to the skin. Individuals should never apply essential oils directly to the skin unless directed to do so by a trained healthcare professional and/or aromatherapist.

Colonic irrigation should only be performed by a healthcare professional. Pregnant women should never douche, as the practice can introduce bacteria into the vagina and uterus. They should also avoid using hot tubs without the consent of their healthcare provider.

The vagina is self-cleansing, and douches have been known to upset the balance of vaginal pH and flora, promoting vaginitis and other infections. Some studies have linked excessive vaginal douching to increased incidence of **pelvic inflammatory disease** (PID).

Side effects

Most forms of hydrotherapy are well tolerated. There is a risk of allergic reaction (also known as **contact dermatitis**) for some patients using essential oils and herbs in their bath water. These individuals may want to test for allergic sensitization to herbs by performing a skin patch test (i.e., rubbing a small amount of diluted herb on the inside of their elbow and observing the spot for redness and irritation). People who experience an allergic reaction to an essential oil should discontinue its use and contact their healthcare professional for further guidance.

The most serious possible side effect of hydrotherapy is overheating, which may occur when an individual spends too much time in a hot tub or jacuzzi. However, when properly supervised, this is a minimal risk.

Research and general acceptance

Hydrotherapy treatments are used by both allopathic and complementary medicine to treat a wide variety of discomforts and disorders. Not as well accepted are invasive hydrotherapy techniques, such as colonic irrigation, **enemas**, and douching. These internal cleansing techniques can actually harm an individual by upsetting the natural balance of the digestive tract and the vagina. Most conventional medical professionals agree that vaginal douches are not necessary to promote hygiene in most women, and can actually do more harm than good.

Resources

BOOKS

Cameron, Michelle H. *Physical Agents in Rehabilitation: From Research to Practice*. 3rd ed. St. Louis, MO: Saunders/Elsevier, 2009.

Sinclair, Marybetts. *Modern Hydrotherapy for the Massage Therapist*. Philadelphia: Wolters Kluwer Health/Lippincott Williams & Wilkins, 2008.

PERIODICALS

Baird, Carol L. "First-Line Treatment for Osteoarthritis: Part 2: Nonpharmacologic Interventions and Evaluation." *Orthopaedic Nursing* 20 (November-December 2001): 13–20.

Barker, K. L., H. Dawes, P. Hansford, and D. Shamley. "Perceived and Measured Levels of Exertion of Patients with Chronic Back Pain Exercising in a Hydrotherapy Pool." *Archives of Physical Medicine and Rehabilitation* 84 (September 2003): 1319–1323.

Cider, A., M. Schaufelberger, K. S. Sunnerhagen, and B. Andersson. "Hydrotherapy—A New Approach to Improve Function in the Older Patient with Chronic Heart Failure." *European Journal of Heart Failure* 5 (August 2003): 527–535.

Keegan, L. "Therapies to Reduce Stress and Anxiety." *Critical Care Nursing Clinics of North America* 15 (September 2003): 321–327.

Mayhall, C. G. "The Epidemiology of Burn Wound Infections: Then and Now." *Clinical Infectious Diseases* 37 (August 15, 2003): 543–550.

Molter, N. C. "Creating a Healing Environment for Critical Care." *Critical Care Nursing Clinics of North America* 15 (September 2003): 295–304.

Taylor, S. "The Ventilated Patient Undergoing Hydrotherapy: A Case Study." *Australian Critical Care* 16 (August 2003): 111–115.

ORGANIZATIONS

American Association of Naturopathic Physicians, 4435 Wisconsin Avenue, NW, Suite 403 , Washington, DC, 20016, (202) 237-8150, (202) 237-8152, (866) 538-2267, member.services@naturopathic.org, http://naturopathic.org/.

Canadian Association of Naturopathic Doctors, 20 Holly St., Ste. 200, Toronto, Ontario, M4S 3B1, Canada, (416) 496-8633, (416) 496-8634, (800) 551-4381, http://www.cand.ca.

Paula Anne Ford-Martin
Rebecca J. Frey, PhD

Hydroxzine *see* **Anti-itch drugs**

Hyperactivity *see* **Attention deficit hyperactivity disorder (ADHD)**

Hyperaldosteronism

Definition

Hyperaldosteronism is a disorder which is defined by the body's overproduction of aldosterone, a hormone that controls **sodium** and potassium levels in the blood. Its overproduction leads to retention of salt and loss of potassium, which leads to **hypertension** (high blood pressure).

Description

Also known as Conn's syndrome, primary aldosteronism, and secondary aldosteronism, this disorder takes several forms. It often begins with a tumor that produces aldosterone. In fact, approximately 60–70% of the cases of primary aldosteronism result from tumors in the adrenal gland area. Aldosterone is normally produced by the adrenal cortex, or the outer portion of the gland that rests on top of each kidney. Primary aldosteronism is due to adenoma, a typically benign tumor in which the cells form to act as glands or cause the glands on which they rest to overproduce. It can cause a number of problems, most notably hypertension. In secondary aldosteronism, factors outside the adrenal gland may cause overproduction of aldosterone, or overproduction of renin, an enzyme stored in the kidney area that stimulates aldosterone and raises blood pressure. Obstructive renal artery disease may also cause hypertension from elevated renin stimulating aldosterone. **Oral contraceptives** have been known to increase the secretion of aldosterone in some patients. This disorder is more common in women.

Causes and symptoms

Hyperaldosteronism is most often caused by the invasion of adenoma. Other adrenal cancers and hyperplasia, or the increase in the bulk of an organ due to increased cell production, may also cause hyperaldosteronism. Those diseases and factors influencing the adrenal and kidney functions may lead to secondary aldosteronism. The primary symptom of hyperaldosteronism is moderate hypertension, or high blood pressure. In addition, a patient may experience **orthostatic hypotension**, or reduced blood pressure when a person stands after lying down. **Constipation**, muscle weakness (sometimes to the point of **periodic paralysis**), excessive urination, excessive thirst, **headache**, and personality changes are also possible symptoms. Some patients will show no obvious symptoms.

Diagnosis

Screening tests can be conducted to pinpoint a diagnosis of hyperaldosteronism. If a patient is taking drugs to reduce high blood pressure, the physician may order these drugs stopped for a time period before conducting tests, since these drugs will affect results. Blood and urine tests may be conducted to check for levels of aldosterone, potassium levels, or renin activity. A computed tomography scan (CT scan) may be ordered to detect tumors as small as 5–7 mm. These combined tests approach 95% accuracy for detecting aldosterone-producing adenoma. Laboratory findings recording blood pressure, **edema**, and aldosterone and **plasma renin activity** can help the physician differentiate between primary aldosteronism and secondary aldosteronism.

Treatment

Once the physician has made a diagnosis of hyperaldosteronism, the adrenal glands should be checked for possible adenomas. This can be done through imaging or with a surgical dissection of the gland. Surgical or ablative treatment will vary depending on the number of tumors found. Since more than 60% of hyperaldosteronism cases are caused by these tumors, treatment of the tumors will help eliminate the resulting high blood pressure in many patients. Some patients will receive **antihypertensive drugs**, like **calcium channel blockers**, to control high blood pressure. The use of **diuretics** can help control hypertension by reducing volume. Potassium levels should be considered in the type of diuretic ordered and the levels should be checked throughout treatment. The most widely used drug for treatment of hyperaldosteronism is spironolactone. This drug helps control aldosterone, but should not be prescribed for some patients, especially those with certain kidney diseases. Spironolactone has several possible adverse effects, depending on the dosage. In all cases of hyperaldosteronism, the treatment should be carefully based on the specific type or underlying cause of the disorder.

Alternative treatment

Patients may choose to work with their physician or alternative provider to control hypertension with diet, **stress reduction** (including massage, **meditation**, **biofeedback**, and **yoga**), and other remedies. Blood pressure elevation needs to be controlled and monitored by frequent blood pressure measurements. There is no alternative treatment known for the underlying adenoma.

Prognosis

Hyperaldosteronism carries with it all the possible complications of high blood pressure, including thickening of arterial walls and a higher risk of **angina**, kidney failure, **stroke**, or **heart attack**. Another possible, and less reversible complication than hypertension, is kidney damage. When primary aldosteronism is caused by a solitary adenoma, the prognosis is good. Once this tumor is removed, blood pressure will drop, and 70% of these patients have full remission. Patients whose hyperaldosteronism results from adrenal hyperplasia will remain hypertensive. However, in up to 70% of patients, blood pressure can be reduced somewhat with drug therapy. Many patients will be faced with the prospect of controlling their hypertension for the remainder of their lives.

Prevention

There is no known prevention for most causes of hyperaldosteronism.

Resources

OTHER

Hypertension Network. http://www.bloodpressure.com.

ORGANIZATIONS

American Heart Association National Center, 7272 Greenville Avenue, Dallas, TX, 75231, (800) 242-8721, Review.personal.info@heart.org.

American Society of Hypertension, 148 Madison Avenue, Fifth Floor, New York, NY, 10016, (212) 696-9099, (212) 696-0711, ash@ash-us.org, http://www.ash-us. org/.

National Heart Lung and Blood Institute Health Informa tion Center, P.O. Box 30105, Bethesda, MD, 20824-0105, (301) 592-8573, (240) 629-3246, http://www.nhlbi.nih.gov.

Teresa Odle

Hyperbaric chamber

Definition

A hyperbaric chamber is a room that allows an individual to breathe 100% pure oxygen at greater than 1 standard atmosphere of pressure.

Purpose

Hyperbaric chambers are used to deliver hyperbaric **oxygen therapy** (HBOT). HBOT was developed

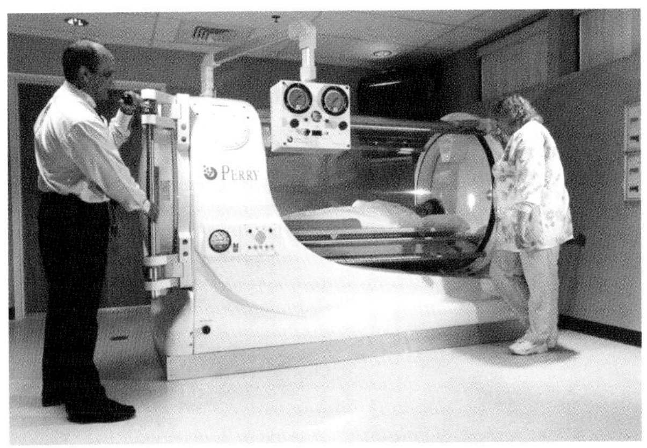

Patient lying in a hyperbaric chamber. *(© Chuck Mason/ Alamy.)*

to treat underwater divers suffering from **decompression sickness** (the bends). It has since been approved by the Undersea and Hyperbaric Medical Society for 13 conditions including:

- air or gas embolism
- carbon monoxide (CO) poisoning
- smoke inhalation
- gas gangrene caused by certain bacteria
- decompression sickness
- radiation tissue damage
- thermal burns
- non-healing skin grafts
- crush injuries
- wounds that fail to heal through conventional treatment
- serious blood loss
- intracranial abscess

Although hyperbaric therapy has become increasingly popular for other uses, especially in sports medicine, its use is controversial. Terrell Owens of the Philadelphia Eagles used HBOT for an ankle injury prior to playing in the Super Bowl in 2005, but medical professionals questioned the appropriateness of this treatment.

Precautions

Individuals who have lung disease, including **asthma**, **emphysema**, obstructive lung disease, or any condition in which air is trapped in the lungs, are poor candidates for this therapy and should discuss the relative benefits and drawbacks of HBOT with their doctor. Individuals who have had chest surgery or who have had a central venous catheter implanted are also at higher risk for complications. People with seizure disorders should be carefully monitored, as this treatment may increase the risk and severity of seizures. People with colds or clogged ears may want to wait to undergo HBOT, as they may experience difficulties with pressure equalization that can cause damage to the middle or inner ear. HBOT in **pregnancy** is controversial. Individuals with diabetes may need to adjust their glucose and insulin balance, since HBOT slows the absorption of insulin.

Description

At normal atmospheric pressure, oxygen binds with a molecule in red blood cells called hemoglobin. The oxygen is carried through the body to tissues where it is needed as the blood circulates. Under normal conditions, almost all (about 97%) of the available hemoglobin carries oxygen. Increasing the atmospheric pressure does little to increase the oxygen-carrying capacity of the blood. However, under normal conditions, only a small amount of oxygen is dissolved in the fluid that carries the red blood cells (blood plasma). Increasing the atmospheric pressure to two to three times normal and breathing 100% oxygen forces more oxygen to dissolve into the blood plasma. In this way, hyperbaric chambers increase the amount of oxygen circulating in the body. This can promote healing in areas that are not receiving adequate oxygen. The extra oxygen can also help to cure certain infections caused by anerobic bacteria that can live only in the absence of oxygen.

There are two types of hyperbaric chambers—monoplace and multiplace. Monoplace chambers accommodate a single person. The patient enters the chamber, then it is closed and the pressure is increased. The advantages of a monoplace chamber are that the patient does not have to wear a mask or a hood to receive the oxygen and the treatment regimen is designed specifically for each individual. The major disadvantages are that the patient is inaccessible to the staff during treatment should an emergency arise, and the pure oxygen atmosphere creates an increased fire hazard. In multiplace chambers, several patients use the same chamber simultaneously. Each person is given oxygen through a face mask or hood, but all patients receive the same treatment. A staff member remains in the chamber throughout the procedure.

Hyperbaric chambers can be associated with hospitals, but are increasingly part of free-standing clinics. Insurance may cover the cost of treatment for approved indications such as **carbon monoxide poisoning**, but may reject payment for uses that are considered experimental or controversial. The American Board of Medical Specialists certifies physician competency in the undersea medicine, including the use of hyperbaric chambers. The Baromedical Nurses Association offers three levels of certification for hyperbaric nurses, and the National Board of Hyperbaric Medicine Technology certifies hyperbaric technicians. Individuals considering hyperbaric therapy should seek facilities run by health care providers credentialed by these organizations.

Preparation

No special preparation is needed to use a hyperbaric chamber other than educating patients about what to expect during treatment.

Aftercare

After HBOT is complete, a period of decompression in the chamber is required until the pressure in the chamber is equal to the pressure outside. Serious complications can occur if decompression occurs suddenly.

Risks

Hyperbaric chambers, because of their use of 100% oxygen, present a potential fire risk. In addition, although hyperbaric oxygen therapy is very safe when used correctly, complications can occur. Oxygen **poisoning**, also called oxygen toxicity, can occur when an individual is exposed to high doses of oxygen for a prolonged period. Excess oxygen causes chemical changes in the body that negatively affect cells and metabolic processes. Symptoms of oxygen poisoning include **nausea**, **vomiting**, dry **cough**, seizures, chest **pain**, sweating, muscle twitching, ringing of the ears, **hallucinations**, **dizziness**, **shortness of breath** and a decreased level of consciousness.

Other complications can occur as the result of increased pressure within the chamber. These include pain and bloody discharge from congested sinuses, ear pain, rupture of the eardrum, and bleeding from the ear if the Eustachian tube that connects the ear to the back of the throat is clogged and pressure on either side of the eardrum is not equalized. Teeth that are infected or have been repaired may become painful or explode if gas is trapped within them. A few individuals develop **pneumothorax**. This is a serious condition where air is trapped between the lungs and the chest cavity.

Normal results

HBOT is expected to promote healing and improve the health of individuals with conditions for which it is approved.

Abnormal results

Under some conditions HBOT fails to cause improvement or complications occur.

Resources

OTHER

Moder, Cheryl. *Hyperbaric Oxygen Therapy: Where Medicine Meets the Deep Blue Sea*. February 20, 2005 [cited February 20, 2005]. http://www.emedicine.com/plastic/topic526.htm.

Neumeister, Michael. *Hyperbaric Oxygen Therapy*. November 11, 2004 [cited February 16, 2005]. http://www.emedicine.com/plastic/topic526.htm.

Prince, Mark. *Hyperbaric Oxygen*. October 27, 2004 [cited February 16, 2005]. http://www.emedicine.com/ent/topic733.htm.

ORGANIZATIONS

Undersea and Hyperbaric Medical Society, 21 West Colony Place, Suite 280, Durham, NC, 27705, (919) 490-5140, (919) 490-5149, (877) 533-UHMS (8467), uhms@uhms@org, http://www.uhms.org.

Tish Davidson, A. M.

Hyperbaric oxygenation *see* **Oxygen/ozone therapy**

Hyperbilirubinemia *see* **Neonatal jaundice**

Hypercalcemia

Definition

Hypercalcemia is an abnormally high level of **calcium** in the blood, usually more than 10.5 milligrams per deciliter of blood.

Description

Calcium plays an important role in the development and maintenance of bones in the body. It is also needed in tooth formation and is important in other body functions. Normally, the body maintains a balance between the amount of calcium in food sources and the calcium already available in the body's tissues. The balance can be upset if excess amounts of calcium are eaten or if the body is unable to process the mineral because of disease.

Calcium is one of the most important and most abundant **minerals** in the human body. Dairy products are the major source of calcium. Eggs, green leafy vegetables, broccoli, legumes, nuts, and whole grains provide smaller amounts. Only about 10–30% of the calcium in food is absorbed into the body. Most calcium is found in combination with other dietary components and must be broken down by the digestive system before it can be used. Calcium is absorbed into the body in the small intestine. Its absorption is influenced by such factors as the amount of vitamin D hormone available to aid the process and the levels of calcium already present in the body. As much as 99% of the body's calcium is stored in bone tissue. A healthy person experiences a constant turnover of calcium as bone tissue is built and reshaped. The remaining 1% of the body's calcium circulates in the blood and other body fluids. Circulating calcium plays an important role in the control of many body functions, such as blood clotting, transmission of nerve impulses, muscle contraction, and other metabolic activities. In the bloodstream, calcium maintains a constant balance with another mineral, phosphate.

Two main control agents are vital in maintaining calcium levels, vitamin D hormone and parathyroid hormone. A hormone is a chemical substance that is formed in one organ or part of the body and carried in the blood to another organ. It can alter the function, and sometimes the structure, of one or more organs.

- Parathyroid hormone (PTH). The four parathyroid glands are endocrine glands located next to the thyroid gland in the neck. A gland is a cell or group of cells that produces a material substance (secretion). When the level of calcium circulating in the blood drops, the parathyroid gland releases its hormone. PTH then acts in three ways to restore the normal blood calcium level. It stimulates the absorption of more calcium in the intestine; it takes more calcium from the bone tissue, and it causes the kidneys to excrete more phosphate.
- Vitamin D hormone. This hormone works with parathyroid hormone to control calcium absorption and affects the deposit of calcium and phosphate in the bone tissue.

The kidneys also help to control calcium levels. Healthy kidneys can increase calcium excretion almost fivefold to maintain normal concentrations in the body. Hypercalcemia can occur when the concentration of calcium overwhelms the ability of the kidneys to maintain balance.

Causes and symptoms

Causes of hypercalcemia

Many different conditions can cause hypercalcemia; the most common are **hyperparathyroidism** and **cancer**.

PRIMARY HYPERPARATHYROIDISM. Primary hyperparathyroidism is the excessive secretion of parathyroid hormone by one or more of the parathyroid glands. It is the most common cause of hypercalcemia in the general population. Women have this condition more frequently than men do, and it is more common in older people. It can appear 30 or more years after radiation treatments to the neck. Ninety percent of the cases of primary hyperparathyroidism are caused by a nonmalignant growth on the gland.

Hyperparathyroidism can also occur as part of a rare hereditary disease called multiple endocrine neoplasia. In this disease, tumors develop on the parathyroid gland.

CANCER. People with cancer often have hypercalcemia. In fact, it is the most common life-threatening metabolic disorder associated with cancer. Ten to 20 percent of all persons with cancer have hypercalcemia. Cancers of the breast, lung, head and neck, and kidney are frequently associated with hypercalcemia. It also occurs frequently in association with certain cancers of the blood, particularly malignant myeloma. It is seen most often in patients with tumors of the lung (25–35%) and breast (20–40%), according to the National Cancer Institute. Cancer causes hypercalcemia in two ways. When a tumor grows into the bone, it destroys bony tissue (osteolysis). When the bone is not involved, factors secreted by cancer cells can increase calcium levels (humoral hypercalcemia of malignancy). The two mechanisms may operate at the same time.

Because immobility causes an increase in the loss of calcium from bone, cancer patients who are weak and spend most of their time in bed are more prone to hypercalcemia. Cancer patients are often dehydrated because they take in inadequate amounts of food and fluids and often suffer from **nausea and vomiting**. **Dehydration** reduces the ability of the kidneys to remove excess calcium from the body. Hormones and **diuretics** that increase the amount of fluid released by the body can also trigger hypercalcemia.

OTHER CAUSES. Other conditions can cause hypercalcemia. Excessive intake of vitamin D increases intestinal absorption of calcium. During therapy for peptic ulcers, abnormally high amounts of calcium **antacids** are sometimes taken. Over use of antacids can cause milk-alkali syndrome and hypercalcemia. Diseases such as Paget's, in which bone is destroyed or reabsorbed, can also cause hypercalcemia. As in cancer or **paralysis** of the arms and legs, any condition in which the patient is immobilized for long periods of time can lead to hypercalcemia due to bone loss.

Common symptoms

Many patients with mild hypercalcemia have no symptoms and the condition is discovered during routine laboratory screening. Gastrointestinal symptoms include loss of appetite, **nausea**, **vomiting**, **constipation**, and abdominal **pain**. There may be a blockage in the bowel. If the kidneys are involved, the individual will have to urinate frequently during both the day and night and will be very thirsty. As the calcium levels rise, the symptoms become more serious. Stones may form in the kidneys and waste products can build up. Blood pressure rises. The heart rhythm may change. Muscles become increasingly weak. The individual may experience mood swings, confusion, **psychosis**, and eventually, **coma** and **death**.

Diagnosis

High levels of calcium in the blood are a good indication of hypercalcemia, but these levels may fluctuate. Calcium levels are influenced by other compounds in the blood that may combine with calcium. Higher calcium and lower phosphate levels may suggest primary hyperparathyroidism. The blood levels of protein (serum albumin) and parathyroid hormone (PTH) are also measured in the diagnosis of hypercalcemia. Too much PTH in the blood may indicate primary hyperparathyroidism. Levels of calcium and phosphate in the urine should also be measured. The medical history and physical condition of the individual must be taken into consideration, especially in the early stages of hypercalcemia when symptoms are mild.

Treatment

The treatment of hypercalcemia depends on how high the calcium level is and what is causing the elevation. Hypercalcemia can be life-threatening and rapid reduction may be necessary. If the patient has normal kidney function, fluids can be given by vein (intravenously) to clear the excess calcium. The amount of fluid taken in and eliminated must be carefully monitored. If the patient's kidneys are not working well, acute hemodyalysis is probably the safest and most effective method to reduce dangerous calcium levels. In this procedure, blood is circulated through tubes made of semi-permeable membranes against a special solution that filters out unwanted substances before returning the blood to the body.

Drugs such as furosemide, called loop diuretics, can be given after adequate fluid intake is established. These drugs inhibit calcium reabsorption in the kidneys and promote urine production. Drugs that inhibit bone loss, such as calcitonin, biphosphates, and plicamycin, are helpful in achieving long-term control. Phosphate pills help lower high calcium levels caused by a deficiency in phosphate. Anti-inflammatory agents such as **steroids** are helpful with some cancers and toxic levels of vitamin D.

Treatment of the underlying cause of the hypercalcemia will also correct the imbalance. Hyperparathyroidism is usually treated by surgical removal of one or more of the parathyroid glands and any tissue, other than the glands themselves, that is producing excessive amounts of the hormone.

The hypercalcemia caused by cancer is difficult to treat without controlling the cancer. Symptoms can be alleviated with fluids and drug therapy as outlined above.

Prognosis

Surgery to remove the parathyroid glands and any misplaced tissue that is producing excessive amounts of hormone succeeds in about 90% of all cases. Outcome is also influenced by whether any damage to the kidneys can be reversed.

Mild hypercalcemia can be controlled through good fluid intake and the use of effective drugs.

Hypercalcemia generally develops as a late complication of cancer and the expected outlook is grim without effective anticancer therapy.

Prevention

People with cancer who are at risk of developing hypercalcemia should be familiar with early symptoms and know when to see a doctor. Good fluid intake (up to four quarts of liquid a day if possible), controlling nausea and vomiting, paying attention to fevers, and keeping physically active as much as possible can help prevent problems. Dietary calcium restriction is not necessary because hypercalcemia reduces absorption of calcium in the intestine.

Resources

OTHER

"Hypercalcemia." *National Cancer Institute Page*. http://www.nci.nih.gov.

Karen Ericson, RN

Hypercholesterolemia

Definition

Hypercholesterolemia refers to levels of cholesterol in the blood that are higher than normal.

Description

Cholesterol circulates in the blood stream. It is an essential molecule for the human body. Cholesterol is a molecule from which hormones and **steroids** are made. It is also used to maintain nerve cells. Between 75 and 80% of the cholesterol that circulates in a person's bloodstream is made in that person's liver. The remainder is acquired from outside sources. Cholesterol is found in animal sources of food. It is not found in plants.

Normal blood cholesterol level is a number derived by laboratory analysis. A normal or desirable cholesterol level is defined as less than 200 mg of cholesterol per deciliter of blood (mg/dL). Blood cholesterol is considered to be borderline when it is in the range of 200 to 239 mg/dL. Elevated cholesterol level is 240 mg/dL or above. Elevated blood cholesterol is considered to be hypercholesterolemia.

Cholesterol has been divided into two major categories: low-density lipoprotein (LDL), the so-called "bad" cholesterol, and high-density lipoprotein (HDL), the so-called "good" cholesterol. Diet, **exercise**, **smoking**, alcohol, and certain illnesses can affect the levels of both types of cholesterol. Eating a high fat diet will increase one's level of LDL cholesterol. Exercising and reducing one's weight will both increase HDL cholesterol and lower LDL cholesterol.

The most common cause of elevated serum cholesterol is eating foods that are rich in saturated fats or contain high levels of cholesterol. Elevated cholesterol also can be caused by an underlying disease that raises blood cholesterol levels such as **diabetes mellitus**, **kidney disease**, **liver disease**, or **hypothyroidism**. It also can be caused by an inherited disorder in which cholesterol is not metabolized properly by the body. **Obesity**, which generally results from eating a diet high in fat, also can lead to elevated cholesterol levels in the blood. This is because obesity itself leads the body to produce excessive amounts of cholesterol.

Hypercholesterolemia increases the risk of heart disease. Elevated levels of circulating cholesterol cause deposits to form inside blood vessels. These deposits, called plaque, are composed of fats deposited from the bloodstream. When the deposits become sufficiently large, they block blood vessels and decrease the flow of blood. These deposits result in a disease process called **atherosclerosis**, which can cause **blood clots** to form that will ultimately stop blood flow. If this happens in the arteries supplying the heart, a **heart attack** will occur. If it happens in the brain, the result is a **stroke** where a portion of brain tissue dies. Atherosclerosis causes more deaths from heart disease than any other single condition. Heart disease has been the leading cause of **death** in the United States for the past half century.

There is a syndrome called familial hypercholesterolemia. Affected persons have consistently high levels of LDL. This leads to early clogging of the coronary arteries. In turn this leads to a heart attack. Among affected males, a first heart attack typically occurs in their 40s to 50s. Approximately 85% of men with this disorder have experienced a heart attack by the time they reach 60 years of age. The incidence of heart attacks among women with this disorder also is increased. However, it is delayed 10 years compared to men. The incidence of familial hypercholesterolemia is seven out of 1,000 people.

Causes and symptoms

Hypercholesterolemia is silent. There are no symptoms that are obvious to the naked eye. It is diagnosed by a blood test or after a heart attack or stroke occurs.

Diagnosis

Hypercholesterolemia is diagnosed by using a blood test. A blood specimen is obtained after the patient does not eat or drink anything (except water) for 12 hours. The **fasting** is done to measure the LDL and HDL cholesterol, which can only be determined accurately in a fasting state. Some experts agree that an acceptable limit for LDL cholesterol as 130 mg/dL, though the National Cholesterol Education Program Adult Treatment Panel III recommended a goal of less than 100mg/dL. Total cholesterol of under 200 mg/dL is thought to be an acceptable range.

Treatment

If an individual's cholesterol is elevated, discussions with a physician should be scheduled to determine what course of treatment may be needed. Initial treatment for hypercholesterolemia usually requires dietary changes to reduce the intake of total fat, saturated fat, and cholesterol. Most health care professionals will recommend that a person's weight and height be proportionate. In addition to diet, guidelines recommend exercise to help bring weight and cholesterol to acceptable levels. Further, experts counsel persons with elevated blood cholesterol levels to increase their intake of soluble fiber. Sources of soluble fiber include bran, foods containing whole grains and other sources of indigestible fiber such as lignin. Physicians also recommend that patients with high cholesterol stop smoking as part of first-line therapy for hypercholesterolemia.

The reason for treating elevated cholesterol is to reduce an individual's risk of complications. If a diet low in cholesterol and saturated fats doesn't significantly reduce a person's cholesterol level, medication may be required. For every 1 percent reduction in cholesterol level, the risk of heart disease is reduced by 2 percent. It also is possible to partially reverse atherosclerosis that has already occurred by aggressively lowering cholesterol levels with diet and medications.

Prescription drugs are available to help lower cholesterol levels in the blood. These may be used as first-line therapy in high-risk patients or after about three months of dietary and lifestyle therapy. Cholestyramine, cholestipol, lovastatin, simvastatin, pravastatin, fluvaststin, rosuvastatin, and gemfibrazol are some of the drugs approved for use in the United States. The most often prescribed group of drugs are the statins, which also have been shown in some studies to reduce risk of depression and **dementia**.

Alternative treatment

There are advocates of treatment using **vitamins**, **minerals** and antioxidant substances in relatively high amounts. These amounts generally exceed those provided by the Food and Drug Administration in its Minimum Daily Requirements (MDR). Advocates of such therapies also emphasize increased levels of exercise, attaining an ideal body weight and increasing levels of fiber in one's diet.

Some people have advocated the use of garlic, soy and isoflavones to lower serum cholesterol levels. In 2003, enriched green tea was found to be an effective addition to a low-fat diet for lowering LDL cholesterol in adults.

Prognosis

The prognos is in direct proportion to serum cholesterol levels. People with hypercholesterolemia are at high risk of dying from heart disease.

Many studies have looked at the relationship between elevated cholesterol levels, increased risk for heart attack and death. In one investigation of relatively young males who had no known heart disease, cholesterol levels were measured and participants were followed for six years. During this time, all heart attacks and deaths that occurred among participants were recorded. As serum cholesterol levels increased, so did the risk of experiencing a fatal heart attack. The risk of a fatal heart attack was approximately five times higher among persons having cholesterol levels of 300 mg/dL or more compared to those with cholesterol levels below 200 mg/dL.

The Framingham Heart Study is an ongoing research effort. Cholesterol levels, smoking habits, heart attack rates, and deaths in the population of an entire town have been recorded for over 40 years. After 30 years, more than 85% of persons with cholesterol levels of 180 mg/dL or less were still alive; almost a third of those with cholesterol levels greater than 260 mg/dL had died.

Prevention

Experts suggest the following steps to maintain serum cholesterol within normal limits: an important component is to maintain a normal weight for height and to reduce one's weight if it is inappropriate for height. Changing dietary habits by reducing the amount of fat and cholesterol consumed is advised. Doctors recommend avoiding smoking by not starting or quitting if currently a smoker. Increasing levels of fiber in the diet by including foods such as beans, raw fruits, whole grains and vegetables is receommended. It is important to exercise on a regular basis. Aerobic exercise is especially helpful in reducing serum cholesterol levels.

People from families with a strong history of early heart attacks should be evaluated with a lipid screen. Proper diet, exercise and the use of effective drugs can reduce serum lipid levels.

Nutrition and cardiac experts offer the following suggestions:

- purchasing low-fat or fat-free dairy products such as milk, cheese, sour cream, and yogurt
- eating lean red meats, chicken without skin, and fish
- reducing consumption of foods high in saturated fat such as french fries
- avoiding foods that are rich sources of cholesterol such as eggs, liver, cheese, and bacon
- eating smaller servings

- keeping a food journal and writing down everything eaten each day
- preparing food by microwaving, boiling, broiling, or baking food instead of frying
- trimming the fat from meat before cooking it.

Resources

BOOKS

Burke, Allen, and Fabio Tavora. *Practical Cardiovascular Pathology: An Atlas*. Philadelphia: Wolters Kluwer Health/Lippincott Williams & Wilkins, 2011.

Cecil, Russell L., Lee Goldman, and D. A. Audiello. *Cecil Medicine*. 23rd ed., Philadelphia: Saunders Elsevier, 2008.

Jennings, C. S., et al. *Preventive Cardiology: A Practical Manual*. Oxford, UK; New York: Oxford University Press, 2009.

Libby, Peter, et al. *Heart Disease: A Textbook of Cardiovascular Medicine*. 8th ed. Philadelphia: Elsevier/Saunders, 2008.

PERIODICALS

Aronow, Wilbert S. "Hypercholesterolemia: The Evidence Supports Use of Statins." *Geriatrics* August 2003: 18.

"Cholesterol-lowering Effect of Green Tea." *Nutraceuticals International* September 2003.

Jackson, P.R. "Cholesterol-lowering Therapy for Smokers." *The Lancet* 357, no. 9260 (2001): 960–961.

"Link to Cholesterol Drugs Disputed." *Cardiovascular Week* September 29, 2003: 73.

Mechcatie, Elizabeth. "FDA Okays Rosuvastatin for Hypercholeterolemia: Most Potent Statin to Date." *Internal Medicine News*. September 1, 2003: 30–31.

OTHER

American Academy of Family Practice. http://www.aafp.org/afp/20000201/675.html.

"Hyperlipidemia." American Heart Association. http://www.americanheart.org/presenter.jhtml?identifier=4600.

Merck Manual. http://www.merck.com/pubs/mmanual/section2/chapter15/15c.htm.

National Library of Medicine: http://www.nlm.nih.gov/medlineplus/ency/article/000403.htm.

ORGANIZATIONS

American Heart Association National Center, 7272 Greenville Avenue, Dallas, TX, 75231, (800) 242-8721, Review.personal.info@heart.org.

American Medical Association, 515 N. State St., Chicago, IL, 60654, (800) 621-8335, http://www.ama-assn.org/.

American Society of Nuclear Cardiology, 4550 Montgomery Ave., Suite 780 North, Bethesda, MD, 20814-3304, (301) 215-7575, (301) 215-7113, info@asnc.org, http://www.asnc.org.

L. Fleming Fallon, Jr., MD, DrPH
Teresa G. Odle

Hypercoagulation disorders

Definition

Hypercoagulation disorders (or hypercoagulable states or disorders) have the opposite effect of the more common **coagulation disorders**. In hypercoagulation, there is an increased tendency for clotting of the blood, which may put a patient at risk for obstruction of veins and arteries (phlebitis or **pulmonary embolism**).

Description

In normal hemostasis, or the stoppage of bleeding, clots form at the site of the blood vessel's injury. The difference between that sort of clotting and the clotting present in hypercoagulation is that these clots develop in circulating blood.

This disorder can cause clots throughout the body's blood vessels, sometimes creating a condition known as thrombosis. Thrombosis can lead to infarction, or **death** of tissue, as a result of blocked blood supply to the tissue. However, hypercoagulability does not always lead to thrombosis. In **pregnancy** and other hypercoagulable states, the incidence of thrombosis is higher than that of the general population, but is still under 10%. In association with certain genetic disorders, hypercoagulation disorders may be more likely to lead to thrombosis. Hypercoagulation disorders are also known as hyperhomocystinemia, antithrombin III deficiency, factor V leyden, and protein C or protein S deficiency.

Causes and symptoms

Hypercoagulation disorders may be acquired or hereditary. Some of the genetic disorders that lead to hypercoagulation are abnormal clotting factor V, variations in fibrinogen, and deficiencies in proteins C and S. Other body system diseases may lead to these disorders, including diabetes, sickle cell anemia, **congenital heart disease**, lupus, **thalassemia**, polycythemia rubra vera, and others.

Antithrombin III deficiency is a hereditary hypercoagulation disorder that affects both sexes. Symptoms include obstruction of a blood vessel by a clot (thromboembolic disease), vein inflammation (phlebitis), and ulcers of the lower parts of the legs.

The role of proteins C and S is a complex one. In order for coagulation to occur, platelets (small, round fragments in the blood) help contract blood vessels to

KEY TERMS

Blood clot—A thickening of the blood into a jelly-like substance that helps stop bleeding. Clotting of the blood within a blood vessel can lead to blockage of blood flow.

Embolism—The blockage of a blood vessel by air, blood clot, or other foreign body.

Embolus—An embolus is a clot that has formed in a blood vessel somewhere in the body, often in the heart. It can break away from the wall of the vessel where it was formed, travel through the circulatory system, and become wedged in the brain, causing an embolic stroke. Ischemic strokes can be caused by the formation of a blood clot in one of the cerebral arteries (arteries supplying blood to the brain). If the clot grows large enough it will block blood flow.

Plaque—A deposit, usually of fatty material, on the inside wall of a blood vessel.

Thrombosis—The formation or development of a blood clot or thrombus.

lessen blood loss and to help plug damaged blood vessels. The conversion of platelets into actual clots is a complicated web involving proteins that are identified clotting factors. The factors are carried in the plasma, or liquid portion of the blood. Proteins C and S are two of the clotting factors present in the plasma to help regulate or activate parts of the clotting process. Protein C is considered an anticoagulant. Mutation defects in the proteins may decrease their concentrations in the blood, and may or may not affect their resulting anticoagulant activity.

Factor V is an unstable clotting factor present in plasma. Abnormal factor V resists the changes that normally occur through the influence of protein C, which can also lead to hypercoagulability. Prothrombin, a glycoprotein that converts to thrombin in the early stage of the clotting process, is affected by the presence of these proteins, as well as other clotting factors.

Diagnosis

Examination

The diagnosis of hypercoagulation disorders is completed with a combination of **physical examination**, medical history, and blood tests. An accurate medical history is important to determine possible symptoms and causes of hypercoagulation disorders.

Tests

There are a number of blood tests that can determine the presence or absence of proteins, clotting factors, and platelet counts in the blood. Among the tests used to detect hypercoagulation is the Antithrombin III assay. Protein C and Protein S concentrations can be diagnosed with immunoassay or plasma antigen level tests.

Treatment

Warfarin (Coumadin) and heparin anticoagulants may be administered to reduce the clotting effects and maintain fluidity in the blood. Heparin is an anticoagulant that prevents thrombus formation and is used primarily for liver and lung clots. Heparin works right away, keeping **blood clots** from growing. It usually is injected. In recent years, more physicians have been prescribing low-molecular weight heparin, purified versions of the drug that can be given with less monitoring such as enoxaparin (Lovenox). Warfarin often is used for long-term treatment of blood clots and is taken orally. Patients must work closely with their physicians to constantly monitor its effects and adjust dose if necessary. Too little warfarin can lead to clotting, but too much can thin the blood so much that life-threatening bleeding can occur. The same can be true of low-molecular weight heparin when used on a long-term, at-home basis.

Prognosis

The prognosis for patients with hypercoagulation disorders varies depending on the severity of the clotting and thrombosis. If undetected and untreated, thrombosis could lead to recurrent thrombosis and pulmonary **embolism**, a potentially fatal problem.

Prevention

Hereditary hypercoagulation disorders may not be prevented. Genetic and blood testing may help determine a person's tendency to develop these disorders.

Resources

BOOKS

Lipsky, Martin S., et al. *American Medical Association Guide to Preventing and Treating Heart Disease: Essential Information You and Your Family Need to Know About Having a Healthy Heart*. Hoboken, NJ: Wiley, 2008.

Rokavec, Kathleen A. *The Hospital Book*. Raleigh, NC: lulu.com., 2009.

Wallach, Jacques. *Interpretation of Diagnostic Tests*. 8th ed. Philadelphia: Lippincott Williams & Wilkins, 2006.

Zimring, Michael P. *Healthy Travel: Don't Travel Without It!* Laguna Beach, CA: Basic Health Publications, 2009.

OTHER

Bren, Linda. "Travel: Avoiding Deep Vein Thrombosis (DVT)." *MedicineNet*. November 15, 2004. www.medicinenet.com/script/main/art.asp?articlekey=40582 (accessed October 10, 2010).

ORGANIZATIONS

American Heart Association, 7272 Greenville Ave., Dallas, TX, 75231, (301) 223-2307, (800) 242-8721, http://www.americanheart.org.

National Heart, Lung, and Blood Institute, P.O. Box 30105, Bethesda, MD, 20824-0105, (301) 592-8573, (204) 629-3246, nhlbiinfo@nhlbi.nih.gov, http://www.nhlbi.nih.gov.

National Hemophilia Foundation, 116 West 32nd St., 11th Floor, New York, NY, 10001, (800) 424-2634, http://www.hemophilia.org.

Teresa G. Odle
Laura Jean Cataldo, RN, EdD

Hyperemesis gravidarum

Definition

Hyperemesis gravidarum means excessive **vomiting** during **pregnancy**.

Description

In pregnant women, **nausea and vomiting** (morning sickness) are common, affecting up to 80% of pregnancies. Hyperemesis, or extreme nausea and excessive vomiting, occur in about 1% of pregnancies. This condition causes uncontrollable vomiting, severe **dehydration**, and weight loss for the mother. However, hyperemesis gravidarum rarely causes problems for the unborn baby.

Causes and symptoms

The cause of nausea and vomiting during pregnancy is unknown but may be related to the level of certain hormones produced during pregnancy. Hyperemesis is seen more often in first pregnancies and multiple pregnancies (twins, triplets, etc.). The main symptom of hyperemesis is severe vomiting, which causes dehydration and weight loss.

Diagnosis

Although many women with morning sickness feel like they are vomiting everything they eat, they continue to gain weight and are not dehydrated; they do not have hyperemesis gravidarum. Women with this condition will start to show signs of **starvation**, including weight loss. **Physical examination** and laboratory tests of blood and urine samples will be used to help diagnose the condition. One of the most common tests used to help diagnosis and monitor hyperemesis gravidarum is a test for ketones in the urine. Excessive ketones in the urine (ketonuria) indicate that the body is not using carbohydrates from food as fuel and is inadequately trying to break down fat as fuel. Ketonuria is a sign that the body is beginning to operate in starvation mode.

Treatment

Hospitalization is often required. Intravenous fluids with substances that help the body conduct nerve signals (electrolytes) may be given to correct the dehydration and excessive acid in the blood (acidosis). Anti-nausea or sedative medications may be given by injection to stop the vomiting. In some cases, oral medication may be prescribed to control the nausea and vomiting while food is reintroduced. If food cannot be tolerated at all, intravenous **nutritional supplements** may be necessary. Injections of vitamin B_6, in particular, may help overcome nutritional deficiencies that often occur.

Alternative treatment

The severe vomiting associated with hyperemesis gravidarum requires medical attention. Milder episodes of nausea or vomiting may be reduced with deep breathing and relaxation exercises. The use of herbal remedies should be done with extreme caution during pregnancy, especially in the first trimester. Natural remedies to reduce nausea include a teaspoon of cider vinegar in a cup of warm water, or tea made from anise (*Pinpinella anisum*), fennel seed (*Foeniculum vulgare*), red raspberry (*Rubus idaeus*), or ginger (*Zingiber officinale*). Wristbands can be positioned over **acupressure** points on both wrists. **Aromatherapy** with lavender, rose, or chamomile can be soothing, as can smelling ground ginger. Homeopathic remedies—which use extremely diluted solutions as treatments—can be safe and effective for controlling symptoms in some women.

Prognosis

In virtually all cases, the pregnancy can continue to the successful delivery of a healthy baby.

Prevention

Although there is no evidence that hyperemesis gravidarum can be prevented, vomiting during pregnancy sometimes may be lessened. Maintaining a healthy diet, getting adequate sleep, and controlling **stress** may contribute to prevention or improvement of symptoms. Several strategies may help lessen the nausea and vomiting. Eating dry foods and limiting fluid intake may also be helpful. Small meals should be eaten frequently throughout the day, with a protein snack at night. Eating soda crackers before rising from bed in the morning may help prevent early morning nausea. Iron supplements may cause nausea and can be eliminated until the nausea is controlled. Sitting upright for 45 minutes after meals may also help.

Resources

OTHER

Levy, B. T., and P. L. Brown. "Nausea and Vomiting in Pregnancy." *The Virtual Hospital Page*. University of Iowa. http://www.vh.org.

"Natural Remedies During Pregnancy: Frequently Asked Questions." *Childbirth.Org*. http://www.childbirth.org/articles/remedy.html.

Altha Roberts Edgren

Hyperhidrosis

Definition

Hyperhidrosis is a disorder marked by excessive sweating. It usually begins at **puberty** and affects the palms, soles, and armpits.

Description

Sweating is the body's way of cooling itself and is a normal response to a hot environment or intense **exercise**. Excessive sweating unrelated to these conditions can be a problem for some people. Those with constantly moist hands may feel uncomfortable shaking hands or touching, while others with sweaty armpits and feet may have to contend with the unpleasant odor that results from the bacterial breakdown of sweat and cellular debris (bromhidrosis). People with hyperhidrosis often must change their clothes at least once a day, and their shoes can be ruined by the excess moisture. Hyperhidrosis may contribute to such skin diseases as **athlete's foot** (tinea pedis) and **contact dermatitis**.

In addition to excessive sweat production, the texture and color of the skin itself may be affected by hyperhidrosis. The skin may turn pink or bluish white. Severe hyperhidrosis of the soles of the feet may produce cracks, fissures, and scaling of the skin.

Hyperhidrosis in general and axillary hyperhidrosis (excessive sweating in the armpits) in particular are more common in the general population than was previously thought. A group of dermatologists in Virginia reported in 2004 that 2.8% of the United States population, or about 7.8 million persons, have hyperhidrosis. Of this group, slightly more than half (4 million persons) have axillary hyperhidrosis. One-third of the latter group, or about 1.3 million persons, find that the condition significantly interferes with daily activities and is barely tolerable. Only 38% had ever discussed their excessive sweating with their doctor.

Causes and symptoms

There are three basic forms of hyperhidrosis: emotionally induced; localized; and generalized. Emotionally induced hyperhidrosis typically affects the palms of the hands, soles of the feet, and the armpits. Localized hyperhidrosis typically affects the palms, armpits, groin, face, and the area below the breasts in women, while generalized hyperhidrosis may affect the entire body.

Hyperhidrosis may be either idiopathic (of unknown cause) or secondary to **fever**, metabolic disorders, **alcoholism**, **menopause**, **Hodgkin's lymphoma**, **tuberculosis**, various types of **cancer**, or the use of certain medications. The medications most commonly associated with hyperhidrosis are propranolol, venlafaxine, **tricyclic antidepressants**, pilocarpine, and physostigmine.

Most cases of hyperhidrosis begin during childhood or adolescence. Hyperhidrosis that begins in adult life should prompt the doctor to look for a systemic illness, medication side effect, or metabolic disorder.

Hyperhidrosis affects both sexes equally and may occur in any age group. People of any race may be affected; however, for some unknown reason, Japanese are affected 20 times more frequently than members of other ethnic groups.

Diagnosis

Hyperhidrosis is diagnosed by patient report and a **physical examination**. In many cases the physician can directly observe the excessive sweating.

Tests

The doctor may perform an iodine starch test, which involves spraying the affected areas of the patient's body with a mixture of 500 g of water-soluble

KEY TERMS

Dermatitis—A skin condition characterized by a red, itchy rash. It may occur when the skin comes in contact with something to which it is sensitive.

starch and 1 g iodine crystals. Areas of the skin producing sweat turn black.

The doctor will order other laboratory or imaging tests if he or she suspects that the sweating is associated with another disease or disorder.

Treatment

Most over-the-counter antiperspirants are not strong enough to effectively prevent hyperhidrosis. To treat the disorder, doctors prescribe 20% aluminum chloride hexahydrate solution (Drysol). It is applied at night to the affected areas and then wrapped in a plastic film until morning. Drysol works by blocking the sweat pores. Formaldehyde and glutaraldehyde-based solutions can also be prescribed; however, formaldehyde may trigger an allergic reaction and glutaraldehyde can stain the skin (for this reason it is primarily applied to the soles).

Drugs

Anticholinergic drugs may be given. These drugs include such medications as propantheline, oxybutynin, and benztropine.

Injections of botulinum toxin (Botox) under the skin work well for some patients. Botox works to stop the excessive sweating by preventing the transmission of nerve impulses to the sweat glands. These injections must be repeated every 4–12 months.

Alternative

An electrical device that emits low-voltage current can be held against the skin to reduce sweating. These treatments are usually conducted in a doctor's office on a daily basis for several weeks, followed by weekly visits. Dermatologists recommend that patients wear clothing made of natural or absorbent fabrics, avoid high-buttoned collars, use talc or cornstarch, and keep underarms shaved.

The only permanent cure for hyperhidrosis of the palms is a surgical procedure known as a **sympathectomy**. To treat severe excessive sweating, a surgeon can remove a portion of the nerve near the top of the spine that controls palm sweat. Few neurosurgeons in the United States will perform the procedure because it often results in compensatory sweating in other regions of the body. Alternatively, it is possible to surgically remove the sweat gland-bearing skin of the armpits, but this is a major procedure that may require skin grafts.

More recently, **liposuction** under the armpits has been successfully used to treat hyperhidrosis in this region of the body. The liposuction removes some of the excess sweat glands responsible for axillary hyperhidrosis. The procedure also has the advantage of leaving smaller **scars** and being less disruptive to the overlying skin.

Prognosis

Hyperhidrosis is not associated with increased mortality; it primarily affects the patient's quality of life rather than longevity. While the condition cannot be cured without radical surgery, it can usually be controlled effectively.

Resources

BOOKS

Mooney, Jean. *Illustrated Dictionary of Podiatry and Foot Science*. St Louis: Churchill Livingstone Elsevier, 2009.

Willoughby, William Franklin. *Regulation of the Sweating System*. New York: Nabu Press, 2010.

PERIODICALS

Licht, P.B., and H.K. Pilegaard. "Severity of Compensatory Sweating after Thoracoscopic Sympathectomy." *Annals of Thoracic Surgery* 78 (August 2004): 427–431.

Strutton, D.R., J.W. Kowalski, D.A. Glaser, and P.E. Stang. "U.S. Prevalence of Hyperhidrosis and Impact on Individuals with Axillary Hyperhidrosis: Results from a National Survey." *Journal of the American Academy of Dermatology* 51 (August 2004): 241–248.

OTHER

Altman, Rachel, and Robert Schwartz. "Hyperhidrosis." *eMedicine*. March 12, 2010. http://emedicine.medscape.com/article/1073359-overview (accessed October 10, 2010).

ORGANIZATIONS

American Academy of Dermatology (AAD), P.O. Box 4014, Schaumburg, IL, 60168-4014, (847) 330-0230, http://www.aad.org.

Carol A. Turkington
Rebecca J. Frey, PhD
Laura Jean Cataldo, RN, EdD

Hyperhomocystinemia *see* **Hypercoagulation disorders**

Hypericum perforatum see **St. Johns wort**

Hyperkalemia

Definition

Hyperkalemia refers to serum or plasma levels of potassium ions above 5.5 mEq/L. The concentration of potassium is often expressed in units of milliequivalents per liter (mEq/L). The normal concentration of potassium in the serum is in the range of 3.5–5.0 mEq/L.

Description

A normal adult who weighs about 150 lb (70 kg) contains a total of about 3,500 mEq of potassium stores in the body. Most of this potassium (about 98%) occurs inside various cells (intracellular) and organs, where its concentration is about 150 mEq/L. This level is in contrast to the much lower concentration found in the blood serum, where only about 0.4% of the body's potassium resides. Hyperkalemia can be caused by an overall excess of body potassium, or by a shift from inside to outside cells. For example, hyperkalemia can be caused by the sudden release of potassium ions from muscle into the surrounding fluids.

In a normal person, hyperkalemia from too much potassium in the diet is prevented by at least three types of regulatory processes. First, various cells and organs act to prevent hyperkalemia by taking up potassium from the blood. It is also prevented by the action of the kidneys, which excrete potassium into the urine. A third protective mechanism is **vomiting**. Consumption of a large dose of potassium ions, such as potassium chloride, induces a vomiting reflex to expel most of the potassium before it can be absorbed.

Causes and symptoms

Hyperkalemia can occur from a variety of causes, including the consumption of too much of a potassium salt; failure of the kidneys to normally excrete potassium ions into the urine; leakage of potassium from cells and tissues into the bloodstream; and from acidosis. The most common cause of hyperkalemia is kidney (or renal) disease, which accounts for about three-quarters of all cases. Kidney function is measured by the glomerular filtration rate, the rate at which each kidney performs its continual processing and cleansing of blood. The normal glomerular filtration rate is about 100 mL/min. If the kidney is damaged so that the glomerular filtration rate is only 5 mL/min or less, hyperkalemia may result, especially if high-potassium foods are consumed. The elderly are at particular risk, since many regulatory functions of the body may not work as efficiently in this population. Elderly patients who are being treated with certain drugs for high blood pressure, such as spironolactone (Aldactone) and triamterene (Dyazide), must be monitored for possible hyperkalemia as these medications promote the retention of potassium by the kidneys.

Hyperkalemia can also be caused by a disease of the adrenal gland called **Addison's disease**. The adrenal gland produces the hormone aldosterone that promotes the excretion of potassium into the urine by the kidney.

Injury to muscle or other tissues, including severe **burns** or infections, can also lead to hyperkalemia. Since most of the potassium in the body is contained in muscle, a severe trauma that crushes muscle cells results in an immediate increase in the concentration of potassium in the blood.

Acidic blood plasma, or acidosis, is an occasional cause of hyperkalemia. Acidosis, which occurs in a number of diseases, is defined as an increase in the concentration of hydrogen ions in the bloodstream. In the body's attempt to correct the situation, hydrogen is taken up by muscle cells out of the blood in an exchange mechanism involving the transfer of potassium ions into the bloodstream. This can abnormally elevate the plasma's concentration of potassium ions. When acidosis is the cause of hyperkalemia, treating the patient for acidosis has two benefits: a reversal of both the acidosis and the hyperkalemia.

Symptoms of mild to moderate hyperkalemia are often vague. Many cases of hyperkalemia are discovered incidentally as a result of routine blood laboratory testing. Heart abnormalities of mild hyperkalemia (5.5 to 6.0 mEq/L potassium) can be detected by an electrocardiogram (ECG or EKG). With severe hyperkalemia (over 7.0 mEq/L potassium), the heart may beat at a dangerously rapid rate (fibrillation) or stop beating entirely (cardiac arrest). Patients with moderate or severe hyperkalemia may also develop nervous system symptoms such as **tingling** of the skin, **numbness** of the hands or feet, weakness, or a flaccid **paralysis**, which is characteristic of both hyperkalemia and **hypokalemia** (low plasma potassium).

Diagnosis

The patient's medical history is often an invaluable tool in helping to diagnose hyperkalemia. A history of kidney problems, trauma that involves crushing injuries, burns, consumption of medications that cause the body to retain potassium, and/or consumption of high potassium foods, particularly if kidney function is impaired, may prompt a diagnosis of hyperkalemia.

KEY TERMS

Acidosis—A medical condition caused by an increase in the concentration of hydrogen ions in the blood. The result of this increase is a lowered (acidic) blood pH level.

Potassium—A chemical element; also referred to as an electrolyte, which is predominantly found inside cells of the body (intracellular). Small changes in potassium levels can have pronounced effects on the cardiovascular and neuromuscular systems.

Tests

Hyperkalemia can be measured by acquiring a sample of blood to measure the concentration of potassium ions in the bloodstream.

Procedures

Since high or low potassium levels result in abnormalities in heart function, an electrocardiogram is usually the method of choice for the diagnosis of both hyperkalemia and hypokalemia. Specific EKG changes often correlate with the level of hyperkalemia.

Treatment

Traditional

Patients with severe or symptomatic hyperkalemia should be have intravenous access initiated, should be placed on a cardiac monitor for observation of EKG changes, and should be admitted to an intensive care unit (ICU) for continuous observation and treatment to quickly lower potassium levels.

Drugs

If life-threatening EKG abnormalities are noted, a rapid reduction in potassium levels can be achieved by treatment with **electrolyte supplementscalcium** chloride or calcium gluconate. Onset of action is typically within five minutes. Patients receiving this treatment should be monitored continually by means of a cardiac monitor.

Insulin injections are used to treat hyperkalemia in emergency situations. Insulin is a hormone well-known for its ability to stimulate the entry of sugar (glucose) into cells. It also provokes the uptake of potassium ions by cells, decreasing potassium ion concentration in the blood. When insulin is used to treat hyperkalemia, glucose is also injected. Serum potassium levels begin to decline within 30 to 60 minutes and remain low for several hours.

In non-emergency situations, hyperkalemia can be treated with a low potassium diet in some individuals. If this does not succeed, the patient can be given a special resin to bind potassium ions. One such resin, **sodium** polystyrene sulfonate (Kayexalate), remains in the intestines where it absorbs potassium and forms a complex of resin and potassium. This complex is excreted in the feces. A typical dose of resin is 15 g, taken one to four times per day. The correction of hyperkalemia with resin treatment takes at least 24 hours. However, recent research seems to indicate that use of sodium polystyrene sulfonate to treat hyperkalemia may not as effective as once thought in lowering potassium levels and may increase risk for necrosis in the large intestine.

Prognosis

The prognosis for specifically correcting hyperkalemia is excellent. However, hyperkalemia is usually caused by kidney failure, an often irreversible and eventually fatal condition.

Prevention

Most healthy people are not at risk for hyperkalemia. Patients with renal disease and those on certain diuretic medications must be monitored to prevent its occurrence.

Resources

PERIODICALS

Einhorn, L.M., et al. "The Frequency of Hyperkalemia and its Significance in Chronic Kidney Disease." *Archives of Internal Medicine* 169, no. 12 (June 22, 2009): 1156–62.

Khanna, A., and W.B. White. "The Management of Hyperkalemia in Patients with Cardiovascular Disease." *American Journal of Medicine* 122, no. 3 (March 2009): 215–21.

Sterns, R.H., et al. "Ion-exchange Resins for the Treatment of Hyperkalemia: Are They Safe and Effective?" *Journal of the American Society of Nephrology* 21, no. 5 (May 2010): 733–5.

Weisberg, L.S. "Management of Severe Hyperkalemia." *Critical Care Medicine* 36, no. 12 (December 2008): 3246–51.

OTHER

Garth, David. "Hyperkalemia." *eMedicine*. July 16, 2010. http://www.emedicine.medscape.com/article/766479-overview (accessed October 6, 2010).

Tom Brody, PhD
Melinda Granger Oberleitner
RN, DNS, APRN, CNS

Hyperkinetic disorder *see* **Attention-deficit/ Hyperactivity disorder (ADHD)**

Hyperlipemia *see* **Hyperlipoproteinemia**

Hyperlipidemia *see* **Hyperlipoproteinemia**

Hyperlipoproteinemia

Definition

Hyperlipoproteinemia occurs when there is too much lipid (fat) in the blood. Shorter terms that mean the same thing are hyperlipidemia and hyperlipemia. Dyslipidemia refers to a redistribution of cholesterol from one place to another that increases the risk of **vascular disease** without increasing the total amount of cholesterol. When more precise terms are needed, **hypercholesterolemia** and hypertriglyceridemia are used.

Description

It is commonly known that oil and water do not mix unless another substance like a detergent is added. Yet the body needs to transport both lipids (fats) and water-based blood within a single circulatory system. There must be a way to mix the two so that essential fatty nutrients can be transported in the blood and so that fatty waste products can be carried away from tissues. The solution is to combine the lipids with protein to form water-soluble packages that can be transported in the blood.

These packages of fats are called lipoproteins. They are a complex mixture of **triglycerides**, cholesterol, phospholipids, and special proteins. Some of these chemicals are fatty nutrients absorbed from the intestines on their way to being made part of the body. Cholesterol is a waste product on its way out of the body through the liver, the bile, and ultimately the bowel for excretion. The proteins and phospholipids make the packages water-soluble.

There are five different sizes of these chemical packages. Each package needs all four chemicals in it to hold everything in solution. They differ in how much of each they contain. If blood serum is spun very rapidly in an ultracentrifuge, these five packages will layer out according to their density. They have, therefore, been named according to their densities—high-density lipoproteins (HDL), low-density lipoproteins (LDL), intermediate-density lipoproteins (IDL), very low density lipoproteins (VLDL), and chylomicrons. Only the HDLs and the LDLs will be discussed in the rest of this article.

If there is not enough detergent in the laundry, the oily stains will remain in the clothes. In the same way, if the balance of chemicals in these packages is not right, cholesterol will stay in tissues rather than being excreted from the body. What is even worse, if the chemical composition of these packages changes, the cholesterol can fall out of the blood and stay where it lands. On the other hand, a different change in the balance can remove cholesterol from tissues where there is too much. This appears to be exactly what is going on in **atherosclerosis**. The lesions contain lots of cholesterol.

The LDLs are overloaded with cholesterol. A minor change in the other chemicals in this package will leave cholesterol behind. The HDLs have a third to a half as much cholesterol. They seem to be able to pick up cholesterol left behind by the LDLs. It seems that atherosclerosis begins with tiny tears at stressed places in the walls of the arteries. Low density lipoproteins from the blood enter these tears, where their chemistry changes enough to leave cholesterol behind. The cholesterol causes irritation; the body responds with inflammation; damage and scarring follow. Eventually the artery gets so diseased blood cannot flow through it. Strokes and heart attacks are the result.

However, if there are lots of HDLs in the blood, the cholesterol is rapidly picked up and not allowed to cause problems. Women before **menopause** have estrogen (the female hormone), which encourages the formation of HDLs. This is the reason they have so little vascular disease and why they rapidly catch up to men after menopause, when estrogen levels fall. Replacement of estrogen after menopause has been prescribed for protection through the later years. However, in 2003, the Women's Health Initiative, a large clinical trial involving postmenopausal women, was halted in July 2002 because of the many detrimental effects of combined estrogen and progesterone therapy (called **hormone replacement therapy**). Among the effects was increased risk of heart disease, sometimes within the first year of use.

Cholesterol is the root of the problem, but like any other root it cannot just be eliminated. Ninety percent of the cholesterol in the body is created there as a waste product of necessary processes. The solution lies in getting it out to the body without clogging the arteries.

Of course the story is much more complex. The body has dozens of chemical processes that make up, break down, and reconfigure all these chemicals. It is these processes that are the targets of intervention in the effort to cure vascular disease.

Diseases

Near the dawn of concern over cholesterol and vascular disease a family of hereditary diseases was identified, all of which produced abnormal quantities of blood fats. These diseases were called dyslipoproteinemias and came in both too many and too little varieties. The hyperlipoproteinemias found their way into five categories, depending on which chemical was in excess.

- Type 1 has a pure elevation of triglycerides in the chylomicron fraction. These people sometimes get pancreatitis and abdominal pains, but they do not seem to have an increase in vascular disease.
- Type 2 appears in two distinct genetic patterns and a third category, which is by far the most important kind, because everyone is at risk for it. All Type 2s have elevated cholesterol. Some have elevated triglycerides also. The familial (genetic) versions of Type 2 often develop xanthomas, which are yellow fatty deposits under the skin of the knuckles, elbows, buttocks or heels. They also may have xanthelasmas, smaller yellow patches on the eyelids.
- Type 3 appears in one in 10,000 people and elevates both triglycerides and cholesterol with consequent vascular disease. In 2003, researchers discovered the molecular mechanism that contributes to high triglycerides in those with this type of hyperlipopoproteinemia.
- Type 4 elevates only triglycerides and does not increase the risk of vascular disease.
- Type 5 is similar to Type 1.
- Dyslipidemia refers to a normal amount of cholesterol that is mostly in LDLs, where it causes problems.

All but Type 2 are rare and of interest primarily because they give insight into the chemistry of blood fats.

In addition to the above genetic causes of blood fat disorders, a number of acquired conditions can raise lipoprotein levels:

- Diabetes mellitus, because it alters the way the body handles its energy needs, and also affects the way it handles fats. The result is elevated triglycerides and reduced HDL cholesterol. This effect is amplified by obesity.
- Hypothyroidism is a common cause of lipid abnormalities. The thyroid hormone affects the rate of many chemical processes in the body, including the clearing of fats from the blood. The consequence usually is an elevation of cholesterol.
- Kidney disease affects the blood's proteins and consequently the composition of the fat packages. It usually raises the LDLs.
- Liver disease, depending on its stage and severity, can raise or lower any of the blood fats.
- Alcohol raises triglycerides. In moderate amounts (if they are very moderate) it raises HDLs and can be beneficial.
- Cigarette smoking lowers HDL cholesterol, as does malnutrition and obesity.

Certain medications elevate blood fat levels. Because some of these medications are used to treat heart disease, it has been necessary to reevaluate their usefulness:

- Thiazides, water pills used to treat high blood pressure, can raise both cholesterol and triglycerides.
- Beta-blockers, another class of medication used to treat high blood pressure, cortisone-like drugs, and estrogen can raise triglycerides.
- Progesterone, the pregnancy hormone, raises cholesterol.

Not all of these effects are necessarily bad, nor are they necessarily even significant. For instance, estrogen is clearly beneficial. Each effect must be considered in the overall goal of treatment.

Causes and symptoms

A combination of heredity and diet is responsible for the majority of fat disorders. It is not so much the cholesterol in the diet that is the problem, because that accounts for only 10% of the body's store. It is the other fats in the diet that alter the way the body handles its cholesterol. There is a convincing relation between fats in the diet and the incidence of atherosclerosis. The guilty fats are mostly the animal fats, but palm and coconut oil also are harmful. These fats are called saturated fats for the chemical reason that most of their carbon atoms have as many hydrogen atoms attached as they can accommodate. More important than the kind of fat is the amount of fat. For many people, fat is half of their diet. One-fifth to one-fourth is a much healthier fraction, the rest of the diet being made up of complex carbohydrates and protein.

This disease is silent for decades, until the first episode of heart disease or **stroke**.

Diagnosis

It would be easier if simple cholesterol and triglyceride tests were all it took to assess the risk of atherosclerosis. However, the important information is which package the cholesterol is in—the LDLs or the HDLs. That takes a more elaborate testing process. To complicate matters further, the amount of fats in the blood varies greatly in relation to the last meal—how long ago it was and what kind of food was eaten. A true estimate of the risk comes from several tests several weeks apart, each done after at least 12 hours of **fasting**.

Treatment

Diet and lifestyle change are the primary focus for most cholesterol problems. It is a mistake to think that a pill will reverse the effects of a bad diet, **obesity**, **smoking**, excess alcohol, **stress**, and inactivity. Reducing the amount of fat in the diet by at least half is the most important move to make. Much of the food eaten to satisfy a "sweet tooth" is higher in fat than in sugar. A switch away from saturated fats is the next step, but the rush to polyunsaturated fats was ill-conceived. These, particularly the hydrogenated fats in margarine, have problems of their own. They raise the risk of **cancer** and are considered more dangerous than animal fat by many experts. Theory supports population studies that suggest monounsaturated olive oil may be the healthiest of all.

There was a tremendous push at the end of the 20th century to use lipid-lowering medications. The most popular and most expensive agents, the "statins," hinder the body's production of cholesterol and sometimes damage the liver as a side effect. Their full name is 3-hydroxy-3-methylglutaryl-coemzyme A *(HMG-CoA)* reductase inhibitors. Their generic names are cervistatin, fluvastatin, lovastatin, pravastatin, simvastatin, and the newest and most powerful as of 2010, rosuvastatin. Studies show that these drugs lower cholesterol. Only recently, though, has any evidence appeared that this affects health and longevity. Earlier studies showed, in fact, an increased **death** rate among users of the first class of lipid-altering agents—the fibric acid derivatives. The chain of events connecting raised HDL and lowered LDL cholesterol to longer, healthier lives is still to be forged.

High-tech methods of rapidly reducing very high blood fat levels are performed for those rare disorders that require it. There are resins that bind cholesterol in the intestines. They taste awful, feel like glue and routinely cause gas, bloating, and **constipation**. For acute cases, there is a filtering system that takes fats directly out of the blood.

Niacin (nicotinic acid) lowers cholesterol effectively and was the first medication proven to improve overall life expectancy. It also can be liver toxic, and the usual formulation causes a hot flash in many people. This can be overcome by taking a couple of aspirins 30 minutes before the niacin, or by taking a special preparation called "flush free," "inositol-bound" or inositol hexanicotinate.

Alternative treatment

Omega-3 oil is a special kind found mostly in certain kinds of fish. It is beneficial in lowering cholesterol. An herbal alternative called guggulipid, *Commiphora mukul*, an extract of an Indian plant, has been touted as working the same way as the expensive and liver toxic cholesterol-lowering medications. However, a 2003 clinical trial found that the supplement did not meet these claims. In fact, guggul did not lower total cholesterol, LDL cholesterol, or triglycerides. Most patients tolerated the supplement, but some developed a hypersensitivity rash.

To lower cholesterol, **naturopathic medicine**, **traditional Chinese medicine**, and **ayurvedic medicine** may be considered. Some herbal therapies include alfalfa (*Medicago sativa*), Asian **ginseng** (*Panax ginseng*), and fenugreek (*Trigonella foenum-graecum*). Garlic (*Allium sativum*) and onions are also reported to have cholesterol-lowering effects. In naturopathic medicine, the liver is considered to be an organ that needs cleansing and rebalancing. The liver often is treated with a botanical formula that will act as a bitter to stimulate bile flow in the liver. Before initiating alternative therapies, medical consultation is strongly advised.

Prognosis

The prognosis is good for Type 1 hyperlipoproteinemia with treatment; without treatment, death may result. For Type 2 the prognosis is poor even with treatment. The prognosis for Type 3 is good when the prescribed diet is strictly followed. For Types 4 and 5 the prognosis is uncertain, due to the risk of developing premature **coronary artery disease** and **pancreatitis**, respectively.

Prevention

Genetic inheritance cannot be changed, but its effects may be modified with proper treatment. Family members of an individual with hyperlipoproteinemia should consider having their blood lipids assessed. The sooner any problems are identified, the better the chances of limiting or preventing the associated health risks. Anyone with a family history of disorders leading to hyperlipoproteinemia also may benefit from **genetic testing** and counseling to assist them in making reproductive decisions.

Resources

PERIODICALS

Brunk, Doug. "Three Studies Further Confirm Ill Effects of HRT: Heart Disease Risk Rises First Year of Use:

Continuing Analysis of WHI Data." *Family Practice News* 33, no. 17 (September 1, 2003): 1–2.
Dowhower Karpa, Kelly. "New Statin Said to be More Powerful than Others." *Drug Topics* 147, no. 17 (September 1, 2003): 27.
"Herbal Extract Not Effective in Treating High Cholesterol." *Drug Week* August 29, 2003: 197.
Kyperos, Kyriakos E., et al. "Molecular Mechanisms of Type III Hyperlipoproteinemia: the Contribution of the Carboxy-terminal Domain of ApoE Can Account for the Dyslipidemia that is Associated With the E2/E2 Phenotype." *Biochemistry* 42, no. 33 (August 26, 2003): 9841–9853.

J. Ricker Polsdorfer, MD
Teresa G. Odle

Hypermagnesemia *see* **Magnesium imbalance**

Hypermenorrhea *see* **Dysfunctional uterine bleeding**

Hypermetropia *see* **Hyperopia**

Hypernatremia

Definition

The normal concentration of **sodium** in the blood plasma is 136–145 mEq/L. Hypernatremia is defined as a serum sodium level over 145 mEq/L. Severe hypernatremia, with serum sodium above 152 mEq/L, is a rare disorder in patients with an intact thirst response that can result in seizures and **death** if left untreated.

Description

Sodium is an atom, or ion, that carries a single positive charge. The sodium ion may be abbreviated as Na^+ or as simply Na. Sodium can occur as a salt in a crystalline solid. Sodium chloride (NaCl), sodium phosphate (Na_2HPO_4) and sodium bicarbonate ($NaHCO_3$) are commonly occurring salts. These salts can be dissolved in water or in juices of various foods. Dissolving involves the complete separation of ions, such as sodium and chloride, in common table salt (NaCl).

About 40% of the body's sodium is contained in bone. Approximately 2–5% occurs within organs and cells and the remaining 55% is in blood plasma and other extracellular fluids. The amount of sodium in blood plasma is typically 140 mEq/L, a much higher amount than is found in intracellular sodium (about 5 mEq/L). This asymmetric distribution of sodium ions is essential for human life. It makes possible proper nerve conduction, the passage of various nutrients into cells, and the maintenance of blood pressure.

The body continually regulates its handling of sodium. When dietary sodium is too high or low, the intestines and kidneys respond to adjust concentrations to normal. During the course of a day, the intestines absorb dietary sodium while the kidneys excrete a nearly equal amount of sodium into the urine. If a low sodium diet is consumed, the intestines increase their efficiency of sodium absorption, and the kidneys reduce its release into urine.

The concentration of sodium in the blood plasma depends on two things: the total amount of sodium and water in arteries, veins, and capillaries (the circulatory system). The body uses separate mechanisms to regulate sodium and water, but they work together to correct blood pressure when it is too high or too low. Too high a concentration of sodium, or hypernatremia, can be corrected either by decreasing sodium or by increasing body water. The existence of separate mechanisms that regulate sodium concentration account for the fact that there are numerous diseases that can cause hypernatremia, including diseases of the kidney, pituitary gland, and hypothalamus.

Causes and symptoms

Vasopressin, also called anti-diuretic hormone, is made by the hypothalamus and released by the pituitary gland into the bloodstream. There it travels to the kidney where it reduces the release of water into the urine. With less vasopressin production, the body fails to conserve water, and the result is a trend toward higher plasma sodium concentrations. Hypernatremia may occur in **diabetes insipidus**, a disease that causes excessive urine production. (It is not the same disease as **diabetes mellitus**, a disease resulting from impaired insulin production.) The defect involves either the failure of the hypothalamus to make vasopressin or the failure of the kidney to respond to vasopressin. In either case, the kidney is able to conserve and regulate the body's sodium levels, but is unable to conserve and retain the body's water. Hypernatremia does not occur in diabetes insipidus if the patient is able to drink enough water to keep up with urinary loss, which may be as high as 10 L per day.

Hypernatremia may occur in unconscious (or comatose) patients due to the inability to drink water. Water is continually lost by evaporation from the lungs and in the urine. If the patient is not given

KEY TERMS

Acidosis—A medical condition caused by an increase in the concentration of hydrogen ions in the blood. The result of this increase is a lowered (acidic) blood pH level.

mEq/L—Abbreviation for milliequivalents per liter. Some medical tests results are reported in mEq/L.

Plasma—Clear, yellow- or straw-colored fluid that is the liquid component of blood and lymphatic fluid.

water via infusion, the sodium concentration in the blood may increase and hypernatremia could develop.

Hypernatremia can occur in individuals in which the thirst impulse is impaired or who cannot satisfy the thirst impulse on their own. Hypernatremia induced by these mechanisms is most likely to occur in infants, in psychiatric patients, and in elderly patients, especially those confined to institutionalized care settings.

Hypernatremia can occur accidentally in the hospital when patients are infused with solutions containing sodium, such as sodium bicarbonate for the treatment of acidosis (acidic blood). It can also be accidentally induced with sodium chloride infusions, especially in elderly patients with impaired kidney function.

Hypernatremia can cause neurological damage due to shrinkage of brain cells. Neurological symptoms include confusion, **coma**, **paralysis** of the lung muscles, and death. The severity of the symptoms is related to how rapidly the hypernatremia developed. Hypernatremia that comes on rapidly does not allow the cells of the brain time to adapt to their new high-sodium environment. Hypernatremia is especially dangerous for children and the elderly.

Diagnosis

Tests

Hypernatremia is diagnosed by acquiring a blood sample and then measuring the concentration of sodium ions in the blood. Other tests that may be ordered in the diagnosis of hypernatremia include urine osmolality, urine sodium, and serum glucose tests. A head CT scan or **magnetic resonance imaging** test (MRI) may be ordered in patients with severe hypernatremia. Less frequently ordered tests that may be utilized include a water deprivation test and an antidiuretic hormone (ADH) simulation test.

Treatment

Hypernatremia is treated with infusions of a solution of water containing 0.9% sodium chloride (0.9 g NaCl/100 mL water), which is the normal concentration of sodium chloride in the blood plasma. The infusion is performed over many hours or days to prevent abrupt and dangerous changes in brain cell volume. When possible, patients should be encouraged to drink water unless contraindicated for other medical reasons. In emergencies, such as when hypernatremia is causing neurological symptoms, infusions may be conducted with salt solutions containing 0.45% sodium chloride, which is half the normal physiologic level.

Prognosis

The prognosis for treating hypernatremia is excellent, except if neurological symptoms are severe or if overly rapid attempts are made to treat and reverse the condition. Some patients may be left with permanent neurological damage despite treatment.

Prevention

Hypernatremia occurs only in unusual circumstances that are not normally under a person's control. Monitoring the fluid consumption of vulnerable individuals, particularly those in institutionalized care settings, is strongly recommended. As hypernatremia in infants is most often caused by not receiving enough breast milk from the mother or from inaccurate formula preparation, educating new parents to these possibilities is important before the infant leaves the hospital.

Resources

BOOKS

Verbalis, J.G., and T. Berl. "Disorders of Water Balance." In *Brenner and Rector's The Kidney*. 8th Ed. B.M. Brenner, ed. Philadelphia: Saunders Elsevier, (2008).

PERIODICALS

Herrod, P.J., et al. "Hypo-and Hypernatremia in Surgical Patients: Is There Room for Improvement?" *World Journal of Surgery* 34, no. 3 (March 2010): 495–9.

Leung, C., W.C. Chang, and S.J. Yeh. "Hypernatremic Dehydration Due to Concentrated Infant Formula: Report of Two Cases." *Pediatric Neonatology* 50, no. 2 (2009): 70–3.

O'Connor, K.A., et al. "The Pattern of Plasma Sodium Abnormalities in an Acute Elderly Care Ward: A Cross-Sectional Study." *Irish Journal of Medical Sciences* 175, no. 3 (July–September 2006): 28–31.

OTHER

Lukitsch, Ivo, and Trung Pham. "Hypernatremia." *eMedicine*. April 19, 2010. http://emedicine.medscape.com/article/241094-overview (accessed October 10, 2010).

Semenovskaya, Zina, Richard Sinert, and Steven Stephanides. "Hypernatremia." *eMedicine* Aug 18, 2009. http://emedicine.medscape.com/article/766683-overview (accessed October 10, 2010).

Tom Brody, PhD
Melinda Granger RN, DNS, APRN, CNS

Hypernephroma *see* **Kidney cancer**

Hyperopia

Definition

Hyperopia (farsightedness) is the condition of the eye where incoming rays of light reach the retina before they converge into a focused image.

Description

When light goes through transparent but dense material like the materials of the eye's lens system (the lens and cornea), its velocity decreases. If the surface of the dense material is not perpendicular to the incoming light, as is the case with the curved surfaces on lenses and corneas, the direction of the light changes. The greater the curvature of the lens system, the greater the change in the direction of the light.

When parallel light rays from an object go through the lens system of the eye, they are bent so they converge at a point some distance behind the lens. With perfect vision this point of convergence, where the light rays are focused, is on the retina. This happens when the cumulative curvature of the lens plus cornea and the distance from the lens to the retina are just right for each other. The condition where the point of focus of parallel light rays from an object is behind the retina is called hyperopia. This condition exists when the combined curvature of the lens and cornea is insufficient (e.g., flatter than needed for the length of the eyeball). This condition can be equivalently described by saying hyperopia exists when the eyeball is too short for the curvature of its lens system.

There is a connection between the focusing of the lens of the eye (accommodation) and convergence of the eyes (the two eyes turning in to point at a close object). The best example is during reading. The lens accommodates to make the close-up material clear and the eyes turn in to look at the print and keep it single. Because of this connection between accommodation and convergence, if the lens needs to accommodate to focus for distance (to bring the image back onto the retina) the eyes may appear to turn in even when looking at the distance. This can cause a condition known as accommodative esotropia in children. The eyes turn in and the cause is accommodation because of hyperopia.

Causes and symptoms

Babies are generally born slightly hyperopic. This tends to decrease with age. There is normal variation in eyeball length and curvature of the lens and cornea. Some combinations of these variables give rise to eyes where the cornea is too flat for the distance between

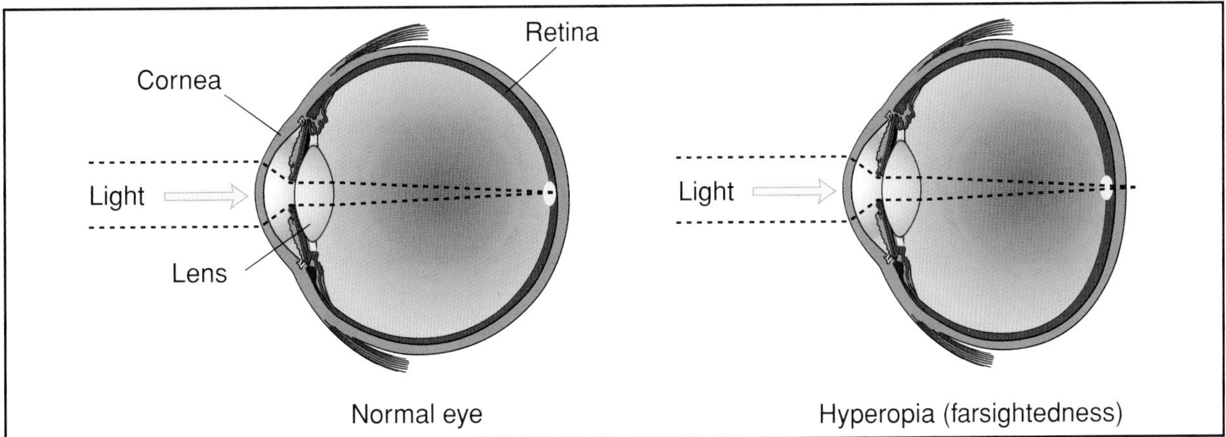

Hyperopia, or farsightedness, is a condition of the eye where incoming rays of light impinge on the retina before converging into a focused image, resulting in difficulty seeing nearby objects clearly. *(Illustration by Electronic Illustrators Group. Reproduced by permission of Gale, a part of Cengage Learning.)*

the cornea and the retina. If the hyperopia is not too severe the lens may be able to accommodate and bring the image back onto the retina. This would result in clear distance vision, but the constant focusing might result in headaches or eyestrain. If the lens cannot accommodate for the full amount of the hyperopia the distance image would be blurry.

If the eyes are focusing for distance and now the person is looking at a near object, the eyes need to accommodate further. This may result in blurry near by objects or headaches during close work.

Depending upon the amount of hyperopia, symptoms can range from none to clear distance vision but blurry near vision, to blurry distance and near vision. Headaches and eyestrain may also occur, particularly when doing near tasks. An eye turned in (esotropia) may be a result of hyperopia, particularly in children. However, because a turned eye may be a result of more serious causes it is very important to have it checked out.

Diagnosis

Because it is possible to have good visual acuity with some degree of hyperopia it is important to relax accommodation before the eye exam. This is done with the use of eyedrops and is called a cycloplegic exam or cycloplegic refraction. The drops relax the accommodation (thus making reading blurry until the drops wear off). Patients will usually be asked to have someone drive them home because of the blurriness. The doctor can then determine the patient's visual status with a hand-held instrument called a retinoscope and/or have the patient read from an eye chart while placing different lenses in front of the patient's eyes. Refractive error is measured in units called diopters (D).

Treatment

The usual treatment for hyperopia is corrective lenses (spectacles or **contact lenses**).

Different surgical methods to correct hyperopia are under investigation. One approach is to implant corrective contact lenses behind the patient's iris. The first experimental implantable contact lenses were implanted in 1997. Another approach is to surgically increase the curvature of the eye's existing cornea or lens. Although there have been many reports of success using different kinds of lasers to increase corneal curvature, there are still problems with stability and predictability. The introduction of light-activated biologic tissue glue in 1997 holds promise for improvements in those areas.

Prognosis

The prognosis for fully corrected vision is excellent for patients with low to moderate amounts of hyperopia. Patients with very high hyperopia (+10.00D or more) may not achieve full correction. Moreover, surgery to correct hyperopia will probably be perfected and approved in the near future.

Hyperopia increases the chances of chronic glaucoma, but vision loss from glaucoma is preventable.

Prevention

Hyperopia is usually present at birth, and there is no known way to prevent it.

ORGANIZATIONS

American Academy of Ophthalmology (AAO), P. O. Box 7424, San Francisco, CA, 94120-7424, (415) 561-8500, (415) 561-8500, http://www.aao.org.

American Optometric Association, 243 North Lindbergh Blvd., St. Louis, MO, 63141, (314) 991-4100, (314) 991-4101, (800) 365-2219, http://www.aoa.org/.

Lorraine Lica, PhD

Hyperparathyroidism

Definition

Parathyroid glands are four pea-sized glands located just behind the thyroid gland in the front of the neck. The function of parathyroid glands is to produce a hormone called parathyroid hormone (parathormone), which helps regulate **calcium** and phosphate in the body. Hyperparathyroidism is the overproduction of this hormone.

Description

Thyroid glands and parathyroid glands, despite their similar name and proximity, are entirely separate, and each produces hormones with different functions. Hyperparathyroidism may be primary or secondary. It most often occurs in those over age 30, and most commonly in patients 50 to 60 years old. It rarely occurs in children or the elderly. Women are affected by the disease up to three times more often than men. It is estimated that 28 of every 100,000 people in the United States will develop hyperparathyroidism each year.

Normally, parathyroid glands produce the parathormone as calcium levels drop and lower to meet the demands of a growing skeleton, **pregnancy**, or

lactation. However, when one or more parathyroid glands malfunctions, it can lead to overproduction of the hormone and elevated calcium level in the blood. Therefore, a common result of hyperparathyroidism is **hypercalcemia**, or an abnormally high level of calcium in the blood. Primary hyperparathyroidism occurs as a malfunction of one of the glands, usually as a result of a benign tumor called an adenoma. Secondary hyperparathyroidism occurs as the result of a metabolic abnormality outside the parathyroid glands, which causes a resistance to the function of the parathyroid hormones. Primary hyperparathyroidism is one of the most common endocrine disorders, led only by diabetes and **hyperthyroidism**.

Causes and symptoms

Often, there are no obvious symptoms or suspicion of hyperparathyroidism, and it is first diagnosed when a patient is discovered to be hypercalcemic during a routine blood chemistry profile. Patients may believe they have felt fine, but realize improvements in sleep, irritability, and memory following treatment. When symptoms are present, they may include development of gastric ulcers or **pancreatitis** because high calcium levels can cause inflammation and **pain** in the linings of the stomach and pancreas.

Most of the symptoms of hyperparathyroidism are those present as a result of hypercalcemia, such as **kidney stones**, **osteoporosis**, or bone degradation resulting from the bones giving up calcium. Muscle weakness, central nervous system disturbances such as depression, psychomotor and personality disturbances, and rarely, even **coma** can occur. Patients may also experience **heartburn**, **nausea**, **constipation**, or abdominal pain. In secondary hyperparathyroidism, patients may show signs of calcium imbalance such as deformities of the long bones. Symptoms of the underlying disease may also be present.

Most commonly, hyperparathyroidism occurs as the result of a single adenoma, or benign tumor, in one of the parathyroid glands. About 90% of all cases of hyperparathyroidism are caused by an adenoma. The tumors are seldom cancerous. They will grow to a much larger size than the parathyroid glands, often to the size of a walnut. Genetic disorders or multiple endocrine tumors can also cause a parathyroid gland to enlarge and oversecrete hormone. In 10% or fewer of patients with primary hyperparathyroidism, there is enlargement of all four parathyroid glands. This condition is called parathyroid hyperplasia.

Diagnosis

Diagnosis of hyperparathyroidism is most often made when a blood test (radioimmunoassay) reveals high levels of parathyroid hormone and calcium. A blood test that specifically measures the amount of parathyroid hormone has made diagnosis simpler. X ray examinations may be performed to look for areas of diffuse bone demineralization, bone cysts, outer bone absorption and erosion of the long bones of the fingers and toes. Hypercalcemia is mild or intermittent in some patients, but is an excellent indicator of primary hyperparathyroidism. Dual energy x ray absorptiometry (DEXA or DXA), a tool used to diagnose and measure osteoporosis, is used to show reduction in bone mass for primary hyperparathryroidism patients. Once a diagnosis of hyperparathyroidism is reached, the physician will probably order further tests to evaluate complications. For example, abdominal radiographs might reveal kidney stones.

For secondary hyperparathyroidism, normal or slightly decreased calcium levels in the blood and variable phosphorous levels may be visible. Patient history of familial **kidney disease** or convulsive disorders may suggest a diagnosis of secondary hyperparathyroidism. Other tests may reveal a disease or disorder, which is causing the secondary hyperparathyroidism.

Treatment

Hyperparathyroidism cases will usually be referred to an endocrinologist, a physician specializing in hormonal problems, or a nephrologist, who specializes in kidney and mineral disorders.

Patients with mild cases of hyperparathyroidism may not need immediate treatment if they have only slight elevations in blood calcium level and normal kidneys and bones. These patients should be regularly checked, probably as often as every six months, by **physical examination** and measurement of kidney function and calcium levels. A bone densitometry measurement should be performed every one or two years. After several years with no worsened symptoms, the length of time between exams may be increased.

Patients with more advanced hyperparathyroidism will usually have all or half of the affected parathyroid gland or glands surgically removed. This surgery is relatively safe and effective. The primary risks are those associated with **general anesthesia**. There are some instances when the surgery can be performed with the patient under regional, or cervical block, anesthesia. Often studies such as ultrasonography prior to surgery help pinpoint the affected areas.

Alternative treatment

Forcing fluids and reducing intake of calcium-rich foods can help decrease calcium levels prior to surgery or if surgery is not necessary.

Prognosis

Removal of the enlarged parathyroid gland or glands cures the disease 95% of the time and relief of bone pain may occur in as few as three days. In up to 5% of patients undergoing surgery, chronically low calcium levels may result, and these patients will require a calcium supplement or vitamin D treatment. Damage to the kidneys as a result of hyperparathyroidism is often irreversible. Prognosis is generally good, however complications of hyperparathyroidism such as osteoporosis, bone **fractures**, kidney stones, peptic ulcers, pancreatitis, and nervous system difficulties may worsen the prognosis.

Prevention

Secondary hyperparathyroidism may be prevented by early treatment of the disease causing it. Early recognition and treatment of hyperparathyroidism may prevent hypercalcemia. Since the cause of primary hyperparathyroidism, or the adenoma which causes parathyroid enlargement, is largely unknown, there are no prescribed prevention methods.

Resources

OTHER

"Endocrine Disorder and Endocrine Surgery." Endocrine Web Page. http://www.endocrineweb.com.

ORGANIZATIONS

Osteoporosis and Related Bone Diseases—National Resource Center, 2 AMS Circle, Bethesda, MD, 20892-3676, (202) 223-0344, (202) 293-2356, NIAMSBoneInfo@mail.nih .gov, http://www.niams.nih.gov/Health _Info/bone/ default.asp.

Paget Foundation, 120 Wall Street, Ste. 1602, New York, NY, 10005-4035, (212) 509-5335, (212) 509-8492, (800) 237-2438, Pagetfdn@aol.com, http://www.paget.org.

Teresa Odle

Hyperpigmentation

Definition

Hyperpigmentation is the increase in the natural color of the skin.

Description

Melanin, a brown pigment manufactured by certain cells in the skin called melanocytes, is responsible for skin color. Mela1nin production is stimulated by a pituitary hormone called melanocyte stimulating hormone (MSH). Other pigments appear in the skin much less often.

Causes and symptoms

Darkened spots on the skin come in several varieties. The most ominous is **malignant melanoma**, a very aggressive **cancer** that begins as an innocent mole. The majority of **moles** (nevus), however, are and remain benign (harmless). The average person has several dozen, and certain people with a hereditary excess may have hundreds. Freckles, age spots, and cafe au lait spots, known as ephelides, are always flat and not as dark. Cafe au lait spots are seen mostly in people with another hereditary disorder called **neurofibromatosis**. "Port wine stains" are congenital dark red blotches on the skin. Other common dark colorations on the skin are called keratosis and consist of locally overgrown layers of skin that are dark primarily because there is more tissue than normal. A few of these turn into skin cancers of a much less dangerous kind than melanoma.

Darkened regions of the skin occur as a result of abnormal **tanning** when the skin is sensitive to sunlight. Several diseases and many drugs can cause **photosensitivity**. Among the common drugs responsible for this uncommon reaction are birth control pills, **antibiotics** (**sulfonamides** and **tetracyclines**), **diuretics**, **nonsteroidal anti-inflammatory drugs** (NSAID), **pain** relievers, and some psychoactive medications. Some of the same drugs may also cause patches of discolored skin known as localized drug reactions and representing an allergy to that drug. Sunlight darkens an abnormal chemical in the skin of patients with porphyria cutanea tarda. Several endocrine diseases, some cancers, and several drugs abnormally stimulate melanocytes, usually through an overproduction of MSH. Arsenic **poisoning** and **Addison's disease** are among these causes. A condition known as acanthosis nigricans is a velvety darkening of skin in folded areas (arm pits, groin, and neck) that can signal a cancer or hormone imbalance.

Of particular note is a condition called melasma (dark pigmentation of the skin), caused by the female hormone estrogen. Normal in **pregnancy**, this brownish discoloration of the face can also happen with birth control pills that contain estrogen.

Overall darkening of the skin may be due to pigmented chemicals in the skin. Silver, gold, and iron each have a characteristic color when visible in the skin. Several drugs and body chemicals, like bilirubin, can end up as deposits in the skin and discolor it.

There are a number of other rare entities that color the skin, each in its own peculiar way. Among these are strange syndromes that seem to be **birth defects** and vitamin and nutritional deficiencies.

Diagnosis

The pattern of discoloration is immediately visible to the trained dermatologist, a physician specializing in skin diseases, and may be all that is required to name and characterize the discoloration. Many of these pigment changes are signs of internal disease that must be identified. Pigmentation changes may also be caused by medication, and the drug responsible for the reaction must be identified and removed.

Treatment

Skin sensitive to sunlight must be protected by shade or **sunscreens** with an SPF of 15 or greater. Skin cancers must be, and unsightly benign lesions may be, surgically removed. **Laser surgery** is an effective removal technique for many localized lesions. Because it spreads so rapidly, melanoma should be immediately removed, as well as some of the surrounding tissue to prevent regrowth.

Prevention

Sunlight is the leading cause of dark spots on the skin, so shade and sunscreens are necessary preventive strategies, especially in people who burn easily.

Resources

PERIODICALS

Bernstein L. J., et al. "The Short- and Long-term Side Effects of Carbon Dioxide Laser Resurfacing." *Dermatologic Surgery* 23 (July 1997): 519-525.

J. Ricker Polsdorfer, MD

Hyperprolactation *see* **Galactorrhea**

Hypersensitivity pneumonitis

Definition

Hypersensitivity pneumonitis refers to an inflammation of the lungs caused by repeated breathing in of a foreign substance, such an organic dust, a fungus, or a mold. The body's immune system reacts to these substances, called antigens, by forming antibodies, molecules that attack the invading antigen and try to destroy it. The combination of antigen and antibody produces acute inflammation, or pneumonitis (a hypersensitivity reaction), which later can develop into chronic lung disease that impairs the lungs' ability to take oxygen from the air and eliminate carbon dioxide.

Description

Hypersensitivity pneumonitis (HP) is sometimes called "allergic alveolitis." "Allergic" refers to the antigen-antibody reaction, and "alveolitis" means an inflammation of the tiny air sacs in the lungs where oxygen and CO_2 are exchanged, the alveoli. It also is known as "extrinsic" allergic alveolitis, meaning that the antigen that sets up the allergic reaction (also called an allergen) comes from the outside. Most of the antigens that cause this disease come from plant or animal proteins or microorganisms, and many of those affected are exposed either at work or in the course of some hobby or other activity. The first known type of HP, farmer's lung, is caused by antigens from tiny microorganisms living on moldy hay. An example of disease connected with a hobby is pigeon breeder's lung, caused by inhaling protein material from bird droppings or feathers. After a time, very little of the allergenic material is needed to set off a reaction in the lungs.

Roughly one in every 10,000 persons develops some form of HP. A mysterious aspect of this condition is that, even though many persons may be exposed to a particular antigen, only a small number of them will develop the disease. Genetic differences may determine who becomes ill; this remains unclear. Probably between 5% and 15% of all persons who are regularly exposed to organic materials develop HP. Most of those who do get it do *not* smoke (**smoking** may create the type of cells that take up antigens and neutralize them). The amount of antigen is an important factor in whether HP will develop and what form it will take. Sudden heavy exposure can produce symptoms in a matter of hours, whereas mild but frequent exposures tend to produce a long-lasting, "smoldering" illness. HP may be more likely to develop in persons exposed to polluted air or industrial fumes.

Typical changes occur in the lungs of persons with HP. In the acute stage, large numbers of inflammatory cells are found throughout the lungs and the air sacs may be filled by a thick fluid mixed with these cells. In the subacute stage, disease extends into the small breathing tubes, or bronchioles, and the inflammatory cells collect into tiny granules called granulomas. Finally, in the chronic stage of HP, the previously inflamed parts of the lungs become scarred and unable to function, as in **pulmonary fibrosis**.

Causes and symptoms

A number of different types of HP are known, since a wide range of allergens may produce an allergic reaction in the lungs. Many of them produce similar symptoms and abnormal physical findings, but some have their own typical features. Some of the more common forms are:

- Farmer's lung. This can affect any farmer who works with wet hay or other moldy dust. Small farmers who have to directly thresh and handle their hay are most at risk, as are those living in cold and humid areas where damp weather is common.
- Pigeon breeder's lung. Also called "bird fancier's lung," it is second to farmer's lung as the best known type of HP. A substance has been found in pigeon droppings that may cause the allergic reaction, but there may be more than one such substance. Besides pigeons, the disorder may follow exposure to ducks, geese, pheasants, and even canaries. Parakeets produce an especially severe form of disease. Most patients are middle-aged women, who usually care for birds either at home or on bird breeding farms.
- Bagassosis. Caused by bagasse, a substance produced when juice is extracted from sugar cane and is used in making paper and explosives. A fungus is probably responsible. Young and middle-aged men who work in the sugar industry are at risk.
- Byssinosis. A similar condition affecting workers who inhale dust from cotton, flax, or hemp.
- Humidifier lung. An acute form of HP caused by inhaling actinomycetes, the same organisms that cause farmer's lung, which grow in contaminated humidifier vents, air conditioners, heating systems, and even saunas.
- Other antigens. HP has been seen in persons working with detergents, silicone, mushrooms, cheese, wood dust, maple bark, coffee, and furs.

In the acute stage, patients with HP begin coughing, develop **fever**, and note tightness in the chest as well as extreme tiredness and aching, four to eight hours after the most recent exposure. Most patients are well aware of the connection between their work (or an activity) and their symptoms. After a time, patients may have trouble breathing. They also may lose their appetite, lose weight, and generally feel ill. Finally, in the chronic stage, the patient will have increasing trouble breathing and may sometimes wheeze. With advanced disease, the skin may appear bluish (because too little oxygen is getting into the blood). When a physician listens to the patient's chest with a stethoscope, there may be crackling sounds or loud **wheezing**. In the late stages, club-shaped fingertips are a sign that the patient has not been getting enough oxygen for an extended period of time.

Diagnosis

No single test can make a definite diagnosis of HP. The key is to relate some specific exposure or activity to episodes of symptoms. A **chest x ray** may be normal in the acute stage, but later may show a hazy appearance that looks like "ground glass." There may be linear or rounded shadows in the central parts of the lungs. Studies of lung function in the acute stage typically show abnormally small lung volume. The ability to breathe at a fast rate is impaired. Blood from an artery typically has a low level of oxygen. Later, when the lungs have begun to scar, the airways (breathing tubes) are obstructed and the rate of air flow is reduced.

Some experts believe that skin testing can help diagnose HP and show which particular antigen is causing the symptoms. Small amounts of several suspect antigens are injected just beneath the surface of the skin, usually on the arm or back, and the reactions compared to that caused by injecting a harmless salt solution. Another diagnostic test is to place a thin tube into the airways, inject a small amount of fluid, and draw it back up (bronchoalveolar lavage). A very large number of cells called lymphocytes is typical of HP, and mast cells, which are part of the immune system, may also be seen. Rarely, a tissue sample (biopsy) of lung tissue may be taken through a tube placed in the airways and examined under a microscope. Finally, a patient may be "challenged" by actually inhaling a particular antigen in the form of an aerosol and noting whether lung function suddenly becomes worse. This test is usually not necessary.

Treatment

Treatment of HP requires identifying the offending antigen and avoiding further exposure. Although it may sometimes be necessary for a patient to find a totally different type of work, often it is possible to simply perform different duties or switch to a work site where exposure is minimal. In some cases, (like pigeon breeder's lung), wearing a mask can prevent exposure. If acute symptoms are severe, the patient may be treated with a steroid hormone for two to six weeks. This often suppresses the inflammatory response and allows the lungs a chance to recover. In the chronic stage, steroid treatment can delay further damage to the lungs and help preserve their function.

Prognosis

In general, most of the symptoms of HP disappear when the patient is no longer exposed to the causative allergen. The actual chances of complete recovery depend in part on what form of HP is present. Older patients and those exposed repeatedly for long periods after initially developing symptoms tend to have a poorer long-term outlook. The worst outcome is that long repeated episodes of exposure will cause chronic lung inflammation, scar the lungs, and permanently make then unable to properly provide oxygen to the blood. Rarely, a patient will become permanently disabled.

Prevention

It is often not possible to prevent initial episodes of HP because there is no way of predicting which individuals (such as farmers) will have an allergic reaction to a particular allergen. Once the connection is made between a type of exposure and definite hypersensitivity symptoms, prevention of further episodes is simple as long as further exposure can be avoided.

Exactly how to avoid exposure depends on a person's work or activities and what is causing the reaction. People with farmer's lung can dry hay thoroughly before storing it. For pigeon breeder's lung (and many other types of HP), a mask can be worn. In many industrial settings, it is possible to take precautions that will limit the amount of allergen that workers will inhale. If it is not possible to avoid exposure altogether, exposure can be timed and strictly minimized.

ORGANIZATIONS

American Lung Association, 1301 Pennsylvania Ave. NW, Suite 800, Washington, DC, 20001, (202) 758-3355, (202) 452-1805, (800) 548-8252, info@lungusa.org, http://www.lungusa.org/.

Asthma and Allergy Foundation of America, 8201 Corporate Drive, Suite 1000, Landover, MD, 20785, (800) 727-8462, info@aafa.org, http://www.aafa.org/.

David A. Cramer, MD

Hypersomnia *see* **Sleep disorders**

Hypersplenism

Definition

Hypersplenism is a type of disorder that causes the spleen to rapidly and prematurely destroy blood cells.

Description

The spleen is located in the upper left area of the abdomen. One of this organ's major functions is to remove blood cells from the body's bloodstream. In hypersplenism, its normal function accelerates, and it begins to automatically remove cells that may still be normal in function. Sometimes the spleen will temporarily hold onto up to 90% of the body's platelets and 45% of the red blood cells. Hypersplenism may occur as a primary disease, leading to other complications, or as a secondary disease, resulting from an underlying disease or disorder. Hypersplenism is sometimes referred to as enlarged spleen (splenomegaly). An enlarged spleen is one of the symptoms of hypersplenism. What differentiates hypersplenism is its premature destruction of blood cells.

Causes and symptoms

Hypersplenism may be caused by a variety of disorders. Sometimes, it is brought on by a problem within the spleen itself and is referred to as primary hypersplenism. Secondary hypersplenism results from another disease such as chronic **malaria**, **rheumatoid arthritis**, **tuberculosis**, or **polycythemia vera**, a blood disorder. Spleen disorders in general are almost always secondary in nature. Hypersplenism may also be caused by tumors.

Symptoms of hypersplenism include easy bruising, easy contracting of bacterial diseases, **fever**, weakness, heart **palpitations**, and ulcerations of the mouth, legs, and feet. Individuals may also bleed unexpectedly and heavily from the nose or other mucous membranes and from the gastrointestinal or urinary tracts. Most patients will develop an enlarged spleen, anemia, leukopenia, or abnormally low white blood cell counts, or **thrombocytopenia**, a deficiency of circulating platelets in the blood. Other symptoms may be present that reflect the underlying disease that has caused hypersplenism.

An enlarged spleen can be caused by a variety of diseases, including **hemolytic anemia**, liver **cirrhosis**, leukemia, malignant lymphoma and other infections and inflammatory diseases. Splenomegaly occurs in about 10% of **systemic lupus erythematosus** patients. Sometimes it is caused by recent viral infection, such as mononucleosis. An enlarged spleen may cause **pain** in the upper left side of the abdomen and a premature feeling of fullness at meals.

Diagnosis

Diagnosis of hypersplenism begins with review of symptoms and patient history and careful feeling (palpation) of the spleen. Sometimes, a physician can feel an enlarged spleen. X ray studies, such as ultrasound and computed tomography scan (CT scan), may help diagnose an enlarged spleen and possible underlying causes, such as tumors. Blood tests indicate decreases in white blood cells, red blood cells, or platelets. Another test measures red blood cells in the liver and spleen after injection of a radioactive substance and indicates areas where the spleen is holding on to large numbers of red cells or is destroying them.

Enlarged spleens are diagnosed using a combination of patient history; **physical examination**, including palpation of the spleen, if possible; and diagnostic tests. A history of fever and systemic symptoms may be present because of infection, malaria, or an inflammatory disorder. A **complete blood count** is taken to check counts of young red blood cells. **Liver function tests**, CT scans, and ultrasound exams can also help to detect an enlarged spleen.

Treatment

In secondary hypersplenism, the underlying disease must be treated to prevent further sequestration or destruction of blood cells, and possible spleen enlargement. Those therapies will be tried prior to removal of the spleen (**splenectomy**), which is avoided if possible. In severe cases, the spleen must be removed. Splenectomy will correct the effects of low blood cell concentrations in the blood.

Prognosis

Prognosis depends on the underlying cause and progression of the disease. Left untreated, spleen enlargement can lead to serious complications. Hypersplenism can also lead to complications due to decreased blood cell counts.

Prevention

Some of the underlying causes of hypersplenism or enlarged spleen can be prevented, such as certain forms of anemia and cirrhosis of the liver due to alcohol use. In other cases, the hypersplenism may not be preventable, as it is a complication to an underlying disorder.

ORGANIZATIONS

American Liver Foundation, 75 Maiden Lane, Suite 603, New York, NY, 10038, (212) 668-1000, (212) 483-8179, http://www.liverfoundation.org/.

American Society of Hematology, 2021 L St. NW, Suite 900, Washington, DC, 20036, (202) 776-0544, (202) 776-0545, http://www.hematology.org.

National Heart Lung and Blood Institute Health Information Center, P.O. Box 30105, Bethesda, MD, 20824-0105, (301) 592-8573, (240) 629-3246, http://www.nhlbi.nih.gov.

Teresa Norris, RN

Hypertension

Definition

Hypertension is high blood pressure. Blood pressure is the force of blood pushing against the walls of arteries as it flows through them. Arteries are the blood vessels that carry oxygenated blood from the heart to the body's tissues.

Demographics

Hypertension is a major health problem, especially because it has no symptoms. Many people have hypertension without knowing it. In the United States, about 50 million people age six and older have high blood pressure. Hypertension is more common in men than women and in people over the age of 65 than in younger persons. More than half of all Americans over the age of 65 have hypertension. It also is more common in African Americans than in white Americans.

Description

As blood flows through arteries it pushes against the inside of the artery walls. The more pressure the blood exerts on the artery walls, the higher the blood pressure will be. The size of small arteries also affects the blood pressure. When the muscular walls of arteries are relaxed, or dilated, the pressure of the blood flowing through them is lower than when the artery walls narrow, or constrict.

Blood pressure is highest when the heart beats to push blood out into the arteries. When the heart relaxes to fill with blood again, the pressure is at its

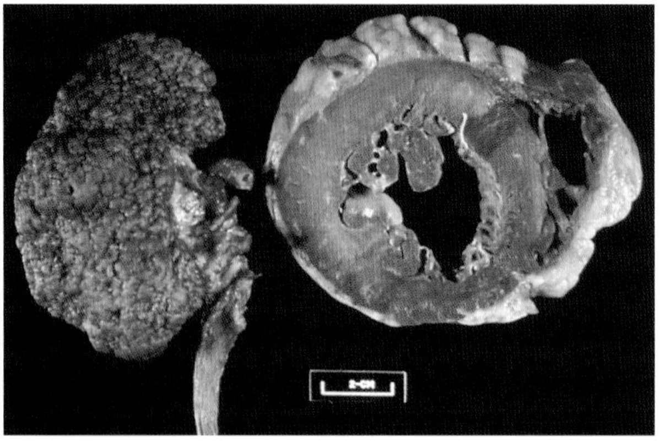

The effects of hypertension on the heart and kidney. Hypertension has caused renal atrophy and scarring, and left ventricular hypertrophy in the sectioned heart (at right). *(Dr. E. Walker/Photo Researchers, Inc.)*

lowest point. Blood pressure when the heart beats is called systolic pressure. Blood pressure when the heart is at rest is called diastolic pressure. When blood pressure is measured, the systolic pressure is stated first and the diastolic pressure second. Blood pressure is measured in millimeters of mercury (mm Hg). For example, if a person's systolic pressure is 120 and diastolic pressure is 80, it is written as 120/80 mm Hg. The American Heart Association has long considered blood pressure less than 140 over 90 normal for adults. However, the National Heart, Lung, and Blood Institute in Bethesda, Maryland, released new clinical guidelines for blood pressure in 2003, lowering the standard normal readings. A normal reading was lowered to less than 120 over less than 80.

Hypertension is serious because people with the condition have a higher risk for heart disease and other medical problems than people with normal blood pressure. Serious complications can be avoided by getting regular blood pressure checks and treating hypertension as soon as it is diagnosed.

If left untreated, hypertension can lead to the following medical conditions:

- arteriosclerosis, also called atherosclerosis
- heart attack
- stroke
- enlarged heart
- kidney damage

Arteriosclerosis is hardening of the arteries. The walls of arteries have a layer of muscle and elastic tissue that makes them flexible and able to dilate and constrict as blood flows through them. High blood pressure can make the artery walls thicken and harden. When artery walls thicken, the inside of the blood vessel narrows. Cholesterol and fats are more likely to build up on the walls of damaged arteries, making them even narrower. **Blood clots** also can get trapped in narrowed arteries, blocking the flow of blood.

Arteries narrowed by arteriosclerosis may not deliver enough blood to organs and other tissues. Reduced or blocked blood flow to the heart can cause a **heart attack**. If an artery to the brain is blocked, a **stroke** can result.

Hypertension makes the heart work harder to pump blood through the body. The extra workload can make the heart muscle thicken and stretch. When the heart becomes too enlarged it cannot pump enough blood. If the hypertension is not treated, the heart may fail.

The kidneys remove the body's wastes from the blood. If hypertension thickens the arteries to the kidneys, less waste can be filtered from the blood. As the condition worsens, the kidneys fail and wastes build up in the blood. Dialysis or a kidney transplant are needed when the kidneys fail. About 25% of people who receive **kidney dialysis** have kidney failure caused by hypertension.

Risk factors

Even though the cause of most hypertension is not known, some people have risk factors that increase their chance of developing hypertension. Many of these risk factors can be avoided to lower the chance of developing hypertension or as part of a treatment program to lower blood pressure.

Risk factors for hypertension include:

- age over 60
- male sex
- race
- heredity
- salt sensitivity
- obesity
- inactive lifestyle
- heavy alcohol consumption
- use of oral contraceptives

Some people inherit a tendency for hypertension. People with family members who have hypertension are more likely to develop it than those whose relatives are not hypertensive. People with these risk factors can avoid or eliminate other risk factors to lower their chance of developing hypertension. A 2003 report found that the rise in incidence of high blood pressure among children is most likely due to an increase in the number of overweight and obese children and adolescents.

Causes and symptoms

Many different actions or situations can normally raise blood pressure. Physical activity can temporarily raise blood pressure. Stressful situations can make blood pressure go up; when the **stress** goes away, blood pressure usually returns to normal. These temporary increases in blood pressure are not considered hypertension. A diagnosis of hypertension is made only when a person has multiple high blood pressure readings over a period of time.

The cause of hypertension is not known in 90–95% of the people who have it. Hypertension without a known cause is called primary or essential hypertension.

When a person has hypertension caused by another medical condition, it is called secondary hypertension. Secondary hypertension can be caused by a number of different illnesses. Many people with kidney disorders have secondary hypertension. The kidneys regulate the balance of salt and water in the body. If the kidneys cannot rid the body of excess salt and water, blood pressure goes up. Kidney infections, a narrowing of the arteries that carry blood to the kidneys, called **renal artery stenosis**, and other kidney disorders can disturb the salt and water balance.

Cushing's syndrome and tumors of the pituitary and adrenal glands often increase levels of the adrenal gland hormones cortisol, adrenalin, and aldosterone, which can cause hypertension. Other conditions that can cause hypertension are blood vessel diseases, thyroid gland disorders, some prescribed drugs, **alcoholism**, and **pregnancy**.

One of the most dangerous features of hypertension is the fact that it does not usually cause any symptoms. Individuals may not be aware that they have the condition, or they may mistakenly downplay its importance, simply because it is not causing any discernible problems. Without treatment, the deleterious effects of hypertension progress unchecked.

When blood pressure becomes extremely high, for example over 180/110 mmHg (termed malignant hypertension), symptoms such as **headache**, visual disturbances, **anxiety**, and **shortness of breath** may occur. If left untreated, stroke may supervene, or a hypertensive crisis, in which organs cannot receive an adequate blood supply and begin to fail, may occur.

Diagnosis

Examination

Because hypertension does not cause symptoms, it is important to have blood pressure checked regularly. Blood pressure is measured with an instrument called a sphygmomanometer. A cloth-covered rubber cuff is wrapped around the upper arm and inflated. When the cuff is inflated, an artery in the arm is squeezed to momentarily stop the flow of blood. Then, the air is let out of the cuff while a stethoscope placed over the artery is used to detect the sound of the blood spurting back through the artery. This first sound is the systolic pressure, the pressure when the heart beats. The last sound heard as the rest of the air is released is the diastolic pressure, the pressure between heart beats. Both sounds are recorded on the mercury gauge on the sphygmomanometer.

Normal blood pressure is defined by a range of values. Blood pressure lower than 120/80 mm Hg is considered normal. A number of factors such as **pain**, stress, or anxiety can cause a temporary increase in blood pressure. For this reason, hypertension is not diagnosed on one high blood pressure reading. If a blood pressure reading is 120/80 or higher for the first time, the physician will have the person return for another blood pressure check. Diagnosis of hypertension usually is made based on two or more readings after the first visit.

Systolic hypertension of the elderly is common and is diagnosed when the diastolic pressure is normal or low, but the systolic is elevated, e.g., 170/70 mm Hg. This condition usually co-exists with hardening of the arteries (**atherosclerosis**).

Blood pressure measurements are classified in stages, according to severity:

- normal blood pressure: less than 120/80 mm Hg
- pre-hypertension: 120–129/80–89 mm Hg
- Stage 1 hypertension: 140–159/90–99 mm Hg
- Stage 2 hypertension: at or greater than 160–179/100–109 mm Hg

A typical **physical examination** to evaluate hypertension includes:

- medical and family history
- physical examination
- ophthalmoscopy: Examination of the blood vessels in the eye
- chest x ray
- electrocardiograph (ECG)
- blood and urine tests

The medical and family history help the physician determine if the patient has any conditions or disorders that might contribute to or cause the hypertension. A family history of hypertension might suggest a genetic predisposition for hypertension.

The physical exam may include several blood pressure readings at different times and in different positions. The physician uses a stethoscope to listen to sounds made by the heart and blood flowing through the arteries. The pulse, reflexes, and height and weight are checked and recorded. Internal organs are palpated, or felt, to determine if they are enlarged.

Because hypertension can cause damage to the blood vessels in the eyes, the eyes may be checked with a instrument called an ophthalmoscope. The physician will look for thickening, narrowing, or hemorrhages in the blood vessels.

Tests

A **chest x ray** can detect an enlarged heart, other vascular (heart) abnormalities, or lung disease.

An electrocardiogram (ECG) measures the electrical activity of the heart. It can detect if the heart muscle is enlarged and if there is damage to the heart muscle from blocked arteries.

Urine and blood tests may be done to evaluate health and to detect the presence of disorders that might cause hypertension.

Treatment

Traditional

There is no cure for primary hypertension, but blood pressure can almost always be lowered with the correct treatment. The goal of treatment is to lower blood pressure to levels that will prevent heart disease and other complications of hypertension. In secondary hypertension, the disease that is responsible for the hypertension is treated in addition to the hypertension itself. Successful treatment of the underlying disorder may cure the secondary hypertension.

Guidelines advise that clinicians work with patients to agree on blood pressure goals and develop a treatment plan for the individual patient. Actual combinations of medications and lifestyle changes will vary from one person to the next. Treatment to lower blood pressure may include changes in diet, getting regular **exercise**, and taking antihypertensive medications. Patients falling into the pre-hypertension range who do not have damage to the heart or kidneys often are advised to make lifestyle changes only. A 2003 report of a clinical trial showed that adults with elevated blood pressures lowered them as much as 38% by making lifestyle changes and participating in the DASH diet, which encourages eating more fruit and vegetables.

Drugs

Patients with stage 1 hypertension may be advised to take antihypertensive medication. Numerous drugs have been developed to treat hypertension. The choice of medication depends on the stage of hypertension, side effects, other medical conditions the patient may have, and other medicines the patient is taking.

If treatment with a single medicine fails to lower blood pressure enough, a different medicine may be tried or another medicine may be added to the first. Patients with more severe hypertension may initially be given a combination of medicines to control their hypertension. Combining antihypertensive medicines with different types of action often controls blood pressure with smaller doses of each drug than would be needed for just one.

Antihypertensive medicines fall into several classes of drugs:

- diuretics
- beta-blockers
- calcium channel blockers
- angiotensin converting enzyme inhibitors (ACE inhibitors)
- alpha-blockers
- alpha-beta blockers
- vasodilators
- peripheral acting adrenergic antagonists
- centrally acting agonists

Diuretics help the kidneys eliminate excess salt and water from the body's tissues and the blood. This reduces the swelling caused by fluid buildup in the tissues. The reduction of fluid dilates the walls of arteries and lowers blood pressure. Diuretics are recommended as the first drug of choice for most patients with high blood pressure and as part of any multi-drug combination.

Beta-blockers lower blood pressure by acting on the nervous system to slow the heart rate and reduce the force of the heart's contraction. They are used with caution in patients with **heart failure**, **asthma**, diabetes, or circulation problems in the hands and feet.

Calcium channel blockers block the entry of **calcium** into muscle cells in artery walls. Muscle cells need calcium to constrict, so reducing their calcium keeps them more relaxed and lowers blood pressure.

ACE inhibitors block the production of substances that constrict blood vessels. They also help reduce the build-up of water and salt in the tissues. They often are given to patients with heart failure, **kidney disease**, or diabetes. ACE inhibitors may be used together with diuretics.

Alpha-blockers act on the nervous system to dilate arteries and reduce the force of the heart's contractions.

Alpha-beta blockers combine the actions of alpha and **beta blockers**.

Vasodilators act directly on arteries to relax their walls so blood can move more easily through them. They lower blood pressure rapidly and are injected in hypertensive emergencies when patients have dangerously high blood pressure.

Peripheral acting adrenergic antagonists act on the nervous system to relax arteries and reduce the force of the heart's contractions. They usually are prescribed together with a diuretic. Peripheral acting adrenergic antagonists can cause slowed mental function and lethargy.

Centrally acting agonists also act on the nervous system to relax arteries and slow the heart rate. They are usually used with other antihypertensive medicines.

Home remedies

Lifestyle changes that may reduce blood pressure by 5 to 10 mm Hg include:

- reducing salt intake
- reducing fat intake
- losing weight
- getting regular exercise
- quitting smoking
- reducing alcohol consumption
- managing stress

Prognosis

There is no cure for hypertension. However, it can be well controlled with proper treatment. Therapy with a combination of lifestyle changes and antihypertensive medicines can keep blood pressure at levels that will not cause damage to the heart or other organs. The key to avoiding serious complications of hypertension is to detect and treat it before damage occurs. Because antihypertensive medicines control blood pressure, but do not cure it, patients must continue taking the medications to maintain reduced blood pressure levels and avoid complications.

Prevention

Prevention of hypertension centers on avoiding or eliminating known risk factors. Even persons at risk because of age, race, or sex or those who have an inherited risk can lower their chance of developing hypertension.

The risk of developing hypertension can be reduced by:

- reducing salt intake
- reducing fat intake
- losing weight
- getting regular exercise
- quitting smoking
- reducing alcohol consumption
- managing stress

Resources

BOOKS

Goldman, L., and D. Ausiello, eds. *Cecil Textbook of Internal Medicine*, 23rd ed. Philadelphia: Saunders, 2008.

Libby, P., et al. *Braunwald's Heart Disease*, 8th ed. Philadelphia: Saunders, 2007.

PERIODICALS

McNamara, Damian. "Obesity Behind Rise in Incidence of Primary Hypertension." *Family Practice News*, April 1, 2003: 45-51.

McNamara, Damian. "Trial Shows Efficacy of Lifestyle Changes for BP: More Intensive Than Typical Office Visit." *Family Practice News*, July 1, 2003: 1-2.

"New BP Guidelines Establish Diagnosis of Pre-hypertension: Level Seeks to Identify At-risk Individuals Early." *Case Management Advisor*, July 2003: S1.

"New Hypertension Guidelines: JNC-7." *Clinical Cardiology Alert*, July 2003: 54-63.

ORGANIZATIONS

American Heart Association, 7272 Greenville Avenue, Dallas, TX, 75231, (800) 242-8721, http://www.americanheart.org.

National Heart, Lung and Blood Institute, P.O. Box 30105, Bethesda, MD, 20824-0105, (301) 592-8573, (240) 629-3246, nhlbiinfo@nhlbi.nih.gov, http://www.nhlbi.nih.gov.

Texas Heart Institute, P.O. Box 20345, Houston, TX, 77225-0345, (800) 292-2221, hic@heart.thi.tmc.edu, http://www.texasheart.org.

Toni Rizzo
Teresa G. Odle

Hyperthermia *see* **Fever**

Hyperthyroidism

Definition

Hyperthyroidism is the overproduction of **thyroid hormones** by an overactive thyroid gland. More specifically, the thyroid gland produces too much of a hormone called thyroxine.

The term *hyperthyroidism* covers any disease which results in overabundance of thyroid hormone. Other names for hyperthyroidism, or specific diseases within the category, include Graves' disease, diffuse toxic **goiter**, Basedow's disease, Parry's disease, and thyrotoxicosis.

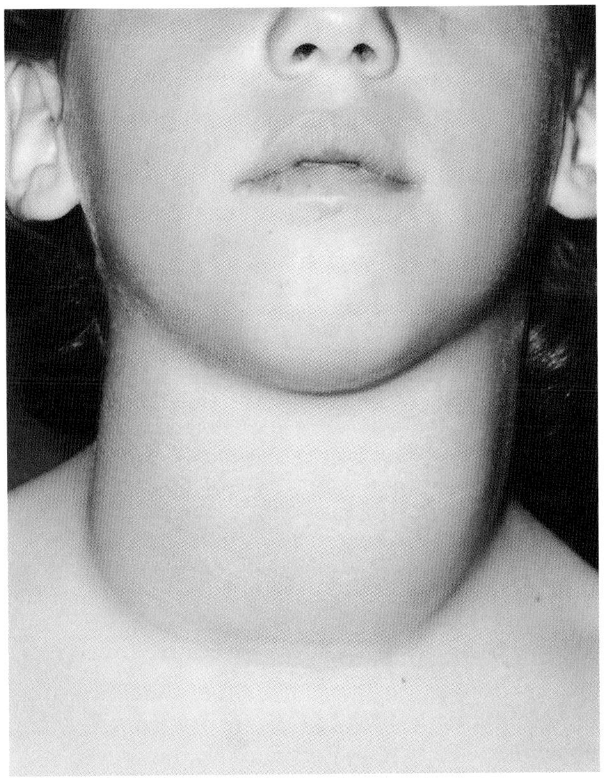

A symptom of hyperthyroidism is the enlargement of the thyroid gland. *(© Lester V. Bergman/Corbis.)*

Demographics

Hyperthyroidism is a fairly common disorder; the National Institute of Diabetes and Digestive and Kidney Diseases (NIDDK) estimates that about 1% of the population of the United States and Canada has some form of hyperthyroidism. It is primarily a disease of adults; most patients are 35 or older at the time of diagnosis. Only about 5% of patients are younger than 15 years of age. The peak age for hyperthyroidism caused by Graves' disease is 35 to 40 years; hyperthyroidism caused by multinodular goiter is more common in adults over 50 than in younger adults.

The disease is 10 times more common in women than in men, and the annual incidence of hyperthyroidism in the United States is about 1 per 1,000 women. About 7% of women of childbearing age develop postpartum **thyroiditis** in the year after they give birth. Between 3% and 7% of adults in the United States develop thyroid nodules. Occult hyperthyroidism may occur in patients over 65 and is characterized by a distinct lack of typical symptoms. Diffuse toxic goiter occurs in as many as 80% of patients with hyperthyroidism.

Among children, about five times as many girls as boys develop hyperthyroidism. Almost all cases of pediatric hyperthyroidism are the form called Graves' disease. There is a form of hyperthyroidism called neonatal Graves' disease, which occurs in infants born of mothers with Graves' disease. Children with such other conditions as trisomy 21 (**Down syndrome**), **Addison's disease**, diabetes, **systemic lupus erythematosus**, **rheumatoid arthritis**, **myasthenia gravis**, **vitiligo**, **pernicious anemia**, and immune thrombocytopenic purpura are more likely to develop Graves' disease.

Hyperthyroidism is equally common among Caucasians, Asians, and Hispanics in the United States but is less common among African Americans. The reason for this difference was not known as of 2009.

Description

Located in the front of the neck, the thyroid gland is a butterfly-shaped structure lying between the Adam's apple and the collarbone. It takes its name from a Greek word meaning "shield." It consists of two lobes about 2 inches in length (in adults) connected by a thin strip of tissue called the isthmus. The thyroid gland weighs about a tenth of an ounce in newborns and 0.6–1.5 ounces in adults. One of the largest endocrine glands in the body, the thyroid controls the rate at which the body burns energy, its sensitivity to other hormones, and its manufacture of proteins.

The thyroid gland produces two hormones: thyroxine (T_4) and triiodothyronine (T_3, which regulate the body's metabolic rate by helping to form protein ribonucleic acid (RNA) and increasing oxygen absorption in every cell. In turn, the production of these hormones is controlled by thyroid-stimulating hormone (TSH), which is produced by the pituitary gland. Hyperthyroidism occurs when production of the thyroid hormones increases despite the level of TSH being produced. The excessive amount of thyroid hormones in the blood increases the body's metabolism, producing both mental and physical symptoms.

Risk factors

Risk factors for hyperthyroidism include:

- Female sex
- Age over 60
- Family history of thyroid disorders. Some genes have been identified as of 2009 that increase a person's susceptibility to autoimmune thyroid disease.
- Personal history of thyroid surgery or goiter
- Having type 1 diabetes, pernicious anemia, or primary adrenal insufficiency
- Pregnancy
- Giving birth within the past 6 months

- Eating large amounts of iodine-containing foods.
- Use of medications containing iodine, particularly amiodarone (Cordarone), a drug given to treat irregular heart rhythms.

Causes and symptoms

Causes

Hyperthyroidism is often associated with the body's production of autoantibodies in the blood that cause the thyroid to grow and secrete excess thyroid hormone. This condition, as well as other forms of hyperthyroidism, may be inherited. It accounts for 70–75% of cases of hyperthyroidism.

Other causes of hyperthyroidism include multinodular goiter or Plummer's disease (about 15–20% of cases of hyperthyroidism), a condition in which adenomas (nodules or lumps) form within the thyroid gland and cause it to secrete a larger than normal amount of thyroid hormone, and thyroiditis, a condition in which a malfunction of the immune system or a viral infection causes the thyroid gland to leak thyroid hormone. Last, hyperthyroidism can be caused by taking too much thyroid hormone in tablet form. In a few very rare cases, hyperthyroidism can be caused by a malignant (cancerous) tumor in the thyroid gland.

Symptoms

Regardless of the cause or age of the patient, hyperthyroidism produces the same symptoms, including sudden weight loss with increased appetite, **shortness of breath** and **fatigue**, intolerance of heat, heart **palpitations**, increased frequency of bowel movements, warm and smooth skin, weak muscles, **tremors**, **anxiety**, and difficulty sleeping. Women of childbearing age may also notice decreased menstrual flow and irregular menstrual cycles.

The symptoms of hyperthyroidism are often less noticeable in older adults, and may consist mainly of an increased heart rate, heat intolerance, and a tendency to become tired during ordinary activities. In addition, **beta blockers** (a type of heart medication) can mask the symptoms of hyperthyroidism in seniors.

Patients with Graves' disease often have a goiter (visible enlargement of the thyroid gland), although as many as 10 percent do not. These patients may also have bulging eyes. Thyroid storm, a serious form of hyperthyroidism, may show up as sudden and acute symptoms, some of which mimic typical hyperthyroidism, as well as the addition of **fever** (104°F or higher), substantial weakness, extreme restlessness, confusion, emotional swings or **psychosis**, or **coma**. Fortunately, such a fulminant course of Graves' disease is rare in children and adolescents.

Babies with neonatal Graves' disease may suffer from **prematurity**, airway obstruction, and **heart failure**. **Death** occurs in as many as 16 percent of these babies, and other complications from which survivors may suffer include craniosynostosis (early closure of the sutures of the skull, which can result in compression of the growing brain), and developmental delay.

Diagnosis

The diagnosis of hyperthyroidism is based on a combination of patient history, a **physical examination**, and the results of laboratory and imaging tests. In most cases, patients are evaluated and treated by an endocrinologist rather than a family doctor.

Examination

Patients concerned that they may have nodules in their thyroid or an enlarged thyroid can conduct a "neck check" at home by examining their neck below the Adam's apple and above the collarbone while swallowing water and looking in a handheld mirror. Detailed instructions for the neck check can be found at the AACE link under the "Other" Resources listed for this article.

An endocrinologist will look for physical signs and symptoms indicated by the patient's history during an office examination. The patient will typically be asked to lift the head and swallow several times while the doctor feels the part of the neck containing the thyroid gland. On inspection, the physician may note such symptoms as a goiter, warm, smooth, and moist skin, eye bulging or a staring gaze, high blood pressure, irregular heart rhythm, hyperactivity, overactive reflexes, tremor, and muscle weakness. **Pregnancy** or recent **childbirth** or a family history of thyroid disorders may also be clues to a diagnosis of hyperthyroidism.

Tests

A simple blood test can be performed to determine the amount of thyroid hormone in the patient's blood. The American Thyroid Association recommends that adults, particularly women, have this blood test to detect thyroid problems every five years starting at age 35. The diagnosis is usually straightforward with this combination of clinical history, physical examination, and routine blood hormone tests. Radioimmunoassay, a test to show concentrations of thyroid hormones with the use of a radioisotope mixed with fluid samples, helps confirm the diagnosis.

A thyroid scan is a nuclear medicine procedure involving injection of a radioisotope dye that will tag the thyroid and help produce a clear image of inflammation or involvement of the entire thyroid. Other

KEY TERMS

Adenoma—The medical term for a benign (noncancerous) tumor that originates in a gland. Thyroid nodules are one type of adenoma.

Endocrine gland—Any gland that makes hormones and secretes them directly into the bloodstream.

Endocrinologist—A doctor who specializes in diagnosing and treating disorders of the endocrine glands and the hormones they secrete.

Fulminant—Referring to a disease process that is explosive in onset, severe, and potentially deadly.

Goiter—Chronic enlargement of the thyroid gland.

Gonads—Organs that produce gametes (eggs or sperm), such as the ovaries and testes.

Graves' disease—An autoimmune disorder of the thyroid gland, in which the gland swells to twice its normal size and secretes too much thyroid hormone. Graves' disease accounts for 70–75% of cases of hyperthyroidism. It is named for an Irish doctor named Robert James Graves, who described a case of the disorder in 1835.

Hormone—A chemical released by specialized cells that affects cells in other parts of the body. Hormones regulate such body processes as growth, metabolism, the immune system, reproduction, hunger, and mood.

Multinodular goiter—A condition in which benign lumps of tissue (nodules) form within the thyroid gland and cause it to secrete too much thyroid hormone. It is also called Plummer's disease.

Palpitations—Rapid and forceful heartbeat.

Postpartum—After childbirth.

Radioisotope—One of two or more atoms with the same number of protons but a different number of neutrons with a nuclear composition. In nuclear scanning, radioactive isotopes are used as a diagnostic agent.

Thyroid storm—A rare but potentially life-threatening complication of hyperthyroidism, characterized by fever over 104°F, irregular heart rhythm, vomiting, diarrhea, dehydration, coma, and death.

Thyroidectomy—Surgical removal of the thyroid gland.

Thyroiditis—Inflammation of the thyroid gland. It can be caused by a viral infection, a malfunction of the immune system, or certain medications.

Thyrotoxicosis—Another term for hyperthyroidism.

Vitiligo—A chronic skin disorder that causes loss of pigmentation (color) from patches of skin, most often on the face, hands, and wrists.

tests can determine thyroid function and thyroid-stimulating hormone levels. Ultrasonography, **computed tomography scans** (CT scan), and **magnetic resonance imaging** (MRI) may provide visual confirmation of a diagnosis or help to determine the extent of involvement.

Procedures

The doctor may also order a fine needle aspiration biopsy (FNAB), a procedure in which the doctor inserts a thin needle into a suspected thyroid nodule to extract a sample of cells for examination under a microscope. The doctor usually uses an ultrasound monitor to guide the needle. A FNAB can be performed in an outpatient clinic or a doctor's office; it is safer and less invasive than an open surgical biopsy.

Treatment

Traditional

Treatment of hyperthyroidism will depend on the specific disease and individual circumstances such as age, severity of disease, and other conditions affecting a patient's health. No single approach to treatment works for all patients.

Drugs

Hyperthyroidism is usually treated with medications whenever possible. The two types of drugs most often prescribed are antithyroid drugs and radioactive iodine.

ANTITHYROID DRUGS. Antithyroid drugs are often administered to help the patient's body cease overproduction of thyroid hormones. The antithyroid drugs most commonly prescribed are methimazole (Tapazole) and propylthiouracil (PTU). About 20% to 30% of patients with Graves' disease will have long-term remission of hyperthyroidism after treatment with antithyroid drugs for a period of 12–18 months. It takes several weeks or months for antithyroid drugs to bring the patient's level of thyroid hormone into the normal range. Patients may be given beta blockers for symptom relief during this period.

Antithyroid drugs are also used in preparation for either radioiodine treatment or surgery in patients diagnosed with multinodular goiter. These medications may work for young adults, pregnant women, and others. Women who are pregnant should be treated with the lowest dose required to maintain thyroid function in order to minimize the risk of **hypothyroidism** in the infant.

Antithyroid drugs can have unpleasant side effects, such as **rashes**, **itching**, or increased susceptibility to infection due to a decreased level of white blood cells. In rare cases these medications can lead to liver failure.

RADIOACTIVE IODINE. Radioactive iodine (iodine-131) is often prescribed to damage cells that make thyroid hormone. The cells need iodine to make the hormone, so they will absorb any iodine found in the body. The patient may take an iodine capsule daily for several weeks, resulting in the eventual shrinkage of the thyroid in size, reduced hormone production and a return to normal blood levels. Some patients may receive a single larger oral dose of radioactive iodine to treat the disease more quickly. This should only be done for patients who are not of reproductive age or are not planning to have children, since a large amount can concentrate in the reproductive organs (gonads). The risk of long-term side effects is low, however, as radioactive iodine has been used for over 60 years to treat patients with hyperthyroidism and doctors have followed these patients carefully.

Most patients who are given iodone-131 eventually develop hypothyroidism, which is an abnormally low level of thyroid hormone. Most endocrinologists do not consider this side effect of iodine-131 to be a major problem, however, because hypothyroidism is easier to treat and has fewer long-term complications than hyperthyroidism.

BETA BLOCKERS. Beta blockers may be used in the treatment of patients with hyperthyroidism even though they do not suppress the activity of the thyroid gland. They are useful in regulating the patient's heart rhythm and reducing such symptoms as palpitations, tremor, and nervousness until antithyroid medications can begin to take effect. The beta blockers most often prescribed for hyperthyroidism are the longer-acting drugs like atenolol (Tenormin), metoprolol (Lopressor), and nadolol (Corgard).

Surgery

Some patients may undergo surgery to treat hyperthyroidism. Surgery is usually recommended when the results of a FNAB indicate that the patient has a malignancy in the thyroid, or when the thyroid gland is so enlarged that it is putting pressure on the patient's windpipe or esophagus.

Most commonly, patients treated with **thyroidectomy** in the form of partial or total removal of the thyroid suffer from large goiter and have suffered relapses, even after repeated attempts to address the disease through drug therapy. Some patients may be candidates for surgery because they were not good candidates for iodine therapy, or refused iodine administration. Patients receiving thyroidectomy or iodine therapy must be carefully monitored for years to watch for signs of hypothyroidism, or insufficient production of thyroid hormones, which can occur as a complication of thyroid production suppression.

Alternative

Consumption of such foods as broccoli, Brussels sprouts, cabbage, cauliflower, kale, rutabagas, spinach, turnips, peaches, and pears can help naturally suppress thyroid hormone production. Caffeinated drinks and dairy products should be avoided. Under the supervision of a trained physician, high dosages of certain vitamin/mineral combinations can help to alleviate hyperthyroidism.

Prognosis

Hyperthyroidism is generally treatable and carries a good prognosis. Most patients lead normal lives with proper treatment. Thyroid storm, however, can be life-threatening and can lead to heart, liver, or kidney failure. Luckily, this form of fulminant hyperthyroidism is rare in children and adolescents.

Hyperthyroidism is associated with an increased risk of **Alzheimer's disease** in later life even when the thyroid dysfunction has been successfully treated. The reason for this association was not fully understood as of 2009.

Prevention

Although a periodic neck check at home cannot prevent hyperthyroidism in the strict sense of prevention, it can help in detecting the condition earlier rather than later.

There are no known prevention methods for hyperthyroidism, since its causes were either inherited or not completely understood as of 2009. The best prevention tactic is knowledge of family history and close attention to symptoms and signs of the disease. Careful attention to prescribed therapy can prevent complications of the disease.

Resources

BOOKS

Cooper, David S. *Medical Management of Thyroid Disease*, 2nd ed. New York: Informa Healthcare, 2009.

Mertens, Lionel, and Jeremy Bogaert, eds. *Handbook of Hyperthyroidism: Etiology, Diagnosis, and Treatment.* Hauppauge, NY: Nova Science, 2009.

Shannon, Joyce Brennfleck. *Endocrine and Metabolic Disorders Sourcebook*, 2nd ed. Detroit, MI: Omnigraphics, 2007.

PERIODICALS

Baloch, Z.W., and V.A. LiVolsi. "Fine-needle Aspiration of the Thyroid: Today and Tomorrow." *Best Practice and Research: Clinical Endocrinology and Metabolism* 22 (December 2008): 929–39.

Brown, R.S. "Autoimmune Thyroid Disease: Unlocking a Complex Puzzle." *Current Opinion in Pediatrics* 21 (August 2009): 523–28.

Hegedüs, L. "Treatment of Graves' Hyperthyroidism: Evidence-based and Emerging Modalities." *Endocrinology and Metabolism Clinics of North America* 38 (June 2009): 355–71.

Kaguelidou, F., et al. "Graves' Disease in Childhood: Advances in Management with Antithyroid Drug Therapy." *Hormone Research* 71 (June 2009): 310–317.

Kharlip, J., and D.S. Cooper. "Recent Developments in Hyperthyroidism." *Lancet* 373 (June 6, 2009): 1930–32.

Kohl, B.A., and S. Schwartz. "Surgery in the Patient with Endocrine Dysfunction." *Medical Clinics of North America* 93 (September 2009): 1031–47.

Mistry, N., et al. "When to Consider Thyroid Dysfunction in the Neurology Clinic." *Practical Neurology* 9 (June 2009): 145–56.

Tan, Z.S., and R.S. Vasan. "Thyroid Function and Alzheimer's Disease." *Journal of Alzheimer's Disease* 16 (March 2009): 503–07.

Yildizhan, R., et al. "Fetal Death Due to Upper Airway Compromise Complicated by Thyroid Storm in a Mother with Uncontrolled Graves' Disease: A Case Report." *Journal of Medical Case Reports* 28 (May 2009): 7297.

OTHER

American Association of Clinical Endocrinologists (AACE). "How to Take the Thyroid 'Neck Check'." http://www.aace.com/public/awareness/tam/2006/pdfs/NeckCheckCard.pdf.

American Thyroid Association (ATA). *Hyperthyroidism.* http://www.thyroid.org/patients/patient_brochures/hyperthyroidism.html.

Hormone Foundation. *Hyperthyroidism.* http://www.hormone.org/Thyroid/hyperthyroidism.cfm.

Lee, Stephanie L., and Sonia Ananthakrishnan. "Hyperthyroidism." *eMedicine*, June 8, 2009. http://emedicine.medscape.com/article/121865-overview.

Mayo Clinic. *Hyperthyroidism.* http://www.mayoclinic.com/health/hyperthyroidism/DS00344.

National Institute of Diabetes and Digestive and Kidney Diseases (NIDDK). *Hyperthyroidism.* http://endocrine.niddk.nih.gov/pubs/Hyperthyroidism/index.htm.

Reid, Jeri R., and Stephen F. Wheeler. "Hyperthyroidism: Diagnosis and Treatment." *American Family Physician* 72 (August 15, 2005): 623–36. http://www.aafp.org/afp/20050815/623.html.

ORGANIZATIONS

American Academy of Otolaryngology—Head and Neck Surgery, 1650 Diagonal Road, Alexandria, VA, 22314, 703-836-4444, http://www.entnet.org/.

American Association of Clinical Endocrinologists (AACE), 245 Riverside Ave., Suite 200, Jacksonville, FL, 32202, 904-353-7878, http://www.aace.com/.

American Thyroid Association (ATA), 6066 Leesburg Pike, Suite 550, Falls Church, VA, 22041, 703-998-8890, 703-998-8893, thyroid@thyroid.org, http://www.thyroid.org/.

Hormone Foundation, 8401 Connecticut Avenue, Suite 900, Chevy Chase, MD, 20815, 800–HORMONE, 301-941-0259, hormone@endo-society.org, http://www.hormone.org/.

National Institute of Diabetes and Digestive and Kidney Diseases (NIDDK), Building 31. Rm 9A06, 31 Center Drive, MSC 2560, Bethesda, MD, 20892-2560, 301-496-3583, http://www2.niddk.nih.gov/Footer/Contact NIDDK.htm, http://www2.niddk.nih.gov/.

Teresa G. Odle
Rosalyn Carson-DeWitt, MD
Rebecca J. Frey, PhD

Hypertrophic cardiomyopathy

Definition

Cardiomyopathy is an ongoing disease process that damages the muscle wall of the lower chambers of the heart. Hypertrophic cardiomyopathy is a form of cardiomyopathy in which the walls of the heart's chambers thicken abnormally. Other names for hypertrophic cardiomyopathy are idiopathic hypertrophic subaortic stenosis and asymmetrical septal hypertrophy.

Description

Hypertrophic cardiomyopathy usually appears in young people, often in athletes. For this reason it is sometimes called athletic heart muscle disease. However, people of any age can develop hypertrophic cardiomyopathy. Often there are no symptoms of hypertrophic cardiomyopathy. Sudden **death** can occur, caused by a heart arrhythmia. The American Heart Association

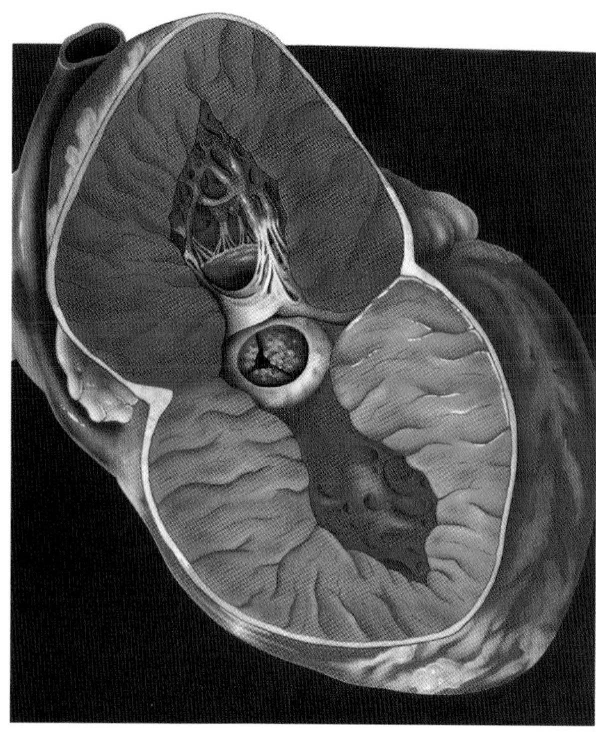

This illustration shows hypertrophic muscle in the heart. The abnormally thick wall of muscle prevents the chambers from stretching to fill up with blood, making the heart less efficient. The extra tissue may also push on the heart valve (center), causing it to leak. *(Custom Medical Stock Photo, Inc. Reproduced by permission.)*

reports that 36% of young athletes who die suddenly have probable or definite hypertrophic cardiomyopathy.

Hypertrophic cardiomyopathy is the result of abnormal growth of the heart muscle cells. The wall between the heart's chambers (the septum) may become so thickened that it blocks the flow of blood through the lower left chamber (left ventricle). The thickened wall may push on the heart valve between the two left heart chambers (mitral valve), making it leaky. The thickened muscle walls also prevent the heart from stretching as much as it should to fill with blood.

Causes and symptoms

The cause of hypertrophic cardiomyopathy is not known. In about one-half of cases, the disease is inherited. An abnormal gene has been identified in these patients. In cases that are not hereditary, a gene that was normal at birth may later become abnormal.

Often people with hypertrophic cardiomyopathy have no symptoms. Unfortunately, the first sign of the condition may be sudden death caused by an abnormal heart rhythm. When symptoms do appear, they include **shortness of breath** on exertion, **dizziness**, **fainting**, **fatigue**, and chest **pain**.

Diagnosis

The diagnosis is based on the patient's symptoms (if any), a complete **physical examination**, and tests that detect abnormalities of the heart chambers. Usually, there is an abnormal heart murmur that worsens with the **Valsalva maneuver**. The electrocardiogram (ECG), which provides a record of electrical changes in the heart muscle during the heartbeat, also is typically abnormal.

Sometimes, a routine **chest x ray** may show that the heart is enlarged. **Echocardiography**, a procedure that produces images of the heart's structure, is usually done. These images can show if the heart wall is thickened and if there are any abnormalities of the heart valves.

Treatment

Treatment of hypertrophic cardiomyopathy usually consists of taking medicines and restricting strenuous **exercise**. Drugs called **beta blockers** and **calcium channel blockers** are usually prescribed. Beta blockers reduce the force of the heart's contractions. **Calcium** channel blockers can help improve the flexibility of the heart muscle walls, allowing them to stretch more. **Antiarrhythmic drugs** may also be given to prevent abnormal heart rhythms.

Patients with hypertrophic cardiomyopathy are also told to avoid strenuous exercise to reduce the risk of passing out or sudden death.

In some cases, if the medications do not help relieve symptoms, surgery may help. In an operation called myotomy-myectomy a piece of the septum is removed to improve blood flow through the heart chamber.

Some patients have **pacemakers** and/or defibrillators implanted to help control the heart rate and rhythm. Pacemakers and defibrillators provide electrical impulses to the heart, which can return the heart beat to a normal rhythm.

If these treatment methods fail and a patient develops **heart failure**, a heart transplant may be necessary.

Prognosis

Some people with hypertrophic cardiomyopathy may not have obstructed blood flow and may never experience symptoms. Others may only experience mild symptoms. With treatment, symptoms may improve. In some patients, the disease may progress to heart failure.

Prevention

While hypertrophic cardiomyopathy cannot be prevented, precautionary measures may prevent sudden deaths. Anyone planning to take part in a program of strenuous competitive exercise should have a checkup by a physician first. A physical examination before athletic participation can usually, but not always, detect conditions like hypertrophic cardiomyopathy. Anyone who experiences symptoms of shortness of breath, tiredness, or fainting with exercise should see a physician.

ORGANIZATIONS

American Heart Association National Center, 7272 Greenville Avenue, Dallas, TX, 75231, (800) 242-8721, Review.personal.info@heart.org.

National Heart Lung and Blood Institute Health Information Center, P.O. Box 30105, Bethesda, MD, 20824-0105, (301) 592-8573, (240) 629-3246, http://www.nhlbi.nih.gov.

Texas Heart Institute. Heart Information Service, MC 3-116, PO Box 20345, Houston, TX, 77225, (832) 355-4011, (800) 292-2221, http://www.texasheart.org.

Toni Rizzo

Hypervitaminosis *see* **Vitamin toxicity**

Hyphema

Definition

A hyphema is an accumulation of blood in the front (anterior) chamber of the eye. It is usually caused by blunt eye trauma.

Description

The anterior chamber (AC) is located behind the front of the eye. The AC is filled with a fluid called aqueous humor. This fluid helps form a cushion for the eye and provides an important route for nutrient and waste transport. Contusive forces from high velocity projectiles (approximately 34% of emergency room cases) such as a rock, crab apples, ice balls, badminton birds, and bungee cords can tear local blood vessels in the eye. Blunt impact from a basketball or racketball accounts for about 62% of cases. Tearing a small blood vessel can cause seepage of blood into a visible layer portion of the AC, causing the affected person to have a red eye.

Causes and symptoms

Hyphema is caused by blunt, projectile, or explosion (about 4% of cases) injuries. These injuries cause a local blood vessel in the eye to tear, filling the front portion of the AC with blood. The initial complaint is a dramatic decrease in vision that eventually gets better as blood seeps towards the back of the eye. Patients will have extreme **pain**, an increase in intraocular pressure (the pressure inside the eye), and **nausea**. Patients usually will show a red eye and a recent history of trauma. Patients are vulnerable to more bleeding three to five days post injury.

Diagnosis

All persons with hyphema must be examined by an ophthalmologist (a physician who specializes in the medical and surgical care of the eye). Usually the clinician will use an ophthalmoscope to visualize the internal structures and damage. In some cases there may be small microscopic bleeds that may form clots (microhyphema) and require specialized instrumentation (a slit lamp) for visualization.

Treatment

Bloodthinners, such as **aspirin** and **nonsteroidal anti-inflammatory drugs**, should be avoided. In most cases the affected person can be medically managed on an outpatient basis. The eye should be shielded, but not patched. The patient should be placed on bed rest with the head elevated 45°. This position allows blood to leave the AC allowing for better vision. Several studies suggest administering medications (aminocaproic acid) that stabilize clot formation, reducing the possibility of increased bleeding.

Prognosis

The outcome depends on the severity of the trauma. Most cases progress well with conservative treatment. Some cases may develop an increase in the pressure within the eye (glaucoma). If this develops the hyphema must be surgically removed by an ophthalmologist. In patients who have a preexisting blood disorder, surgical evacuation should be considered to prevent damage to the optic nerve (the nerve that transmits impulses for processing in the brain).

Prevention

The American Academy of Ophthalmology recommends special eyewear made of polycarbonate lenses when at risk of eye injury. This type of lens has sufficient impact resistance.

Resources

BOOKS

Kliegman, Robert M., and Waldo Emerson Nelson. *Nelson Textbook of Pediatrics*. 18th ed. Philadelphia: Saunders, Elsevier, 2007.

Yanoff, Myron, et al, eds. *Ophthalmology*. 3rd ed. Edinburgh: Mosby International, 2009.

Laith Farid Gulli, M.D.

Hypnosis *see* **Hypnotherapy**

Hypnotherapy

Definition

Hypnotherapy is the treatment of a variety of health conditions by hypnotism or by inducing prolonged sleep.

Pioneers in this field, such as James Braid and James Esdaile, discovered that hypnosis could be used to successfully anesthetize patients for surgeries. James Braid accidentally discovered that one of his patients began to enter a hypnotic state while staring at a fixed light as he waited for his **eye examination** to begin. Since mesmerism had fallen out of favor, Braid coined the term hypnotism, which is derived from the Greek word for sleep. Braid also used the techniques of monotony, rhythm, and imitation to assist in inducing a hypnotic state. These techniques are still in use.

Around 1900, there were very few preoperative anesthetic drugs available. Patients were naturally apprehensive when facing surgery. One out of four hundred patients would die, not from the surgical procedure, but from the anesthesia. Dr. Henry Munro was one of the first physicians to use hypnotherapy to alleviate patient fears about having surgery. He would get his patients into a hypnotic state and discuss their fears with them, telling them they would feel a lot better following surgery. Ether was the most common anesthetic at that time, and Dr. Munro found that he was able to perform surgery using only about 10% of the usual amount of ether.

Purpose

Hypnotherapy is used in a number of fields including **psychotherapy**, surgery, dentistry, research, and medicine. Hypnotherapy is commonly used as an alternative treatment for a wide range of health conditions, including weight control, **pain management**, and **smoking** cessation. It is also used to control **pain** in a variety of conditions such as **headache**, facial **neuralgia**, arthritis, **burns**, musculoskeletal disorders, **childbirth**, and many more. Hypnotherapy is being used in place of anesthesia, particularly in patients who prove to be allergic to anesthetic drugs, for surgeries such as hysterectomies, cesarean sections, certain cardiovascular procedures, **thyroidectomy**, and others. Dentistry is using hypnotherapy with success on patients who are allergic to all types of novocaine drugs. Hypnotherapy is also useful in helping patients overcome **phobias**.

Hypnotherapy is used for nonmedical patients as well as those who wish to overcome bad habits. Hypnotherapy has been shown to help those who suffer from performance **anxiety**, such as in sports, and speaking in public. In academic applications, it has also been shown to help with learning, participating in the classroom, concentrating, studying, focusing attention span, improving memory, and helping remove mental blocks about particular subjects.

In more general areas, hypnotherapy has been found to be beneficial for problems such as motivation, procrastination, decision making, personal achievement and development, job performance, buried or repressed memories, relaxation, and **stress** management.

Description

Origins

Hypnotherapy is thought to date back to the healing practices of ancient Greece and Egypt. Many religions such as Judaism, Christianity, Islam, and others have attributed trance-like behavior to spiritual or divine possession.

Austrian physician, Franz Mesmer (1734–1815), is credited with being the first person to scientifically investigate the idea of hypnotherapy, in 1779, to treat a variety of health conditions. Mesmer studied medicine at the University of Vienna and received his medical degree in 1766. Mesmer is believed to have been the first doctor to understand the relationship of psychological trauma to illness. He induced a trance-like state, which became known as mesmerism, in his patients to successfully treat nervous disorders. These techniques became the foundation for modern-day hypnotherapy.

Mesmer's original interest was in the effect of celestial bodies on human lives. He later became interested in the effects of magnetism, and found that magnets could have tremendous healing effects on the human body. Mesmer believed that the human body contained a magnetic fluid that promoted health and well being. It was thought that any blockage to the normal flow of this magnetic fluid would result in illness, and that the use of the mesmerism technique could restore the normal flow.

Mesmer performed his technique by passing his hands up and down the patient's body. The technique was supposed to transmit magnetic fluid from his hands to the bodies of his patients. During this time, there was no clear delineation between health conditions that were physical or psychological in nature. Although Mesmer did not realize it at that time, his treatments were most effective for those conditions that were primarily psychosomatic.

Mesmer's technique appeared to be quite successful in the treatment of his patients, but he was the subject of scorn and ridicule from the medical profession. Because of all the controversy surrounding mesmerism, and because Mesmer's personality was quite eccentric, a commission was convened to investigate his techniques and procedures. A very distinguished panel of investigators included Benjamin Franklin, the French chemist Antoine-Laurent Lavoisier, and physician Jacques Guillotin. The commission acknowledged that patients did seem to obtain noticeable relief from their conditions, but the whole idea was dismissed as being medical quackery.

It took more than 200 years for hypnotherapy to be incorporated into medical treatment. In 1955, the British Medical Association approved the use of hypnotherapy as a valid medical treatment, with the American Medical Association (AMA) giving its approval in 1958.

Hypnotherapy involves achieving a psychological state of awareness that is different from the ordinary state of consciousness. While in a hypnotic state, a variety of phenomena can occur. These phenomena include alterations in memory, heightened susceptibility to suggestion, **paralysis**, sweating, and blushing. All of these changes can be produced or removed in the hypnotic state. Many studies have shown that roughly 90% of the population is capable of being hypnotized.

This state of awareness can be achieved by relaxing the body, focusing on breathing, and shifting attention away from the external environment. In this state, the patient has a heightened receptivity to suggestion. The usual procedure for inducing a hypnotic trance in another person is by direct command repeated in a soothing, monotonous tone of voice.

Preparations

Ideally, the following conditions should be present to successfully achieve a state of hypnosis:

- willingness to be hypnotized
- rapport between the patient or client and the hypnotherapist
- a comfortable environment that is conducive to relaxation

Precautions

Hypnotherapy can have negative outcomes. When used as entertainment, people have been hypnotized to say or do things that would normally embarrass them. There have been instances where people already dangerously close to psychological breakdown have been pushed into an emotional crisis during what was supposed to be a harmless demonstration of hypnosis. A statement from the World Hypnosis Organization (WHO) warns against performing hypnosis on patients suffering from **psychosis**, organic psychiatric conditions, or antisocial **personality disorders**. Because there are no standard licensing requirements, in the wrong hands, there is a risk that the hypnotist will have difficulty in controlling or ending a hypnotic state that has been induced in the patient.

There is a commonly held belief that a person cannot be coerced into doing things that they would not normally do while under hypnosis. The hynotherapist should take care however, not to give suggestions during hypnosis that are contrary to the patient's moral code.

Many religions do not condone the practice of hypnotherapy. Leaders of the Jehovah's Witnesses and Christian Science religions oppose the use of hypnotherapy and advise their members to avoid it completely, whether for entertainment or therapy. The Church of Jesus Christ of Latter-Day Saints approves it for medical purposes, but cautions members against allowing themselves to be hypnotized for entertainment or demonstration purposes.

In 1985, The AMA convened a commission that warned against using hypnotherapy to aid in recollection of events. The commission cited studies that showed the possibility of hypnotic recall resulting on confabulation or an artificial sense of certainty about the course of events. As a result, many states limit or prohibit testimony of hypnotized witnesses or victims.

Side effects

Experiments have been conducted to determine any side effects of hypnotherapy. Some subjects have reported side effects such as headache, stiff neck, drowsiness, cognitive distortion or confusion, **dizziness**, and anxiety. However, most of these effects cleared up within several hours of the hypnotherapy session.

Research and general acceptance

Research on the effectiveness of hypnotherapy on a variety of medical conditions is extensive. In one study, the use of hypnotherapy did not seem to alter the core symptoms in the treatment of attention-deficit hyperactivity disorder (**ADHD**); however, it did seem to be useful in managing the associated symptoms including sleep disturbances and tics.

Hypnotherapy is being studied in children who have common, chronic problems and to aid in relieving pain. Children are particularly good candidates for hypnotherapy because their lack of worldly experience enables them to move easily between the rational world and their imagination. Studies with children have shown responses to hypnotherapy ranging from diminished pain and anxiety during a number of medical procedures, a 50% range in reduction of symptoms or a complete resolution of a medical condition, and a reduction in use of anti-nausea medication and **vomiting** during **chemotherapy** for childhood cancers.

The use of hypnotherapy with **cancer** patients is another area being investigated. A meta-analysis of 116 studies showed very positive results of using hypnotherapy with cancer patients. Ninety-two percent showed a positive effect on depression; 93% showed a positive effect on physical well-being; 81% showed a positive effect on **vomiting**; and 92% showed a positive effect on pain.

ORGANIZATIONS

American Board of Hypnotherapy, P.O. Box 531605, Henderson, NV, 89053, (702) 456-3267, (702) 436-3267, Candace@abh-abnlp.com, http://www.abh-abnlp.com/.

American Psychotherapy & Medical Hypnosis Association, 3430 Creekwood Drive, Brownsville, TX, 78526, (956) 465-1581, admin@apmha.com, http://apmha.com/.

American Society of Clinical Hypnosis, 140 N. Bloomingdale Rd, Bloomingdale, IL, 60108, (630) 980-4740, (630) 351-8490, info@asch.net, http://www.asch.net/.

Hypnotherapy Society, PO Box 131, Arundel, UK, BN18 8BR, secretary@hypnotherapysociety.com, http://www.hypnotherapysociety.com.

International Council for Medical and Clinical Therapists, 7361 McWhorter Place, Suite 300, Annandale, VA, 2203-5649, (703) 658-2014, http://www.seec-icmct.com/icmct.htm.

International Medical and Dental Hypnotherapy Association, 8852 SR 3001, Laceyville, PA, 18623, (570) 869-1021, (570) 869-1249, (800) 553-6886, info@imdha.com, http://www.imdha.com/.

Society for Clinical and Experimental Hypnosis, 728 Old McLean Village Drive, McLean, VA, 22101.

World Hypnosis Organization, Inc, 2521 W. Montrose Avenue, Chicago, IL, 60618, (773) 267-6677, copal@anet-chi.com, http://www.worldhypnosis.org.

Kim A. Sharp, M.Ln.

Hypoactive sexual desire disorder

Definition

Hypoactive sexual desire disorder (HSDD) is a persistent or recurrent extreme aversion to or avoidance of genital sexual contact with a partner. HSDD is also called sexual aversion, inhibited sexual desire, sexual apathy, or sexual anorexia.

Demographics

HSDD is one of the most common sexual disorders. However the incidence of HSDD is difficult to estimate since as many as 40% of adults report a loss of sexual desire at some point in their lives. HSDD has traditionally been associated with women; however 30% of women report that they have more interest in sex than their male partners. Estimates of the incidence of HSDD in both males and females range from 5 to more than 20 percent.

Description

People with HSDD have a low level of sexual interest and desire that is manifested by the failure to initiate sexual activity or to respond to a partner's sexual overtures. However sexual desire normally fluctuates over the course of person's life. Often sexual desire is high at the beginning of a relationship and low as a relationship wanes. Illness can affect sexual desire, as can life changes such as **pregnancy** and **menopause** in women. According to the American Psychiatric Association's *Diagnostic and Statistical Manual of Mental Disorders*, fourth edition, text revision (*DSM–IV–TR*), a diagnosis of HSDD requires a persistent or recurrent lack of sexual desire that causes marked distress or interpersonal instability. In the most extreme form of HSDD, the patient not only lacks sexual desire, but may find sex to be distasteful, repulsive, or revolting.

HSDD can take various forms:

- Primary HSDD is a condition in which the patient has never felt much sexual interest or desire.

- Secondary or acquired HSDD occurs in patients who formerly had normal sexual desires but no longer have any interest in sex.
- Generalized HSDD is a lack of sexual desire in all situations and with any partner.
- Situational or selective HSDD is an aversion directed at a specific partner or only under certain circumstances.

Risk factors

Because HSDD is caused by so many different physiological, psychological, and emotional factors, it is difficult to delineate risk factors. However people who have experienced sexual trauma or were raised to have negative attitudes toward sex may be at greater risk for primary HSDD.

Causes and symptoms

The major symptom of HSDD is a lack of interest in sex, even under circumstances that are usually erotic, such as viewing pornography. Sexual activity is infrequent or nonexistent, causing distress or discord within relationships.

HSDD can result from physical, emotional, and/or psychological factors. Lifelong or primary HSDD can be a consequence of sexual trauma such as incest, **sexual abuse**, or **rape**. It can result from repressive family attitudes towards sex, which are sometimes reinforced by rigid religious training. HSDD occasionally occurs after initial attempts at sexual intercourse result in **pain** or sexual failure.

Acquired or situational HSDD in an adult is commonly associated with boredom in a sexual relationship. In such cases, as sexual frequency with the partner decreases, real or fantasized sexual desire for others remains normal or even increases. In addition to boredom, relationship issues that can cause situational HSDD include:

- lack of emotional connection with a sexual partner
- frequent quarrelling or unresolved conflicts with a partner
- poorly communicated sexual needs and preferences
- incompatible sexual interest, often because the unaffected partner is sexually demanding
- infidelity or other breach of trust

Psychological causes of HSDD include:

- a history of physical abuse
- depression
- anxiety
- stress
- poor body image
- low self–esteem

Physical causes of HSDD can include:

- hormonal changes due to pregnancy or breastfeeding
- estrogen deficiency due to female menopause
- low levels of the male sex hormone testosterone, which can also be deficient in postmenopausal women
- other hormonal abnormalities
- illnesses, such as cancer, arthritis, diabetes, high blood pressure, coronary artery disease, or neurological diseases
- surgery of the breasts or genital tract
- obesity
- drug or alcohol abuse
- impairment of sexual function, especially male erectile dysfunction or female vaginismus—an involuntary contraction or spasm of the lower vaginal muscles—which prevents vaginal penetration
- the inability to have an orgasm (aorgasmia)
- infertility
- fatigue

Various medications can cause HSDD including:

- selective serotonin reuptake inhibitors (SSRIs), including the antidepressants sertraline (Zoloft), paroxetine (Paxil), and fluoxetine (Prozac)
- blood pressure medications
- antihistamines
- birth control pills
- chemotherapy drugs
- HIV/AIDS drugs
- some hair–loss remedies

Painful intercourse (**dyspareunia**) is more common in women than in men, but can cause HSDD in either sex. Dyspareunia usually has a physical cause, such as an allergic reaction to a spermicidal preparation, lubricant, or condom. Female dyspareunia can be caused by **vaginismus**, urogenital trauma or infection, inflammatory conditions of the labia or vagina, or vaginal injuries. Male dyspareunia can result from infections of the prostate gland, urethra, or testes. Painful erections can be a consequence of **Peyronie's disease**, which is characterized by fibrotic changes in the shaft of the penis that prevent a normal erection.

Delayed sexual maturation is another potential cause of HSDD. In girls delayed sexual maturation is characterized by a lack of breast enlargement by age 13 or by more than a five–year lapse between the initiation of breast growth and the onset of menstruation. Boys

KEY TERMS

Dyspareunia—Difficult or painful sexual intercourse.

Estrogen—Any of several naturally occurring or synthetic steroid hormones that promote the growth and maintenance of the female reproductive system.

Kegel exercises—Repetitive contractions to tone the pubococcygeal muscle of the pelvic floor for enhancing sexual response during intercourse or controlling incontinence.

Labia—The fatty folds of the vulva.

Priapism—A prolonged erection lasting more than four hours.

Prolactinoma—A benign (noncancerous) tumor of the pituitary gland that secretes the hormone prolactin.

Sexual anhedonia—The inability to experience sexual pleasure.

Testosterone—The primary male sex hormone, which is also produced at low levels in females.

Urethra—The tube that discharges urine from the bladder to the outside of the body.

Vaginismus—A painful spasmodic vaginal contraction.

who have no testicular enlargement by 13.5 years of age or who experience more than a five–year lapse between initial and completed growth of the genitalia are considered to have delayed maturation. Delayed **puberty** can result from:

- familial constitutional disorders
- genetic defects such as Turner's syndrome in females or Klinefelter's syndrome in males
- central nervous system disorders, such as pituitary conditions that interfere with the secretion of gonadotropic hormones
- chronic illnesses such as diabetes mellitus, chronic renal failure, or cystic fibrosis

A rare but important cause of HSDD is a functional prolactin–secreting tumor of the pituitary gland, called a prolactinoma. Although prolactinomas are benign tumors, they can cause visual disturbances by enlarging and exerting pressure on the optic nerves. In females prolactinomas are associated with **galactorrhea (lactation** in the absence of pregnancy), **amenorrhea** (lack of a menstrual period), symptoms of estrogen deficiency, and dyspareunia. Males with prolactinomas typically have no interest in sex, although they can achieve an erection.

The pain that accompanies **priapism** can cause HSDD in males. Priapism is an erection lasting more than four hours and occurring in the absence of sexual stimulation. It is not associated with sexual excitement, and the erection does not subside after ejaculation. Although priapism can occur at any age, it is common in boys between the ages of 5 and 10 and in men between the ages of 20 and 50. Priapism in children is commonly associated with leukemia and **sickle cell disease** or occurs secondary to trauma. The most common cause in adults is the intrapenile injection of agents to correct **erectile dysfunction**. Priapism can also be caused by the use of psychotropic drugs, such as chlorpromazine and prazosin.

Sexual anhedonia is a rare type of male HSDD, in which the man experiences erection and ejaculation but derives no pleasure from orgasm. This is attributed to penile anesthesia, caused by psychogenic factors in a hysterical or obsessive person. Loss of tactile sensation in the penis is rarely due to physical factors unless there are associated anesthetized areas around the anus or scrotum.

Diagnosis

Examination

Diagnosis of HSDD will include a complete physical exam, a gynecological exam for women, a psychological evaluation, and medical and sexual histories, as well as an evaluation of prescribed and over–the–counter medications. Any physical causes of HSDD—such as abnormalities of the genitalia, prolactinoma, chronic renal disease, **diabetes mellitus**, a genetic disorder, or a family history of the disorder—must be identified.

Tests

Screening tests or questionnaires may be used to evaluate a patient's degree of sexual desire. Other testing may include:

- blood pressure
- estrogen levels in females, particularly in pre– and post–menopausal women
- testosterone levels in both males and females
- blood prolactin levels
- glucose tolerance to test for diabetes

- thyroid function
- iron deficiency

Procedures

Imaging techniques may be used in the diagnosis of physical causes of HSDD. Enlargement of the pituitary gland can be detected by **magnetic resonance imaging** (MRI) or computerized axial tomography (CAT or CT) scanning.

Treatment

Traditional

Any medical conditions underlying HSDD must be addressed; for example, genitourinary infections, poorly controlled diabetes, **substance abuse**, or suspect medications. Psychological causes of HSDD are addressed through behavioral or dynamic **psychotherapy**. HSDD often requires referral to a specialized counselor or sex therapist. Sexual anhedonia requires psychiatric referral unless there is evidence of **spinal cord injury** or **peripheral neuropathy**. Any other sexual disorders that can contribute to HSDD, such as erectile dysfunction, must be addressed. If the HSDD appears to be of a temporary or transient interpersonal nature, couples therapy may be beneficial. This requires the patience, support, and understanding of the sexual partner.

Drugs

In addition to any necessary adjustments in current medications, HSDD is sometimes treated with drugs:

- Systemic or local estrogen or estrogen/progesterone therapy can treat low hormone levels in menopausal women.
- A blood testosterone level of less than 300 nanograms (ng) per deciliter (dL) in males or 10 ng/dL in females may suggest testosterone replacement therapy. However this is controversial for women and may have adverse side effects.
- Prescription testosterone creams or gels for women may improve sexual desire.
- Tricyclic antidepressants (TCAs) or monoamine oxidase inhibitors (MAOIs) may be used to treat depression or panic symptoms accompanying HSDD.
- Some studies have reported that non–depressed younger women with HSDD may respond favorably to sustained–release tablets of the antidepressant bupropion hydrochloride (Wellbutrin). Women have reported significant increases in frequency of sexual arousal, sexual fantasies, and desire to engage in sexual activities. Bupropion enhances the activity of the neurotransmitters norepinephrine and dopamine, which affect sexual desire.
- Dopamine–stimulating drugs also have been found to increase sexual desire in some men.
- Flibanserin, an antidepressant–type drug, is being marketed as a treatment for female HSDD, but in June 2010, a U.S. Food and Drug Administration (FDA) advisory committee voted 10 to 1 against approving the drug for this purpose.

Alternative

Alternative remedies for HSDD include:

- vitamin E applied to the vagina
- Zestra genital massage oil, a proprietary blend of botanicals that includes borage seed and evening primrose oils, Angelica root, and vitamins C and E
- ArginMax, a nutritional supplement

Home remedies

Some sex therapists recommend a period of abstinence from genital sex and an increased emphasis on non–genital sex for the treatment of HSDD. Other methods for treating HSDD include:

- sexual lubricants
- experimenting with different sexual positions and settings, sex toys, and fantasies
- scheduling time for intimacy
- practicing open and honest communication with sexual partners
- regular aerobic exercise and strength–training to improve mood, body image, and libido
- stress management techniques
- for women, practicing Kegel (pelvic floor muscle) exercises for increasing pleasurable sexual sensations and libido

Prognosis

Prognosis depends primarily on the underlying causes of HSDD. For certain medical conditions the prognosis for the development or recovery of sexual interest is good. Examples include testosterone therapy for **hypogonadism** or appropriate treatment of a prolactin–secreting pituitary tumor. However with certain genetic defects, such as Turner's and Klinefelter's syndromes, attainment of sexual function is impossible.

In general, psychotherapy has proved to be only minimally effective in the treatment of HSDD. However the vast majority of HSDD cases are situational in nature, usually due to dissatisfaction or loss of interest in a sexual partner. In cases of marital discord, couples counseling by a healthcare professional trained in the field can be of significant assistance. However cases in which both partners are dissatisfied often do not respond to such therapy and these situations frequently culminate in separation, finding new sexual partners, or divorce.

Prevention

Since the majority of HSDD cases are situational, they are difficult to predict or prevent. However, open and honest communication between sexual partners is an important step.

Resources

BOOKS

American Psychiatric Association. *Diagnostic and Statistical Manual of Mental Disorders*, 4th ed., text rev. Arlington, VA: American Psychiatric Association, 2007.

Balon, Richard. *Sexual Dysfunction: The Brain–Body Connection*. New York: Karger, 2008.

Hertlein, Katherine M., Gerald R. Weeks, and Nancy Gambescia, eds. *Systemic Sex Therapy*. New York: Routledge, 2009.

PERIODICALS

Bergner, Daniel. "Women Who Want To Want." *New York Times Magazine* (November 29, 2009): 42–7.

Brotto, Lori A. "The DSM Diagnostic Criteria for Hypoactive Sexual Desire Disorder in Women." *Archives of Sexual Behavior* (April 2010) 39(2): 221.

Davis, Susan R., et al. "Testosterone for Low Libido in Postmenopausal Women Not Taking Estrogen." *New England Journal of Medicine* (November 6, 2008) 359(19): 2005.

Jutel, Annemarie. "Framing Disease: The Example of Female Hypoactive Sexual Desire Disorder." *Social Science & Medicine* (April 2010) 70(7): 1084.

OTHER

Bouchez, Colette. "A Woman's Guide to Reviving Sex Drive." WebMD. http://www.webmd.com/menopause/guide/sex–drive–and–menopause (accessed September 26, 2010).

DeNoon, Daniel J. "'Female Viagra' May Treat Low Sexual Desire." WebMD Health News. http://www.webmd.-com/sexual–conditions/news/20100518/female–viagra–may–tr eat–low–sexual–desire (accessed September 26, 2010).

DeNoon, Daniel J. "When a Man's Sex Drive Is Too Low." WebMD The Magazine. http://www.webmd.com/sex–relationships/features/when–a–mans–sex–drive–is–too–low (accessed September 26, 2010).

Mayo Clinic Staff. "Low Sex Drive in Women." MayoClinic.com. http://www.mayoclinic.com/health/low–sex–drive–in–women/DS01043/ (accessed September 26, 2010).

Norton, Amy. "Antidepressant Shows Benefits for Low Sex Drive." Reuters Health. http://www.nlm.nih.gov/medlineplus/news/fullstory_95762.html (accessed September 26, 2010).

ORGANIZATIONS

American Academy of Family Physicians (AAFP), 11400 Tomahawk Creek Pkwy., Leawood, KS, 66211–2680, (913) 906–6000, (800) 274–6000, (913) 906–6075, http://www.aafp.org/online/en/home.html.

American Association of Sex Educators, Counselors, and Therapists (AASECT), PO Box 1960, Ashland, VA, 23005–1960, (804) 752–0026, (804) 752–0056, aacect@aasect.org, http://www.aasect.org.

American College of Obstetricians and Gynecologists (ACOG), PO Box 96920, Washington, DC, 20090–6920, (202) 638–5577, (800) 673–8444, resources@acog.org, http://www.acog.org.

Ralph Myerson, MD
Margaret Alic, PhD

Hypocalcemia

Definition

Hypocalcemia, a low blood **calcium** level, occurs when the level of total calcium in the blood falls below 8.5 mg/dL. The normal concentration of calcium in the blood serum is 8.7–10.4 mg/dL.

Description

Calcium is an important mineral for maintaining human health. It is not only a component of bones and teeth, but is also essential for normal blood clotting and necessary for normal muscle and nerve functions. The calcium ion (Ca^{2+}) has two positive charges. In bone, where 99% of calcium is found, calcium ions occur as a complex with phosphate to form crystals of calcium phosphate. In the bloodstream, calcium ions also occur in complexes, and here calcium is found combined with proteins and various nutrients. However, in the bloodstream, calcium also occurs in a free form. Normally, about 47% of the calcium in the blood plasma is free, 40% is bound to protein, and about 10% occurs in a complex form. Although all calcium in the bloodstream serves a useful purpose, only the concentration of free calcium ions has a direct influence on the functioning of nerves and muscles. For this reason, the

KEY TERMS

Albumin—A type of protein made by the liver and found in the blood.

Cardiac dysrhythmias—Abnormal heart rate, rhythm, or sequence of rhythms.

Ion—A particle that has a positive or negative charge.

measurement of the concentration of free calcium is more important in the diagnosis of disease than measuring the level of total calcium or complexed calcium. The level of total calcium in the blood serum is normally 8.7–10.4 mg/dL, while the level of free calcium is normally 4–5 mg/dL.

Causes and symptoms

Hypocalcemia can be caused by **hypoparathyroidism**, failure to produce 1,25-dihydroxyvitamin D, low levels of plasma magnesium, or by failure to get adequate amounts of calcium or vitamin D in the diet. Hypoparathyroidism involves the failure of the parathyroid gland to make parathyroid hormone. Parathyroid hormone controls and maintains plasma calcium levels. The hormone exerts its effect on the kidneys, where it triggers the synthesis of 1,25-dihydroxyvitamin D. Thus, hypocalcemia can be independently caused by damage to the parathyroid gland or to the kidneys. 1,25-Dihydroxyvitamin D stimulates the uptake of calcium from the diet and the mobilization of calcium from the bone. Bone mobilization means the natural process by which the body dissolves part of the bone in the skeleton in order to maintain or raise the levels of plasma calcium ions.

Low plasma magnesium levels (hypomagnesia) can result in hypocalcemia. Hypomagnesia can occur with **alcoholism** or with diseases characterized by an inability to properly absorb fat. Magnesium is required for parathyroid hormone to play its part in maintaining plasma calcium levels. For this reason, any disease that results in lowered plasma magnesium levels may also cause hypocalcemia.

Hypocalcemia may also result from the consumption of toxic levels of phosphate. Phosphate is a constituent of certain enema formulas. An enema is a solution used to cleanse the intestines via a device inserted into the rectum. Cases of hypocalcemia have been documented where people swallowed enema formulas, or where an enema has been administered to an infant.

Symptoms of severe hypocalcemia include **numbness** or **tingling** around the mouth or in the feet and hands, as well as **muscle spasms** in the face, feet, and hands. Hypocalcemia can result in depression, **memory loss**, or **hallucinations**. Long-term hypocalcemia can also result in dry skin and outbreaks of **psoriasis**. Chronic (lasting more than one year) and moderate hypocalcemia can result in **cataracts** (damage to the eyes).

Diagnosis

Tests

Hypocalcemia is diagnosed by acquiring a sample of blood and then measuring the calcium level in the blood. Hypocalcemia has several causes, and a full diagnosis requires assessment of the parathyroid gland, kidneys, and the plasma magnesium concentration. Other tests that may be ordered include magnesium level, phosphate level, and tests to determine the blood levels of other electrolytes. The physician may also order tests to determine renal function such as the blood urea nitrogen (BUN) and creatinine level blood tests. Blood testing for PTH level, albumin level, liver function, and coagulation capability may be done as well.

The patient may be placed on cardiac monitoring to assess for cardiac dysrhythmias that can be triggered as a result of low calcium levels.

Treatment

The method chosen for treatment depends on the exact cause and on the severity of the hypocalcemia.

Drugs

Severe hypocalcemia requires intravenous replacement of calcium ions, usually in the form of calcium gluconate or calcium chloride. Oral calcium supplements are prescribed for long term treatment (nonemergency) of hypocalcemia. The oral supplements may take the form of calcium citrate, calcium carbonate, calcium chloride, or calcium gluconate. Hypocalcemia resulting from kidney failure is treated with injections of 1,25-dihydroxyvitamin D. Oral vitamin D supplements can increase gastrointestinal absorption of calcium. If hypocalcemia results from hypoparathyroidism, treatment may include oral calcium, 1,25-dihydroxyvitamin D, or other drugs. When low serum magnesium levels occur with hypocalcemia, the magnesium deficiency must be corrected to effectively treat the hypocalcemia.

Prognosis

The prognosis for correcting hypocalcemia is excellent. Damage to the eye that may result from chronic hypocalcemia cannot be reversed.

Prevention

The first, and most obvious, way to help prevent hypocalcemia is to ensure that adequate amounts of calcium and vitamin D are consumed each day, either in the diet or as supplements. The hypocalcemia that may occur with damage to the parathyroid gland or to the kidneys cannot be prevented. Hypocalcemia resulting from overuse of **enemas** can be prevented by reducing enema usage. Hypocalcemia resulting from magnesium deficiency tends to occur in chronic alcoholics, and this type of hypocalcemia can be prevented by reducing alcohol consumption and increasing the intake of healthy foods.

Resources

PERIODICALS

Sarko, J. "Bone and Mineral Metabolism." *Emergency Medicine Clinics of North America* 23, no. 3 (August 2005): 703–21, viii.

OTHER

Beach, Christopher "Hypocalcemia." *eMedicine*. March 29, 2010. http://emedicine.medscape.com/article/767260-overview.

Tom Brody, PhD
Melinda Granger RN, DNS, APRN, CNS

Hypochondriac *see* **Hypochondriasis**

Hypochondriasis

Definition

Hypochondriasis is a mental disorder characterized by excessive fear of or preoccupation with a serious illness, despite medical testing and reassurance to the contrary. It was formerly called hypochondriacal neurosis.

Description

Although hypochondriasis is often considered a disorder that primarily affects adults, it is now increasingly recognized in children and adolescents. In addition, hypochondriasis may develop in elderly people without previous histories of health-related fears. The disorder accounts for about 5% of psychiatric patients and is equally common in men and women.

Causes and symptoms

The causes of hypochondriasis are not precisely known. Children may have physical symptoms that resemble or mimic those of other family members. In adults, hypochondriasis may sometimes reflect a self-centered character structure or a wish to be taken care of by others; it may also have been copied from a parent's behavior. In elderly people, hypochondriasis may be associated with depression or grief. It may also involve biologically based hypersensitivity to internal stimuli.

Most hypochondriacs are worried about being physically sick, although some express fear of insanity. The symptoms reported can range from general descriptions of a specific illness to unusual complaints. In many instances the symptoms reflect intensified awareness of ordinary body functions, such as heartbeat, breathing, or stomach noises. It is important to understand that a hypochondriac's symptoms are not "in the head" in the sense of being delusional. The symptoms are real, but the patient misinterprets bodily functions and attributes them to a serious or even lethal cause.

Diagnosis

The diagnosis is often complicated by the patient's detailed understanding of symptoms and medical terminology from previous contacts with doctors. If a new doctor suspects hypochondriasis, he or she will usually order a complete medical workup in order to rule out physical disease.

Psychological evaluation is also necessary to rule out other disorders that involve feelings of **anxiety** or complaints of physical illness. These disorders include depression, **panic disorder**, and **schizophrenia** with somatic (physical) **delusions**. The following features are characteristic of hypochondriasis:

- The patient is not psychotic (out of touch with reality or hallucinating).
- The patient gets upset or blames the doctor when told there is "nothing wrong," or that there is a psychological basis for the problem.
- There is a correlation between episodes of hypochondriacal behavior and stressful periods in the patient's life.
- The behavior has lasted at least six months.

Evaluation of children and adolescents with hypochondriasis should include the possibility of **abuse** by family members.

Treatment

The goal of therapy is to help the patient (and family) live with the symptoms and to modify thinking and behavior that reinforces hypochondriacal symptoms. This treatment orientation is called supportive, as distinct from insight-oriented, because hypochondriacs usually resist psychological interpretations of their symptoms. Supportive treatment may include medications to relieve anxiety. Some clinicians look carefully for "masked" depression and treat with antidepressants.

Follow-up care includes regular physical checkups because about 30% of patients with hypochondriasis will eventually develop a serious physical illness. The physician also tries to prevent unnecessary medical testing and "doctor shopping" on the patient's part.

Prognosis

Between 33% and 55% of patients with hypochondriasis can expect significant improvement from the current methods of treatment.

Resources

BOOKS

McPhee, Stephen, and Maxine Papadakis. *Current Medical Diagnosis and Treatment. 2010*. 49th ed. New York: McGraw–Hill Medical, 2009.

Rebecca J. Frey, PhD

Hypoesthesias *see* **Numbness and tingling**

Hypoglycemia

Definition

The condition called hypoglycemia is literally translated as low blood sugar. Hypoglycemia occurs when blood sugar (or blood glucose) concentrations fall below a level necessary to properly support the body's need for energy and stability throughout its cells.

Demographics

Attempts at quantifying the incidence of hypoglycemia is challenging, as many individuals do not regularly record, nor report the occurrence of this condition to their healthcare provider. It is thought to affect as many as 1 out of 1,000 people and can occur for a variety of reasons. Episodes of hypoglycemia occurring at night (nocturnal hypoglycemia) are commonly undetected by patients, and it is believed that about 6% of all deaths in diabetes are due to unrecognized nocturnal hypoglycemia.

Description

Carbohydrates are the main dietary source of the glucose that is manufactured in the liver and absorbed into the bloodstream to fuel the body's cells and organs. Glucose concentration is controlled by hormones, primarily insulin and glucagon. Glucose concentration also is controlled by epinephrine (adrenalin) and norepinephrine, as well as growth hormone. If these regulators are not working properly, levels of blood sugar can become either excessive (as in hyperglycemia) or inadequate (as in hypoglycemia). If a person has a blood sugar level of 50 mg/dL or less, he or she is considered hypoglycemic, although glucose levels vary widely from one person to another.

Hypoglycemia can occur in several ways.

Drug-induced hypoglycemia

Drug-induced hypoglycemia, a complication of diabetes, is the most commonly seen and most dangerous form of hypoglycemia.

Hypoglycemia occurs most often in diabetics who must inject insulin periodically to lower their blood sugar. While other diabetics also are vulnerable to low blood sugar episodes, they have a lower risk of a serious outcome than insulin-dependent diabetics. Unless recognized and treated immediately, severe hypoglycemia in the insulin-dependent diabetic can lead to generalized convulsions followed by **amnesia** and unconsciousness. **Death**, though rare, is a possible outcome.

In insulin-dependent diabetics, hypoglycemia known as an insulin reaction or insulin **shock** can be caused by several factors. These include overmedicating with manufactured insulin, missing or delaying a meal, eating too little food for the amount of insulin taken, exercising too strenuously, drinking too much alcohol, or any combination of these factors.

Reactive hypoglycemia

Reactive hypoglycemia (also called postprandial hypoglycemia) occurs about 2–4 hours after eating a meal. A number of reasons for this reaction have been proposed, but no single cause has been identified.

In some cases, this form of hypoglycemia appears to be associated with malfunctions or diseases of the liver, pituitary, adrenals, liver, or pancreas. These conditions are unrelated to diabetes. Children intolerant of a natural sugar (fructose) or who have inherited defects that affect digestion also may experience hypoglycemic attacks. Some children with a negative reaction to **aspirin** also experience reactive hypoglycemia. It sometimes occurs among people with an intolerance to the sugar found in milk (galactose), and it also often begins before diabetes strikes later in life.

Fasting hypoglycemia

Fasting hypoglycemia sometimes occurs after long periods without food, but it also happens occasionally following strenuous **exercise**, such as running in a marathon.

Other factors sometimes associated with hypoglycemia include:

- pregnancy
- a weakened immune system
- a poor diet high in simple carbohydrates
- prolonged use of drugs, including antibiotics
- chronic physical or mental stress
- heartbeat irregularities (arrhythmias)
- allergies
- breast cancer
- high blood pressure treated with beta-blocker medications (after strenuous exercise)
- upper gastrointestinal tract surgery

Causes and symptoms

When carbohydrates are eaten, they are converted to glucose that goes into the bloodstream and is distributed throughout the body. Simultaneously, a combination of chemicals that regulate how our body's cells absorb that sugar is released from the liver, pancreas, and adrenal glands. These chemical regulators include insulin, glucagon, epinephrine (adrenalin), and norepinephrine. The mixture of these regulators released following digestion of carbohydrates is never the same, since the amount of carbohydrates that are eaten is never the same.

Interactions among the regulators are complicated. Any abnormalities in the effectiveness of any one of the regulators can reduce or increase the body's absorption of glucose. Gastrointestinal enzymes such as amylase and lactase that break down carbohydrates may not be functioning properly. These abnormalities may produce hyperglycemia or hypoglycemia and can be detected when the level of glucose in the blood is measured.

Cell sensitivity to these regulators can be changed in many ways. Over time, a person's **stress** level, exercise patterns, advancing age, and dietary habits influence cellular sensitivity. For example, a diet consistently overly rich in carbohydrates increases insulin requirements over time. Eventually, cells can become less receptive to the effects of the regulating chemicals, which can lead to glucose intolerance.

Diet is both a major factor in producing hypoglycemia as well as the primary method for controlling it. **Diets** typical of Western cultures contain excess carbohydrates, especially in the form of simple carbohydrates such as sweeteners, which are more easily converted to sugar. In developing parts of the world, the typical diet contains even higher levels of carbohydrates. Fewer dairy products and meats are eaten, and grains, vegetables, and fruits are consumed. This dietary trend is balanced, however, since people in these cultures eat small meals and usually use carbohydrates efficiently through physical labor.

Early symptoms of severe hypoglycemia, particularly in the drug-induced type of hypoglycemia, resemble an extreme shock reaction. Symptoms include:

- cold and pale skin
- numbness around the mouth
- apprehension
- heart palpitations
- emotional outbursts
- hand tremors
- mental cloudiness
- dilated pupils
- sweating
- fainting

Mild attacks, however, are more common in reactive hypoglycemia and are characterized by extreme tiredness. Patients first lose their alertness, then their muscle strength and coordination. Thinking grows fuzzy, and finally the patient becomes so tired that he or she becomes "zombie-like," awake but not functioning. Sometimes the patient will actually fall asleep. Unplanned naps are typical of the chronic hypoglycemic patient, particularly following meals.

Additional symptoms of reactive hypoglycemia include headaches, double vision, staggering or inability to walk, a craving for salt and/or sweets, abdominal distress, premenstrual tension, chronic **colitis**, **allergies**, ringing in the ears, unusual patterns in the frequency of urination, skin eruptions and inflammations, **pain** in the neck and shoulder muscles, memory problems, and sudden and excessive sweating.

Unfortunately, a number of these symptoms mimic those of other conditions. For example, the depression, **insomnia**, irritability, lack of concentration, crying spells, **phobias**, forgetfulness, confusion, unsocial behavior, and suicidal tendencies commonly seen in nervous system and psychiatric disorders also may be hypoglycemic symptoms. It is very important that anyone with symptoms that may suggest reactive hypoglycemia see a doctor.

Because all of its possible symptoms are not likely to be seen in any one person at a specific time, diagnosing hypoglycemia can be difficult. One or more of its many symptoms may be due to another illness. Symptoms may persist in a variety of forms for long periods of time. Symptoms also can change over time within the same person. Some of the factors that can influence symptoms include physical or mental activities, physical or mental state, the amount of time passed since the last meal, the amount and quality of sleep, and exercise patterns.

Diagnosis

Drug-induced hypoglycemia

Once diabetes is diagnosed, the patient monitors his or her blood sugar level with a portable machine called a glucometer. The diabetic places a small blood sample on a test strip that the machine can read. If the test reveals that the blood sugar level is too low, the diabetic can make a correction by eating or drinking an additional carbohydrate.

Reactive hypoglycemia

Reactive hypoglycemia only can be diagnosed by a doctor. Symptoms usually improve after the patient has gone on an appropriate diet. Reactive hypoglycemia was diagnosed more frequently in the late twentieth century than at the end of the first decade of the twenty-first century. Studies have shown that most people suffering from its symptoms test normal for blood sugar, leading many doctors to suggest that actual cases of reactive hypoglycemia are quite rare. Some doctors think that people with hypoglycemic symptoms may be particularly sensitive to the body's normal postmeal release of the hormone epinephrine, or are actually suffering from some other physical or mental problem. Other doctors believe reactive hypoglycemia actually is the early onset of diabetes that occurs after a number of years. There continues to be disagreement about the cause of reactive hypoglycemia.

A common test to diagnose hypoglycemia is the extended oral glucose tolerance test. Following an overnight fast, a concentrated solution of glucose is drunk and blood samples are taken hourly for five to six hours. Though this test remains helpful in early identification of diabetes, its use in diagnosing chronic reactive hypoglycemia has lost favor because it can trigger hypoglycemic symptoms in people with otherwise normal glucose readings. Some doctors now recommend that blood sugar be tested at the actual time a person experiences hypoglycemic symptoms.

Treatment

Treatment of the immediate symptoms of hypoglycemia can include eating sugar. For example, a patient can eat a piece of candy, drink milk, or drink fruit juice. Glucose tablets can be used by patients, especially those who are diabetic. Effective treatment of hypoglycemia over time requires the patient to follow a modified diet. Patients usually are encouraged to eat small, but frequent, meals throughout the day, avoiding excess simple sugars (including alcohol), fats, and fruit drinks. Those patients with severe hypoglycemia may require fast-acting glucagon injections that can stabilize their blood sugar within approximately 15 minutes.

Alternative treatment

A holistic approach to reactive hypoglycemia is based on the belief that a number of factors may create the condition. Among them are heredity, the effects of other illnesses, emotional stress, too much or too little exercise, bad lighting, poor diet, and environmental pollution. Therefore, a number of alternative methods have been proposed as useful in treating the condition. **Homeopathy**, **acupuncture**, and **applied kinesiology**, for example, have been used, as have herbal remedies. One of the herbal remedies commonly suggested for hypoglycemia is a decoction (an extract made by boiling) of gentian (*Gentiana lutea*). It should be drunk warm 15–30 minutes before a meal. Gentian is believed to help stimulate the endocrine (hormone-producing) glands.

In addition to dietary modifications, people with hypoglycemia may benefit from supplementing their diet with chromium, which is believed to help improve blood sugar levels. Chromium is found in whole grain breads and cereals, cheese, molasses, lean meats, and brewer's yeast. Hypoglycemics should avoid alcohol, **caffeine**, and cigarette smoke, since these substances can cause significant swings in blood sugar levels.

Prevention

Drug-induced hypoglycemia

Preventing hypoglycemic insulin reactions in diabetics requires taking glucose readings through frequent blood sampling. Insulin then can be regulated based on those readings. Continuous glucose monitoring sensors have been developed to help diabetics remain more aware of possible hypoglycemic episodes. These monitors even can check for episodes while the patient sleeps, when many will experience severe hypoglycemia but not know it. Those who don't pay attention to severe hypoglycemia events or who have had previous severe hypoglycemia are the most likely to have future severe hypoglycemia. An audible alert can let the patient know immediately that he or she needs to take care of his or her blood sugar level. Continuous monitoring has proved particularly helpful in pediatric patients with Type 1 diabetes.

Maintaining proper diet also is a factor. Programmable insulin pumps implanted under the skin have proven useful in reducing the incidence of hypoglycemic episodes for insulin-dependent diabetics. Clinical studies continue to seek additional ways to control diabetes and drug-induced hypoglycemia. Tests of a substance called pramlintide indicate that it may help improve glycemic control in diabetics.

Reactive hypoglycemia

The onset of reactive hypoglycemia can be avoided or at least delayed by following the same kind of diet used to control it. While not as restrictive as the diet diabetics must follow to keep tight control over their disease, it is quite similar.

There are a variety of diet recommendations for the reactive hypoglycemic. Patients should:

- avoid overeating
- never skip breakfast
- include protein in all meals and snacks, preferably from sources low in fat, such as the white meat of chicken or turkey, most fish, soy products, or skim milk
- restrict intake of fats (particularly saturated fats, such as animal fats), and avoiding refined sugars and processed foods
- be aware of the differences between some vegetables, such as potatoes and carrots. These vegetables have a higher sugar content than others (like squash and broccoli). Patients should be aware of these differences and note any reactions they have to them.
- be aware of differences found in grain products. White flour is a carbohydrate that is rapidly absorbed into the bloodstream, while oats take much longer to break down in the body.
- keep a "food diary." Until the diet is stabilized, a patient should note what and how much he/she eats and drinks at every meal. If symptoms appear following a meal or snack, patients should note them and look for patterns.
- eat fresh fruits, but restrict the amount they eat at one time. Patients should remember to eat a source of protein whenever they eat high sources of carbohydrate like fruit. Apples make particularly good snacks because, of all fruits, the carbohydrate in apples is digested most slowly.
- follow a diet that is high in fiber. Fruit is a good source of fiber, as are oatmeal and oat bran. Fiber slows the buildup of sugar in the blood during digestion.

A doctor can recommend a proper diet, and there are many cookbooks available for diabetics. Recipes found in such books are equally effective in helping to control hypoglycemia.

Prognosis

Like diabetes, there is no cure for reactive hypoglycemia, only ways to control it. While some chronic cases will continue through life (rarely is there complete remission of the condition), others will develop into type II (age onset) diabetes. Hypoglycemia appears to have a higher-than-average incidence in families where there has been a history of hypoglycemia or diabetes among their members, but whether hypoglycemia is a controllable warning of oncoming diabetes has not yet been determined by clinical research.

A condition known as hypoglycemia unawareness can develop in those who do not control their blood glucose, particularly in people with Type 1 diabetes. These people may lose notice of the automatic warning symptoms of hypoglycemia that normally occur as their bodies become so used to frequent periods of hypoglycemia. It is not a permanent event, but can be treated by careful avoidance of hypoglycemia for about two weeks.

Resources

BOOKS

Colbert, Don, M.D. *The New Bible Cure for Diabetes*. Lake Mary, FL: Siloam Press, 2009.

Kenrose, Stephanie. *The Reactive Hypoglycemia Cookbook*. Charleston, SC: CreateSpace, 2010.

Kenrose, Stephanie. *The Reactive Hypoglycemia Sourcebook*. Raleigh, NC: Lulu, 2009.

Pierce, Dino Paul, CFT, CPT, RD, CDE. *The Diabetes Handbook: Create Awareness and a New You*. Charleston, SC: CreateSpace, 2009.

Vaughn, Richard, A. *Beating The Odds: 64 Years of Diabetes Health*. Charleston, SC: CreateSpace, 2010.

PERIODICALS

Brauker, James, et al. "Use of Continuous Glucose Monitoring Alerts to Better Predict, Prevent and Treat Postprandial Hyperglycemia." *Diabetes*, June 2003: 90-91.

Gertzman, Jerilyn, et al. "Severity of Hypoglycemia and Hypoglycemia Unawareness Are Associated with the

Extent of Unsuspected Nocturnal Hypoglycemia." *Diabetes*, June 2003:146-151.

Kumar, Rajeev, and Miles Fisher. "Impaired Hypoglycemia Awareness: Are we Aware?" *Diabetes and Primary Care*, Summer 2004: 33–38.

Ludvigsson, Johnny, and Ragnar Hanas. "Continuous Subcutaneous Glucose Monitoring Improved Metabolic Control in Pediatric Patients With Type 1 Diabetes: A Controlled Crossover Study." *Pediatrics*, May 2003: 933-936.

ORGANIZATIONS

American Diabetes Association, 1701 North Beauregard St., Alexandria, VA, 22311, (800) 342–2383, AskADA@diabetes.org, http://www.diabetes.org.

Hypoglycemia Association, Inc., 18008 New Hampshire Ave., PO Box 165, Ashton, MD, 20861-0165

National Hypoglycemia Association, Inc., PO Box 120, Ridgewood, NJ, 07451, (201) 670-1189

The Hypoglycemia Support Foundation, Inc., http://www.hypoglycemia.org/default.asp.

Martin W. Dodge, Ph.D.
Teresa G. Odle
Ken R. Wells
Laura Jean Cataldo, RN, Ed.D.

Hypogonadism

Definition

Hypogonadism is the condition more prevalent in males in which the production of sex hormones and germ cells are inadequate.

Description

Gonads are the organs of sexual differentiation—in the female, they are ovaries; in the male, the testes. Along with producing eggs and sperm, they produce sex hormones that generate all the differences between men and women. If they produce too little sex hormone, then either the growth of the sexual organs or their function is impaired.

The gonads are not independent in their function, however. They are closely controlled by the pituitary gland. The pituitary hormones are the same for males and females, but the gonadal hormones are different. Men produce mostly androgens, and women produce mostly estrogens. These two hormones regulate the development of the embryo, determining whether it is a male or a female. They also direct the adolescent maturation of sex organs into their adult form. Further, they sustain those organs and their function throughout the reproductive years. The effects of estrogen reach beyond that to sustain bone strength and protect the cardiovascular system from degenerative disease.

Hormones can be inadequate during or after each stage of development—embryonic and adolescent. During each stage, inadequate hormone stimulation will prevent normal development. After each stage, a decrease in hormone stimulation will result in failed function and perhaps some shrinkage. The organs affected principally by sex hormones are the male and female genitals, both internal and external, and the female breasts. Body hair, fat deposition, bone and muscle growth, and some brain functions are also influenced.

Causes and symptoms

Sex is determined at the moment of conception by sex chromosomes. Females have two X chromosomes, while males have one X and one Y chromosome. If male sperm with a Y chromosome fertilizes an egg, the baby will be male. This is true throughout the animal kingdom. Genetic defects sometimes result in changes in the chromosomes. If sex chromosomes are involved, there is a change in the development of sexual characteristics.

Female is the default sex of the embryo, so most of the sex organ deficits at birth occur in boys. Some, but not all, are due to inadequate androgen stimulation. The penis may be small, the testicles undescended (cryptorchidism), or various degrees of "feminization" of the genitals may be present.

After birth, sexual development does not occur until **puberty**. Hypogonadism most often shows up as an abnormality in boys during puberty. Again, not every defect is due to inadequate hormones. Some are due to too much of the wrong ones. Kallmann's syndrome is a birth defect in the brain that prevents release of hormones and appears as failure of male puberty. Some boys have adequate amounts of androgen in their system but fail to respond to them, a condition known as androgen resistance.

Female problems in puberty are not caused by too little estrogen. Even female reproductive problems are rarely related to a simple lack of hormones, but rather to complex cycling rhythms gone wrong. All the problems with too little hormone happen during **menopause**, which is a normal hypogonadism.

A number of adverse events can damage the gonads and result in decreased hormone levels. The childhood disease **mumps**, if acquired after puberty, can infect and destroy the testicles—a disease called viral **orchitis**. Ionizing radiation and **chemotherapy**, trauma, several drugs (spironolactone, a diuretic and ketoconazole, an antifungal agent), alcohol, **marijuana**, heroin, **methadone**, and environmental toxins can all damage testicles and decrease their hormone production. Severe diseases in the liver or kidneys, certain infections, sickle cell anemia, and some cancers also affect gonads. To treat some male cancers, it is necessary to remove the testicles, thereby preventing the androgens from stimulating **cancer** growth. This procedure, called castration or *orchiectomy*, removes androgen stimulation from the whole body.

For several reasons the pituitary can fail. It happens rarely after **pregnancy**. It used to be removed to treat advanced breast or **prostate cancer**. Sometimes the pituitary develops a tumor that destroys it. Failure of the pituitary is called **hypopituitarism** leaves the gonads with no stimulation to produce hormones.

Besides the tissue changes generated by hormone stimulation, the only other symptoms relate to sexual desire and function. Libido is enhanced by testosterone, and male sexual performance requires androgens. The role of female hormones in female sexual activity is less clear, although hormones strengthen tissues and promote healthy secretions, facilitating sexual activity.

Diagnosis

There are accurate blood tests for most of the hormones in the body, including those from the pituitary and even some from the hypothalamus. Chromosomes can be analyzed, and gonads can be, but rarely are, biopsied.

Treatment

Replacement of missing body chemicals is much easier than suppressing excesses. Estrogen replacement is recommended for nearly all women after menopause for its many beneficial effects. Estrogen can be taken by mouth, injection, or skin patch. It is strongly recommended that the other female hormone, progesterone, be taken as well, because it prevents overgrowth of uterine lining and uterine cancer. Testosterone replacement is available for males who are deficient.

Resources

BOOKS

Fauci, Anthony S., et al., eds. *Harrison's Principles of Internal Medicine*. 17th ed. New York: McGraw–Hill Professional, 2008.

J. Ricker Polsdorfer, MD

Hypokalemia

Definition

Hypokalemia is a condition of below-normal levels of potassium in the blood serum. Potassium, a necessary electrolyte, facilitates nerve impulse conduction and the contraction of skeletal and smooth muscles, including the heart. It also facilitates cell membrane function and proper enzyme activity. Levels must be kept in a proper (homeostatic) balance for the maintenance of health. The normal concentration of potassium in the serum is in the range of 3.5–5.0 mEq/L. Hypokalemia means serum or plasma levels of potassium ions that fall below 3.5 mEq/L. Moderate hypokalemia may be defined as serum potassium between 2.5 and 3.0 mEq/L, while severe hypokalemia is defined as serum potassium under 2.5 mEq/L. (Potassium concentrations are often expressed in units of milliequivalents per liter [mEq/L], rather than in units of millimolarity [mM], however, both units are identical and mean the same thing when applied to concentrations of potassium ions.)

Hypokalemia can result from two general causes: either from an overall depletion in the body's potassium or from excessive uptake of potassium by muscle from surrounding fluids.

Description

A normal adult weighing about 154 lb (70 kg) has about 3.6 **moles** of potassium ions in his body. Most of this potassium (about 98%) occurs inside various cells and organs, where normal concentrations are about 150 mEq/L. Blood serum concentrations are much lower—only about 0.4% of the body's potassium is found in blood serum. Hypokalemia can be caused by the sudden uptake of potassium ions from the bloodstream by muscle or other organs or by an overall depletion of the body's potassium. Hypokalemia due to overall depletion tends to be a chronic phenomenon, while hypokalemia due to a shift in location tends to be a temporary disorder.

Causes and symptoms

Hypokalemia is most commonly caused by the use of **diuretics**. Diuretics are drugs that increase the excretion of water and salts in the urine. Diuretics are used to treat a number of medical conditions, including **hypertension** (high blood pressure), congestive **heart failure**, **liver disease**, and **kidney disease**. Diuretic treatment can have the side effect of producing hypokalemia. In fact, the most common cause of hypokalemia in the elderly is the use of diuretics. The use of furosemide and thiazide, two commonly used diuretic drugs, can lead to hypokalemia. In contrast, spironolactone and triamterene are diuretics that do not provoke hypokalemia.

Other common causes of hypokalemia are excessive **diarrhea** or **vomiting**. Diarrhea and **vomiting** can be produced by infections of the gastrointestinal tract. Caused by a variety of organisms, including bacteria, protozoa, and viruses, diarrhea is a major world health problem. It is responsible for about a quarter of the 10 million infant deaths that occur each year. Although nearly all of these deaths occur in the poorer parts of Asia and Africa, diarrheal diseases are a leading cause of infant **death** in the United States. Diarrhea results in various abnormalities, such as **dehydration** (loss in body water), **hyponatremia** (low **sodium** level in the blood), and hypokalemia.

Because of the need for potassium to control muscle action, hypokalemia can cause the heart to stop beating. Young infants are especially at risk for death from this cause, especially where severe diarrhea continues for two weeks or longer. Diarrhea due to laxative **abuse** is an occasional cause of hypokalemia in the adolescent or adult. Enema abuse is a related cause of hypokalemia. Laxative abuse is especially difficult to diagnose and treat, because patients usually deny the practice. Up to 20% of persons complaining of chronic diarrhea practice laxative abuse. Laxative abuse is often part of **eating disorders**, such as **anorexia nervosa** or **bulimia nervosa**. Hypokalemia that occurs with these eating disorders may be life-threatening.

The potassium loss that accompanies vomiting is only partly due to loss of potassium from the vomit. Vomiting also has the effect of provoking an increase in potassium loss in the urine. It expels acid from the mouth, and this loss of acid results in alkalization of the blood. (Alkalization of the blood means that the pH of the blood increases slightly.) An increased blood pH has a direct effect on the kidneys. Alkaline blood provokes the kidneys to release excessive amounts of potassium in the urine. Severe and continual vomiting can cause excessive losses of potassium from the body and hypokalemia.

A third general cause of hypokalemia is prolonged **fasting** and **starvation**. In most people, after three weeks of fasting, blood serum potassium levels decline to below 3.0 mEq/L and result in severe hypokalemia. In some persons, serum potassium may be naturally maintained at about 3.0 mEq/L, even after 100 days of fasting. During fasting, muscle is naturally broken down, and the muscle protein is converted to sugar (glucose) to supply to the brain the glucose that is essential for its functioning. Other organs are able to survive with a mixed supply of fat and glucose. The potassium within the muscle cell is released during the gradual process of muscle breakdown that occurs with starvation, and this can help counteract the trend to hypokalemia during starvation. Eating an unbalanced diet does not cause hypokalemia because most foods, such as fruits (especially bananas, oranges, and melons), vegetables, meat, milk, and cheese, are good sources of potassium. Only foods such as butter, margarine, vegetable oil, soda water, jelly beans, and hard candies are extremely poor in potassium.

Alcoholism occasionally results in hypokalemia. About one-half of alcoholics hospitalized for withdrawal symptoms experience hypokalemia. The hypokalemia of alcoholics occurs for a variety of reasons, usually poor **nutrition**, vomiting, and diarrhea. Hypokalemia can also be caused by **hyperaldosteronism**; **Cushing's syndrome**; hereditary kidney defects, such as Liddle's syndrome, Bartter's syndrome, and Franconi's syndrome; and eating too much licorice.

Symptoms

Mild hypokalemia usually results in no symptoms, while moderate hypokalemia results in confusion, disorientation, weakness, and discomfort of muscles. On occasion, moderate hypokalemia causes cramps during **exercise**. Another symptom of moderate hypokalemia is a discomfort in the legs that is experienced while sitting still. The patient may experience an annoying feeling that can be relieved by shifting the positions of the legs or by stomping the feet on the floor. Severe hypokalemia results in extreme weakness of the body and, on occasion, in **paralysis**. The paralysis that occurs is "flaccid paralysis," or limpness. Paralysis of the muscles of the lungs results in death. Other signs of severe hypokalemia include low blood pressure (hypokalemia), low heart rate, and signs of an **ileus**. Another dangerous result of severe hypokalemia is abnormal heart beat (arrhythmia) that can lead to death from cardiac arrest (cessation of heart beat).

Diagnosis

Hypokalemia can be measured by acquiring a sample of blood and by then measuring the concentration of potassium ions in the blood. Since hypokalemia results in abnormalities in heart rhythm, an electrocardiogram is usually used in the diagnosis of hypokalemia. The diagnosis of the cause of hypokalemia can be done by measuring the potassium content of the urine. Where urinary potassium is under 25 mEq/L per day, it means that the patient has experienced excessive losses

KEY TERMS

Cardiac arrhythmia—An abnormality in the rate or rhythm of the heartbeat.

Ileus—A blockage of the intestine. Ileus caused by hypokalemia is often termed paralytic ileus because peristalsis, the rhythmic contractions within the bowel that propels digested food through the intestinal tract, ceases.

of potassium due to diarrhea. The urinary potassium test is useful in cases where the patient is denying the practice of laxative or enema abuse. In contrast, where hypokalemia is due to the use of diuretic drugs, the content of potassium in the urine will be high—over 40 mEq/L per day.

Treatment

In emergency situations, when severe hypokalemia is suspected, the patient should be placed on a cardiac monitor, and respiratory status should be assessed. If laboratory test results show potassium levels below 2.5 mEq/L, intravenous potassium should be given. Patients with severe hypokalemia may receive intravenous potassium in the emergency department or may need to be admitted to an inpatient facility to continue replacement therapy under close observation.

In less urgent cases, potassium can be given orally in pill form. Oral potassium chloride is the safest and most effective treatment for hypokalemia. Generally, the consumption of 40–80 mEq/L of KCl per day is sufficient to correct the hypokalemia that results from diuretic therapy. For many people taking diuretics, potassium supplements are not necessary as long as they eat a balanced diet containing foods rich in potassium.

Prognosis

The prognosis for correcting hypokalemia is excellent. In emergency situations where potassium is administered intravenously, the physician must be careful not to give too much potassium. The administration of potassium at high levels, or at a high rate, can lead to abnormally high levels of serum potassium, which can result in cardiac **arrhythmias**.

Prevention

Hypokalemia is not a concern for healthy persons, since potassium is present in a great variety of foods. For patients taking diuretics, the American Dietetic Association recommends use of a high potassium diet. The American Dietetic Association states that if hypokalemia has already occurred, use of the high potassium diet alone may not reverse hypokalemia. Useful components of a high potassium diet include bananas, tomatoes, cantaloupes, figs, raisins, kidney beans, potatoes, and milk.

Resources

PERIODICALS

Assadi, F. "Diagnosis of Hypokalemia: A Problem-Solving Approach to Clinical Cases." *Iranian Journal of Kidney Disease* (July 2008) 2, no. 3: 115–22.

Ingram, T.C., and J.M. Olsson. "In Brief: Hypokalemia." *Pediatric Review* (September 2008) 29, no. 9: e50–1.

OTHER

Garth, David. "Hypokalemia." *eMedicine*. April 2, 2010. http://emedicine.medscape.com/article/767448-overview (accessed October 10, 2010).

Tom Brody, PhD
Melinda Granger Oberleitner
RN, DNS, APRN, CNS

Hypolipoproteinemia

Definition

Hypolipoproteinemia (or hypolipidemia) is the lack of fat in the blood.

Description

Although quite rare, hypolipoproteinemia is a serious condition. Blood absorbs fat from food in the intestine and transports it as a combined package with proteins and other chemicals like cholesterol. Much of the fat goes straight into the liver for processing. The cholesterol, a waste product, ends up in the bile. The proteins act as vessels, carrying the other chemicals around. These packages of fat, cholesterol, and proteins are called lipoproteins.

Causes and symptoms

Low blood fats can be the result of several diseases, or they can be a primary genetic disease with other associated abnormalities.

- Malnutrition is a lack of food, including fats, in the diet.
- Malabsorption is the inability of the bowel to absorb food, causing malnutrition.

- Anemia (too few red blood cells) and hyperthyroidism (too much thyroid hormone) also reduce blood fats.
- Rare genetic conditions called hypobetalipoproteinemia and abetalipoproteinemia cause malabsorption plus nerve, eye, and skin problems in early childhood.
- Tangier disease, causes only the cholesterol to be low. It also produces nerve and eye problems in children.

Symptoms are associated more closely with the cause rather than the actual low blood fats.

Diagnosis

Blood studies of the various fat particles help identify both the low and high fat diseases. These tests are often done after an overnight fast to prevent interference from fat just being absorbed from food. Fats and proteins are grouped together and described by density—high-density lipoproteins (HDL), low-density lipoproteins (LDL), and very low-density lipoproteins (VLDL). There are also much bigger particles called chylomicrons. Each contain different proportions of cholesterol, fats, and protein.

Treatment

Supplemental vitamin E helps children with betalipoprotein deficiencies. There is no known treatment for Tangier disease. Treatment of the causes of the other forms of low blood fats reverses the condition.

Resources

BOOKS

Fauci, Anthony S., et al., eds.*Harrison's Principles of Internal Medicine*. 17th ed. New York: McGraw–Hill Professional, 2008.

J. Ricker Polsdorfer, MD

Hypomagnesemia *see* **Magnesium imbalance**

Hyponatremia

Definition

The normal concentration of **sodium** in the blood plasma is 136–145 mEq/L. Hyponatremia, the most commonly observed electrolyte imbalance, occurs when sodium falls below 130 mEq/L. Plasma sodium levels of 125 mEq/L or less are dangerous and can result in seizures and **coma**.

Description

Sodium is an atom, or ion, that carries a single positive charge. The sodium ion may be abbreviated as Na^+ or as simply Na. Sodium can occur as a salt in a crystalline solid. Sodium chloride (NaCl), sodium phosphate (Na_2HPO_4), and sodium bicarbonate ($NaHCO_3$) are commonly occurring salts. These salts can be dissolved in water or in juices of various foods. Dissolving involves the complete separation of ions, such as sodium and chloride, in common table salt (NaCl).

About 40% of the body's sodium is contained in bone. Approximately 2–5% occurs within organs and cells and the remaining 55% is in blood plasma and other extracellular fluids. The amount of sodium in blood plasma is typically 140 mEq/L, a much higher amount than is found in intracellular sodium (about 5 mEq/L). This asymmetric distribution of sodium ions is essential for human life. It makes possible proper nerve conduction, the passage of various nutrients into cells, and the maintenance of blood pressure.

The body continually regulates its handling of sodium. When dietary sodium is too high or low, the intestines and kidneys respond to adjust concentrations to normal. During the course of a day, the intestines absorb dietary sodium while the kidneys excrete a nearly equal amount of sodium into the urine. If a low sodium diet is consumed, the intestines increase their efficiency of sodium absorption, and the kidneys reduce its release into urine.

The concentration of sodium in the blood plasma depends on two things: 1) the total amount of sodium and, 2) water in arteries, veins, and capillaries (the circulatory system). The body uses separate mechanisms to regulate sodium and water, but they work together to correct blood pressure when it is too high or too low. Too low a concentration of sodium, or hyponatremia, can be corrected either by increasing sodium or by decreasing body water. The existence of separate mechanisms that regulate sodium concentration account for the fact that there are numerous diseases that can cause hyponatremia, including diseases of the kidney, pituitary gland, and hypothalamus.

Causes and symptoms

Hyponatremia can be caused by abnormal consumption or excretion of dietary sodium or water and by diseases that impair the body's ability to regulate them. Maintenance of a low salt diet for many months or excessive sweat loss during a race on a hot day can present a challenge to the body to conserve adequate sodium levels. While these conditions alone are not likely to cause hyponatremia, it can occur under special circumstances. For example, hyponatremia often occurs in patients taking diuretic drugs who maintain a low sodium diet. This is especially of concern in elderly patients, who have a reduced ability to regulate the concentrations of various nutrients in the bloodstream. Diuretic drugs that frequently cause hyponatremia include furosemide (Lasix), bumetanide (Bumex), and most commonly, the thiazide **diuretics**. Diuretics enhance the excretion of sodium into the urine, with the goal of correcting high blood pressure; too much sodium excretion can result in hyponatremia. Usually only mild hyponatremia occurs in patients taking diuretics, but when combined with a low sodium diet or with the excessive drinking of water, severe hyponatremia can develop.

Severe and prolonged **diarrhea** can cause hyponatremia. Severe diarrhea, causing the daily output of 8–10 L of fluid from the large intestines, results in the loss of large amounts of water, sodium, and various nutrients. Some diarrheal diseases release particularly large quantities of sodium and are most likely to cause hyponatremia.

Drinking excess water sometimes causes hyponatremia because the absorption of water into the bloodstream can dilute the sodium in the blood. This cause of hyponatremia is rare, but has been found in psychotic patients who compulsively drink more than 5 gal (20 L) of water per day. Excessive drinking of beer, which is mainly water and low in sodium, can also produce hyponatremia when combined with a poor diet.

Marathon running, under certain conditions, leads to hyponatremia. Races of 25–50 miles can result in the loss of great quantities (2–2.6 gal; 8–10 L) of sweat, which contains both sodium and water. Studies show that about 30% of marathon runners experience mild hyponatremia during a race. Runners who consume only pure water during a race can develop severe hyponatremia because the drinking water dilutes the sodium in the bloodstream. Such runners may experience neurological disorders as a result of the severe hyponatremia and require emergency treatment.

Hyponatremia also develops from disorders in organs that control the body's regulation of sodium or water. The adrenal gland secretes a hormone called aldosterone that travels to the kidney, where it causes the kidney to retain sodium by not excreting it into the urine. **Addison's disease** causes hyponatremia as a result of low levels of aldosterone due to damage to the adrenal gland. The hypothalamus and pituitary gland are involved in sodium regulation by making and releasing vasopressin, known as anti-diuretic hormone, into the bloodstream. Like aldosterone, vasopressin acts in the kidney, but it causes it to reduce the amount of water released into urine. With more vasopressin production, the body conserves water, resulting in a lower concentration of plasma sodium. Certain types of **cancer** cells produce vasopressin, leading to hyponatremia.

KEY TERMS

Cerebral edema—Movement of water into brain cells causing the cells to swell, which disrupts normal functioning of the cells.

Diuretic—Medication that enhances the functioning of the kidney. Typically results in increased elimination of urine from the body.

Plasma—Clear, yellow- or straw-colored fluid that is the liquid component of blood and lymphatic fluid.

Hyponatremia can be acute, developing over 48 hours or less, or chronic, taking days or sometimes weeks to develop. Patient symptoms are often milder if the hyponatremia occurs over time because the body, particularly the brain, has time to compensate for the lower serum (blood) sodium concentration. When hyponatremia occurs rapidly, there is less time for the brain to adjust to the lowered sodium level and clinical manifestations related to cerebral **edema** are common. If the cerebral edema is severe enough, the result may be herniation of the brainstem and **death**. Rapid identification and treatment of the hyponatremic state is critical in averting these serious complications.

Symptoms of moderate hyponatremia include tiredness, disorientation, **headache**, **muscle cramps**, and **nausea**. Severe hyponatremia can lead to seizures and coma. These neurological symptoms are thought to result from the movement of water into brain cells, causing them to swell and disrupt their functioning (cerebral edema).

In most cases of hyponatremia, doctors are primarily concerned with discovering the underlying disease causing the decline in plasma sodium levels. Death that occurs during hyponatremia is usually due to other features of the disease rather than to hyponatremia itself.

Diagnosis

Tests

Hyponatremia is diagnosed by acquiring a blood sample and then measuring the concentration of sodium ions in the blood. Unless the cause is obvious, a variety of tests are subsequently run to determine if sodium was lost from the urine, diarrhea, or from **vomiting**. Tests are also used to determine abnormalities in aldosterone or vasopressin levels. The patient's diet and use of diuretics must be considered.

Treatment

The goals of treatment of acute hyponatremia are to raise the sodium level above 120 mEq/L and to raise the sodium level rapidly by 4–6 mEq/L within the first 1–2 hours of initiation of treatment. Patients with severe hyponatremia should be treated with an infusion of hypertonic (3%) saline to raise the serum sodium level by 4–6 mEq/L. Further correction could be dangerous and is avoided in most patients unless serious neurological symptoms are present.

Patients exhibiting mild symptoms as a result of chronic hyponatremia should be treated cautiously to avoid serious and irreversible damage to the central nervous system that could be precipitated by rapid and overcorrection of hyponatremia. The goals of therapy in these patients is slow and cautious correction of serum sodium levels and identification of the cause of the hyponatremia.

Prognosis

Hyponatremia is just one manifestation of a variety of disorders. While hyponatremia can easily be corrected, the prognosis for the underlying condition that causes it varies.

Prevention

Patients who take diuretic medications must be checked regularly for the development of hyponatremia.

Hyponatremia is more likely to occur in infants and in the elderly. Individuals in these groups are less able to express thirst and are also less able to independently regulate their fluid intake. Caregivers of infants and the elderly should be educated regarding the importance of adequate and appropriate fluid intake.

Resources

PERIODICALS

Sajadieh, A., et al. "Mild Hypnatremia Carries a Poor Prognosis in Community Subjects." *American Journal of Medicine* (July 2009) 122, no. 7: 679–86.

Waikar, S.S., D.B. Mount, and G.C. Curhan. "Mortality After Hospitalization with Mild, Moderate, and Severe Hyponatremia." *American Journal of Medicine* (September 2009) 122, no. 9: 857–65.

OTHER

Craig, Sandy. "Hyponatremia." *eMedicine*. April 13, 2009. http://emedicine.medscape.com/article/767624-overview (accessed October 10, 2010).

Tom Brody, PhD
Melinda Granger Oberleitner
RN, DNS, APRN, CNS

Hypoparathyroidism

Definition

Hypoparathyroidism is the result of a decrease in production of parathyroid hormones by the parathyroid glands located behind the thyroid glands in the neck. The result is a low level of **calcium** in the blood.

Description

Parathyroid glands consist of four pea-shaped glands located on the back and side of the thyroid gland. The gland produces parathyroid hormone which, along with vitamin D and calcitonin, are important for the regulation of the calcium level in the body. Hypoparathyroidism affects both males and females of all ages.

Causes and symptoms

The accidental removal of the parathyroid glands during neck surgery is the most frequent cause of hypoparathyroidism. Complications of surgery on the parathyroid glands is another common cause of this disorder. There is the possibility of autoimmune genetic disorders causing hypoparathyroidism such as Hashimoto's **thyroiditis**, **pernicious anemia**, and **Addison's disease**. The destruction of the gland by radiation is a rare cause of hypoparathyroidism. Occasionally, the parathyroids are absent at birth causing low calcium levels and possible convulsions in the newborn. Symptoms in the advanced and continuous stages of hypoparathyroidism include splitting of the nails, inadequate tooth development and **mental retardation** in children, and seizures.

Abnormal low levels of calcium result in irritability of nerves, causing **numbness and tingling** of the hands and feet, with painful-cramp like **muscle spasms** known as tetany. Laryngeal spasms may also occur causing respiratory obstruction.

Diagnosis

Diagnostic measures begin with the individual's own observation of symptoms. A thorough medical history and **physical examination** by a physician is always required for an accurate diagnosis. The general practitioner may refer the individual to an endocrinologist, a medical specialist who studies the function of the parathyroid glands as well as other hormone producing glands. Laboratory studies include blood and urine tests to help determine phosphate and calcium levels. X rays are useful to determine any abnormalities in bone density associated with abnormal calcium levels. These **autoimmune disorders** may accompany hypoparathyroidism, but are not an actual cause of it.

Treatment

In the event of severe muscle spasms, hospitalization may be warranted for calcium injections. Raising carbon-dioxide levels in the blood, which can decrease muscle spasms, may be achieved in immediate situations by placing a paper bag over the mouth and blowing into it to "reuse" each breath. It is critical to obtain timely periodic laboratory tests to check calcium levels. A high calcium, low-phosphorous diet may be of significance and is directed by the physician or dietitian.

Prognosis

Presently hypoparathyroidism is considered incurable. The disorder requires lifelong replacement therapy to control symptoms. Medical research however, continues to search for a cure.

Prevention

There are no specific preventive measures for hypoparathyroidism. However, careful surgical techniques are critical to reduce the risk of damage to the gland during surgery.

ORGANIZATIONS

American Medical Association, 515 N. State St., Chicago, IL, 60654, (800) 621-8335, http://www.ama-assn.org/.

Jeffrey P. Larson, RPT

Hypophysectomy

Definition

Hypophysectomy or hypophysis is the removal of the pituitary gland.

Purpose

The pituitary gland is in the middle of the head. Removing this master gland is a drastic step that was taken in the extreme circumstance of two cancers that had escaped all other forms of treatment. Cancers of the female breast and male prostate grow faster in the presence of sex hormones. It used to be that sex hormones could be suppressed only by removing their source, the glands that made them. After the gonads were removed, some cancers continued to grow, so other stimulants to their growth had to removed. At this point, some **cancer** specialists turned to the pituitary.

With the development of new therapeutic agents and methods, especially new ways to manipulate hormones without removing their source, this type of endocrine surgery has been largely relegated to history. However, tumors develop in the pituitary gland that require removal of the tumor but partially preserving the gland.

Description

There are several surgical approaches to the pituitary. The surgeon will choose the best one for the specific procedure. The pituitary lies directly behind the nose, and access through the nose or the sinuses is often the best approach. Opening the skull and lifting the frontal lobe of the brain will expose the delicate neck of the pituitary gland. This approach works best if tumors have extended above the pituitary fossa (the cavity in which the gland lies).

Newer surgical methods using technology have made other approaches possible. Stereotaxis is a three-dimensional aiming technique using x rays or scans for guidance. Instruments can be placed in the brain with pinpoint accuracy through tiny holes in the skull. These instruments can then manipulate brain tissue, either to destroy it or remove it. Stereotaxis is also used to direct radiation with similar precision using a gamma knife. Access to some brain lesions can be gained through the blood vessels using tiny tubes and wires guided by x rays.

Preparation

Pituitary surgery is performed by neurosurgeons deep inside the skull. All the patient can do to prepare is keep as healthy as possible and trust that the surgeon will do his usual excellent job. Informed surgical consent is important so that the patient is fully confident of the need for surgery and the expected outcome.

Aftercare

Routine post-operative care is required. In addition, pituitary function will be assessed.

Risks

The risks of surgery are multiple. Procedures are painstakingly selected to minimize risk and maximize benefit. Unique to surgery on the pituitary is the risk of destroying the entire gland and leaving the entire endocrine system without guidance. This used to be the whole purpose of hypophysectomy. After the procedure, the endocrinologist, a physician specializing in the study and care of the endocrine system, would provide the patient with all the hormones needed. Patients with no pituitary function did and still do quite well because of the available hormone replacements.

Normal results

Complete removal of the pituitary was the goal for cancer treatment. In the early twenty-first century, removal of tumors with preservation of the gland is the goal.

Abnormal results

Tumors may not be completely removed, due to their attachment to vital structures.

Resources

BOOKS

Fauci, Anthony S., et al., eds. *Harrison's Principles of Internal Medicine*. 17th ed. New York: McGraw–Hill Professional, 2008.

J. Ricker Polsdorfer, MD

Hypopigmentation *see* **Albinism; Vitiligo**

Hypopituitarism

Definition

Hypopituitarism is loss of function in an endocrine gland due to failure of the pituitary gland to secrete hormones which stimulate that gland's function. The pituitary gland is located at the base of the brain. Patients diagnosed with hypopituitarism may be deficient in one single hormone, several hormones, or have complete pituitary failure.

Description

The pituitary is a pea-sized gland located at the base of the brain, and surrounded by bone. The hypothalamus, another endocrine organ in the brain, controls the function of the pituitary gland by providing "hormonal orders." In turn, the pituitary gland regulates the many hormones that control various functions and organs within the body. The posterior pituitary acts as a sort of storage area for the hypothalamus and passes on hormones that control function of the muscles and kidneys. The anterior pituitary produces its own hormones which help to regulate several endocrine functions.

In hypopituitarism, something interferes with the production and release of these hormones, thus affecting the function of the target gland. Commonly affected hormones may include:

Gonadotropin deficiency

Gonadotropin deficiency involves two distinct hormones affecting the reproductive system. Luteinizing hormone (LH) stimulates the testes in men and the ovaries in women. This deficiency can affect fertility in men and women and menstruation in women. Follicle-stimulating hormone (FSH) has similar effects to LH.

Thyroid stimulating hormone deficiency

Thyroid stimulating hormone (TSH) is involved in stimulation of the thyroid gland. A lack of stimulation in the gland leads to **hypothyroidism**.

Adrenocorticotopic hormone deficiency

Also known as corticotropin, adrenocorticotopic hormone (ACTH) stimulates the adrenal gland to produce a hormone similar to cortisone, called cortisol. The loss of this hormone can lead to serious problems.

Growth hormone deficiency

Growth hormone (GH) regulates the body's growth. Patients who lose supply of this hormone before physical maturity will suffer impaired growth. Loss of the hormone can also affect adults.

Other hormone deficiencies

Prolactin stimulates the female breast to produce milk. A hormone produced by the posterior pituitary, antidiuretic hormone (ADH), controls the function of the kidneys. When this hormone is deficient, **diabetes insipidus** can result. However, patients with hypopituitarism rarely suffer ADH deficiency, unless the hypopituitarism is the result of hypothalamus disease.

Multiple hormone deficiencies

Deficiency of a single pituitary hormone occurs less commonly than deficiency of more than one hormone. Sometimes referred to as progressive pituitary hormone deficiency or partial hypopituitarism, there is usually a predictable order of hormone loss. Generally, growth hormone is lost first, then luteinizing hormone deficiency follows. The loss of follicle-stimulating hormone, thyroid stimulating hormone and adrenocorticotopic hormones follow much later. The progressive loss of pituitary hormone secretion is usually a slow process, which can occur over a period of months or years. Hypopituitarism does occasionally start suddenly with rapid onset of symptoms.

Panhypopituitarism

This condition represents the loss of all hormones released by the anterior pituitary gland. Panhypopituitarism is also known as complete pituitary failure.

Causes and symptoms

There are three major mechanisms that lead to the development of hypopituitarism. The first involves decreased release of hypothalamic hormones that stimulate pituitary function. The cause of decreased hypothalamic function may be congenital or acquired through interference such as tumors, inflammation, infection, mass lesions or interruption of blood supply. A second category of causes is any event or mass which interrupts the delivery of hormones from the hypothalamus. These may include particular tumors and aneurysms. Damage to the pituitary stalk from injury or surgery can also lead to hypopituitarism.

The third cause of hypopituitarism is damage to the pituitary gland cells. Destroyed cells can not produce the pituitary hormones that would normally be secreted by the gland. Cells may be destroyed by a number of tumors and diseases. Hypopituitarism is often caused by tumors, the most common of which is pituitary adenoma.

Symptoms of hypopituitarism vary with the affected hormones and severity of deficiency. Frequently, patients have had years of symptoms that were nonspecific until a major illness or **stress** occurred. Overall symptoms may include **fatigue**, sensitivity to cold, weakness, decreased appetite, weight loss and abdominal **pain**. Low blood pressure, **headache** and visual disturbances are other associated symptoms.

Gonadotropin deficiency

Symptoms specific to this hormone deficiency include decreased interest in sex for women and **infertility** in women and men. Women may also have premature cessation of menstruation, hot flashes, vaginal dryness and pain during intercourse. Women who are postmenopausal will not have obvious symptoms such as these and may first present with headache or loss of vision. Men may also suffer **sexual dysfunction** as a result of gonadotropin deficiency. In acquired gonadotropin deficiency, both men and women may notice loss of body hair.

Thyroid stimulating hormone deficiency

Intolerance to cold; fatigue; weight gain; **constipation**; and pale, waxy, and dry skin indicate thyroid hormone deficiency.

Adrenocorticotopic hormone deficiency

Symptoms of ACTH deficiency include fatigue, weakness, weight loss, and low blood pressure. **Nausea**, pale skin, and loss of pubic and armpit hair in women may also indicate deficiency of ACTH.

Growth hormone deficiency

In children, growth hormone deficiency will result in short stature and growth retardation. Symptoms such as **obesity** and skin wrinkling may or may not show in adults and normal release of growth hormone normally declines with age.

Other hormone deficiencies

Prolactin deficiency is rare and is the result of partial or generalized anterior pituitary failure. When present, the symptom is absence of milk production in women. There are no known symptoms for men. ADH deficiency may produce symptoms of diabetes insipidus, such as excessive thirst and frequent urination.

Multiple hormone deficiencies

Patients with multiple hormone deficiencies will show symptoms of one or more specific hormone deficiencies or some of the generalized symptoms listed in this article.

Panhypopituitarism

The absence of any pituitary function should show symptoms of one or all of the specific hormone deficiencies. In addition to those symptoms, patients may have dry, pale skin that is finely textured. The face may appear finely wrinkled and contain a disinterested expression.

Diagnosis

Once the diagnosis of a single hormone deficiency is made, it is strongly recommended that tests for other hormone deficiencies be conducted.

Gonadotropin deficiency

The detection of low levels of gonadotropin can be accomplished through simple blood tests which measure luteinizing hormone and follicle-stimulating hormone, simultaneously with gonadal steroid levels. The combination of results can indicate to a physician if the cause of decreased hormone levels or function belongs to hypopituitarism or some sort of primary gonadal failure. Diagnosis will vary among men and women.

Thyroid stimulating hormone deficiency

Laboratory tests measuring thyroid function can help determine a diagnosis of TSH deficiency. The commonly used tests are T4 and TSH measurement done simultaneously to determine the reserve, or pool, of thyroid-stimulating hormone.

Adrenocorticotopic hormone deficiency

An insulin tolerance test may be given to determine if cortisol levels rise when **hypoglycemia** is induced. If they do not rise, there is insufficient reserve of cortisol, indicating an ACTH deficiency. If the insulin tolerance test is not safe for a particular patient, a glucagon test offers similar results. A CRH (corticotropin-releasing hormone) test may also be given. It involves injection of CRH to measure, through regularly drawn blood samples, a resulting rise in ACTH and cortisol. Other tests which stimulate ACTH may be ordered.

Growth hormone deficiency

Growth hormone deficiency is measured through the use of insulin-like growth factor I tests, which measure growth factors that are dependent on growth hormones. Sleep and **exercise** studies may also be used to test for growth hormone deficiency, since these activities are known to stimulate growth hormone secretion. Several drugs also induce secretion of growth hormone and may be given to measure hormone response. The standard test for growth hormone deficiency is the insulin-induced hypoglycemia test. This test does carry some risk from the induced hypoglycemia. Other tests include an arginine infusion test, clonidine test and growth-hormone releasing hormone test.

Other hormone deficiencies

If a test calculates normal levels of prolactin, deficiency of the hormone is eliminated as a diagnosis. A TRH (thyrotropin-releasing hormone) simulation test can determine prolactin levels. A number of tests are available to detect ADH levels and to determine diagnosis of diabetes insipidus.

Multiple and general hypopituitarism tests

Physicians should be aware that nonspecific symptoms can indicate deficiency of one or more hormones and should conduct a thorough clinical history. In general, diagnosis of hypopituitarism can be accomplished with a combination of dynamic tests and simple blood tests, as well as imaging exams. Most of these tests can be conducted in an outpatient lab or radiology facility. **Magnetic resonance imaging** (MRI) exams with gadolinium contrast enhancement are preferred imaging exams to study the region of the hypothalamus and pituitary gland. When an MRI is not available, a properly conducted computed tomography scan (CT scan) exam can take its place. These exams can confirm a tumor or other mass, which may be interfering with pituitary function.

Panhypopituitarism

The insulin-induced hypoglycemia, or insulin tolerance test, which is used to determine specific hormone deficiencies, is an excellent test to diagnose panhypopituitarism. This test can reveal levels of growth hormone, ACTH (cortisol) and prolactin deficiency. The presence of insufficient levels of all of these hormones is a good indication of complete pituitary failure. Imaging studies and clinical history are also important.

Treatment

Treatment differs widely, depending on the age and sex of the patient, severity of the deficiency, the number of hormones involved, and even the underlying cause of the hypopituitarism. Immediate hormone replacement is generally administered to replace the specific deficient hormone. Patient education is encouraged to help patients manage the impact of their hormone deficiency on daily life. For instance, certain illnesses, accidents or surgical procedures may have adverse complications due to hypopituitarism.

Gonadotropin deficiency

Replacement of gonadal **steroids** is common treatment for LH and FSH deficiency. Estrogen for women and testosterone for men will be prescribed in the lowest effective dosage possible, since there can be complications to this therapy. To correct women's loss of libido, small doses of androgens may be prescribed. To restore fertility in men, regular hormone injections may be required. Male and female patients whose hypopituitarism results from hypothalamic disease may be successfully treated with a hypothalamic releasing hormone (GnRH), which can restore gonadal function and fertility.

Thyroid stimulating hormone deficiency

In patients who have hypothyroidism, the function of the adrenal glands will be tested and treated with steroids before administering thyroid hormone replacement.

Adrenocorticotopic hormone deficiency

Hydrocortisone or cortisone in divided doses may be given to replace this hormone deficiency. Most patients require 20 mg or less of hydrocortisone per day.

Growth hormone deficiency

It is essential to treat children suffering from growth hormone deficiency. The effectiveness of growth hormone therapy in adults, particularly elderly adults, is not as well documented. It is thought to help restore normal muscle to fat ratios. Growth hormone is an expensive and cautiously prescribed treatment.

Treatment of multiple deficiencies and panhypopituitarism

The treatment of hypopituitarism is usually very straightforward, but must normally continue for the remainder of the patient's life. Some patients may receive treatment with GnRH, the hypothalamic hormone. In most cases, treatment will be based on the specific deficiency demonstrated. Patients with hypopituitarism should be followed regularly to measure treatment effectiveness and to avoid overtreatment with hormone therapy. If the cause of the disorder is a tumor or lesion, radiation or surgical removal are treatment options. Successful removal may reverse the hypopituitarism. However, even after removal of the mass, **hormone replacement therapy** may still be necessary.

Prognosis

The prognosis for most patients with hypopituitarism is excellent. As long as therapy is continued, many experience normal life spans. However, hypopituitarism is usually a permanent condition and the prognosis depends on the primary cause of the disorder. It can be potentially life threatening, particularly when acute hypopituitarism occurs as a result of a large pituitary tumor. Morbidity from the disease has increased, although the cause is not known. It is possible that increased morbidity and **death** are due to overtreatment with hormones. Any time that recovery of pituitary function can occur is preferred to lifelong hormone therapy.

Prevention

There is no known prevention of hypopituitarism, except for prevention of damage to the pituitary/hypothalamic area from injury.

ORGANIZATIONS

Genetic Alliance, Inc., 4301 Connecticut Ave., NW, Suite 404, Washington, DC, 20008-2369, (202) 966-5557, (202) 966-8553, info@geneticalliance.org, http://www.geneticalliance.org.

The Human Growth Foundation, 997 Glen Cove Ave., Suite 5, Glen Head, NY, 11545, (516) 671-4055, (800) 451-6434, http://www.hgfound.org/.

Teresa Norris, RN

Hypoplastic anemia *see* **Aplastic anemia**

Hypospadias and epispadias

Definition

Hypospadias is a congenital defect, primarily of males, in which the urethra opens on the underside (ventrum) of the penis. It is one of the most common congenital abnormalities in the United States, occurring in about 1 of every 125 live male births. The corresponding defect in females is an opening of the urethra into the vagina and is rare.

Epispadias (also called bladder exstrophy) is a congenital defect of males in which the urethra opens on the upper surface (dorsum) of the penis. The corresponding defect in females is a fissure in the upper wall of the urethra and is quite rare.

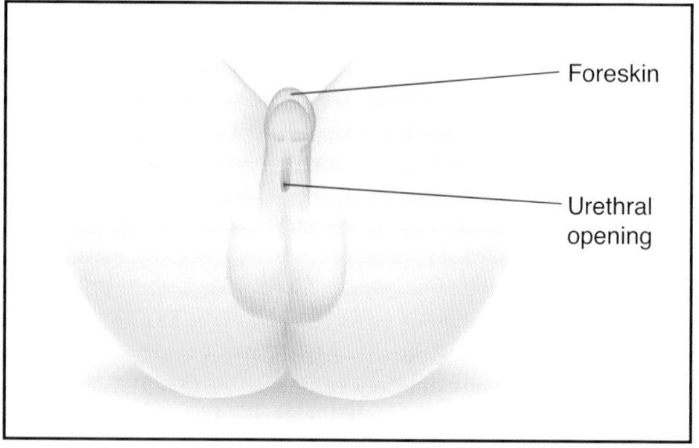

In hypospadias, the urethra opens along the penile shaft rather than at the penile tip. *(Illustration by Argosy, Inc. Reproduced by permission of Gale, a part of Cengage Learning.)*

Description

In a male, the external opening of the urinary tract (external meatus) is normally located at the tip of the penis. In a female, it is normally located between the clitoris and the vagina.

In males with hypospadias, the urethra opens on the inferior surface or underside of the penis. In females with hypospadias, the urethra opens into the cavity of the vagina.

In males with epispadias, the urethra opens on the superior surface or upper side of the penis. In females with epispadias, there is a crack or fissure in the wall of the urethra and out of the body through an opening in the skin above the clitoris.

During the embryological development of males, a groove of tissue folds inward and then fuses to form a tube that becomes the urethra. Hypospadias occurs when the tube does not form or does not fuse completely. Epispadias is due to a defect in the tissue that folds inward to form the urethra.

During the development of a female, similar processes occur to form the urethra. The problem usually is insufficient length of the tube that becomes the urethra. As a result, the urethra opens in an abnormal location, resulting in a hypospadias. Occasionally, fissures form in the bladder. These may extend to the surface of the abdomen and fuse with the adjacent skin. This condition is most commonly identified as a defect in the bladder although it is technically an epispadias.

Hypospadias in males generally occur alone. Female hypospadias may be associated with abnormalities of the genital tract, since the urinary and genital tracts are formed in the same embryonic process.

Because it represents incomplete development of the penis, some experts think that insufficient male hormone may be responsible for hypospadias.

In males, the incidence of hypospadias is approximately one per 250 to 300 live births. Epispadias is much less common, having an incidence of about one per 100,000 live male births.

In females, hypospadias is much less common than in males. It appears about once in every 500,000 live female births. Epispadias is even more rare. Reliable estimates of the prevalence of epispadias in females are not available. Epispadias in females is often diagnosed and recorded as a bladder anomaly.

Causes and symptoms

Hypospadias and epispadias are congenital defects of the urinary tract. This means they occur during intrauterine development. There is no genetic basis for the defects. Specific causes for hypospadias are not known. This means that blood relatives do not have increased chances of developing them. Reports have shown some rise in prevalence of hypospadias among offspring of mothers who work in certain occupations where they may be exposed to chemicals that disrupt the endocrine system. However, a large trial ending in 2003 showed that aside from a slight increased risk among women who were hairdressers from 1992–1996, there is no evidence that maternal occupation or certain chemical exposure increases risk of hypospadias. The role of chemicals in the development of the defect remains uncertain.

Concern was once raised that use of the antihistamine loratadine (Claritin) early in **pregnancy** might cause hypospadias. However, a national clinical trial revealed in 2004 that there was no link between the drug and risk of second or third–degree hypospadias.

Hypospadias usually is not associated with other defects of the penis or urethra. In males, it can occur at any site along the underside of the penis. In females, the urethra exits the body in an abnormal location. This usually is due to inadequate length of the urethra.

Epispadias is associated with bladder abnormalities. In females, the front wall of the bladder does not fuse or close. The bladder fissure may extend to the external abdominal wall. In such a rare case, the front of the pelvis also is widely separated. In males, the bladder fissure extends into the urethra and simply becomes an opening somewhere along the upper surface of the penis.

Hypospadias is associated with difficulty in assigning gender to babies. This occurs when gender is not obvious at birth because of deformities in the sex organs.

Diagnosis

Male external urinary tract defects are discovered at birth during the first detailed examination of the newborn. Female urethral defects may not be discovered for some time due to the difficulty in viewing the infant vagina.

Treatment

Surgery is the treatment of choice for both hypospadias and epispadias. All surgical repairs should be undertaken early and completed without delay. This minimizes psychological trauma.

In males with hypospadias, one surgery usually is sufficient to repair the defect. With more complicated hypospadias (more than one abnormally situated

KEY TERMS

Continence—Control of urination or bowel movement.

Urethra—The tube through which urine passes from the bladder to the outside of the body.

urethral opening), multiple surgeries may be required. In females with hypospadias, surgical repair technically is more complicated but can usually be completed in a brief interval of time.

Repairing an epispadias is more difficult. In males, this may involve other structures in the penis. Males should not be circumcised since the foreskin often is needed for the repair. Unfortunately, choices may be required that affect the ability to inseminate a female partner. Reproduction requires that the urethral meatus be close to the tip of the penis. Cosmetic appearance and ability to urinate (urinary continence) usually are the primary goals. Surgery for these defects is successful 70 to 80% of the time. Modern treatment of complete male epispadias allows for an excellent genital appearance and achievement of urinary continence.

In females, repair of epispadias may require multiple surgical procedures. Urinary continence and cosmetic appearance are the usual primary considerations. Urinary continence usually is achieved although cosmetic appearance may be somewhat compromised. Fertility is not usually affected. Repair rates that are similar or better than those for males usually can be achieved for females.

Hypospadias in both males and females is more of a nuisance and hindrance to reproduction than a threat to health. If surgery is not an option, the condition may be allowed to persist. This usually leads to an increased risk of infections in the lower urinary tract.

Prognosis

With adequate surgical repair, most males with simple hypospadias can lead normal lives with a penis that appears and functions in a normal manner. This includes fathering children. Females with simple hypospadias also have normal lives, including conceiving and bearing children.

The prognosis for epispadias depends on the extent of the defect. Most males with relatively minor epispadias lead normal lives, including fathering children. As the extent of the defect increases, surgical reconstruction generally is acceptable. However, many of these men are unable to conceive children. Most epispadias in females can be surgically repaired. The chances of residual disfigurement increase as the extent of the epispadias increases. Fertility in females is not generally affected by epispadias.

Resources

BOOKS

Dhar, Panchali. *Before the Scalpel: What Everyone Should Know About Anesthesia*. New Haven, CT: Tell Me Press, LLC, 2010.

Liebmann–Smith, Joan, and Jacqueline Egan. *Baby Body Signs: The Head–to–Toe Guide to Your Child's Health, from Birth Through the Toddler Years*. New York, NY: Bantam, 2010.

PERIODICALS

Kubetin, Sally Koch. "Hypospadias, Loratadine Use in Pregnancy: No Link." *Pediatric News*, July 2004.

"Molecular Epidemiology of Hypospadias: Genetic and Environmental Risk Factors." *Health & Medicine Week*, December 15, 2003: 424.

Vrijheid, M., et al. "Risk of Hypospadias in Relation to Maternal Occupational Exposure to Potential Endocrine Disrupting Chemicals." *Occupational and Environmental Medicine*, August 2003: 543–548.

OTHER

Hatch, David A. "Abnormal Development of the Penis and Male Urethra." Genitourinary Development. http://www.meddean.luc.edu/lumen/MedEd/urology/abnpendv.htm (accessed September 11, 2010).

The Penis.com. www.the–penis. com/hypospadias.html. (accessed September 11, 2010).

Society for Pediatric Urology. www.spuonline.org. (accessed September 11, 2010).

ORGANIZATIONS

Association for the Bladder Exstrophy Community, 3075 First St., La Salle, MI, 48145, (866) 300–2222, http://www.bladderexstrophy.com.

Hypospadias and Epispadias Association, 240 W. 44th St., Suite 2, New York, NY, 10036, (212) 382–3471, http://heainfo.org.

L. Fleming Fallon, Jr., MD, PhD.
Teresa G. Odle
Laura Jean Cataldo, RN, Ed.D.

Hypotension

Definition

Hypotension is the medical term for low blood pressure.

Description

The pressure of the blood in the arteries rises and falls as the heart and muscles handle demands of daily living, such as **exercise**, sleep, and **stress**. Some healthy people have blood pressure well below the average for their age, even though they have a completely normal heart and blood vessels. This is often true of athletes who are in superior shape. The term "hypotension" is usually used only when blood pressure has fallen so far that enough blood can no longer reach the brain, causing **dizziness** and **fainting**.

Causes and symptoms

Postural hypotension is the most common type of low blood pressure. In this condition, symptoms appear after a person sits up or stands quickly. In normal people, the cardiovascular system must make a quick adjustment to raise blood pressure slightly to account for the change in position. For those with postural hypotension, the blood pressure adjustment is not adequate or it doesn't happen. Postural hypotension may occur if someone is taking certain drugs or medicine for high blood pressure. It also happens to diabetics when nerve damage has disrupted the reflexes that control blood pressure.

Many people have a chronic problem with low blood pressure that is not particularly serious. This may include people who require certain medications, who are pregnant, have bad veins, or have arteriosclerosis (hardening of the arteries).

The most serious problem with low blood pressure occurs when there is a sudden drop, which can be life-threatening due to widespread **ischemia** (insufficient supply of blood to an organ due to blockage in an artery). This type of low blood pressure may be due to a wide variety of causes, including:

- trauma with extensive blood loss
- serious burns
- shock from various causes (e.g. anaphylaxis)
- heart attack
- adrenal failure (Addisonian crisis)
- cancer
- severe fever
- serious infection (septicemia)

Diagnosis

Blood pressure is a measure of the pressure in the arteries created by the heart contracting. During the day, a normal person's blood pressure changes constantly, depending on activity. Low blood pressure can be diagnosed by taking the blood pressure with a sphygmomanometer. This is a device with a soft rubber cuff that is inflated around the upper arm until it's tight enough to stop blood flow. The cuff is then slowly deflated until the health care worker, listening to the artery in the arm with a stethoscope, can hear the blood first as a beat forcing its way along the artery. This is the systolic pressure. The cuff is then deflated more until the beat disappears and the blood flows steadily through the open artery; this gives the diastolic pressure.

Blood pressure is recorded as systolic (higher) and diastolic (lower) pressures. A healthy young adult has a blood pressure of about 110/75, which typically rises with age to about 140/90 by age 60 (a reading now considered mildly elevated).

Treatment

Treatment of low blood pressure depends on the underlying cause, which can usually be resolved. For those people with postural hypotension, a medication adjustment may help prevent the problem. These individuals may find that rising more slowly, or getting out of bed in slow stages, helps the problem. Low blood pressure with no other symptoms does not need to be treated.

Prognosis

Low blood pressure as a result of injury or other underlying condition can usually be successfully treated if the trauma is not too extensive or is treated in time. Less serious forms of chronic low blood pressure have a good prognosis and do not require treatment.

Resources

BOOKS

Smeltzer, Suzanne C., et al. *Brunner and Suddarth's Textbook of Medical–Surgical Nursing*. 12th ed. Philadelphia:Lippincott Williams & Wilkins, 2009.

Carol A. Turkington

Hypothermia

Definition

Hypothermia, a potentially fatal condition, occurs when body temperature falls below 95°F (35°C).

Description

Although hypothermia is an obvious danger for people living in cold climates, many cases have occurred when the air temperature is well above the freezing mark. Elderly people, for instance, have succumbed to hypothermia after prolonged exposure to indoor air temperatures of 50–65°F (10–18.3°C). In the United States, hypothermia is primarily an urban phenomenon associated with **alcoholism**, drug **addiction**, mental illness, and cold—water immersion accidents. The victims are often homeless male alcoholics. Officially, 11,817 deaths were attributed to hypothermia in the United States from 1979 to 1994, but experts suspect that many fatal cases go unrecognized. Nearly half the victims were 65 or older, with males dominating every age group. Nonwhites were also overrepresented in the statistics. Among males 65 and older, nonwhites outnumbered whites by more than four to one.

Causes and symptoms

Measured orally, a healthy person's body temperature can fluctuate between 97°F (36.1°C) and 100°F (37.8°C). Survival depends on maintaining temperature stability within this range by balancing the heat produced by metabolism with the heat lost to the environment through (for the most part) the skin and lungs. When environmental or other changes cause heat loss to outpace heat production, the brain triggers physiological and behavioral responses to restore the balance. The involuntary muscular activity of shivering, for example, aids heat production by accelerating metabolism. But if the cold stress is too great and the body's defenses are overwhelmed, body temperature begins to fall. Hypothermia is considered to begin once body temperature reaches 95°F (35°C), though even smaller drops in temperature can have an adverse effect.

Hypothermia is divided into two types: primary and secondary. Primary hypothermia occurs when the body's heat-balancing mechanisms are working properly but are subjected to extreme cold, whereas secondary hypothermia affects people whose heat-balancing mechanisms are impaired in some way and cannot respond adequately to moderate or perhaps even mild cold. Primary hypothermia typically involves exposure to cold air or immersion in cold water. The cold air variety usually takes at least several hours to develop, but immersion hypothermia will occur within about an hour of entering the water, since water draws heat away from the body much faster than air does. In secondary hypothermia, the body's heat-balancing mechanisms can fail for any number of reasons, including strokes, diabetes, **malnutrition**, bacterial infection, thyroid disease, spinal cord injuries (which prevent the brain from receiving crucial temperature-related information from other parts of the body), and the use of medications and other substances that affect the brain or spinal cord. Alcohol is one such substance. In smaller amounts it can put people at risk by interfering with their ability to recognize and avoid cold-weather dangers. In larger amounts it shuts down the body's heat-balancing mechanisms.

Secondary hypothermia is often a threat to the elderly, who may be on medications or suffering from illnesses that affect their ability to conserve heat. Malnutrition and immobility can also put the elderly at risk. Some medical research suggests as well that shivering and blood vessel narrowing—two of the body's defenses against cold—may not be triggered as quickly in older people. For these and other reasons, the elderly can, over a period of days or even weeks, fall victim to hypothermia in poorly insulated homes or other surroundings that family, friends, and caregivers may not recognize as life threatening. Another risk for the elderly is the fact that hypothermia can easily be misdiagnosed as a **stroke** or some other common illness of old age.

The signs and symptoms of hypothermia follow a typical course, though the body temperatures at which they occur vary from person to person depending on age, health, and other factors. The impact of hypothermia on the nervous system often becomes apparent quite early. Coordination, for instance, may begin to suffer as soon as body temperature reaches 95°F (35°C). The early signs of hypothermia also include cold and pale skin and intense shivering; the latter stops between 90°F (32.2°C) and 86°F (30°C). As body temperature continues to fall, speech becomes slurred, the muscles go rigid, and the victim becomes disoriented and experiences eyesight problems. Other harmful consequences include **dehydration** as well as liver and kidney failure. Heart rate, respiratory rate, and blood pressure rise during the first stages of hypothermia, but fall once the 90°F (32.2°C) mark is passed. Below 86°F (30°C) most victims are comatose, and below 82°F (27.8°C) the heart's rhythm becomes dangerously disordered. However, even at very low body temperatures, people can survive for several hours and be successfully revived, though they may appear to be dead.

Diagnosis

Information on the patient's prior health and activities often helps doctors establish a correct diagnosis and treatment plan. Pulse, blood pressure, temperature, and respiration require immediate monitoring. Because the temperature of the mouth is not an accurate guide to the body's core temperature, readings are taken at other sites, usually the ear, rectum, or esophagus. Other diagnostic tools include **electrocardiography**, which is used to evaluate heart rhythm, and blood and urine tests, which provide several kinds of key information; a **chest x ray** is also required. A computed tomography scan (CT scan) or **magnetic resonance imaging** (MRI) may be needed to check for head and other injuries.

Treatment

Emergency medical help should be summoned whenever a person appears hypothermic. The danger signs include intense shivering; stiffness and **numbness** in the arms and legs; stumbling and clumsiness; sleepiness, confusion, disorientation, **amnesia**, and irrational behavior; and difficulty speaking. Until emergency help arrives, a victim of outdoor hypothermia should be brought to shelter and warmed by removing wet clothing and footwear, drying the skin, and wrapping him or her in warm blankets or a sleeping bag. Gentle handling is necessary when moving the victim to avoid disturbing the heart. Rubbing the skin or giving the victim alcohol can be harmful, though warm drinks such as clear soup and tea are recommended for those who can swallow. Anyone who aids a victim of hypothermia should also look for signs of **frostbite** and be aware that attempting to rewarm a frostbitten area of the body before emergency help arrives can be extremely dangerous. For this reason, frostbitten areas must be kept away from heat sources such as campfires and car heaters.

Rewarming is the essence of hospital treatment for hypothermia. How rewarming proceeds depends on the body temperature. Different approaches are used for patients who are mildly hypothermic (the patient's body temperature is 90–95°F [32.2–35°C]), moderately hypothermic (86–90°F [30–32.2°C]), or severely hypothermic (less than 86°F [30°C]). Other considerations, such as the patient's age or the condition of the heart, can also influence treatment choices.

Mild hypothermia is reversed with passive rewarming. This technique relies on the patient's own metabolism to rewarm the body. Once wet clothing is removed and the skin is dried, the patient is covered with blankets and placed in a warm room. The goal is to raise the patient's temperature by 0.5–2°C an hour.

Moderate hypothermia is often treated first with active external rewarming and then with passive rewarming. Active external rewarming involves applying heat to the skin, for instance by placing the patient in a warm bath or wrapping the patient in electric heating blankets.

Severe hypothermia requires active internal rewarming, which is recommended for some cases of moderate hypothermia as well. There are several types of active internal rewarming. Cardiopulmonary bypass, in which the patient's blood is circulated through a rewarming device and then returned to the body, is considered the best, and can raise body temperature by 1–2°C every 3–5 minutes. However, many hospitals are not equipped to offer this treatment. The alternative is to introduce warm oxygen or fluids into the body.

Hypothermia treatment can also include, among other things, insulin, **antibiotics**, and fluid replacement therapy. When the heart has stopped, both **cardiopulmonary resuscitation** (CPR) and rewarming are necessary. Once a patient's condition has stabilized, he or she may need treatment for an underlying problem such as alcoholism or thyroid disease.

Prognosis

Victims of mild or moderate hypothermia usually enjoy a complete recovery. In regard to severely hypothermic patients, the prognosis for survival varies due to differences in people's physiological responses to cold.

Prevention

People who spend time outdoors in cold weather can reduce heat loss by wearing their clothing loosely and in layers and by keeping their hands, feet, and head well covered (30–50% of body heat is lost through the head). Because water draws heat away from the body so easily, staying dry is important, and wet clothing and footwear should be replaced as quickly as possible. Wind- and water-resistant outer garments are also crucial. Alcohol should be avoided because it promotes heat loss by expanding the blood vessels that carry body heat to the skin.

Preventing hypothermia among the elderly requires vigilance on the part of family, friends, and caregivers. An elderly person's home should be properly insulated and heated, with living areas kept at a temperature of 70°F (21.1°C). Warm clothing and bedding are essential, as are adequate food, rest, and **exercise**; warming the bed and bedroom before going to sleep is also recommended. Older people who live alone should be visited regularly—at least once a day during very cold weather—to ensure that their health remains sound and that they are taking good care of themselves. For help and advice, family members and others can turn to government and social service agencies. Meals on Wheels and visiting nurse programs, for instance, may be available, and it may be possible to obtain financial aid for winterizing and heating homes.

Resources

BOOKS

Fauci, Anthony S., et al., eds.*Harrison's Principles of Internal Medicine*. 17th ed. New York: McGraw–Hill Professional, 2008.

Howard Baker

Hypothyroidism

Definition

Hypothyroidism is a condition in which a person's thyroid gland is not producing enough hormone. It may be caused by an autoimmune disorder, a genetic defect in a newborn, certain medications, surgical removal of the thyroid gland, **radiation therapy** for **cancer**, and other reasons.

There are three main types of hypothyroidism. The most common is primary hypothyroidism, in which the thyroid doesn't produce an adequate amount of T_4. Secondary hypothyroidism develops when the pituitary gland does not release enough of the thyroid-stimulating hormone (TSH) that prompts the thyroid to manufacture T_4. Tertiary hypothyroidism results from a malfunction of the hypothalamus, the part of the brain that controls the endocrine system. Drug-induced hypothyroidism, an adverse reaction to medication, occurs in 2 of every 10,000 people, but rarely causes severe hypothyroidism.

Demographics

According to the National Institute of Diabetes and Digestive and Kidney Diseases (NIDDK), between 3 and 5% of the general population in the United States and Canada has some form of hypothyroidism. Apart from cretinism, which affects one child in every 3,000–4,000, hypothyroidism is largely a disease of adults. The most common form of primary hypothyroidism in North America is Hashimoto's disease, an autoimmune disorder that is diagnosed in about 14 women out of every 1000 and 1 man in every 2000.

Caucasians and Hispanics (particularly Mexican Americans) in North America have higher rates of hypothyroidism than African Americans. The reason for this difference was not known as of 2009.

Internationally, however, the most common cause of hypothyroidism is a lack of iodine in the diet. The prevalence of hypothyroidism caused by iodine deficiency in developing countries is 2–5%, increasing to 15% by age 75.

Description

Hypothyroidism is an endocrine disorder; that is, it is caused by underfunctioning of a gland that is part of the endocrine system—a group of small organs located throughout the body that regulate growth, metabolism, tissue function, and emotional mood. The thyroid gland itself is a butterfly-shaped organ weighing between half an ounce and 1.5 ounces in adults that lies at the base of the throat below the Adam's apple and above the collarbone. It takes its name from a Greek word meaning "shield." The thyroid consists of two lobes about 2 inches in length (in adults) connected by a thin strip of tissue called the isthmus.

Hypothyroidism develops when the thyroid gland fails to produce or secrete as much thyroxine (T_4) as the body needs. Because T_4 regulates such essential functions as heart rate, digestion, physical growth, and mental development, an insufficient supply of this hormone can slow life-sustaining processes, damage organs and tissues in every part of the body, and lead to life-threatening complications.

Hypothyroidism is not easy to diagnose because its symptoms are found in a number of other diseases; it often comes on slowly; and it may produce few or no symptoms in younger adults. In general, hypothyroidism is characterized by a slowing down of both physical and mental activities.

Risk factors

Risk factors for hypothyroidism include:

- Sex. Women are at greater risk of hypothyroidism than men. The female/male ratio among adults is between 2:1 and 8:1, depending on the age group being studied.
- Age over 50. In one Massachusetts study, 6 percent of women over 60 and 2.5 percent of men over 60 were found to be hypothyroid.
- Race. According to the National Institutes of Health (NIH), the rates of hypothyroidism in the United States are highest among Caucasians (5.1 percent) and Hispanics (4.1 percent) and lowest among African Americans (1.7 percent).
- Obesity.
- Having a small body size at birth and low body mass index during childhood.
- Family history of autoimmune disease.
- Having Turner syndrome, a genetic disorder in which a girl is born with only one X chromosome

instead of the normal two. Turner syndrome affects 1 in every 2500 girls.

Causes and symptoms

Causes

The most common causes of hypothyroidism are:

- Hashimoto's disease. This is an autoimmune disorder in which the patient's immune system attacks the thyroid gland, leading to tissue destruction.
- Treatment for hyperthyroidism. People who have been treated for an oversupply of thyroid hormone (hyperthyroidism) with radioactive iodine (iodine-131) may lose their ability to produce enough thyroid hormone.
- Surgery on the thyroid gland.
- Radiation therapy for the treatment of head or neck cancer.
- Medications. Lithium, given to treat some psychiatric disorders, and certain heart medications may affect the functioning of the thyroid gland. Other drugs known to suppress thyroid function include amiodarone, a heart medication; interferon alpha, given to treat cancer; and stavudine, a drug used to treat HIV infection.
- Pregnancy. As many as 10% of women may become hypothyroid in the first year after childbirth, particularly if they have diabetes.
- Viral infections. These can cause a short-term inflammation of the thyroid gland known as thyroiditis in some people.
- A tumor in the pituitary gland. The pituitary gland produces a hormone called thyroid-stimulating hormone or TSH. Low levels of TSH can lead to secondary hypothyroidism.
- Congenital. About 1 baby in every 3,000–4,000 is born with a defective thyroid gland or no gland at all.
- Too little iodine in the diet. This cause of hypothyroidism is most common in developing countries; it is rare in North America and Europe.

Symptoms

Not every patient with an underactive thyroid has the same symptoms or has them with the same severity. Common symptoms of hypothyroidism, however, include the following:

- Increased sensitivity to cold weather.
- Dry, itchy skin and a pale or yellowish complexion.
- Dry brittle hair that falls out easily and nails that break or split.
- Constipation.
- Goiter (swelling in the front of the neck caused by thyroid enlargement).
- Hoarse voice and puffy facial skin.
- Unexplained weight gain of 10–20 pounds, most of which is fluid.
- Sore and aching muscles, most commonly in the shoulders and hips.
- In women, extra-long menstrual periods or unusually heavy bleeding.
- Weak leg muscles.
- Decreased sweating.
- Arthritis.
- Memory loss or difficulty concentrating.
- Slowed heart rate (less than 60 beats per minute) and lowered blood pressure.
- Depression.

Diagnosis

Adults

Hypothyroidism in adults can be difficult to diagnose because many of its early symptoms are not unique to it. In addition, the symptoms typically come on gradually; the person may simply feel tired or less energetic than usual, or develop dry, itchy skin and brittle hair that falls out easily. Hypothyroidism is sometimes referred to as a "silent" disease precisely because the early symptoms may be so mild that no one realizes anything is wrong. The classic symptoms of hypothyroidism—sensitivity to cold, puffy complexion, decreased sweating, and coarse skin—may occur in only 60 percent of patients. In addition, the patient's loss of energy and low mood may be misdiagnosed as a psychiatric disorder, most commonly major depression. It may take months to years before the person or their doctor begins to suspect a problem with the thyroid gland.

It's important to see a doctor if any of these symptoms appear unexpectedly. People whose hypothyroidism remains undiagnosed and untreated may eventually develop myxedema. Symptoms of this rare but potentially deadly complication include enlarged tongue, swollen facial features, hoarseness, and physical and mental sluggishness.

Myxedema **coma** can cause unresponsiveness; irregular, shallow breathing; and a drop in blood pressure and body temperature. The onset of this medical emergency can be sudden in people who are elderly or have been ill, injured, or exposed to very cold temperatures; have recently had surgery; or use

KEY TERMS

Congenital—Present at birth.

Cretinism—A form of hypothyroidism found in some newborns.

Endocrine system—A system of small organs located throughout the body that regulate metabolism, growth and puberty, tissue function, and mood. The thyroid gland is part of the endocrine system.

Endocrinologist—A doctor who specializes in diagnosing and treating disorders of the endocrine glands and the hormones they secrete.

Goiter—A swelling in the neck caused by an enlarged thyroid gland.

Hashimoto's disease—An autoimmune disorder that is the most common cause of primary hypothyroidism. It was the first disease to be recognized as an autoimmune disorder. It is named for a Japanese doctor, Hakaru Hashimoto, who first described it in 1912.

Hormone—A chemical released by specialized cells that affects cells in other parts of the body. Hormones regulate such body processes as growth, metabolism, the immune system, reproduction, hunger, and mood.

Hyperthyroidism—A disease condition in which the thyroid gland produces too much thyroid hormone.

Hypothyroidism—A disease condition in which the thyroid gland does not produce enough thyroid hormone.

Metabolism—The chemical changes in living cells in which new materials are taken in and energy is provided for vital processes,

Myxedema—A synonym for hypothyroidism. Myxedema coma is a condition in which a person with untreated hypothyroidism loses consciousness. It is potentially fatal.

Thyroid-stimulating hormone (TSH)—A hormone produced by the pituitary gland that stimulates the thyroid gland to produce the hormones that regulate metabolism. Also called thyrotropin.

Thyroiditis—Inflammation of the thyroid gland. It can be caused by a viral infection, a malfunction of the immune system, or certain medications.

Thyroxine (T_4)—The thyroid hormone that regulates many essential body processes.

Triiodothyronine (T_3)—A thyroid hormone similar to thyroxine but more powerful. Preparations of triiodothyronine are used in treating hypothyroidism.

sedatives or antidepressants. Without immediate medical attention, myxedema coma can be fatal.

Children

In the United States, newborn infants between 24 and 72 hours old are tested for congenital thyroid deficiency (cretinism) using a test that measures the levels of thyroxine in the infant's blood. If the levels are low, the physician will likely repeat the blood test to confirm the diagnosis. The physician may take an x ray of the infant's legs. In an infant with hypothyroidism, the ends of the bones have an immature appearance. Treatment within the first few months of life can prevent **mental retardation** and physical abnormalities.

Older children who develop hypothyroidism may suddenly stop growing. If the child was above average height before the disease occurred, he or she may now be short compared to other children of the same age. Therefore, the most important feature of hypothyroidism in a child is a decrease in the rate of growth in height. If the disease is recognized early and adequately treated, the child will grow at an accelerated rate until reaching the same growth percentile where the child measured before the onset of hypothyroidism. Diagnosis of hypothyroidism in school-age children is based on the patient's observations, medical history, **physical examination**, and **thyroid function tests**.

Examination

The doctor may notice such signs of hypothyroidism during an office examination as dry skin, facial puffiness, a **goiter** in the neck, thin or brittle hair, poor muscle tone, pale complexion, and a slower than normal heart rate. As previously mentioned, however, it is possible for a person with hypothyroidism not to have these symptoms.

Tests

The diagnosis of hypothyroidism is usually made by tests of the patient's thyroid function following a careful history of the patient's symptoms. The first test is a blood test for thyroid-stimulating hormone, or TSH. TSH is a hormone produced by the pituitary gland in the brain that stimulates the thyroid gland to produce thyroid hormone. When the thyroid gland is not producing enough hormone, the pituitary gland secretes more TSH; thus a high level of TSH in the blood indicates that the thyroid gland is not as active as it should be.

The TSH test, however, does not always detect borderline cases of hypothyroidism. The doctor may order additional tests to measure the levels of thyroid hormone as well as TSH in the patient's blood. If the doctor thinks that the patient may have Hashimoto's disease, he or she may test for the presence of abnormal antibodies in the blood. Because Hashimoto's disease is an autoimmune disorder, there will be two or three types of anti-thyroid antibodies in the patient's blood in about 90 percent of cases

A woman being tested for hypothyroidism should let her doctor know if she is pregnant or **breastfeeding** and all patients should be sure their doctors are aware of any recent procedures involving radioactive materials or contrast media.

Procedures

In some cases, the doctor may also order an ultrasound study of the patient's neck in order to evaluate the size of the thyroid gland or take a small sample of thyroid tissue in order to make sure that the gland is not cancerous. The usual procedure for obtaining the tissue sample is a fine-needle aspiration biopsy or FNAB. To perform a FNAB, the doctor inserts a thin needle into the thyroid to extract a sample of cells for examination under a microscope. The doctor usually uses an ultrasound monitor to guide the needle. A FNAB can be performed in an outpatient clinic or a doctor's office; it is safer and less invasive than an open surgical biopsy.

Treatment

Traditional

Medications are the treatment of choice for hypothyroidism.

Drugs

Treatment for hypothyroidism consists of a daily dose of a synthetic form of thyroid hormone sold under the trade names of Synthroid, Levothroid, or Levoxyl. The patient is told that the drug must be taken as directed for the rest of his or her life.

In the early weeks of treatment, the patient will need to see the doctor every four to six weeks to have their TSH level checked and the dose of medication adjusted. After the doctor is satisfied with the dosage level and the patient's overall health, checkups are done every six to 12 months. The reason for this careful measurement of the medication is that too much of the synthetic hormone increases the risk of **osteoporosis** in later life or abnormal heart rhythms in the present. **Aging**, other medications, and changes in weight and general health can also affect how much replacement hormone a patient needs, and regular TSH tests are used to monitor hormone levels. Patients should not switch from one brand of thyroid hormone to another without a doctor's permission.

Medications and over-the-counter preparations that can affect the body's absorption of synthetic thyroid hormone include cholestyramine (Questran), **antacids** that contain aluminum hydroxide, **calcium** supplements, and iron supplements. A high intake of soy products or a diet high in fiber can also affect the body's absorption of the hormone, and the patient's doctor may need to adjust the dosage.

Congenital hypothyroidism or cretinism is also treated with synthetic thyroid hormone. It Most hospitals now screen newborns for thyroid problems, because untreated cretinism can lead to lifelong physical and mental developmental disorders.

Regular **exercise** and a high-fiber diet can help maintain thyroid function and prevent **constipation**.

Alternative

Alternative treatments are primarily aimed at strengthening the thyroid and will not eliminate the need for thyroid hormone medications. Herbal remedies to improve thyroid function and relieve symptoms of hypothyroidism include bladder wrack (*Fucus vesiculosus*), which can be taken in capsule form or as a tea. Some foods, including cabbage, peaches, radishes, soybeans, peanuts, and spinach, can interfere with the production of **thyroid hormones**. Anyone with hypothyroidism may want to avoid these foods.

The Shoulder Stand **yoga** position (at least once daily for 20 minutes) is believed to improve thyroid function.

One alternative treatment for hypothyroidism that should *not* be used is coconut oil. There is no evidence that coconut oil stimulates the thyroid gland, and a few studies suggest that it may actually lower thyroid function.

Prognosis

The prognosis for patients with hypothyroidism is very good, provided they take their medication as directed. They can usually live a normal life with a normal life expectancy. Children with cretinism have a good prognosis if the disorder is caught and treated early; some develop **learning disorders**, however, in spite of early treatment.

The chief risks to health are related to lack of treatment for hypothyroidism. If low levels of thyroid hormone are not diagnosed and treated, patients are at increased risk of goiter, an enlarged heart, and severe depression. In addition, women with untreated hypothyroidism have a higher risk of giving birth to babies with **cleft palate** and other **birth defects**.

One rare but potentially life-threatening complication of long-term untreated hypothyroidism is myxedema coma. In this condition, which is usually triggered by **stress** or illness, the person becomes extremely sensitive to cold, may be unusually drowsy, or lose consciousness. Heart rate, blood pressure, and breathing may all be abnormally low. Myxedema coma requires emergency treatment in a hospital with intravenous thyroid hormone and intensive care nursing.

Prevention

There were no proven ways to prevent hypothyroidism as of 2009 because the disorder has so many possible causes.

Resources

BOOKS

Cooper, David S. *Medical Management of Thyroid Disease*, 2nd ed. New York: Informa Healthcare, 2009.

Pratt, Maureen. *The First Year—Hypothyroidism: An Essential Guide for the Newly Diagnosed*, 2nd ed., revised and updated. New York: Marlowe and Co., 2007.

Rone, James K. *The Thyroid Paradox: How to Get the Best Care for Hypothyroidism*. Laguna Beach, CA: Basic Health Publications, 2007.

Shannon, Joyce Brennfleck. *Endocrine and Metabolic Disorders Sourcebook*, 2nd ed. Detroit, MI: Omnigraphics, 2007.

Skugor, Mario. *Thyroid Disorders: A Cleveland Clinic Guide*. Cleveland, OH: Cleveland Clinic Press, 2006.

PERIODICALS

Alexander, E.K. "Thyroid Function: The Complexity of Maternal Hypothyroidism During Pregnancy." *Nature Reviews: Endocrinology* 5 (September 2009): 480–81.

Baloch, Z.W., and V.A. LiVolsi. "Fine-needle Aspiration of the Thyroid: Today and Tomorrow." *Best Practice and Research: Clinical Endocrinology and Metabolism* 22 (December 2008): 929–39.

Brown, R.S. "Autoimmune Thyroid Disease: Unlocking a Complex Puzzle." *Current Opinion in Pediatrics* 21 (August 2009): 523–28.

Carson, M. "Assessment and Management of Patients with Hypothyroidism." *Nursing Standard* 23 (January 7–13, 2009): 48–56.

Counts, D., and S.K. Varma. "Hypothyroidism in Children." *Pediatrics in Review* 30 (July 2009): 251–58.

Miller, M.C., and A. Agrawal. "Hypothyroidism in Postradiation Head and Neck Cancer Patients: Incidence, Complications, and Management." *Current Opinion in Otolaryngology and Head and Neck Surgery* 17 (April 2009): 111–115.

Mistry, N., et al. "When to Consider Thyroid Dysfunction in the Neurology Clinic." *Practical Neurology* 9 (June 2009): 145–56.

Wirsing, N., and A. Hamilton. "How Often Should You Follow Up on a Patient with Newly Diagnosed Hypothyroidism?" *Journal of Family Practice* 58 (January 2009): 40–41.

OTHER

American Thyroid Association. *Hypothyroidism*. http://www.thyroid.org/patients/brochures/Hypo_brochure.pdf.

Bharaktiya, Shikha, et al. "Hypothyroidism." *eMedicine*. July 23, 2009. http://emedicine.medscape.com/article/122393-overview

Mayo Clinic. *Hypothyroidism (Underactive Thyroid)*. http://www.mayoclinic.com/health/hypothyroidism/DS00353

National Institute of Diabetes and Digestive and Kidney Diseases (NIDDK). *Hypothyroidism*. http://endocrine.niddk.nih.gov/pubs/Hypothyroidism/index.htm

ORGANIZATIONS

American Academy of Otolaryngology—Head and Neck Surgery, 1650 Diagonal Road, Alexandria, VA, 22314, 703-836-4444, http://www.entnet.org/.

American Association of Clinical Endocrinologists (AACE), 245 Riverside Ave., Suite 200, Jacksonville, FL, 32202, 904-353-7878, http://www.aace.com/.

American Thyroid Association (ATA), 6066 Leesburg Pike, Suite 550, Falls Church, VA, 22041, 703-998-8890, 703-998-8893, thyroid@thyroid.org, http://www.thyroid.org/.

Hormone Foundation, 8401 Connecticut Avenue, Suite 900, Chevy Chase, MD, 20815, 800–HORMONE, 301-941-0259, hormone@endo-society.org, http://www.hormone. org/.

National Institute of Diabetes and Digestive and Kidney Diseases (NIDDK), Building 31. Rm 9A06, 31 Center Drive, MSC 2560, Bethesda, MD, 20892-2560, 301-496-3583, http://www2.niddk.nih.gov/Footer/Contact NIDDK.htm, http://www2.niddk.nih.gov/.

Judith Sims, M.S.
Rebecca J. Frey, PhD

Hypotonic duodenography

Definition

Hypotonic duodenography is an x ray procedure that produces images of the duodenum. The duodenum is the first part of the small intestine.

Purpose

Hypotonic duodenography may be ordered to detect tumors of the head of the pancreas or the area where the pancreatic and bile ducts meet the small intestine. Lesions causing upper abdominal **pain** may be demonstrated by duodenography, and the procedure can aid in the diagnosis of chronic **pancreatitis**.

Precautions

Some patients with narrowing of the tubes in the upper gastrointestinal tract should not receive duodenography. Patients with certain heart disorders and glaucoma are cautioned against receiving an agent called anticholinergic, which is administered during the procedure to lessen intestinal **muscle spasms**. A hormone called glucagon may also be used to relax the intestines, but its use is not recommended in patients with most forms of diabetes.

Description

Hypotonic duodenography is also referred to as x ray of the duodenum or simply as duodenography. The patient is seated while the radiologist places a catheter in the nose and down into the stomach. Then the patient lies down and the tube is continued to the duodenum. The radiologist is guided in this placement by a fluoroscopic image. (Fluoroscopic equipment shows an immediate x ray. In this case, the x ray shows the location of the catheter as it is moved into the stomach and duodenum.) Next, either the glucagon is administered intravenously or anticholinergic is injected into the patient to relax the muscles of the intestine.

After several minutes, the physician will administer barium through the catheter. Barium is a contrast agent that will help highlight the area on the fluoroscopy screen and x rays. After a few films are taken, some of the barium is withdrawn and air is sent in through the catheter. Additional images are acquired and the catheter is then removed. The procedure takes from 30–60 minutes.

Preparation

Patients are required to fast from midnight before the test until after the test, or about 6–12 hours. Just prior to the exam, patients should remove dentures, glasses, and other objects that may interfere with the procedure. The patient may be instructed to empty his or her bladder just prior to duodenography.

Aftercare

The barium should be expelled within two to three days. Extra fluids and/or an agent given by the physician to help encourage bowel movement may aid in barium elimination. Physicians and patients should watch for possible reactions to the anticholinergic or glucagon. If an anticholinergic is used, patients are advised to empty their bladder within a few hours after the exam and to wait two hours for clearing of vision or have someone drive them home. Patients will notice that their stools are chalky white from the barium for one to three days following the procedure.

Risks

Abdominal cramping may occur when the physician instills air into the duodenum, but aside from the discomfort, there are few risks associated with this procedure. Side effects from the contrast, hormones or agents may occur. Those patients with diabetes, heart disease, or glaucoma run the highest risk of reaction and should not receive anticholinergic or glucagon, depending on their specific conditions. Elderly patients or those who are extremely ill, must be closely monitored during the procedure for possible return of fluid, or gastric reflux.

Normal results

The linings of the duodenum and surrounding tissues will look smooth and even. The shape of the head of the pancreas will appear normal and near the duodenal wall.

Abnormal results

Any masses or irregular nodules on the wall of the duodenum may indicate tumors or abnormality of tissue. Tumors of the head of the pancreas or of the opening into the intestine from the pancreatic and bile ducts may be seen. Chronic pancreatitis may be indicated on the x rays. In many instances, follow-up laboratory or imaging studies may be ordered to further study the abnormal findings and confirm a diagnosis.

ORGANIZATIONS

American College of Radiology, 1891 Preston White Drive, Reston, VA, 20191, (703) 648-8900, (800) 227-5463, info@acr.org, www.acr.org.

National Cancer Institute (National Institutes of Health), NCI Office of Communications and Education, 6116 Executive Blvd. Suite 300, Bethesda, MD, 20892-8322, (800) 4-CANCER (422-6237), cancergovstaff@mail.nih.gov, http://www.cancer.gov/.

Teresa Odle

Hypovolemic shock *see* **Shock**

Hysterectomy

Definition

Hysterectomy is the surgical removal of all or part of the uterus. In a total hysterectomy, the uterus and cervix are removed. In some cases, the fallopian tubes and ovaries are removed along with the uterus, which is a hysterectomy with bilateral **salpingo-oophorectomy**. In a subtotal hysterectomy, only the uterus is removed. In a radical hysterectomy, the uterus, cervix, ovaries, oviducts, lymph nodes, and lymph channels are removed. The type of hysterectomy performed depends on the reason for the procedure. In all cases, menstruation permanently stops and a woman loses the ability to bear children.

Purpose

The most frequent reason for hysterectomy in American women is to remove fibroid tumors, accounting for 30% of these surgeries. Fibroid tumors are noncancerous (benign) growths in the uterus that can cause pelvic, **low back pain**, and heavy or lengthy menstrual periods. They occur in 30–40% of women over age 40 and are three times more likely to be present in African-American women than in Caucasian women. Fibroids do not need to be removed unless they are causing symptoms that interfere with a woman's normal activities.

Treatment of **endometriosis** is the reason for 20% of hysterectomies. The endometrium is the lining of the uterus. Endometriosis occurs when the cells from the endometrium begin growing outside the uterus. The outlying endometrial cells respond to the hormones that control the menstrual cycle, bleeding each month the way the lining of the uterus does. This causes irritation of the surrounding tissue, leading to **pain** and scarring.

Twenty percent of hysterectomies are done because of heavy or abnormal vaginal bleeding that cannot be linked to any specific cause and cannot be controlled by other means. Another 20% are performed to treat prolapsed uterus, **pelvic inflammatory disease**, or endometrial hyperplasia, a potentially precancerous condition.

About 10% of hysterectomies are performed to treat **cancer** of the cervix, ovaries, or uterus. Women with cancer in one or more of these organs almost always have the organ(s) removed as part of their cancer treatment.

Demographics

Hysterectomy is the second most common operation performed on women in the United States. About 556,000 of these surgeries are done annually. By age 60, approximately one out of every three American women will have had a hysterectomy. It is estimated that 30% of hysterectomies are unnecessary.

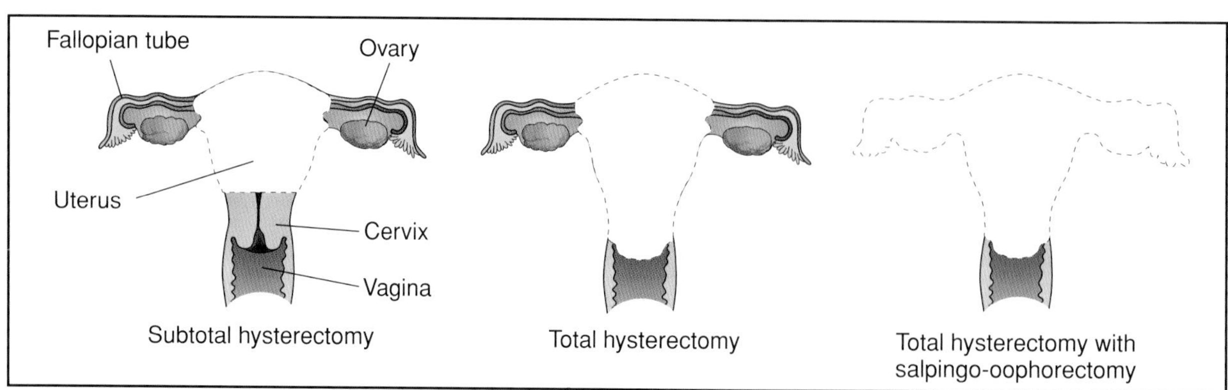

Three types of hysterectomies: subtotal, total, and total with salpingo-oophorectomy. *(Illustration by Electronic Illustrators Group. Reproduced by permission of Gale, a part of Cengage Learning.)*

KEY TERMS

Cervix—The lower part of the uterus extending into the vagina.

Fallopian tubes—Slender tubes that carry eggs (ova) from the ovaries to the uterus.

Lymph nodes—Small, compact structures lying along the channels that carry lymph, a yellowish fluid. Lymph nodes produce white blood cells (lymphocytes), which are important in forming antibodies that fight disease.

Pap smear—The common term for the Papanicolaou test, a simple smear method of examining stained cells to detect cancer of the cervix.

Prolapsed uterus—A uterus that has slipped out of place, sometimes protruding down through the vagina.

The frequency with which hysterectomies are performed in the United States has been questioned in recent years. It has been suggested that a large number of hysterectomies are performed unnecessarily. The United States has the highest rate of hysterectomies of any country in the world. Also, the frequency of this surgery varies across different regions of the United States. Rates are highest in the South and Midwest and are higher for African-American women. In the early twenty-first century, although the number of hysterectomies performed has declined, the number of hysterectomies performed on younger women in their 30s and 40s is increasing, and 55% of all hysterectomies are performed on women ages 35–49.

Description

A hysterectomy is classified according to what structures are removed during the procedure and what method is used to remove them.

Total hysterectomy

A total hysterectomy, sometimes called a simple hysterectomy, removes the entire uterus and the cervix. The ovaries are not removed and continue to secrete hormones. Total hysterectomies are usually performed in the case of uterine and **cervical cancer**. This is the most common kind of hysterectomy.

In addition to a total hysterectomy, a procedure called a bilateral salpingo-oophorectomy is sometimes performed. This surgery removes the ovaries and the fallopian tubes. Removal of the ovaries eliminates the main source of the hormone estrogen, so **menopause** occurs immediately. Removal of the ovaries and fallopian tubes is performed in about one-third of hysterectomy operations, often to reduce the risk of **ovarian cancer**.

Subtotal hysterectomy

If the reason for the hysterectomy is to remove **uterine fibroids**, treat abnormal bleeding, or relieve pelvic pain, it may be possible to remove only the uterus and leave the cervix. This procedure is called a subtotal hysterectomy (or partial hysterectomy), and removes the least amount of tissue. The opening to the cervix is left in place. Some women believe that leaving the cervix intact aids in their achieving sexual satisfaction. This procedure, which used to be rare, is now performed more frequently.

Subtotal hysterectomy is easier to perform than a total hysterectomy, but leaves a woman at risk for cervical cancer. She will still need to get yearly Pap smears.

Radical hysterectomy

Radical hysterectomies are performed on women with cervical cancer or **endometrial cancer** that has spread to the cervix. A radical hysterectomy removes the uterus, cervix, above part of the vagina, ovaries, fallopian tubes, lymph nodes, lymph channels, and tissue in the pelvic cavity that surrounds the cervix. This type of hysterectomy removes the most tissue and requires the longest hospital stay and a longer recovery period.

Methods of hysterectomy

There are two ways that hysterectomies can be performed. The choice of method depends on the type of hysterectomy, the doctor's experience, and the reason for the hysterectomy.

ABDOMINAL HYSTERECTOMY. About 75% of hysterectomies performed in the United States are abdominal hysterectomies. The surgeon makes a 4–6-in (10–15-cm) incision either horizontally across the pubic hair line from hip bone to hip bone or vertically from navel to pubic bone. Horizontal incisions leave a less noticeable scar, but vertical incisions give the surgeon a better view of the abdominal cavity. The blood vessels, fallopian tubes, and ligaments are cut away from the uterus, which is lifted out.

Abdominal hysterectomies take from one to three hours. The hospital stay is three to five days, and it takes four to eight weeks to return to normal activities.

The advantages of an abdominal hysterectomy are that the uterus can be removed even if a woman has internal scarring (**adhesions**) from previous surgery or her fibroids are large. The surgeon has a good view of the abdominal cavity and more room to work. Also, surgeons tend to have the most experience with this type of hysterectomy. The abdominal incision is more painful than with vaginal hysterectomy, and the recovery period is longer.

VAGINAL HYSTERECTOMY. With a vaginal hysterectomy, the surgeon makes an incision near the top of the vagina. The surgeon then reaches through this incision to cut and tie off the ligaments, blood vessels, and fallopian tubes. Once the uterus is cut free, it is removed through the vagina. The operation takes one to two hours. The hospital stay is usually one to three days, and the return to normal activities takes about four weeks.

The advantages of this procedure are that it leaves no visible scar and is less painful. The disadvantage is that it is more difficult for the surgeon to see the uterus and surrounding tissue. This makes complications more common. Large fibroids cannot be removed using this technique. It is very difficult to remove the ovaries during a vaginal hysterectomy, so this approach may not be possible if the ovaries are involved.

Vaginal hysterectomy can also be performed using a laparoscopic technique. With this surgery, a tube containing a tiny camera is inserted through an incision in the navel. This allows the surgeon to see the uterus on a video monitor. The surgeon then inserts two slender instruments through small incisions in the abdomen and uses them to cut and tie off the blood vessels, fallopian tubes, and ligaments. When the uterus is detached, it is removed though a small incision at the top of the vagina.

This technique, called laparoscopic-assisted vaginal hysterectomy, allows surgeons to perform a vaginal hysterectomy that might otherwise be too difficult. The hospital stay is usually only one day. Recovery time is about two weeks. The disadvantage is that this operation is relatively new and requires great skill by the surgeon.

Any vaginal hysterectomy may have to be converted to an abdominal hysterectomy during surgery if complications develop.

Diagnosis/Preparation

Before surgery the doctor will order blood and urine tests. The woman may also meet with the anesthesiologist to evaluate any special conditions that might affect the administration of anesthesia. On the evening before the operation, the woman should eat a light dinner and then have nothing to eat or drink after midnight.

Aftercare

After surgery, a woman will feel some degree of discomfort; this is generally greatest in abdominal hysterectomies because of the incision. Hospital stays vary from about two days (laparoscopic-assisted vaginal hysterectomy) to five or six days (abdominal hysterectomy with bilateral salpingo-oophorectomy). During the hospital stay, the doctor will probably order more blood tests.

Return to normal activities such as driving and working takes anywhere from two to eight weeks, again depending on the type of surgery. Some women have emotional changes following a hysterectomy. Women who have had their ovaries removed will probably start **hormone replacement therapy**.

Risks

Hysterectomy is a relatively safe operation, although like all major surgery it carries risks. These include unanticipated reaction to anesthesia, internal bleeding, **blood clots**, damage to other organs such as the bladder, and post-surgery infection.

Other complications sometimes reported after a hysterectomy include changes in sex drive, weight gain, **constipation**, and pelvic pain. Hot flashes and other symptoms of menopause can occur if the ovaries are removed. Women who have both ovaries removed and who do not take estrogen replacement therapy run an increased risk for heart disease and **osteoporosis** (a condition that causes bones to be brittle). Women with a history of psychological and emotional problems before the hysterectomy are likely to experience psychological difficulties after the operation.

As in all major surgery, the health of the patient affects the risk of the operation. Women who have chronic heart or lung diseases, diabetes, or iron-deficiency anemia may not be good candidates for this operation. Heavy **smoking**, **obesity**, use of steroid drugs, and use of illicit drugs add to the surgical risk.

Normal results

Although there is some concern that hysterectomies may be performed unnecessarily, there are many conditions for which the operation improves a woman's quality of life. In the Maine Woman's Health Study, 71% of women who had hysterectomies to correct moderate or severe painful symptoms reported feeling better mentally, physically, and sexually after the operation.

Morbidity and mortality rates

The rate of complications differs by the type of hysterectomy performed. Abdominal hysterectomy is associated with a higher rate of complications (9.3%), while the overall complication rate for vaginal hysterectomy is 5.3%, and 3.6% for laparoscopic vaginal hysterectomy. The risk of **death** from hysterectomy is about one in every 1,000 women. The rates of some of the more commonly reported complications are:

- excessive bleeding (hemorrhaging): 1.8–3.4%
- fever or infection: 0.8–4.0%
- accidental injury to another organ or structure: 1.5–1.8%

Alternatives

Women for whom a hysterectomy is recommended should discuss possible alternatives with their doctor and consider getting a second opinion, since this is major surgery with life-changing implications. Whether an alternative is appropriate for any individual woman is a decision she and her doctor should make together. Some alternative procedures to hysterectomy include:

- Embolization. During uterine artery embolization, interventional radiologists put a catheter into the artery that leads to the uterus and inject polyvinyl alcohol particles right where the artery leads to the blood vessels that nourish the fibroids. By killing off those blood vessels, the fibroids have no more blood supply, and they die off. Severe cramping and pain after the procedure is common, but serious complications are less than 5% and the procedure may protect fertility.
- Myomectomy. A myomectomy is a surgery used to remove fibroids, thus avoiding a hysterectomy. Hysteroscopic myomectomy, in which a surgical hysteroscope (telescope) is inserted into the uterus through the vagina, can be done on an outpatient basis. If there are large fibroids, however, an abdominal incision is required. Patients typically are hospitalized for two to three days after the procedure and require up to six weeks recovery. Laparoscopic myomectomies are also being done more often. They only require three small incisions in the abdomen and have much shorter hospitalization and recovery times. Once the fibroids have been removed, the surgeon must repair the wall of the uterus to eliminate future bleeding or infection.
- Endometrial ablation. In this surgical procedure, recommended for women with small fibroids, the entire lining of the uterus is removed. After undergoing endometrial ablation, patients are no longer fertile. The uterine cavity is filled with fluid and a hysteroscope is inserted to provide a clear view of the uterus. Then, the lining of the uterus is destroyed using a laser beam or electric voltage. The procedure is typically done under anesthesia, although women can go home the same day as the surgery. Another newer procedure involves using a balloon, which is filled with superheated liquid and inflated until it fills the uterus. The liquid kills the lining, and after eight minutes the balloon is removed.
- Endometrial resection. The uterine lining is destroyed during this procedure using an electrosurgical wire loop (similar to endometrial ablation).

Resources

BOOKS

Katz, V. L., et al. *Comprehensive Gynecology*. 5th ed. St. Louis: Mosby, 2007.

Khatri, Vijay P., and J. A. Asensio. *Operative Surgery Manual*. Philadelphia: Saunders, 2002.

Townsend, Courtney M., et al. *Sabiston Textbook of Surgery*. 18th ed. Philadelphia: Saunders, 2007.

PERIODICALS

"Hysterectomy." Medline Plus, February 19, 2009. http://www.nlm.nih.gov/medlineplus/ency/article/002915.htm

"Hysterectomy (abdominal): Discharge." Medline Plus, February 18, 2009. http://www.nlm.nih.gov/medlineplus/ency/patientinstructions/000275.htm

ORGANIZATIONS

American Cancer Society, 1599 Clifton Road NE, Atlanta, GA, 30329-4251, (800) 227-2345, http://www.cancer.org.

American College of Obstetricians and Gynecologists, 409 Twelfth Street SW, P.O. Box 96920, Washington, DC, 20090-6920, (202) 638-5577, http://www.acog.org.

National Cancer Institute, Building 31, Room 10A31, 31 Center Drive, MSC 2580, Bethesda, MD, 20892-2580, (800) 422-6237, http://www.nci.nih.gov.

Debra Gordon
Stephanie Dionne Sherk
brenda w. lerner

Hysteria

Definition

The term "hysteria" has been in use for more than 2,000 years, and its definition has become broader and more diffuse over time. In modern psychology and psychiatry, hysteria is a feature of hysterical disorders in which a patient experiences physical symptoms that have a psychological, rather than an organic, cause. It

JEAN MARTIN CHARCOT (1825–1893)

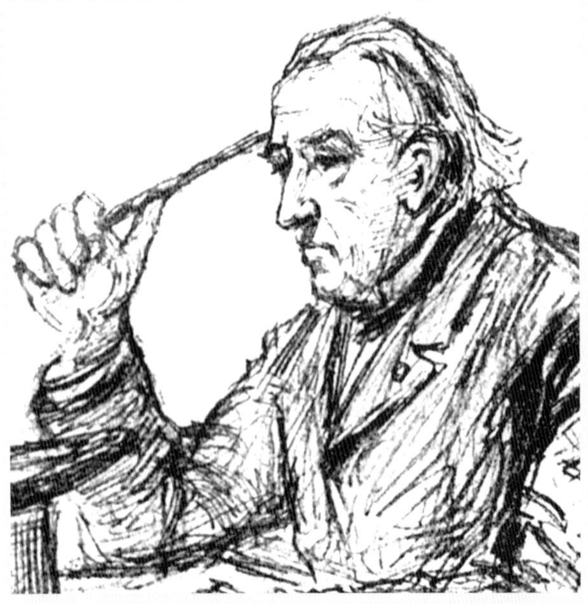

(The Library of Congress.)

Jean Martin Charcot was born to a carriage maker on November 29, 1825, in Paris, France. Charcot attended the University of Paris, earning his medical degree in 1853. In 1860, he accepted a position at the university as a professor of pathological anatomy until 1862, when he was named senior physician at the Salpêtrière, a hospital for the treatment of mental illness.

Charcot's research and work on psychoneuroses and hysterical disorders untimately helped to dispell the belief that hysteria was a disorder found only in women. Charcot also explored the possibility that physiological abnormalities of the nervous system played a part when behavioral problems were exhibited. He became known for his ability to diagnose and locate these abnormalities of the central nervous system. Finally, Charcot's most notable contribution to the field of psychiatry was his successful use of hypnotism in the diagnosis and treatment of hysteria. He found that, while hypnotized, the patient recalled details, which were not readily available to the individual in a conscious state. In addition, Charcot found that the therapist could more easily influence the hypnotized patient during therapy. In 1882, Charcot presented his research findings to the French Academy of Sciences with favorable results.

Charcot was a prolific writer and a talented artist. Between 1888 and 1894, his complete works were compiled into nine volumes. His most noted work *Lectures on the Diseases of the Nervous System* was published in 1877. Charcot died on August 16, 1893.

is defined as an histrionic personality disorder characterized by excessive emotions, dramatics, and attention–seeking behavior.

Description

Hysterical disorders

Patients with hysterical disorders, such as conversion and somatization disorder experience physical symptoms that have no organic cause. Conversion disorder affects motor and sensory functions, while somatization affects the gastrointestinal, nervous, cardiopulmonary, or reproductive systems. These patients are not "faking" their ailments, as the symptoms are very real to them. Disorders with hysteric features typically begin in adolescence or early adulthood.

Histrionic personality disorder

Histrionic personality disorder has a prevalence of approximately 2-3 percent in the general population. It begins in early adulthood and has been diagnosed more frequently in women than in men. Histrionic personalities are typically self–centered and attention seeking. They operate on emotion, rather than fact or logic, and their conversation is full of generalizations and dramatic appeals. While the patient's enthusiasm, flirtatious behavior, and trusting nature may make them appear charming, their need for immediate gratification, mercurial displays of emotion, and constant demand for attention often alienates them from others.

Causes and symptoms

Hysterical disorders

Hysteria may be a defense mechanism to avoid painful emotions by unconsciously transferring this distress to the body. There may be a symbolic function for this behavior. For example a **rape** victim may develop paralyzed legs. Symptoms may mimic a number of physical and neurological disorders which must be ruled out before a diagnosis of hysteria is made.

Histrionic personality disorder

According to the *Diagnostic and Statistical Manual of Mental Disorders,* Fourth Edition (*DSM–IV*),

KEY TERMS

Psychiatrist—A medical doctor who has completed specialized training in the diagnosis and treatment of mental illness. Psychiatrists can diagnose mental illnesses, provide mental health counseling, and prescribe medications.

Psychologist—A mental health professional who treats mental and behavioral disorders by support and insight to encourage healthy behavior patterns and personality growth. Psychologists also study the brain, behavior, emotions, and learning.

Psychotherapy—The treatment of mental and behavioral disorders by support and insight to encourage healthy behavior patterns and personality growth.

individuals with histrionic personality possess at least five of the following symptoms or personality features:

- a need to be the center of attention
- inappropriate, sexually seductive, or provocative behavior while interacting with others
- rapidly changing emotions and superficial expression of emotions
- vague and impressionistic speech (gives opinions without any supporting details)
- easily influenced by others
- believes relationships are more intimate than they are

Diagnosis

Hysterical disorders frequently prove to be actual medical or neurological disorders, which makes it important to rule these disorders out before diagnosing a patient with hysterical disorders. In addition to a patient interview, several clinical inventories may be used to assess the patient for hysterical tendencies, such as the Minnesota Multiphasic Personality Inventory–2 (MMPI–2) or the Millon Clinical Multiaxial Inventory–III (MCMI–III). These tests may be administered in an outpatient or hospital setting by a psychiatrist or psychologist.

Treatment

Hysterical disorders

For people with hysterical disorders, a supportive healthcare environment is critical. Regular appointments with a physician who acknowledges the patient's physical discomfort are important. **Psychotherapy** may be attempted to help the patient gain insight into the cause of their distress. Use of behavioral therapy can help to avoid reinforcing symptoms.

Histrionic personality disorder

Psychotherapy is generally the treatment of choice for histrionic personality disorder. It focuses on supporting the patient and on helping develop the skills needed to create meaningful relationships with others.

Prognosis

Hysterical disorders

The outcome for hysterical disorders varies by type. Somatization is typically a lifelong disorder, while conversion disorder may last for months or years. Symptoms of hysterical disorders may suddenly disappear, only to reappear in another form later.

Histrionic personality disorder

Individuals with histrionic personality disorder may be at a higher risk for suicidal gestures, attempts, or threats in an effort to gain attention. Providing a supportive environment for patients with both hysterical disorders and histrionic personality disorder is key to helping these patients.

Resources

BOOKS

Borch–Jacobsen, Mikkel. *Making Minds and Madness: From Hysteria to Depression*. New York, NY: Cambridge University Press, 2009.

Graham, George. *The Disordered Mind: An Introduction to Philosophy of Mind and Mental Illness*. New York, NY: Routledge, 2010.

North, Carol, and Sean Yutzy. *Goodwin and Guze's Psychiatric Diagnosis*. New York, NY: Oxford University Press, 2010.

Shams, K. *Human Relation and Personified Relational Disorders*. Raleigh, NC: lulu.com, 2009.

ORGANIZATIONS

American Academy of Child and AdolescentPsychiatry, 3615 Wisconsin Ave., NW, Washington, DC, 20016–3007, (202) 966–7300, http://www.aacap.org .

American Psychiatric Association, 1000 Wilson Blvd., Suite 1825, Arlington, VA, 22209, (703) 907–7300, apa@psych.org, http://www.psych.org/.

National Alliance on Mental Illness (NAMI), 3803 N. Fairfax Dr., Suite 100, Arlington, VA, 22201, (703) 524–7600, (800) 950–NAMI (6264), (703) 524–9094, http://www.nami.org/Hometemplate.cfm.

National Institute of Mental Health (NIMH), 6001 Executive Blvd., Room 8184, MSC 9663, Bethesda, MD, 20892, (301) 443–4513, (866) 615–6464, (301) 443–4279, nimhinfo@nih.gov, http://www.nimh.nih.gov/index.shtml.

National Mental Health Association (NMHA), 2000 N. Beauregard St., 6th floor, Alexandria, VA, 22311, (703) 684–7722, (800) 969–NMHA, (703) 684–5968, http://www1.nmha.org/.

Paula Anne Martin–Ford
Laura Jean Cataldo, RN, Ed.D.

Hysterosalpingography

Definition

Hysterosalpingography is a procedure where x rays are taken of a woman's reproductive tract after a dye is injected. *Hystero* means uterus and *salpingo* means tubes, so hysterosalpingography literally means to take pictures of the uterus and fallopian tubes. This procedure may also be called hysterography (or HSG).

Purpose

Hysterosalpingography is used to determine if the fallopian tubes are open, or if there are any apparent abnormalities or defects in the uterus. It can be used to detect tumors, scar tissue, or tears in the lining of the uterus. This procedure is often used to help diagnose **infertility** in women. The fallopian tubes are the location where an egg from the ovary joins with sperm to produce a fertilized ovum. If the fallopian tubes are blocked or deformed, the egg may not be able to descend or the sperm may be blocked from moving up to meet the egg. Up to 30% of all cases of infertility are due to damaged or blocked fallopian tubes.

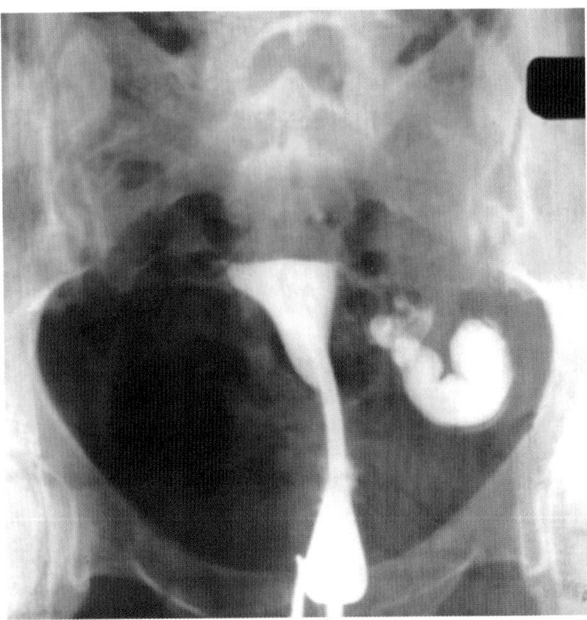

A hysterosalpingogram of the abdomen of a woman whose fallopian tubes are blocked. The fallopian tube (right on image) is blocked near the uterus, the triangular shape at center. The other fallopian tube is obstructed at a point further from the uterus where dilatation has occurred. *(Photo Researchers, Inc.)*

Precautions

This procedure should not be done on women who suspect they might be pregnant or who may have a pelvic infection. Women who have had an allergic reaction to dye used in previous x-ray procedures should inform their doctor.

Description

As with other types of pelvic examinations, the woman will lie on her back on an examination table with her legs sometimes raised in stirrups. The x ray equipment is placed above the abdomen.

A speculum is inserted into the vagina and a catheter (a thin tube) is inserted into the uterus through the cervix (the opening to the uterus). A small balloon in the catheter is inflated to hold it in place. A liquid water-based or oil-based dye is then injected through the catheter into the uterus. This process can cause cramping, **pain**, and uterine spasms.

As the dye spreads through the reproductive tract, the doctor may watch for blockages or abnormalities on an x ray monitor. Several x rays will also be taken. The procedure takes approximately 15–30 minutes. The x rays will be developed while the patient waits, but the final reading and interpretation of the x rays by a radiologist (a doctor who specializes in x rays) may not be available for a few days.

Interestingly, sometimes the hysterosalpingography procedure itself can be considered a treatment. The dye used can sometimes open up small blockages in the fallopian tubes. The need for additional test procedures or surgical treatments to deal with infertility should be discussed with the doctor.

Preparation

This procedure is generally done in the x-ray department of a hospital or large clinic. **General anesthesia** is not needed. A pain reliever may be taken prior to the procedure to lessen the severity of cramping.

Aftercare

While no special aftercare is required after a hysterosalpingography, the woman may be observed for some period after the procedure to ensure that she does not have any allergic reactions to the dye. A sanitary napkin may be worn after the procedure to absorb dye that will flow out through the vaginal opening. If a blockage is seen in a tube, the patient may be given an antibiotic. A woman should notify her doctor if she experiences excessive bleeding, extensive pelvic pain, **fever**, or an unpleasant vaginal odor after the procedure. These symptoms may indicate a pelvic infection. Counseling may be necessary to interpret the results of the x rays, and to discuss any additional procedures to treat tubal blockages or uterine abnormalities found.

Risks

Cramps during the procedure are common. Complications associated with hysterosalpingography include abdominal pain, pelvic infection, and allergic reactions. It is also possible that abnormalities of the fallopian tubes and uterus will not be detected by this procedure.

Normal results

A normal hysterosalpingography will show a healthy, normally shaped uterus and unblocked fallopian tubes.

Abnormal results

Blockage of one or both of the fallopian tubes or abnormalities of the uterus may be detected.

ORGANIZATIONS

American Society for Reproductive Medicine, 1209 Montgomery Highway, Birmingham, AL, 35216-2809, (205) 978-5000, (205) 978-5005, asrm@asrm.org, http://www.asrm.org.

Altha Roberts Edgren

Hysteroscopy

Definition

Hysteroscopy is a procedure that allows a physician to look through the vagina and neck of the uterus (cervix) to inspect the cavity of the uterus. A telescope-like instrument called a hysteroscope is used. Hysteroscopy is used as both a diagnostic and a treatment tool.

Purpose

Diagnostic hysteroscopy may be used to evaluate the cause of **infertility**, to determine the cause of repeated miscarriages, or to help locate polyps and fibroids.

The procedure is also used to treat gynecological conditions, often instead of or in addition to **dilatation and curettage** (D&C). A D&C is a procedure for scraping the lining of the uterus. A D&C can be used to take a sample of the lining of the uterus for analysis. Hysteroscopy is an advance over D&C because the doctor can take tissue samples of specific areas or actually see fibroids, polyps, or structural abnormalities.

When used for treatment, the hysteroscope is used with other devices to remove polyps, fibroids, or IUDs that have become embedded in the wall of the uterus.

Precautions

The procedure is not performed on women with **cervical cancer**, **endometrial cancer**, or acute pelvic inflammation.

Description

Diagnostic hysteroscopy is performed in either a doctor's office or hospital. Before inserting the hysteroscope, the doctor injects a local anesthetic around the cervix. Once it has taken effect, the doctor dilates the cervix and then inserts a narrow lighted tube (the hysteroscope) through the cervix to reveal the inside of the uterus. Ordinarily, the walls of the uterus are touching each other. In order to get a better view, the uterus is inflated with carbon dioxide gas or fluid. Hysteroscopy takes about 30 minutes, and can cost anywhere from $750 to $4,000 depending on the extent of the procedure.

Treatment involving the use of hysteroscopy is usually performed as a day surgical procedure with regional or **general anesthesia**. Tiny surgical instruments are inserted through the hysteroscope, and are used to remove polyps or fibroids. A small sample of tissue lining the uterus is often removed for examination, especially if there is any abnormal bleeding.

Preparation

If the procedure is done in the doctor's office, the patient will be given a mild **pain** reliever before the procedure to ease cramping. The doctor will wash the vagina and cervix with an antiseptic solution.

If the procedure is done in the hospital under general anesthesia, the patient should not eat or drink

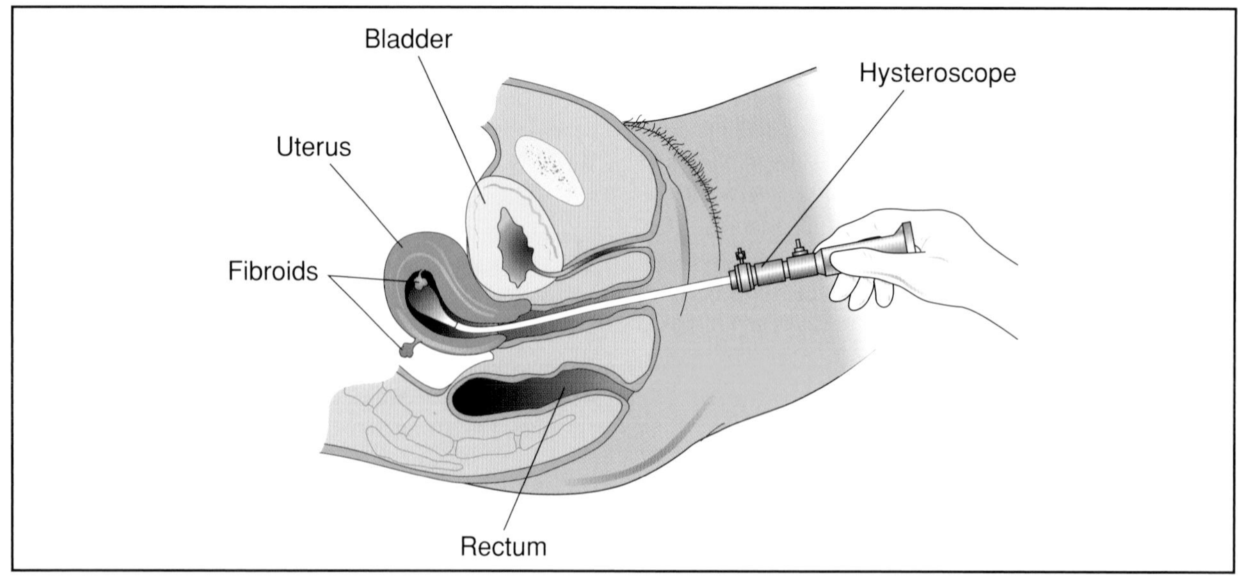

Hysteroscopy is a procedure that allows inspection of the uterus by using a telescope-like instrument called a hysteroscope. *(Illustration by Electronic Illustrators Group. Reproduced by permission of Gale, a part of Cengage Learning.)*

anything (even water) after midnight the night before the procedure.

Aftercare

Many women experience light bleeding for several days after surgical hysteroscopy. Mild cramping or pain is common after operative hysteroscopy, but usually fades away within eight hours. If carbon dioxide gas was used, there may also be some shoulder pain. Nonprescription pain relievers may help ease discomfort. Women may want to take the day off and relax after having hysteroscopy.

Risks

Diagnostic hysteroscopy is a fairly safe procedure that only rarely causes complications. The primary risk is prolonged bleeding or infection, usually following surgical hysteroscopy to remove a growth.

Very rare complications include perforation of the uterus, bowel, or bladder. Surgery under general anesthesia causes the additional risks typically associated with anesthesia.

Patients should alert their health care provider if they develop any of these symptoms:

- abnormal discharge
- heavy bleeding
- fever over 101°F (38.3°C)
- severe lower abdominal pain

Normal results

A uterus with no fibroids or other growths would be considered normal and healthy.

Abnormal results

Using hysteroscopy, the doctor may find **uterine fibroids** or polyps (often the cause of abnormal bleeding) or a septum (extra fold of tissue down the center of the uterus) that can cause infertility. Sometimes, precancerous or malignant growths are discovered.

Resources

PERIODICALS

Anon. "Looking Inside the Uterus." *Harvard Women's Health Watch* 4, no. 5 (January 1997): 4-5.

Carol A. Turkington

Hysterosonography

Definition

Hysterosonography, which is also called sonohysterography, is a new noninvasive technique that involves the slow infusion of sterile saline solution into a woman's uterus during ultrasound imaging. Hysterosonography allows the doctor to evaluate abnormal growths inside the uterus; abnormalities of the tissue lining the uterus (the endometrium); or disorders affecting deeper tissue layers. Hysterosonography does not require either radiation or contrast media, or invasive surgical procedures

Purpose

Hysterosonography is used to evaluate patients in the following groups:

- peri- or postmenopausal women with unexplained vaginal bleeding
- women whose endometrium appears abnormal during baseline ultrasound imaging
- women with fertility problems. Infertility is sometimes related to polyps, leiomyomas (fibroids), or adhesions inside the uterus. Adhesions are areas of tissue that have grown together to form bands or membranes across the inside of the uterus.
- women receiving tamoxifen therapy for breast cancer

Hysterosonography is useful as a screening test to minimize the use of more invasive diagnostic procedures, such as tissue biopsies and dilatation and curettage (D&C). Hysterosonography can also be used as a follow-up after uterine surgery to evaluate its success.

Precautions

Hysterosonography is difficult to perform in patients with certain abnormalities, including:

- Cervical stenosis. Cervical stenosis means that the lower end of the uterus is narrowed or tightened. It complicates the insertion of a tube (catheter).
- Adhesions or large fibroids. These growths sometimes block the flow of saline fluid into the uterus.

Patients with active **pelvic inflammatory disease** (PID) should not be tested with hysterosonography until the disease is brought under control. Women with chronic PID or heart problems are given **antibiotics** before the procedure.

Description

A hysterosonography is preceded by a baseline ultrasound examination performed through the vagina. This allows the doctor to detect an unsuspected **pregnancy** and to assess the thickness and possible abnormalities of the patient's endometrium. The doctor then inserts a catheter into the uterus and injects sterile saline fluid while ultrasound imaging is recorded on film or videotape. The procedure takes about 10 to 15 minutes.

Preparation

Patients do not require special preparation apart from the timing of the procedure. Patients with fertility problems are examined during the first 10 days of the menstrual cycle. Patients who may have polyps are usually examined at a later phase in the cycle. The best time for examining women with fibroids is still under discussion.

Aftercare

Aftercare consists of advising the patient to contact her doctor in case of abnormal bleeding, **fever**, or abdominal **pain**. Some spotting or cramping is common, however, and can usually be treated with **nonsteroidal anti-inflammatory drugs**, such as ibuprofen.

Risks

The chief risks are mild spotting and cramping after the procedure.

Normal results

Normal findings include a symmetrical uterus with a normal endometrium and no visible masses or tumors.

Abnormal results

Abnormal findings include **adhesions**; polyps; leiomyomas; abnormal thickening of the endometrium; or tissue changes related to tamoxifen (Nolvadex), which is a drug given for **breast cancer**.

Resources

PERIODICALS

Cullinan, Joanne, et al. "Sonohysterography: A Technique for Endometrial Evaluation." *RadioGraphics* 15 (May 1995): 501-514.

Rebecca J. Frey, PhD

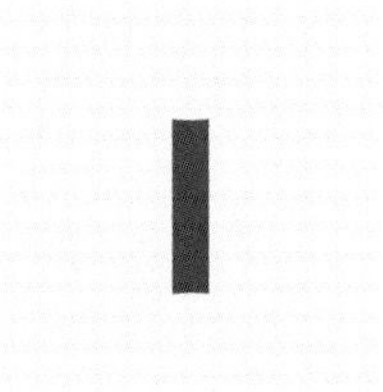

IBS *see* **Irritable bowel syndrome**

Ibuprophen *see* **Nonsteroidal anti-inflammatory drugs**

Ichthyosis

Definition

Derived from two Greek words meaning "fish" and "disease," ichthyosis is a congenital (meaning present at birth) dermatological (skin) disease that is represented by thick, scaly skin.

Description

The ichthyoses are a group of skin diseases caused by an abnormality in skin growth that results in drying and scaling. There are at least 20 types of ichthyosis. Ichthyosis can be more or less severe, sometimes accumulating thick scales and cracks that are painful and bloody. Ichthyosis is not contagious. Some forms of ichthyosis are inherited while others are acquired in later life as a symptom of systemic disorders.

The most common form of ichthyosis, accounting for 95% of all cases of ichthyosis, is called ichthyosis vulgaris (*vulgaris* is the Latin word for "common"), and occurs in approximately one person in every 250. It is inherited in an autosomal dominant manner. The most rare types of ichthyosis occur in fewer than one person in one million and are inherited in an autosomal recessive manner. Ichthyosis occurs regardless of the part of the world the child is from, or the ethnic background of the parents.

Acquired ichthyosis is extremely rare; neither its incidence in the United States nor its incidence in the rest of the world are known.

Both inherited and acquired ichthyoses affect males and females equally.

Causes and symptoms

Inherited ichthyoses

Depending on the specific type of ichthyosis, the inheritance can be autosomal recessive, autosomal dominant, X-linked recessive, X-linked dominant, or sporadic. Autosomal recessive means that the altered gene for the disease or trait is located on one of the first 22 pairs of chromosomes, which are also called "autosomes." Males and females are equally likely to have an autosomal recessive disease or trait. Recessive means that two copies of the altered gene are necessary to express the condition. Therefore, a child inherits one copy of the altered gene from each parent, who are called carriers (because they have only one copy of the altered gene). Since carriers do not express the altered gene, parents usually do not know they carry the altered gene that causes ichthyosis until they have an affected child. Carrier parents have a 1-in-4 chance (or 25%) with each **pregnancy**, to have a child with ichthyosis.

Autosomal dominant inheritance also means that both males and females are equally likely to have the disease but only one copy of the altered gene is necessary to have the condition. An individual with ichthyosis has a 50/50 chance to pass the condition to his or her child.

The skin is made up of several layers, supported underneath by a layer of fat that is thicker or thinner depending on location. The lower layers contain blood vessels, the middle layers contain actively growing cells, and the upper layer consists of dead cells that serve as a barrier to the outside world. This barrier is nearly waterproof and highly resistant to infection. Scattered throughout the middle layers are hair follicles, oil and sweat glands, and nerve endings. The upper layer is constantly flaking off and being replaced from beneath by new tissue. In ichthyosis, the skin's natural shedding process is slowed or inhibited; and in some types, skin cells are produced too rapidly.

The abnormality in skin growth and hydration called ichthyosis may present with symptoms at birth or in early childhood. Ichthyosis can itch relentlessly, leading to such complications of scratching as lichen simplex (**dermatitis** characterized by raw patches of skin). Either the cracking or the scratching can introduce infection, bringing with it discomfort and complications.

Acquired ichthyoses

The mildest form of acquired ichthyosis is called xeroderma, or dry flaky skin. It is not associated with any systemic diseases. Xeroderma occurs most often on the lower legs of middle-aged and elderly adults during cold weather, or on the lower legs of people who bathe too often. It is characterized chiefly by mild or moderate **itching**.

Ichthyosis may also be an early symptom of such disorders as **AIDS**, lymphoma, **hypothyroidism**, or **leprosy**. In these cases the ichthyosis is most noticeable on the patient's trunk and legs.

A few rare cases of acquired ichthyosis have been attributed to the use of certain drugs, specifically cimetidine (Tagamet), triparanol (Metasqualene), dixyrazine (a phenothiazine derivative used as an antipsychotic), nicotinic acid (vitamin B_3, butyrophenone antipsychotics (Haldol, Inapsine, Orap), and clofazimine (Lamprene).

Diagnosis

A dermatologist will often make the diagnosis of ichthyosis based on findings from a clinical examination. However, a **skin biopsy**, or DNA study (from a small blood sample) is necessary to confirm the diagnosis. Evaluation for associated problems is done by a complete physical medical examination.

For some types of ichythyosis, the abnormal gene has been identified and prenatal testing is available. At present this is true for the autosomal recessive congenital ichythoses, which include: lamellar ichthyosis (LI), autosomal recessive lamellar ichthyosis (ARLI), congenital ichthyosiform erythroderma (CIE), and nonbullous congenital ichthyosiform erythroderma (NBCIE).

There are four different genes that have been located for the autosomal recessive congenital ichthyoses. Testing, however, is available for only one gene, known as transglutaminase-1 (TGM1). This gene is located on chromosome 14. Once a couple has had a child with ichthyosis, and they have had the genetic cause identified by DNA studies (performed from a small blood sample), prenatal testing for future pregnancies may be considered. (Note that prenatal testing may not be possible if both mutations cannot be identified.) Prenatal diagnosis is available via either **chorionic villus sampling** (CVS) or **amniocentesis**. CVS is a biopsy of the placenta performed in the first trimester of pregnancy under ultrasound guidance. Ultrasound is the use of sound waves to visualize the developing fetus. The genetic makeup of the placenta is identical to the fetus and therefore the TGM1 gene can be studied from this tissue. There is approximately a one in 100 chance for **miscarriage** with CVS. Amniocentesis is a procedure done under ultrasound guidance in which a long thin needle is inserted through the mother's abdomen into the uterus, to withdraw a couple of tablespoons of amniotic fluid (fluid surrounding the developing baby) to study. The TGM1 gene can be studied using cells from the amniotic fluid. Other genetic tests, such as a chromosome analysis, may also be performed through either CVS or amniocentesis.

Acquired ichthyosis is usually diagnosed in the course of identifying the underlying disorder. With the exception of acquired ichthyosis related to lymphoma, a doctor cannot tell the difference between inherited and acquired ichthyosis by examining skin samples through a microscope.

Treatment

Most treatments for ichthyosis are topical, which means that they are applied directly to the skin, not taken internally. Xeroderma is eaily treated by minimizing bathing and applying an emollient cream or mineral oil after bathing while the skin is still moist. Some forms of ichthyosis require two forms of treatment—a reduction in the amount of scale buildup and moisturizing of the underlying skin. Several agents are available for each purpose. Reduction in the amount of scale is achieved by keratolytics. Among this class of drugs are urea, lactic acid, and salicylic acid. Petrolatum, 60% propylene glycol, and glycerin are successful moisturizing agents, as are many commercially available products. Increased humidity of the ambient air is also helpful in preventing skin dryness.

Because the skin acts as a barrier to the outside environment, medicines have a hard time penetrating, especially through the thick skin of the palms of the hands and the soles of the feet. This resistance is diminished greatly by maceration (softening the skin). Soaking hands in water macerates skin so that

KEY TERMS

Amniocentesis—A procedure performed at 16–18 weeks of pregnancy in which a needle is inserted through a woman's abdomen into her uterus to draw out a small sample of the amniotic fluid from around the baby. Either the fluid itself or cells from the fluid can be used for a variety of tests to obtain information about genetic disorders and other medical conditions in the fetus.

Amniotic fluid—The fluid that surrounds a developing baby during pregnancy.

Autosomal dominant—A pattern of genetic inheritance where only one abnormal gene is needed to display the trait or disease.

Autosomal recessive inheritance—A pattern of genetic inheritance where two abnormal genes are needed to display the trait or disease.

Dermatologist—A physician who specializes in diagnosing and treating disorders of the skin.

Emollients—Petroleum or lanolin-based skin lubricants.

Keratin—A tough, nonwater-soluble protein found in the nails, hair, and the outermost layer of skin. Human hair is made up largely of keratin.

Keratinocytes—Skin cells.

Keratolytic—An agent that dissolves or breaks down the outer layer of skin (keratins).

Retinoids—A derivative of synthetic Vitamin A.

Sporadic—Isolated or appearing occasionally with no apparent pattern.

X-linked dominant inheritance—The inheritance of a trait by the presence of a single gene on the X chromosome in a male or female, passed from an affected female who has the gene on one of her X chromosomes.

X-linked recessive inheritance—The inheritance of a trait by the presence of a single gene on the X chromosome in a male, passed from a female who has the gene on one of her X chromosomes, and who is referred to as an unaffected carrier.

it looks like prune skin. Occlusion (covering) with rubber gloves or plastic wrap will also macerate skin. Applying medicines and then covering the skin with an occlusive dressing will facilitate entrance of the medicine and greatly magnify its effect.

Secondary treatments are necessary to control pruritus (itching) and infection. Commercial products containing camphor, menthol, eucalyptus oil, aloe, and similar substances are very effective as antipruritics. If the skin cracks deeply enough, a pathway for infection is created. **Topical antibiotics** like bacitracin are effective in prevention and in the early stages of these skin infections. Cleansing with hydrogen peroxide inhibits infection as well.

Finally, there are topical and internal derivatives of vitamin A called retinoids that improve skin growth and are used for severe cases of **acne**, ichthyosis, and other skin conditions. Tazarotene (Tazorac), a retinoid that was originally developed to treat **psoriasis** and acne, appears to give good results in treating ichthyosis with fewer side effects than other retinoids.

Prognosis

This condition requires continuous care throughout a lifetime. Properly treated, in most cases it is a cosmetic problem. There are a small number of lethal forms, such as harlequin fetus.

Resources

BOOKS

Beers, Mark H., Robert S. Porter, and Thomas V. Jones, eds. *The Merck Manual of Diagnosis and Therapy*. 18th ed. Whitehouse Station, NJ: Merck Research Laboratories, 2006.

PERIODICALS

Fleckman, P. "Management of the Ichthyoses." *Skin Therapy Letter* 8 (September 2003): 3–7.

Hatsell, S. J., H. Stevens, A. P. Jackson, et al. "An Autosomal Recessive Exfoliative Ichthyosis with Linkage to Chromosome 12q13." *British Journal of Dermatology* 149 (July 2003): 174–180.

Lefevre, C., S. Audebert, F. Jobard, et al. "Mutations in the Transporter ABCA12 Are Associated with Lamellar Ichthyosis Type 2." *Human Molecular Genetics* 12 (September 15, 2003): 2369–2378.

Marulli, G. C., E. Campione, M. S. Chimenti, et al. "Type I Lamellar Ichthyosis Improved by Tazarotene 0.1% Gel." *Clinical and Experimental Dermatology* 28 (July 2003): 391–393.

OTHER

Immune Deficiency Foundation Website. www.primaryimmune.org.

ORGANIZATIONS

Foundation for Ichthyosis and Related Skin Types (FIRST), 2616 North Broad Street, Colmar, PA, 18915, 215 997-9400, 215 997-9403, 800 545-3286, info@firstskinfoundation. org, http://www.firstskinfoundation.org/.

Genetic Alliance, Inc., 4301 Connecticut Ave., NW, Suite 404, Washington, DC, 20008-2369, 202 966-5557, 202 966-8553, info@geneticalliance.org, http://www.geneticalliance.org.

National Organization for Rare Disorders, P.O. Box 8923, New Fairfield, CT, 06812-8923, (800) 999-6673, http://www.rarediseases.org.

Catherine L. Tesla, MS, CGC
Rebecca J. Frey, PhD

Icterus *see* **Jaundice**

Idiopathic hypertrophic subaortic stenosis *see* **Hypertrophic cardiomyopathy**

Idiopathic infiltrative lung diseases

Definition

The term *idiopathic* means "cause unknown." The idiopathic infiltrative lung diseases, also known as interstitial lung diseases, are a group of more than a hundred disorders seen in both adults and (less often) in children, whose cause is unknown but which tend to spread, or "infiltrate" through much or all of the lung tissue. They range from mild conditions that respond well to treatment, to progressive, nonresponsive disease states that severely limit lung function and may cause **death**.

Description

The body produces inflammatory cells in response to a variety of conditions, including a number of different diseases, pollutants, certain infections, exposure to organic dust or toxic fumes and vapors, and various drugs and poisons. When white blood cells and tissue fluid rich in protein collect in the small air sacs of the lungs, or alveoli, the sacs become inflamed (alveolitis). In time, the fluid may solidify and cause scar formation that replaces the normal lung tissue. This process is known as **pulmonary fibrosis**. In about half of all patients, no specific cause is ever found; they are said to have idiopathic pulmonary fibrosis.

Some patients have special types of interstitial lung disease that may occur in certain types of patients, or feature typical pathological changes when a sample of lung tissue is examined under a microscope. They include:

- Usual interstitial pneumonitis. Disease occurs in a patchy form throughout the lungs. Parts of the lungs can appear normal while others have dense scar tissue and lung cysts, often the end result of pulmonary fibrosis. This disease progresses quite slowly. Both children and adults may be affected.
- Desquamative interstitial pneumonitis. Similar-appearing lesions are present throughout the lungs. Both inflammatory cells and cells that have separated from the air sac linings ("desquamated") are present. Some researchers believe this is an early form of usual interstitial pneumonitis.
- Lymphocytic interstitial pneumonitis. Most of the cells infiltrating the lungs are the type of white blood cells called lymphocytes. Both the breathing tubes (bronchi) and blood vessels of the lungs become thickened. In children, this condition tends to occur when the immune system is not operating properly as occurs with Acquired Immune Deficiency Syndrome (AIDS).

Causes and symptoms

By definition, the causes of *idiopathic* infiltrative lung diseases are not known. Some forms of pulmonary fibrosis, however, do have specific causes and these may provide a clue as to what may cause idiopathic diseases. Known causes of pulmonary fibrosis include diseases that impair the body's immune function; infection by viruses and the bacterium causing **tuberculosis**; and exposure to such mineral dusts as silica or asbestos, or such organic materials as bird droppings. Other cases of pulmonary fibrosis result from exposure to fumes and vapors, radiation (in industry or medically), and certain drugs used to treat disease.

Patients with interstitial lung disease usually have labored breathing when exerting themselves. Often they **cough** and feel overly tired ("no stamina"). **Wheezing** is uncommon. When the physician listens to the patient's chest with a stethoscope, dry, crackling sounds may be heard. Some patients have vague chest **pain**. When disease progresses, the patient may breathe very rapidly, have mottled blue skin (because of getting too little oxygen), and lose weight. The fingertips may appear thick or club-shaped.

Diagnosis

Both **scars** in the lung and cysts (air-filled spaces) can be seen on a **chest x ray**. Up to 10% of patients, however, may have normal x rays even if their symptoms

KEY TERMS

Bronchoalveolar lavage—A way of obtaining a sample of fluid from the airways by inserting a flexible tube through the windpipe. Used to diagnose the type of lung disease.

Desquamation—Shedding of the cells lining the insides of the air sacs. A feature of desquamative interstitial pneumonitis.

Idiopathic—A disease whose cause is unknown.

Immune system—A set of body chemicals and specialized cells that attack an invading agent (such as a virus) by forming antibodies that can engulf and destroy it.

Infiltrative—A process whereby inflammatory or other types of disease spread throughout an organ such as the lungs.

Interstitial—Refers to the connective tissue that supports the "working parts" of an organ, in the case of the lungs the air sacs.

Pulmonary fibrosis—A scarring process that is the end result of many forms of long-lasting lung disease.

are severe. A special type of x ray, high-resolution computed tomography scan (CT scan), often is helpful in adult patients. Tests of lung function will show that the lungs cannot hold enough air with each breath, and there is too little oxygen in the blood, especially after exercising. In a procedure called bronchoalveolar lavage, a tube is placed through the nose and windpipe into the bronchi and a small amount of saline is released and then withdrawn. This fluid can then be analyzed for cells. A tiny piece of lung tissue can be sampled using the same instrument. If necessary, a larger sample (a biopsy) is taken through an incision in the chest wall and examined under a microscope.

Treatment

The first medication given, providing scarring is not too extensive, is usually a steroid drug such as prednisone. An occasional patient will improve dramatically if steroid therapy stops the inflammation. Most patients, however, improve to a limited extent. It may take 6–12 weeks for a patient to begin to respond. Patients must be watched closely for a gain in body weight, high blood pressure, and depression. **Steroids** can also result in diabetes, ulcer disease, and cataract. Patients treated with steroids are at risk of contracting serious infection. If steroids have not proved effective or have caused serious side effects, other anti-inflammatory drugs, such as cyclophosphamide (Cytoxan) or azathioprine (Imuran), can be tried. Cytoxan sometimes is combined with a steroid, but it carries its own risks, which include bladder inflammation and suppression of the bone marrow. Some patients will benefit from a bronchodilator drug that relaxes the airway and makes breathing easier.

Some patients with interstitial lung disease, especially children, will need **oxygen therapy**. Usually oxygen is given during sleep or **exercise**, but if the blood oxygen level is very low it may be given constantly. A program of conditioning, training in how to breathe efficiently, energy-saving tips, and a proper diet will help patients achieve the highest possible level of function given the state of their illness. All patients should be vaccinated each year against **influenza**. A last resort for those with very advanced disease who do not respond to medication is **lung transplantation**. This operation is being done more widely, and it is even possible to replace both lungs.

Prognosis

A scoring system based on lung function and x ray appearances has been designed to help monitor a patient's course. In general, idiopathic forms of interstitial lung disease cause a good deal of illness, and a significant number of deaths. A majority of patients get worse over time, although survival for many years is certainly possible. An estimated one in five affected children fail to survive. In different series, survival times average between four and ten years. Early diagnosis gives the best chance of a patient recovering or at least stabilizing. Once the lungs are badly scarred, nothing short of lung transplantation offers hope of restoring lung function. Patients with desquamative interstitial pneumonitis tend to respond well to steroid treatment, and live longer than those with other types of infiltrative lung disease.

Prevention

Since we do not understand what causes idiopathic interstitial lung diseases, there is no way to prevent them. What can be done is to prevent extensive scarring of the lungs by making the diagnosis shortly after the first symptoms develop, and trying steroids or other drugs in hope of suppressing lung inflammation. Every effort should be made to avoid exposure to dusts, gases, chemicals, and even pets. Keeping fit and learning how to breathe efficiently will help maintain lung function as long as possible.

ORGANIZATIONS

American Lung Association, 1301 Pennsylvania Ave. NW, Suite 800, Washington, DC, 20001, 202 758-3355, 202 452-1805, 800 548-8252, info@lungusa.org, http://www.lungusa.org/.

David A. Cramer, MD

Idiopathic primary renal hematuric/proteinuric syndrome

Definition

This syndrome includes a group of disorders characterized by blood and protein in the urine and by damage to the kidney glomeruli (filtering structures) that may lead to kidney failure.

Description

This syndrome, also known as Berger's disease or IgA nephropathy, arises when internal kidney structures called glomeruli become inflamed and injured. It can occur at any age, but the great majority of patients are 16–35 when diagnosed. Males seem to be affected more often than females, and whites are more often affected than blacks. Blood in the urine (hematuria), either indicated by a visible change in the color of the urine or detected by laboratory testing, is a hallmark of this syndrome, and it may occur continuously or sporadically. The pattern of occurrence is not indicative of the severity of kidney damage.

Causes and symptoms

The glomeruli are the kidney structures that filter the blood and extract waste, which is then excreted as urine. The barrier between the blood and the urine side of the filter mechanism is a membrane only one cell layer thick. Anything that damages the membrane will result in hematuria. Symptoms of idiopathic primary renal hematruic/proteinuric syndrome are caused by inflammation of the glomeruli and deposit of IgA antibodies in kidney tissue. Although a genetic basis for this syndrome is suspected, this has not been proven. Symptoms often appear 24–48 hours after an upper respiratory or gastrointestinal infection. Symptoms of the syndrome include:

- blood in the urine (hematuria)
- protein in the urine (proteinuria)
- pain in the lower back or kidney area
- elevated blood pressure (20–30% of cases)
- nephrotic syndrome (less than 10% of cases)
- swelling (occasionally)

This condition usually does not get worse with time, although renal failure occasionally results. In patients with large amounts of IgA deposits in their glomeruli, the long-term prognosis may not be favorable. The syndrome can go into remission spontaneously, although this is more common in children than in adults.

Diagnosis

One of the objectives of diagnosis is to distinguish glomerular from non-glomerular kidney diseases. Idiopathic primary hematuric/proteinuric syndrome involves the glomeruli. The presence of fragmented or distorted red blood cells in the urine is evidence of glomerular disease. A high concentration of protein in the urine is also evidence for glomerular disease. The hematuria associated with this syndrome must be distinguished from that caused by urinary tract diseases, which can also cause a loss of blood into the urine. Biopsy of the patient's kidney shows deposits of IgA antibodies. Detecting IgA-antibody deposits rules out thin membrane disease as the cause of the hematuria and proteinuria. Test values are normal for ASO, complement, rheumatoid factor, antinuclear antibodies, anti-DNase, and cryoglobulins, all of which are associated with different types of **kidney disease**. A diagnosis of idiopathic primary renal hematuric/proteinuric syndrome is largely made by ruling out other diseases and their causes, leaving this syndrome as the remaining possible diagnosis.

Treatment

Many patients do not need specific treatment, except for those who have symptoms indicating a poor prognosis. Oral doses of **corticosteroids** are effective in patients with mild proteinuria and good kidney function. Other treatments, such as medications to lower blood pressure, are aimed at slowing or preventing kidney damage. If kidney failure develops, dialysis or **kidney transplantation** is necessary.

Prognosis

Idiopathic primary renal hematuric/proteinuric syndrome progresses slowly and in many cases does not progress at all. Risk for progression of the disorder is considered higher if there is:

KEY TERMS

Glomeruli (singular, glomerulus)—Filtering structures in the kidneys.

Hematuria—The presence of hemoglobin or red blood cells in the urine.

Idiopathic—Refers to a disease that arises from an obscure or unknown cause.

Nephrotic syndrome—A kidney disorder characterized by fluid retention (edema) and proteinuria. It is caused by damage to the kidney glomeruli.

Proteinuria—The presence of protein in the urine exceeding normal levels.

- high blood pressure
- large amounts of protein in the urine
- increased levels of urea and creatinine in the blood (indications of kidney function)

About 25–35% of patients may develop kidney failure within about 25 years.

Prevention

Since the underlying causes of this syndrome are so poorly understood, there is no known prevention.

Resources

BOOKS

Greenberg, Arthur, et al.*Primer on Kidney Diseases*. 5th ed. Philadelphia: Saunders/Elsevier, 2009.

ORGANIZATIONS

IgA Nephropathy Support Network, 89 Ashfield Road, Shelburne Falls, MA, 01370, 413 625-9339,.

National Kidney Foundation, Inc. , 30 East 33rd Street, New York, NY, 10016, 212 889-2210, 212 689-9261, 800 622-9010, http://www.kidney.org/.

John T. Lohr, PhD

Idiopathic thrombocytopenic purpura

Definition

Idiopathic thrombocytopenic purpura, or ITP, is a bleeding disorder caused by an abnormally low level of platelets in the patient's blood. Platelets are small plate-shaped bodies in the blood that combine to form a plug when a blood vessel is injured. The platelet plug then binds certain proteins in the blood to form a clot that stops bleeding. ITP's name describes its cause and two symptoms. Idiopathic means that the disorder has no apparent cause. ITP is now often called immune thrombocytopenic purpura rather than idiopathic because of recent findings that ITP patients have autoimmune antibodies in their blood. **Thrombocytopenia** is another word for a decreased number of blood platelets. Purpura refers to a purplish or reddish-brown skin rash caused by the leakage of blood from broken capillaries into the skin. Other names for ITP include purpura hemorrhagica and essential thrombocytopenia.

Demographics

ITP may be either acute or chronic. The acute form is most common in children between the ages of one and six years; the chronic form is most common in adult females between 30 and 40. ITP is uncommon in adults older than age 60. Between 10% and 20% of children with ITP have the chronic form. ITP does not appear to be related to race, lifestyle, climate, or environmental factors.

In the United States, annual incidence of ITP is difficult to determine because it is thought that most cases of ITP are so mild that medical attention is not needed. Estimates are that ITP affects 5 in every 100,000 children and 2 in every 100,000 adults in the U.S. every year.

Description

ITP is a disorder that affects the overall *number* of blood platelets rather than their function. The normal platelet level in adults is between 150,000 and 450,000/mm^3. Platelet counts below 50,000 mm^3 increase the risk of dangerous bleeding from trauma; counts below 20,000/mm^3 increase the risk of spontaneous bleeding.

Causes and Symptoms

In adults, ITP is considered an autoimmune disorder, which means that the body produces antibodies that damage some of its own products–in this case, blood platelets. Some adults with chronic ITP also have other immune system disorders, such as **systemic lupus erythematosus** (SLE) or acute or chronic leukemia. ITP is usually triggered by a viral infection such as infection with **rubella**, **chickenpox**, **measles**, cytomegalovirus, **Epstein-Barr virus**, or hepatitis virus

KEY TERMS

Autoimmune disorder—A disorder in which the patient's immune system produces antibodies that destroy some of the body's own products. ITP in adults is thought to be an autoimmune disorder.

Idiopathic—Of unknown cause. Idiopathic refers to a disease that is not preceded or caused by any known dysfunction or disorder in the body.

Petechiae—Small pinpoint hemorrhages in skin or mucous membranes caused by the rupture of capillaries.

Platelet—A blood component that helps to prevent blood from leaking from broken blood vessels. ITP is a bleeding disorder caused by an abnormally low level of platelets in the blood.

Prednisone—A corticosteroid medication that is used to treat ITP. Prednisone works by decreasing the effects of antibody on blood platelets. Long-term treatment with prednisone is thought to decrease antibody production.

Purpura—A skin discoloration of purplish or brownish red spots caused by bleeding from broken capillaries.

Splenectomy—Surgical removal of the spleen.

Thrombocytopenia—An abnormal decline in the number of platelets in the blood.

(A, B, C). It usually begins about two or three weeks after the infection. ITP may also occur as a result of infection with the human **immunodeficiency** virus (HIV). However, most commonly, ITP follows a viral upper respiratory infection or **gastroenteritis**.

Some medications are also linked to the development of ITP. These medications include:

- quinidine or quinine medications
- heparin
- antibiotics such as cephalosporin drugs and rifampicin
- analgesics
- diuretics
- antihypertensives

ITP is also associated with acute and chronic alcohol ingestion and is also seen in individuals with chronic **liver disease**.

In children, most cases of ITP are acute while in adults, most cases are chronic.

Acute ITP

Acute ITP is characterized by bleeding into the skin or from the nose, mouth, digestive tract, or urinary tract. The onset is usually sudden. Bleeding into the skin takes the form of purpura or petechiae. Purpura is a purplish or reddish-brown rash or discoloration of the skin; petechiae are small round pinpoint hemorrhages. Both are caused by the leakage of blood from tiny capillaries under the skin surface. In addition to purpura and petechiae, the patient may notice that he or she **bruises** more easily than usual. In extreme cases, patients with ITP may bleed into the lungs, brain, or other vital organs.

Chronic ITP

Chronic ITP has a gradual onset and may have minimal or no external symptoms. The low **platelet count** may be discovered in the course of a routine blood test. Most patients with chronic ITP, however, will consult their primary care doctor because of the purpuric skin rash, nosebleeds, or bleeding from the digestive or urinary tract. Women sometimes go to their gynecologist for unusually heavy or lengthy menstrual periods.

Diagnosis

ITP is usually considered a diagnosis of exclusion, which means that the doctor arrives at the diagnosis by a process of ruling out other possible causes. If the patient belongs to one or more of the risk groups for chronic ITP, the doctor may order a blood test for autoantibodies in the blood early in the diagnostic process.

Physical examination

If the doctor suspects ITP, he or she will examine the patient's skin for bruises, purpuric areas, or petechiae. If the patient has had nosebleeds or bleeding from the mouth or other parts of the body, the doctor will examine these areas for other possible causes of bleeding. Patients with ITP usually look and feel healthy except for the bleeding.

The most important features that the doctor will be looking for during the **physical examination** are the condition of the patient's spleen and the presence of **fever**. Patients with ITP do not have fever, whereas patients with lupus and some other types of thrombocytopenia are usually feverish. The doctor will have the patient lie flat on the examining table in order to feel the size of the spleen. If the spleen is noticeably enlarged, ITP is usually excluded as the diagnosis.

Laboratory testing

The doctor will order a **complete blood count** (CBC), a test of clotting time, a bone marrow test, and a test for antiplatelet antibodies if it is available in the hospital laboratory. Patients with ITP usually have platelet counts below 20,000/mm^3 and prolonged **bleeding time**. The size and appearance of the platelets may be abnormal. The red blood cell count (RBC) and **white blood cell count** (WBC) are usually normal, although about 10% of patients with ITP are also anemic. The blood marrow test yields normal results. Detection of antiplatelet antibodies in the blood is considered to confirm the diagnosis of ITP.

In most children, examination of the bone marrow is not required to diagnose acute ITP.

Treatment

General care and monitoring

There is no specific treatment for ITP. In most cases, the disorder will resolve without medications or surgery within two to six weeks. Nosebleeds can be treated with ice packs when necessary.

General care includes explaining ITP to the patient and advising him or her to watch for bruising, petechiae, or other signs of recurrence. Children should be discouraged from rough contact sports or other activities that increase the risk of trauma. Patients are also advised to avoid using **aspirin** or ibuprofen (Advil, Motrin) as **pain** relievers because these drugs lengthen the clotting time of blood.

Treatment with **corticosteroids** such as oral prednisone or IV methylprednisone are the initial drugs of choice for the treatment of ITP.

Emergency treatment

Patients with acute ITP who are losing large amounts of blood or bleeding into their central nervous system require emergency treatment. This includes transfusions of platelets, intravenous immunoglobulins, or treatment with corticosteroids such as methylprednisone. Prednisone is a steroid medication that decreases the effects of antibody on platelets and eventually lowers antibody production. If the patient has a history of ITP that has not responded to prednisone or immunoglobulins, the surgeon may remove the patient's spleen. This operation is called a **splenectomy**. The reason for removing the spleen when ITP does not respond to other forms of treatment is that the spleen sometimes keeps platelets out of the general blood circulation.

Medications and transfusions

Patients with chronic ITP can be treated with prednisone, immune globulin, or large doses of intravenous **gamma globulin**. Although 90% of patients respond to immunoglobulin treatment, it is very expensive. About 80% of patients respond to prednisone therapy. Platelet transfusions are not recommended for routine treatment of ITP. If the patient's platelet level does not improve within one to four months, or requires high doses of prednisone, the doctor may recommend splenectomy. All medications for ITP are given either orally or intravenously; intramuscular injection is avoided because of the possibility of causing bleeding into the skin.

Newer medications which may be used in the treatment of ITP include the monoclonal antibody rituximab (Rituxan) which can be combined with the corticosteroid dexamethasone to treat chronic ITP and thrombopoietin-receptor agonists romiplostim (Nplate) and eltrombopag (Promacta) which work by directly stimulating the bone marrow to increase platelet production.

Surgery

Between 80% and 85% of adults with ITP have a remission of the disorder after the spleen is removed. Splenectomy is usually avoided in children younger than five years because of the increased risk of a severe infection after the operation. In older children, however, splenectomy is recommended if the child has been treated for 12 months without improvement; if the ITP is very severe or the patient is getting worse; if the patient begins to bleed into the head or brain; and if the patient is an adolescent female with extremely heavy periods. Relapse of ITP is more common after splenectomy in patients with chronic ITP as compared to those with acute ITP.

Prognosis

The prognosis for recovery from acute ITP is good; 80% of patients recover without special treatment. The prognosis for chronic ITP is also good; most patients experience long-term remissions. In rare instances, however, ITP can cause life-threatening hemorrhage or bleeding into the central nervous system.

Prevention

In most individuals, ITP occurs as a manifestation of another disease or as a consequence of a viral infection. Therefore, at this time ITP cannot be entirely prevented.

Resources

PERIODICALS

Danese, M.D., Lindquist, K., Gleeson, M., Deuson, R., & Mikhael, J. "Cost and Mortality Associated with Hospitalizations in Patients with Immune Thrombocytopenic Purpera."*American Journal of Hematology* (Jul 16, 2009).

Fogarty, P.F. & Segal, J.B. "The Epidemiology of Thrombocytopenia Purpera."*Current Opinion in Hematology* (Sep 2007); 14(5):515–9.

Stasi, R., Evangelista, M.L., Stipa, E., et al. "Idiopathic Thrombocytopenia Purpura: Current Concepts in Pathophysiology and Management." *Journal of Thrombosis and Haemostasis* (Jan 2008); 99(1): 4–13.

OTHER

Sandler, S.G. & Bhanji, R. "Immune Thrombocytopenia Purpera."eMedicine. May 10, 2010 [cited July 24, 2010]. http://www.emedicine.medscape.com/article/202158

Rebecca J. Frey, PhD
Melinda Granger Oberleitner
RN, DNS APRN, CNS

IHSS *see* **Hypertrophic cardiomyopathy**

Ileal conduit *see* **Urinary diversion surgery**

Ileocol *see* **Crohn's disease**

Ileostomy *see* **Enterostomy**

Ileus

Definition

Ileus is a partial or complete non–mechanical blockage of the small and/or large intestine. When this blockage occurs the bowel becomes full of gases and fluids. Consequently, patients often report mild abdominal **pain** and bloating. They may also experience poor appetite, **nausea**, and, sometimes, **vomiting**. The term "ileus" comes from the Latin word for **colic**. Ileus is sometimes also called bowel obstruction, intestinal volvulus, colonic ileus, and other such terms.

Demographics

The blockage of the intestines from the condition called ileus can occur at any age. In infants and children, it is the major cause of bowel obstruction. In adults, abdominal surgery can often bring about ileus. It occurs throughout the human population, regardless of one's ethnic background or other factors.

Description

There are two types of **intestinal obstructions** (when the bowel does not work correctly), mechanical and non–mechanical. Mechanical obstructions occur because the bowel is physically (structurally) blocked and its contents cannot pass the point of the obstruction. This happens when the bowel twists on itself (volvulus) or as the result of hernias, impacted feces, abnormal tissue growth, or the presence of foreign bodies in the intestines.

Unlike mechanical obstruction, non–mechanical obstruction, called ileus or paralytic ileus, occurs when there is not a structural problem within the bowel but, instead, because peristalsis stops. Peristalsis is the rhythmic contraction that moves material through the bowel. Thus, ileus occurs when the muscles of the bowel wall have failed, and they are unable to transport contents through the intestinal tract. Ileus is most often associated with an infection of the peritoneum (the membrane lining the abdomen). It is one of the major causes of bowel obstruction in infants and children.

Another common cause of ileus is a disruption or reduction of the blood supply to the abdomen. Handling the bowel during abdominal surgery can also cause peristalsis to stop, so people who have had abdominal surgery are more likely to experience ileus. When ileus results from abdominal surgery, the condition known as postoperative ileus, the condition is often temporary and usually lasts from 48 to 72 hours.

Ileus sometimes occurs as a complication of surgery on other parts of the body, including **joint replacement** or chest surgery.

Ileus can also be caused by kidney diseases, especially when potassium levels decrease. Ileus can also be caused by heart disease and certain **chemotherapy** drugs such as vinblastine (Velban, Velsar) and vincristine (Oncovin, Vincasar PES, Vincrex). Infants with **cystic fibrosis** are more likely to experience meconium ileus (a dark green material in the intestine). Over all, the total rate of bowel obstruction due both to mechanical and non–mechanical causes is one in one thousand people (1/1,000).

Causes and symptoms

The major cause of ileus is operations occurring within and about the intestines. However, normal activity of the intestines usually returns within hours to days after such operations. Other causes of ileus include:

- drugs, such as antacids, chlorpromazine, opioids, warfarin, and amitriptline
- metabolic changes, such as those caused by low levels of iron, potassium magnesium, or sodium
- pneumonia
- heart attack (myocardial infarction)
- trauma, such as injuries to the head and spinal column
- pneumonia

When the bowel stops functioning, the following symptoms can occur:

- abdominal cramping
- abdominal distension, discomfort, and tenderness
- poor appetite
- nausea and vomiting, especially after eating
- excessive belching
- constipation
- failure to pass gas (flatulence) or to have a bowel movement (defecation)
- absence of abdominal cramping

Diagnosis

When a doctor listens with a stethoscope to the abdomen, there will be few or no bowel sounds, indicating that the intestine has stopped functioning. Ileus can be confirmed by x rays of the abdomen, **computed tomography scans** (CT scans), or ultrasound. It may be necessary to do more invasive tests, such as a **barium enema** or upper gastrointestinal (GI) series, if the obstruction is mechanical. Blood tests also are useful in diagnosing paralytic ileus.

Barium studies are used in cases of mechanical obstruction, but may cause problems by increasing pressure or intestinal contents if used in ileus. Also, in cases of suspected mechanical obstruction involving the gastrointestinal tract (from the small intestine downward) use of barium x rays are contraindicated, since they may contribute to the obstruction. In such cases a barium enema should always be performed first.

Treatment

Patients may be treated with supervised bed rest in a hospital and bowel rest. Bowel rest means that nothing is taken by mouth and patients are fed intravenously or through the use of a nasogastric tube. (A nasogastric tube provides relief for patients with **vomiting** and distension; however, it has not been found helpful with treating ileus itself.) A nasogastric tube is a tube inserted through the nose, down the throat, and into the stomach. A similar tube can be inserted in the intestine. The contents are then suctioned out. In some cases, especially where there is a mechanical obstruction, surgery may be necessary.

Narcotics are often used after surgery for pain relief but can be replaced over time with nonsteroidal anti–inflammatory drugs (NSAIDs), which also help with reducing inflammation. Drug therapies that promote intestinal motility (ability of the intestine to move spontaneously), such as cisapride (Prepulsid, Propulsid) and vasopressin (Pitressin), are sometimes prescribed.

Alternative treatment

Alternative practitioners offer few treatment suggestions, but focus on prevention by keeping the bowels healthy through eating a good diet that is high in fiber and low in fat. If the case is not a medical emergency, homeopathic treatment and **traditional Chinese medicine** can recommend therapies that may help to reinstate peristalsis.

Prognosis

The outcome of ileus varies depending on its cause. Complications may occur, including infection, **jaundice** (yellow skin discoloration), perforation (hole) in the intestine, or electrolyte imbalances (any of a number of free–ion substances in the body that are not in normal concentrations).

Prevention

Most cases of ileus are not preventable. Surgery to remove a tumor or other mechanical obstruction will help prevent a recurrence.

KEY TERMS

Bowel—The part of the intestines that is connected to the anus.

Computed tomography scan (or CT scan)—A computer enhanced x–ray study performed to detect abnormalities that do not show up on normal x rays.

Meconium—A greenish fecal material that forms the first bowel movement of an infant.

Peritoneum—The transparent membrane lining the abdominal cavity that holds internal organs in place.

Some measures that have been recommended to minimize the severity of postoperative ileus or shorten its duration include making sure that any electrolyte imbalances are corrected, and using nonopioid medications to relieve pain, as opioid drugs (including morphine, oxycodone, and codeine) tend to cause **constipation**. One group of drugs that shows promise for treating abdominal pain is a class of medications known as kappa–opioid agonists. As of 2008, however, these drugs are still under investigation for controlling visceral pain in humans. Further clinical studies are needed to determine their ability to treat such pain.

Resources

BOOKS

Beers, Mark H., et al., ed. *The Merck Manual of Diagnosis and Therapy*, 18th ed. Whitehouse Station, NJ: Merck Research Laboratories, 2006.

Feldman, Mark., et al., ed. *Sleisenger and Fordtran's Gastrointestinal and Liver Disease: Pathophysiology/Diagnosis/Management*. Philadelphia: Saunders/Elsevier, 2006.

Townsend, C. M, et al. ed. *Sabiston Textbook of Surgery: The Biological Basis of Modern Surgical Practice*, 18th ed. Philadelphia: Saunders/Elsevier, 2008.

PERIODICALS

Chang, Howard Y., and Anthony J. Lembo. "Opioid–induced Bowel Dysfunction." *Current Treatment Options in Gastroenterology*. 11(1) (February 2008): 11–18.

OTHER

Heller, Jacob L. "Intestinal Obstruction." Medline Plus, U.S. National Library of Medicine and National Institutes of Health. July 23, 2008. http://www.nlm.nih.gov/medlineplus/ency/article/000260.htm (accessed September 4, 2010).

Mukherjee, Sandeep, et al. "Ileus." eMedicine, WebMD. December 28, 2009, http://emedicine.medscape.com/article/178948-overview (accessed September 4, 2010).

ORGANIZATIONS

ITP Foundation, 40 West Chesapeake Ave., Suite 308, Towson, MD, 21204, (203) 655–6954, itpf@itpfoundation.org, http://www.itpfoundation.org/.

Tish Davidson, A. M.
Rebecca J. Frey, PhD

Immobilization

Definition

Immobilization refers to the process of holding a joint or bone in place with a splint, cast, or brace. This is done to prevent an injured area from moving while it heals.

Purpose

Splints, casts, and braces support and protect broken bones, dislocated joints, and such injured soft tissue as tendons and ligaments. Immobilization restricts motion to allow the injured area to heal. It can help reduce **pain**, swelling, and muscle spasm. In some cases, splints and casts are applied after surgical procedures that repair bones, tendons, or ligaments. This allows for protection and proper alignment early in the healing phase.

Precautions

There are no special precautions for immobilization.

Description

When an arm, hand, leg, or foot requires immobilization, the cast, splint, or brace will generally extend from the joint above the injury to the joint below the injury. For example, an injury to the mid-calf requires immobilization from the knee to the ankle and foot. Injuries of the hip and upper thigh or shoulder and upper arm require a cast that encircles the body and extends down the injured leg or arm.

Casts and splints

Casts are generally used for immobilization of a broken bone. Once the doctor makes sure the two broken ends of the bone are aligned, a cast is put on to keep them in place until they are rejoined through natural healing. Casts are applied by a physician, a nurse, or an assistant. They are custom-made to fit each person, and are usually made of plaster or fiberglass. Fiberglass weighs less than plaster, is more durable, and allows the skin more adequate airflow than plaster. A layer of cotton or synthetic padding is first wrapped around the skin to cover the injured area and protect the skin. The plaster or fiberglass is then applied over this.

Most casts should not be gotten wet. However, some types of fiberglass casts use Gore-tex padding that is waterproof and allows the person to completely immerse the cast in water when taking a shower or bath. There are some circumstances when this type of cast material can not be used.

A splint is often used to immobilize a dislocated joint while it heals. Splints are also often used for finger injuries, such as **fractures** or baseball finger. Baseball finger is an injury in which the tendon at the end of the finger is separated from the bone as a result of trauma. Splinting also is used to immobilize an

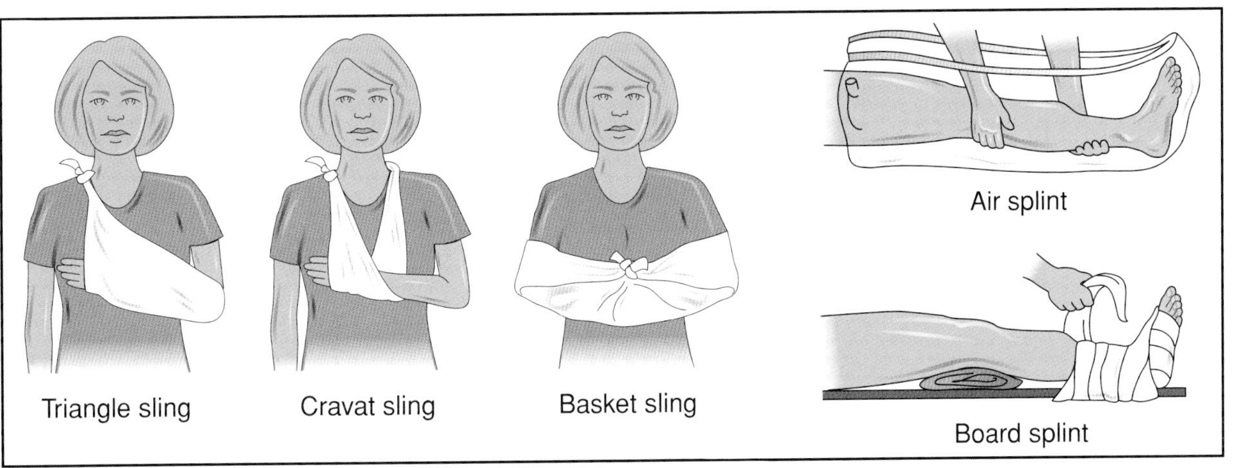

Immobilization refers to the process of immobilizing or fixating the position of a joint, bone, extremity, or torso with a splint, cast, or brace. Immobilization can help reduce pain, swelling, and muscle spasms. The illustrations above feature several types of immobilization techniques. *(Illustration by Electronic Illustrators Group. Reproduced by permission of Gale, a part of Cengage Learning.)*

injured arm or leg immediately after an injury. Before moving a person who has injured an arm or leg some type of temporary splint should be applied to prevent further injury to the area. Splints may be made of acrylic, polyethylene foam, plaster of paris, or aluminum. In an emergency, a splint can be made from a piece of wood or rolled magazine.

Slings

Slings are often used to support the arm after a fracture or other injury. They are generally used along with a cast or splint, but sometimes are used alone as a means of immobilization. They can be used in an emergency to immobilize the arm until the person can be seen by a doctor. A triangular bandage is placed under the injured arm and then tied around the neck.

Braces

Braces are used to support, align, or hold a body part in the correct position. Braces are sometimes used after a surgical procedure is performed on an arm or leg. They can also be used for an injury. Since some braces can be easily taken off and put back on, they are often used when the person must have **physical therapy** or **exercise** the limb during the healing process. Many braces can also be adjusted to allow for a certain amount of movement.

Braces can be custom-made, or a ready-made brace can be used. The off-the-shelf braces are made in a variety of shapes and sizes. They generally have Velcro straps that make the brace easy to adjust, and to put on and take off. Both braces and splints offer less support and protection than a cast and may not be a treatment option in all circumstances.

Collars

A collar is generally used for neck injuries. A soft collar can relieve pain by restricting movement of the head and neck. They also transfer some of the weight of the head from the neck to the chest. Stiff collars are generally used to support the neck when there has been a fracture in one of the bones of the neck. Cervical collars are widely used by emergency personnel at the scene of injuries when there is a potential neck or **head injury**.

Traction

Immobilization may also be secured by **traction**. Traction involves using a method for applying tension to correct the alignment of two structures (such as two bones) and hold them in the correct position. For example, if the bone in the thigh breaks, the broken ends may have a tendency to overlap. Use of traction will hold them in the correct position for healing to occur. The strongest form of traction involves inserting a stainless steel pin through a bony prominence attached by a horseshoe-shaped bow and rope to a pulley and weights suspended over the end of the patient's bed.

Traction must be balanced by countertraction. This is obtained by tilting the bed and allowing the patient's body to act as a counterweight. Another technique involves applying weights pulling in the opposite direction.

Traction for neck injuries may be in the form of a leather or cotton cloth halter placed around the chin and lower back of the head. For very severe neck injuries that require maximum traction, tongs that resemble ice tongs are inserted into small holes drilled in the outer skull.

All traction requires careful observation and adjustment by doctors and nurses to maintain proper balance and alignment of the traction with free suspension of the weights.

Immobilization can also be secured by a form of traction called skin traction. This is a combination of a splint and traction that is applied to the arms or legs by strips of adhesive tape placed over the skin of the arm or leg. Adhesive strips, moleskin, or foam rubber traction strips are applied on the skin. This method is effective only if a moderate amount of traction is required.

Preparation

There are many reasons for immobilization using splints, casts, and braces. Each person should understand his or her diagnosis clearly.

Aftercare

After a cast or splint has been put on, the injured arm or leg should be elevated for 24 to 72 hours. It is recommended that the person lie or sit with the injured arm or leg raised above the level of the heart. Rest combined with elevation will reduce pain and speed the healing process by minimizing swelling.

Fingers or toes can be exercised as much as can be tolerated after casting. This has been found to decrease swelling and prevent stiffness. If excessive swelling is noted, the application of ice to the splint or cast may be helpful.

After the cast, splint, or brace is removed, gradual exercise is usually performed to regain muscle strength and motion. The doctor may also recommend **hydrotherapy**, **heat treatments**, and other forms of physical therapy.

Risks

For some people, such as those in traction, immobilization will require long periods of bedrest. Lying in one position in bed for an extended period of time can result in sores on the skin (decubitus ulcers) and skin infection. Long periods of bedrest can also cause a buildup of fluid in the lungs or an infection in the lungs (**pneumonia**). Urinary infection can also be a result of extended bedrest.

KEY TERMS

Decubitus ulcers— A pressure sore resulting from ulceration of the skin occurring in persons confined to bed for long periods of time

Ligament—Ligaments are structures that hold bones together and prevent excessive movement of the joint. They are tough, fibrous bands of tissue.

Pneumonia—An acute or chronic disease characterized by inflammation of the lungs and caused by viruses, bacteria, or other microorganisms.

Tendon—Tendons are structures that attach bones to muscles and muscles to other muscles.

People who have casts, splints, or braces on their arms or legs will generally spend several weeks not using the injured arm or leg. This lack of use can result in decreased muscle tone and shrinkage of the muscle (atrophy). Much of this loss can usually be regained, however, through **rehabilitation** after the injury has healed.

Immobility can also cause psychological **stress**. An individual restricted to a bed with a traction device may become frustrated and bored, and perhaps even depressed, irritable, and withdrawn.

There is the possibility of decreased circulation if the cast, splint, or brace fits too tightly. Excessive pressure over a nerve can cause irritation or possible damage if not corrected. If the cast, splint, or brace breaks or malfunctions, the healing process of the bone or soft tissue can be disrupted and lead to deformity.

Normal results

Normally, the surgical or injured area heals appropriately with the help of immobilization. The form of immobilization can be discontinued, which is followed by an appropriate rehabilitation program under the supervision of a physical therapist to regain range of motion and strength.

Resources

OTHER

"Casts & Splints." *The Center for Orthopaedics and Sports Medicine*. http://www.arthroscopy.com.

Jeffrey P. Larson, RPT

Immune complex detection *see* **Immune complex test**

Immune complex test

Definition

These tests evaluate the immune system, whose function is to defend the body against such invaders as bacteria and viruses. The immune system also plays a role in the control of **cancer**, and is responsible for the phenomena of allergy, hypersensitivity, and rejection problems when organs or tissue are transplanted.

One of the ways the immune system protects the body is by producing proteins called antibodies. Antibodies are formed in response to another type of protein called an antigen (anything foreign or different from a natural body protein). Immune complex reactions occur when large numbers of antigen-antibody complexes accumulate in the body.

KEY TERMS

Antibody—A (immunoglobulin) molecule that interacts with a specific antigen. Antibodies provide protection from microscopic invaders like bacteria.

Antigen—Any substance that is capable under certain circumstances of producing an immune response either from antibodies or T-cells; bacteria are often antigens.

Autoimmune disorder—A disorder caused by a reaction of an individual's immune system against the organs or tissues of the body. Autoimmune processes can have different results: slow destruction of a particular type of cell or tissue, stimulation of an organ into excessive growth, or interference in function.

Biopsy—The removal and examination, usually under a microscope, of tissue from the living body. Used for diagnosis.

Systemic lupus erythematosus—A chronic disease of the connective tissues in the body; characterized by involvement of the skin, joints, kidneys, and serosal membranes (membranes that form the outer covering of organs in the abdomen or chest).

Purpose

The purpose of the immune complex test is to demonstrate circulating immune complexes in the blood, to estimate the severity of immune complex disease, and to monitor response to therapy.

Precautions

Because this test is requested when the physician suspects that a patient's immune system is not functioning properly, special care should be taken during and after blood is drawn. For example, the venipuncture site should be kept clean and dry to avoid any chance of infection.

Description

Immune complexes are normally not detected in the blood. However, when immune complexes are produced faster than they can be cleared by the system, immune complex disease may occur. Examples of such disorders are drug sensitivity, **rheumatoid arthritis**, and a disease called **systemic lupus erythematosus**, or SLE.

The method generally used for detecting immune complexes is examination of a tissue obtained by biopsy (removal and examination of tissue sample) and the subsequent use of different staining techniques with specific antibodies. However, since tissue biopsies do not provide information about the level of complexes still in the circulatory system, serum assays obtained from blood samples which indirectly detect circulating immune complexes are useful. However, due to the variability of these complexes, several test methods may be used. Also, as most immune complex assays have not been standardized, more than one test may be required to achieve accurate results.

Preparation

This test requires a blood sample. It is not necessary for the patient to be in a **fasting** (nothing to eat or drink) state before the test.

Risks

Risks for this test are minimal, but may include slight bleeding from the blood-drawing site, **fainting** or feeling lightheaded after venipuncture, or hematoma (blood accumulating under the puncture site).

Normal results

Normally, immune complexes are not detected in the blood.

Abnormal results

The presence of detectable immune complexes in the blood is important in the diagnosis of autoimmune diseases, such as SLE and rheumatoid arthritis. However, for definitive diagnosis, the results of other studies must be considered with the presence of any immune complex. For example, immune complexes are associated with high numbers of a component called antinuclear antibodies in the diagnosis of systemic lupus erythematosus. A different example is the kidneys. Because of their filtering functions, elements in the kidneys called renal glomeruli can be affected by immune complexes. In such cases, renal biopsy is used to provide conclusive evidence for immune complex.

Resources

BOOKS

Brunner, Lillian Sholtis. *Brunner and Suddarth's Handbook of Laboratory and Diagnostic Tests.* Philadelphia: Wolters Kluwer/Lippincott Williams & Wilkins, 2010.

Janis O. Flores

Immunodeficiency

Definition

Immunodeficiency disorders are a group of disorders in which part of the immune system is missing or defective. Therefore, the body's ability to fight infections is impaired. As a result, the person with an immunodeficiency disorder has frequent infections—thus, are at greater susceptibility to infection—that are generally more severe and last longer than usual. The infections involving immunodeficiency disorders commonly reside in the skin, throat, ears, sinuses, lungs, brain, spinal cord, urinary tract, and intestines.

Demographics

These disorders are caused by genetic or hereditary defects and, as such, can happen to anyone regardless of age or gender. While some immunodeficiency disorders are commonly scattered within the human population, other types are only infrequently found. Even though numerous types of such disorders exist they all have one feature in common: each involves a defect of a specific function of body's overall immune system.

Description

The immune system is the body's main method for fighting infections. Any defect in the immune system decreases a person's ability to fight infections. A person with an immunodeficiency disorder may get more frequent infections, heal more slowly, and have a higher incidence of some cancers.

The normal immune system involves a complex interaction of certain types of cells that can recognize and attack "foreign" invaders (called antigens), such as bacteria, viruses, toxins, fungi, and blood or tissues from other humans or species. It also plays a role in fighting **cancer**. The immune system has both innate and adaptive components. Innate immunity is made up of immune protections people are born with. Adaptive immunity develops throughout life. It adapts to fight off specific invading organisms. Adaptive immunity is divided into two components: humoral immunity and cellular immunity.

The innate immune system is made up of the skin (which acts as a barrier to prevent organisms from entering the body), white blood cells called phagocytes, a system of proteins called the complement system, and chemicals called interferons. When phagocytes encounter an invading organism, they surround and engulf it to destroy it. The complement system also attacks bacteria. The elements in the complement system create a hole in the outer layer of the target cell, which leads to the **death** of the cell.

The adaptive component of the immune system is extremely complex, and is still not entirely understood. Basically, it has the ability to recognize an organism or tumor cell as not being a normal part of the body, and to develop a response to attempt to eliminate it.

The humoral response of adaptive immunity involves a type of cell called B lymphocytes. B lymphocytes manufacture proteins called antibodies (which are also called immunoglobulins). Antibodies attach themselves to the invading foreign substance. This allows the phagocytes to begin engulfing and destroying the organism. The action of antibodies also activates the complement system. The humoral response is particularly useful for attacking bacteria.

The cellular response of adaptive immunity is useful for attacking viruses, some parasites, and possibly cancer cells. The main type of cell in the cellular response is T lymphocytes. There are helper T lymphocytes and killer T lymphocytes. The helper T lymphocytes play a role in recognizing invading organisms, and they also help killer T lymphocytes to multiply. As the name suggests, killer T lymphocytes act to destroy the target organism.

Defects can occur in any component of the immune system or in more than one component (combined immunodeficiency). Different immunodeficiency diseases involve different components of the immune system. The defects can be inherited and/or present at birth (congenital) or acquired.

Congenital immunodeficiency disorders

Congenital (primary) immunodeficiency is present at the time of birth, and is the result of genetic defects. These immunodeficiency disorders are also called primary immunodeficiencies. The disorders are generally classified according to the part of the immune system that is improperly functioning. The World Health Organization (WHO) estimates that over 70 primary immunodeficiency disorders are present around the world. In the United States, the National Institute of Child Health and Human Development estimates about 400 children are born annually with a primary immunodeficiency disorder. It also states that roughly 25,000 to 50,000 people are living in any given year with such a disorder. The number of new cases is rising in the United Sates as new laboratory tests become more commonly available. Congenital immunodeficiencies may occur because of defects in B lymphocytes, T lymphocytes, or both. They also can occur in the innate immune system.

HUMORAL IMMUNITY DISORDERS. Bruton's agammaglobulinemia, also known as **X–linked agammaglobulinemia**, is a congenital immunodeficiency disorder. The defect results in a decrease or absence of B lymphocytes, and therefore a decreased ability to make antibodies. People with this disorder are particularly susceptible to infections of the throat, skin, middle ear, and lungs. It is seen only in males because it is caused by a genetic defect on the X chromosome. Since males have only one X chromosome, they always have the defect if the gene is present. Females can have the defective gene, but since they have two X chromosomes, there will be a normal gene on the other X chromosome to counter it. Women may pass the defective gene on to their male children.

B LYMPHOCYTE DEFICIENCES. If there is an abnormality in either the development or function of B lymphocytes, the ability to make antibodies will be impaired. This allows the body to be susceptible to recurrent infections.

A type of B lymphocyte deficiency involves a group of disorders called selective immunoglobulin deficiency syndomes. Immunoglobulin is another name for antibody, and there are five different types of immunoglobulins (called IgA, IgG, IgM, IgD, and IgE). The most common type of immunoglobulin deficiency is selective IgA deficiency, occurring in about one in every 500 white (Caucasian) persons. The amounts of the other antibody types are normal. Some patients with selective IgA deficiency experience no symptoms, while others have occasional lung infections and **diarrhea**. In another immunoglobulin disorder, IgG and IgA antibodies are deficient and there is increased IgM. People with this disorder tend to get severe bacterial infections.

Common variable immunodeficiency is another type of B lymphocyte deficiency. In this disorder, the production of one or more of the immunoglobulin types is decreased and the antibody response to infections is impaired. It generally develops around the age of 10 to 20 years. The symptoms vary among affected people. Most people with this disorder have frequent infections, and some of them also experience anemia and **rheumatoid arthritis**. Many people with common variable immunodeficiency develop cancer.

T LYMPHOCYTE DEFICIENCIES. Severe defects in the ability of T lymphocytes to mature results in impaired immune responses to infections with antigens, such as viruses, fungi, and certain types of bacteria. These infections are usually severe and can be fatal.

DiGeorge syndrome is a T lymphocyte deficiency that starts during fetal development and is the result of a deletion in a particular chromosome. Children with DiGeorge syndrome either do not have a thymus or have an underdeveloped thymus. Since the thymus is a major organ that directs the production of T–lymphocytes, these patients have very low numbers of T–lymphocytes. They are susceptible to recurrent infections, and usually have physical abnormalities as well. For example, they may have low–set ears, a small receding jawbone, and wide–spaced eyes. People with DiGeorge syndrome are particularly susceptible to viral and fungal infections.

In some cases, no treatment is required for DiGeorge syndrome because T lymphocyte production improves. Either an underdeveloped thymus begins to produce more T lymphocytes or organ sites other than the thymus compensate by producing more T lymphocytes.

COMBINED IMMUNODEFICIENCIES. Some types of immunodeficiency disorders affect both B lymphocytes and T lymphocytes. For example, **severe combined immunodeficiency** disease (SCID), sometimes commonly called Bubble Boy Syndrome, is caused by the defective development or function of these two types of lymphocytes. It results in impaired humoral and cellular immune responses. SCID usually is recognized during the first year of life. It tends to cause a fungal infection of the mouth (thrush), diarrhea, **failure to thrive**, and serious infections. If not treated with a bone marrow transplant, a person with SCID will generally die from infections before age two. It is reported that the prevalence of SCID is one in 100,000 births, although that figure is regularly considered an underestimate. In some local populations, this figure is much greater. For instance, in the Navajo population within the United States, it is reported that one in 2,000 babies inherit SCID.

DISORDERS OF INNATE IMMUNITY. Disorders of innate immunity affect phagocytes or the complement system. These disorders also result in recurrent infections.

Acquired immunodeficiency disorders

Acquired (secondary) immunodeficiency is more common than congenital immunodeficiency. It is frequently the result of an infectious process or other disease, **malnutrition**, medications/drugs, or **aging**. For example, the human immunodeficiency virus (HIV) is the virus that causes acquired immunodeficiency syndrome (**AIDS**). However, this is not the most common cause of acquired immunodeficiency.

Acquired immunodeficiency often occurs as a complication of other conditions and diseases. For example, the most common causes of acquired immunodeficiency are malnutrition, some types of cancer, and infections. People who weigh less than 70% of the average weight of persons of the same age and gender are considered to be malnourished. Examples of types of infections that can lead to immunodeficiency are **chickenpox**, cytomegalovirus, German **measles**, measles, **tuberculosis**, **infectious mononucleosis** (Epstein–Barr virus), chronic hepatitis, lupus, and bacterial and fungal infections.

In 2003, a new infection emerged that produces immunodeficiency. **Severe acute respiratory syndrome (SARS)** mysteriously appeared in a hospital in China. It eventually affected 8,000 people in Asia and Canada, killing 800 altogether. **Fever**, lower respiratory tract symptoms, and abnormal chest x rays characterize the disease. However, it also produces immunodeficiency. No cases of the disease were reported from July 2003 through December 2003, but scientists feared it would reappear. Thus, the World Health Organization (WHO) set up a network of medical and research professionals to deal with SARS. As of May 2006, the SARS infection has been completely contained. However, it is not considered eradicated, so could possibility return to infect the human population.

Sometimes, acquired immunodeficiency is brought on by drugs used to treat another condition. For example, patients who have an organ transplant are given drugs to suppress the immune system so the body will not reject the organ. Also, some **chemotherapy** drugs, which are given to treat cancer, have the side effect of killing cells of the immune system. During the period of time that these drugs are being taken, the risk of infection increases. It usually returns to normal after the person stops taking the drugs.

Causes and symptoms

Congenital immunodeficiency is caused by genetic defects, which generally occur while the fetus is developing in the womb. These defects affect the development and/or function of one or more of the components of the immune system, such as lymphoid tissue within bone marrow, thymus, lymph nodes, tonsils, spleen, and gastrointestinal tract. Acquired immunodeficiency is the result of a disease process, and it occurs later in life. The causes, as described above, can be diseases, infections, or the side effects of drugs given to treat other conditions.

People with an immunodeficiency disorder tend to become infected by organisms that do not usually cause disease in healthy persons. The major symptoms of most immunodeficiency disorders are repeated infections that heal slowly. These chronic infections cause symptoms that persist for long periods of time. People with chronic infection tend to be pale and thin. They may have skin **rashes**. Their lymph nodes tend to be larger than normal and their liver and spleen may be enlarged, too. The lymph nodes are small organs that house antibodies and lymphocytes. Broken blood vessels, especially near the surface of the skin, may be seen. This can result in black–and–blue marks in the skin. The person may lose hair from their head. Sometimes, a red inflammation of the lining of the eye (**conjunctivitis**) is present. They may have a crusty appearance in and on the nose from chronic nasal dripping.

Diagnosis

Usually, the first sign that a person might have an immunodeficiency disorder is that they do not improve rapidly when given **antibiotics** to treat an infection. Strong indicators that an immunodeficiency disorder may be present are when rare diseases occur or the patient gets ill from organisms that do not normally cause diseases, especially if the patient repeatedly is infected. If this happens in very young children, it is an indication that a genetic defect may be causing an immunodeficiency disorder. When this situation occurs in older children or young adults, their medical history will be reviewed to determine if childhood diseases may have caused an immunodeficiency disorder. Other possibilities will then be considered, such as recently acquired infections—for example, HIV, hepatitis, tuberculosis, etc.

Laboratory tests are used to determine the exact nature of the immunodeficiency. Most tests are performed on blood samples. Blood contains antibodies, lymphocytes, phagocytes, and complement components—all of the major immune components that might cause immunodeficiency. A blood cell count will determine if the number of phagocytic cells or lymphocytes is below normal. Lower than normal counts of either of these two cell types correlates with immunodeficiencies. The blood cells also are checked for their appearance. Sometimes a person may have normal cell counts, but the cells are structurally defective. If the lymphocyte cell count is low, further testing is usually done to determine whether any particular type of lymphocyte is lower than normal. A lymphocyte proliferation test is done to determine if the lymphocytes can respond to stimuli. The failure to respond to stimulants correlates with immunodeficiency. A process called electrophoresis can measure antibody levels. Complement levels can be determined by immunodiagnostic tests.

Treatment

There is no cure for immunodeficiency disorders. Therapy is aimed at controlling infections and, for some disorders, replacing defective or absent components.

Patients with Bruton's agammaglobulinemia must be given periodic injections of a substance called **gamma globulin** throughout their lives to make up for their decreased ability to make antibodies. The gamma globulin preparation contains antibodies against common invading bacteria. If left untreated, the disease usually is fatal.

Common variable immunodeficiency also is treated with periodic injections of gamma globulin throughout life. Additionally, antibiotics are given when necessary to treat infections.

Patients with selective IgA deficiency usually do not require any treatment. Antibiotics can be given for frequent infections.

In some cases, treatment is not required for DiGeorge syndrome because T lymphocyte production improves on its own. Either an underdeveloped thymus begins to produce more T lymphocytes or organ sites other than the thymus compensate by producing more T lymphocytes. In some severe cases, a bone marrow transplant or thymus transplant can be done to correct the problem.

For patients with SCID, **bone marrow transplantation** is necessary. In this procedure, healthy bone marrow from a donor who has a similar type of tissue (usually a relative, such as a brother or sister) is removed. The bone marrow is a substance that resides in the cavity of bones. Such marrow produces blood including some of the white blood cells that make up the immune system. The bone marrow of the person receiving the transplant is destroyed, and is then replaced with marrow from the donor.

Treatment of the HIV infection that causes AIDS consists of drugs called antiretrovirals. These drugs attempt to inhibit the process that the virus goes through to kill T lymphocytes. Several of these drugs used in various combinations with one another can prolong the time period before the disease becomes apparent. However, this treatment is not a cure. Other treatments for people with AIDS are aimed at the particular infections and conditions that arise because of the impaired immune system. SARS is a relatively new acquired disease. Treatment to date involves combination therapy with **steroids** and interferon and supplemental oxygen for breathing difficulties. In 2004, the U.S. Food and Drug Administration approved the drug octagam 5% (Immune Globulin Intravenous (Human) 5%), an intravenous immunoglobulin product from the company Octapharma AG, to treat primary immunodeficiency diseases. At that time, the drug had been used in Europe for over ten years for the same purpose.

In most cases, immunodeficiency caused by malnutrition is reversible. The health of the immune system is directly linked to the nutritional status of the patient. Among the essential nutrients required by the immune system are proteins, **vitamins**, iron, and zinc.

For people being treated for cancer, periodic relief from chemotherapy drugs can restore the function of the immune system.

In general, people with immunodeficiency disorders should maintain a healthy diet because malnutrition can aggravate immunodeficiencies. They also should avoid being near people who have colds or

KEY TERMS

Agammaglobulinemia—The lack of gamma globulins in the blood. Antibodies are the main gamma globulins of interest, so this term means a lack of antibodies.

are sick because they can easily acquire new infections. For the same reason, they should practice good personal hygiene, especially dental care. People with immunodeficiency disorders also should avoid eating undercooked food because it might contain bacteria that could cause infection. This food would not cause infection in persons with healthy immune systems, but in someone with an immunodeficiency, food is a potential source of infectious organisms. People with immunodeficiency should be given antibiotics at the first indication of an infection.

Prognosis

The prognosis depends on the type of immunodeficiency disorder. People with Bruton's agammaglobulinemia who are given injections of gamma globulin generally live into their 30s or 40s. They often die from chronic infections, usually of the lung. People with selective IgA deficiency generally live normal lives. They may experience problems if given a blood **transfusion**, and therefore they should wear a Medic Alert bracelet or have some other way of alerting any physician who treats them that they have this disorder.

SCID is the most serious of the immunodeficiency disorders. If a bone marrow transplant is not successfully performed, the child usually will not live beyond two years old.

People with HIV/AIDS are living longer than in the past because of **antiretroviral drugs** that became available in the mid-1990s. However, AIDS still is a fatal disease. People with AIDS usually die of opportunistic infections, which are infections that occur because the impaired immune system is unable to fight them.

Some complications that can occur include frequent or persistent illnesses and the increased risk from certain cancers. Infections are also much more likely with people having immunodeficiency disorders.

Prevention

There is no way to prevent a congenital immunodeficiency disorder. However, individuals with a congenital immunodeficiency disorder might want to consider getting **genetic counseling** before having children to find out if there is a chance they will pass the defect on to their children.

Some of the infections associated with acquired immunodeficiency can be prevented or treated before they cause problems. For example, there are effective treatments for tuberculosis and most bacterial and fungal infections. HIV infection can be prevented by practicing "safer sex" and not using illegal intravenous drugs. These are the primary routes of transmitting the virus. For people who do not know the HIV status of the person with whom they are having sex, safer sex involves using a condom.

Malnutrition can be prevented by getting adequate **nutrition**. Malnutrition tends to be more of a problem in developing countries.

Resources

BOOKS

Abbas, Abul K., and Andrew H. Lichtman. *Basic Immunology: Functions and Disorders of the Immune System.* Philadelphia: Saunders/Elsevier, 2009.

Beers, Mark H., et al., eds. *The Merck Manual of Diagnosis and Therapy,* 18th ed. Whitehouse Station, NJ: Merck Research Laboratories, 2006.

Elgert, Klaus D. *Immunology: Understanding the Immune System,* 2nd ed. Hoboken, NJ: Wiley–Blackwell, 2009.

OTHER

Buckley, Rebecca H. "Immunodeficiency Disorders." Merck Manuals Online Medical Library. (September 2008), http://www.merck.com/mmhe/sec16/ch184/ch184a.html (accessed September 4, 2010).

Dugdale, David C., III, and Stuart I. Henochowicz. "Immunodeficiency disorders." Medline Plus, U.S. National Library of Medicine and National Institutes of Health. (May 2, 2008), http://www.nlm.nih.gov/medlineplus/ency/article/000818.htm (accessed September 4, 2010).

Fonseca, Felicia. "A Rare and Once–baffling Disease Forces Navajo Parents to Cope." Indian Country News. (December 2007), http://indiancountrynews.net/index.php?option = com_content&task = view&id = 2109&Itemid = 1 (accessed September 4, 2010).

"Primary Immunodeficiency." National Institute of Child Health and Human Development. (April 7, 2008), http://www.nichd.nih.gov/publications/pubs/primary_immuno.cfm (accessed September 4, 2010).

ORGANIZATIONS

Immune Deficiency Foundation, 30 Old Kings Hwy. South, Suite 275, Darien, CT, 06820, (800) 296–4433, idf@primaryimmune.org, http://www.primaryimmune.org.

John T. Lohr, PhD
Teresa G. Odle

Immunoelectrophoresis

Definition

Immunoelectrophoresis, also called **gamma globulin** electrophoresis, or immunoglobulin electrophoresis, is a method of determining the blood levels of three major immunoglobulins: immunoglobulin M (IgM), immunoglobulin G (IgG), and immunoglobulin A (IgA).

Purpose

Immunoelectrophoresis is a powerful analytical technique with high resolving power as it combines separation of antigens by electrophoresis with immunodiffusion against an antiserum. The increased resolution is of benefit in the immunological examination of serum proteins. Immunoelectrophoresis aids in the diagnosis and evaluation of the therapeutic response in many disease states affecting the immune system. It is usually requested when a different type of electrophoresis, called a serum **protein electrophoresis**, has indicated a rise at the immunoglobulin level. Immunoelectrophoresis is also used frequently to diagnose **multiple myeloma**, a disease affecting the bone marrow.

Precautions

Drugs that may cause increased immunoglobulin levels include therapeutic gamma globulin, hydralazine, isoniazid, phenytoin (Dilantin), procainamide, **oral contraceptives**, **methadone**, **steroids**, and **tetanus** toxoid and antitoxin. The laboratory should be notified if the patient has received any vaccinations or immunizations in the six months before the test. This is mainly because prior immunizations lead to the increased immunoglobulin levels resulting in false positive results.

It should be noted that, because immunoelectrophoresis is not quantitative, it is being replaced by a procedure called immunofixation, which is more sensitive and easier to interpret.

Description

Serum proteins separate in agar gels under the influence of an electric field into albumin, alpha 1, alpha 2, and beta and gamma globulins. Immunoelectrophoresis is performed by placing serum on a slide containing a gel designed specifically for the test. An electric current is then passed through the gel, and immunoglobulins, which contain an electric charge, migrate through the gel according to the difference in their individual electric charges. Antiserum is placed alongside the slide to identify the specific type of immunoglobulin present. The results are used to identify different disease entities, and to aid in monitoring the course of the disease and the therapeutic response of the patient to such conditions as immune deficiencies, autoimmune disease, chronic infections, chronic viral infections, and intrauterine fetal infections.

There are five classes of antibodies: IgM, IgG, IgA, IgE, and IgD.

IgM is produced upon initial exposure to an antigen. For example, when a person receives the first tetanus **vaccination**, antitetanus antibodies of the IgM class are produced 10 to 14 days later. IgM is abundant in the blood but is not normally present in organs or tissues. IgM is primarily responsible for ABO blood grouping and rheumatoid factor, yet is involved in the immunologic reaction to other infections, such as hepatitis. Since IgM does not cross the placenta, an elevation of this immunoglobulin in the newborn indicates intrauterine infection such as **rubella**, cytomegalovirus (CMV) or a sexually transmitted disease (STD).

IgG is the most prevalent type of antibody, comprising approximately 75% of the serum immunoglobulins. IgG is produced upon subsequent exposure to an antigen. As an example, after receiving a second tetanus shot, or booster, a person produces IgG antibodies in five to seven days. IgG is present in both the blood and tissues, and is the only antibody to cross the placenta from the mother to the fetus. Maternal IgG protects the newborn for the first months of life, until the infant's immune system produces its own antibodies.

IgA constitutes approximately 15% of the immunoglobulins within the body. Although it is found to some degree in the blood, it is present primarily in the secretions of the respiratory and gastrointestinal tract, in saliva, colostrum (the yellowish fluid produced by the breasts during late **pregnancy** and the first few days after **childbirth**), and in tears. IgA plays an important role in defending the body against invasion of germs through the mucous membrane-lined organs.

IgE is the antibody that causes acute allergic reactions; it is measured to detect allergic conditions. IgD, which constitutes the smallest portion of the immunoglobulins, is rarely evaluated or detected, and its function is not well understood.

Preparation

This test requires a blood sample.

Aftercare

Because this test is ordered when either very low or very high levels of immunoglobulins are suspected,

KEY TERMS

Antibody—A protein manufactured by the white blood cells to neutralize an antigen in the body. In some cases, excessive formation of antibodies leads to illness, allergy, or autoimmune disorders.

Antigen—A substance that can cause an immune response, resulting in production of an antibody, as part of the body's defense against infection and disease. Many antigens are foreign proteins not found naturally in the body, and include germs, toxins, and tissues from another person used in organ transplantation.

Autoimmune disorder—A condition in which antibodies are formed against the body's own tissues; for example, in some forms of arthritis.

the patient should be alert for any signs of infection after the test, including **fever**, chills, rash, or skin ulcers. Any bone **pain** or tenderness should also be immediately reported to the physician.

Risks

Risks for this test are minimal, but may include slight bleeding from the blood-drawing site, **fainting** or feeling lightheaded after venipuncture, or bruising.

Normal results

Reference ranges vary from laboratory to laboratory and depend upon the method used. For adults, normal values are usually found within the following ranges (1mg = approximately 0.000035 oz. and 1dL = approximately 0.33 oz.):

- IgM: 60–290 mg/dL
- IgG: 700–1,800 mg/dL
- IgA: 70–440 mg/dL

Abnormal results

Increased IgM levels can indicate **Waldenström's macroglobulinemia**, a malignancy caused by secretion of IgM at high levels by malignant lymphoplasma cells. Increased IgM levels can also indicate chronic infections, such as hepatitis or mononucleosis and autoimmune diseases, like **rheumatoid arthritis**.

Decreased IgM levels can be indicative of **AIDS**, immunosuppression caused by certain drugs like steroids or dextran, or leukemia.

Increased levels of IgG can indicate chronic **liver disease**, autoimmune diseases, hyperimmunization reactions, or certain chronic infections, such as **tuberculosis** or **sarcoidosis**.

Decreased levels of IgG can indicate **Wiskott-Aldrich syndrome**, a genetic deficiency caused by inadequate synthesis of IgG and other immunoglobulins. Decreased IgG can also be seen with AIDS and leukemia.

Increased levels of IgA can indicate chronic liver disease, chronic infections, or inflammatory bowel disease.

Decreased levels of IgA can be found in ataxia, a condition affecting balance and gait, limb or eye movements, speech, and telangiectasia, an increase in the size and number of the small blood vessels in an area of skin, causing redness. Decreased IgA levels are also seen in conditions of low blood protein (hypoproteinemia), and drug immuno-suppression.

Resources

BOOKS

Fischbach, Frances Talaska, and Marshall Barnett Dunning. *A Manual of Laboratory and Diagnostic Tests*. 8th ed. Philadelphia: Wolters Kluwer Health/Lippincott Williams & Wilkins, 2009.

Pagana, Kathleen Deska, and Timothy J. Pagana. *Mosby's Manual of Diagnostic and Laboratory Tests*. 4th ed. St. Louis: Mosby, 2009.

Janis O. Flores

Immunoglobulin *see* **Gammaglobulin**

Immunoglobulin deficiency syndromes

Definition

Immunoglobulin deficiency syndromes are a group of **immunodeficiency** disorders in which the patient has a reduced number of or lack of antibodies.

Demographics

The disorders can appear in anyone, from newborn babies to the elderly.

Description

Immunoglobulins (Ig), also commonly known as antibodies, are **gamma globulin** proteins. That is, they are a type of protein found in the blood and other fluids of humans and other vertebrates. Immunoglobulins are used to neutralize bacteria, viruses, and other invading foreign substances. There are five major classes of antibodies: IgG, IgM, IgA, IgD, and IgE. Each differs in its functional location, physical properties, and ability to counter foreign substances within the body.

- IgG is the most abundant of the classes of immunoglobulins. It is the antibody for viruses, bacteria, and antitoxins. In addition, it is found in most tissues and plasma. It is also the only Ig that is able to help provide immunity to a mother's fetus.
- IgM is the first antibody present in an immune response.
- IgA is an early antibody for bacteria and viruses. It is found in saliva, tears, and all other mucous secretions such as within respiratory and urogenital tracts.
- IgD activity is not well understood. However, research has shown that it functions primarily as a receptor on B–cells that have yet to be subjected to antigens.
- IgE is present in respiratory secretions. It is an antibody for parasitic diseases (such as those caused by parasitic worms), Hodgkin's disease, hay fever, atopic dermatitis, and allergic asthma.

All antibodies are made by B–lymphocytes (B–cells). Any disease that harms the development or function of B–cells causes a decrease in the amount of antibodies produced. Since antibodies are essential in fighting infectious diseases, people with immunoglobulin deficiency syndromes become ill more often than those without the disorder. However, the cellular immune system is still functional, so these patients are more prone to infection caused by organisms usually controlled by antibodies. Most of these invading germs (microbes) make capsules, a mechanism used to confuse the immune system. In a healthy body, antibodies can bind to the capsule and overcome the bacteria's defenses. The bacteria that make capsules include the streptococci, meningococci, and *Haemophilus influenzae*. These organisms cause such diseases as otitis, **sinusitis**, **pneumonia**, **meningitis**, **osteomyelitis**, septic arthritis, and **sepsis**. Patients with immunoglobulin deficiencies are also prone to some viral infections, including echovirus, enterovirus, and **hepatitis B**. They may also have a bad reaction to the attenuated version of the **polio** virus vaccine.

There are two types of immunodeficiency diseases: secondary and primary. Secondary disorders occur in normally healthy bodies that are suffering from an underlying disease. Once the disease is treated, the immunodeficiency is reversed.

Primary immunodeficiency diseases occur because of defective B–cells or antibodies. They account for approximately 50% of all immunodeficiencies, and they are, therefore, the most prevalent type of immunodeficiency disorders. These disorders include:

- X–linked agammaglobulinemia is an inherited disease. The defect is on the X chromosome and, consequently, this disease is seen more frequently in males than females. The defect results in a failure of B–cells to mature. Mature B–cells are capable of making antibodies and developing "memory," a feature in which the B–cell rapidly recognizes and responds to an infectious agent the next time it is encountered. Thus, patients with x–linked agammaglobulinemia do not generate mature B–cells. All classes of antibodies are decreased in agammaglobulinemia. It occurs in about one in 100,000 newborn males, without a predisposition to ethnic origin.
- Selective IgA deficiency, a mild but very common deficiency, is an inherited disease, resulting from a failure of B–cells to switch from making IgM, the early antibody, to IgA. Although the number of B–cells is normal, and the B–cells are otherwise normal (they can still make all other classes of antibodies), the amount of IgA produced is limited. This results in more infections of mucosal surfaces, such as the nose, mouth, throat, lungs, digestive tract, and intestines. Roughly no more than one in 333 people is inflicted by the deficiency; however its frequency is dependent on various populations.
- Transient hypogammaglobulinemia of infancy is a temporary disease of unknown cause. Normally, it appears after birth of a child with increased infections but, sometimes, without any symptoms. It is believed to be caused by a defect in the development of T–helper cells (cells that recognize foreign antigens and activate T– and B–cells in an immune response). As the child ages, the number and condition of T–helper cells normally improves and this situation usually corrects itself. Hypogammaglobulinemia is characterized by low levels of gammaglobulin (antibodies) in the blood. During the disease

period, patients have decreased levels of IgG antibodies, and sometimes of IgA and IgM antibodies. In laboratory tests, the antibodies that are present do not react well with infectious bacteria. The incidence of the disease varies widely in infants.

- Common variable immunodeficiency, which includes a group of primary immunodeficiencies, is a defect in both B cells and T–lymphocytes. The differences of its members are the result of the underlying causes. Most causes are unknown. However, all result in a near complete lack of antibodies in the blood, and all occur very frequently with respect to other such related diseases.
- Ig heavy chain deletions is a genetic disease in which part of the antibody molecule is not produced. It results in the loss of several antibody classes and subclasses, including most IgG antibodies and all IgA and IgE antibodies. The disease occurs because part of the gene for the heavy chain has been lost.
- Selective IgG subclass deficiencies is a group of genetic diseases in which some of the subclasses of IgG are not made. There are four subclasses in the IgG class of antibodies. As the B–cell matures, it can switch from one subclass to another. In these diseases there is a defect in the maturation of the B–cells that results in a lack of switching.
- IgG deficiency with hyper–IgM is a disease that results when the B–cell fails to switch from making IgM to IgG. This produces an increase in the amount of IgM antibodies present and a decrease in the amount of IgG antibodies. This disease is the result of a genetic mutation.
- Severe combined immunodeficiency (SCID) is not strictly a deficiency of immunoglobulin, although it is often categorized within this group. It occurs due to the absence or dysfunction of important immune cells called T–cells, or of both T– and B–cells. The condition can be X–linked, in which case more males than females are affected, or it can be inherited in an autosomal fashion (in which case males and females can be equally affected). In SCID, the thymus gland (which produces T–cell) may be abnormal.

Causes and symptoms

Immunoglobulin deficiencies are the result of congenital defects affecting the development and function of B lymphocytes (B–cells). There are two main points in the development of B–cells when defects can occur. First, B–cells can fail to develop into antibody–producing cells. **X–linked agammaglobulinemia** is an example of this disease. Secondly, B–cells can fail to make a particular type of antibody or fail to switch classes during maturation. Initially, when B–cells start making antibodies for the first time, they make IgM. As they mature and develop memory, they switch to one of the other four classes of antibodies. Failures in switching or failure to make a subclass of antibody leads to immunoglobulin deficiency diseases. Another mechanism that results in decreased antibody production is a defect in T–helper cells. Generally, defects in T–helper cells are listed as severe combined immunodeficiencies.

Symptoms are persistent and frequent infections, **diarrhea**, **failure to thrive**, and malabsorption (of nutrients).

KEY TERMS

Antibody—Another term for immunoglobulin. A protein molecule that specifically recognizes and attaches to infectious agents.

T–helper cell—A type of cell that recognizes foreign antigens and activates T– and B–cells in an immune response.

Diagnosis

An immunodeficiency disease is suspected when children become ill frequently, especially from the same organisms, or from organisms that don't usually cause infection. Standard treatments may also fail. The profile of organisms that cause infection in patients with immunoglobulin deficiency syndrome is unique and is preliminary evidence for this disease. Laboratory tests are performed to verify the diagnosis. Antibodies can be found in the blood. Blood is collected and analyzed for the content and types of antibodies present. Depending on the type of immunoglobulin deficiency the laboratory tests will show a decrease or absence of antibodies or specific antibody subclasses.

Treatment

Immunodeficiency diseases cannot be cured. Intravenous administration of immunoglobulin may temporarily boost immunity, but these treatments may need to be repeated at regular intervals. Acute or chronic bacterial infections are treated with **antibiotics**; antifungal drugs are also available. Very few drugs are effective against viral diseases. In severe cases, **bone marrow transplantation** may be considered and can cure some cases of immunodeficiency

Bone marrow transplantation can, in most cases, completely correct the immunodefiency.

Prognosis

Patients with immunoglobulin deficiency syndromes must practice impeccable health maintenance and care, paying particular attention to optimal dental care, in order to stay in good health.

Prevention

There is not a known way to prevent immunoglobulin deficiency syndromes.

Resources

BOOKS

Abbas, Abul K. et al. *Basic Immunology: Functions and Disorders of the Immune System*. Philadelphia: Saunders/Elsevier, 2011.

Berkow, Robert, ed. *Merck Manual of Medical Information*. Whitehouse Station, NJ: Merck Research Laboratories, 2004.

Coico, Richard. *Immunology: A Short Course*. Hoboken, NJ: Wiley–Blackwell, 2009.

Massoud, Mahmoudi. *Allergy and Asthma: Practical Diagnosis and Management*. New York: McGraw-Hill Medical, 2008.

OTHER

Bascom, Rebecca, and Marina Y Dolina. "Immunoglobulin A Deficiency." eMedicine, WebMD. (September 29, 2009), http://emedicine medscape.com/article/136580–overview (accessed September 5, 2010).

Buckley, Rebecca H. "IgA Deficiency." Merck Manuals Online Medical Library. (September 2008), http://www.merck. com/mmpe/sec13/ch164/ch164k.html (accessed September 5, 2010).

Buckley, Rebecca H. "Selective Immunoglobulin Deficiency." Merck Manuals Online Medical Library. (September 2008), http://www.merck.com/mmhe/sec16/ch184/ch184h.html?qt= Immunoglobulin deficiency&alt=sh (accessed September 5, 2010).

Dibbern, Donald A., and John M. Routes. "Immunoglobulin D Deficiency." eMedicine, WebMD. (December 2, 2009), http://emedicine.medscape.com/article/136803–overview (accessed September 5, 2010).

Hussain, Iftikhar, and Srividya Sridhara. "Immunoglobulin M Deficiency." eMedicine, WebMD. (July 21, 2009), http://emedicine.medscape.com/article/137693–overview (accessed September 5, 2010).

Lin, Robert Y., and Robert A. Schwartz. "Immunoglobulin G Deficiency." eMedicine, WebMD. (July 9, 2009), http://emedicine.medscape.com/article/136897–overview (accessed September 5, 2010).

"Merck Manuals Online Medical Library." Merck. http://www.merck.com/mmhe/index.html. (accessed September 5, 2010).

Jacqueline L. Longe

Immunoglobulin electrophoresis *see* **Immunoelectrophoresis**

Immunoglobulins G, A, and M test *see* **Immunoelectrophoresis**

Immunologic therapies

Definition

Immunologic therapy is the treatment of disease using medicines that boost the body's natural immune response.

Purpose

Immunologic therapy is used to improve the immune system's natural ability to fight diseases such as **cancer**, hepatitis and **AIDS**. These drugs may also be used to help the body recover from immunosuppression resulting from treatments such as **chemotherapy** or **radiation therapy**.

Description

Most drugs in this category are synthetic versions of substances produced naturally in the body. In their natural forms, these substances help defend the body against disease. For example, aldesleukin (Proleukin) is an artificially made form of interleukin-2, which helps white blood cells work. Aldesleukin is administered to patients with kidney cancers and skin cancers that have spread to other parts of the body. Filgrastim (Neupogen) and sargramostim (Leukine) are versions of natural substances called colony stimulating factors, which drive the bone marrow to make new white blood cells. Another type of drug, epoetin (Epogen, Procrit), is a synthetic version of human erythropoietin that stimulates the bone marrow to make new red blood cells. Thrombopoietin stimulates the production of platelets, disk-shaped bodies in the blood that are important in clotting. Interferons are substances the body produces naturally using immune cells to fight infections and tumors. The synthetic interferons carry brand names such as Alferon, Roferon or Intron A. Some of the interferons that are currently in use as drugs are Recombinant Interferon Alfa-2a,

Recombinant Interferon Alfa-2b, interferon alfa-n1 and Interferon Alfa-n3. Alfa interferons are used to treat **hairy cell leukemia**, **malignant melanoma** and AIDs-related **Kaposi's sarcoma**. In addition interferons are also used for other conditions such as laryngeal papillomatosis, **genital warts** and certain types of hepatitis.

Recommended dosage

The recommended dosage depends on the type of immunologic therapy. For some medicines, the physician will decide the dosage for each patient, taking into account a patient's weight and whether he/she is taking other medicines. Some drugs used in immunologic therapy are given only in a hospital, under a physician's supervision. For those that patients may give themselves, check with the physician who prescribed the medicine or the pharmacist who filled the prescription for the correct dosage.

Most of these drugs come in injectable form. These drugs are generally administered by the cancer care provider.

Precautions

Aldesleukin

This medicine may temporarily increase the chance of getting infections. It may also lower the number of platelets in the blood, and thus possibly interfering with the blood's ability to clot. Taking these precautions may reduce the chance of such problems:

- Avoid people with infections, if possible.
- Be alert to signs of infection, such as fever, chills, sore throat, pain in the lower back or side, cough, hoarseness, or painful or difficulty with urination. If any of these symptoms occur, get in touch with a physician immediately.
- Be alert to signs of bleeding problems, such as black, tarry stools, tiny red spots on the skin, blood in the urine or stools, or any other unusual bleeding or bruising.
- Take care to avoid cuts or other injuries. Be especially careful when using knives, razors, nail clippers and other sharp objects. Check with a dentist for the best ways to clean the teeth and mouth without injuring the gums. Do not have dental work done without checking with a physician.
- Wash hands frequently, and avoid touching the eyes or inside of the nose unless the hands have just been washed.

Aldesleukin may make some medical conditions worse, such as **chickenpox**, **shingles** (herpes zoster), **liver disease**, lung disease, heart disease, underactive thyroid, **psoriasis**, immune system problems and mental problems. The medicine may increase the chance of seizures (convulsions) in people who are prone to having them. Also, the drug's effects may be greater in people with **kidney disease**, because their kidneys are slow to clear the medicine from their bodies.

Colony stimulating factors

Certain drugs used in treating cancer reduce the body's ability to fight infections. Although colony stimulating factors help restore the body's natural defenses, the process takes time. Getting prompt treatment for infections is important, even while taking this medicine. Call the physician at the first sign of illness or infection, such as a **sore throat**, **fever** or chills.

People with certain medical conditions could have problems if they take colony stimulating factors. People who have kidney disease, liver disease or conditions caused by inflammation or immune system problems can worsen these problems with colony stimulating factors. Those who have heart disease may be more likely to experience side effects such as water retention and heart rhythm problems while taking these drugs. Finally, patients who have lung disease might increase their chances of suffering from **shortness of breath**. Those who have any of these medical conditions should check with their personal physicians before using colony stimulating factors.

Epoetin

Epoetin is a medicine that may cause seizures (convulsions), especially in people who are prone to having them. No one who takes these drugs should drive, use machines or do anything considered dangerous in case of a seizure.

Epoetin helps the body make new red blood cells, but it is not effective unless there is adequate iron in the body. The physician may recommend taking iron supplements or certain **vitamins** that help supply the body with iron. It is necessary to follow the physician's advice in this instance—recommendations for iron in this case, as with any supplements should only come from a physician.

In studies of laboratory animals, epoetin taken during **pregnancy** caused **birth defects**, including damage to the bones and spine. However, the drug has not been reported to cause problems in human babies whose mothers take it. Women who are pregnant or who may become pregnant should check with their physicians for the most up-to-date information on the safety of taking this medicine during pregnancy.

People with certain medical conditions may have problems if they take this medicine. For example, the chance of side effects may be greater in people with high blood pressure, heart or blood vessel disease or a history of **blood clots**. Epoetin may not work properly in people who have bone problems or sickle cell anemia.

Interferons

Interferons can add to the effects of alcohol and other drugs that slow down the central nervous system, such as **antihistamines**, cold medicine, allergy medicine, sleep aids, medicine for seizures, tranquilizers, some **pain** relievers, and **muscle relaxants**. They may also add to the effects of anesthetics, including those used for dental procedures. Those taking interferons should check with their physicians before taking any of the above.

Some people experience **dizziness** or unusual **fatigue**, or become less alert than usual while being treated with these drugs. Because of these possible problems, anyone who takes these drugs should not drive, use machines or do anything else considered dangerous until they have determined how the drugs affect them.

Interferons often cause flu-like symptoms, including fever and chills. The physician who prescribes this medicine may recommend taking **acetaminophen** (Tylenol) before—and sometimes after—each dose to keep the fever from getting too high. If the physician recommends this, follow instructions carefully.

Like aldesleukin, interferons may temporarily increase the chance of getting infections and lower the number of platelets in the blood, leading to clotting problems. To help prevent these problems, follow the precautions for reducing the risk of infection and bleeding listed for aldesleukin.

People who have certain medical conditions may have problems if they take interferons. For example, the drugs may worsen some medical conditions, including heart disease, kidney disease, liver disease, lung disease, diabetes, bleeding problems and mental problems. In people who have overactive immune systems, these drugs can even increase the activity of the immune system. People who have shingles or chickenpox, or who have recently been exposed to chickenpox may increase their risk of developing severe problems in other parts of the body if they take interferons. People with a history of seizures or mental problems could at risk if taking interferon.

In teenage women, interferons may cause changes in the menstrual cycle. Young women should discuss this possibility with their physicians. Older people may be more sensitive to the effects of interferons. This may increase the chance of side effects.

These drugs are not known to cause fetal **death**, birth defects or other problems in humans when taken during pregnancy. Women who are pregnant or who may become pregnant should ask their physicians for the latest information on the safety of taking these drugs during pregnancy.

Women who are **breastfeeding** their babies may need to stop while taking this medicine. Whether interferons pass into breast milk is not known. Because of the chance of serious side effects to the baby, breastfeeding while taking interferon is discouraged. Check with a physician for advice.

General precautions for all types of immunologic therapy

Regular physician visits are necessary during immunologic therapy treatment. This gives the physician a chance to make sure the medicine is working and to check for unwanted side effects.

Anyone who has had unusual reactions to drugs used in immunologic therapy should let the physician know before resuming the drugs. Any **allergies** to foods, dyes, preservatives, or other substances should also be reported.

Side effects

Aldesleukin

In addition to its helpful effects, this medicine may cause serious side effects. Generally, it is given only in a hospital, where medical professionals can watch for early signs of problems. Medical tests might be performed to check for unwanted effects.

Anyone who has breathing problems, fever or chills while being given aldesleukin should check with a physician immediately.

Other side effects should be brought to a physician's attention as soon as possible:

- dizziness
- drowsiness
- confusion
- agitation
- depression

- nausea and vomiting
- diarrhea
- sores in the mouth and on the lips
- tingling of hands or feet
- decrease in urination
- unexplained weight gain of five or more pounds

Some side effects are usually temporary and do not need medical attention unless they are bothersome. These include dry skin; itchy or burning skin; rash or redness followed by peeling; loss of appetite; and a general feeling of illness or discomfort.

Colony stimulating factors

As this medicine starts to work, the patient might experience mild pain in the lower back or hips. This is nothing to cause undue concern, and will usually go away within a few days. If the pain is intense or causes discomfort, the physician may prescribe a painkiller.

Other possible side effects include **headache**, joint or muscle pain and skin rash or **itching**. These side effects tend to disappear as the body adjusts to the medicine, and do not need medical treatment. If they continue, or they interfere with normal activities, check with a physician.

Epoetin

This medicine may cause flu-like symptoms, such as muscle aches, bone pain, fever, chills, shivering, and sweating, within a few hours after it is taken. These symptoms usually go away within 12 hours. If they do not, or if they are troubling, check with a physician. Other possible side effects that do not need medical attention are **diarrhea**, **nausea** or **vomiting** and fatigue or weakness.

Certain side effects should be brought to a physician's attention as soon as possible. These include headache, vision problems, increased blood pressure, fast heartbeat, weight gain and swelling of the face, fingers, lower legs, ankles or feet.

Anyone who has chest pain or seizures after taking epoetin should seek professional emergency medical attention immediately.

Interferons

This medicine may cause temporary hair loss (**alopecia**). While upsetting, it is not a sign that something is seriously wrong. The hair should grow back normally after treatment ends.

As the body adjusts to the medicine many other side effects usually go away during treatment. These include flu-like symptoms, taste alteration, loss of appetite (anorexia), **nausea and vomiting**, skin rash, and unusual fatigue. If these problems persist, or if they interfere with normal life, check with a physician.

A few more serious side effects should be brought to a physician's attention as soon as possible:

- confusion
- difficulty thinking or concentrating
- nervousness
- depression
- sleep problems
- numbness or tingling in the fingers, toes and face

General caution regarding side effects for all types of immunologic therapy

Other side effects are possible with any type of immunologic therapy. Anyone who has unusual symptoms during or after treatment with these drugs should should contact the physician immediately.

Interactions

Anyone who has immunologic therapy should let the physician know all other medicines being taken. Some combinations of drugs may interact, that can increase or decrease the effects of one or both drugs or can increase the likelihood of side effects. Consultation with a physician is highly recommended to get the insight on whether the possible interactions can interfere with drug therapy or cause harmful effects.

Immunoprevention

Considering that most of the biological modifiers such as cytokines elicit immune response that inhibit incipient tumors before they are clinically evident, immunoprevention has been proposed as a recent strategy for combating cancer. Treatment involving immune molecules (such as cytokines) prepared synthetically or that are not produced by the patients themselves is called as passive immunotherapy. Conversely, a vaccine is a form of active immune therapy because it elicits an immune response in patients. A cancer vaccine may be made of whole tumor cell or of substances or fragments contained in the tumor called antigens.

Newer types of immunologic therapy that are still considered investigational include cell-based therapies. Instead of using synthetic chemicals that resemble substances produced by the body, cell-based

KEY TERMS

AIDS—Acquired immune deficiency syndrome. A disease caused by infection with the human immunodeficiency virus (HIV). In people with this disease, the immune system breaks down, increasing vulnerability to other infections and some types of cancer.

Bone marrow—Soft tissue that fills the hollow centers of bones. Blood cells and platelets (disk-shaped bodies in the blood that are important in clotting) are produced in the bone marrow.

Chemotherapy—Treatment of an illness with chemical agents. The term usually is used to describe the treatment of cancer with drugs.

Clot—A hard mass that forms when blood coagulates.

Fetus—A developing baby inside the womb.

Hepatitis—Inflammation of the liver caused by a virus, chemical, or drug.

Immune response—The body's natural protective reaction to disease and infection.

Immune system—The system that protects the body against disease and infection through immune responses.

Inflammation—Pain, redness, swelling, and heat that usually develop in response to injury or illness.

Psoriasis—A skin disease that manifests itself with itchy, scaly, red patches on the skin.

Seizure—A sudden attack, spasm, or convulsion.

Shingles—A disease caused by an infection with the herpes zoster virus—the same virus that causes chickenpox. Symptoms of shingles include pain and blisters along one nerve, usually on the face, chest, stomach, or back.

Sickle cell anemia—An inherited disorder in which red blood cells contain an abnormal form of hemoglobin, a protein that carries oxygen. The abnormal form of hemoglobin causes the red cells to become sickle-shaped. The misshapen cells may clog blood vessels, preventing oxygen from reaching tissues and leading to pain, blood clots and other problems. Sickle cell anemia is most common in people of African descent and in people from Italy, Greece, India, and the Middle East.

therapies use modified stem cells or dendritic cells as vaccines against cancer. Stem cells are undifferentiated cells whose daughter cells can develop into various types of specialized cells, while dendritic cells are cells that are able to initiate and modify the immune system's responses to cancer by activating B cells and T cells. Dendritic cells appear to offer a promising new form of immunotherapy for cancer.

Another investigational form of treatment is the development of cell-free tumor-specific peptide vaccines. Peptides are subunits of protein molecules that contain two or more amino acids. Peptide vaccines are intended to induce responses in the patient's T cells that inhibit tumor growth. As of late 2003, however, peptide-based tumor vaccines have been shown to shrink cancerous tumors only in patients with limited disease.

Adoptive immunotherapy

Adoptive immunotherapy involves stimulating T lymphocytes by exposing them to tumor antigens. These modified cells are grown in the laboratory and then injected into patients. Since the cells taken from a different individual for this purpose often results in rejection, patients serve both as donor and recipient of their own T cells. Adoptive immunotherapy is particularly effective in patients who have received massive doses of radiation and chemotherapy. In such patients, therapy results in immunosuppression (weakened immune systems), making them vulnerable to viral infections. For example, CMV-specific T cells can reduce the risk of cytomegalovirus (CMV) infection in transplant patients.

Resources

PERIODICALS

Fishman, M. N., and S. J. Antonia. "Cell-Based Immune Therapy for Metastatic Renal Cancer." *Expert Review of Anticancer Therapy* 3 (December 2003): 837–849.

Nieda, M., M. Tomiyama, and K. Egawa. "Ex Vivo Enhancement of Antigen-Presenting Function of Dendritic Cells and Its Application for DC-Based Immunotherapy." *Human Cell* 16 (December 2003): 199–204.

Paczesny, S., H. Ueno, J. Fay, et al. "Dendritic Cells as Vectors for Immunotherapy of Cancer." *Seminars in Cancer Biology* 13 (December 2003): 439–447.

Rosenberg, S. A. "Progress in Human Tumor Immunology and Immunotherapy." *Nature* 411, no. 6835 (2001): 380–385.

Scheibenbogen, C., A. Letsch, A. Schmittel, et al. "Rational Peptide-Based Tumour Vaccine Development and T Cell Monitoring." *Seminars in Cancer Biology* 13 (December 2003): 423–429.

Nancy Ross-Flanigan
Kausalya Santhanam, PhD
Teresa G. Odle
Rebecca J. Frey, PhD

Immunosuppressant drugs

Definition

Immunosuppressant drugs, also called **anti-rejection drugs**, are used to prevent the body from rejecting a transplanted organ.

Purpose

When an organ, such as a liver, a heart or a kidney, is transplanted from one person (the donor) into another (the recipient), the immune system of the recipient triggers the same response against the new organ it would have to any foreign material, setting off a chain of events that can damage the transplanted organ. This process is called rejection and it can occur rapidly (acute rejection), or over a long period of time (chronic rejection). Rejection can occur despite close matching of the donated organ and the transplant patient. Immunosuppressant drugs greatly decrease the risks of rejection, protecting the new organ and preserving its function. These drugs act by blocking the immune system so that it is less likely to react against the transplanted organ. A wide variety of drugs are available to achieve this aim but work in different ways to reduce the risk of rejection.

In addition to being used to prevent organ rejection, immunosuppressant drugs are also used to treat such severe skin disorders as **psoriasis** and such other diseases as **rheumatoid arthritis**, **Crohn's disease** (chronic inflammation of the digestive tract) and patchy hair loss (**alopecia** areata). Some of these conditions are termed "autoimmune" diseases, indicating that the immune system is acting against the body itself.

Description

Immunosuppressant drugs can be classified according to their specific molecular mode of action. The three main immunosuppressant drugs currently used in organ transplantations are the following:

- Cyclosporins (Neoral, Sandimmune, SangCya). These drugs act by inhibiting T-cell activation, thus preventing T-cells from attacking the transplanted organ.
- Azathioprines (Imuran). These drugs disrupt the synthesis of DNA and RNA and cell division.
- Corticosteroids such as prednisolone (Deltasone, Orasone). These drugs suppress the inflammation associated with transplant rejection.

Most patients are prescribed a combination of drugs after their transplant, one from each of the above main groups; for example cyclosporin, azathioprine and prednisolone. Over a period of time, the doses of each drug and the number of drugs taken may be reduced as the risks of rejection decrease. However, most patients need to take at least one immunosuppressive for the rest of their lives.

Immunosuppressants can also be classified depending on the specific transplant:

- basiliximab (Simulect) is also used in combination with such other drugs as cyclosporin and corticosteroids, in kidney transplants
- daclizumab (Zenapax) is also used in combination with such other drugs as cyclosporin and corticosteroids, in kidney transplants
- muromonab CD3 (Orthoclone OKT3) is used, along with cyclosporin, in kidney, liver and heart transplants
- tacrolimus (Prograf) is used in liver transplants and is under study for kidney, bone marrow, heart, pancreas, pancreatic island cell, and small bowel transplantation

Some immunosuppressants are also used to treat a variety of autoimmune diseases:

- Azathioprine (Imuran) is used not only to prevent organ rejection in kidney transplants, but also in treatment of rheumatoid arthritis. It has been used to treat chronic ulcerative colitis, but it has been of limited value for this use.
- Cyclosporin (Sandimmune, Neoral) is used in heart, liver, kidney, pancreas, bone marrow and heart/lung transplantation. The Neoral form has been used to treat psoriasis and rheumatoid arthritis. The drug has also been used for many other conditions including multiple sclerosis, diabetes and myesthenia gravis.
- Glatiramer acetate (Copaxone) is used in treatment of relapsing-remitting multiple sclerosis. In one study, glatiramer reduced the frequency of multiple sclerosis attacks by 75% over a two-year period.

- Mycopehnolate (CellCept) is used along with cyclosporin in kidney, liver and heart transplants. It has also been used to prevent the kidney problems associated with lupus erythematosus.
- Sirolimus (Rapamune) is used in combination with other drugs including cyclosporin and corticosteroids, in kidney transplants. The drug is also used for the treatment of psoriasis.

Recommended dosage

Immunosuppressant drugs are available only with a physician's prescription. They come in tablet, capsule, liquid and injectable forms.

The recommended dosage depends on the type and form of immunosuppressant drug and the purpose for which it is being used. Doses may be different for different patients. The prescribing physician or the pharmacist who filled the prescription will advise on correct dosage.

Taking immunosuppressant drugs exactly as directed is very important. Smaller, larger or more frequent doses should never be taken, and the drugs should never be taken for longer than directed. The physician will decide exactly how much of the medicine each patient needs. Blood tests often are necessary to monitor the action of the drug.

The prescribing physician should be consulted before stopping an immunosuppressant drug.

Precautions

Seeing a physician regularly while taking immunosuppressant drugs is important. These regular check-ups will allow the physician to make sure the drug is working as it should and to watch for unwanted side effects. These drugs are very powerful and can cause serious side effects, such as high blood pressure, kidney problems and liver problems. Some side effects may not show up until years after the medicine is used. Anyone who has been advised to take immunosuppressant drugs should thoroughly discuss the risks and benefits with the prescribing physician

Immunosuppressant drugs lower a person's resistance to infection and can make infections harder to treat. The drugs can also increase the chance of uncontrolled bleeding. Anyone who has a serious infection or injury while taking immunosuppressant drugs should get prompt medical attention and should make sure that the treating physician knows about the immunosuppressant prescription. The prescribing physician should be immediately informed if signs of infection, such as **fever** or chills, **cough** or hoarseness, **pain** in the lower back or side, or painful or difficult urination, bruising or bleeding, blood in the urine, bloody or black, tarry stools occur. Other ways of preventing infection and injury include washing the hands frequently, avoiding sports in which injuries may occur, and being careful when using knives, razors, fingernail clippers or other sharp objects. Avoiding contact with people who have infections is also important. In addition, people who are taking or have been taking immunosuppressant drugs should not have immunizations, such as **smallpox** vaccinations, without checking with their physicians. Because of their low resistance to infection, people taking these drugs might get the disease that the vaccine is designed to prevent. People taking immunosuppressant drugs also should avoid contact with anyone who has taken the oral **polio** vaccine, as there is a chance the virus could be passed on to them. Other people living in their home should not take the oral polio vaccine.

Immunosuppressant drugs may cause the gums to become tender and swollen or to bleed. If this happens, a physician or dentist should be notified. Regular brushing, flossing, cleaning and gum massage may help prevent this problem. A dentist can provide advice on how to clean the teeth and mouth without causing injury.

Special conditions

People who have certain medical conditions or who are taking certain other medicines may have problems if they take immunosuppressant drugs. Before taking these drugs, the prescribing physician should be informed about any of these conditions:

ALLERGIES. Anyone who has had unusual reactions to immunosuppressant drugs in the past should let his or her physician know before taking the drugs again. The physician should also be told about any **allergies** to foods, dyes, preservatives, or other substances.

PREGNANCY. Azathioprine may cause **birth defects** if used during **pregnancy**, or if either the male or female is using it at time of conception. Anyone taking this medicine should use a barrier method of birth control, such as a diaphragm or **condoms**. Birth control pills should not be used without a physician's approval. Women who become pregnant while taking this medicine should check with their physicians immediately.

The medicine's effects have not been studied in humans during pregnancy. Women who are pregnant or who may become pregnant and who need to take this medicine should check with their physicians.

KEY TERMS

Antibody—Protein produced by the immune system in response to the presence in the body of an antigen.

Antigen—Any substance or organism that is foreign to the body. Examples of antigens are: bacteria, bacterial toxins, viruses, or other cells or proteins.

Autoimmune disease—A disease in which the immune system is overactive and has lost the ability to distinguish between self and non-self.

Chronic—A word used to describe a long-lasting condition. Chronic conditions often develop gradually and involve slow changes.

Corticosteroids—A class of drugs that are synthetic versions of the cortisone produced by the body. They rank among the most powerful anti-inflammatory agents.

Cortisone—Glucocorticoid produced by the adrenal cortex in response to stress. Cortisone is a steroid with anti-inflammatory and immunosuppressive properties.

Inflammation—A process occurring in body tissues, characterized by increased circulation and the accumulation of white blood cells. Inflammation also occurs in such disorders as arthritis and causes harmful effects.

Inflammatory—Pertaining to inflammation.

Immune response—Physiological response of the body controlled by the immune system that involves the production of antibodies to fight off specific foreign substances or agents (antigens).

Immune system—The network of organs, cells, and molecules that work together to defend the body from foreign substances and organisms causing infection and disease such as: bacteria, viruses, fungi and parasites.

Immunosuppressant—Any chemical substance that suppresses the immune response.

Immunosuppressive—Any agent that suppresses the immune response of an individual.

Immunosuppressive cytotoxic drugs—A class of drugs that function by destroying cells and suppressing the immune response.

Lymphocyte—Lymphocytes are white blood cells that participate in the immune response. The two main groups are the B cells that have antibody molecules on their surface and T cells that destroy antigens.

Psoriasis—A skin disease characterized by itchy, scaly, red patches on the skin.

Rejection—Rejection occurs when the body recognizes a new transplanted organ as "foreign" and turns on the immune system of the body.

T cells—Any of several lymphocytes that have specific antigen receptors, and that are involved in cell-mediated immunity and destruction of antigen-bearing cells.

Transplantation—The removal of tissue from one part of the body for implantation to another part of the body; or the removal of tissue or an organ from one individual and its implantation in another individual by surgery.

BREASTFEEDING. Immunosuppressant drugs pass into breast milk and may cause problems in nursing babies whose mothers take it. **Breastfeeding** is not recommended for women taking this medicine.

OTHER MEDICAL CONDITIONS. People who have certain medical conditions may have problems if they take immunosuppressant drugs. For example:

- People who have shingles (herpes zoster) or chickenpox, or who have recently been exposed to chickenpox, may develop severe disease in other parts of their bodies when they take these medicines.
- The medicine's effects may be greater in people with kidney disease or liver disease, because their bodies are slow to get rid of the medicine.
- The effects of oral forms of this medicine may be weakened in people with intestinal problems, because the medicine cannot be absorbed into the body.

Before using immunosuppressant drugs, people with these or other medical problems should make sure their physicians are aware of their conditions.

USE OF CERTAIN MEDICINES. Taking immunosuppressant drugs with certain other drugs may affect the way the drugs work or may increase the chance of side effects.

Side effects

Increased risk of infection is a common side effect of all the immunosuppressant drugs. The immune system protects the body from infections and when the immune system is suppressed, infections are more likely. Taking such **antibiotics** as co-trimoxazole prevents some of these infections. Immunosuppressant drugs are also associated with a slightly increased risk of **cancer** because the immune system also plays a role in protecting the body against some forms of cancer. For example, long-term use of immunosuppressant drugs carries an increased risk of developing skin cancer as a result of the combination of the drugs and exposure to sunlight.

Other side effects of immunosuppressant drugs are minor and usually go away as the body adjusts to the medicine. These include loss of appetite, **nausea** or **vomiting**, increased hair growth, and trembling or shaking of the hands. Medical attention is not necessary unless these side effects continue or cause problems.

The treating physician should be notified immediately if any of the following side effects occur:

- unusual tiredness or weakness
- fever or chills
- frequent need to urinate

Interactions

Immunosuppressant drugs may interact with other medicines. When this happens, the effects of one or both drugs may change or the risk of side effects may be greater. Other drugs may also have an adverse effect on immunosuppressant therapy. This is particularly important for patients taking cyclosporin or tacrolimus. For example, some drugs can cause the blood levels to rise, while others can cause the blood levels to fall and it is important to avoid such contraindicated combinations. Other examples are:

- The effects of azathioprine may be greater in people who take allopurinol, a medicine used to treat gout.
- A number of drugs, including female hormones (estrogens), male hormones (androgens), the antifungal drug ketoconazole (Nizoral), the ulcer drug cimetidine (Tagamet) and the erythromycins (used to treat infections), may increase the effects of cyclosporine.
- When sirolimus is taken at the same time as cyclosporin, the blood levels of sirolimus may be increased to a level where there are severe side effects. Although these two drugs are usually used together, the sirolimus should be taken four hours after the dose of cyclosporin.
- Tacrolimus is eliminated through the kidneys. When the drug is used with other drugs that may harm the kidneys, such as cyclosporin, the antibiotics gentamicin and amikacin, or the antifungal drug amphotericin B, blood levels of tacrolimus may be increased. Careful kidney monitoring is essential when tacrolimus is given with any drug that might cause kidney damage.
- The risk of cancer or infection may be greater when immunosuppressant drugs are combined with certain other drugs which also lower the body's ability to fight disease and infection. These drugs include corticosteroids such as prednisone; the anticancer drugs chlorambucil (Leukeran), cyclophosphamide (Cytoxan) and mercaptopurine (Purinethol); and the monoclonal antibody muromonab-CD3 (Orthoclone), which also is used to prevent transplanted organ rejection.

Not every drug that may interact with immunosuppressant drugs is listed here. Anyone who takes immunosuppressant drugs should let the physician know all other medicines he or she is taking and should ask whether the possible interactions can interfere with treatment.

Resources

BOOKS

Abbas, Abul K., and Andrew H. Lichtman. *Basic Immunology: Functions and Disorders of the Immune System.* 3rd ed. Updated. Philadelphia: Saunders/Elsevier, 2011.

Janeway, Charles, et al. *Immunobiology: The Immune System in Health and Disease*. 6th ed. New York: Garland Science, 200.

Sompayrac, Lauren. *How the Immune System Works*. 3rd ed. Malden, MA: Blackwell, 2009.

Nancy Ross-Flanigan

Immunotherapy *see* **Immunologic therapies**

Impacted tooth

Definition

An impacted tooth is any tooth that is prevented from reaching its normal position in the mouth by tissue, bone, or another tooth.

Description

The teeth that most commonly become impacted are the third molars, also called wisdom teeth. These large teeth are the last to develop, beginning to form when a person is about nine years old, but not breaking through the gum tissue until the late teens or early twenties. By this time, the jaws have stopped growing and may be too small to accommodate these four additional teeth. As the wisdom teeth continue to move, one or more may become impacted, either by running into the teeth next to them or becoming blocked within the jawbone or gum

KEY TERMS

Dry socket—A painful condition following tooth extraction in which a blood clot does not properly fill the empty socket, leaving the bone underneath exposed to air and food.

Eruption—The process of a tooth breaking through the gum tissue to grow into place in the mouth.

Extraction—The removal of a tooth from its socket in the bone.

Pericoronitis—A gum condition in which irritation and inflammation are produced by the crown of an incompletely erupted tooth.

Wisdom tooth—One of the four last teeth on the top and bottom rows of teeth. Also called a third molar.

tissue. An impacted tooth can cause further dental problems, including infection of the gums, displacement of other teeth, or decay. At least one wisdom tooth becomes impacted in nine of every ten people.

Causes and Symptoms

The movement of an erupting wisdom tooth and any subsequent impaction may produce **pain** at the back of the jaw. Pain may also be the result of infection, either from decay in any exposed portion of the tooth or from trapped food and plaque in the surrounding gum tissue. Infection typically produces an unpleasant taste when biting down and **bad breath**. Another source of pain may be pericoronitis, a gum condition in which the crown of the incompletely erupted tooth produces inflammation, redness, and tenderness of the gums. Less common symptoms of an impacted tooth are swollen lymph nodes in the neck, difficulty opening the mouth, and prolonged **headache**.

Diagnosis

Upon visual examination, the dentist may find signs of infection or swelling in the area where the tooth is present or only partially erupted. **Dental x rays** are necessary to confirm tooth impaction.

Treatment

Because impacted teeth may cause dental problems with few if any symptoms to indicate damage, dentists commonly recommend the removal of all wisdom teeth, preferably while the patient is still a young adult. A dentist may perform an extraction with forceps and local anesthetic if the tooth is exposed and appears to be easily removable in one piece. However, he or she may refer a difficult extraction to an oral surgeon, a specialist who administers either nitrous oxide-oxygen (commonly called "laughing gas"), an intravenous sedative, or a general anesthetic to alleviate any pain or discomfort during the surgical procedure. Extracting an impacted tooth typically requires cutting through gum tissue to expose the tooth, and may require removing portions of bone to free the tooth. The tooth may have to be removed in pieces to minimize destruction to the surrounding structures. The extraction site may or may not require one or more stitches to help the incision heal.

Prognosis

The prognosis is very good when impacted teeth are removed from young healthy adults without complications. Potential complications include postoperative infection, temporary **numbness** from nerve irritation, jaw fracture, and jaw joint pain. An additional condition which may develop is called dry socket: when a blood clot does not properly form in the empty tooth socket, or is disturbed by an oral vacuum (such as from drinking through a straw or **smoking**), the bone beneath the socket is painfully exposed to air and food, and the extraction site heals more slowly.

ORGANIZATIONS

American Association of Oral & Maxillofacial Surgeons, 9700 West Bryn Mawr Avenue, Rosemont, IL, 60018-5701, 847 678-6200, 847 678-6286, 800 822-6637, http://www.aaoms.org.

Bethany Thivierge

Impedance phlebography

Definition

Impedance phlebography is a noninvasive test that uses electrical monitoring to measure blood flow in veins of the leg. Information from this test helps a doctor to detect **deep vein thrombosis** (**blood clots** or **thrombophlebitis**).

Purpose

Impedance phlebography may be done in order to:

- detect blood clots lodged in the deep veins of the leg

- screen patients who are likely to have blood clots in the leg
- detect the source of blood clots in the lungs (pulmonary emboli)

Blood clots in the legs can lead to more serious problems. If a clot breaks loose from a leg vein, it may travel to the lungs and lodge in a blood vessel in the lungs. Blood clots are more likely to occur in people who have recently had leg injuries, surgery, **cancer**, or a long period of bed rest.

Precautions

Because this test is not invasive, it can be done on all patients. However, the accuracy of the results will be affected if the patient does not breathe normally or keep the leg muscles relaxed. Compression of the veins because of pelvic tumors or decreased blood flow, due to **shock** or any condition that reduces the amount of blood the heart pumps, may also change the test results.

Description

Impedance phlebography works by measuring the resistance to the transmission of electrical energy (impedance). This resistance changes depending on the volume of blood flowing through the veins. By graphing the impedance, a doctor or technician can tell whether a clot is obstructing blood flow.

Using conductive jelly, the examiner puts electrodes on the patient's calf. These electrodes are connected to an instrument called a plethysmograph, which records the changes in electrical resistance that occur during the test.

The patient lies down and raises one leg at a 30° angle, so that the calf is above the level of the heart. The examiner wraps a pressure cuff around the patient's thigh and inflates it to a pressure of 45–60 cm of water for 45 seconds. The plethysmograph records the electrical changes that correspond to changes in the volume of blood in the vein at the time the pressure is exerted and again three seconds after the cuff is deflated. This procedure is repeated several times in both legs.

This test takes 30 to 45 minutes. Impedance phlebography is also called an impedance test of blood flow or impedance plethysmography.

Preparation

Patients undergoing this test do not need to alter their diet, change their normal activities, or stop taking any medications. They will wear a surgical gown during the test, and be asked to urinate before the test starts. If keeping the legs elevated causes discomfort, mild **pain** medication will be given.

KEY TERMS

Thrombophlebitis—Inflammation of a vein, associated with the formation of a blood clot.

Aftercare

The patient may resume normal or postoperative activities after the test.

Risks

Impedance phlebography is painless and safe. It presents no risk to the patient.

Normal results

Normally, inflating the pressure cuff will cause a sharp rise in the pressure in the veins of the calf because blood flow is blocked. When the cuff is released, the pressure decreases rapidly as the blood flows away.

Abnormal results

If a clot is present, the pressure in the calf veins will already be high. It does not become sharply higher when the pressure cuff is tightened. When the pressure cuff is deflated, the clot blocks the flow of blood out of the calf vein. The decrease in pressure is not as rapid as when no clot is present, and the shape of the resulting graph is different.

Resources

OTHER

Griffith, H. Winter. "Complete Guide to Medical Tests." *ThriveOnline*. http://thriveonline.oxygen.com.

Tish Davidson, A.M.

Impedance plethysmography *see* **Impedance phlebography**

Impedance test of blood flow *see* **Impedance phlebography**

Impetigo

Definition

Impetigo refers to a very localized bacterial infection of the skin. There are two types, bullous and epidemic.

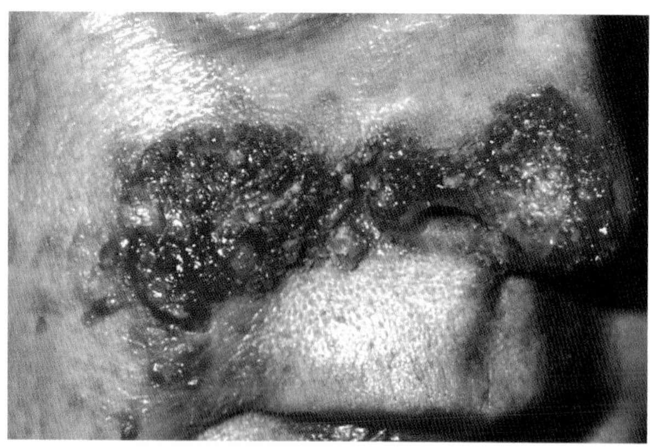

Impetigo is a contagious bacterial skin infection that mostly affects the area around the nose and mouth. Usually caused by staphylococci, this person's impetigo was triggered by herpes simplex. *(Photo Researchers, Inc.)*

KEY TERMS

Systemic—Involving the whole body; the opposite of localized.

Ulcer—An irritated pit in the surface of a tissue.

Vesicle—A bump on the skin filled with fluid.

Description

Impetigo is a skin infection that tends primarily to afflict children. Impetigo caused by the bacterium *Staphylococcus aureus* (also known as staph) affects children of all ages. Impetigo caused by the bacteria called group A streptococci (also know as strep) are most common in children ages two to five.

The bacteria that cause impetigo are very contagious. They can be spread by a child from one part of his or her body to another by scratching, or contact with a towel, clothing, or stuffed animal. These same methods can pass the bacteria on from one person to another.

Impetigo tends to develop in areas of the skin that have already been damaged through some other mechanism (a cut or scrape, burn, insect bite, or vesicle from **chickenpox**).

Causes and symptoms

The first sign of bullous impetigo is a large bump on the skin with a clear, fluid-filled top (called a vesicle). The bump develops a scab-like, honey-colored crust. There is usually no redness or **pain**, although the area may be quite itchy. Ultimately, the skin in this area will become dry and flake away. Bullous impetigo is usually caused by staph bacteria.

Epidemic impetigo can be caused by staph or strep bacteria, and (as the name implies) is very easily passed among children. Certain factors, such as heat and humidity, crowded conditions, and poor hygiene increase the chance that this type of impetigo will spread rapidly among large groups of children. This type of impetigo involves the formation of a small vesicle surrounded by a circle of reddened skin. The vesicles appear first on the face and legs. When a child has several of these vesicles close together, they may spread to one another. The skin surface may become eaten away (ulcerated), leaving irritated pits. When there are many of these deep, pitting ulcers, with pus in the center and brownish-black scabs, the condition is called ecthyma. If left untreated, the type of bacteria causing this type of impetigo has the potential to cause a serious **kidney disease** called **glomerulonephritis**. Even when impetigo is initially caused by strep bacteria, the vesicles are frequently secondarily infected with staph bacteria.

Impetigo is usually an uncomplicated skin condition. Left untreated, however, it may develop into a serious disease, including **osteomyelitis** (bone infection), septic arthritis (joint infection), or **pneumonia**. If large quantities of bacteria are present and begin circulating in the bloodstream, the child is in danger of developing an overwhelming systemic infection known as **sepsis**.

Diagnosis

Characteristic appearance of the skin is the usual method of diagnosis, although fluid from the vesicles can be cultured and then examined in an attempt to identify the causative bacteria.

Treatment

Uncomplicated impetigo is usually treated with a topical antibiotic cream called mupirocin. In more serious, widespread cases of impetigo, or when the child has a **fever** or **swollen glands**, **antibiotics** may be given by mouth or even through a needle placed in a vein (intravenously).

Prognosis

Prognosis for a child with impetigo is excellent. The vast majority of children recover quickly, completely, and uneventfully.

Prevention

Prevention involves good hygiene. Handwashing; never sharing towels, clothing, or stuffed animals; and keeping fingernails well-trimmed are easy precautions to take to avoid spreading the infection from one person to another.

Resources

OTHER

Rockoff, Alan. "Impetigo (Impetigo Contagiosa)." MedicineNet. com. http://www.medicinenet.com/impetigo/article.htm (accessed November 22, 2010).

Rosalyn Carson-DeWitt, MD

Implant therapy *see* **Radioactive implants**

Implantable cardioverter-defibrillator

Definition

The implantable cardioverter-defibrillator is an electronic device to treat life-threatening heartbeat irregularities. It is surgically implanted.

Purpose

The implantable cardioverter-defibrillator is used to detect and stop serious ventricular **arrhythmias** and restore a normal heartbeat in people who are at high risk of sudden **death**. The American Heart Association recommends that implantable cardioverter-defibrillators only be considered for patients who have a life-threatening arrhythmia. A recent study by the National Heart, Lung, and Blood Institute demonstrated that implantable cardioverter-defibrillators are the treatment of choice instead of drug therapy for patients who have had a cardiac arrest or **heart attack** and are at risk for developing **ventricular tachycardia**, which is a very rapid heartbeat, or **ventricular fibrillation**, which is an ineffective, irregular heart activity. Other studies suggest that 20% of these high risk patients would die within two years without an implantable cardioverter-defibrillator. With the device, the five-year risk of sudden death drops to five percent.

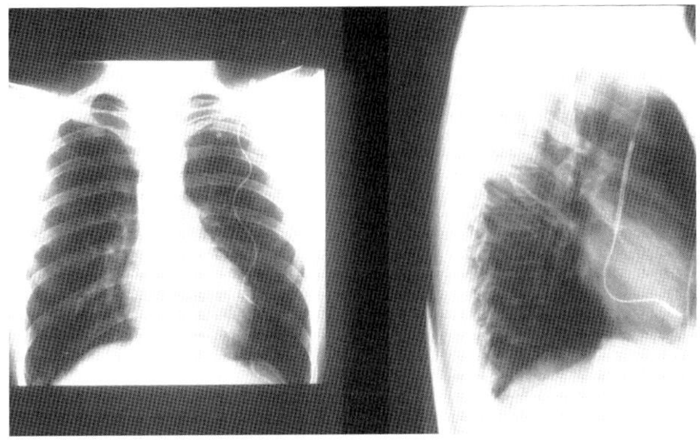

X ray of implanted cardioverter-defibrillator. *(Custom Medical Stock Photo, Inc. Reproduced by permission.)*

Precautions

The implantable cardioverter-defibrillator should not be used on patients who faint from causes other than a known life-threatening ventricular arrhythmia, to treat slow heart rates, or during an emergency.

Description

According to the American College of Cardiology, more than 80,000 Americans currently have an implantable cardioverter-defibrillator; 17,000 of these were implanted in 1995 alone. The battery-powered device rescues the patient from a life-threatening arrhythmia by rapid pacing and/or delivering electrical shock(s) to suspend heart activity and then allow it to initiate a normal rhythm. Before the development of the implantable cardioverter-defibrillator, most people who experienced ventricular fibrillation and were not near a hospital with a well equipped emergency team died within minutes.

The implantable cardioverter-defibrillator is like a mini computer connected to the patient's heart. Newer models weigh less than 10 ounces and can be implanted beneath the skin of the chest in the pectoral region, without major surgery. A lead from the device is then inserted into the heart through a vein. The procedure is performed in an operating room under **general anesthesia**. Earlier versions of implantable cardioverter-defibrillators were implanted in the abdomen and required open-chest surgery to connect the electrodes to the left and right ventricles.

The implantable cardioverter-defibrillator is set above the patient's **exercise** heart rate. Once the device is in place, many tests will be conducted to ensure that the device is sensing and defibrillating properly. The newer implantable cardioverter-defibrillators last seven or eight years. Technology and procedures continue to evolve.

KEY TERMS

Arrhythmia—A variation of the normal rhythm of the heartbeat.

Cardioverter—A device to apply electric shock to the chest to convert an abnormal heartbeat into a normal heartbeat.

Defibrillation—An electronic process which helps re-establish a normal heart rhythm.

Ventricles—The two large lower chambers of the heart which pump blood to the lungs and the rest of the human body.

Ventricular fibrillation—An arrhythmia in which the heart beats very fast but blood is not pumped out to the body. Ventricular fibrillation can quickly become fatal if not corrected.

Ventricular tachycardia—An arrhythmia in which the heart rate is more than 100 beats per minute.

Preparation

Before the procedure, a complete medical history and physical exam will be done. **Electrocardiography**, special electrophysiologic testing, **chest x ray**, **urinalysis**, and a blood test are usually also required.

Aftercare

The patient is monitored for arrhythmias and to ensure that the implantable cardioverter-defibrillator is working properly. The physician also watches for signs of infection. Before the patient leaves the hospital, the device is tested again. Anti-arrhythmia drug therapy is necessary in more than half of all patients with implantable cardioverter-defibrillators, but the number of drugs and the dosages are usually reduced. Any time a significant change in anti-arrhythmia medication is made, the device will be tested again.

The patient is taught how the device works, and that the shock it delivers will feel like a punch or kick in the chest. The patient is told to notify his/her physician when the implantable cardioverter-defibrillator delivers a shock, and to go to the emergency room if multiple shocks are sent within a short period of time.

Although most patients with implantable cardioverter-defibrillators are glad that they have the device and feel that it has extended their lives, they do experience fear and **anxiety**. This stems from the sensation of the shock(s), the unpredictable circumstances under which shock(s) occurs, and unknown outcomes.

Risks

There can be serious complications to the implantation of a cardioverter-defibrillator. These include inflammation of the pericardium, the sac that surrounds the heart; heart attack; congestive **heart failure**; and post-operative **stroke**. Serious infections can develop in the area around the device while the patient is initially hospitalized or up to several months later. Death due to the device's failure while being tested during surgery is an uncommon risk. The risk of death from the implantation procedure is about the same as that for a pacemaker, less than one percent. There are also potentially serious risks associated with the device's improper functioning once it is in place.

ORGANIZATIONS

American Heart Association National Center, 7272 Greenville Avenue, Dallas, TX, 75231, 800 242-8721, Review.personal.info@heart.org.

Texas Heart Institute. Heart Information Service, MC 3-116, PO Box 20345, Houston, TX, 77225, 832 355-4011, 800 292-2221, http://www.texasheart.org.

Lori De Milto

Impotence

Definition

Impotence, often called **erectile dysfunction**, is the inability to achieve or maintain an erection long enough to engage in sexual intercourse.

Description

Under normal circumstances, when a man is sexually stimulated, his brain sends a message down the spinal cord and into the nerves of the penis. The nerve endings in the penis release chemical messengers, called neurotransmitters, that signal the corpora cavernosa (the two spongy rods of tissue that span the length of the penis) to relax and fill with blood. As they expand, the corpora cavernosa close off other veins that would normally drain blood from the penis. As the penis becomes engorged with blood, it enlarges and stiffens, causing an erection. Problems with blood vessels, nerves, or tissues of the penis can interfere with an erection.

Causes and symptoms

It is estimated that up to 20 million American men frequently suffer from impotence and that it strikes up to half of all men between the ages of 40 and 70. Doctors used to think that most cases of impotence were psychological in origin, but they now recognize that, at least in older men, physical causes may play a primary role in 60% or more of all cases. In men over the age of 60, the leading cause is **atherosclerosis**, or narrowing of the arteries, which can restrict the flow of blood to the penis. Injury or disease of the connective tissue, such as **Peyronie's disease**, may prevent the corpora cavernosa from completely expanding. Damage to the nerves of the penis, from certain types of surgery or neurological conditions, such as Parkinson's disease or **multiple sclerosis**, may also cause impotence. Men with diabetes are especially at risk for impotence because of their high risk of both atherosclerosis and a nerve disease called **diabetic neuropathy**.

Certain types of blood pressure medications, antiulcer drugs, **antihistamines**, tranquilizers (especially before intercourse), antifungals (hetoconazole), antipsychotics, **antianxiety drugs**, and antidepressants, known as **selective serotonin reuptake inhibitors** (SSRIs, including Prozac and Paxil), can interfere with erectile function. **Smoking**, excessive alcohol consumption, and illicit drug use may also contribute. In rare cases, low levels of the male hormone testosterone may contribute to erectile failure. Finally, psychological factors, such as **stress**, guilt, or anxiety, may also play a role, even when the impotence is primarily due to organic causes.

Diagnosis

The doctor also obtains a thorough medical history to find out about past pelvic surgery, diabetes, cardiovascular disease, **kidney disease**, and any medications the man may be taking. The **physical examination** should include a genital examination, a measurement of blood flow through the penis, hormone tests, and a glucose test for diabetes.

In some cases, nocturnal penile tumescence testing is performed to find out whether the man has erections while asleep. Healthy men usually have about four or five erections throughout the night. The man applies a device to the penis called a Rigiscan before going to bed at night, and the device can determine whether he has had erections. (If a man is able to have normal erections at night, this suggests a psychological cause for his impotence.)

Treatment

Years ago, the standard treatment for impotence was an implantable penile prosthesis or long-term **psychotherapy**. Although physical causes are now more readily diagnosed and treated, individual or marital counseling is still an effective treatment for impotence when emotional factors play a role. Fortunately, other approaches are now available to treat the physical causes of impotence.

Medications

The first line and by far the most common treatment today is with the prescription drug **sildenafil citrate**, sold under the brand name Viagra. An estimated 20 million prescriptions for the pill have been filled since it was approved by the FDA in March 1998. It is also the most effective treatment with a success rate of more than 60%. The drug boosts levels of a substance called cyclic GMP, which is responsible for widening the blood vessels of the penis. In clinical studies, Viagra produced headaches in 16% of men who took it, and other side effects included flushing, **indigestion**, and stuffy nose.

The primary drawback to Viagra, which works about an hour after it is taken, it that the FDA cautions men with heart disease or low blood pressure to be thoroughly examined by a physician before obtaining a prescription.

In the summer of 2002, two investigational drugs were announced to become available in the near future to also treat erectile dysfunction. Vardenafil and tadalafil both helped men who also had such conditions as diabetes, high blood pressure and benign prostatic hypertrophy. The drugs are now available via prescription.

Vardenafil and tadalafil belong to the same group of chemical compounds as sildenafil, namely phosphodiesterase type 5 (PDE-5) inhibitors. Some men cannot benefit from sildenafil or the two newer PDE-5 inhibitors because they have low levels of nitric oxide. British investigators reported in late 2002 that three different types of compounds are being studied as possible medications for men with low levels of nitric oxide. They are Rho-kinase inhibitors, soluble guanylate cyclase activators, and nitric oxide-releasing PDE-5 inhibitors.

Other medications under investigation as treatments for impotence are topical agents. Topical means that they are applied externally to the skin rather than being injected or taken by mouth. If approved, these drugs would provide a noninvasive

KEY TERMS

Alprostadil—A smooth muscle relaxant sometimes injected into the penis or applied to the urethral opening to treat impotence.

Atherosclerosis—A disorder in which plaques of cholesterol, lipids, and other debris build up on the inner walls of arteries, narrowing them.

Corpus cavernosum (plural, corpora cavernosa)—One of two rods of spongy tissue in the penis that become engorged with blood in order to produce an erection.

Gene therapy—A method of treating a disorder by replacing damaged or abnormal genes with normal ones. Some researchers think that gene therapy may offer a new way to treat impotence.

Neurotransmitters—Chemicals that modify or help transmit impulses between nerve synapses.

Papaverine—A smooth muscle relaxant sometimes injected into the penis as a treatment for impotence.

Peyronie's disease—A disease resulting from scarring of the corpus cavernosa, causing painful erections.

Topical—A type of medication that is applied to a specific and limited area of skin, and affects only the area to which it is applied.

Urethra—The small tube that drains urine from the bladder, as well as serving as a conduit for semen during ejaculation in men.

Viagra—Trade name of an orally administered drug for erectile failure first cleared for marketing in the United States in March 1998. Its generic name is sildenafil citrate.

alternative for men who cannot take sildenafil or other oral medications for impotence.

Injection therapy involves injecting a substance into the penis to enhance blood flow and cause an erection. The Food and Drug Administration (FDA) approved a drug called alprostadil (Caverject) for this purpose in July of 1995. Alprostadil relaxes smooth muscle tissue to enhance blood flow into the penis. It must be injected shortly before intercourse. Another, similar drug that is sometimes used is papaverine—not yet been approved by the FDA for this use. Either drug may sometimes cause painful erections or **priapism** (uncomfortable, prolonged erections) that must be treated with a shot of epinephrine.

Alprostadil may also be administered into the urethral opening of the penis. In MUSE (medical urethral system for erection), the man inserts a thin tube the width of a vermicelli noodle into his urethral opening and presses down on a plunger to deliver a tiny pellet containing alprostadil into his penis. The drug takes about 10 minutes to work and the erection lasts about an hour. The main side effect is a sensation of **pain** and burning in the urethra, which can last about five to 15 minutes.

Mechanical and surgical treatments

Another approach is vacuum therapy. The man inserts his penis into a clear plastic cylinder and uses a pump to force air out of the cylinder. This forms a partial vacuum around the penis, which helps to draw blood into the corpora cavernosa. The man then places a special ring over the base of the penis to trap the blood inside it. The only side effect with this type of treatment is occasional bruising if the vacuum is left on too long.

Implantable **penile prostheses** are usually considered a last resort for treating impotence. They are implanted in the corpora cavernosa to make the penis rigid without the need for blood flow. The semi-rigid type of prosthesis consists of a pair of flexible silicone rods that can be bent up or down. This type of device has a low failure rate but, unfortunately, it causes the penis to always be erect, which can be difficult to conceal under clothing.

The inflatable type of device consists of cylinders that are implanted in the corpora cavernosa, a fluid reservoir implanted in the abdomen, and a pump placed in the scrotum. The man squeezes the pump to move fluid into the cylinders and cause them to become rigid. (He reverses the process by squeezing the pump again.) While these devices allow for intermittent erections, they have a slightly higher malfunction rate than the silicon rods.

Men can return to sexual activity six to eight weeks after implantation surgery. Since implants affect the corpora cavernosa, they permanently take away a man's ability to have a natural erection.

In rare cases, if narrowed or diseased veins are responsible for impotence, surgeons may reroute the blood flow into the corpus cavernosa or remove leaking vessels. However, the success rate with these procedures has been very low, and they are still considered experimental.

Gene therapy

A newer investigational approach to the treatment of erectile dysfunction is **gene therapy**. As of late 2002, several preclinical studies have shown promise, but none of the gene-based strategies so far have yet been tested for safety.

Alternative treatment

A number of herbs have been promoted for treating impotence. The most widely touted herbs for this purpose are *Coryanthe yohimbe* (available by prescription as yohimbine, with the trade name Yocon) and gingko (*Gingko biloba*), although neither has been conclusively shown to help the condition in controlled studies. In addition, gingko carries some risk of abnormal blood clotting and should be avoided by men taking blood thinners such as coumadin. Other herbs promoted for treating impotence include true unicorn root (*Aletrius farinosa*), **saw palmetto** (*Serenoa repens*), **ginseng** (*Panax ginseng*), and Siberian ginseng (*Eleuthrococcus senticosus*). *Strychnos Nux vomica* has been recommended, especially when impotence is caused by excessive alcohol, cigarettes, or dietary indiscretions, but it can be very toxic if taken improperly, so it should be used only under the strict supervision of a physician trained in its use.

Prognosis

With proper diagnosis, impotence can nearly always be treated or managed successfully. Unfortunately, fewer than 10% of impotent men seek treatment.

Prevention

There is no specific treatment to prevent impotence. Perhaps the most important measure is to maintain general good health and avoid atherosclerosis by exercising regularly, controlling weight, controlling **hypertension** and high cholesterol levels, and avoiding smoking. Avoiding excessive alcohol intake may also help.

Resources

BOOKS

Beers, Mark H., Robert S. Porter, and Thomas V. Jones, eds. *The Merck Manual of Diagnosis and Therapy*. 18th ed. Whitehouse Station, NJ: Merck Research Laboratories, 2006.

McVary, Kevin T.*Contemporary Treatment of Erectile Dysfunction: A Clinical Guide*. Totowa, NJ: Humana, 2010.

Tsertsvadze, Alexander.*Diagnosis and Treatment of Erectile Dysfunction*. Rockville, MD: Agency for Healthcare Research and Quality, 2009.

PERIODICALS

Campbell, Adam. "Soft Science: The Exclusive World on Which Sex Supplements May Help and Which Won't." *Men's Health* May 2002: 100.

Cellek, S., R. W. Rees, and J. Kalsi. "A Rho-Kinase Inhibitor, Soluble Guanylate Cyclase Activator and Nitric Oxide-Releasing PDE5 Inhibitor: Novel Approaches to Erectile Dysfunction." *Expert Opinion on Investigational Drugs* 11 (November 2002): 1563–1573.

Christ, G. J. "Gene Therapy for Erectile Dysfunction: Where Is It Going?" *Current Opinion in Urology* 12 (November 2002): 497–501.

Gresser, U., and C. H. Gleiter. "Erectile Dysfunction: Comparison of Efficacy and Side Effects of the PDE-5 Inhibitors Sildenafil, Vardenafil and Tadalafil—Review of the Literature." *European Journal of Medical Research* 7 (October 29, 2002): 435–446.

"Is Viagra Safe?" *Internal Medicine Alert* June 29, 2002: 90.

Norton, Patrice G.W. "Investigational Drugs in Erectile Dysfunction. (Vardenafil, Tadalafil)." *Internal Medicine News* June 1, 2002: 50.

Yap, R. L., and K. T. McVary. "Topical Agents and Erectile Dysfunction: Is There a Place?" *Current Urology Reports* 3 (December 2002): 471–476.

ORGANIZATIONS

American Urological Association (AUA), 1000 Corporate Boulevard, Linthicum, MD, 21090, 410 689-3700, 410 689-3800, 866 746-4282, aua@AUAnet.org, http://www.auanet.org.

American Urological Association Foundation, 1000 Corporate Blvd., Linthicum, MD, 21090, 410 689-3700, 410 689-3800, 866 746-4282, auafoundation@auafoundation.org, http://www.urologyhealth.org/.

Center for Biologics Evaluation and Research (CBER), U. S. Food and Drug Administration (FDA), 10903 New Hampshire Ave, Silver Spring, MD, 20993-0002, 888 463-6332, http://www.fda.gov/BiologicsBloodVaccines.

National Institute of Diabetes and Digestive and Kidney Diseases (NIDDK) NIH Bldg 31, Rm 9A06 31 Center Drive, MSC 2560, Bethesda, MD, 20892-2560, 301 496.3583, http://www2.niddk.nih.gov.

Ken R. Wells
Rebecca J. Frey, PhD

Impulse control disorders

Definition

Impulse control disorders are characterized by an individual's inability to resist the impulse to perform an action that is harmful to one's self or others. This condition is a relatively new class of **personality disorders**. Medical researchers surmise that at the root of the problem, the afflicted person desires small, short–term pleasures or gains—often performed impulsively and without the ability to resist such behaviors—over the likelihood of much larger, long–term loses. Some of the most common types of these disorders are **intermittent explosive disorder**, kleptomania, pyromania, compulsive gambling disorder, and trichotillomania.

Demographics

Such disorders are found in both genders of the population. They usually begin to appear in children in and around the ages of seven to 15 years of age.

Description

All of these impulse control disorders involve the loss or lack of control in certain specific situations. The hallmark of these disorders is the individual's inability to stop impulses that may cause harm to themselves or others. Affected individuals often feel **anxiety** or tension in considering these behaviors. This anxiety or tension is relieved or diminished once the action is performed.

Intermittent explosive disorder (IED) is more common among males, and involves repeated and aggressive, violet outbursts that lead to assaults on others or destruction of property. These outbursts, often only ten to twenty minutes in duration, are unprovoked or seem to be out of proportion to the event that precedes them. Afterwards, such people often feel remorse and regret from such actions. The outbursts may happen in several separate incidents over a few hours or days or may occur as one or more every so many weeks or months. Examples of intermittent explosive disorder commonly found in daily life include road rage and domestic violence and **abuse**.

Kleptomania is more common among females, and involves the theft of objects that are seemingly worthless. The act of stealing relieves tension and anxiety, and increases personal gratification during the act. Once the act is accomplished, individuals feel relieved of their tensions. In addition, they do not steal for the sense of monetary gain. The actual stealing is not preplanned, and the concept of punishment for the crime does not occur to these individuals, although they are aware that what they are doing is wrong. The people afflicted with kleptomania are often very ashamed of their actions afterwards, but are unable to stop themselves and oftentimes unwilling to seek medical or psychological help.

Pyromania is more common among males, and involves setting fires in order to feel pleasure and relieve tension. It is classified by the deliberate setting of fires more than once. Pyromaniacs do not start fires for the same reasons as do arsonists. They are not looking for revenge, monetary gain, or political reasons, only feelings of relief or gratification. They do not start fires as direct part of criminal behavior or due to **hallucinations** (such as with drug use). The individual exhibits a fascination and attraction to fire and any objects associated with it. Pryomanics often direct their actions toward fire stations and other buildings associated with fire control and prevention.

Pathological gambling occurs in roughly one to three percent of the population, and involves excessive (compulsive) gambling despite heavy monetary losses. This disorder typically begins in youth, and affected individuals are often competitive, easily bored, restless, and generous. Their losses actually act as a motivating factor in continuing gambling in order to recoup some of what was lost. Pathological gamblers often use lies, theft, and fraud to continue their compulsive gambling habit. They often gamble more during periods of high **stress** or anxiety in order to counter their feelings. Often they gamble for the excitement and not for the money. However, many of them lose large amounts of money, which only makes them more anxious and, in turn, more likely to place larger and riskier bets.

Trichotillomania, also commonly called hair–pulling disorder, involves the uncontrollable, nearly continuous pulling of hair from one's own scalp, face, or other areas of the body, and is more common in females. It often begins in childhood, and is often associated with major depression or attention deficit/hyperactivity disorder. There is an increased sense of tension before pulling the hair, which is relieved once it is pulled out. Recurrent pulling out of one's hair may result in noticeable hair loss. It can be a mild problem for some people and in others, quite devastating. For all of them, the disorder is very emotional, especially when large amounts of hair are pulled from visible parts of the body, such as from the head. Affected individuals can undergo significant distress and impaired social, occupational, and functional behavior.

Causes and symptoms

The exact causes of impulse control disorders are not fully understood as of 2010. Individuals who have had serious head injuries, however, can be at a higher risk for developing impulse control disorders, as are those with **epilepsy**.

Some cases of impulse control disorders appear to be side effects of general medical conditions. Several groups of researchers have noted that some older adults with Parkinson's disease become compulsive gamblers as the disease progresses. It is thought that this gambling behavior is a side effect of dopaminergic drugs, as it does not respond to standard treatments for compulsive gambling but only to changes in the patient's medication. A study performed in 2007, headed by a medical researcher from the U.S. National Institute of Neurological Disorders and Stroke, found that pathological gamblers who received dopamine agonists developed Parkinson's disease at a younger age than those without the disorder. Those with the disorder also scored lower on an impulsivity scale than did other people.

Another medical condition that is associated with impulse control disorders is carcinoid syndrome. In one group of 20 patients with the syndrome, 75% met DSM–IV diagnostic criteria for one or another impulse control disorder. The researchers attribute the connection to the high levels of serotonin (a neurotransmitter) produced by carcinoid tumors.

The cause of intermittent explosive disorder may be due to environmental, genetic, or biological factors, but the exact cause is still undetermined.

Numerous symptoms of intermittent explosive disorder are:

- irritability
- rage and anger
- tingling
- increased energy
- tremors and palpitations
- tightness of the chest
- headache or pressure in or about the head

The cause of kleptomania is not known for sure in the medical community. Some researchers have suggested that certain chemicals in the brain may be linked to the condition. However, additional research is needed before a determination of the cause of the disorder can be announced.

Some of the symptoms of kleptomania are:

- strong urges to steal even though the items are not needed
- tension and anxiety leading up to the act of stealing
- feelings of pleasure and satisfaction while in the act of the theft
- feelings of guilt, embarrassment, and shame afterwards

Although not known for sure, genetic and environmental factors are considered to be possible causes for pathological gambling. Certain natural occurring chemicals in the brain, such as dopamine, norepinephrine, and serotonin indicate possible associations with the disorder. Sometimes, medications taken (external to the disorder) may bring on the disorder. Serious injuries, such as brain trauma, can also contribute to pathological gambling.

Several symptoms of pathological gambling are:

- extreme excitement from taking large gambling bets
- being preoccupied with gambling
- increasing the number and/or amount of gambling bets
- showing more interest in gambling than other personal and professional interests
- lying about gambling
- feelings of remorse and guilt after gambling
- large debts and financial problems; also, some legal difficulties may develop
- problems holding onto job and career, and difficulties coping with family responsibilities

For trichotillomania, mutations in the gene SLITRK1 have been associated with the disorder. Tourette syndrome—in which people make unusual movements and sounds—is also linked to the disorder. Problems with natural chemicals in the brain, such as dopamine and serotonin, are suggested as a possible cause of trichotillomania.

Symptoms of trichotillomania include:

- bald or patchy spots on the scalp or other parts of the body
- excessive playing with hair or pulled–out hair, including chewing of hair
- thin or missing eyebrows and eyelashes
- pulling hair across the face, especially the lips

Diagnosis

A diagnosis of any of these impulse control disorders can be made only after other medical and psychiatric disorders that may cause the same symptoms have been ruled out. Once this is done a medical

KEY TERMS

Carcinoid syndrome—The pattern of symptoms (often including asthma and diarrhea) associated with carcinoid tumors of the digestive tract or lungs.

Compulsive gambling disorder—An impulse control disorder in which an individual cannot resist gambling despite repeated losses.

Intermittent explosive disorder—A personality disorder in which an individual is prone to intermittent explosive episodes of aggression during which he or she causes bodily harm or destroys property.

Kleptomania—An impulse control disorder in which one steals objects that are of little or no value.

Pyromania—An impulse control disorder in which one sets fires.

Trichotillomania—An impulse or compulsion to pull out one's own hair.

professional analyzes the physical and mental problems apparent to the patient.

In addition, many doctors administer questionnaires or similar psychiatric screeners as part of the differential diagnosis. Two instruments that were devised in the early 2000s to specifically target impulsive behavior are the Gambling Urge Scale (GUS) and the Lifetime History of Impulsive Behaviors (LHIB) Interview.

For instance, in a medical diagnosis of pathological gambling, five or more of the following symptoms must be present:

- a preoccupation with gambling
- a need to gamble with more money to achieve the thrill of winning
- repeated attempts to control or stop gambling
- irritability or restlessness due to repeated attempts of control
- gambling as an escape from stress
- lying to cover up gambling
- conducting illegal activities, such as embezzling or fraud, to finance gambling
- losing a job or personal relationship due to gambling
- borrowing money to fund gambling

Treatment

A combination of psychological counseling and medication are the preferred treatments for impulse control disorders. For kleptomania, pyromania, and trichotillomania, behavior modification is usually the treatment of choice. Children with trichotillomania are often helped by antidepressant medication. For pathological gambling, treatment usually involves an adaptation of the model set forth by Alcoholics Anonymous. Individuals are counseled with the goal of eventual responding to appropriate social limits. In the case of intermittent explosive disorder, anger management and medication may be used in extreme cases of aggression.

Prognosis

These disorders can usually be controlled with medication, although the medication may need to be continued long–term to help prevent further aggressive outbursts. Long–term counseling is usually necessary as well. Support groups and meetings may also help these individuals.

The prognosis for intermittent explosive disorder, kleptomania, and pyromania is fair. Little is known about the prognosis for trichotillomania, and studies have shown that the condition can disappear for long periods (months to years) without any psychological counseling. For pathological gambling, the prognosis varies greatly from person to person. While total cure for this condition is unlikely, much like **alcoholism**, long periods of abstinence or continuous abstinence are possible.

Prevention

There are no known preventive treatments or measures for impulse control disorders.

Resources

BOOKS

Aboujaoude, Elias, and Lorrin M. Koran. *Impulse Control Disorders*. New York: Cambridge University Press, 2010.

Grant, Jon E. *Impulse Control Disorders: A Clinician's Guide to Understanding and Treating Behavioral Addictions*. New York: W. W. Norton, 2008.

Hollander, Eris, and Dan J. Stein, eds. *Clinical Manual of Impulse–Control Disorders*. Arlington, VA: American Psychiatric, 2006.

OTHER

"Characteristics Of Increased Risk For Compulsive Gambling Linked To Parkinson's Disease Medications" Science Daily. (February 15, 2007). http://www.sciencedaily.com/releases/2007/02/070212184152.htm. (accessed September 4, 2010).

"Compulsive Gambling" Mayo Clinic. (April 8, 2010). http://www.mayoclinic.com/health/compulsive–gambling/DS00443 (accessed September 4, 2010).

"Intermittent Explosive Disorder." Mayo Clinic. (June 10, 2010). http://www.mayoclinic.com/health/intermittent-explosive-disorder/DS00730 (accessed September 4, 2010).

"Kleptomania." Mayo Clinic. (October 30, 2009). http://www.mayoclinic.com/health/kleptomania/DS01034 (accessed September 4, 2010).

"Trichotillomania." Mayo Clinic. (April 8, 2010). http://www.mayoclinic.com/health/trichotillomania/DS00895 (accessed September 4, 2010).

ORGANIZATIONS

American Psychiatric Association (APA), 1000 Wilson Blvd., Suite 1825, Arlington, VA, 22209, (888) 357–7924, http://www.psych.org.

Gamblers Anonymous International Service Office, PO Box 17173, Los Angeles, CA, 90017, (213) 386–8789, (213) 386–0030, isomain@gamblersanonymous.org, http://www.gamblersanonymous.org.

National Institute of Mental Health (NIMH), 6001 Executive Blvd., Room 8184, MSC 9663, Bethesda, MD, 20892–9663, (301) 443–4513, http://www.nimh.nih.gov.

Trichotillomania Learning Center, Inc., 207 McPherson St., Suite H, Santa Cruz, CA, 95060–5863, (831) 457–1004, (831) 426–4383, info@trich.org, http://www.trich.org.

Liz Meszaros
Rebecca Frey, PhD

In vitro fertilization

Definition

In vitro fertilization (IVF) is a procedure in which eggs (ova) from a woman's ovary are removed. They are fertilized with sperm in a laboratory procedure, and then the fertilized egg (embryo) is returned to the woman's uterus.

Purpose

IVF is one of several assisted reproductive techniques (ART) used to help infertile couples to conceive a child. If after one year of having sexual intercourse without the use of birth control a woman is unable to get pregnant, **infertility** is suspected. Some of the reasons for infertility are damaged or blocked fallopian tubes, hormonal imbalance, or **endometriosis** in the woman. In the man, low sperm count or poor quality sperm can cause infertility.

IVF is one of several possible methods to increase the chance for an infertile couple to become pregnant. Its use depends on the reason for infertility. IVF may be an option if there is a blockage in the fallopian tube or endometriosis in the woman or low sperm count or poor quality sperm in the man. There are other possible treatments for these conditions, such as surgery for blocked tubes or endometriosis, which may be tried before IVF.

IVF will not work for a woman who is not capable of ovulating or a man who is not able to produce at least a few healthy sperm.

Precautions

The screening procedures and treatments for infertility can become a long, expensive, and sometimes, disappointing process. Each IVF attempt takes at least an entire menstrual cycle and can cost $5,000-$10,000, which may or may not be covered by health insurance. The **anxiety** of dealing with infertility can challenge both individuals and their relationship. The added **stress** and expense of multiple clinic visits, testing, treatments, and surgical procedures can become overwhelming. Couples may want to receive counseling and support throughout the process.

Description

In vitro fertilization is a procedure where the joining of egg and sperm takes place outside of the woman's body. A woman may be given fertility drugs before this procedure so that several eggs mature in the ovaries at the same time. Eggs (ova) are removed from a woman's ovaries using a long, thin needle. The physician gains access to the ovaries using one of two possible procedures. One procedure involves inserting the needle through the vagina (transvaginally). The physician guides the needle to the location of the ovaries with the help of an ultrasound machine. In the other procedure, called **laparoscopy**, a small thin tube with a viewing lens is inserted through an incision in the navel. This allows the physician to see inside the patient, and locate the ovaries, on a video monitor.

Once the eggs are removed, they are mixed with sperm in a laboratory dish or test tube. (This is where the term *test tube baby* comes from.) The eggs are monitored for several days. Once there is evidence that fertilization has occurred and the cells begin to divide, they are then returned to the woman's uterus.

PATRICK CHRISTOPHER STEPTOE (1913–1988)

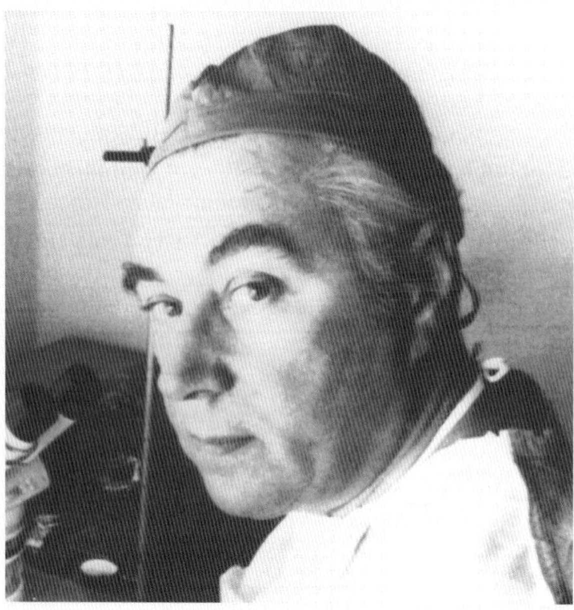

(AP Images.)

Patrick Christopher Steptoe was born in Oxfordshire, England, on June 9, 1913. His mother was a social worker and his father was a church organist. Steptoe entered the University of London's St. George Hospital Medical School, earning his physician's license in 1939 and becoming a member of the Royal College of Surgeons. When Steptoe volunteered as a naval surgeon during World War II, he was captured and held as a prisoner until his release in 1943. Following his release, Steptoe studied obstetrics and gynecology and moved to Manchester to start a private practice in 1948. In 1951, Steptoe accepted a position at Oldham General and District Hospital in England.

During his time at Oldham, Steptoe continued his study of fertility problems. Using a laparoscope, he developed a method to remove eggs from a woman's ovaries. In 1966, Steptoe teamed with physiologist Robert G. Edwards who had successfully fertilized eggs outside of the body. In 1968, the pair had a breakthrough when Edwards successfully fertilized an egg that Steptoe had removed, but their attempts to implant the embryo failed repeatedly. However, Steptoe and Edwards experienced success when a fertilized egg was implanted into the uterus of Leslie Brown. Brown gave birth to a healthy baby girl, Louise, on July 25, 1978.

Steptoe retired and built a clinic in Cambridge. He and Edwards were named Commanders of the British Empire, and Steptoe was honored with fellowship in the Royal Society. He and his wife had two children. Steptoe died on March 21, 1988.

In the procedure to remove eggs, enough may be gathered to be frozen and saved (either fertilized or unfertilized) for additional IVF attempts. A 2004 study from the Mayo Clinic found that frozen sperm was as effective as fresh sperm for IVF.

IVF has been used successfully since 1978, when the first child to be conceived by this method was born in England. Over the past 20 years, thousands of couples have used this method of ART or similar procedures to conceive.

Other types of assisted reproductive technologies might be used to achieve **pregnancy**. A procedure called intracytoplasmic sperm injection (ICSI) uses a manipulation technique that must be performed using a microscope to inject a single sperm into each egg. The fertilized eggs can then be returned to the uterus, as in IVF. In gamete intrafallopian tube transfer (GIFT) the eggs and sperm are mixed in a narrow tube and then deposited in the fallopian tube, where fertilization normally takes place. Another variation on IVF is zygote intrafallopian tube transfer (ZIFT). As in IVF, the fertilization of the eggs occurs in a laboratory dish. And, similar to GIFT, the embryos are placed in the fallopian tube (rather than the uterus as with IVF).

Preparation

Once a woman is determined to be a good candidate for in vitro fertilization, she will generally be given "fertility drugs" to stimulate ovulation and the development of multiple eggs. These drugs may include gonadotropin releasing hormone agonists (GnRHa), Pergonal, Clomid, or human chorionic gonadotropin (hcg). The maturation of the eggs is then monitored with ultrasound tests and frequent blood tests. If enough eggs mature, the physician will perform the procedure to remove them. The woman may be given a sedative prior to the procedure. A local anesthetic agent may also be used to reduce discomfort during the procedure.

Aftercare

After the IVF procedure is performed the woman can resume normal activities. A pregnancy test can be

KEY TERMS

Fallopian tubes—In a woman's reproductive system, a pair of narrow tubes that carry the egg from the ovary to the uterus.

GIFT—Stands for gamete intrafallopian tube transfer. This is a process where eggs are taken from a woman's ovaries, mixed with sperm, and then deposited into the woman's fallopian tube.

ICSI—Stands for intracytoplasmic sperm injection. This process is used to inject a single sperm into each egg before the fertilized eggs are put back into the woman's body. The procedure may be used if the male has a low sperm count.

ZIFT—Stands for zygote intrafallopian tube transfer. In this process of in vitro fertilization, the eggs are fertilized in a laboratory dish and then placed in the woman's fallopian tube.

done approximately 12–14 days later to determine if the procedure was successful.

Risks

The risks associated with in vitro fertilization include the possibility of **multiple pregnancy** (since several embryos may be implanted) and **ectopic pregnancy** (an embryo that implants in the fallopian tube or in the abdominal cavity outside the uterus). There is a slight risk of ovarian rupture, bleeding, infections, and complications of anesthesia. If the procedure is successful and pregnancy is achieved, the pregnancy would carry the same risks as any pregnancy achieved without assisted technology.

Normal results

Success rates vary widely between clinics and between physicians performing the procedure and implantation does not guarantee pregnancy. Therefore, the procedure may have to be repeated more than once to achieve pregnancy. However, success rates have improved in recent years, up from 20% in 1995 to 27% in 2001.

Abnormal results

An ectopic or multiple pregnancy may abort spontaneously or may require termination if the health of the mother is at risk. The number of multiple pregnancies has decreased in recent years as technical advances and professional guidelines have led to implanting of fewer embryos per attempt.

Resources

PERIODICALS

"Frozen, Fresh Sperm Both Effective for In Vitro Fertilization." *Obesity, Fitness & Wellness Week* June 5, 2004: 1059.

"Multiple Births Via In Vitro Fertilization Are Declining." *Women's Health Weekly* May 6, 2004: 16.

OTHER

"Infertility." *HealthWorld Online Page*. http://www.healthy.net.

"In vitro Fertilization: A Teacher's Guide from Newton's Apple." *PBS Page*. http://www.pbs.org/ktca/newtons/11/invitro.html.

ORGANIZATIONS

American Society for Reproductive Medicine, 1209 Montgomery Highway, Birmingham, AL, 35216-2809, 205 978-5000, 205 978-5005, asrm@asrm.org, http://www.asrm.org.

Center for Fertility and In Vitro Fertilization Loma Linda University, 11370 Anderson St, Loma Linda, CA, 92354, 909 558-2851, 909 558-2450, amarta@llu. edu, http://lomalindahealth.org/health-care/our-services/fertility/index.page?.

Resolve, 1310 Broadway, Somerville, MA, 02144-1731, 617 623-0744, http://www.resolve.org.

Altha Roberts Edgren
Teresa G. Odle

Inclusion blennorrhea *see* **Inclusion conjunctivitis**

Inclusion conjunctivitis

Definition

Inclusion **conjunctivitis** is an inflammation of the conjunctiva (the membrane that lines the eyelids and covers the white part, or sclera, of the eyeball) by the bacterium *Chlamydia trachomatis*. Chlamydia is a sexually transmitted organism. Chlamydia was originally called "chlamydozoa" by Polish dermatologist Ludwig Halberstaedter and Czech zoologist Stanislaus von Prowazek in 1907 when they discovered *Chlamydia trachomatis*. Chlamydozoa is the Greek word for "mantle."

Demographics

The disease usually affects teenagers and young adults who are sexually active. In fact, persons with the disease often times also have genital chlamydia (an infection of the genitals). The disease also occurs in newborn infants. Women are usually more susceptible to the disease than are men, and people in urban areas frequently acquire it more than do rural people.

Description

Inclusion conjunctivitis, known as neonatal inclusion conjunctivitis in the newborn and adult inclusion conjunctivitis in the adult, is also called inclusion blennorrhea, chlamydial conjunctivitis, or swimming pool conjunctivitis. It usually occurs from poor personal hygiene, specifically from the transmission of contaminated genital secretions to the eye. This disease affects four of 1,000 (0.4%) live births. Approximately half of the infants born to untreated infected mothers will develop the disease.

Causes and symptoms

Inclusion conjunctivitis in the newborn, called neonatal conjunctivitis, results from passage through an infected birth canal and develops from 5 to 12 days after birth. Both eyelids and conjunctivae are swollen and red in color. There may be a discharge of pus from the eyes, swelling of the eyelids, and redness around the eye. Irritation, infection, or blocked tear ducts are three primary causes of inclusion conjunctivitis. In infants, the disease can become very serious.

Most instances of adult inclusion conjunctivitis result from exposure to infected genital secretions. It is transmitted to the eye by fingers and occasionally by the water in swimming pools, poorly chlorinated hot tubs, or by sharing makeup. In adult inclusion conjunctivitis, one eye is usually involved, with a stringy discharge of mucus and pus. There may be little bumps called follicles inside the lower eyelid and the eye is red. Occasionally, the condition damages the cornea, causing cloudy areas and a growth of new blood vessels (neovascularization). Women sometimes report genito-urinary symptoms.

Diagnosis

Inclusion conjunctivitis is usually considered when the patient has a follicular conjunctivitis that will not go away, even after using **topical antibiotics**. Diagnosis depends upon tests performed on the discharge from the eye. Gram stains determine the type of microorganism, while culture and sensitivity tests determine which antibiotic will kill the harmful microorganism. Conjuntival scraping determines whether chlamydia is present in cells taken from the conjunctiva.

KEY TERMS

Cervicitis—Cervicitis is an inflammation of the cervix or neck of the uterus.

Conjunctiva—The conjunctiva is the membrane that lines the eyelids and covers the white part of the eyeball (sclera).

Cornea—The clear dome-shaped structure that covers the colored part of the eye (iris).

Neovascularization—Neovascularization is the growth of new blood vessels.

Urethritis—Urethritis is an inflammation of the urethra, the canal for the discharge of urine that extends from the bladder to the outside of the body.

Treatment

Treatment in the newborn consists of administration of tetracycline ointment to the conjunctiva and erythromycin orally or through intravenous therapy for fourteen days. Infants can also be given erythromycin ophthalmic ointment for one week, and erythromycin or azithromycin elixir for two to three weeks. The mother should be treated for **cervicitis** (inflammation of the uterine cervix) and the father for **urethritis** (inflammation of the urethra), even if they do not have symptoms of these diseases.

In adults, tetracycline ointment or drops should be applied to the conjunctiva and oral tetracycline, amoxacillin, or erythromycin should be taken for up to three weeks, or doxycycline for one week. A single oral dose of azithromycin helps to control redness in and around the eye, along with mucous discharge. In severe cases, intravenous **antibiotics** may also be used, together with topical antibiotics. If a blocked tear duct is to blame, warm and gently massages are given between the nasal area and the eye. They help to reduce swelling and irritation. If the blocked tear duct does not heal within one year, surgery may be necessary.

Patients should have weekly checkups so the doctor can monitor the healing.

Oral tetracycline should not be administered to children whose permanent teeth have not erupted. It should also not be given to nursing or pregnant women.

Prognosis

Untreated inclusion conjunctivitis in the newborn persists for 3 to 12 months and usually heals; however, there may be scarring or neovascularization. The occurrence of it in infants has decreased over the past few decades as more women are screened and treated before they become pregnant. In the adult, if left untreated, the disease may continue for months and cause corneal neovascularization. Even if treated, antibiotics usually do not reverse damage that may have occurred, but they may help prevent it if given early enough. The infection can spread to the nasopharynx and the lower respiratory tract. **Pneumonia** can result if left untreated.

Prevention

The neonatal infection may be prevented by instilling erythromycin drops or ointment into the eye's conjunctival cul-de-sac at the baby's birth. Many state laws require medical professionals perform such preventative measures to babies born in hospitals. However, it is not prevented by silver nitrate, which was a treatment in the past. Instead, antibiotic eye drops are used.

Chlamydia is a contagious, sexually transmitted disease. Some systemic symptoms include a history of vaginitis, **pelvic inflammatory disease**, or urethritis. Patients with symptoms of these diseases should be treated by a physician.

Resources

BOOKS

Reinhard, Thomas, and Frank Larkin, eds. *Cornea and External Eye Disease*. Berlin: Springer, 2008.

Yanoff, Myron, and Jay J. Kuker. *Ophthalmology*. 3rd ed. Edinburgh, Scotland: Mosby Elsevier, 2009.

OTHER

"Conjunctivitis (Pink Eye) in Newborns" Centers for Disease Control and Prevention. (June 4, 2010), http://www.cdc.gov/conjunctivitis/newborns.html. (accessed July 1, 2010).

"The Many Faces of Chlamydial Infection " Review of Ophthalmology. (April 1, 2008), http://www.revophth.com/index.asp?page=1_13785.htm. (accessed July 1, 2010).

ORGANIZATIONS

American Academy of Ophthalmology, 655 Beach Street, San Francisco, CA, 94109, (415) 561-8500, eyenet@aao.org, http://www.eyenet.org.

American Optometric Association, 243 North Lindbergh Blvd., St. Louis, MO, 63141, (800) 365-2219, eyenet@aao.org, http://www.aoanet.org.

Lorraine Steefel, RN

Incompetent cervix

Definition

A cervix (the structure at the bottom of the uterus) that is incompetent is abnormally weak, and therefore it can gradually widen during **pregnancy**. Left untreated, this can result in repeated pregnancy losses or premature delivery.

Description

Incompetent cervix is the result of an anatomical abnormality. Normally, the cervix remains closed throughout pregnancy until labor begins. An incompetent cervix gradually opens due to the pressure from the developing fetus after about the 13th week of pregnancy. The cervix begins to thin out and widen without any contractions or labor. The membranes surrounding the fetus bulge down into the opening of the cervix until they break, resulting in the loss of the baby or a very premature delivery.

Causes and symptoms

Some factors that can contribute to the chance of a woman having an incompetent cervix include trauma to the cervix, physical abnormality of the cervix, or having been exposed to the drug diethylstilbestrol (DES) in the mother's womb. Some women have cervical incompetence for no obvious reason.

Diagnosis

Incompetent cervix is suspected when a woman has three consecutive spontaneous pregnancy losses during the second trimester (the fourth, fifth and sixth months of the pregnancy). The likelihood of this happening by random chance is less than 1%. Spontaneous losses due to incompetent cervix account for 20–25% of all second trimester losses. A spontaneous second trimester pregnancy loss is different from a **miscarriage**, which usually happens during the first three months of pregnancy.

The physician can check for abnormalities in the cervix by performing a manual examination or by an ultrasound test. The physician can also check to see if the cervix is prematurely widened (dilated). Because incompetent cervix is only one of several potential causes for this, the patient's past history of pregnancy losses must also be considered when making the diagnosis.

KEY TERMS

Diethylstilbestrol (DES)—DES is a drug given to women a generation ago to prevent miscarriage. At that time it was not known that female children born of women who had been given DES would show a higher rate for cervical and other reproductive abnormalities, as well as a rare form of vaginal cancer, when they reached reproductive age.

Effacement—The thinning out of the cervix that normally occurs along with dilation shortly before delivery.

Preterm labor—Labor before the thirty-seventh week of pregnancy.

Treatment

Treatment for incompetent cervix is a surgical procedure called cervical cerclage. A stitch (suture) is used to tie the cervix shut to give it more support. It is most effective if it is performed somewhere between 14–16 weeks into the pregnancy. The stitch is removed near the end of pregnancy to allow for a normal birth.

Cervical cerclage can be performed under spinal, epidural, or **general anesthesia**. The patient will need to stay in the hospital for one or more days. The procedure to remove the suture is done without the need for anesthesia. The vagina is held open with an instrument called a speculum and the stitch is cut and removed. This may be slightly uncomfortable, but should not be painful.

Some possible risks of cerclage are premature rupture of the amniotic membranes, infection of the amniotic sac, and preterm labor. The risk of infection of the amniotic sac increases as the pregnancy progresses. For a cervix that is dilated 3 centimeters (cm), the risk is 30%.

After cerclage, a woman will be monitored for any preterm labor. The woman needs to consult her obstetrician immediately if there are any signs of contractions.

Cervical cerclage can not be performed if a woman is more than 4 cm dilated, if the fetus has already died in her uterus, or if her amniotic membranes are torn and her water has broken.

Prognosis

The success rate for cerclage correction of incompetent cervix is good. About 80-90% of the time women deliver healthy infants. The success rate is higher for cerclage done early in pregnancy.

Resources

OTHER

"Cervical insufficiency (incompetent cervix)." Babycenter.com (April 2005). http://www.babycenter.com/0_cervical-insufficiency-incompetent-cervix_1425796.bc. (accessed November 22, 2010).

Tish Davidson, A.M.

Incontinence *see* **Urinary incontinence**

Indigestion

Definition

Indigestion, which is sometimes called **dyspepsia** or an upset stomach, is a general term covering a group of nonspecific symptoms in the digestive tract. It is not considered a disease but, rather, several symptoms that are experienced due to impaired digestion of consumed foods. Indigestion is often described as an uncomfortable feeling of fullness, bloating, **nausea**, **heartburn**, or gassy discomfort in the chest or upper abdomen. The symptoms develop during meals or shortly afterward. In most cases, indigestion is a minor problem that often clears up without professional treatment.

Demographics

Indigestion is a widespread condition that can occur at any age, for both men and women. It is estimated to occur at some time in 25% of the adult population of the United States.

Description

Most people with indigestion do not feel sick enough to see a doctor; nonetheless, it is a common reason for office visits. About 3% of visits to primary care doctors are for indigestion. Indigestion may only occur occasionally in some people, while others may have it daily.

Causes and symptoms

Physical causes

The symptoms associated with indigestion have a variety of possible physical and lifestyle causes, ranging from commonplace food items to serious systemic disorders:

- Diet. Milk, milk products, alcoholic beverages, tea, and coffee cause indigestion in some people because they stimulate the stomach's production of acid. Chocolate, carbonated beverages, and spicy foods can also cause indigestion.
- Medications. Certain prescription drugs as well as over-the-counter medications can irritate the stomach lining. These medications include aspirin, nonsteroidal anti-inflammatory drugs (NSAIDs), some antibiotics, digoxin, theophylline, corticosteroids, iron (ferrous sulfate), oral contraceptives, and tricyclic antidepressants.
- Disorder of the stomach. Inflammation of the stomach (gastritis).
- Disorders of the pancreas and gallbladder. These include inflammation of the gallbladder or pancreas, cancer of the pancreas, and gallstones.
- Intestinal parasites. Parasitic infections that cause indigestion include amebiasis, fluke and tapeworm infections, giardiasis, and strongyloidiasis.
- Systemic disorders, including diabetes, thyroid disease, collagen vascular disease.
- Cancers of the digestive tract, such as stomach cancer.
- Conditions associated with women's reproductive organs. These conditions include menstrual cramps, pregnancy, and pelvic inflammatory disease.

Psychological and emotional causes

Indigestion often accompanies an emotional upset, because the part of the nervous system involved in the so-called "fight-or-flight" response also affects the digestive tract. People diagnosed with **anxiety**, nervousness, or **somatoform disorders** frequently have problems with indigestion. Many people in the general population, however, will also experience heartburn, "butterflies in the stomach," or stomach cramps when they are in upsetting situations—such as school examinations, arguments with family members, crises in their workplace, and other such emotional traumas. Some people's digestive systems appear to react more intensely to emotional **stress** due to hypersensitive nerve endings in their intestinal tract.

Symptoms

The most common symptoms include:

- Uncomfortable fullness in the stomach during and/or after meals, which lasts longer then normal, especially when not eating much food
- Awareness, mild discomfort, or even more severe pain, in the upper abdominal area, what is called the epigastric area
- Burning sensation in the upper abdomen (epigastric area)

Less common symptoms are:

- Bloating, with an uncomfortable feeling of tightness in the stomach
- Nausea, with a feeling that vomiting may occur
- Belching or burping

Specific gastrointestinal disorders

In some cases, the patient's description of the symptoms suggests a specific digestive disorder as the cause of the indigestion. Some doctors classify these cases into three groups.

ESOPHAGITIS TYPE. Esophagitis is an inflammation of the tube that carries food from the throat to the stomach (the esophagus). The tissues of the esophagus can become irritated by the flow (reflux) of stomach acid backward into the lower part of the esophagus. If the patient describes the indigestion in terms of frequent or intense heartburn, the doctor will consider **gastroesophageal reflux disease** (GERD) as a possible cause. GERD is a common disorder in the general population, affecting about 30% of adults.

PEPTIC ULCER TYPE. Patients who smoke and are over 45 years of age are more likely to have indigestion of the peptic ulcer type. This group also includes people who find that their indigestion is relieved by taking **antacids** or eating a small amount of food at each meal. Patients in this category are often found to have *Helicobacter pylori* infections. *H. pylori* is a rod-shaped bacterium that lives in the tissues of the stomach and causes irritation of the mucous lining of the stomach walls. Most people with *H. pylori* infections do not develop chronic indigestion, but the organism appears to cause peptic ulcer disease (PUD) in a vulnerable segment of the population.

NONULCER TYPE. Most cases of chronic indigestion—as many as 65%—fall into this third category. Nonulcer dyspepsia is sometimes called functional dyspepsia because it appears to be related to abnormalities in the way that the stomach empties its contents into the intestine. In some people, the stomach empties either too slowly or too rapidly. In others, the stomach's muscular contractions are irregular and uncoordinated as it receives, digests, and moves foods into the small intestine. These disorders of stomach movement (motility) may be caused by hypersensitive nerve endings in the stomach tissues. Patients in this group are likely to be younger than 45 years and have a history of taking medications for anxiety or depression.

Diagnosis

Patient history

Because indigestion is a nonspecific set of symptoms, patients who feel sick enough to seek medical attention are likely to go to their primary care doctor. The history does not always point to an obvious diagnosis. The doctor can, however, use the process of history-taking to evaluate the patient's mood or emotional state in order to assess the possibility of a psychiatric disturbance. In addition, asking about the location, intensity, timing, and recurrence of the indigestion can help the doctor weigh the different diagnostic possibilities.

An important part of the history-taking is asking about symptoms that may indicate a serious illness. These warning symptoms include:

- Weight loss
- Persistent vomiting
- Difficulty or pain in swallowing
- Vomiting blood or passing blood in the stools
- Anemia.

Imaging studies

If the doctor thinks that the indigestion should be investigated further, he or she will order an endoscopic examination of the stomach. An endoscope is a slender tube-shaped instrument that allows the doctor to look at the lining of the patient's stomach. If the patient has indigestion of the esophagitis type or nonulcer type, the stomach lining will appear normal. If the patient has PUD (peptic ulcer disease) the doctor will be able to see abnormal breaks or ulcerated areas in the tissue. He or she may also order ultrasound imaging of the abdomen, or a radionuclide scan to evaluate the motility of the stomach. Blood, breath, or stool tests may also be ordered to show if a bacterium is causing the problem. In addition, a biopsy may be required to analyze pieces of the affected tissue for damage.

Laboratory tests

BLOOD TESTS. If the patient is over 45 years of age, the doctor will have the patient's blood analyzed for a complete blood cell count, measurements of liver enzyme levels, electrolyte and serum **calcium** levels, and thyroid function.

TESTS FOR *HELICOBACTER PYLORI*. Doctors can now test patients for the presence of *H. pylori* without having to take a tissue sample from the stomach. One of these noninvasive tests is a blood test and the other is a breath test.

Treatment

Since most cases of indigestion are not caused by serious disorders, many doctors prefer to try medications and other treatment measures before ordering an **endoscopy**.

Diet and stress management

Many patients benefit from the doctor's reassurance that they do not have a serious or fatal disorder. Cutting out alcoholic beverages, drinks containing **caffeine**, and carbonated beverages often helps. Eliminating tobacco products is also helpful. The patient may also be asked to keep a record of food intake, daily schedule, and symptom severity. Food diaries sometimes reveal psychological or dietary factors that influence indigestion. Eating smaller but more frequent meals can also be beneficial, especially when eaten slowly.

Medications

Patients with the esophagitis type of indigestion are often treated with H_2 antagonists. H_2 antagonists are drugs that block the secretion of stomach acid. They include ranitidine (Zantac), cimetidine (Tagamet), nizatidine (Axid), and famotidine (Pepcid).

Antacid-type medicines, some found over-the-counter and others with a prescription, are commonly taken to reduce acid production in the stomach. Most of these include different combinations of magnesium, aluminum, and calcium. These medicines are usually found over-the-counter, and include Maalox, Rolaids, Tums, and Mylanta.

Some patients take **proton pump inhibitors** (PPIs). They are usually given to people who have both indigestion and GERD. PPIs, which also reduce stomach acid, include omeprazole (Prilosec), lansoprazole (Prevacid), and exomeprazole (Nexium).

Patients with motility disorders may be given prokinetic drugs. Prokinetic medications speed up the emptying of the stomach and increase intestinal motility. They include metoclopramide (Reglan) and cisapride (Propulsid). These drugs relieve symptoms in about 75% of patients.

KEY TERMS

Dyspepsia—Another name for indigestion.

Endoscope—A slender tubular instrument used to examine the inside of the stomach.

Gastroesophageal reflux disease (GERD)—A disorder of the lower end of the esophagus, caused by stomach acid flowing backward into the esophagus and irritating the tissues.

H_2 antagonist—A type of drug that relieves indigestion by reducing the production of stomach acid.

Heartburn—A popular term for an uncomfortable burning sensation in the stomach and lower esophagus, sometimes caused by the reflux of small amounts of stomach acid.

Helicobacter pylori—A gram-negative rod-shaped bacterium that lives in the tissues of the stomach and causes inflammation of the stomach lining.

Motility—The movement or capacity for movement of an organism or body organ. Indigestion is sometimes caused by abnormal patterns in the motility of the stomach.

Peptic ulcer disease (PUD)—A stomach disorder marked by corrosion of the stomach lining due to the acid in the digestive juices.

Prokinetic—A drug that works to speed up the emptying of the stomach and the motility of the intestines.

Reflux—The backward flow of a body fluid or secretion. Indigestion is sometimes caused by the reflux of stomach acid into the esophagus.

Removal of H. pylori

It is not clear that patients with *H. pylori* infections who have *not* developed gastric ulcers need to have the bacterium removed. Some studies indicate, however, that these patients may benefit from antibiotic therapy.

Alternative treatment

HERBAL MEDICINES. Practitioners of Chinese traditional herbal medicine might recommend medicines derived from peony (*Paeonia lactiflora*), hibiscus (*Hibiscus sabdariffa*), or hare's ear (*Bupleurum chinense*) to treat indigestion. Western herbalists are likely to prescribe fennel (*Foeniculum vulgare*), lemon balm (*Melissa officinalis*), or peppermint (*Mentha piperita*) to relieve stomach cramps and heartburn.

HOMEOPATHY. Homeopaths tailor their remedies to the patient's overall personality profile as well as the specific symptoms. Depending on the patient's reaction to the indigestion and some of its likely causes, the homeopath might choose *Gelsemium* (*Gelsemium sempervirens*), *Carbo vegetalis*, *Nux vomica*, or *Pulsatilla* (*Pulsatilla nigricans*).

Other treatments

Some alternative treatments are aimed at lowering the patient's stress level or changing attitudes and beliefs that contribute to indigestion. These therapies and practices include **Reiki**, **reflexology**, **hydrotherapy**, therapeutic massage, **yoga**, and **meditation**.

Prognosis

Most cases of mild indigestion do not need medical treatment. For patients who consult a doctor and are given an endoscopic examination, 5 to 15% are diagnosed with GERD and 15 to 25% with PUD. About 1% of patients who are endoscoped have **stomach cancer**. Most patients with functional dyspepsia do well on either H_2 antagonists or prokinetic drugs, depending on the cause of their indigestion.

Prevention

Indigestion can often be prevented by attention to one's diet, general stress level, and ways of managing stress. Specific preventive measures include:

- Stop smoking.
- Cutting down on or eliminating alcohol, tea, or coffee.
- Avoiding foods that are highly spiced or loaded with fat.
- Eating slowly and keeping mealtimes relaxed.
- Practicing yoga or meditation.
- Not taking aspirin or other medications on an empty stomach.
- Keeping one's weight within normal limits.

Resources

OTHER

"Indigestion" Mayo Clinic. (April 8, 2010), http://www.mayoclinic.com/health/indigestion/DS01141. (accessed July 5, 2010).

"Indigestion" Medline Plus, U.S. National Library of Medicine and National Institutes of Health. (July 2, 2010), http://www.nlm.nih.gov/medlineplus/indigestion.html. (accessed July 5, 2010).

"Indigestion" National Digestive Diseases Information Clearinghouse, National Institute of Diabetes and Digestive and Kidney Diseases, National Institutes of Health. (November 2008), http://digestive.niddk.nih.gov/ddiseases/pubs/indigestion/. (accessed July 5, 2010).

ORGANIZATIONS

American Gastroenterological Association , 4930 Del Ray Avenue, Bethesda, MD, 20814, (301) 654-2055, (800) 296-4433, (301) 654-5920, member@gastro.org, http://www.gastro.org/.

Rebecca J. Frey, PhD

Indinavir *see* **Protease inhibitors**

Indirect Coombs' test *see* **Coombs' tests**

Indium scan of the body

Definition

A scanning procedure in which a patient's white blood cells are first labeled with the radioactive substance indium, and then the patient's body is scanned as a way of tracking the white blood cells at the site of possible infection.

Purpose

The procedure is used to detect inflammatory processes in the body such as infections. By labelling the leukocytes (white blood cells), radiologists or nuclear medicine specialists can then watch their migration toward an **abscess** or other infection.

Description

A nuclear medicine technologist withdraws about 50 mL of blood. White blood cells are collected, exposed to indium, and reinjected by IV back into the patient.

The scan is scheduled for between 18 and 24 hours after the white blood cells have been labelled with indium. (In some cases, more scanning may be scheduled 48 hours after labelling).

For the scan, the patient lies on a special scanning table, as either a single camera passing underneath the table or two cameras (one above the table and one underneath) are placed as close as possible to the body, slowly scanning the person's body.

The radiologist may need extra pictures, but these take only a few minutes each.

While the patient must remain perfectly still during the scan, there should be no discomfort.

KEY TERMS

Indium—A silvery metallic element with some nonmetallic chemical properties used to label white blood cells prior to scanning.

Leukocyte—A white blood cell protects the body against infection and fight infection when it occurs. They are bigger than red blood cells.

Aftercare

After the scan, the patient should be able to continue with normal daily activities with no problems.

Risks

The only risk during this scanning procedure could be to a patient who is pregnant, as with any type of injectable radioactive substance. If the woman is pregnant, the radiologist must be notified; if the scan is cleared, the radiologist may use a lower dosage of indium.

Normal results

The scan should reveal no infection or pathology.

Abnormal results

The scan will reveal details, such as location, about an infection in the patient's body.

Carol A. Turkington

Induction of labor

Definition

Induction of labor involves using artificial means to assist the mother in delivering her baby.

KEY TERMS

Cesarean section—Delivery of a baby through an incision in the mother's abdomen instead of through the vagina; also called a C-section.

Preeclampsia—Hypertension (high blood pressure) experienced during pregnancy.

Rh blood incompatibility—A blood type problem between mother (who is Rh negative) and baby (who is Rh positive), making the immune system of the mother attack her unborn baby. During delivery of the first pregnancy, the mother's immune system becomes sensitive to the Rh positive blood of the baby. The mother's system may then attack later pregnancies and cause severe illness or death to those babies.

Vasoconstriction—Constriction of a blood vessel.

Purpose

Labor is brought on, or induced, when the **pregnancy** has extended significantly beyond the expected delivery date and the mother shows no signs of going into labor. Generally, if the unborn baby is more than two weeks past due, labor will be induced. In most cases, a mother delivers her baby between 38–42 weeks of pregnancy. This usually means that labor is induced if the pregnancy has lasted more than 42 weeks. Labor is also induced if the mother is suffering from diseases (**preeclampsia**, chronic **hypertension**), if there is an Rh blood incompatibility between the baby and the mother, or if the mother or baby has a medical problem that requires delivery of the baby (like a premature rupture of the membranes).

Description

The uterus is the hollow female organ that supports the development and nourishment of the unborn baby during pregnancy. Sometimes labor is induced by the rupturing the amniotic membrane to release amniotic fluid. This is an attempt to mimic the normal process of "breaking water" that occurs early in the normal birth process. This method is sometimes enough stimulation to induce contractions in the mother's uterus. If labor fails to start, drugs are used.

Most labor is induced by using the drug Pitocin, a synthetic form of oxytocin. Oxytocin is a natural hormone produced in the body by the pituitary gland. During normal labor, oxytocin causes contractions. When labor does not occur naturally, the doctor may give the mother Pitocin to start the contractions. Pitocin makes the uterus contract with strength and force almost immediately. This drug is given through a vein in a steady flow that allows the doctor to control the amount the mother is given.

Sometimes vaginal gels are used to induce labor. Normally, the baby will pass through the opening of the uterus (the cervix) into the birth canal during delivery. Because of this, the cervix softens and begins to enlarge (dilate) during the early part of labor to make room for the baby to pass through. The cervix will continue to dilate, and the contractions will eventually push the baby out of the mother's body. When labor needs to be induced, the cervix is often small, hard, and not ready for the process. The doctor may need to prepare or "ripen" the cervix to induce labor. The hormone prostaglandin in a gel form may be applied high in the vagina to soften and dilate the cervix, making the area ready for labor. This may be enough to stimulate contractions on its own. More often, prostaglandin gel is used in conjunction with Pitocin.

If all attempts to induce labor fail, a **cesarean section** is performed.

Risks

Once labor has been induced, the unborn baby is monitored to guard against a reduction in its oxygen supply, or hypoxia. The drugs used to induce labor cause vasoconstriction, which can decrease blood supply to the unborn baby. Throughout the process, the baby's heart rate is monitored by an electronic device placed on top of the mother's abdomen. The heart rate is one sign that the unborn baby is getting enough oxygen and remains healthy. Once the membranes are broken, prolonged labor may result in infection to either the newborn or the mother.

Normal results

Once labor is induced and the cervix has dilated, labor usually proceeds normally. When performed properly, induced labor is a safe procedure for both mother and baby.

Resources

BOOKS

Beers, Mark H., Robert S. Porter, and Thomas V. Jones, eds. *The Merck Manual of Diagnosis and Therapy*. 18th ed. Whitehouse Station, NJ: Merck Research Laboratories, 2006.

John T. Lohr, PhD

Infant massage

Definition

Infant massage refers to **massage therapy** as specifically applied to infants. In most cases, oil or lotion is used as it would be on an adult subject by a trained and licensed massage therapist. Medical professionals caring for infants might also use massage techniques on infants born prematurely, on those with motor or gastrointestinal problems, or on those who have been exposed to **cocaine** in utero.

Description

Various techniques are used in infant massage, with the different strokes specific to a particular therapy. Special handling is used for treating a baby with gas and **colic**. Some of the strokes are known as "Indian milking," which is a gentle stroking of the child's legs; and the "twist and squeeze" **stroke**, a gentle squeeze of the muscles in the thigh and calf. The light "feather" strokes often employed in regular Swedish massage are applied at the end of a massage. The procedure is not unlike certain forms of adult massage, but with extra care taken for the fragility of the infant.

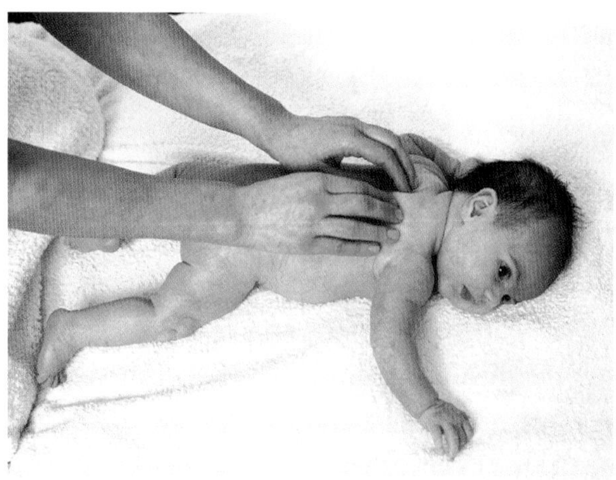

Infant receiving a massage. *(Photo Researchers, Inc.)*

There are also specific Chinese techniques of pediatric massage, including massage of children with special needs. In China, these forms of massage can be given by medical professionals, but parents are often taught how to do the simpler forms for home treatment of their children.

Origins

The practice of massaging infants dates back to ancient times, particularly in Asian and Pacific Island cultures; that is, massage was a component of the baby's regular bath routine among the Maoris of New Zealand and the natives of the Hawaiian Islands. Touch in these cultures is considered healthful both physically and spiritually. Infant massage was also recommended by practitioners of Ayurveda in ancient India. It is likely that early humans practiced infant massage, as many other species of mammals, such as cats, dogs, horses, and monkeys lick or groom their young after birth to cleanse and stimulate them.

In the West, however, infant massage has received more attention in recent years in conjunction with the popularity of natural **childbirth** and midwife-assisted births. Dr. Frédéric Leboyer, a French physician who was one of the leaders of the natural childbirth movement, helped to popularize infant massage through his photojournalistic book on the Indian art of baby massage.

Infant massage was introduced formally into the United States in 1978 when Vimala Schneider McClure, a **yoga** practitioner who had served in an orphanage in Northern India, developed a training program for instructors at the request of childbirth educators. An early research study by R. Rice in 1976 had showed that premature babies who were massaged surged ahead in weight gain and neurological development over those who were not massaged. From McClure's training in India, her knowledge of Swedish massage and **reflexology**, along with her knowledge of yoga postures that she had already adapted for babies, she became the foremost authority on infant massage. In 1986 she founded the International Association of Infant Massage (IAIM), which has chapters in 26 countries around the world as of 2010. Another group, the International Institute of Infant Massage, has trained instructors in 40 countries.

KEY TERMS

Ayurveda—The traditional medical system of India, considered a form of alternative medicine in Western countries.

Linoleic acid—An unsaturated omega-6 fatty acid found in many plant oils that humans need in their diet. Plant oils rich in linoleic acid are beneficial to the skin when used in massage.

Oxytocin—A hormone secreted in the brains of mammals that acts as a neurotransmitter in the brain and also functions in sexual arousal, maternal behavior, and emotional bonding in humans. Synthetic oxytocin is used to induce or support labor in difficult childbirths.

Benefits

According to the IAIM, the benefits of infant massage include:

- relaxation
- relief from stress
- interaction with adults, including fathers as well as mothers
- stimulation of the nervous system
- improved digestion and elimination
- improved blood circulation and skin condition
- relief of teething pains
- stimulation of oxytocin secretion in the person giving the massage. The IAIM states, "[Oxytocin] is useful as a pain reliever and has a calming effect on the person."

The results of several studies showed that infant massage alleviates the **stress** that newborns experience as a result of the enormous change that birth brings about in their lives after the 6–9 months they have spent in the womb. Both premature infants and full-term babies need the relaxation that comes from massaging and moving their limbs and muscles. In infants with colic, massage provides the relief necessary to disperse gas, ease **muscle spasms**, tone the digestive system and help it work efficiently. Some techniques even help bring relief from **teething** and emotional stress. The stimulation an infant receives from massage can aid circulation, strengthen muscles, help digestion, and relieve **constipation**. The bonding that occurs with massage between a parent and child enhances the entire process of bonding that comes with contact through all of the senses, including touch, voice, and sight. It affords a physical experience of quality time between the parents and the child as well as with any significant others in a baby's life.

Precautions

Extreme caution is necessary when performing infant massage. Strokes are made with the greatest delicacy in order not to harm the infant in any way. Proper techniques are taught by licensed massage therapists or IAIM instructors, ensuring that the infant is treated with appropriate physical touch. Anyone who is unfamiliar with handling a baby should receive appropriate instruction before beginning infant massage.

Practitioners of infant massage advise the use of sunflower seed oil or other oils rich in linoleic acid for infant massage, and avoid the use of mustard oil. Mustard oil is used in some traditional societies for infant massage but can harm the baby's skin.

Preparation

If lotions or oils are used, care is taken to ensure their safety on a baby's delicate skin. The most important consideration is to use vegetable oils rather than mineral oils, which can clog the pores in the skin. The oil that is used should be warmed in the caregiver's hands before applying it to the baby's skin. The environment in which the massage is given to an infant should be comfortably warm, and as calm and nonthreatening as possible.

Aftercare

No specific aftercare is required after infant massage.

Risks

No adverse side effects have been reported when infant massage is done properly after careful instruction, or by a licensed massage therapist who specializes in infant care.

Research and general acceptance

In addition to the study already noted regarding touch therapy, a website devoted to infant massage lists research published as early as 1969, and cites hundreds of individual projects that have been conducted throughout the world focusing on infant massage. Many of the studies are related to the benefits of massage and touch for premature infants and others born with such risk factors as drug dependence. Conclusions regarding the benefits are overwhelmingly positive. The proliferation of therapists licensed in infant massage across the United States and worldwide indicates that infant massage is increasingly recognized as a legitimate health care treatment. According to the International Institute of Infant Massage, as of 2010 instructors in the field "include OTs and PTs, child-life specialists, nurses, developmental specialists, childbirth educators, social workers, early interventionists, speech pathologists, case workers, doctors, massage therapists, midwives, **lactation** consultants, and of course parents."

As of 2010 there are 10 research studies of infant massage registered with the National Institutes of Health (NIH). The studies are investigating the benefits of massage for preterm infants, including weight gain, strengthening of the immune system, and development of the central nervous system; sensitivity training for parents; the use of **aromatherapy** together with massage in relieving distress in infants; and the role of infant massage in preventing mother/infant relational disturbances.

Training and certification

The IAIM offers four-day workshops in the countries where it has chapters for the training and certification of instructors in infant massage. Certified instructors (CIMIs) receive their certification after completing "practice teachings with families," passing an examination at the end of the workshop, and passing a clinical evaluation by a registered IAIM trainer. The International Institute of Infant Massage offers a similar four-day program "which includes participation in the four-day training and successful completion of a peer review take-home exam, which includes a practicum of teaching five families during the following four-month period." Tuition for the training as of 2010 is $595.

The licensing of massage therapists varies from state to state, as infant massage qualifies for consideration as medical treatment. Infant massage is becoming an increasingly popular discipline within the field. Numerous websites provide listings for infant massage specialists throughout the United States. The IAIM course is recognized as the official course for infant massage, while the National Certification Board for Therapeutic Massage and Bodywork (NTCTMB) has approved the International Institute of Infant Massage as an approved provider of continuing education. Completion of the institute's course in infant massage is credited as 30 hours of continuing education.

Resources

BOOKS

Ady, Mary. *An Infant Massage Guidebook: For Well, Premature, and Special Needs Babies*. Bloomington, IN: AuthorHouse, 2008.

McClure, Vimala Schneider. *Infant Massage: A Handbook for Loving Parents*, 3rd rev. ed. New York: Bantam Books, 2000.

Reese, Suzanne P. *Baby Massage: Soothing Strokes for Healthy Growth*. New York: Viking Studio, 2006.

Schneider, Elaine Fogel. *Massaging Your Baby: The Joy of Touch Time*. Garden City Park, NY: Square One Publishers, 2006.

PERIODICALS

Field, T., et al. "Preterm Infant Massage Therapy Research: A Review." *Infant Behavior and Development* 33 (April 2010): 115–24.

Gonzalez, A.P., et al. "Weight Gain in Preterm Infants Following Parent-administered Vimala Massage: A Randomized Controlled Trial." *American Journal of Perinatology* 26 (April 2009): 247–52.

Massaro, A.N., et al. "Massage with Kinesthetic Stimulation Improves Weight Gain in Preterm Infants." *Journal of Perinatology* 29 (May 2009): 352–57.

Maulik, P.K., and G.L. Darmstadt. "Community-based Interventions to Optimize Early Childhood Development in Low Resource Settings." *Journal of Perinatology* 29 (August 2009): 531–42.

McGrath, J.M. "Touch and Massage in the Newborn Period: Effects on Biomarkers and Brain Development." *Journal of Perinatal and Neonatal Nursing* 23 (October-December 2009): 304–06.

Procianoy, R.S., et al. "Massage Therapy Improves Neurodevelopment Outcome at Two Years Corrected Age for Very Low Birth Weight Infants." *Human Development* 85 (January 2010): 7–11.

Vinaver, N. "What Is a Birth without Loving Touch?" *Midwifery Today with International Midwife* 92 (Winter 2009-2010): 9–10.

OTHER

International Association of Infant Massage (IAIM). *Benefits of Infant Massage*. http://iaim.net/benefits.php

International Institute of Infant Massage. *Why Infant Massage?*. http://infantmassageinstitute.com/InfantMassageInfo.html

Luther Midelfort Hospital. *Infant Massage, parts 1, 2, 3, and 4*. This is a four-part series of videos on infant massage. The instructor is certified by the IAIM and the sponsoring hospital is part of the Mayo Health System. Each video takes between 5 and 8 minutes to play. Part 1, Part 2, Part 3, Part 4.

The Pregnancy Show. This is a 3-1/2 minute video on the techniques of infant massage. http://www.youtube.com/watch?v=kZ4HPREfBgo

ORGANIZATIONS

American Massage Therapy Association (AMTA), 500 Davis Street, Suite 900, Evanston, IL, 60201, 847-864-0123 , 877-905-2700, 847-864-5196, info@amtamassage.org, http://www.amtamassage.org/.

National Center for Complementary and Alternative Medicine (NCCAM), 9000 Rockville Pike, Bethesda, MD, 20892, info@nccam.nih.gov, http://nccam.nih.gov/.

Touch Research Institute, University of Miami, Miller School of Medicine, Miami, FL, 33136, tfield@med. miami.edu, http://www6.miami.edu/touch-research/.

International Association of Infant Massage (IAIM), Heidenstams Gata 9, Hisings Backa, Gothenburg, Sweden, S-422 47, +46 (0)31-528980, http://www.iaim.net/.

International Institute of Infant Massage, 605 Bledsoe Road, NW, AlbuquerqueNM, United States, 87107, 505-341-9381, 505-341-9386, info@infantmassage.com, http://infantmassageinstitute.com/.

Jane Spehar
Rebecca J. Frey, PhD

Infant respiratory distress syndrome *see* **Respiratory distress syndrome**

Infantile paralysis *see* **Polio**

Infarct avid imaging *see* **Technetium heart scan**

Infarction *see* **Stroke**

ELIZABETH LEE HAZEN (1885–1975)

Elizabeth Lee Hazen was born on August 24, 1885, in Rich, Mississippi. Hazen, born the middle of three children to Maggie (Harper) and William Edgar Hazen, was orphaned before she turned four. She and her sister went to live with their aunt and uncle shorly after her younger brother died. Hazen attended the Mississippi Industrial Institute and College at Columbus, receiving her B.S. degree in 1910. During college, Hazen became interested in science and she studied biology at Columbia University, earning her M.S. in 1917. After working in the U.S. Army laboratories during World War I, she returned to Columbia where she received her Ph.D. in microbiology in 1927. Following her work as an instructor at Columbia, Hazen accepted a position with the New York Department of Health where she researched bacterial diseases.

In 1948, Hazen and Rachel Brown began researching fungal infections found in humans due to antibiotic treatments and diseases. Some of the antibiotics they discovered did indeed kill the fungus; however, they also killed the test mice. Finally, Hazen located a microorganism on a farm in Virginia, and Brown's tests indicated that the microorganism produced two antibiotics, one of which proved effective for treating fungus and candidiasis in humans. Brown purified the antibiotic which was patented under the name *nystatin.* In 1954, the antibiotic became available in pill form. Hazen and Brown continued their research and discovered two other antibiotics. Hazen received numerous awards individually and with her research partner, Rachel Brown. Elizabeth Hazen died on June 24, 1975.

Infection control

Definition

Infection control refers to policies and procedures used to minimize the risk of spreading infections, especially in hospitals and human or animal health care facilities.

Purpose

The purpose of infection control is to reduce the occurrence of infectious diseases. These diseases are usually caused by bacteria or viruses and can be spread by human to human contact, animal to human contact, human contact with an infected surface, airborne transmission through tiny droplets of infectious agents suspended in the air, and, finally, by such common vehicles as food or water. Diseases that are spread from animals to humans are known as zoonoses; animals that carry disease agents from one host to another are known as vectors.

Infection control in hospitals and other health care settings

Infections contracted in hospitals are also called nosocomial infections. They occur in approximately 5% of all hospital patients. These infections result in increased time spent in the hospital and, in some cases, **death**. There are many reasons nosocomial infections are common, one of which is that many hospital patients have a weakened immune system which makes them more susceptible to infections. This weakened immune system can be caused either by the patient's diseases or by treatments given to the patient. Second, many medical procedures can increase the risk of infection by introducing infectious agents into the patient. Thirdly, many patients are admitted to

Selected infectious diseases and corresponding treatment

Disease	Symptoms	Transmittal	Treatment
Chicken pox	Rash, low-grade fever	Person to person	None; acetaminophen may treat fever or discomfort
Common cold/influenza	Runny nose, sore throat, cough, fever, headache, muscle aches	Person to person	None, although various remedies may help relieve symptoms
Hepatitis A	Jaundice, flu-like symptoms	Sexual contact with an infected person or contact with contaminated blood, food, or water	None; acetaminophen may treat fever or pain
H1N1 influenza	Fever, cough, sore throat, body aches, loss of appetite, fatigue	Person to person	Antiviral drugs
Measles	Skin rash, runny nose and eyes, fever, cough	Person to person	None; acetaminophen may treat fever or discomfort
Meningitis	Neck pain, headache, pain caused by exposure to light, fever, nausea, drowsiness	Person to person	Antibiotics for bacterial meningitis, hospital care for viral meningitis
Methicillin-resistant Staphylococcus aureus (MRSA)	Rash, shortness of breath, fever, chest pain, headache	Person to person or contact with contaminated surfaces	Antibiotics
Mumps	Swelling of salivary glands	Person to person	Anti-inflammatory drugs
Ringworm	Skin rash	Contact with infected animal or person	Antifungal drugs applied topically or taken orally
Tetanus	Lockjaw, other spasms	Soil infection of wounds	Antibiotics, antitoxins, muscle relaxants

(Table by PreMediaGlobal. Reproduced by permission of Gale, a part of Cengage Learning.)

hospitals because of **infectious disease**. These infectious agents can then be transferred from patient to patient by hospital workers or visitors.

Infection control has become a formal discipline in the United States since the 1950s, due to the spread of **staphylococcal infections** in hospitals. Because there is both the risk of health care providers acquiring infections themselves, and of their passing infections on to patients, the Centers for Disease Control and Prevention (CDC) established guidelines for infection control procedures. In addition to hospitals, infection control is important in nursing homes, clinics, child care centers, and restaurants, as well as in the home.

To lower the risk of nosocomial infections, the CDC began a national program of hospital inspection in 1970 known as the National Nosocomial Infections Surveillance system, or NNIS. The CDC reported that over 300 hospitals participate in the NNIS system as of the early 2000s. Data collected from the participating hospitals show that infection control programs can siginificantly improve patient safety, lower infection rates, and lower patient mortality.

Dental health care settings are similar to hospitals in that both personnel and equipment can transmit infection if proper safeguards are not observed. The CDC issued new guidelines in 2003 for the proper maintenance and sterilization of dental equipment, hand hygiene for dentists and dental hygienists, dental radiology, medications, and oral surgery, environmental infection control, and standards for dental laboratories.

The newest addition to the infection control specialist's resources is molecular typing, which speeds up the identification of a disease agent. Rapid identification in turn allows for timely containment of a disease outbreak.

Threat of emerging infectious diseases

Due to constant changes in our lifestyles and environments, new diseases are constantly appearing that people are susceptible to, making protection from the threat of infectious disease urgent. Many new contagious diseases have been identified in the past 30 years, such as **AIDS**, Ebola, and hantavirus. Increased travel between continents makes the worldwide spread of disease a bigger concern than it once was. Additionally, many common infectious diseases have become resistant to known treatments.

The emergence of the **severe acute respiratory syndrome (SARS)** epidemic in Asia in February

KEY TERMS

Acquired immune deficiency syndrome (AIDS)—A disease that weakens the body's immune system. It is also known as HIV infection.

Antibiotic—A substance, such as a drug, that can stop a bacteria from growing or destroy the bacteria.

Antibiotic resistance—The ability of infectious agents to change their biochemistry in such a way as to make an antibiotic no longer effective.

Bioterrorism—The intentional use of disease-causing microbes or other biologic agents to intimidate or terrorize a civilian population for political or military reasons.

Ebola—The disease caused by the newly described and very deadly Ebola virus found in Africa.

Epidemiology—The branch of medicine that deals with the transmission of infectious diseases in large populations and with detection of the sources and causes of epidemics.

Hantavirus—A group of arboviruses that cause hemorrhagic fever (characterized by sudden onset, fever, aching and bleeding in the internal organs).

Immunization—Immunity refers to the body's ability to protect itself from a certain disease after it has been exposed to that disease. Through immunization, also known as vaccination, a small amount of an infectious agent is injected into the body to stimulate the body to develop immunity.

Immunocompromized—Refers to the condition of having a weakened immune system. This can happen due to genetic factors, drugs, or disease.

Nosocomial infection—An infection acquired in a hospital setting.

Staphylococcal infection—An infection caused by the organism *Staphlococcus.* Infection by this agent is common and is often resistant to antibiotics.

Vector—An animal carrier that transfers an infectious organism from one host to another.

Zoonosis (plural, zoonoses)—Any disease of animals that can be transmitted to humans under natural conditions. Lyme disease, rabies, psittacosis (parrot fever), cat-scratch fever, and monkeypox are examples of zoonoses.

2003 was a classic instance of an emerging disease that spread rapidly because of the increased frequency of international and intercontinental travel. In addition, the SARS outbreak demonstrated the vulnerability of hospitals and health care workers to emerging diseases. Clusters of cases within hospitals occurred in the early weeks of the epidemic when the disease had not yet been recognized and the first SARS patients were admitted without **isolation** precautions.

The SARS epidemic also raised a number of ethical and legal questions regarding current attitudes toward infection control.

Problems of antibiotic resistance

Because of the overuse of **antibiotics**, many bacteria have developed a resistance to common antibiotics. This means that newer antibiotics must continually be developed in order to treat an infection. However, further resistance seems to come about almost simultaneously. This indicates to many scientists that it might become more and more difficult to treat infectious diseases. The use of antibiotics outside of medicine also contributes to increased antibiotic resistance. One example of this is the use of antibiotics in animal husbandry. These negative trends can only be reversed by establishing a more rational use of antibiotics through treatment guidelines.

Bioterrorism

The events of September 11, 2001, and the **anthrax** scare that followed in October 2001 alerted public health officials as well as the general public to the possible use of infectious disease agents as weapons of terrorism. The Centers for Disease Control and Prevention (CDC) now has a list of topics and resources related to bioterrorism on its web site.

Description

The goals of infection control programs are: immunizing against preventable diseases, defining precautions that can prevent exposure to infectious agents, and restricting the exposure of health care workers to an infectious agent. An infection control practitioner is a specially trained professional, oftentimes a nurse, who oversees infection control programs.

Commonly recommended precautions to avoid and control the spread of infections include:

- Vaccinate people and pets against diseases for which a vaccine is available. The vaccines used against infectious diseases are very safe compared to most drugs.
- Wash hands often.
- Cook food thoroughly.
- Use antibiotics only as directed.
- See a doctor for infections that do not heal.
- Avoid areas with a lot of insects.
- Be cautious around wild or unfamiliar animals, or any animals that are unusually aggressive. Do not purchase exotic animals as pets.
- Do not engage in unprotected sex or in intravenous drug use.
- Find out about infectious diseases when you make travel plans. Travelers' advisories and adult vaccination recommendations are available on the CDC web site or by calling the CDC's telephone service at 404-332-4559.

Because of the higher risk of spreading infectious disease in a hospital setting, higher levels of precautions are taken there. Typically, health care workers wear gloves with all patients, since it is difficult to know whether a transmittable disease is present or not. Patients who have a known infectious disease are isolated to decrease the risk of transmitting the infectious agent to another person. Hospital workers who come in contact with infected patients must wear gloves and gowns to decrease the risk of carrying the infectious agent to other patients. All articles of equipment that are used in an isolation room are decontaminated before reuse. Patients who are immunocompromised may be put in protective isolation to decrease the risk of infectious agents being brought into their room. Any hospital worker with infections, including colds, are restricted from that room.

Hospital infections can also be transmitted through the air. Thus care must be taken when handling infected materials so as to decrease the numbers of infectious agents that become airborne. Special care should also taken with hospital ventilation systems to prevent recirculation of contaminated air.

Resources

BOOKS

Beers, Mark H., Robert S. Porter, and Thomas V. Jones, eds. *The Merck Manual of Diagnosis and Therapy*. 18th ed. Whitehouse Station, NJ: Merck Research Laboratories, 2006.

PERIODICALS

Ashford, D. A., R. M. Kaiser, M. E. Bales, et al. "Planning Against Biological Terrorism: Lessons from Outbreak Investigations." *Emerging Infectious Diseases* 9 (May 2003): 515–519.

Gostin, L. O., R. Bayer, and A. L. Fairchild. "Ethical and Legal Challenges Posed by Severe Acute Respiratory Syndrome: Implications for the Control of Severe Infectious Disease Threats." *Journal of the American Medical Association* 290 (December 24, 2003): 3229–3237.

Ho, P. L., X. P. Tang, and W. H. Seto. "SARS: Hospital Infection Control and Admission Strategies." *Respirology* 8, Supplement (November 2003): S41–S45.

Jacobson, R. M., K. S. Zabel, and G. A. Poland. "The Overall Safety Profile of Currently Available Vaccines Directed Against Infectious Diseases." *Expert Opinion on Drug Safety* 2 (May 2003): 215–223.

Jarvis, W. R. "Benchmarking for Prevention: the Centers for Disease Control and Prevention's National Nosocomial Infections Surveillance (NNIS) System Experience." *Infection* 31, Supplement 2 (December 2003): 44–48.

Kohn, W. G., A. S. Collins, J. L. Cleveland, et al. "Guidelines for Infection Control in Dental Health-Care Settings—2003." *Morbidity and Mortality Weekly Reports: Reports and Recommendations* 52, RR-17 (December 19, 2003): 1–61.

Peng, P. W., D. T. Wong, D. Bevan, and M. Gardam. "Infection Control and Anesthesia: Lessons Learned from the Toronto SARS Outbreak." *Canadian Journal of Anaesthesiology* 50 (December 2003): 989–997.

Petrak, R. M., D. J. Sexton, M. L. Butera, et al. "The Value of an Infectious Diseases Specialist." *Clinical Infectious Diseases* 36 (April 15, 2003): 1013–1017.

Sehulster, L., and R. Y. Chinn. "Guidelines for Environmental Infection Control in Health-Care Facilities. Recommendations of CDC and the Healthcare Infection Control Practices Advisory Committee (HICPAC)." *Morbidity and Mortality Recommendations and Reports* 52, RR-10 (June 6, 2003): 1–42.

Subramanian, D., J. A. Sandoe, V. Keer, and M. H. Wilcox. "Rapid Spread of Penicillin-Resistant *Streptococcus pneumoniae* Among High-Risk Hospital Inpatients and the Role of Molecular Typing in Outbreak Confirmation." *Journal of Hospital Infection* 54 (June 2003): 99–103.

ORGANIZATIONS

American College of Epidemiology, 1500 Sunday Drive, Suite 102, Raleigh, NC, 27607, 919 861-5573, 919 787-4916, info@acepidemiology.org, http://www.acepidemiology.org/.

American Public Health Association (APHA), 800 I Street NW, Washington, DC, 20001-3710, 202 777-APHA, 202 777-2534, http://www.apha.org.

American Veterinary Medical Association (AVMA), 1931 North Meacham Road, Suite 100, Schaumburg, IL,

60173-4360, 847 925-1329, 800 248-2862, http://www.avma.org/.

Centers for Disease Control and Prevention (CDC), 1600 Clifton Road, Atlanta, GA, 30333, 800 232-4636, cdcinfo@cdc.gov, http://www.cdc.gov.

National Institute of Allergies and Infectious Diseases, 6610 Rockledge Drive, MSC 6612, Bethesda, MD, 20892-6612, 301 496-5717, 301 402-3573, 866 284-4107, ocpostoffice@niaid.nih.gov, http://www.niaid.nih.gov.

Cindy L. A. Jones, PhD
Rebecca J. Frey, PhD

Infectious arthritis

Definition

Infectious arthritis, which is sometimes called septic arthritis or pyogenic arthritis, is a serious infection of the joints characterized by **pain**, **fever**, occasional chills, inflammation and swelling in one or more joints, and loss of function in the affected joints. It is considered a medical emergency.

Description

Infectious arthritis can occur in any age group, including newborns and children. In adults, it usually affects the wrists or one of the patient's weight-bearing joints–most often the knee–although about 20% of adult patients have symptoms in more than one joint. Multiple joint infection is common in children and typically involves the shoulders, knees, and hips.

Some groups of patients are at greater risk for developing infectious arthritis. These high-risk groups include:

- Patients with chronic rheumatoid arthritis.
- Patients with certain systemic infections, including gonorrhea and HIV infection. Women and male homosexuals are at greater risk for gonorrheal arthritis than are male heterosexuals.
- Patients with certain types of cancer.
- IV drug abusers and alcoholics.
- Patients with artificial (prosthetic) joints.
- Patients with diabetes, sickle cell anemia, or systemic lupus erythematosus (SLE).
- Patients with recent joint injuries or surgery, or patients receiving medications injected directly into a joint.

Causes and symptoms

In general, infectious arthritis is caused by the spread of a bacterial, viral, or fungal infection through the bloodstream to the joint. The disease agents may enter the joint directly from the outside as a result of an injury or a surgical procedure, or they may be carried to the joint by the blood from infections elsewhere in the body. The specific organisms vary somewhat according to age group. Newborns are most likely to acquire gonococcal infections of the joints from a mother with **gonorrhea**. Children may also acquire infectious arthritis from a hospital environment, often as a result of catheter placement. The organisms involved are usually either *Haemophilus influenzae* (in children under two years of age) or *Staphylococcus aureus*. In older children or adults, the infectious organisms include *Streptococcus pyogenes* and *Streptococcus viridans* as well as *Staphylococcus aureus*. *Staphylococcus epidermidis* is usually involved in joint infections related to surgery. Sexually active teenagers and adults frequently develop infectious arthritis from *Neisseria gonorrhoeae* infections. Older adults are often vulnerable to joint infections caused by gram-negative bacilli, including *Salmonella* and *Pseudomonas*.

Infectious arthritis often has a sudden onset, but symptoms sometimes develop over a period of three to 14 days. The symptoms include swelling in the infected joint and pain when the joint is moved. Infectious arthritis in the hip may be experienced as pain in the groin area that becomes much worse if the patient tries to walk. In 90% of cases, there is some leakage of tissue fluid into the affected joint. The joint is sore to the touch; it may or may not be warm to the touch, depending on how deep the infection lies within the joint. In most cases the patient will have fever and chills, although the fever may be only low-grade. Children sometimes develop **nausea and vomiting**.

Septic arthritis is considered a medical emergency because of the damage it causes to bone as well as cartilage, and its potential for creating **septic shock**, which is a potentially fatal condition. *Staphylococcus aureus* is capable of destroying cartilage in one or two days. Destruction of cartilage and bone in turn leads to **dislocations** of the joints and bones. If the infection is caused by bacteria, it can spread to the blood and surrounding tissues, causing abscesses or even blood poisoning. The most common complication of infectious arthritis is **osteoarthritis**.

Diagnosis

The diagnosis of infectious arthritis depends on a combination of laboratory testing with careful

KEY TERMS

Arthrocentesis—A procedure in which the doctor inserts a needle into the patient's joint to withdraw fluid for diagnostic testing or to drain infected fluid from the joint.

Pyogenic arthritis—Another name for infectious arthritis. Pyogenic means that pus is formed during the disease process.

Sepsis—Invasion of the body by disease organisms or their toxins. Generalized sepsis can lead to shock and eventual death.

Septic arthritis—Another name for infectious arthritis.

Synovial fluid (SF)—A fluid secreted by tissues surrounding the joints that lubricates the joints.

history-taking and **physical examination** of the affected joint. It is important to keep in mind that infectious arthritis can coexist with other forms of arthritis, **gout**, **rheumatic fever**, **Lyme disease**, or other disorders that can cause a combination of joint pain and fever. In some cases, the doctor may consult a specialist in orthopedics or rheumatology to avoid misdiagnosis.

Patient history

The patient's history will tell the doctor whether he or she belongs to a high-risk group for infectious arthritis. Sudden onset of joint pain is also important information.

Physical examination

The doctor will examine the affected joint for swelling, soreness, warmth, and other signs of infection. Location is sometimes a clue to diagnosis; infection of an unusual joint, such as the joints between the breastbone and collarbone, or the pelvic joints, often occurs in drug abusers.

Laboratory tests

Laboratory testing is necessary to confirm the diagnosis of infectious arthritis. The doctor will perform an arthrocentesis, which is a procedure that involves withdrawing a sample of synovial fluid (SF) from the joint with a needle and syringe. SF is a lubricating fluid secreted by tissues surrounding the joints. Patients should be warned that arthrocentesis is a painful procedure. The fluid sample is sent for culture in the sealed syringe. SF from infected joints is usually streaked with pus or looks cloudy and watery. Cell counts usually indicate a high level of white cells; a level higher than 100,000 cells/mm^3 or a neutrophil proportion greater than 90% suggests septic arthritis. A Gram's stain of the culture obtained from the SF is usually positive for the specific disease organism.

Doctors sometimes order a biopsy of the synovial tissue near the joint if the fluid sample is negative. Cultures of other body fluids, such as urine, blood, or cervical mucus, may be taken in addition to the SF culture.

Diagnostic imaging

Diagnostic imaging is not helpful in the early stages of infectious arthritis. Destruction of bone or cartilage does not appear on x rays until 10–14 days after the onset of symptoms. Imaging studies are sometimes useful if the infection is in a deep-seated joint.

Treatment

Infectious arthritis requires usually requires several days of treatment in a hospital, with follow-up medication and **physical therapy** lasting several weeks or months.

Medications

Because of the possibility of serious damage to the joint or other complications if treatment is delayed, the patient will be started on intravenous **antibiotics** before the specific organism is identified. After the disease organism has been identified, the doctor may give the patient a drug that targets the specific bacterium or virus. **Nonsteroidal anti-inflammatory drugs** are usually given for viral infections.

Intravenous antibiotics are given for about two weeks, or until the inflammation has disappeared. The patient may then be given a two- to four-week course of oral antibiotics.

Surgery

In some cases, surgery is necessary to drain fluid from the infected joint. Patients who need surgical drainage include those who have not responded to antibiotic treatment, those with infections of the hip or other joints that are difficult to reach with arthrocentesis, and those with joint infections related to gunshot or other penetrating **wounds**.

Patients with severe damage to bone or cartilage may need **reconstructive surgery**, but it cannot be performed until the infection is completely gone.

Monitoring and supportive treatment

Infectious arthritis requires careful monitoring while the patient is in the hospital. The doctor will drain the joint on a daily basis and remove a small sample of fluid for culture to check the patient's response to the antibiotic.

Infectious arthritis often causes intense pain. Patients are given medications to relieve pain, together with hot compresses or ice packs on the affected joint. In some cases the patient's arm or leg is put in a splint to protect the sore joint from accidental movement. Recovery can be speeded up, however, if the patient practices range-of-motion exercises to the extent that the pain allows.

Prognosis

The prognosis depends on prompt treatment with antibiotics and drainage of the infected joint. About 70% of patients will recover without permanent joint damage. However, many patients will develop osteoarthritis or deformed joints. Children with infected hip joints sometimes suffer damage to the growth plate. If treatment is delayed, infectious arthritis has a mortality rate between 5% and 30% due to septic shock and **respiratory failure**.

Prevention

Some cases of infectious arthritis are preventable by lifestyle choices. These include avoidance of self-injected drugs; sexual abstinence or monogamous relationships; and prompt testing and treatment for suspected cases of gonorrhea. Patients receiving corticosteroid injections into the joints for osteoarthritis may want to weigh this treatment method against the increased risk of infectious arthritis.

Resources

BOOKS

McPhee, Stephen, and Maxine Papadakis.*Current Medical Diagnosis and Treatment, 2010*, 49th ed. New York: McGraw-Hill Medical, 2009.

Rebecca J. Frey, PhD

Infectious disease

Definition

Infectious disease—also called communicable disease—is any illness caused by an infective agent—a germ, microbe, or parasite. Infective agents include bacteria, viruses, fungi, parasitic protozoa, and worms.

Demographics

Virtually all children contract infectious disease, especially during infancy and early childhood. Respiratory and gastrointestinal infections are the most common causes of illness in children. Respiratory infections affect as many as 32% of all infants. Up to 26% of infants contract gastrointestinal infections.

Worldwide, more children and adults die from infectious disease than any other single cause. The vast majority of these deaths occur in poorer counties with limited access to prevention, medical care, and drugs. In 2008, infectious disease killed 5,970,000 children under the age of five, accounting for 68% of all deaths in that age group: an estimated 18% died of **pneumonia**, 15% of **diarrhea**, and eight percent of **malaria**. According to the World Health Organization (WHO), more than 800,000 children under five die every year from **pneumococcal pneumonia** and **meningitis**. Children under age two are at particular risk for serious pneumococcal infections. Children with HIV/AIDS are 20–40 more likely than others to contract pneumococcal infections. Pneumococcal meningitis is disabling or fatal in 40–70% of affected children.

Among American children, the frequency and severity of infectious disease has declined dramatically in recent decades, primarily due to the development of vaccines for common childhood infections. The United States is one of the few places in the world where **polio** has been completely eradicated. Childhood pneumococcal infections caused by vaccine–targeted bacterial strains have been almost completely eliminated.

Description

When an infective agent enters the body and begins to multiply, the immune system responds with various defensive mechanisms that protect against most infectious disease. However when an infective agent temporarily evades or overwhelms the immune system and begins to damage tissues, signs and symptoms of disease develop.

The most common infectious diseases are contagious—they spread via direct transfer of an infective agent from one person to another. Shaking hands, kissing, or coughing or sneezing on someone can directly transmit contagious diseases such as colds, flu, or **tuberculosis** (TB). Some infective agents, including cold viruses, can be contracted by indirect contact with a contaminated surface such as a faucet, doorknob, or computer keyboard. International airplane travel is responsible for the spread of contagious diseases around the world. Infant diarrhea caused by rotavirus or the protozoan *Giardia lamblia* often spreads among babies and young children through the accidental transferring of feces from hand to mouth after diaper changes. Some infectious diseases can be passed from a mother to her unborn child across the placenta or during birth.

Other infectious diseases can be transmitted from animals or animal waste to humans. Dog and cat saliva may contain more than 100 different types of infective agents. *Pasteurella* bacteria are the most common microbes transmitted via pet **bites**. These bacteria can cause serious—sometimes fatal—infectious diseases such as meningitis, an inflammation of the lining of the brain and spinal cord. **Toxoplasmosis** is a bacterial infection that is transmitted via cat feces. Pet reptiles, such as turtles, snakes, and iguanas, can transmit *Salmonella* bacteria. Wild animals can directly or indirectly transmit a wide variety of infectious disease.

Some infectious diseases are transferred between human hosts by insect vectors:

- Mosquitoes transfer the protozoan that causes malaria, as well as West Nile virus, dengue fever, and viral encephalitis.
- Body lice can transmit typhus.
- Fleas can transmit typhus and transfer plague bacteria from rodents to humans.
- Deer ticks—which are actually more closely related to crabs than to insects—can transfer the bacterium that causes Lyme disease from mice to humans.
- Ticks can also transmit the bacterium that cause Rocky Mountain spotted fever and tularemia and the protozoan that causes babesiosis.

Some infectious diseases are spread from a single source to many people through contaminated food or water. For example, the bacterium ***Escherichia coli*** (*E. coli*) can be transmitted via unwashed fruit or vegetables or undercooked meat.

Some infectious diseases have recently emerged, re–emerged, or become much more widespread and dangerous by acquiring drug resistance. Examples include:

- methicillin–resistant *Staphylococcus aureus* (MRSA) bacteria
- multi– and extensively drug–resistant TB bacteria
- 2009 H1N1 influenza virus
- H5N1 avian influenza virus
- West Nile virus
- Ebola virus
- Marburg virus
- Nipah virus
- SARS virus
- dengue virus
- polio virus
- malaria parasite

Risk factors

Risk factors for respiratory or gastrointestinal infectious diseases in babies include:

- premature birth
- low birth weight
- low socioeconomic status
- multiple siblings
- daycare
- parental smoking

Children with weakened immune systems are at increased risk for infectious disease. Infection can occur if a child:

- has HIV/AIDS
- has an autoimmune disease
- is taking steroids or anti–rejection drugs for a transplanted organ
- is being treated for cancer

In 2010, scientists reported the discovery of mutations that increase susceptibility to infectious disease. The mutations are in a gene called CISH that encodes a protein that regulates the immune system's response to infectious disease. A child who inherits one of these mutations from a parent has an 18% increased risk for infectious disease. Inheriting four or more of the mutations increases the risk to 81%.

Causes and symptoms

Although most bacteria are not harmful—and some types are essential for proper functioning of the human body—some bacteria produce toxins that cause infectious disease. *Streptococcus* can cause infections ranging from relatively mild ear infections to

KEY TERMS

Bacteria—Single–celled microorganisms that live in soil, water, organic matter, plants, and animals, and are associated with a number of infectious diseases.

Fungi—A kingdom of saprophytic and parasitic spore–producing organisms that include mushrooms and yeast.

Helminths—Parasitic worms, such as tapeworms or liver flukes, that can live in the human body.

Immunization—Treatment, usually by vaccination, to produce immunity to a specific infective agent.

Meningitis—An infection or inflammation of membranes surrounding the brain and spinal cord.

Pneumococcal—Infection by the bacterium *Streptococcus pneumoniae* that causes acute pneumonia.

Pneumonia—Inflammation of the lungs, usually caused by infection with a bacterium, virus, or fungus.

Protozoa—Single–celled microorganisms of the Kingdom Protista, some of which can cause infectious disease in humans.

Vaccine—A preparation of live, weakened, or killed microorganisms that is administered to produce or increase immunity to specific diseases.

strep throat to potentially fatal pneumococcal pneumonia, meningitis, and **sepsis** or blood poisoning. Children can be especially vulnerable to bacteria that cause:

- diphtheria
- pertussis or whooping cough
- tetanus
- urinary tract infections

Viruses cause many childhood diseases including:

- common colds
- influenzas
- diarrhea from rotaviruses
- measles
- mumps
- rubella (German measles)
- chicken pox
- polio
- hepatitis
- human papillomavirus (HPV)
- herpes
- HIV/AIDS

Fungi cause various infectious diseases including:

- thrush, a mouth and throat infection in infants caused by *Candida albicans*
- skin conditions, such as ringworm and athlete's foot
- pneumonia caused by *Pneumocystis carinii*

Protozoan parasites cause infectious diseases such as malaria, **giardiasis**, and toxoplasmosis. Helminths are larger parasites—such as tapeworms and roundworms—that can infect the intestinal tract, lungs, liver, skin, or brain.

Symptoms of infectious disease vary with the type of infection. However many infectious diseases have symptoms that include:

- fever and chills
- loss of appetite
- muscle aches
- fatigue

Diagnosis

Examination

A medical history and physical exam—including the child's breathing pattern and respiratory rate, body temperature, and other symptoms—may be sufficient for diagnosing an infectious disease. Sometimes an infectious organism in a blood or urine sample can be seen under a microscope.

Tests

Blood, urine, throat swabs, or other bodily secretions may be cultured in a laboratory to identify the infective agent. Diagnosis of some infectious diseases requires a **lumbar puncture** or spinal tap to obtain a sample of cerebrospinal fluid.

Procedures

Diagnostic procedures may include:

- a chest x ray to diagnose pneumonia
- computerized tomography (CT) scans or magnetic resonance imaging (MRI)
- a biopsy—the removal of a tiny amount of tissue from an infected area, such as the lung for diagnosing fungal pneumonia

Treatment

Traditional

Treatment depends on the type of infectious disease. Some diseases resolve on their own without any treatment other than possibly relieving symptoms.

Drugs

- Bacterial infections are treated with antibiotics.
- A very few antiviral drugs, such as acyclovir, are available for treating viral infections such as flu and herpes.
- Various drugs may be used to treat hepatitis B and C.
- HIV/AIDS is treated with a combination of drugs known as highly active antiretroviral therapy (HAART).
- Fungal infections of the skin and nails may be treated with over–the–counter or prescription medications applied directly to the affected area.
- Oral antifungal medications are used to treat systemic fungal infections, such as histoplasmosis, or severe infections of the mouth and throat in children with weakened immune systems.
- Only a very few anti–parasitic drugs are available and some of these are either very toxic or are becoming less effective with the spread of drug–resistant parasites.

Alternative

A wide variety of alternative therapies are used to treat infectious disease, although bacterial infections usually require **antibiotics**. Yogurt containing healthy gut bacteria can ease gastrointestinal symptoms and has been shown to reduce the incidence of some common infections in children.

Home remedies

Many mild infectious diseases respond well to home remedies. Bed rest and drinking plenty of fluids are the most common remedies.

Prognosis

Prognosis varies greatly depending on the type of infectious disease. Some, such as the **common cold**, usually resolve quickly without medical treatment, and most infectious diseases have only minor complications. However some—such as pneumonia or meningitis—can be life–threatening. Even some common and usually mild infectious diseases—such as **measles**, **mumps**, chicken pox, or seasonal flu—can be dangerous or life–threatening in very young children.

Prevention

Many common infectious diseases are preventable with good hygiene and vaccines. The best protection is frequent and thorough hand washing:

- before, during, and after handling food
- before eating
- after using the toilet
- after changing diapers
- after touching animals or their toys, leashes, or waste
- after touching trash, cleaning rags, drains, or soil
- after contact with body fluids, including blood, vomit, saliva, or nasal secretions
- before cleaning a wound, administering medicine, or inserting contact lenses
- more often, if someone in the home is ill

Hands should be washed by:

- wetting with water and applying soap
- rubbing them together vigorously to lather and scrub all surfaces for 20 seconds
- rinsing well under running water
- drying with a paper towel or air dryer
- turning off the faucet with a paper towel
- using alcohol–based disposable hand wipes or sanitizers if soap and water are not available

Other practices for preventing infectious disease include:

- breastfeeding, which helps protect infants from respiratory and gastrointestinal infections
- avoiding touching one's eyes, nose, and mouth
- covering one's mouth and nose when coughing or sneezing
- rinsing fresh fruit and vegetables under running water and scrubbing firm–skinned produce with a vegetable brush
- keeping meat, poultry, seafood, and eggs separated from other foods at all times
- refrigerating foods promptly at a constant temperature of 40°F (4°C) or below, with enough room for cold air to circulate freely
- freezing foods at 0°F (–18°C) or below
- using separate cutting boards for produce and meat, poultry, seafood, or eggs
- washing cutting boards, dishes, utensils, and counter tops with hot, soapy water between preparation of each food item
- never reusing marinades from raw foods without boiling first

- thoroughly cooking all foods, especially meat, at the correct temperature
- cleaning with disposable paper towels or sanitizing wipes, cloth towels that are washed in hot water, or sponges that are washed in the dishwasher or microwaved daily for 30 seconds
- cleaning and disinfecting all bathroom surfaces, especially when someone in the home has an infectious disease
- avoiding sharing personal items, including toothbrushes, combs, drinking glasses, and eating utensils
- keeping children home when they are sick
- not flying when ill
- practicing safer sex or abstaining from sex entirely to avoid sexually transmitted infections that can be passed to unborn children

Precautions against contracting infectious disease from animals include:

- adopting pets from an animal shelter or purchasing from a reputable store or breeder
- obtaining routine care and immunizations for your pet from a veterinarian
- obeying leash laws
- cleaning litter boxes daily, except when a person is pregnant
- keeping children away from pet waste
- keeping sandboxes covered
- washing one's hands thoroughly after contact with animals
- keeping wild animals away from the house
- using insect repellent and routinely checking for ticks and removing them immediately by applying gentle, steady pressure with tweezers

Children should be immunized as follows:

- at birth or as soon as possible: hepatitis B (HBV)
- at one–four months: HBV
- at two months: diphtheria, tetanus, and acellular pertussis (DTaP); haemophilus influenza type b (Hib); inactivated poliovirus (IPV); pneumococcal conjugate (PCV); rotavirus (RV)
- four months: DTaP; Hib; IPV; PCV; RV
- six months: DTaP; Hib; PCV; RV
- six months and annually: seasonal flu
- six to 18 months: HBV; IPV
- 12–15 months: varicella (chicken pox, Var); Hib; PCV; measles, mumps, and rubella (MMR)
- 12–23 months: hepatitis A (HepA)
- 15–18 months: DTaP
- four–six years: IPV; Var; DTaP; MMR
- 11–12 years: DTaP booster; meningitis (MCV)
- girls at 11–12 years: human papillomavirus (HPV) to prevent genital warts and cervical cancer
- additional immunizations for foreign travel

Resources

BOOKS

Finn, Adam, and Andrew J. Pollard, eds. *Hot Topics in Infection and Immunity in Children IV*. New York: Springer, 2008.

Shah, Samir S., ed. *Pediatric Practice: Infectious Diseases*. New York: McGraw-Hill Medical, 2009.

Shannon, Joyce Brennfleck. *Contagious Diseases Sourcebook: Basic Consumer Information About Disease Spread from Person to Person*, 2nd ed. Detroit: Omnigraphics, 2010.

PERIODICALS

Black, Robert E., et al. "Global, Regional, and National Causes of Child Mortality in 2008: A Systematic Analysis." *Lancet* 375(9730) (June 5–11, 2010): 1969–87.

Khor, Chiea C., et al. "CISH and Susceptibility to Infectious Diseases." *New England Journal of Medicine* 362(22) (June 3, 2010): 2092.

Rockoff, Jonathan D. "More Parents Seek Vaccine Exemption." *Wall Street Journal* (July 6, 2010): A19.

"Science and Technology: Mens Sana in Corpore Sano; Disease and Intelligence." *Economist* 396(8689) (July 3, 2010): 75.

OTHER

"Breast Milk Reduces Infections in Babies." HealthDay. (June 21, 2010). http://www.nlm.nih.gov/medlineplus/news/fullstory_100207.html (accessed September 26, 2010).

"Childhood Diseases: What Parents Should Know." MedlinePlus. (Spring 2008). http://www.nlm.nih.gov/medlineplus/magazine/issues/pdf/spring2008.pdf (accessed September 26, 2010).

"Infectious Diseases." MedlinePlus. (June 30, 2010). http://www.nlm.nih.gov/medlineplus/infectiousdiseases.html (accessed September 26, 2010).

Mayo Clinic Staff. "Germs: Understand and Protect Against Bacteria, Viruses and Infection." MayoClinic.com. (April 30, 2009). http://www.mayoclinic.com/health/germs/ID00002/METHOD=print (accessed September 26, 2010).

Mayo Clinic Staff. "Infectious Diseases." MayoClinic.com. (July 21, 2009). http://www.mayoclinic.com/health/infectious-diseases/DS01145 (accessed September 26, 2010).

"An Ounce of Prevention Keeps the Germs Away: Seven Keys to a Safer Healthier Home." Centers for Disease Control and Prevention. http://www.cdc.gov/ounceofprevention/docs/oop_brochure_eng.pdf (accessed September 26, 2010).

"Understanding Microbes in Sickness and in Health." National Institute of Allergy and Infectious Diseases. (September 2009). http://www.niaid.nih.gov/topics/

microbes/documents/microbesbook.pdf (September 26, 2010).

ORGANIZATIONS

National Foundation for Infectious Diseases (NFID), 4733 Bethesda Ave., Suite 750, Bethesda, MD, 20814, (301) 656–0003, (301) 907–0878, info@nfid.org, http://www.nfid.org.

National Institute of Allergy and Infectious Diseases, Office of Communications and Public Liaison (NIAID), 6610 Rockledge Dr., Bethesda, MD, 20892–66123, (866) 284–4107, http://www3.niaid.nih.gov.

U.S. Centers for Disease Control and Prevention (CDC), 1600 Clifton Rd., Atlanta, GA, 30333, (800) CDC–INFO (232–4636), cdcinfo@cdc.gov, http://www.cdc.gov.

Margaret Alic, PhD

Infectious hepatitis *see* **Hepatitis A**

Infectious mononucleosis

Definition

Infectious mononucleosis is a contagious illness caused by the **Epstein-Barr virus** that can affect the liver, lymph nodes, and oral cavity. While mononucleosis is not usually a serious disease, its primary symptoms of **fatigue** and lack of energy can linger for several months.

Description

Infectious mononucleosis, frequently called "mono" or the "kissing disease," is caused by the Epstein-Barr virus (EBV) found in saliva and mucus. The virus affects a type of white blood cell called the B lymphocyte producing characteristic atypical lymphocytes that may be useful in the diagnosis of the disease.

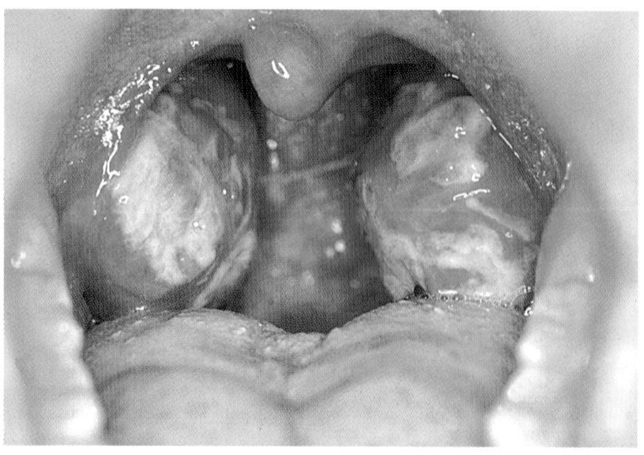

Sore throat and swollen tonsils caused by infectious mononucleosis. *(Dr. P. Marazzi/Photo Researchers, Inc.)*

While anyone, even young children, can develop mononucleosis, it occurs most often in young adults between the ages of 15 and 35 and is especially common in teenagers. The mononucleosis infection rate among college students who have not previously been exposed to EBV has been estimated to be about 15%. In younger children, the illness may not be recognized.

The disease typically runs its course in four to six weeks in people with normally functioning immune systems. People with weakened or suppressed immune systems, such as **AIDS** patients or those who have had organ transplants, are particularly vulnerable to the potentially serious complications of infectious mononucleosis.

Causes and symptoms

The EBV that causes mononucleosis is related to a group of herpes viruses, including those that cause **cold sores**, chicken pox, and **shingles**. Most people are exposed to EBV at some point during their lives. Mononucleosis is most commonly spread by contact with virus-infected saliva through coughing, sneezing, kissing, or sharing drinking glasses or eating utensils.

In addition to general weakness and fatigue, symptoms of mononucleosis may include any or all of the following:

- Sore throat and/or swollen tonsils
- Fever and chills
- Nausea and vomiting, or decreased appetite
- Swollen lymph nodes in the neck and armpits
- Headaches or joint pain
- Enlarged spleen
- Jaundice
- Skin rash.

Complications that can occur with mononucleosis include a temporarily enlarged spleen or inflamed liver. In rare instances, the spleen may rupture, producing sharp **pain** on the left side of the abdomen, a symptom that warrants immediate medical attention. Additional symptoms of a ruptured spleen include light headedness, rapidly beating heart, and difficulty breathing. Other rare, but potentially life-threatening, complications may involve the heart or brain. The infection may also cause significant destruction of the body's red blood cells or platelets.

Symptoms do not usually appear until four to seven weeks after exposure to EBV. An infected

KEY TERMS

Antibody—A specific protein produced by the immune system in response to a specific foreign protein or particle called an antigen.

Herpes viruses—A group of viruses that can cause cold sores, shingles, chicken pox, and congenital abnormalities. The Epstein-Barr virus which causes mononucleosis belongs to this group of viruses.

Reye's syndrome—A very serious, rare disease, most common in children, which involves an upper respiratory tract infection followed by brain and liver damage.

person can be contagious during this incubation time period and for as many as five months after the disappearance of symptoms. Also, the virus will be excreted in the saliva intermittently for the rest of their lives, although the individual will experience no symptoms. Contrary to popular belief, the EBV is not highly contagious. As a result, individuals living in a household or college dormitory with someone who has mononucleosis have a very small risk of being infected unless they have direct contact with the person's saliva.

Diagnosis

If symptoms associated with a cold persist longer than two weeks, mononucleosis is a possibility; however, a variety of other conditions can produce similar symptoms. If mononucleosis is suspected, a physician will typically conduct a **physical examination**, including a "Monospot" antibody blood test that can indicate the presence of proteins or antibodies produced in response to infection with the EBV. These antibodies may not be detectable, however, until the second or third weeks of the illness. Occasionally, when this test is inconclusive, other blood tests may be conducted.

Treatment

The most effective treatment for infectious mononucleosis is rest and a gradual return to regular activities. Individuals with mild cases may not require bed rest but should limit their activities. Any strenuous activity, athletic endeavors, or heavy lifting should be avoided until the symptoms completely subside, since excessive activity may cause the spleen to rupture.

The **sore throat** and **dehydration** that usually accompany mononucleosis may be relieved by drinking water and fruit juices. Gargling salt water or taking throat lozenges may also relieve discomfort. In addition, taking over-the-counter medications, such as **acetaminophen** or ibuprofen, may relieve symptoms, but **aspirin** should be avoided because mononucleosis has been associated with **Reye's syndrome**, a serious illness aggravated by aspirin.

While **antibiotics** do not affect EBV, the sore throat accompanying mononucleosis can be complicated by a streptococcal infection, which can be treated with antibiotics. Cortisone anti-inflammatory medications are also occasionally prescribed for the treatment of severely swollen tonsils or throat tissues.

Prognosis

While the severity and length of illness varies, most people diagnosed with mononucleosis will be able to return to their normal daily routines within two to three weeks, particularly if they rest during this time period. It may take two to three months before a person's usual energy levels return. One of the most common problems in treating mononucleosis, particularly in teenagers, is that people return to their usual activities too quickly and then experience a relapse of symptoms. Once the disease has completely run its course, the person cannot be re-infected.

Prevention

Although there is no way to avoid becoming infected with EBV, paying general attention to good hygiene and avoiding sharing beverage glasses or having close contact with people who have mononucleosis or cold symptoms can help prevent infection.

Resources

OTHER

"Communicable Disease Fact Sheet." New York State Department of Health.

"Mononucleosis." *MayoClinic.com.* http://www.mayoclinic.com/health/mononucleosis/DS00352.

ORGANIZATIONS

National Institute of Allergies and Infectious Diseases, 6610 Rockledge Drive, MSC 6612, Bethesda, MD, 20892-6612, 301 496-5717, 301 402-3573, 866 284-4107, ocpostoffice@niaid.nih.gov, http://www.niaid.nih.gov.

Susan J. Montgomery

Infertility

Definition

Infertility, is the biological failure of a couple to conceive a **pregnancy** after trying to do so frequently and without the use of contraceptives for at least one full year. In primary infertility, pregnancy has never occurred. In secondary infertility, one or both members of the couple has previously conceived, but is unable to conceive again after a full year of trying. The inability to conceive may be due to a single cause or multiple causes, in either the female or the male, or both. However, medical treatments are available that are safe and effective so that many couples can eventually become pregnant.

Demographics

Infertility can occur in both men and women.

Description

Most couples in the United States conceive within the first six months of trying when they do so without contraceptive devices and techniques. In fact, according to the Mayo Clinic, about 85% of couples become pregnant after 12 months of trying, while about half of the remaining 15% become pregnant over the next 36 months. However, according to 2008 statistics, infertility is a problem for about 10 to 15% of couples at any given time. Infertility has increased as a problem over the last 40 years. Some studies pin the blame for this increase on social phenomena, including the tendency for marriage to occur at a later age, which means that couples are trying to start families at a later age. It is well known that fertility in women decreases with increasing age, as illustrated by the following statistics:

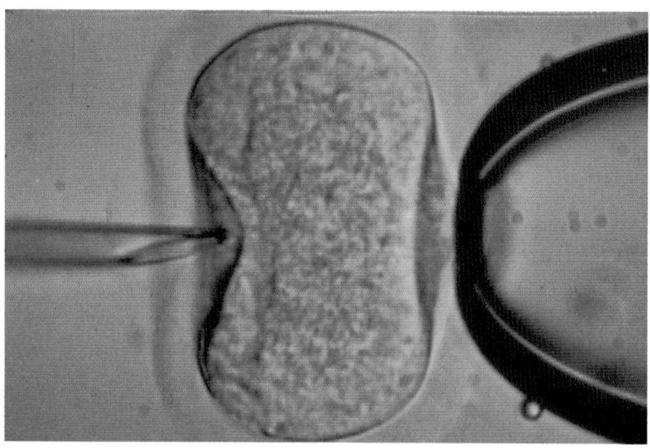

A microscopic image of a needle (left) injecting sperm cells directly into a human egg (center). The broad object at right is a pipette used to hold the ovum steady. *(Hank Morgan/Photo Researchers, Inc.)*

- Infertility in married women ages 16–20 = 4.5%
- Infertility in married women ages 35–40 = 31.8%
- Infertility in married women over the age of 40 = 70%.

Today, individuals often have multiple sexual partners before they marry and try to have children. This increase in numbers of sexual partners has led to an increase in sexually transmitted infections. Scarring from these infections, especially from **pelvic inflammatory disease** (a serious infection of the female reproductive organs, most commonly caused by **gonorrhea**) seems to be in part responsible for the increase in infertility. Furthermore, use of some forms of a contraceptive called the intrauterine device (**IUD**) contributed to an increased rate of pelvic inflammatory disease, with subsequent scarring. However, newer IUDs do not lead to this increased rate of infection.

To understand issues of infertility, it is first necessary to understand the basics of human reproduction. Fertilization occurs when a sperm from the male merges with an egg (ovum) from the female, creating a zygote that contains genetic material from both the father and the mother. If pregnancy is then established, the zygote will develop into an embryo, then a fetus, and ultimately a baby will be born.

The male contribution to fertilization and the establishment of pregnancy is the sperm. Sperm are small cells that carry the father's genetic material. This genetic material is contained within the oval head of the sperm. The sperm are mixed into fluid called semen, which is discharged from the penis during sexual intercourse. The whip–like tail of the sperm allows the sperm to swim up the female reproductive tract, in search of the egg it will try to fertilize.

The female makes many contributions to fertilization and the establishment of pregnancy. The ovum (plural: ova) is the cell that carries the mother's genetic material. These ova develop within the ovaries. Once a month, a single mature ovum is produced, which leaves the ovary in a process called ovulation. This ovum enters a tube (the Fallopian tube) leading to the uterus. The ovum needs to meet up with the sperm in the Fallopian tube if fertilization is to occur.

When fertilization occurs, the resulting cell (which now contains genetic material from both the mother and the father) is called the zygote. This single cell divides into multiple cells within the Fallopian tube, and the resulting cluster of cells (called a blastocyst)

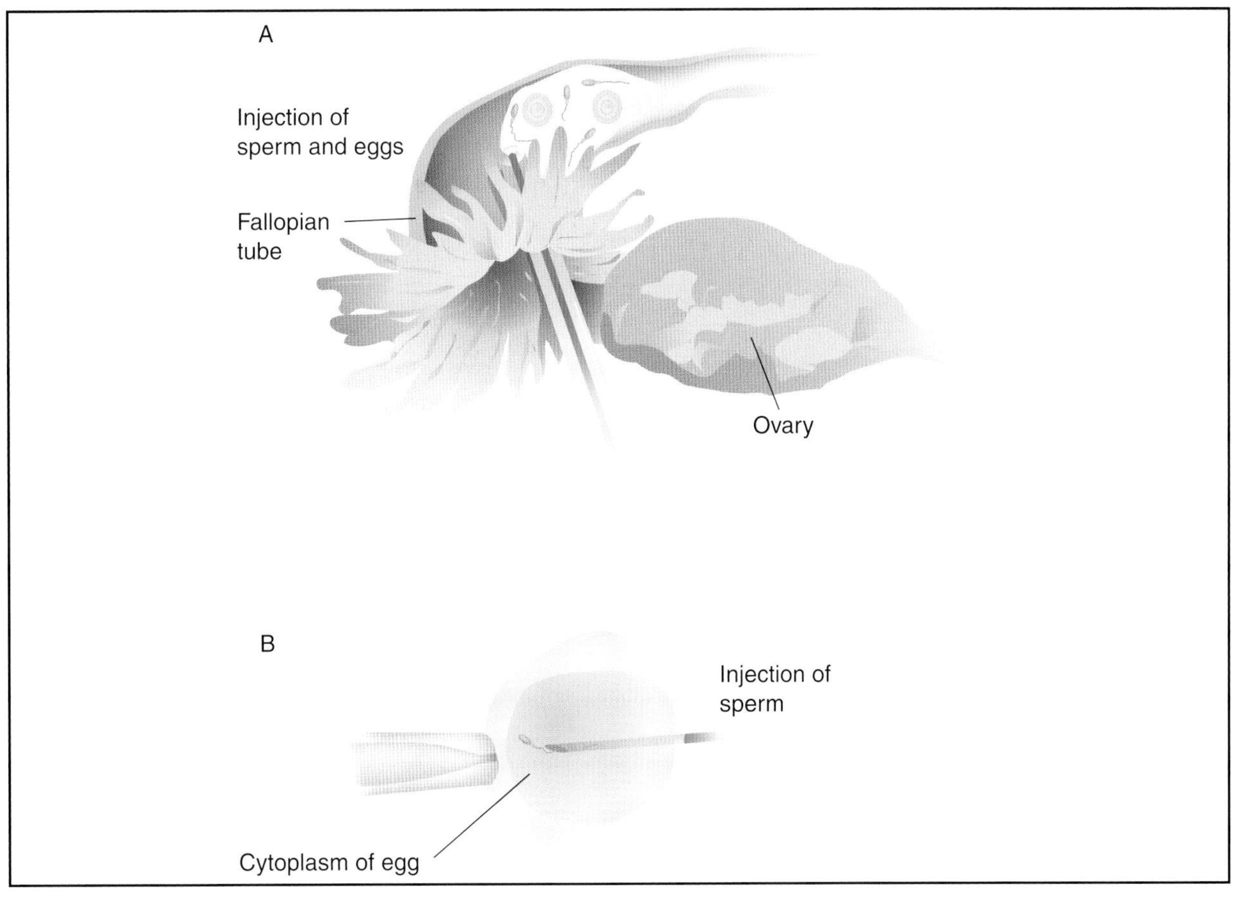

A. An egg and sperm are injected into the fallopian tube to encourage natural fertilization in a procedure called gamete intrafallopian transfer (GIFT). B. An alternative to GIFT is the injection of sperm directly into an egg using microscopic needles. *(Illustration by Argosy, Inc. Reproduced by permission of Gale, a part of Cengage Learning.)*

then moves into the womb (uterus). The uterine lining (endometrium) has been preparing itself to receive a pregnancy by growing thicker. If the blastocyst successfully reaches the inside of the uterus and attaches itself to the wall of the uterus, implantation and pregnancy have been achieved.

Causes and symptoms

Unlike most medical problems, infertility is an issue requiring the careful evaluation of two separate individuals, as well as an evaluation of their interactions with each other. In about three to four percent of couples, no cause for infertility is discovered. Medical studies have shown that **smoking** adds to infertility problems for both men and women. In addition, men and women who smoke are less likely to respond to infertility treatment.

The main factors involved in causing infertility, listing from the most to the least common, include:

- Male problems: 20%
- Male and female problems: 30–40%
- Female problems: 40–50%. (In these cases the problem is likely to come from conditions such as ovulation problems, pelvic adhesions and endometriosis, or cervical factors.)

Male factors

Male infertility can be caused by a number of different characteristics of the sperm. To check for these characteristics, a sample of semen is obtained and examined under the microscope, a procedure known as **semen analysis**. Four basic characteristics are usually evaluated:

- Sperm count refers to the number of sperm present in a semen sample. The normal number of sperm present in one milliliter (mL) of semen is more than 20 million. An individual with only five to 20 million sperm per milliliter of semen is considered subfertile, an individual with fewer than five million sperm per milliliter of semen is considered infertile.

- Sperm are also examined to see how well they swim (sperm motility) and to be sure that most have normal structure.
- Not all sperm within a specimen of semen will be perfectly normal. Some may be immature, and some may have abnormalities of the head or tail. A normal semen sample will contain no more than 25% abnormal forms of sperm.
- Volume of the semen sample is important. An abnormal amount of semen could affect the ability of the sperm to successfully fertilize an ovum.

Another test can be performed to evaluate the ability of the sperm to penetrate the outer coat of the ovum. This test is conducted by observing whether sperm in a semen sample can penetrate the outer coat of a guinea pig ovum. Fertilization cannot occur, of course, but this test is useful in predicting the ability of the individual's sperm to penetrate a human ovum.

Any number of conditions result in abnormal findings in the semen analysis. Genetic problems at birth can lead to improper growth of the testicles and, thus, infertility. Men can be born with one or both testicles that have not descended properly from the abdominal cavity (where testicles develop originally) into the scrotal sac, or may be born with only one instead of the normal two testicles. When testicles have not descended from the abdominal cavity, they are exposed to a higher body temperature than when they are descended. The higher temperature reduces the production of sperm. Testicle size can be smaller than normal. Past infections (including **mumps**) can affect testicular function, as can a past injury. For instance, exposure to sexually transmitted infections (STIs), such as gonorrhea and chlamydia, can result in infertility. The presence of abnormally large veins (varicocele) in the testicles can increase testicular temperature, which decreases sperm count.

History of having been exposed to various toxins, drug use, excess alcohol use, use of anabolic **steroids**, certain medications, diabetes, thyroid problems or other endocrine disturbances, and prostate problems can have direct effects on the formation of sperm (spermatogenesis). Problems with the male anatomy can cause sperm to be ejaculated not out of the penis, but into the bladder (a process known as retrograde ejaculation). Diabetes is a medical disorder and prostate, urethral, and bladder surgeries are three procedures that can lead to retrograde ejaculation. In addition, scarring from past infections can interfere with ejaculation. A condition called **hypospadias** can also cause infertility. Hypospadias occurs when the urinary opening on a man' penis is incorrectly located on its underside so that sperm cannot reach the cervix of a woman.

Sexual issues, such as **erectile dysfunction**, **premature ejaculation**, and **dyspareunia** (painful intercourse), can contribute to a male's infertility. Various psychological problems can also lead to a diminished level of fertility. **Stress** and depression can interfere with hormones that help to produce sperm. Men with long–term depression may have reduced sperm count. Physically, a man who is underweight so that he has been denied certain nutrients, such as vitamin C, zinc, and folate, may lead to infertility. On the other hand, **obesity** (being extremely overweight) in males can also be a contributing factor in infertility.

Treatment of male infertility includes addressing known reversible factors first; for example, discontinuing any medication known to have an effect on spermatogenesis or ejaculation, as well as decreasing alcohol intake, and treating thyroid or other endocrine disease. Varicoceles can be treated surgically. Testosterone in low doses can improve sperm motility.

Other treatments of male infertility include collecting semen samples from multiple ejaculations, after which the semen is put through a process that allows the most motile sperm to be sorted out. These motile sperm are pooled together to create a concentrate that can be deposited into the female partner's uterus at a time that coincides with ovulation. In cases where the male partner's sperm is proven to be absolutely unable to cause pregnancy in the female partner, and with the consent of both partners, donor sperm may be used for this process. Depositing the male partner's sperm or donor sperm by mechanical means into the female partner are both forms of artificial insemination.

Ovulatory problems

The first step in diagnosing ovulatory problems in women is to make sure that an ovum is being produced each month. A woman's morning body temperature is slightly higher around the time of ovulation. A woman can measure and record her temperatures daily and a chart can be drawn to show whether or not ovulation has occurred. Luteinizing hormone (LH) is released just before ovulation. A simple urine test can be done to check if LH has been released around the time that ovulation is expected.

Treatment of ovulatory problems depends on the cause. If a thyroid or pituitary problem is responsible, simply treating that problem can restore fertility. (The thyroid and pituitary glands release hormones that also are involved in regulating a woman's menstrual cycle.) Medication can also be used to stimulate fertility. The most commonly used of these medications are clomiphene (Clomid) and menotropin (Pergonal). These drugs increase the risk of multiple births (twins, triplets, etc.). Other possible medications include gonadotropin medications, which are injected medications made up of hormones produced in the pituitary glands. They may directly stimulate the ovaries to produce eggs. Follicle stimulating hormone (FSH) has a 95% chance of simulating ovulation in women with an ovulatory problem. However, its use does not guarantee a successful pregnancy and may lead to multiple pregnancies.

Pelvic adhesions and endometriosis

Pelvic **adhesions** and **endometriosis** can cause infertility by preventing the sperm from reaching the egg or interfering with fertilization. Pelvic adhesions are fibrous **scars**. These scars can be the result of past infections, such as pelvic inflammatory disease, or infections following abortions or prior births. Previous surgeries can also leave behind scarring.

Endometriosis may lead to pelvic adhesions. Endometriosis is the abnormal location of uterine tissue outside of the uterus. When uterine tissue is planted elsewhere in the pelvis, it still bleeds on a monthly basis with the start of the normal menstrual period. This leads to irritation within the pelvis around the site of this abnormal tissue and bleeding, and may cause scarring, along with pelvic **pain**.

Pelvic adhesions cause infertility by blocking the Fallopian tubes. The ovum may be prevented from traveling down the Fallopian tube from the ovary or the sperm may be prevented from traveling up the Fallopian tube from the uterus.

A hysterosalpingogram (HSG) can show if the Fallopian tubes are blocked. This is an x–ray examination that tests whether dye material can travel through the patient's Fallopian tubes. A few women become pregnant following this x–ray exam. It is thought that the dye material in some way helps flush out the tubes, decreasing any existing obstruction. Scarring also can be diagnosed by examining the pelvic area with a scope that can be inserted into the abdomen through a tiny incision made near the naval. This scoping technique is called **laparoscopy**.

Pelvic adhesions can be treated during laparoscopy. The adhesions are cut using special instruments. Endometriosis can be treated with certain medications, but may also require surgery to repair any obstruction caused by adhesions.

Cervical factors

The cervix is the opening from the vagina into the uterus through which the sperm must pass. Mucus produced by the cervix helps to transport the sperm into the uterus. Injury to the cervix or scarring of the cervix after surgery or infection can result in a smaller than normal cervical opening, making it difficult for the sperm to enter. Injury or infection can also decrease the number of glands in the cervix, leading to a smaller amount of cervical mucus. In other situations, the mucus produced is the wrong consistency (perhaps too thick) to allow sperm to travel through the cervix. In addition, some women produce antibodies (immune cells) that are specifically directed to identify sperm as foreign invaders and to kill them.

Cervical mucus can be examined under a microscope to diagnose whether cervical factors are contributing to infertility. The interaction of a live sperm sample from the male partner and a sample of cervical mucus from the female partner can also be examined. This procedure is called a post–coital test.

Treatment of cervical factors includes **antibiotics** in the case of an infection, steroids to decrease production of anti–sperm antibodies, and artificial insemination techniques to completely bypass the cervical mucus.

Other causes of female infertility include: Fallopian tube damage or blockage (usually caused by inflammation), elevated prolactin (hyperprolactinemia), **polycystic ovary syndrome** (which results in the production of too much androgen hormone), early **menopause** (premature ovarian failure), **uterine fibroids** (benign tumors on the wall of the uterus), and various other medical problems (such as **sickle cell disease**, **kidney disease**, and diabetes).

Treatment

Couples can naturally increase the chances of becoming pregnant by having sexual intercourse as frequently as possible. However, it is especially important to have it between the tenth day and eighteen day after the beginning of a woman's menstrual period. Ovulation normally occurs, when menstruation periods are regularly spaced apart, about fourteen days before menstruation begins. Therefore, sexual activity should be especially frequent from three days before to three days after ovulation. For additional help, a physician may recommend using an ovulation prediction test kit to help determine the best times for intercourse.

KEY TERMS

Blastocyst—A cluster of cells representing multiple cell divisions that have occurred in the Fallopian tube after successful fertilization of an ovum by a sperm. This is the developmental form which must leave the Fallopian tube, enter the uterus, and implant itself in the uterus to achieve actual pregnancy.

Cervix—The opening from the vagina, which leads into the uterus.

Embryo—The stage of development of a baby between the second and eighth weeks after conception.

Endometrium—The lining of the uterus.

Fallopian tube—The tube leading from the ovary into the uterus. Just as there are two ovaries, there are two Fallopian tubes.

Fetus—A baby developing in the uterus from the third month to birth.

Ovary—The female organ in which eggs (ova) are stored and mature.

Ovum (plural: ova)—The reproductive cell of the female, which contains genetic information and participates in the act of fertilization. Also popularly called the egg.

Semen—The fluid that contains sperm, which is ejaculated by the male.

Sperm—The reproductive cell of the male, which contains genetic information and participates in the act of fertilization of an ovum.

Spermatogenesis—The process by which sperm develop to become mature sperm, capable of fertilizing an ovum.

Zygote—The result of the sperm successfully fertilizing the ovum. The zygote is a single cell that contains the genetic material of both the mother and the father.

Assisted reproductive techniques include **in vitro fertilization** (IVF), gamete intrafallopian transfer (GIFT), and zygote intrafallopian tube transfer (ZIFT). These are usually used after other techniques to treat infertility have failed.

In vitro fertilization involves the use of a drug to induce the simultaneous release of many eggs from the female's ovaries, which are retrieved surgically. Meanwhile, several semen samples are obtained from the male partner, and a sperm concentrate is prepared. The ova and sperm are then combined in a laboratory, where several of the ova may be fertilized. Cell division is allowed to take place up to the embryo stage. While this takes place, the female may be given drugs to ensure that her uterus is ready to receive an embryo. Three or four of the embryos are transferred to the female's uterus, and the wait begins to see if any or all of them implant and result in an actual pregnancy.

Success rates of IVF are still rather low. Most centers report pregnancy rates between 10–20%. Since most IVF procedures put more than one embryo into the uterus, the chance for a multiple birth (twins or more) is greatly increased in couples undergoing IVF.

GIFT involves retrieval of both multiple ova and semen, and the mechanical placement of both within the female partner's Fallopian tubes, where one hopes that fertilization will occur. ZIFT involves the same retrieval of ova and semen, and fertilization and growth in the laboratory up to the zygote stage, at which point the zygotes are placed in the Fallopian tubes. Both GIFT and ZIFT seem to have higher success rates than traditional IVF.

Prognosis

It is very difficult to obtain statistics regarding the prognosis of infertility because many different problems may exist within an individual or couple trying to conceive. In general, it is believed that of all couples who undergo a complete evaluation of infertility followed by treatment and therapies, about half will ultimately have a successful pregnancy. Of those couples who do not choose to undergo evaluation or treatment, about five percent go on to conceive after a year or more of infertility.

Prevention

Having fewer sexual partners and using contraceptive devices (such as **condoms**) that reduce the chances of contracting sexually transmitted infections, such as chlamydia and gonorrhea, can reduce the chances of becoming infertile. Getting a mumps **vaccination** is also an effective way to prevent infertility. Maintaining a healthy lifestyle with respect to diet and **exercise** is also helpful. Advice from your family doctor or a medical professional is beneficial in learning more about how to prevent infertility.

Resources

BOOKS

Infertility. Rockville, MD: Food and Drug Administration (FDA) Office on Women's Health, 2007.

Piehl, Norah. *Infertility*. Detroit: Greenhaven Press, 2008.

OTHER

"Infertility" Mayo Clinic. (April 8, 2010), http://www.mayoclinic.com/health/infertility/DS00310. (accessed September 5, 2010).

"Infertility" Medline Plus, U.S. National Library of Medicine and National Institutes of Health. (July 2, 2010), http://www.nlm.nih.gov/medlineplus/infertility.html. (accessed September 5, 2010).

ORGANIZATIONS

American Society for Reproductive Medicine, 1209 Montgomery Hwy., Birmingham, AL, 35216–2809, (205) 978–5000, (205) 978–5005, asrm@asrm.org, http://www.asrm.com.

International Center for Infertility Information Dissemination, PO Box 6836, Arlington, VA, 22206, (703) 379–9178, (703) 379–1593, http://www.inciid.org.

Rosalyn Carson–DeWitt, MD
Teresa G. Odle

Infertility drugs

Definition

Infertility drugs are medicines that help bring about **pregnancy**.

Purpose

Infertility is the inability of a man and woman to achieve pregnancy after at least a year of having regular sexual intercourse without any type of birth control. There are many possible reasons for infertility, and finding the most effective treatment for a couple may involve many tests to find the problem. For pregnancy to occur, the woman's reproductive system must release eggs regularly—a process called ovulation. The man must produce healthy sperm that are able to reach and unite with an egg. And once an egg is fertilized, it must travel to the woman's uterus (womb), become implanted and remain there to be nourished.

If a couple is infertile because the woman is not ovulating, infertility drugs may be prescribed to stimulate ovulation. The first step usually is to try a drug such as clomiphene. If that does not work, human chorionic gonadotropin (hCG) may be tried, usually in combination with other infertility drugs.

Clomiphene and hCG may also be used to treat other conditions in both males and females.

Description

Clomiphene (Clomid, Milophene, and Serophene)) comes in tablet form and is available only with a physician's prescription. Human chorionic gonadotropin is given as an injection, only under a physician's supervision.

Clomiphene citrate is used to increase the natural production of the hormones that stimulate ovulation in otherwise healthy women. When clomiphene is administered, the body produces higher levels of luteinizing hormone (LH), follicle stimulating hormone (FSH), and gonadotropins. These hormones induce ovulation.

Human chorionic gonadotropin (hCG) is sold under many brand names including Gonic, Pregnyl, Ovidrel, Chorex, Chorigon, and Profasi. This hormone stimulates the gonads in both men and women. In men, hCG increases androgen production. In women, it increases the levels of progesterone. Human chorionic gonadotropin can help stimulate ovulation in women.

Although some people believe that hCG can help lose weight, there is no evidence that this hormone offers any benefit in weight loss programs. Many medical organizations, such as the American Medical Association (AMA), warn about using hCG for such a purpose. Consequently, it should not be used for this purpose.

A number of other natural and synthetic hormones are used to induce ovulation. Urofollitropin (Bravelle, Fertinex) is a concentrated preparation of human hormones, while follitropin alfa (Gonal–F) and follitropin beta (Follistim) are human FSH preparations of recombinant DNA (deoxyribonucleic acid) origin. Developments in this field are continuous. For example, in June 2004, the U.S. Food and Drug Administration (FDA) approved a follitropin beta injection, called Follistim AQ Cartridge, in individualized doses for women to self–inject. Then, in 2008, the FDA approved SpermCheck Fertility test kit, made by ContraVac, which tests for sperm count in men.

Menotropins (Pergonal, Humegon, Repronex) are often given with human chorionic gonadotropin to stimulate ovulation in women and sperm production in men.

Recommended dosage

Dosage may be different for different patients. The physician who prescribed the drug or the pharmacist who filled the prescription will recommend the correct dosage.

Clomiphene must be taken at certain times during the menstrual cycle and patients should follow directions exactly. It is usually taken once a day for five days, beginning on or about day five of the menstrual cycle. However, this dosage and the times in which it is taken may be different for various individuals. Consequently, do not take it in dosages that are more or less than what is prescribed by the doctor. Go strictly by what the doctor says.

Precautions

Seeing a physician regularly while taking infertility drugs is important because side effects and complications can occur.

Treatment with infertility drugs increases the chance of multiple births. Although this eventuality may seem like a good thing to couples who want children very badly, multiple fetuses can cause problems during pregnancy and delivery and can even threaten the babies' survival.

Having intercourse at the proper time in the woman's menstrual cycle helps increase the chance of pregnancy. The physician may recommend using an ovulation prediction test kit to help determine the best times for intercourse.

Some people feel dizzy or lightheaded, or less alert when using clomiphene. The medicine may also cause blurred vision and other vision changes. Individuals who take clomiphene should not drive, use machines, or do anything else that might be dangerous until they have found out how the drugs affect them.

Questions remain about the safety of long–term treatment with clomiphene. Women should not have more than six courses of treatment with this drug and should ask their physicians for the most up–to–date information about its use.

Special conditions

People who have certain medical conditions or who are taking certain other medicines may have problems if they take infertility drugs. Before taking these drugs, patients should tell the physician about any of these conditions:

ALLERGIES. Anyone who has had unusual reactions to infertility drugs in the past should let his or her physician know before taking the drugs again. The physician should also be told about any **allergies** to foods, dyes, preservatives, or other substances.

PREGMAMCY. Clomiphene may cause **birth defects** if taken during pregnancy. Women who think they have become pregnant while taking clomiphene should stop taking the medicine immediately and check with their physicians.

OTHER MEDICAL CONDITIONS. Infertility drugs may make some medical conditions worse. Before using infertility drugs, people with any of these medical problems should make sure their physicians are aware of their conditions:

- Endometriosis
- Fibroid tumors of the uterus
- Unusual vaginal bleeding
- Ovarian cyst
- Enlarged ovaries
- Inflamed veins caused by blood clots
- Liver disease, now or in the past
- Depression.

USE OF CERTAIN MEDICINES. Taking infertility drugs with certain other medicines may affect the way the drugs work or may increase the chance of side effects.

Side effects

When used in low doses for a short time, clomiphene and HCG rarely cause side effects. However, anyone who has stomach or pelvic **pain** or bloating while taking either medicine should check with a physician immediately. Infertility drugs may also cause less serious symptoms such as hot flashes, breast tenderness or swelling, heavy menstrual periods, bleeding between menstrual periods, **nausea** or **vomiting**, **dizziness**, lightheadedness, irritability, nervousness, restlessness, **headache**, tiredness, sleep problems, or depression. These problems usually go away as the body adjusts to the drug and do not require medical treatment unless they continue or they interfere with normal activities.

KEY TERMS

Endometriosis—A condition in which tissue like that normally found in the lining of the uterus is present outside the uterus. The condition often causes pain and bleeding.

Fetus—A developing baby inside the womb.

Fibroid tumor—A noncancerous tumor formed of fibrous tissue.

Ovary—A reproductive organ in females that produces eggs and hormones.

Other side effects are possible. Anyone who has unusual symptoms after taking infertility drugs should contact a physician.

Interactions

Infertility drugs may interact with other medicines. When this happens, the effects of one or both of the drugs may change or the risk of side effects may be greater. Anyone who takes infertility drugs should let the physician know all other medicines she is taking.

Resources

BOOKS

Infertility. Rockville, MD: Food and Drug Administration (FDA) Office on Women's Health, 2007.

Piehl, Norah. *Infertility*. Detroit: Greenhaven Press, 2008.

OTHER

"Infertility" Mayo Clinic. (April 8, 2010).http://www.mayoclinic.com/health/infertility/DS00310 (accessed September 21, 2010).

"Infertility" Medline Plus, U.S. National Library of Medicine and National Institutes of Health. (July 2, 2010). http://www.nlm.nih.gov/medlineplus/infertility.html (accessed September 21, 2010).

"Infertility and Reproduction Overview" Mayo Clinic. http://www.webmd.com/infertility-and-reproduction/default.htm (accessed September 21, 2010).

"U.Va. Start-Up ContraVac Sees First Sales of Revolutionary SpermCheck Product" University of Virginia. (October 18, 2009). http://uvapf.org/live_data/live_site_page.php?page_id=23&article_id=59. (accessed September 21, 2010).

ORGANIZATIONS

American Society for Reproductive Medicine (ASRM), 1209 Montgomery Hwy., Birmingham, AL, 35216-2809, (205) 978-5000, (205) 978-5005, asrm@asrm.org, http://www.asrm.com.

International Center for Infertility Information Dissemination (INCIID), PO Box 6836, Arlington, VA, 22206, (703) 379-9178, (703) 379-1593, INCIIDinfo@inciid.org, http://www.inciid.org.

Nancy Ross-Flanigan
Teresa G. Odle

Infertility therapies

Definition

Infertility is the inability of a man and a woman to conceive a child through sexual intercourse. There are many possible reasons for the problem, which can involve the man, the woman, or both partners. Various treatments, or infertility therapies, are available that enable a woman to become pregnant; the correct one will depend on the specific cause of the infertility.

Purpose

Infertility treatment is aimed at enabling a woman to have a baby by treating the man, the woman, or both partners. During normal conception of a child, the man's sperm travels to the woman's Fallopian tubes, where, if conditions are right, it will encounter an egg that has been released from the ovary. The sperm fertilizes the egg, which will enter the uterus where it implants and begins to divide, forming an embryo. The embryo develops during **pregnancy** into a baby.

Infertility treatment attempts to correct or compensate for any abnormalities in this process that prevent the fertilization of an egg or development of an embryo.

Precautions

It is important for a couple contemplating infertility treatment to examine their own ideas and feelings about the process and consider ethical objections before the woman becomes pregnant from such treatment. Some infertility clinics recommend that couples attend at least one session with a psychologist or psychiatrist before proceeding with infertility therapy. In this way couples can freely express their concerns and learn more about what they are about to experience. It also helps to identify couples that may be having difficulties coping with the situation. Infertility support groups are also available in most areas to help with questions that arise, along with helping to provide an experienced viewpoint about infertility therapy.

Description

About 85% of women who are trying to get pregnant and use no birth control will do so within one year, and half of the other 15% become pregnant within another three years. If after one year of having sexual intercourse with no **contraception** a couple has not conceived, they should seek the advice of a physician. Tests can be performed to look for possible infertility problems.

Treating an underlying infection or illness is the first step in infertility treatment. The physician may also suggest improving general health, changing diet, reducing **stress**, and counseling.

Treatment

Low sperm count treatments

The most common cause of male infertility is failure to produce enough healthy sperm. For fertilization to occur, the number of sperm cells in the man's semen (the fluid ejected during sexual intercourse) must be sufficient, and the sperm cells must have the right shape, appearance, and activity (motility).

Defects in sperm can be caused by an infection resulting from a sexually transmitted infection (STI), a blockage caused by a varicose vein in the scrotum (varicocele), an endocrine imbalance, or problems with other male reproductive organs (such as the testicles, prostate gland, or seminal vesicles).

A **physical examination** of a man's genitals is usually the first step in identifying a low sperm count. The medical history of the man is also collected, especially noting incidences of illnesses, injuries, and recurring health problems. Semen is also examined with a **semen analysis** test. The number of sperm is counted under a microscope.

If low sperm count is the problem, it is possible to restore fertility by:

- treating any underlying infections.
- timing sex to coincide with the time the woman is ovulating, which means that the egg is released from the ovary and is beginning to travel down the Fallopian tube (the site of fertilization).
- having sex less often to build up the number of sperm in the semen.
- treating any endocrine imbalance with drugs.
- having a surgical procedure to remove a varicocele (varicocelectomy).

Fertility drugs

If infertility is due to a woman's failure to release eggs from the ovary (ovulate), fertility drugs can help bring hormone levels into balance, stimulating the ovaries and triggering egg production.

Surgical repair

In some women, infertility is due to blocked Fallopian tubes. The egg is released from the ovary, but sperm is prevented from reaching it because of a physical obstruction in the Fallopian tube. If this is the case, surgery may help repair the damage. Microsurgery can sometimes repair the damage to scarred Fallopian tubes if it is not too severe. Not all tube damage can be repaired, however, and most tubal problems are more successfully treated with **in vitro fertilization**.

Fibroid tumors in the uterus also may cause infertility, and they can be surgically treated. **Endometriosis**, a condition in which parts of the lining of the uterus become imbedded on other internal organs (such as the ovaries or Fallopian tubes) may contribute to infertility. It may be necessary to surgically remove the endometrial tissue to improve fertility.

Artificial insemination

Artificial insemination may be tried if sperm count is low, the man is impotent, or the woman's vagina creates a hostile environment for the sperm. The procedure is not always successful. In this procedure, semen is collected and placed into the woman's cervix with a small syringe at the time of ovulation. From the cervix, sperm can travel to the Fallopian tube where fertilization takes place. If the partner's sperm count is low, it can be mixed with donor sperm before being transferred into the uterus.

If sperm is not present in the male partner's semen, then artificial insemination can be performed using a donor's sperm obtained from a sperm bank.

Assisted reproductive technologies

Some fertility treatments require removal of eggs and/or sperm and manipulation of them in certain ways in a laboratory to assist fertilization. These techniques are called as a group: assisted reproductive technologies (ART). They have helped thousands of women each year in the United States to become pregnant so that couples can have their own biological children.

IN VITRO FERTILIZATION (IVF). When infertility cannot be treated by other means or when the cause is not known, it is still possible to become pregnant through in vitro fertilization (IVF), a costly, complex procedure that achieves pregnancy about 20% of the time. IVF is usually recommended when both Fallopian tubes are blocked, but it can be used for other problems (such as endometriosis, cervical factor infertility, and ovulation disorders).

In this procedure, a woman's eggs are removed by withdrawing them from the woman' ovaries with a special needle. Attempts are then made to fertilize the eggs with sperm from her partner or a donor. This fertilization takes place in a Petri dish in a laboratory. The fertilized egg (embryo) is then returned to the woman's uterus so that it can develop normally from that point.

Often, three to six fertilized eggs are returned at the same time into the uterus. Usually one or two of the embryos survive and grow into fetuses, but sometimes three or more fetuses result.

A child born in this method is popularly known as a "test tube baby," but in fact the child actually develops inside the mother. Only the fertilization of the egg takes place in the laboratory. The birth of the first test tube baby occurred in 1978 in the United Kingdom. As of 2008, around three million babies around the world had been born with the help of in vitro fertilization, with about half a million of them in the United States.

INTRACYTOPLASMIC SPERM INJECTION (ICSI). In a variation of IVF called intracytoplasmic sperm injection (ICSI), single sperm cells are injected directly into each egg with the use of a microscopic technique called micromanipulation. This process, developed in 1991 in Belgium, may be helpful for men with severe infertility (low sperm count) and also when eggs cannot be easily penetrated by sperm.

GAMETE INTERFALLOPIAN TRANSFER (GIFT). In this technique, eggs are removed from the ovaries of a woman and placed directly into one of her two Fallopian tubes to encourage fertilization to occur naturally. At least one normal Fallopian tube must be available for the procedure to work successfully. This procedure, developed by Argentine endocrinologist Ricardo Asch (1947–), is performed by means of **laparoscopy**. In laparoscopy, a small tube with a viewing lens at one end is inserted into the abdomen through a small incision. The lens allows the physician to see inside the patient on a video monitor.

ZYGOTE INTRAFALLOPIAN TRANSFER (ZIFT). If infertility is caused by a low sperm count, zygote intrafallopian transfer (ZIFT) can be tried. This technique combines GIFT and IVF. This procedure is also called a "tubal embryo transfer."

In this technique, in–vitro fertilization is first performed, so that the actual fertilization takes place and is confirmed in the laboratory. Two days later, instead of placing the embryo in the uterus, the physician performs laparoscopy to place the embryos in the Fallopian tube, much as with the GIFT procedure. The success of this technique is usually not known for about five weeks.

A woman must have at least one functioning Fallopian tube in order to participate in ZIFT.

Preparation

Couples who are having fertility problems may want to limit or avoid:

- tobacco
- alcohol
- caffeine
- stress
- tight–fitting undershorts (men)
- hot tubs, saunas and steam rooms (high temperatures can kill sperm).

Risks

Women who take fertility drugs have a higher likelihood of getting pregnant with more than one child at a time, resulting in multiple pregnancies. Such pregnancies also carry the risk of low birth weight for the infants born as a result of this procedure. There are also rare but serious side effects to fertility drugs. **Birth defects** have been shown to be possible when assisted reproductive technologies are used. For instance, ovarian hyperstimulation syndrome (OHSS) may occur at a higher rate in women using infertility therapies than with other women. OHSS is a complication—directly caused by the use of fertility medications—in which the ovaries become enlarged, abdominal swelling occurs, blood pressure decreases, and other symptoms occur. Invasive procedures used with the various types of infertility therapies, as with any type of surgery, carry risk of infection, bleeding, and other complications.

Normal results

Typically, at least half of all couples who are infertile will respond to treatment with a successful pregnancy. For those who cannot become pregnant with treatment or insemination, surrogate parenting or adopting may be other options.

KEY TERMS

Gamete—An egg (ovum) from the female or a mature sperm from the male.

Laparoscopy—A procedure in which a viewing tube is inserted through the abdominal wall to examine a woman's reproductive organs.

Ovulation—The release of an egg from the ovary. Fertilization can occur within a day or two of ovulation.

Zygote—A fertilized egg.

Resources

BOOKS

Infertility. Rockville, MD: Food and Drug Administration (FDA) Office on Women's Health, 2007.

Piehl, Norah. *Infertility*. Detroit: Greenhaven Press, 2008.

OTHER

"Infertility" Mayo Clinic. (April 8, 2010), http://www.mayoclinic.com/health/infertility/DS00310. (accessed September 5, 2010).

"Infertility" Medline Plus, U.S. National Library of Medicine and National Institutes of Health. (July 2, 2010), http://www.nlm. nih.gov/medlineplus/infertility.html (accessed September 5, 2010).

"Infertility and Reproduction Overview" Mayo Clinic. http://www.webmd.com/infertility-and-reproduction/default.htm (accessed September 5, 2010).

"30 Years of Test–tube Babies" New York Daily News. (July 23, 2008), http://www.nydailynews.com/lifestyle/health/2008/07/24/2008-07-24_30_years_of_testtube_babies.html (accessed September 5, 2010).

ORGANIZATIONS

American Society for Reproductive Medicine, 1209 Montgomery Hwy., Birmingham, AL, 35216–2809, (205) 978–5000, (205) 978–5005, asrm@asrm.org, http://www.asrm.com.

RESOLVE: The National Infertility Association, 1760 Old Meadow Rd., Suite 500, McLean, VA, 22102, (703) 556–7172, (703) 506–3266, info@resolve.org, http://www.resolve.org.

Carol A. Turkington

Influenza

Definition

Usually referred to as the flu or grippe, influenza is a highly infectious respiratory disease. The disease is caused by certain strains of the influenza virus. When the virus is inhaled, it attacks cells in the upper respiratory tract, causing typical flu symptoms such as **fatigue**, **fever** and chills, a hacking **cough**, and body aches. Influenza victims are also susceptible to potentially life-threatening secondary infections. Although the stomach or intestinal "flu" is commonly blamed for stomach upsets and **diarrhea**, the influenza virus rarely causes gastrointestinal symptoms. Such symptoms are most likely due to other organisms such as rotavirus, *Salmonella*, *Shigella*, or ***Escherichia coli***.

Description

The flu is considerably more debilitating than the **common cold**. Influenza outbreaks occur suddenly, and infection spreads rapidly. The annual **death** toll attributable to influenza and its complications averages 20,000 in the United States alone.

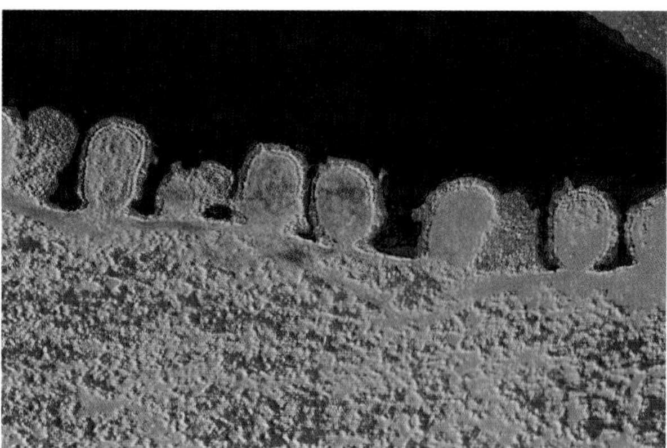

A transmission electron microscopy (TEM) image of influenza viruses budding from the surface of an infected cell. *(SPL/Photo Researchers, Inc.)*

In the 1918-1919 Spanish flu pandemic, the death toll reached a staggering 20–40 million worldwide. Approximately 500,000 of these fatalities occurred in the United States.

Influenza outbreaks occur on a regular basis. The most serious outbreaks are pandemics, which affect millions of people worldwide and last for several months. The 1918–1919 influenza outbreak serves as the primary example of an influenza pandemic. Pandemics also occurred in 1957 and 1968 with the Asian flu and Hong Kong flu, respectively. The Asian flu was responsible for 70,000 deaths in the United States, while the Hong Kong flu killed 34,000.

Epidemics are widespread regional outbreaks that occur every two to three years and affect 5–10% of the population. The Russian flu in the winter of 1977 is an example of an epidemic. A regional epidemic is shorter lived than a pandemic, lasting only several weeks. Finally, there are smaller outbreaks each winter that are confined to specific locales.

The earliest existing descriptions of influenza were written nearly 2500 years ago by the ancient Greek physician Hippocrates. Historically, influenza was ascribed to a number of different agents, including "bad air" and several different bacteria. In fact, its name comes from the Italian word for "influence," because people in eighteenth-century Europe thought that the disease was caused by the influence of bad weather. It was not until 1933 that the causative agent was identified as a virus.

There are three types of influenza viruses, identified as A, B, and C. Influenza A can infect a range of animal species, including humans, pigs, horses, and birds, but only humans are infected by types B and C. Influenza A is responsible for most flu cases, while infection with types B and C virus are less common and cause a milder illness.

In the United States, 90% of all deaths from influenza occur among persons older than 65. Flu-related deaths have increased substantially in the United States since the 1970s, largely because of the **aging** of the American population. In addition, elderly persons are vulnerable because they are often reluctant to be vaccinated against flu.

A new concern regarding influenza is the possibility that hostile groups or governments could use the virus as an agent of bioterrorism. A report published in early 2003 noted that Type A influenza virus has a high potential for use as such an agent because of the virulence of the Type A strain that broke out in Hong Kong in 1997 and the development of laboratory methods for generating large quantities of the virus. The report recommended the stockpiling of present **antiviral drugs** and speeding up the development of new ones.

Causes and symptoms

Approximately one to four days after infection with the influenza virus, the victim is hit with an array of symptoms. "Hit" is an appropriate term, because symptoms are sudden, harsh, and unmistakable. Typical influenza symptoms include the abrupt onset of a **headache**, dry cough, and chills, rapidly followed by overall achiness and a fever that may run as high as 104°F (40°C). As the fever subsides, nasal congestion and a **sore throat** become noticeable. Flu victims feel extremely tired and weak and may not return to their normal energy levels for several days or even a couple of weeks.

Influenza complications usually arise from bacterial infections of the lower respiratory tract. Signs of a secondary respiratory infection often appear just as the victim seems to be recovering. These signs include high fever, intense chills, chest pains associated with breathing, and a productive cough with thick yellowish green sputum. If these symptoms appear, medical treatment is necessary. Other secondary infections, such as sinus or ear infections, may also require medical intervention. Heart and lung problems, and other chronic diseases, can be aggravated by influenza, which is a particular concern with elderly patients.

With children and teenagers, it is advisable to be alert for symptoms of **Reye's syndrome**, a rare, but serious complication. Symptoms of Reye's syndrome are **nausea and vomiting**, and more seriously, neurological problems such as confusion or **delirium**. The syndrome has been associated with the use of **aspirin** to relieve flu symptoms.

Diagnosis

Although there are specific tests to identify the flu virus strain from respiratory samples, doctors typically rely on a set of symptoms and the presence of influenza in the community for diagnosis. Specific tests are useful to determine the type of flu in the community, but they do little for individual treatment. Doctors may administer tests, such as throat cultures, to identify secondary infections.

Since 1999, however, seven rapid diagnostic tests for flu have become commercially available. These tests appear to be especially useful in diagnosing flu in children, allowing doctors to make more accurate treatment decisions in less time.

Treatment

Essentially, a bout of influenza must be allowed to run its course. Symptoms can be relieved with bed rest and by keeping well hydrated. A steam vaporizer may make breathing easier, and **pain** relievers will take care of the aches and pain. Food may not seem very appetizing, but an effort should be made to consume nourishing food. Recovery should not be pushed too rapidly. Returning to normal activities too quickly invites a possible relapse or complications.

Drugs

Since influenza is a viral infection, **antibiotics** are useless in treating it. However, antibiotics are frequently used to treat secondary infections.

Over-the-counter medications are used to treat flu symptoms, but it is not necessary to purchase a medication marketed specifically for flu symptoms. Any medication that is designed to relieve symptoms, such as pain and coughing, will provide some relief. Medications containing alcohol, however, should be avoided because of the dehydrating effects of alcohol. The best medicine for symptoms is simply an analgesic, such as aspirin, **acetaminophen**, or naproxen. Without a doctor's approval, aspirin is generally not recommended for people under 18 owing to its association with Reye's syndrome, a rare aspirin-associated complication seen in children recovering from the flu. To be on the safe side, children should receive acetaminophen or ibuprofen to treat their symptoms.

There are four antiviral drugs marketed for treating influenza. To be effective, treatment should begin no later than two days after symptoms appear. Antivirals may be useful in treating patients who have weakened immune systems or who are at risk for developing serious complications. They include amantadine

(Symmetrel, Symadine) and rimantadine (Flumandine), which work against Type A influenza, and zanamavir (Relenza) and oseltamavir phosphate (Tamiflu), which work against both Types A and B influenza. Amantadine and rimantadine can cause side effects such as nervousness, **anxiety**, lightheadedness, and **nausea**. Severe side effects include seizures, delirium, and hallucination, but are rare and are nearly always limited to people who have kidney problems, seizure disorders, or psychiatric disorders. The new drugs zanamavir and oseltamavir phosphate have few side effects but can cause **dizziness**, jitters, and **insomnia**.

Alternative treatments

There are several alternative treatments that may help in fighting off the virus and recovering from the flu, in addition to easing flu symptoms.

- Acupuncture and acupressure. Both are said to stimulate natural resistance, relieve nasal congestion and headaches, fight fever, and calm coughs, depending on the acupuncture and acupressure points used.
- Aromatherapy. Aromatherapists recommend gargling daily with one drop each of the essential oils of tea tree (*Melaleuca* spp.) and lemon mixed in a glass of warm water. If already suffering from the flu, two drops of tea tree oil in a hot bath may help ease the symptoms. Essential oils of eucalyptus (*Eucalyptus globulus*) or peppermint (*Mentha piperita*) added to a steam vaporizer may help clear chest and nasal congestion.
- Herbal remedies. Herbal remedies can be used to stimulate the immune system (echinacea), as antivirals (*Hydrastis canadensis*) goldenseal and garlic (*Allium sativum*), or directed at whatever symptoms arise as a result of the flu. For example, an infusion of boneset (*Eupatroium perfoliatum*) may counteract aches and fever, and yarrow (*Achillea millefolium*) or elderflower tinctures may combat chills.
- Homeopathy. To prevent flu, a homeopathic remedy called *Oscillococcinum* may be taken at the first sign of flu symptoms and repeated for a day or two. Although oscillococcinum is a popular flu remedy in Europe, a research study published in 2003 found it to be ineffective. Other homeopathic remedies recommended vary according to the specific flu symptoms present. *Gelsemium* (*Gelsemium sempervirens*) is recommended to combat weakness accompanied by chills, a headache, and nasal congestion. *Bryonia* (*Bryonia alba*) may be used to treat muscle aches, headaches, and a dry cough. For restlessness, chills, hoarseness, and achy joints, poison ivy (*Rhus toxicodendron*) is recommended. Finally, for achiness and a dry cough or chills, *Eupatorium perfoliatum* is suggested.
- Hydrotherapy. A bath to induce a fever will speed recovery from the flu by creating an environment in the body where the flu virus cannot survive. The patient should take a bath as hot as he/she can tolerate and remain in the bath for 20–30 minutes. While in the bath, the patient drinks a cup of yarrow or elderflower tea to induce sweating. During the bath, a cold cloth is held on the forehead or at the nape of the neck to keep the temperature down in the brain. The patient is assisted when getting out of the bath (he/she may feel weak or dizzy) and then gets into bed and covers up with layers of blankets to induce more sweating.
- Traditional Chinese medicine (TCM). Practitioners of TCM recommend mixtures of herbs to prevent flu as well as to relieve symptoms once a person has fallen ill. There are several different recipes for these remedies, but most contain ginger and Japanese honeysuckle in addition to other ingredients.
- Vitamins. For adults, 2–3 grams of vitamin C daily may help prevent the flu. Increasing the dose to 5–7 grams per day during the flu can felp fight the infection. (The dose should be reduced if diarrhea develops.)

Prognosis

Following proper treatment guidelines, healthy people under the age of 65 usually suffer no long-term consequences associated with flu infection. The elderly and the chronically ill are at greater risk for secondary infection and other complications, but they can also enjoy a complete recovery.

Most people recover fully from an influenza infection, but it should not be viewed complacently. Influenza is a serious disease, and approximately 1 in 1,000 cases proves fatal.

Prevention

The Centers for Disease Control and Prevention recommend that people get an influenza vaccine injection each year before flu season starts. In the United States, flu season typically runs from late December to early March. Vaccines should be received two to six weeks prior to the onset of flu season to allow the body enough time to establish immunity. Adults only need one dose of the yearly vaccine, but children under nine years of age who have not previously been immunized should receive two doses with a month between each dose.

Each season's flu vaccine contains three virus strains that are the most likely to be encountered in

KEY TERMS

Bioterrorism—The intentional use of disease-causing microbes or other biologic agents to intimidate or terrorize a civilian population for political or military reasons. Type A influenza virus could be used as an agent of bioterrorism.

Common cold—A mild illness caused by a upper respiratory viruses. Usual symptoms include nasal congestion, coughing, sneezing, throat irritation, and a low-grade fever.

Epidemic—A widespread regional disease outbreak.

Guillain-Barré syndrome—Also called acute idiopathic polyneuritis, this condition is a neurologic syndrome that can cause numbness in the limbs and muscle weakness following certain viral infections.

Pandemic—Worldwide outbreak of an infection, afflicting millions of victims.

the coming flu season. When there is a good match between the anticipated flu strains and the strains used in the vaccine, the vaccine is 70–90% effective in people under 65. Because immune response diminishes somewhat with age, people over 65 may not receive the same level of protection from the vaccine, but even if they do contract the flu, the vaccine diminishes the severity and helps prevent complications.

The virus strains used to make the vaccine are inactivated and will not cause the flu. In the past, flu symptoms were associated with vaccine preparations that were not as highly purified as modern vaccines, not to the virus itself. In 1976, there was a slightly increased risk of developing **Guillain-Barré syndrome**, a very rare disorder, associated with the swine flu vaccine. This association occurred only with the 1976 swine flu vaccine preparation and has never recurred.

Serious side effects with modern vaccines are extremely unusual. Some people experience a slight soreness at the point of injection, which resolves within a day or two. People who have never been exposed to influenza, particularly children, may experience one to two days of a slight fever, tiredness, and muscle aches. These symptoms start within 6–12 hours after the **vaccination**.

It should be noted that certain people should not receive an influenza vaccine. Infants six months and younger have immature immune systems and will not benefit from the vaccine. Since the vaccines are prepared using hen eggs, people who have severe **allergies** to eggs or other vaccine components should not receive the influenza vaccine. As an alternative, they may receive a course of amantadine or rimantadine, which are also used as a protective measure against influenza. Other people who might receive these drugs are those who have been immunized after the flu season has started or who are immunocompromised, such as people with advanced HIV disease. Amantadine and rimantadine are 70–90% effective in preventing influenza.

There are two types of influenza vaccines: the flu shot and the flu mist. The flu shot consists of inactivated (killed) influenza viruses and is given by injection into the muscle. With the flu mist, the live, attenuated (weakened) influenza vaccine (LAIV) is sprayed into the nostrils, but this type of vaccination is not recommended for persons over the age of 49. Both injectable and mist vaccine typically contain three influenza viruses, two of type A virus and one of type B virus. The strains of viruses included in the vaccine change yearly based on international surveillance data of influenza cases and estimations by scientists on what types and strains of viruses will be prevalent in the coming influenza season. When the strains included in the vaccine are well matched to the strains present in the community, the vaccine usually can protect seven to nine out of ten vaccinated persons. However, in elderly people, the vaccine may not work as well in preventing influenza, but will result in decrease in severity of symptoms and in the risk of health complications.

In April 2009, the United States Department of Health and Human Services declared a public health emergency regarding human cases of H1N1 influenza A, more commonly called swine flu. Swine flu was of special concern because for several reasons. Experts believed that the virus was a new strain of influenza with a genetic composition different from the familiar viruses that cause seasonal influenza. Because it was radically different, individuals were especially susceptible to developing serious illness. In addition, the virus often caused more intense symptoms in young, healthy people than in the elderly or the very young who are the greatest target of seasonal flu. Because the decision had already been made about which strains of seasonal flu were to be included in the vaccine for the next flu season and manufacture had already begun, a special push was made to make a separate vaccine against the swine flu. Thus, in the winter of 2009 through the 2010 flu season, people were advised to get two separate flu shots, one against seasonal flu and one against the new H1N1 influenza A.

Certain groups are strongly advised to be vaccinated because they are at increased risk for influenza-related complications:

- All people 65 years and older
- Residents of nursing homes and chronic-care facilities, regardless of age
- Adults and children who have chronic heart or lung problems, such as asthma
- Adults and children who have chronic metabolic diseases, such as diabetes and renal dysfunction, as well as severe anemia or inherited hemoglobin disorders
- Children and teenagers who are on long-term aspirin therapy
- Women who will be in their second or third trimester during flu season or women who are nursing
- Anyone who is immunocompromised, including HIV-infected persons, cancer patients, organ transplant recipients, and patients receiving steroids, chemotherapy, or radiation therapy
- Anyone in contact with the above groups, such as teachers, care givers, health-care personnel, and family members
- Travelers to foreign countries.

A person need not be in one of the at-risk categories listed above, however, to receive a flu vaccination. Anyone who wants to forego the discomfort and inconvenience of an influenza attack may receive the vaccine.

Resources

BOOKS

Beers, Mark H., Robert S. Porter, and Thomas V. Jones, eds. *The Merck Manual of Diagnosis and Therapy*. 18th ed. Whitehouse Station, NJ: Merck Research Laboratories, 2006.

Brouwer, Emma S.*Influenza Pandemic: Preparedness and Response to a Health Disaster*. Hauppauge, NY: Nova Science, 2010.

PERIODICALS

Jonas, W. B., T. J. Kaptchuk, and K. Linde. "A Critical Overview of Homeopathy." *Annals of Internal Medicine* 138 (March 4, 2003): 393–399.

Krug, R. M. "The Potential Use of Influenza Virus as an Agent for Bioterrorism." *Antiviral Research* 57 (January 2003): 147–150.

Oxford, J. S., S. Bossuyt, S. Balasingam, et al. "Treatment of Epidemic and Pandemic Influenza with Neuraminidase and M2 Proton Channel Inhibitors." *Clinical Microbiology and Infection* 9 (January 2003): 1–14.

Roth, Y., J. S. Chapnik, and P. Cole. " Feasibility of Aerosol Vaccination in Humans." *Annals of Otology, Rhinology, and Laryngology* 112 (March 2003): 264–270.

Shortridge, K. F., J. S. Peiris, and Y. Guan. "The Next Influenza Pandemic: Lessons from Hong Kong." *Journal of Applied Microbiology* 94, Supplement (2003): 70S–79S.

Storch, G. A. "Rapid Diagnostic Tests for Influenza." *Current Opinion in Pediatrics* 15 (February 2003): 77–84.

Thompson, W. W., D. K. Shay, E. Weintraub, et al. "Mortality Associated with Influenza and Respiratory Syncytial Virus in the United States." *Journal of the American Medical Association* 289 (January 8, 2003): 179–186.

OTHER

NIAID Fact Sheet: Flu. Bethesda, MD: NIAID, January 2003. http://www.niaid.nih.gov/factsheets/flu.htm.

ORGANIZATIONS

Centers for Disease Control and Prevention (CDC), 1600 Clifton Road, Atlanta, GA, 30333, 800 232-4636, cdcinfo@cdc.gov, http://www.cdc.gov.

National Institute of Allergies and Infectious Diseases, 6610 Rockledge Drive, MSC 6612, Bethesda, MD, 20892-6612, 301 496-5717, 301 402-3573, 866 284-4107, ocpostoffice@niaid.nih.gov, http://www.niaid.nih.gov.

Julia Barrett
Rebecca J. Frey, PhD

Influenza vaccination

Definition

An **influenza vaccination** is a vaccination that is used to protect individuals against the viruses that cause influenza, which is also called the flu.

Purpose

Influenza vaccination helps to protect people against getting influenza. Protection is imperfect because the viruses that cause influenza are constantly changing (mutating). Influenza vaccines are updated every year to reflect the current stains of flu that are expected to be most prevalent, and re-vaccination is recommended every year.

KEY TERMS

Guillain-Barre Syndrome—A disorder characterized by progressive symmetrical paralysis and loss of reflexes, usually beginning in the legs. The paralysis characteristically involves more than one limb (most commonly the legs), is progressive, and usually proceeds from the end of an extremity toward the torso. Guillain-Barre usually occurs after a respiratory infection, and it is apparently caused by a misdirected immune response that results in the direct destruction of the myelin sheath surrounding the peripheral nerves or of the axon of the nerve itself.

Influenza —Commonly known as flu; an infectious disease of birds and mammals caused by viruses of the family Orthomyxoviridae (the influenza viruses); common symptoms of the disease are the chills, then fever, sore throat, muscle pains, severe headache, coughing, weakness and general feelings of illness.

Vaccination—Injection of a killed or weakened microbe in order to stimulate the immune system against the microbe, thereby preventing disease. Vaccinations, or immunizations, work by stimulating the immune system, the natural disease-fighting system of the body. The healthy immune system is able to recognize invading bacteria and viruses and produce substances (antibodies) to destroy or disable them. Vaccinations prepare the immune system to ward off a disease. To immunize against viral diseases, the virus used in the vaccine has been weakened or killed.

Description

Every year in the United States about 226,000 people are hospitalized and 36,000 die of influenza-related complications, most often bacterial **pneumonia**, **dehydration**, or a worsening of chronic medical conditions, such as congestive **heart failure**, **asthma**, or diabetes. Ninety% of the deaths occur in individuals 65 years and older. During influenza epidemics, hospitalization rates for older people increase two to five times compared to other seasons of the year and, more than half of the hospitalizations are people 65 and older.

An influenza vaccination is the best way to be protected from contracting influenza. Older Hispanic and African-American adults are much less likely to be vaccinated against influenza than their white counterparts. The rate of vaccination of senior citizens is about 65% in the United States African-Americans 65 years and older lag behind whites by about 21% in getting annual vaccinations, while Hispanic Americans 65 years and older lag behind whites by 19%. In large urban areas with high levels of unvaccinated persons, there is a potential for outbreaks of influenza; thus improving overall immunization coverage rates is essential. Studies have also shown that elderly people who choose to be vaccinated are generally in better health than those who fail to get the vaccine, so influenza control strategies should be developed to target those who are not being vaccinated. The United States Centers for Disease Control and Prevention (CDC) has set a target date of 2010 to increase influenza vaccinations to 90% among all adults aged 65 years and older, with an emphasis on vaccinating minority groups. In the U.S. the influenza vaccination is provided at no cost to all senior citizens covered by Medicare.

There are two types of influenza vaccines: the flu shot and the flu mist. The flu shot consists of inactivated (killed) influenza viruses and is given by injection into the muscle. With the flu mist, the live, attenuated (weakened) influenza vaccine (LAIV) is sprayed into the nostrils, but this type of vaccination is not recommended for persons over the age of 49. Both injectable and mist vaccine typically contain three influenza viruses, two of type A virus and one of type B virus. The strain of viruses included in the vaccine change yearly based on international surveillance data of influenza cases and estimations by scientists on what types and strains of viruses will be prevalent in the coming influenza season. When the strains included in the vaccine are well matched to the strains present in the community, the vaccine usually can protect seven to nine out of ten vaccinated persons. However, in elderly people, the vaccine may not work as well in preventing influenza, but will result in decrease in severity of symptoms and in the risk of health complications.

In April 2009, the United States Department of Health and Human Services declared a public health emergency regarding human cases of H1N1 influenza A, more commonly called swine flu. Swine flu was of special concern because for several reasons. Experts believed that the virus was a new strain of influenza with a genetic composition different from the familiar viruses that cause seasonal influenza. Because it was radically different, individuals were especially susceptible to developing serious illness. In addition, the virus often caused more intense symptoms in young, healthy people than in the elderly or the very young who are the greatest target of seasonal flu. Because the decision had already been made about which strains of seasonal flu were to be included in the vaccine for the next flu season and manufacture had already begun, a special push was made to make a separate vaccine against the swine flu. Thus, in the winter of 2009 through the 2010 flu season, people were advised to get two separate flu shots, one against seasonal flu and one against the new H1N1 influenza A.

Vaccinations against influenza are especially important for those who are not in good health. The vaccination is recommended for persons who have trouble swallowing or breathing, are receiving long term steroid therapy, or who have had heart attacks, heart disease, lung diseases such as asthma, **emphysema**, or chronic **bronchitis**, diabetes, HIV, blood disorders such as sickle cell anemia or other **hemoglobinopathies**, kidney or **liver disease**, or weakened immune systems. Individuals with such conditions are at an increased risk of developing serious influenza-related complications. Those who are at a high risk of complications and who have not received their influenza vaccination the preceding fall or winter should be vaccinated before travel to the tropics, travel with tourist groups, or travel to the Southern Hemisphere during April through September.

Recommended dosage

As of 2010, the United States Centers for Disease Control and Prevention (CDC) recommended that the following groups be vaccinated against seasonal influenza.

- children between the ages of 6 months and 19 years
- pregnant women
- all individuals age 50 or older
- people with certain chronic medical problems
- health care workers
- people caring for or living with children under age 5
- people caring for or living with someone at high risk for complications from influenza
- healthy individuals of any age who wish to reduce their chances of getting the flu, especially those living in group situations such as dormitories or military barracks

All persons 50 years of age and older should receive one dose intramuscularly of the inactivated seasonal influenza vaccine every year. Individuals ages 2–49 may be given flu mist rather than an injection. Ideally vaccination should occur during the period from September to mid-November, but a vaccination received later may still be beneficial. Influenza can occur any time from November through May in the northern hemisphere, with cases usually peaking in January or February. The influenza vaccine can safely be given with other vaccines, including the pneumococcal vaccine.

As of the 2009–2010 influenza season, additional vaccination against H1N1 swine flu was recommended for everyone with first responders, health care workers, and other high-risk individuals given priority.

Precautions

People who should not be vaccinated against influenza without first contacting a physician for advice include:

- those who have a severe allergy to chicken eggs
- those who have had a severe reaction to an influenza vaccination previously
- those who previously developed Guillain-Barre Syndrome (a very rare condition that results in weakness and paralysis of muscles of the body) within six weeks of getting an influenza vaccination

In addition, a person who has a moderate or severe illness with a **fever** should wait to get vaccinated until their symptoms decrease.

It takes up to two weeks to develop protection after the shot, with the protection from the vaccination lasting up to one year.

Side effects

Although the risk of the influenza vaccine causing serious harm or **death** is small and is much less than the health risks from contracting influenza, the vaccine, as with any medicine, can cause problems such as severe allergic reactions. Because the viruses in the vaccine have been killed, no one can get influenza from the vaccine. Mild problems that can occur soon after the vaccination is given and lasting 1 to 2 days include:

- soreness, redness, or swelling where the shot was given
- low grade fever
- aches
- chills
- general feelings of ill health
- runny nose (flu mist only)
- wheezing (flu mist only)
- sore throat (flu mist only)

More severe problems that can be associated with the influenza vaccine are life-threatening allergic reactions. These will occur within a few minutes to a few hours after the shot. A person should stay in the clinic where the shot was given for 15 minutes, in case an immediate reaction occurs. Such reactions could include **hives**, difficulty breathing, or swelling of the throat, tongue, or lips. If a severe reaction occurs after the person leaves the clinic, the affected person should immediately be taken to an emergency health care facility. The chance of such an adverse reaction occurring is estimated at less than one in a million people. Any adverse reaction should be reported to the U.S. Department of Heath and Human Services through the Vaccine Adverse Event Reporting Service. If a person has had a serious reaction to a vaccine, a federal program, the National Vaccine Injury Compensation Program, is available to help pay for the care of the person harmed or injured by the shot.

Interactions

Influenza vaccines are not known to interact with any drugs or foods.

Resources

OTHER

Flu. MedlinePlus. April 7, 2010. http://www.nlm.nih.gov/medlineplus/flu.html

Flu Vaccine (Influenza Immunization). MedicineNet.com. November 2, 2009. http://www.medicinenet.com/flu_vaccination/article.htm

Vaccines. United States Centers for Disease Control and Prevention (CDC). March 30, 2010 http://www.cdc.gov/vaccines

ORGANIZATIONS

United States Centers for Disease Control and Prevention (CDC), 1600 Clifton Road, Atlanta, GA, 30333, (404) 639-3534, 800-CDC-INFO (800-232-4636). TTY: (888) 232-6348, inquiry@cdc.gov, http://www.cdc.gov.

World Health Organization, Avenue Appia 20, 1211 Geneva 27, Switzerland, +22 41 791 21 11, +22 41 791 31 11, info@who.int, http://www.who.int.

Judith L. Sims
Tish Davidson, AM

Infrequent menstruation *see* **Oligomenorrhea**

Inhalants and related disorders

Definition

Inhalants are chemicals that are inhaled through the nose or mouth for a quick "high." They include a broad range of chemicals found in hundreds of different readily available products. Inhalant intoxication, **abuse**, and dependence are classified as substance use disorders.

Demographics

Inhalants are one of the few substance use disorders that more often affect younger children. Because inhalants are inexpensive and readily available, they are often used by children aged 6–16, as well as by people with little money. In 2008, two million Americans aged 12 and over abused inhalants. It has been estimated that 10–20% of youths aged 12–17 have tried inhalants and about 6% of Americans tried inhalants prior to the fourth grade. The peak period for inhalant use appears to be the seventh through ninth grades. However inhalant use among American teens may be on the decline.

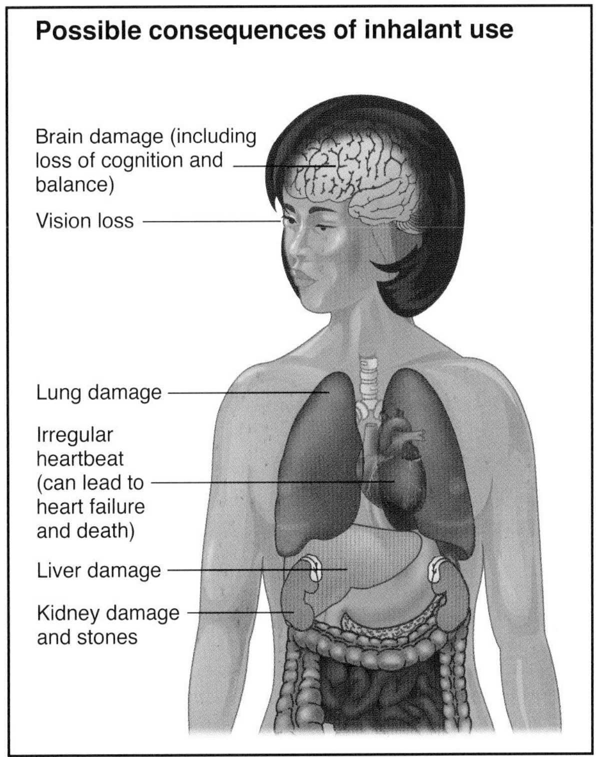

(Illustration by Electronic Illustrators Group. Reproduced by permission of Gale, a part of Cengage Learning.)

Among adults and children younger than 12, inhalant use is more common among males than females. However there are no gender differences in inhalant use in teens between the ages of 12 and 17.

The use of inhalants and inhalant dependence are common among those who do not have access to other drugs or are otherwise isolated, such as prison inmates. As with other substance use disorders, people who have greater access to inhalants are more likely to develop dependence. This group includes workers in industrial settings.

Description

Inhalants include volatile solvents—liquids that vaporize at room temperature—and aerosols—sprays that contain both solvents and propellants. Examples of inhalants include:

- glue
- gasoline
- paint thinner
- hairspray
- lighter fluid
- spray paint
- nail polish remover
- correction fluid
- rubber cement
- felt-tip marker fluids
- vegetable sprays
- certain cleaners

Inhalants are generally used by breathing in the vapors directly from the container ("sniffing"), by inhaling fumes from substances placed in a bag ("bagging"), or by inhaling from a cloth soaked in the substance ("huffing"). Inhalants take effect very quickly because they enter the bloodstream directly from the lungs. The "high" from inhalants is usually brief, so they are often used repeatedly over several hours. This pattern of use can be particularly dangerous, leading to unconsciousness or even **death**.

The American Psychiatric Association's *Diagnostic and Statistical Manual of Mental Disorders*, fourth edition, text revision (*DSM-IV-TR*) does not include use of anesthetic gases (such as nitrous oxide, chloroform, and ether) or nitrites (such as amyl and butyl nitrites) as inhalant-related disorders because they have slightly different intoxication properties. Rather, use of these substances is classified with other substance-related disorders. However the symptoms are very similar to those of inhalants and related disorders.

Although only a small proportion of inhalant use meets the diagnostic criteria for abuse or dependence, all use of chemical inhalants constitutes abuse, since they are not being used for their intended purposes. Unlike all other substance dependencies, inhalants and related disorders may not result in clinically significant **withdrawal syndromes**. Instead inhalants are sometimes considered to be "gateway" drugs, because inhalant use often precedes the use of other substances such as alcohol, **marijuana**, or **cocaine**.

Risk factors

Factors associated with inhalant disorders include poverty, a history of childhood abuse, poor grades, and dropping out of school. However the latter two factors may be a result of inhalant use rather than a cause. Inhalants are often used in group settings and are highly subject to peer influence.

Causes and symptoms

The symptoms of inhalant intoxication differ slightly depending on the type of inhalant, the amount used, and other factors. However in general, intoxication from an inhalant usually occurs within five minutes and lasts for 5–30 minutes. Inhalants typically depress the central nervous system, with effects similar to those of alcohol, and produce euphoria, excitement, **dizziness**, and slurred speech. Inhalant intoxication can cause a feeling of floating or a sense of power.

An overdose of inhalant can result in **coma** or death. The most serious medical risk of inhalant use is "sudden sniffing death." Inhalants, especially repeated use in a single, prolonged session, can cause a rapid and irregular heartbeat or severe breathing difficulties, followed by **heart failure** and death. Sudden sniffing death can occur within minutes. Inhalant use also can cause permanent damage to the brain, lungs, kidneys, muscles, and heart. In addition to damage from the vapors themselves, many inhalants contain dangerously high levels of copper, zinc, and heavy metals.

The *DSM-IV-TR* requires the following criteria for a diagnosis of inhalant intoxication:

- Use: There was recent intentional inhalant use.
- Personality changes: There are significant behavioral or psychological changes during or shortly after inhaling. These might include provoking a fight, assault, using poor judgment, apathy, or impaired functioning at work or school or in a social situation.
- Inhalant-specific intoxication syndrome: Two or more of the following symptoms occur during or shortly after inhalant use or exposure: dizziness;

KEY TERMS

Aerosols—Sprays that contain propellants and solvents, including many household products.

Delusion—A persistent false belief held in the face of strong contradictory evidence.

Euphoria—An exaggerated state of psychological and physical well-being.

Hallucinations—False sensory perceptions; hearing sounds or seeing people or objects that are not there. Hallucinations can also affect the senses of smell, touch, and taste.

Tolerance—The body's adjustment to a drug so that it takes more and more to produce the same physiological or psychological effects.

Volatile solvents—Liquids that vaporize at room temperature, including a variety of industrial and household products and art and office-supply solvents.

involuntary side-to-side eye movements (nystagmus); loss of coordination; slurred speech; unsteady gait (difficulty walking); lethargy (fatigue); slowed reflexes; psychomotor retardation (moving slowly); tremor (shaking); generalized muscle weakness; blurred or double vision; stupor or coma; euphoria.

Inhalant abuse is defined as significant negative consequences from the recurrent use of inhalants without physical dependence on the substance. Abusers typically use inhalants less frequently than those with inhalant dependence, but nevertheless suffer negative consequences. For example inhalant abuse may contribute to poor grades or school truancy. According to the *DSM-IV-TR*, to meet the diagnostic criteria for inhalant abuse, one or more of the following symptoms must occur and cause significant impairment or distress within a 12-month period:

- Interference with role fulfillment: Inhalant use frequently interferes with obligations at work, home, or school. Users may be unable to perform chores or pay attention at school.
- Danger to self: The user repeatedly uses inhalants in physically hazardous situations such as while driving a car.
- Legal problems: The user has recurrent legal problems related to inhalant use, such as assault arrests.
- Social problems: The user continues to use inhalants despite repeated interpersonal or relationship problems caused by or worsened by their use. For example the affected person may have arguments related to inhalant use.

Inhalant dependence or **addiction** is a syndrome in which inhalant use continues despite significant problems caused by or worsened by the use. The problems may involve employment, family relationships, and/or physical impairments such as kidney or liver damage. Users may find it difficult to stop using inhalants despite these problems. Heavy users of inhalants may develop a tolerance to the substance that suggests physical dependence. Dependent users may inhale daily or several times per week. The solitary use of inhalants is associated with heavy, prolonged use and may indicate dependency. To meet the diagnostic criteria for inhalant dependence the *DSM-IV-TR* requires that three or more of the following symptoms occur and cause significant impairment or distress within a 12-month period:

- Tolerance: The user has developed tolerance to the inhalant, as indicated by the same amount having less effect over time or by the need to use increasingly higher amounts to achieve the same effect. After a period of regular inhalant use, users often find that they require at least 50% more than the original amount to achieve the same effect.
- Loss of control: The user repeatedly uses a larger amount of inhalant than planned or uses over a longer period of time than planned; for example using inhalants on school days after initially limiting their use to weekends.
- Inability to stop using: The user has either unsuccessfully attempted to cut down or stop using inhalants or has a persistent desire to stop.
- Time: The user spends large amounts of time obtaining inhalants, using them, being under their influence, and recovering from their effects. Although inhalants may be readily available for very little money, they may be used repeatedly for hours every day.
- Interference with activities: The user either abandons or reduces the amount of time devoted to recreational and social activities and/or occupational activities because of inhalant use. Inhalant use may replace sports, time with friends, or work.
- Harm to self: Inhalant use continues despite physical problems, such as liver or heart damage, or psychological problems, such as depression or memory loss, that are caused by or worsened by the inhalant use.

Diagnosis

Users rarely seek diagnosis and treatment for inhalant abuse or dependence on their own. A child or adolescent may be brought to a doctor by a parent or other relative who is concerned about personality changes, a chemical odor on the child's breath, or other signs of inhalant abuse. The parent may have discovered empty containers of the inhaled substance. Sometimes inhalant use by a child or adolescent is diagnosed in a hospital emergency room after an overdose or accidental injury.

Examination

Inhalant use is sometimes diagnosed by the existence of:

- auditory, visual, or tactile hallucinations
- other perceptual disturbances, such as illusions
- delusions, such as a belief that one can fly

Inhalant disorder may be difficult to diagnose, since intoxication from alcohol, sedatives, hypnotics (medications to induce sleep), or anxiolytics (tranquilizers) can resemble inhalant intoxication. The use of other substances is not uncommon among inhalant abusers and those with inhalant dependency often have other **substance abuse** disorders as well. In the latter case inhalant use is usually secondary to other substance use, since inhalants are only occasionally the primary drug of choice.

Tests

Although inhalants can be detected in blood or urine samples, laboratory tests may not always confirm a diagnosis of inhalant disorder since the substances do not remain in the body for very long.

Treatment

Traditional

Inhalant intoxication is often treated in a hospital emergency room because of serious psychological or medical consequences. The latter may include **headache**, **nausea**, **vomiting**, severe breathing difficulties, heart failure, or injuries sustained while under the influence of inhalants, such as falls or auto accidents. Life-threatening **burns** are common since many inhalants are highly flammable. Users may also require emergency treatment for suffocation from inhaling from a plastic bag placed over the head or from **choking** on inhaled vomit.

Treatment of inhalant and related disorders usually takes a long period and involves:

- family support
- different social networks if the individual uses inhalants with friends
- new coping skills
- increased self-esteem

Prognosis

The course of inhalant use, abuse, and dependence differs somewhat depending on the user's age. Younger children who regularly abuse inhalants, especially after school and on weekends—and even children who are dependent on inhalants—often stop on their own as they get older. They may avoid substance use altogether or move on to other substances. Adults suffering from inhalant abuse or dependence may continue to use regularly for years. Alternatively they may binge frequently—using inhalants much more often for shorter periods of time. This pattern of use can also continue for years. Chronic inhalant users are difficult to treat because they often have other serious personal and social problems, have difficulty avoiding inhalants, and frequently relapse.

Prevention

Comprehensive prevention programs that involve families, schools, communities, and media such as television can be effective in reducing substance abuse. The focus of such programs is the avoidance of any initial contact with abused substances. This is the most effective method for preventing inhalant and related disorders.

Parents and teachers can help prevent inhalant abuse by educating children about the negative effects of inhalants and by recognizing signs of inhalant use including:

1. chemical odors on a child's breath or clothes
2. slurred speech
3. drunken or disoriented behavior
4. nausea or lack of appetite
5. inattentiveness
6. poor coordination

Resources

BOOKS

American Psychiatric Association. *Diagnostic and Statistical Manual of Mental Disorders,* 4th ed., text rev. Arlington, VA: American Psychiatric Association, 2007.

Flynn, Noa. *Inhalants and Solvents: Sniffing Disaster*. Philadelphia: Mason Crest, 2008.

Kuhn, Cynthia, et al. *Buzzed: The Straight Facts About the Most Used and Abused Drugs from Alcohol to Ecstasy*, 3rd ed. New York: W. W. Norton, 2008.
McCage, Crystal. *Inhalants*. San Diego, CA: ReferencePoint Press, 2008.
Robinson, Matthew. *Inhalant Abuse*. New York: Rosen Central, 2008.

PERIODICALS

Magid, Jennifer. "HUFFING: A Deadly High." *Current Health 1* 33(3) (November 2009): 20–22.
Perron, Brian E., and Matthew O. Howard. "Adolescent Inhaler Use, Abuse and Dependence." *Addiction* 104(7) (July 2009): 1185.

OTHER

Balster, Robert. "Inhalant Abuse in the United States." American Psychological Association http://www. apa.org/about/gr/science/spin/2009/10/inhalant-abuse.pdf
"Inhalants." MedlinePlus. http://www.nlm.nih.gov/medlineplus/inhalants.html
"Inhalants." National Institute on Drug Abuse. http://www.drugabuse.gov/drugpages/inhalants.html
NIDA. "Inhalants." drugabuse.gov http://www.inhalants.drugabuse.gov/
"NIDA InfoFacts: Inhalants." National Institute on Drug Abuse. http://www.drugabuse.gov/infofacts/inhalants.html

ORGANIZATIONS

American Psychological Association, 750 First Street, NE , Washington, DC, 20002-4242, (202) 336-5500, (800) 374-2721, http://www.apa.org.
National Clearinghouse for Alcohol and Drug Information, P.O. Box 2345, Rockville, MD, 20847-2345, (877) SAMHSA7, (240) 221-4292, http://ncadi.samhsa.gov/default.aspx.
National Institute on Drug Abuse, 6001 Executive Boulevard, Room 5213, Bethesda, MD, 20892-9561, (301) 443-1124, information@nida.nih.gov, http://www.drugabuse.gov/NIDAHome.html.
Substance Abuse & Mental Health Services Administration (SAMHSA) Health Information Network (SHIN), PO Box 2345, Rockville, MD, 20847-2345, (877) SAMHSA-7 (726-4727), (240) 221-4292, SHIN @samhsa.hhs.gov, http://www.samhsa.gov/shin.

Jennifer Hahn, PhD
Margaret Alic, PhD

Inhalation therapies

Definition

Inhalation therapies are a group of respiratory, or breathing, treatments designed to help restore or improve breathing function in patients with a variety of diseases, conditions, or injuries. The treatments range from at-home **oxygen therapy** for patients with **chronic obstructive pulmonary disease** to mechanical ventilation for patients with acute **respiratory failure**. Inhalation therapies usually include the following categories:

- Oxygen therapy
- Incentive spirometry
- Continuous positive airway pressure (CPAP)
- Oxygen chamber therapy
- Mechanical ventilation
- Newborn life support.

Purpose

Inhalation therapies are ordered for various stages of diseases which are causing progressive or sudden respiratory failure. Although physicians generally follow guidelines to assign specific therapy according the type and stage of a disease, the ultimate decision is based on a number of tests indicating pulmonary function and the presence or absence of oxygen in body organs and tissues.

Oxygen therapy

Oxygen therapy is most commonly ordered to support patients with **emphysema** and other chronic obstructive pulmonary disease (COPD). The oxygen therapy is usually ordered once decreased oxygen saturation in the blood or tissues is demonstrated. Oxygen therapy may also be used in the hospital setting to help return a patient's breathing and oxygen levels to normal.

Incentive spirometry

Spirometry is a diagnostic method for measuring gases and respiratory function. Incentive spirometry may be ordered to help patients practice and improve controlled breathing. It may be ordered after surgery to the abdomen, lungs, neck, or head.

Continuous positive airway pressure (CPAP)

Common uses of continuous positive airway pressure include **sleep apnea**, **respiratory distress syndrome** in infants, and **adult respiratory distress syndrome**. Signs of **atelectasis** (absence of gas from the lungs) or abnormalities of the lower airways may also indicate CPAP.

Oxygen chamber therapy

Oxygen chamber therapy is ordered for various causes that indicate immediate need for oxygen saturation in the blood. Divers with decompression illness, climbers at high altitudes, patients suffering from severe carbon dioxide **poisoning**, and children or adults in acute respiratory distress may require oxygen chamber therapy. In recent years, physicians have also used the forced pressure of oxygen chambers to help heal **burns** and other **wounds**, since the pressure under which the oxygen is delivered can reach areas that are blocked off or suffering from poor circulation.

Mechanical ventilation

Mechanical ventilation is ordered for patients in acute respiratory distress, and is often used in an intensive care situation. In some cases, mechanical ventilation is a final attempt to continue the breathing function in a patient and may be considered "life-sustaining."

Newborn life support

Newborn babies, particularly those who were premature, may require inhalation therapies immediately upon birth, since the lungs are among the last organs to fully develop. Some newborns suffer from serious respiratory problems or birth complications, such as respiratory distress syndrome, neonatal wet lung syndrome, apnea of **prematurity** or persistent fetal circulation, which may require inhalation therapies.

Precautions

There are numerous indications for not prescribing various inhalation therapies.

Oxygen therapy

Patients and family members who smoke should not have oxygen prescribed or should avoid **smoking** in the area to prevent combustion. Sedatives should be avoided for patients on oxygen therapy.

Incentive spirometry

Patients who are unable or unwilling to properly and consistently practice incentive spirometry as prescribed should not receive this form of treatment.

Continuous positive airway pressure (CPAP)

Patients unable or unwilling to comply with the physician's instructions for use of CPAP are not likely to have it prescribed. Extremely obese patients may have less success with this form of therapy for the treatment of sleep apnea.

Oxygen chamber therapy

Complications may arise from this form of treatment and during transport to or from the oxygen chamber. Therefore, some patients may not receive enough benefit to outweigh possible complications. All patients, particularly children, must be carefully monitored.

Mechanical ventilation

Use of mechanical ventilation will be carefully weighed against benefit and possible risks. Some patients will require **sedation** to prevent fighting of the ventilator, which can increase the risk of complications.

Newborn life support

Not all infants with breathing problems will require measures as severe as mechanical ventilation. The physician will make the determination based on weight and condition of the infant. Newborns with patent ductus arteriosis, a handicap affecting the pulmonary artery, are more likely to suffer pulmonary hemorrhage from mechanical ventilation.

Description

Oxygen therapy

Once a patient shows hypoxemia, or decreased oxygen in arterial blood, supplemental oxygen may be ordered. The main purpose of the oxygen is to prevent damage to vital organs resulting from inadequate oxygen supply. The lowest possible saturation will be given to keep the patient's measurements at a minimum acceptable level. The oxygen is administered through a mask or nasal tube, or sometimes directly into the trachea. The amount of oxygen prescribed is measured in liters of flow per minute. Patients with chronic hypoxemia, most likely in late stages of COPD, will often receive long-term oxygen therapy.

Most patients will receive their long-term oxygen therapy through home oxygen use. A physician must prescribe home oxygen and levels will be monitored to ensure that the correct amount of oxygen is administered. Some patients will receive oxygen therapy only at night or when exercising.

The choice of type of home oxygen systems will vary depending on availability, cost considerations, and the mobility of the patient. Those patients who are ambulatory, especially those who work, will need a system with a small portable tank. Depending on the system chosen, frequent deliveries of oxygen and filling of portable tanks will be necessary.

In the case of respiratory distress in newborns or adults, oxygen therapy may be attempted before mechanical ventilation since it is a noninvasive and less expensive choice. Oxygen has been found effective in treating patients with other diseases such as **cystic fibrosis**, chronic congestive **heart failure**, or other lung diseases.

Incentive spirometry

Incentive spirometry is also referred to as sustained maximal inspiration. It is designed to mimic natural sighs and yawns. A device provides positive feedback when a patient inhales at a predetermined rate and sustains the breath for a specific period of time. This helps teach the patient to take long, slow, and deep breaths. A spirometer, or equipment that measures pulmonary function, is provided to the patient and a respiratory therapist will work with the patient to demonstrate and explain the technique. Once patients show mastery of the technique, they are instructed to practice the exercises frequently on their own.

Continuous positive airway pressure (CPAP)

Patients with sleep apnea will receive continuous positive airway pressure to prevent upper airway collapse. It is usually administered through a tight-fitting mask as humidified oxygen. The pressure of flow is constant during both exhaling and inhaling and the level of pressure is determined based on each individual. Most patients undergoing CPAP in a hospital setting will receive continuous monitoring of some vital signs and periodic sampling of blood gas values.

Oxygen chamber therapy

Also known as hyperbaric oxygen chamber or hyperbaric oxygen therapy (HBO), this treatment delivers pure oxygen under pressure equal to that of 2–3 times normal atmospheric pressure. For years, this treatment has been especially effective on scuba divers who suffer from the "bends," or decompression illness. The patient enters the chamber, a plastic cylinder-shaped structure that is normally transparent. In most cases, just one patient will enter by being rolled into the chamber on a type of stretcher. Once inside, the oxygen will be delivered under forced pressure and the patient is free to read, nap, or listen to the radio. The therapy usually lasts one hour, although it can take up to five hours in serious decompression cases. Before exiting the chamber, the pressure will eventually be lowered to normal atmospheric level.

Mechanical ventilation

In general, mechanical ventilation replaces or supports the normal ventilatory lung function of a patient. Although normally delivered in a hospital, often to treat serious illness, mechanical ventilation may be performed at home under the order and supervision of a physician and home health agency. The patient will usually be intubated and the ventilator machine "takes over" the breathing function.

There are several modes and methods of mechanical ventilation, each offering different advantages and disadvantages. In assist/control ventilation, the oldest mode of ventilation, the physician predetermines settings and the ventilator delivers a breath each time the patient makes an effort to inhale. In synchronized intermittent mandatory ventilation, the machine senses a patient's effort to inhale and delivers the preset amount. The amount cannot be increased by the patient's effort. Pressure-control ventilation involves the physician's selection of a peak pressure and this method is most useful for patients suffering from obstructive airways disease. In cases of severe hypoventilation, an endotracheal tube must be inserted. If a patient will be on mechanical ventilation for more than two weeks, a tracheostomy, or surgical incision, will be performed for placement of the breathing tubes.

There are other modes of ventilation that may be used, including high-frequency ventilation, a newer technique that delivers 100 to 200 breaths per minute to the patient. The breaths are delivered through a humidified, high-pressure gas jet. High-frequency ventilation may be ordered when a patient does not respond to conventional mechanical ventilation or for certain conditions and circumstances.

Newborn life support

Premature infants, especially those born before the 28th week of gestation, have underdeveloped breathing muscles and immature structures within the lungs. These infants will require breathing support, often in the form of mechanical ventilation. The support delivers warm, humidified, oxygen-enriched gases either by oxygen hood or through mechanical ventilation. In serious cases, the infant may require mechanical ventilation with CPAP or positive-end expiratory pressure (PEEP) through a tightly fitting face mask or even by endotracheal intubation.

Need for continued resuscitation for newborns depends not only on gestational age, but on signs indicating ineffective breathing, including color, heart rate, and respiratory effort. CPAP will be delivered through nasal or endotracheal tubes with a continuous-flow ventilator specifically designed for infants. An alarm system alerts the neonatal staff to problems and monitoring of breathing and other vital functions will accompany the therapy. As respiratory distress syndrome begins to resolve, usually in four or five days, the type of support will be reduced accordingly and the infant may be weaned from the ventilator and moved to only CPAP or an oxygen hood.

Preparation

Preparation for any of these treatments is normally not necessary, and in fact, these therapies may be administered as a result of an emergency situation. Some of the methods, particularly incentive spirometry, or at-home oxygen or ventilation, will require education and cooperation with a home health agency or respiratory therapist. Pretreatment testing of various indicators of respiratory function and oxygen saturation will be performed to determine exact needs of individual patients.

Aftercare

Pulmonary function tests and other tests will be performed to verify that treatments have been successful or to monitor and adjust treatments. Mechanical ventilation will require weaning from the equipment and may also require care for the area surrounding the intubation.

Risks

Inhalation therapies may carry risks, complications or side effects including:

Oxygen therapy

At-home oxygen therapy carries risk if improper care is taken to follow instructions when handling the oxygen. Patients are cautioned not to smoke near the oxygen supply and to keep the supply away from other sources that may cause electrical spark, flames, or intense heat. Patients on home oxygen therapy should avoid use of sedatives.

Incentive spirometry

The major risk associated with incentive spirometry relates to improper use. Patients must be carefully instructed in the technique and monitored periodically for compliance and improvement. Barotrauma, injury to the middle ear or sinuses caused by imbalance between the affected cavity and the outside, or ambient pressure, can result form incentive spirometry. A patient may also suffer discomfort or **fatigue**.

Continuous positive airway pressure (CPAP)

The effectiveness of CPAP may be limited if patients do not cooperate. Possible side effects of CPAP include skin abrasions from the mask, leakage from the tube or mask, nasal congestion, nasal or oral dryness, or discomfort from the pressure of delivery.

Oxygen chamber therapy

Hyperbaric oxygen therapy is painless. The only risk would be associated with improper administration of the pressure levels, which should not occur, since respiratory staff and the supervising physician should be thoroughly trained in performance of this therapy. The drawback to hyperbaric oxygen treatment is the limited availability of chambers. Many cities do not have readily available chambers.

Mechanical ventilation

The biggest risk of mechanical ventilation is sometimes considered to be a patient's dependence on the machine and the difficulty of weaning the patient. The physician will carefully select and monitor the mode of ventilation, the machine's settings, and the patient's progress to prevent this complication. A patient may therefore be left on a ventilator after sufficient progress is made to gradually wean breathing dependence.

Intubation and mechanical ventilation are frightening and uncomfortable for many patients and they may fight the ventilator. If this occurs, the physician may order a sedative to ensure cooperation and effectiveness of the therapy. Intubation often results in irritation to the trachea and larynx. Tracheostomy is associated with risk of bleeding, **pneumothorax**, local infection, and increased incidence of aspiration.

Newborn life support

Infants are continuously monitored to determine even small changes in breathing function. Mechanical ventilation can result in increases in respiratory distress or other complications. It is possible for the ventilator to be accidentally disconnected and staff is trained to watch for signs or alarms indicating disconnection. Mechanical ventilation increases risk of infection in premature babies. Complications of PEEP or CPAP may include pneumothorax or decreased cardiac output.

Normal results

Oxygen therapy

In the case of COPD, oxygen therapy does not treat the disease but can prolong life, quality of life,

KEY TERMS

Aspiration—Accidental suction of fluids or vomit into the respiratory system.

Cannula—A tube inserted into a cavity to serve as a channel for the transport of fluid.

Endotracheal—Placed within the trachea.

Hypoventilation—Reduced ventilation in the lungs' air sacs resulting in above normal carbon dioxide pressure.

Hypoxemia—A condition in which there is deficient oxygen supply in the blood.

Hypoxia—Low levels of oxygen in blood, tissue, or air.

Intubation—Placement of a tube into a hollow organ (such as the trachea).

Pneumothorax—Presence of gas or air in the hollow space around the lungs.

Trachea—The windpipe, or main channel by which air passes to and from the lungs.

and onset of more serious symptoms. Effective oxygen therapy for any patient should lead to improved or sustained levels of oxygen in arterial blood.

Incentive spirometry

With proper use of incentive spirometry, the physician should observe improved pulse rate, decreased respiratory rate, improved respiratory muscle performance, and other indicators of improved function. Lung function following lung resection should show marked improvement following incentive spirometry.

Continuous positive airway pressure

Successful CPAP will result in reduction in apnea for those suffering from sleep apnea. A study reported on in 1998 demonstrated that CPAP was effective in the majority of patients with sleep apnea, with the exception of significantly obese patients with blood gas values that were worse during waking hours at rest and at **exercise**. Hospitalized patients on CPAP therapy should show improvement in blood gas and other pulmonary measurements as expected by the treating physician.

Oxygen chamber therapy

Divers undergoing emergency treatment in a **hyperbaric chamber** should show immediate improvement in oxygen levels throughout the body, regardless of blood flow restrictions, after one or two treatments. Those patients receiving oxygen chamber therapy for difficult wounds may continue to receive treatments daily for several weeks before satisfactory results are reached. Patients with carbon dioxide poisoning should show improvement in or recovery of neurologic function. Results of hyperbaric chamber therapy depend largely on how quickly the patient was brought to the chamber, as well as the severity of the initial condition.

Mechanical ventilation

Successful mechanical ventilation will result in gradual decrease in dependence on the ventilator and weaning from the machine. Reduction of therapy to another form, such as CPAP or oxygen therapy, indicates that ventilation has worked as expected. In the case of COPD, exacerbation may be successfully treated with mechanical ventilation and the patient may return to home oxygen therapy. Pediatric patients will demonstrate normal growth and development as a normal result of long-term mechanical ventilation at home. Some patients, particularly those in a hospital intensive care unit, will not be able to breathe again without the ventilator and families and physicians will face tough choices about continued **life support**.

Newborn life support

Neonates will be constantly monitored to measure lung function. Those measurements will help caregivers determine if and when mechanical ventilation can be reduced and CPAP or oxygen mask begun. CPAP is considered successful when the infant's respiratory rate is reduced by 30–40%, a chest radiograph shows improved lung volume and appearance, stabilization of oxygen levels is documented and caregivers observe improvement in the infant's comfort. Evidence that there is no infection from ventilation is also considered normal. In some cases, inhalation therapy, including mechanical ventilation, will not work and the infant's parents and physicians will face tough decisions about invasive procedures with associated high risks or cessation of life support.

Resources

OTHER

Hyperbaric Research and Treatment Center Page. http://www.hyperbaricrx.com.

ORGANIZATIONS

American Association for Respiratory Care, 9425 N. MacArthur Blvd, Suite 100, Irving, TX, 75063-4706, 972 243-2272, 972 484-2720, info@aarc.org, http://ww.aarc.org.

American Lung Association, 1301 Pennsylvania Ave. NW, Suite 800, Washington, DC, 20001, 202 758-3355, 202 452-1805, 800 548-8252, info@lungusa.org, http://www.lungusa.org/.

National Heart Lung and Blood Institute Health Information Center, P.O. Box 30105, Bethesda, MD, 20824-0105, 301 592-8573, 240 629-3246, http://www.nhlbi.nih.gov.

Teresa Odle

Inner ear infection *see* **Labyrinthitis**

Insecticide poisoning

Definition

Insecticide **poisoning** is exposure to a group of chemicals designed to eradicate insects that cause affected persons to develop clinical signs that can progress to **death**.

Description

Insecticides belong to a group of chemicals called organophosphates used to protect against insects. Their use is popular since they are effective and do not remain in the environment, disintegrating within a few days. Organophosphates act to inhibit an enzyme in humans called acetyl cholinesterase. This enzyme functions to degrade a chemical called acetylcholine, which excites nerve cells. The resultant effect of organophosphates would be an increase in acetylcholine, thus causing initial excitation of nerve cells.

Poisoning can occur with a broad range of symptoms affecting the functioning of nerves and initial symptoms similar to the flu such as **vomiting**, abdominal **pain**, **dizziness**, and **headache**. Common names for insecticides include dichlorvos, chlorpyrifos, diazinon, fenthion, malathion, parathion, and carbamate. A special type of insecticide called paraquat is very lethal and responsible for approximately 1,000 deaths per year just in Japan. Paraquat poisoning releases oxygen free radicals that destroy lung and kidney tissues. When poisoning is suspected, a comprehensive management and assessment plan should be performed. This initial assessment should include:

- Description of toxins: names of chemical(s).
- Magnitude of exposure: determination of amount of exposure.
- Progression of symptoms: determining the progression of symptoms can provide information concerning life support and overall outcome.

General signs and symptoms of insecticide poisoning

Symptom/sign	Common causative agents	Possible causative agents
Rotten egg odor	Sulfur	
Hypothermia	Creosote Norbormide	
Hyperthermia (fever, pyrexia)	Nitrophenols Pentachlorophenol	Borate Thallium Metaldehyde Inorganic arsenicals Chlorophenoxy compounds Cadmium dusts Naphthalene
Chills	Phosphine Arsine	
Hot sensations	Nitrophenols Chlordimeform	Pentachlorophenol
Myalgia	Paraquat Chlorophenoxy compounds	
Thirst	Pentachlorophenol Nitrophenois Inorganic arsenicals Phosphorus Phosphides Sodium fluoride Cholecalciferol Aminopyridine	Borate Endothall
Anorexia	Organophosphates Carbamate insecticides Nicotine Pentachlorophenol Hexachlorobenzene Chlordimeform Cholecalciferol	Halocarbon fumigants Nitrophenols Inorganic arsenicals Aminopyridine
Alcohol intolerance	Thiram Calcium cyanamide	
Sweet taste in the mouth	Chlordimeform	
Metallic taste in the mouth	Inorganic arsenicals Organic mercury	
Salty, soapy taste in the mouth	Sodium fluoride	

SOURCE: U.S. Environmental Protection Agency, *Recognition and Management of Pesticide Poisoning*, "Index of Signs and Symptoms." Available online at: http://www.epa.gov/oppfead1/safety/healthcare/handbook/handbook.htm (accessed August 18, 2010).

(Table by PreMediaGlobal. Reproduced by permission of Gale, a part of Cengage Learning.)

- Time of exposure: knowing the time of exposure is vital since symptoms may be delayed, and it may assist to develop a management plan.
- Medical history: underlying diseases and therapeutic mediations may worsen toxic manifestations.

KEY TERMS

Acetylcholine—A chemical called a neurotransmitter that functions to excite nerve cells.

Acetylcholinesterase—An enzyme that breaks down acetylcholine.

Central nervous system—Consists of the brain and spinal cord and integrates and processes information.

Enzyme—A protein that speeds up a chemical reaction, but is not consumed during the process.

Oxygen free radicals—Reactive molecules containing oxygen and can cause cell damage.

Causes and symptoms

Exposure to insecticides can occur by ingestion, inhalation, or exposure to skin or eyes. The chemicals are absorbed through the skin, lungs, and gastrointestinal tract and then widely distributed in tissues. Symptoms cover a broad spectrum and affect several organ systems:

- Gastrointestinal: nausea, vomiting, cramps, excess salivation, and loss of bowel movement control
- Lungs: increases in bronchial mucous secretions, coughing, wheezing, difficulty breathing, and water collection in the lungs (this can progress to breathing cessation)
- Skin: sweating
- Eyes: blurred vision, smaller sized pupil, and increased tearing
- Heart: slowed heart rate, block of the electrical conduction responsible of heartbeat, and lowered blood pressure
- Urinary system: urinary frequency and lack of control
- Central nervous system: convulsions, confusion, paralysis, and coma

Diagnosis

The confirmatory diagnosis for insecticide poisoning is the measurement of blood acetyl cholinesterase less than 50% of normal. The chemicals can also be detected by specific urine testing. Signs and symptoms in addition to a comprehensive poisoning assessment are essential for diagnosis. Carbamate insecticide poisoning exhibits symptoms similar to organophosphate poisoning but without central nervous system signs.

Treatment

Decontaminate exposed clothing and wash with soap and water immediately. Emergency measures may focus on ventilator support and heart monitoring. If inhalation is suspected, the patient should be removed from the site of exposure. If the eyes were the entry site, they should be flushed with large amounts of water. If the chemicals were ingested, the stomach may be washed out and **activated charcoal** may be administered. Atropine or glycopyrrolate (Robinul) is the drug of choice for carbamate insecticide poisoning. It reverses many symptoms, but is only partially effective for central nervous symptom effects such as **coma** and convulsions. A medication called Pralidoxime is also commonly indicated to reactivate acetylcholinesterase and to reverse typical symptoms due to organophosphate poisoning. Additionally, the patient is monitored for heart, lung, liver functioning, specific blood tests, and oxygen levels in blood.

Prognosis

Prognosis depends on the specific chemical of exposure, magnitude and time of exposure, progression of symptoms (severity), and onset for medical attention.

Prevention

Adherence to accepted guidelines for handling and management is the key to preventing insecticide poisoning. These may include masks, gowns, gloves, goggles, respiratory breathing machines, or hazardous material suits.

Resources

BOOKS

Cecil, Russell L., Lee Goldman, and D. A. Audiello.*Cecil Medicine*. 23rd ed, Philadelphia: Saunders Elsevier, 2008.

Krieger, Robert Irving, and Wayland J. Hayes.*Hayes' Handbook of Pesticide Toxicology*. Amsterdam; Boston: Elsevier: Academic Press, 2010.

Rakel, Robert E., Edward T. Bope, and Howard F. Conn. *Conn's Current Therapy 2004: Latest Approved Methods of Treatment for the Practicing Physician*. Philadelphia: Saunders, 2004.

PERIODICALS

Blain, P. G. "Effects of Insecticides." *Lancet* 357 (5 May 2001): 1442.

OTHER

Material Safety Data Sheets. http://www.oshweb.com/owd/owd01.nsf/rubriek?openform&rubriek = EHEN-4QHD69.

National Toxicology Program. http://ntp.niehs.nih.gov.

Laith Farid Gulli, M.D.

Insomnia

Definition

Insomnia is the inability to obtain an adequate amount or quality of sleep. The difficulty may be in falling asleep, remaining asleep, or waking up too early. A person may experience one or all of these symptoms. People with insomnia do not feel refreshed when they wake up. Insomnia affects more than 70 million people, according to the National Institutes of Health. The sleeplessness is a symptom that may be caused by physical or mental conditions or circumstances. Furthermore, research indicated that insomnia may also be a medical condition, according to the National Sleep Foundation (NSF).

Description

There are two main types of insomnia. One is acute insomnia (sometimes called transient insomnia). This type occurs when insomnia symptoms exist over a reasonably short period of time. The other type is chronic insomnia, which is diagnosed when the symptoms manifest themselves over a longer period (generally more than one month). Insomnia can also be classified as either primary or secondary. Primary insomnia is a disorder that cannot be attributed to another condition or disorder. Secondary insomnia can be traced back to a source, which may be a medical condition; the use of medications, alcohol, or other substances; or a mental disorder such as severe depression.

Adults need approximately seven to eight hours of sleep each night. Teenagers should get about nine hours of sleep, and infants need to sleep from 16 to 18 hours of sleep each day. Sleep is essential for mental and physical restoration. It is a cycle with two separate states: rapid eye movement (REM), the stage in which most dreaming occurs; and non-REM (NREM). Four stages of sleep take place during NREM: stage I, when the person passes from relaxed wakefulness; stage II, an early stage of light sleep; stages III and IV, which are increasing degrees of deep sleep. Most stage IV sleep (also called delta sleep) occurs in the first several hours of sleep. A period of REM sleep normally follows a period of NREM sleep.

Disrupted sleep

Sleeplessness or insomnia may be caused by a physical condition such as **obesity**, a mental condition such as depression, shift work with irregular hours, or a traumatic event. In the days immediately after the terrorist attacks on September 11, 2001, 47% of Americans rated their sleep as "poor," or "fair," according to NSF's "2002 Sleep in America" poll. In comparison, 27% of poll participants rated sleep as poor or fair for most nights of that year.

The foundation's 2005 poll indicated that women were more likely to experience insomnia than men. NSF explored that demographic in the "2007 Sleep in America" poll of women between the ages of 18 and 64. That study showed that sleep problems such as insomnia were experienced by 72% of working mothers and 68% of single working women. Furthermore, 74% of stay-at-home mothers displayed symptoms of insomnia during a couple nights each week.

That poll paralleled other research that showed that women are 1.3 more likely to report insomnia than men. They may experience sleeplessness before and at the onset of their menstrual cycle, during **pregnancy**, and **menopause**. In addition, the foundation reported that people over the age of 65 are more likely to be bothered by insomnia than younger individuals.

Furthermore, people who are divorced, widowed, or separated are more likely to have the problem than those who are married. In addition, insomnia is more frequently reported by those with lower socioeconomic status.

Insomnia is classified both by its nightly symptoms and its duration. Sleep-onset insomnia refers to difficulty falling asleep. Maintenance insomnia refers to waking frequently during the night or waking early. Insomnia is also classified in relation to the number of sleepless nights. Short-term, or transient, insomnia is a common occurrence and usually lasts only a few days. Long-term, or chronic, insomnia lasts more than three weeks. This condition increases the risk for injuries in the home, at the workplace, and while driving because of the person experiences daytime sleepiness and decreased concentration ability. Chronic insomnia could also lead to **mood disorders** such as depression.

Not all disruptions in the normal pattern of sleeping and waking are considered insomnia. Such factors as **jet lag**, unusually high levels of **stress**, changing work shifts, or other drastic changes in the person's routine can all lead to sleep problems. Unless the problems are ongoing and severe enough that they are causing distress for the person in important areas of life, he or she is not considered to have insomnia.

Causes and symptoms

The symptoms of insomnia can vary greatly from person to person. Some people find that they have trouble falling asleep at night and can lie in bed for hours without being able to drift off. Others find that they fall asleep easily, but wake many times during the night. Other people awaken too early in the morning and are then unable to get back to sleep. Some people even get enough hours of sleep but find that they do not feel rested, often because their sleep is too light.

Not all people experiencing insomnia have symptoms that occur during the daytime, but many do. Some people experience such symptoms as reduced ability to concentrate or pay attention, decreased alertness, and mental sluggishness. Some people have trouble staying awake. More people think that they have these symptoms than actually do. Upon clinical examination, many people who think that they are excessively sleepy during the day actually are not.

Transient insomnia is often caused by a temporary situation in a person's life such as an argument with a loved one, a brief medical illness, or jet lag. When the situation is resolved or the precipitating factor disappears, the condition goes away, usually without medical treatment.

Prescription drugs such as **asthma** medicine, **steroids**, and anti-depressants may cause insomnia. Sleeplessness may also be a side effect of over-the-counter products such as nasal **decongestants** and appetite suppressants.

Chronic insomnia usually has different causes, and there may be more than one factor contributing to sleeplessness. Causes of insomnia include:

- A medical condition or its treatment, including sleep apnea, diabetes, arthritis, a heart condition, and asthma
- Use of substances such as caffeine, alcohol, and nicotine
- Psychiatric conditions such as mood or anxiety disorders
- Stress or depression, such as sadness caused by the loss of a loved one or a job.
- A change in work shift
- A work schedule with nontraditional hours. Shift workers who may experience insomnia include medical professionals, truck drivers, the military, and people working at businesses open 24 hours a day.
- Sleep-disordered breathing, such as snoring
- Periodic jerky leg movements, *nocturnal myoclonus*, which occur just as the individual is falling asleep.
- Restless legs syndrome, which involves the urge to move the legs. The person may also experience feelings such as tingling or cramping.
- Repeated nightmares or panic attacks during sleep

Excessive worrying about whether the person will be able to fall asleep may also cause insomnia. The concern creates so much **anxiety** that the individual's bedtime rituals and behavior actually trigger insomnia, a condition called psychophysiological insomnia.

Symptoms of insomnia

People who have insomnia do not start the day refreshed from a good night's sleep. They are tired. They may have difficulty falling asleep and commonly lie in bed tossing and turning for hours. Or the individual may go to sleep without a problem but wakes in the early hours of the morning. The person is either unable to go back to sleep or drifts into a restless, unsatisfying sleep. This is a common symptom in the elderly and those suffering from depression. Sometimes sleep patterns are reversed and the individual has difficulty staying awake during the day and takes frequent naps. The sleep at night is fitful and frequently interrupted.

Demographics

There are many different opinions about how much of the general American population experiences insomnia. Estimates suggest that around 5–20% of the adult population suffers from some form of insomnia or long-term sleeping problem. Nearly half report at least occasional sleeping problems. Accurate data are difficult to gather, as many people misperceive how much sleep they actually get and how many times they normally wake up during the night. It is generally agreed, however, that women are more likely than men to suffer from insomnia. As people get older, they are also are more likely to experience insomnia. People who are nervous or tense are more likely to have insomnia than those who are not. Lastly, people who live near airports or other sources of nighttime as well as daytime noise have higher rates of insomnia than the general population.

Diagnosis

Insomnia is a disorder that is usually self-reported; that is, patients usually bring up the subject of sleep problems with their doctors rather than the doctor suggesting the diagnosis. There are no laboratory tests for insomnia, but the doctor may suggest keeping a sleep diary, in which the patient notes the time they went to bed, the time(s) at which they got up during the night, their activities before bed, etc. Sleep diaries can be helpful in uncovering specific factors related to the insomnia.

Insomnia, unlike some medical conditions, is easily recognizable, as people know when they are not getting enough sleep. The key to treating insomnia is determining its causes. Some people can identify sleep-inhibiting factors such as a **death** in the family or a hectic work schedule with too much caffeine consumption and not enough **exercise**. A doctor will take factors such as these into account when making a diagnosis.

The physician's diagnosis is based on the patient's reported signs and symptoms. The doctor may review a patient's health history or order tests to determine if a medical condition is causing the insomnia. The physician may ask if the patient is depressed, in **pain**, under stress, or taking medications, according to the National Sleep Foundation. The doctor may ask about disruptions in a patient's life such as working nontraditional shifts or traveling across different time zones.

It may be useful for the patient to keep a daily record for two weeks of sleep patterns, food intake, use of alcohol, **caffeine**, nicotine, medications, exercise, and any other information recommended by the physician. If the patient has a bed partner, information can be obtained about whether the patient snores or is restless during sleep. This information, together with a medical history and **physical examination**, can help confirm the doctor's assessment.

A wide variety of healthcare professionals can recognize and treat insomnia. When a patient with chronic insomnia does not respond to treatment, or the condition is not adequately explained by the patient's physical, emotional, or mental circumstances, then more extensive testing by a specialist in **sleep disorders** may be warranted.

According to the *Diagnostic and Statistical Manual of Mental Disorders-IV-TR(DSM-IV-TR)*, which presents the guidelines used by the American Psychiatric Association for diagnosis of disorders, in order to be diagnosed with primary insomnia, a person must experience the symptoms for at least a month, and the symptoms must cause them distress or reduce their ability to function successfully. The symptoms cannot be caused by a different sleep disorder, a medical condition, or be a side effect of medications or **substance abuse**.

Insomnia may also be comorbid with (occur together with) other psychiatric disorders, including **mania**, depression, and the **anxiety disorders**.

Treatment

In both alternative and conventional medicine, treatment of insomnia includes alleviating or coping with any physical and emotional problems that contribute to the condition. Also effective is exploring changes in lifestyle that will improve the situation.

Many treatments have been explored for treating insomnia in a number of different settings. The patient may wish to consider consulting a sleep clinic or a doctor who specializes in the treatment of sleep disorders as well as their family doctor.

Behavioral and educational therapies are usually tried first, because they do not have side effects and cannot create a chemical dependence the way some sleep medications can. Many different approaches have been designed to help patients whose insomnia is linked to particular factors.

Changes in behavior

Patients can make changes in their daily routine that are simple and effective in treating insomnia. Eating a healthy diet rich in **calcium**, magnesium, and the B **vitamins** is also beneficial.

Patients should go to bed only when sleepy and use the bedroom only for sleep or sex. Activities such as reading, watching television, or snacking should take place elsewhere. If people are unable to go to sleep, they should go into another room and do some quiet activity such as reading. People should return to bed only when sleepy. Patients should set the alarm and get up every morning at the same time, no matter how much they have slept, to establish a regular sleep-wake pattern. Naps during the day should be avoided, but if absolutely necessary, then a 30-minute nap early in the afternoon may not interfere with sleep at night.

Another successful technique is called sleep-restriction therapy, restricting the time in bed to the actual time spent sleeping. This approach allows a slight sleep debt to build up, which increases the individual's ability to fall asleep and stay asleep. If a patient sleeps five hours a night, the time in bed is limited to 5–5.5 hours. The time in bed is gradually increased in small segments, with the individual rising at the same time each morning; at least 85% of the time in bed must be spent sleeping.

Mind and body relaxation

Incorporating relaxation techniques into bedtime rituals helps a person go to sleep faster and improves the quality of sleep. These, alone or in combination with other relaxation techniques, can safely promote sleepiness. Also effective are massage techniques such as **shiatsu**, the traditional Japanese form of body work. Gentle pressure is applied to points of the body to bring on sleep.

Learning to substitute pleasant thoughts for unpleasant ones (imagery training) helps reduce worrying. Another technique is using recordings that combine the sounds of nature with soft relaxing music. **Meditation**, prayer, and breathing exercises could also be effective.

Insomnia may be treated professionally through techniques such as cognitive therapy. The therapist works with the patient to discover attitudes and feelings that disrupt sleep.

Herbal remedies

Many alternative treatments are effective in treating both the symptom of insomnia and its underlying causes. Much treatment is centered on herbal remedies, but the United States Food and Drug Administration does not regulate these treatments, which means that the remedies have not proven to be safe or effective. Furthermore, ingredients are not standardized to comply with regulations. People should consult with their healthcare provider or complementary medicine practitioner before taking herbal remedies. This is especially important because some remedies such as melatonin interact with herbals like valerian and prescription medicines.

Valerian

Research up to the spring of 2008 indicated that valerian may help with insomnia. People who took valerian fell asleep more quickly and experienced improved slumber. Because of the herb's sedative properties, valerian is used to treat insomnia and anxiety. It is an approved remedy in the German Commission E Monographs, a guide to herbal remedies. Approved uses include sleeping disorders caused by nervousness.

Valerian's sedative properties have been studied in animals and people. As of the spring of 2008, valerian was regarded as probably safe when taken at the recommended dosage. The remedy did not appear to disrupt sleep cycles or REM sleep.

Furthermore, a combination of valerian and hops could help with sleeplessness. Other herbs most recommended for treating insomnia include skullcap and **ginseng**. Herbal products are available in capsule, tincture, and powdered form. Some people treat insomnia by sipping a warm cup of tea made with an herb mixture such as valerian, chamomile, hops, lemon balm, passionflower, or **St. John's wort**.

Aromatherapy and hydrotherapy

Aromatherapy involves healing through essential oils, the aromatic extracts of plants. Essential oils may be used for a soothing bath; applied to the face, neck, shoulders, and pillow; or diffused in air.

Hydrotherapy consists of a warm bath, scented with an essence such as rose, lavender, or marjoram. Valerian may also be added to bath water.

Dream pillows

Another form of aromatherapy involves sleeping on a dream pillow. Also known as a sleep pillow, it can be made by sewing together two 8-inch pieces of fabric. There should be an opening to insert a tablespoon. Herbs such as hops, chamomile, and lavender are spooned into the dream pillow, which is placed under the bed pillow.

Melatonin

Melatonin is a natural hormone that is secreted from the brain's pineal gland. The gland regulates a person's biological clock, particularly day and night cycles. Melatonin is generally used as a jet lag remedy. It may also help establish sleep patterns for shift workers. While melatonin may help people fall asleep more quickly, studies indicated limited success when it was used for treating insomnia. Melatonin is not regulated by the FDA, so the long-term effects of taking it are not known.

Traditional Chinese medicine

Traditional Chinese medicine (TCM) treatments for insomnia include **acupuncture** and herbal remedies. Acupuncture involves the insertion of needles to manipulate energy flows around the body. Acupuncture is also applied to the treatment of conditions, including anxiety.

In TCM, herbs are used as remedies in teas and other preparations. Treatments for insomnia include reishi, a medicinal mushroom available in extract form. However, the side effects of reishi could include **dizziness** and nose bleeds, so it is important to consult with a healthcare professional before taking this remedy.

Light therapy

In **light therapy**, natural or artificial light is used to boost serotonin, a neurotransmitter in the brain related to reducing anxiety. This therapy is used to treat **seasonal affective disorder**, a condition that some people experience when there is less sunlight or fewer daylight hours. Some people with this disorder feel depressed during the winter, and their spirits pick up during the summer. Light therapy is used to combat the depression experienced during the winter. There were no known risks as of the spring of 2008.

A study on the use of bright light therapy to treat insomnia was described in the July 2005 edition of the professional journal *Sleep*. The research involved 24 men diagnosed with early-morning waking insomnia. During the two nights of the study, the men were exposed to light while watching television. Some received bright light (2,500-lux white light) from 8 p.m. to midnight the first night and from 9 p.m. to 1 a.m. the following night. The other subjects were in the dim-light control group. The subjects in the bright light group said they tended to sleep longer than they did before the treatment. They woke up later. When they did waken, they went back to sleep more quickly.

Massage therapy

Massage therapy encourages relaxation by relaxing tense muscles throughout the body. It is especially helpful for restless leg syndrome, when this is a cause of insomnia. A massage once a week by a registered massage therapist may help the individual relieve stress that is causing sleeplessness.

Allopathic treatment

A physician may determine that drug therapy is necessary to treat insomnia. Drugs may be prescribed if the patient is undergoing a crisis or insomnia persists after a patient has made lifestyle changes. However, drug therapy is regarded as a short-term remedy, not a solution.

Conventional medications given for insomnia include sedatives, tranquilizers, and anti-anxiety drugs. All require a doctor's prescription and may be habit-forming. They could lose effectiveness over time and can reduce alertness during the day. The medications should be taken up to four times daily or as directed for approximately three to four weeks. The dose will vary with the physician, patient, and medication. If insomnia is related to depression, then an antidepressant medication may be helpful.

Drugs prescribed for improving sleep are called hypnotics. This category includes **benzodiazepines**, which are prescribed for anxiety and insomnia. Benzodiazepines commonly prescribed for insomnia include triazolam (Halcion), tempazepam (Restoril), lorazepam (Ativan), alprazolam (Xanax), fluazepam (Dalmane), and oxazepam (Serax).

Another medication prescribed for insomnia is zolpidem tartrate (Ambien). Recently, two drugs have been approved by the US Food and Drug Administration for long-term use. A drug called ramelteon (brand name Rozerem) has shown no evidence of potential for **abuse**, dependence or withdrawal in clinical studies. Eszopiclone (brand name Lunesta) is also approved for long-term use. Rozerem and Lunesta are currently available by prescription only.

Over-the-counter sleep products include Nytol, Sominex, Unisom Nightime Tablets, and Tylenol PM. While these products are usually not addictive, some experts believe they are not very effective in sustaining stage IV sleep and can affect the quality of sleep.

Nutrition/Dietetic concerns

Calcium and magnesium are recommended as **nutritional supplements** because of their calming effects. Because these essential nutrients must be in balance with each other, they should be taken together daily with a meal. Supplemental B vitamin complex is also recommended to help relieve stress and achieve a restful state. Caffeine and alcohol should be avoided. Relaxing teas containing chamomile and/or catnip (catmint) can be consumed before bed. Herbal tinctures such as skullcap, passionflower, hops, kava kava, or valerian root are considered nerviness and are known to calm the nervous system and promote restful sleep. A natural hormone produced by the body, dehydroepisterone (DHEA), is reduced in older individuals and has been shown to improve sleep when taken as a supplement. It is available in whole food stores and in some pharmacies.

Expected results

Insomnia has numerous causes and treatments, so the amount of time may vary before results are seen. A prescription drug may bring immediate results to someone coping with a spouse's death. An herbal remedy may not work immediately for a person who consumed excessive amounts of caffeine to stay awake at work after a sleepless night. A procedure such as cognitive therapy may take some time as therapist and patient work to resolve issues that hinder sleep.

Research has provided information about when some treatments take effect:

- Valerian is sold commercially in the form of capsules, extracts, and teas. The capsule or extract dosage ranges from 300 to 600 mg. As a sleep aid, it should be taken shortly before bedtime. People who have trouble falling asleep may see results quickly. It could take from two weeks to a month before a person with chronic insomnia experiences improved sleep.
- A combination of hops and valerian at bedtime could provide a good night's sleep.
- Melatonin is taken in a dose of from 0.3 to 3 mg an hour of retiring. When taken as a 3-mg dose one to two hours before bed for a maximum of four to five days per week, the dietary supplement melatonin was said to be effective in shortening the time before a person fell asleep. Side effects could include nightmares and sleepwalking.
- St. John's wort can take two weeks to take effect.
- A combination of alternative therapies should bring a difference in disturbed sleep within two to four days.
- Combinations of treatments could more quickly bring about an uninterrupted night of sleep. The person who reduces caffeine intake, walks for 15 minutes, and enjoys an herbal bath may discover that that combination brings restful sleep.
- Acupuncture is said to bring some people immediate relief. In small studies, people said that after treatment that it was easier to fall asleep and they remained asleep. This treatment is safe when it is done correctly.
- Light therapy proved to be effective in the treatment of men whose insomnia caused them to wake early. In that study, the men said they experienced an immediate benefit. However, no women were studied, and the research did not include people with other types of insomnia.

Prevention

Prevention of insomnia centers around the promotion of a healthy lifestyle. A balance of rest, recreation, and exercise in combination with stress management, regular physical examinations, and a healthy diet can do much to reduce the risk. Walking is also recommended. However, exercise should be done no more than three hours before bedtime.

KEY TERMS

Biofeedback—A training technique that enables an individual to gain some element of control over involuntary body functions.

Mood disorder—A group of mental disorders involving a disturbance of mood, along with either a full or partial excessively happy (manic) or extremely sad (depressive) syndrome not caused by any other physical or mental disorder. Mood refers to a prolonged emotion.

Sleep apnea—A condition in which a person stops breathing while asleep. These periods can last up to a minute or more and can occur many times each hour. In order to start breathing again, the person must become semi-awake. The episodes are not remembered, but the following day the person feels tired and sleepy. If severe, sleep apnea can cause other medical problems.

Sleep disorder—Any condition that interferes with sleep. As of 2008, at least 84 have been identified, according to the American Sleep Disorders Association.

Also to be avoided in the evening are drinks that contain caffeine such as coffee, tea, and colas. Chocolate contains a stimulant and may keep people awake. In addition, alcohol may initially make a person sleepy. However, it could have the opposite effect a few hours later.

Maintaining a comfortable bedroom temperature, reducing noise, and eliminating light are also helpful. The bedroom should be used only for sleeping, not watching television or reading.

Exercise, relaxation, and **nutrition** should be considered ongoing preventive measures. While life brings unexpected stresses and pressures, the person who is familiar with relaxation techniques is more prepared to cope with insomnia.

Prognosis

Insomnia can be prevented or corrected in most adults, although in some cases an underlying illness will require treatment in order to correct related insomnia. **Sleep apnea** is a potentially serious disorder related to breathing difficulties and chronic lung conditions; it can be fatal if not treated.

Untreated insomnia has potentially serious consequences, including an increased risk of motor vehicle accidents, impaired school or job performance, and a high rate of absenteeism from work. Fortunately, insomnia can be treated very effectively in most patients. Treatment using a combination of approaches is usually most effective. Patients who have had insomnia once are at an increased risk for recurrent insomnia.

Caregiver concerns

An individual who is not enjoying regular sleep may become anxious, depressed or irritable during the day, and may also fall asleep for long periods, preventing sleep at night. The caregiver can encourage movement and exercise during the day, which will help the individual gain a good night's sleep. The evening meal should be served early enough to allow two hours for digestion before trying to go to sleep. If the individual is taking sleeping medication, dosage should be checked by the caregiver to avoid overdosing. Activities during the day should be carefully supervised to prevent accidents caused by inattention or drowsiness.

Resources

BOOKS

American Psychiatric Association. *Diagnostic and Statistical Manual of Mental Disorders*. 4th ed. text revised. Washington DC: American Psychiatric Association, 2000.

Currie, Shawn R. "Sleep Dysfunction." *Clinicians's Handbook of Adult Behavioral Assessment*, Ed. Michel Hersen. San Diego, CA: Elsevier Academic Press, 2006: 401–430.

Lee-Chiong, Teofilo L. Ed. *Sleep: A Comprehensive Handbook*. New York: Wiley-Liss, 2006.

Mayo Clinic Book of Alternative Medicine. New York: Time Inc. Home Entertainment, 2007.

PERIODICALS

Irwin, Michael R. and Cole, Jason C. "Comparative Meta-Analysis of Behavioral Interventions for Insomnia and Their Efficacy in Middle-Aged Adults and in Older Adults 55+ Years of Age." *Health Psychology*, 25(1), Jan 2006: 3–14.

Jansson, Markus and Linton, Steven J. "Psychosocial Work Stressors in the Development and Maintenance of Insomnia: A Prospective Study." *Journal of Occupational Health Psychology*, 11(3), Jul 2006: 241–248.

Jansson, Markus and Linton, Steven J. "The Role of Anxiety and Depression in the Development of Insomnia: Cross-Sectional and Prospective Analyses." *Psychology and Health*, 21(3), Jun 2006: 383–397.

Manber, Rachel and Harvey, Allison. "Historical Perspective and Future Directions in Cognitive Behavioral Therapy for Insomnia and Behavioral Sleep Medicine." *Clinical Psychology Review*, 25(5), Jul 2005: 535–538.

Smith, Michael T. and Perlis, Michael L. "Who Is a Candidate for Cognitive-Behavioral Therapy for Insomnia?" *Health Psychology*, 25(1), Jan 2006: 15–19.

"Snooze Alarm: Herbal Sleep Aids Come Up Short." *Environmental Nutrition* (October 2006): 3.

OTHER

"Insomnia." Mayo Foundation for Medical Education and Research. Mayo Clinic, 2007. http://www.mayoclinic.com/health/insomnia/DS00187

Johnston, Smith L., III "Societal and Workplace Consequences of Insomnia, Sleepiness, and Fatigue." Medscape Neurology & Neurosurgery, September 29, 2005. http://www.medscape.com/viewarticle/513572_1

Lack, L., H. Wright, K. Kemp, S. Gibbon, S. "The Treatment of Early-Morning Awakening Insomnia with 2 Evenings of Bright Light." Sleep (July 2005). http://www.ncbi.nlm.nih.gov/pubmed/16171276.

Sleep Disorders Infocenter. Holistic Online.com. http://holisticonline.com/Remedies/Sleep/sleep_home.htm

ORGANIZATIONS

American Academy of Sleep Medicine. 6301 Bandel Road NW, Suite 101, Rochester, MN, 55901. Telephone: (507) 287-6006. www.asda.org

American Medical Association., 515 N. State St., Chicago, IL, 60610, (800) 621-8335, http://www.ama-assn.org.

American Sleep Association, 614 South 8th Street, Suite 282, Philadelphia, PA, 19147, 443-593-2285, sleep@1sleep.com

National Sleep Foundation., 1522 K St. NW, Suite 500, Washington, DC, DC, 20005, (202) 347-3471, http://www.sleepfoundation.org/.

L. Lee Culvert
Tish Davidson, A.M.
Liz Swain
Ruth A. Wienclaw, Ph.D.
Laura Jean Cataldo, RN, Ed.D.

Insulin *see* **Antidiabetic drugs**

Insulin resistance

Definition

Insulin resistance is not a disease as such but rather a state or condition in which a person's body tissues have a lowered level of response to insulin, a hormone secreted by the pancreas that helps to regulate the level of glucose (sugar) in the body. As a result, the person's body produces larger quantities of insulin to maintain normal levels of glucose in the blood. There is considerable individual variation in sensitivity to insulin within the general population, with the most insulin-sensitive persons being as much as six times as sensitive to the hormone as those identified as most resistant. Some doctors use an arbitrary number, defining insulin resistance as a need for 200 or more units of insulin per day to control blood sugar levels. Various researchers have estimated that 3–16 percent of the general population in the United States and Canada is insulin-resistant; another figure that is sometimes given is 70–80 million Americans.

Insulin resistance can be thought of as a set of metabolic dysfunctions associated with or contributing to a range of serious health problems. These disorders include type 2 diabetes (formerly called adult-onset or non-insulin-dependent diabetes), the metabolic syndrome (formerly known as syndrome X), **obesity**, and **polycystic ovary syndrome**. Some doctors prefer the term "insulin resistance syndrome" to "metabolic syndrome."

Description

To understand insulin resistance, it may be helpful for the reader to have a brief account of the way insulin works in the body. After a person eats a meal, digestive juices in the small intestine break down starch or complex sugars in the food into glucose, a simple sugar. The glucose then passes into the bloodstream. When the concentration of glucose in the blood reaches a certain point, the pancreas is stimulated to release insulin into the blood. As the insulin reaches cells in muscle and fatty (adipose) tissues, it attaches itself to molecules called insulin receptors on the surface of the cells. The activation of the insulin receptors sets in motion a series of complex biochemical signals within the cells that allow the cells to take in the glucose and convert it to energy. If the pancreas fails to produce enough insulin or the insulin receptors do not function properly, the cells cannot take in the glucose and the level of glucose in the blood remains high.

The insulin may fail to bind to the insulin receptors for any of several reasons. Some persons inherit a gene mutation that leads to the production of a defective form of insulin that cannot bind normally to the insulin receptor. Others may have one of two types of abnormalities in the insulin receptors themselves. In type A, the insulin receptor is missing from the cell surface or does not function properly. In type B, the person's immune system produces autoantibodies to the insulin receptor.

In the early stages of insulin resistance, the pancreas steps up its production of insulin in order to control the increased levels of glucose in the blood. As a result, it is not unusual for patients to have high blood sugar levels and high blood insulin levels (a condition known as hyperinsulinemia) at the same time. If insulin resistance is not detected and treated, however, the islets of Langerhans (the insulin-secreting groups of cells) in the pancreas may eventually shut down and decrease in number.

Causes and symptoms

Causes

The reasons for the development of insulin resistance are not completely understood as of the early 2000s, but several factors that contribute to it have been identified:

- Genetic factors. Insulin resistance is known to run in families. Genetic mutations may affect the insulin receptor, the signaling proteins within cells, or the mechanisms of glucose transport.
- Obesity. Being overweight keeps the muscles from using insulin properly, as it decreases the number of insulin receptors on cell surfaces.
- Low level of physical activity. Because muscle tissue takes up 95 percent of the glucose that insulin helps the body utilize (brain cells and blood cells do not depend on insulin to help them use glucose), inactivity further reduces the muscles ability to use insulin effectively.
- Aging. The aging process affects the efficiency of glucose transport.
- Other diseases and disorders. Some disorders—most notably Cushing syndrome and cirrhosis—and such stresses on the body as trauma, surgery, malnutrition, or severe infections speed up the breakdown of insulin or interfere with its effects.
- Certain medications. Some drugs, including cyclosporine, niacin, and the protease inhibitors used to treat HIV infection, may contribute to insulin resistance.

Symptoms

The symptoms of insulin resistance vary considerably from person to person. Some people may have no noticeable symptoms until they develop signs of heart disease or are diagnosed with high blood pressure during a routine checkup. Other patients may come to the doctor with extremely high levels of blood sugar (hyperglycemia) and such classical symptoms of diabetes as thirst, frequent urination, and weight loss. A small percentage of patients—most commonly women with polycystic ovary syndrome—

develop a velvet-textured blackish or dark brown discoloration of the skin known as acanthosis nigricans. This symptom, which is most commonly found on the neck, groin, elbows, knees, knuckles, or armpits, is thought to appear when high levels of insulin in the blood spill over into the skin. This spillover activates insulin receptors in the skin and causes it to develop an abnormal texture and color. Acanthosis nigricans occurs more frequently in Hispanic and African American patients than in Caucasians.

Disorders associated with insulin resistance

Insulin resistance became an important field of research in the late 1980s, when doctors first began to understand it as a precondition of several common but serious threats to health. As of the early 2000s, insulin resistance is associated with the following disorders:

- Obesity. Obesity is not only the most common cause of insulin resistance but is a growing health concern in its own right. According to the National Institutes of Health (NIH), the percentage of American adults who meet the criteria for obesity rose from 25 percent to 33 percent between 1990 and 2000—an increase of a third within the space of a decade. Obesity is a risk factor for the development of type 2 diabetes, high blood pressure, and coronary artery disease.
- Pre-diabetes and type 2 diabetes. The NIH estimates that about 6.3 percent of the American population has diabetes. Of these 18.3 million people, 5.2 million are undiagnosed. Type 2 diabetes is much more common than type 1, accounting for 90–95 percent of patients with diabetes. Diabetes increases a person's risk of blindness, kidney disease, heart disease and stroke, disorders of the nervous system, complications during pregnancy, and dental problems; it also worsens the prognosis for such infectious diseases as influenza or pneumonia. About 41 million Americans are thought to have pre-diabetes, which is a condition marked by elevated levels of blood glucose after fasting or after a 2-hour test for glucose tolerance. According to the NIH, a majority of prediabetic people will develop type 2 diabetes within 10 years unless they lose between 5 and 7 percent of their body weight.
- Heart disease. Insulin resistance has been linked to a group of risk factors for heart disease and stroke known as the metabolic syndrome (formerly called syndrome X). The metabolic syndrome, like obesity, has become increasingly prevalent in the United States since the 1990s; as of the early 2000s, about a quarter of the general adult population is thought to have it, with the rate rising to 40 percent for adults over the age of 60. To be diagnosed with the metabolic syndrome, a person must have three or more of the following risk factors: a waist circumference greater than 40 in (102 cm) in men or 35 in (88 cm) in women; a level of blood triglycerides of 150 milligrams per deciliter (mg/dL) or higher; blood pressure of 130/85 Hg or higher; fasting blood sugar level of 110 mg/dL or higher; and a blood level of high-density lipoprotein (HDL) cholesterol (the so-called "good" cholesterol) lower than 50 mg/dL for men or 40 mg/dL for women.
- Polycystic ovary syndrome (PCOS). PCOS is an endocrine disorder that develops in 3–10 percent of premenopausal women as a result of the formation of cysts (small fluid-filled sacs) in the ovaries. Women with PCOS do not have normal menstrual periods; they are often infertile and may develop hirsutism (excess body hair) or other indications of high levels of androgens (male sex hormones) in the blood. This condition is called hyperandrogenism, and has been linked to insulin resistance in women with PCOS. Weight loss in these patients usually corrects hyperandrogenism and often restores normal ovulation patterns and fertility.

Diagnosis

Patient history and physical examination

Because insulin resistance is a silent condition in many people, the National Institute of Diabetes and Digestive and Kidney Diseases (NIDDK) recommends that all adults over the age of 45 be tested for type 2 diabetes. People younger than 45 who are overweight and have one or more of the following risk factors should also visit their doctor to be tested:

- One or more family members with diabetes.
- High levels of triglycerides and low levels of HDL cholesterol as defined by the criteria for metabolic syndrome.
- Hypertension (high blood pressure).
- A history of smoking.
- A history of diabetes during pregnancy (gestational diabetes).
- Giving birth to a baby weighing more than 9 pounds. In addition to increasing the mother's risk of developing type 2 diabetes, children who are large for their gestational age (LGA) at birth have an increased risk of developing insulin resistance and metabolic syndrome in later life.
- Having African American, Hispanic, Native American, or Asian American/Pacific Islander heritage.

Some signs and symptoms associated with insulin resistance can be detected by a primary care physician during a routine office visit. Blood pressure, weight, body shape, and the condition of the skin can be checked, as well as determining whether the patient meets the criteria for obesity or is less severely overweight. Obesity is determined by the patient's body mass index, or BMI. The BMI, which is an indirect measurement of the amount of body fat, is calculated in English units by multiplying a person's weight in pounds by 703.1, and dividing that number by the person's height in inches squared. A BMI between 19 and 24 is considered normal; 25–29 is overweight; 30–34 is moderately obese; 35–39 is severely obese; and 40 or higher is defined as morbidly obese. The doctor may also evaluate the patient for obesity in the office by measuring the thickness of the skinfold at the back of the upper arm.

The distribution of the patient's weight is also significant, as insulin resistance is associated with a so-called "apple-shaped" figure, in which much of the excess weight is carried around the abdomen. People whose excess weight is carried on the hips (the "pear-shaped" figure) or distributed more evenly on the body are less likely to develop insulin resistance. One way of measuring weight distribution is the patient's waist-to-hip ratio; a ratio greater than 1.0 in men or 0.8 in women is strongly correlated with insulin resistance.

Laboratory tests

There is no single laboratory test that can be used to diagnose insulin resistance by itself. Doctors usually evaluate individual patients on the basis of specific symptoms or risk factors. The tests most commonly used include the following:

- Blood glucose tests. A high level of blood glucose may indicate either that the body is not producing enough insulin or is not using it effectively. Two common tests used to screen for insulin resistance are the fasting glucose test and the glucose tolerance test. In the fasting glucose test, the person takes no food after midnight and has their blood glucose level measured early in the morning. Normal blood glucose levels after several hours without food should be below 100 milligrams per deciliter (mg/dL). If the level is between 100 and 125 mg/dL, the person has impaired fasting glucose (IFG) or pre-diabetes. If the level is over 126 and is confirmed by a second test, the person has diabetes. In the glucose tolerance test, the person is given a sugar solution to drink and their blood glucose level is measured 2 hours later. A normal level is 140 mg/dL; 140–199 mg/dL indicates impaired glucose tolerance (IGT) or pre-diabetes, while a level of 200 mg/dL or higher indicates diabetes.
- Tests of blood insulin levels. These help to determine whether high blood glucose levels are the result of insufficient production of insulin or inefficient use of insulin.
- Lipid profile test. This test measures the amount of total cholesterol, high-density lipoprotein (HDL) cholesterol, low-density lipoprotein (LDL) cholesterol, and triglycerides. Patients with insulin resistance will have high levels of LDL cholesterol and triglycerides with low levels of HDL cholesterol.
- Measurement of blood electrolytes and uric acid. Many patients with the metabolic syndrome have high blood levels of uric acid.

A highly accurate technique for measuring insulin resistance is called the euglycemic clamp technique. The patient's blood insulin level is kept ("clamped") at a high but steady level by continual insulin infusion while the blood glucose level is monitored at frequent intervals. Glucose concentrations in the blood are maintained at a normal level by an adjustable-rate glucose drip. The amount of glucose needed to maintain a normal blood glucose level over a given unit of time indicates the degree of insulin resistance. This test, however, requires complex equipment and careful monitoring; it is considered too cumbersome to use in routine screening and is used mostly by researchers.

Treatment

Lifestyle modifications

Lifestyle modifications are the first line of treatment in dealing with insulin resistance:

- Weight reduction. Losing weight increases the body's sensitivity to insulin. It is not necessary, however, for patients to reduce their weight to the ideal levels listed on life insurance charts. In recent years, researchers have found that even a modest weight loss—usually defined as 10 percent of the patient's pretreatment weight—is enough to control or at least improve insulin resistance and other health complications of obesity. Weight reduction is usually accomplished by a combination of reduced calorie intake and increased physical activity. Insulin sensitivity is reported to improve within a few days of lowered calorie intake, even before the patient loses a measurable amount of weight.
- Exercise. Regular exercise improves the body's sensitivity to insulin by increasing the muscles' uptake of glucose from the bloodstream, by increasing the efficiency of the circulatory system and glucose transport,

and by reducing the amount of fat around the patient's abdomen. The American Academy of Family Practice (AAFP) recommends 30 minutes of moderately intense physical activity on most or all days of the week for people diagnosed with insulin resistance. Walking is a very good form of exercise because it does not require any special equipment other than comfortable walking shoes, can be combined with doing errands, and can be done either alone or with a group of friends. Riding a bicycle is another form of exercise recommended for weight control.

- Adding foods high in fiber to the diet. A diet high in natural fiber, found in whole grains and vegetables, lowers the levels of blood insulin as well as lowering the patient's risk of developing high blood pressure.
- Quitting smoking. Giving up smoking lowers the risk of heart disease, stroke, or lung cancer as well as increasing the body's sensitivity to insulin.
- Limiting alcohol consumption. Alcohol is a source of "empty" calories with little nutritional value of its own.

Medications

There are several different types of medications that can be used to treat patients with abnormal blood sugar or insulin levels:

- Biguanides. Biguanides are drugs that improve the body's sensitivity to insulin by lowering the absorption of glucose in the small intestine, decreasing the liver's production of glucose, and increasing the uptake of glucose in muscle and fatty tissues. Metformin (Glucophage), a drug used in the treatment of type 2 diabetes, is the most commonly used biguanide in treating insulin resistance. It has also been studied as a possible treatment in preventing or delaying the onset of type 2 diabetes.
- Thiazolidinediones. These drugs stimulate glucose uptake in the muscles and fatty tissues by activating specific receptors in the cell nucleus. They also lower blood insulin levels in patients with hyperinsulinemia. The thiazolidinediones include pioglitazone (Actos) and rosiglitazone (Avandia).
- Glucocorticoids. These drugs may be given to patients with insulin resistance caused by anti-insulin antibodies produced by their immune system. Prednisone (Deltasone) is the most commonly used glucocorticoid.
- Insulin itself. Some patients with insulin resistance benefit from injectable insulin to reduce their blood sugar levels.

As of early 2005, however, the Food and Drug Administration (FDA) has not approved any drugs for the treatment of insulin resistance by itself. For this reason, the American Diabetes Association does not recommend treating insulin resistance with medications unless the patient has already been diagnosed with diabetes.

The patient's doctor may also prescribe medications to treat specific health problems associated with insulin resistance. These drugs may include **diuretics** and other medications to lower blood pressure; **aspirin** to reduce the risk of **heart attack**; medications to lower the levels of **triglycerides** and LDL cholesterol in the blood; and weight-control drugs. The drugs most frequently prescribed in the early 2000s to help patients lose weight are orlistat (Xenical) and sibutramine (Meridia).

Acanthosis nigricans may be treated with topical preparations containing Retin-A, 20% urea, or salicylic acid; however, many patients find that the skin disorder improves by itself following weight loss.

Surgery

Insulin resistance by itself does not require surgical treatment; however, patients who have already developed heart disease may require coronary artery bypass surgery. In addition, very obese patients—those with a BMI of 40 or higher—may benefit from **bariatric surgery**. Bariatric surgery includes such procedures as vertical banded gastroplasty and **gastric bypass**, which limit the amount of food that the stomach can contain.

Alternative treatment

Some alternative treatments for insulin resistance and type 2 diabetes have been studied by the Agency for Healthcare Research and Quality (AHRQ). One study reported in 2004 that **omega-3 fatty acids**, a dietary supplement commonly derived from fish, canola, or soybean oil, did not appear to have any significant effect on blood sugar levels or blood insulin levels in patients diagnosed with type 2 diabetes or the metabolic syndrome. An earlier study of **Ayurvedic medicine**, the traditional medical system of India, reported in 2001 that certain herbs used to make Ayurvedic medicines, such as fenugreek, holy basil, *Coccinia indica*, and *Gymnema sylvestre* appear to be effective in lowering blood sugar levels and merit further study. The AHRQ report also noted that the Ayurvedic practice of combining herbal medicines with **yoga** and other forms of physical activity should be investigated further.

Other alternative treatments for insulin resistance and type 2 diabetes include chromium supplements, **ginseng**, **biofeedback**, and **acupuncture**. The connection between chromium supplementation and insulin resistance is that the body needs chromium to produce a substance called glucose tolerance factor, which increases the effectiveness of insulin. Further studies need to be done,

KEY TERMS

Acanthosis nigricans—A dark brownish or blackish discoloration of the skin related to overweight and high levels of insulin in the blood. Acanthosis nigricans is most likely to develop in the groin or armpits, or around the back of the neck.

Bariatrics—The branch of medicine that deals with the prevention and treatment of obesity and related disorders.

Body mass index (BMI)—A measurement that has replaced weight as the preferred determinant of obesity. The BMI can be calculated (in English units) as 703.1 times a person's weight in pounds divided by the square of the person's height in inches.

Glucose—A simple sugar produced when carbohydrates are broken down in the small intestine. It is the primary source of energy for the body. Various tests that measure blood glucose levels are used in diagnosing insulin resistance.

Hyperandrogenism—Excessive secretion of androgens (male sex hormones).

Hyperinsulinemia—The medical term for high levels of insulin in the blood.

Insulin—A protein hormone secreted by the islets of Langerhans in the pancreas in response to eating. Insulin carries glucose and amino acids to muscle and adipose cells and promotes their efficient use and storage.

Islets of Langerhans—Special structures in the pancreas responsible for insulin secretion among other functions. They are named for Paul Langerhans, the German researcher who first identified them in 1869.

Lipids—A group of fats and fat-like substances that are not soluble in water, are stored in the body, and serve as a source of fuel for the body.

Metabolic syndrome—A group of risk factors for heart disease, diabetes, and stroke. It includes abdominal obesity, high blood pressure, high blood glucose levels, and low levels of high-density lipoprotein (HDL) cholesterol. The metabolic syndrome is sometimes called the insulin resistance syndrome.

Metabolism—The sum of an organism's physical and chemical processes that produce and maintain living tissue, and make energy available to the organism. Insulin resistance is a disorder of metabolism.

Obesity—Excessive weight gain due to accumulation of fat in the body, sometimes defined as a BMI of 30 or higher, or body weight greater than 30 percent above one's desirable weight on standard height-weight tables.

Pancreas—A large gland located behind the stomach near the spleen that secretes digestive enzymes into the small intestine and insulin into the bloodstream.

Syndrome—In general, a set of symptoms that occur together as signs of a disease or disorder.

Syndrome X—A term that was sometimes used for metabolic syndrome when the syndrome was first identified in the 1960s.

Triglycerides—Fatty compounds synthesized from carbohydrates during the process of digestion and stored in the body's adipose (fat) tissues. High levels of triglycerides in the blood are associated with insulin resistance.

Type 2 diabetes mellitus—One of the two major types of diabetes mellitus, characterized by late age of onset (30 years or older), insulin resistance, high levels of blood sugar, and little or no need for supplemental insulin. It was formerly known as adult-onset or non-insulin-dependent diabetes.

however, before recommendations about dietary chromium as a treatment for insulin resistance can be made.

Prognosis

Since insulin resistance is a condition that precedes the appearance of symptoms of a number of different disorders, its prognosis depends in part on the patient's age, ethnicity, family history, and severity of any current health problems. Some patients diagnosed with insulin resistance eventually develop type 2 diabetes, but it is not yet known why the others do not; for example, some patients do not develop diabetes in spite of a high degree of insulin resistance. What is known at present is that weight reduction and **exercise** can control or even reverse insulin resistance in many people.

Prevention

Genetic factors contributing to insulin resistance cannot be changed as of the early 2000s.

With regard to lifestyle factors, the National Institute of Diabetes and Digestive and Kidney Diseases (NIDDK) reported the findings of a study of the effects of lifestyle changes or metformin on the incidence of diabetes in a group of over 3200 overweight people with impaired glucose tolerance, which is a risk factor for developing type 2 diabetes. The researchers found that the subjects in the lifestyle modification group, who lowered their food intake and took 30-minute walks five days a week, had a 58-percent lower incidence of diabetes. The subjects who received metformin had a 31-percent lower incidence of diabetes. Lifestyle changes were most effective in volunteers over the age of 60, while metformin was most effective in younger subjects. In short, the 2002 study confirmed the beneficial effects of lowered food intake and increased activity as preventive measures against type 2 diabetes.

Another important part of preventing insulin resistance is patient education. A number of resources on weight control and exercise written for the general public are available from the Weight-Control Information Network (WIN) on the NIDDK website at http://win.niddk.nih.gov/publications/physical.htm. Some pamphlets are available in Spanish as well as English. Patient education materials on insulin resistance in relation to heart disease and diabetes can be downloaded free of charge from the American Heart Association and American Diabetes Association websites.

Resources

BOOKS

Beers, Mark H., Robert S. Porter, and Thomas V. Jones, eds. *The Merck Manual of Diagnosis and Therapy*. 18th ed. Whitehouse Station, NJ: Merck Research Laboratories, 2006.

Hart, Cheryle, and Mary Kay Grossman.*The Insulin–Resistance Diet: How to Turn Off Your Body's Fat–Making Machine*. Nerw York: McGraw-Hill, 2007.

Karst, Karlene.*The Metabolic Syndrome Program: How to Lose Weight, Beat Heart Disease, Stop Insulin Resistance and More*. New York: Wiley, 2006.

PERIODICALS

Boney, C. M., A. Verma, R. Tucker, and B. R. Vohr. "Metabolic Syndrome in Childhood: Association with Birth Weight, Maternal Obesity, and Gestational Diabetes Mellitus." *Pediatrics* 115 (March 2005): 290–296.

Diabetes Prevention Program Research Group. "Reduction in the Incidence of Type 2 Diabetes with Lifestyle Intervention or Metformin." *New England Journal of Medicine* 346 (February 7, 2002): 393–403.

Ford, Earl S., Wayne H. Giles, and William H. Dietz. "Prevalence of the Metabolic Syndrome Among US Adults." *Journal of the American Medical Association* 287 (January 16, 2002): 356–359.

Litonjua, P., A. Pinero-Pilona, L. Aviles-Santa, and P. Raskin. "Prevalence of Acanthosis Nigricans in Newly-Diagnosed Type 2 Diabetes." *Endocrine Practice* 10 (March–April 2004): 101–106.

Rao, Goutham. "Insulin Resistance Syndrome." *American Family Physician* 63 (March 15, 2001): 1159–1166.

Scheinfeld, N. S. "Obesity and Dermatology." *Clinical Dermatology* 22 (July-August 2004): 303–309.

Sivitz, William I. "Understanding Insulin Resistance: What Are the Clinical Implications?" *Postgraduate Medicine* 116 (July 2004): 41–48.

OTHER

Agency for Healthcare Research and Quality (AHRQ). Evidence Report/Technology Assessment: Number 41. "Ayurvedic Intervention for Diabetes Mellitus." Rockville, MD: AHRQ, 2001. http://www.ahrq.gov/clinic/epcsums/ayurvsum.htm.

Mayo Clinic Staff. "Metabolic Syndrome." http://www.mayoclinic.com/invoke.cfm?id = DS00522.

National Institute of Diabetes and Digestive and Kidney Diseases (NIDDK) News Brief, 6 February 2002. "Diet and Exercise Delay Diabetes and Normalize Blood Glucose." http://www.niddk.nih.gov/welcome/releases/02-06-02.htm.

ORGANIZATIONS

American Academy of Dermatology, PO Box 4014, Schaumburg, IL, 60168-4014, 847 240-1859, 866 503-SKIN (7546), http://www.aad.org.

American Diabetes Association, 1701 North Beauregard Street, Alexandria, VA, 22311, 800 342-2383, Ask ADA@diabetes.org, http://www.diabetes.org/.

American Heart Association National Center, 7272 Greenville Avenue, Dallas, TX, 75231, 800 242-8721, Review.personal.info@heart.org.

National Diabetes Information Clearinghouse (NDIC), 1 Information Way, Bethesda, MD, 20892-3560, 703 738-4929, 800 860-8747, ndic@info.niddk.nih.gov, http://diabetes.niddk.nih.gov/.

The Obesity Society, 8630 Fenton St., Suite 814, Silver Spring, MD, 20910, 301 563-6526, 301 563-6595, http://www.obesity.org/.

Rebecca Frey, PhD

Intelligence tests *see* **Stanford-Binet intelligence scales; Wechsler intelligence test**

Intention tremor *see* **Tremors**

Interferon *see* **Antiviral drugs; Immunologic therapies**

Interleukin-2 *see* **Immunologic therapies**

Intermittent claudication

Definition

Intermittent claudication is a **pain**, cramping, or weakness in the legs (usually the calf muscle of one or both lower limbs, although it can sometimes occur in the arms), especially when exercising such as walking or climbing stairs. The pain, which occurs because of reduced blood flow through the limbs, is intermittent and goes away when the person rests. It is a type of arterial occlusive disease. Intermittent claudication is also called **angina** cruris or sometimes simply as claudication and is a symptom of peripheral artery disease.

Demographics

People age 50 years or older are at risk of intermittent claudication. The risk increases with age. Statistically, 5% of men and 2.5% of women experience symptoms of this condition, according to the Vascular Disease Foundation (VDF). Many people with this condition have cholesterol plaque build-up in the leg's arteries. **Smoking** raises the risk, as do high blood pressure, **obesity**, lack of **exercise**, and diabetes.

Description

Claudication comes from the Latin word (*claudicare*) that means "to limp," and the condition is characterized by intermittent pain, usually of the leg muscles but not the joints. Poor circulation produces the pain. The legs do not receive the oxygen-rich (oxygenated) blood supply needed for activities like walking and exercising. The decreased blood flow is caused by the narrowing or damage of arteries that bring blood to the legs and feet. Most patients also have cholesterol plaque in the arteries of their legs.

The leg pain produced by claudication is usually experienced as cramping in the thighs, calves, hips, and feet. The pain stops several minutes after the person rests, but returns when the person performs activities that use the leg muscles. If untreated, claudication is no longer intermittent and occurs when a person is resting.

Intermittent claudication is the main symptom of peripheral arterial disease (PAD), which is also known as **peripheral vascular disease** or occlusive arterial disease. Intermittent claudication is an early symptom of the condition that affects peripheral arteries, those blood vessels located outside the heart. PAD is caused by arteriosclerosis, the narrowing and hardening of the arteries. According to the National Heart, Lung, and Blood Institute, about 10% of people with PAD also have intermittent claudication.

Women with diabetes are much more likely to experience PAD as those without diabetes, according to the American Diabetes Association (ADA). Furthermore, intermittent claudication is related to a two to three times increased risk of coronary heart disease, **stroke**, or cardiac failure in men with diabetes, according to the association.

Causes and symptoms

Intermittent claudication is caused by poor circulation and is experienced in a person's muscle groups. It affects the peripheral arteries that convey oxygen-rich blood from the heart to the legs. A person with this condition feels pain shortly after beginning to exercise. Walking may trigger the pain in an inactive person. Activities such as climbing stairs, walking rapidly or dancing can cause the pain to increase.

The person feels the pain as tightness in the calf, thigh, or buttocks. The pain stops after the person rests for several minutes. However, it returns when the person reaches the exertion level that previously produced the pain.

Intermittent claudication is the primary symptom of PAD, the condition causing reduced flow of blood and oxygen to tissues. If the intermittent condition is not treated, the person will find that resting does not relieve pain. As arteries become more clogged, the person could feel pain even when not exercising. Symptoms include cold or numb feet and toes, poor balance when standing, a drop in leg strength, sores that heal slowly, and **erectile dysfunction (impotence)**.

The most common cause of intermittent claudication is **atherosclerosis**. It involves atherosclerotic lesions of the limbs. Such lesions reduce the amount of blood to the muscles of the lower legs. The symptoms of atherosclerosis, and of intermittent claudication, are:

- Cyanosis (blue discoloration of skin, especially toes or fingers).
- Pain, cramping, burning/aching feeling, tightness, or weakness, especially in the low extremities (legs, feet, calves, hips, or buttocks), while walking or exercising.
- Deteriorate changes such as shiny skin and hair loss.
- Decreased body temperature; including a feeling of cold and a look of pallor.
- Sores on lower legs, feet, toes, arms, or elsewhere.
- Impotence (men).

In the advanced stages of PAD, the person experiences pain when resting. This condition, ischemic rest pain, is characterized by symptoms visible on the feet and toes. These include ulcers, loss of hair, and the change to red color when feet are suspended. Other symptoms include blue or purple markings on the legs, feet, and toes. The coloring is a sign that less oxygen is reaching these areas. Furthermore, black skin on the legs and feet is a sign of **gangrene** infection.

Risks

The risk factors for intermittent claudication include:

- High blood pressure.
- Total blood cholesterol over 240 milligrams per deciliter.
- Obesity (being extremely overweight).
- Diabetes.
- Tobacco products, such as smoking.
- Over 70 years of age (over 50 years of age for tobacco users or those with diabetes).
- Family history of peripheral artery disease, atherosclerosis, or intermittent claudication.

Diagnosis

If a person experiences symptoms of intermittent claudication, their doctor will review the patient's medical history and examine the person for signs of the condition. This examination includes checking for a lower pulse or the absence of a pulse behind the knee, on the ankle, foot, and groin.

The doctor may order an ankle-brachial index (ABI) test to determine whether arteries are blocked. This procedure will verify if the person has PAD and provides information on the severity of the condition. The ABI measures blood pressure in the arms and ankle. Readings are taken when the person is at rest and after exercising lightly by walking on a treadmill. The ABI index is found by dividing the ankle blood pressure by the pressure for the arm. An ABI below 0.90 in a person at rest is a sign of PAD.

The physician may also order a Doppler ultrasound examination to measure the flow of blood through the arteries. Cuffs are placed on four places on each leg. The doctor then moves an ultrasound probe over arteries in the foot. The probe detects signals (sound waves) from the artery. Testing can last from 20 minutes to an hour. The results will show the degree of PAD for the patient. The procedures are usually covered by medical insurance.

Treatment

Lifestyle changes are the primary form of treating intermittent claudication. Physicians advise people to quit smoking, exercise, and to follow the American Heart Association's healthy diet guidelines. Other suggestions may be to lower blood pressure and cholesterol levels.

The goal of treatment is stop development of PAD. By exercising, eating a diet that includes fiber and low-fat foods, and not smoking, a person could also reverse the build-up that clogs arteries. After several months of this regimen, many people experience a lessening of leg pain. If pain continues, the doctor may prescribe medication. Furthermore, surgery may be needed in some cases. In most cases, when treated properly, intermittent claudication can be controlled without pain so patients can live an active lifestyle.

Walking

Walking is frequently an important treatment for intermittent claudication. A person experiencing the pain of intermittent claudication may not feel like walking. However, walking can increase the capacity to exercise. Before starting an exercise program, the person should consult with consult with a doctor.

The physician reviews the patient's medical history, does a physical and may order an exercise **stress test** on a treadmill. The test shows how long a person walks before claudication starts. Information such as blood pressure is used to evaluate the person's ability to walk. The findings are also used to develop a medically supervised exercise program.

At the beginning, the treadmill is set to cause claudication symptoms in three to five minutes, according to the Vascular Disease Foundation. The person walks until pain is moderately severe. A rest period is scheduled after the person walks eight to 10 minutes.

The person walks and rests, with the goal of walking for a total of 35 minutes. The person walks at least three times weekly. If a treadmill is not available, VDF recommends that people walk on a track. Generally, a person walking three times weekly will be able to walk longer after three to 12 months.

Medications

People diagnosed with PAD are at a high risk for a stroke and **heart attack**. Regularly taking **aspirin** may reduce this risk. Clopidogrel, a drug marketed as Plavix, has been shown to also reduce such risks. Other medications include angiotensin converting enzyme

(ACE) inhibitors, beta-blockers, pentoxifylline, and cilostazol (selective PDE3 inhibitor).

A doctor may also prescribe cilostazol—sold under the name Pletal—which extends the distance people can walk without pain. One tablet is taken twice daily.

Surgical procedures

Surgical procedures may be necessary in cases where intermittent claudication is disabling. The person experiences pain when resting, has open sores that do not heal, or symptoms of gangrene like dying skin in the leg or foot.

Bypass surgery directs blood through a grafted blood vessel, bypassing the damaged artery. The grafted vessel is either a healthy artery or vein or an artificial vessel.

Angioplasty is a procedure to open blocked blood vessels. A catheter (tube) is inserted in the groin and moved to the artery. Then a tiny balloon is inflated to open the artery. Another angioplasty procedure involves the insertion of a stent, a metal device that keeps the vessel open.

Angioplasty is a minimally invasive procedure. **Local anesthesia** is used, and a person is able to resume normal activities within one to two days. The cost of angioplasty is less than one-half the cost of bypass surgery. A non-invasive procedure is not as risky as surgery. However, a bypass may be needed when multiple sections of blood vessels are blocked.

Once a person is diagnosed with intermittent claudication, health plans usually cover part of treatment costs.

Alternative treatment

Ginkgo biloba extract, an herbal remedy, has been used by people with intermittent claudication. The extract made from the dried leaves of the Gingko tree is thought to improve blood flow, allowing people to walk longer without pain.

However, herbal remedies are not regulated the U.S. Food and Drug Administration, and people should consult with their doctors before taking ginkgo. Furthermore, use of this remedy could interact adversely when taken with vitamin E and vitamin B_3, which are also used as alternative treatments, and some other medications.

Prognosis

If untreated, advanced intermittent claudication can eventually restrict a person's mobility. In later stages, people feel pain when resting. The leg or foot may feel cold. In the extreme stage, the person might need a cane, walker, or wheelchair. There is more risk of gangrene developing, and **amputation** might be necessary. Diabetics face an increased risk of amputation. PAD also increases the risk of heart attacks and strokes.

KEY TERMS

Arthrosclerosis—A condition where fatty deposits cause the arteries to narrow.

Gangrene—The decay of tissue in the body; it is caused by an obstruction to the blood supply.

Prevention

A healthy lifestyle is the best method for preventing intermittent claudication. Cigarette smokers should quit smoking. Regular exercise and a healthy diet may help reduce the risk of this condition. Maintaining healthy blood pressure and cholesterol levels may also help to prevent this condition.

The methods of preventing intermittent claudication are also the means for managing the risks associated with a diagnosis of PAD.

People can learn more about peripheral vascular disease through public education programs like the free Legs for Life screenings held at sites across the nation. The program, started by the Society of Interventional Radiology, features a free ABI testing.

Resources

BOOKS

Mohler III, Emile R., and Alan T. Hirsch. *100 Questions and Answers about Peripheral Artery Disease (PAD)*. Sudbury, MA: Jones and Bartlett Publishers, 2010.

Mohler III, Emile R., and Michael R. Jaff, eds. *Peripheral Arterial Disease*. Philadelphia: American College of Physicians, 2008.

Rajagopalan, Sanjay, Debabrata Mukherjee, and Emile R. Mohler III, eds. *Manual of Vascular Diseases*. Philadelphia: Lippincott Williams and Wilkins, 2005.

OTHER

"Claudication" Mayo Clinic. (April 8, 2010), http://www.mayoclinic.com/health/claudication/DS01052. (accessed July 7, 2010).

"Intermittent Claudication: 8 Ways to Ease the Pain." The Doctors Book of Home Remedies, Rodale. www.mothernature.com/Library/Bookshelf/Books/47/85.cfm. (accessed July 12, 2010).

"Legs For Life" Society of Interventional Radiology. http://www.legsforlife.org/. (accessed July 7, 2010).

"PAD: Intermittent Claudication" Vascular Disease Foundation. (July 10, 2010), http://www.vdf.org/diseaseinfo/pad/claudication.php. (accessed July 7, 2010).

"Peripheral Artery Disease" Mayo Clinic. (April 21, 2010), http://www.mayoclinic.com/health/peripheral-arterial-disease/DS00537. (accessed July 7, 2010).

"Peripheral Artery Disease" National Heart, Lung, and Blood Institute. http://www.nhlbi.nih.gov/health/dci/Diseases/pad/pad_signs.html. (accessed July 7, 2010).

ORGANIZATIONS

American Diabetes Association, 1701 North Beauregard St., Alexandria, VA, 22311, (800) 342–2383, AskADA@diabetes.org, http://www.diabetes.org.

Society of Interventional Radiology, 3975 Fair Ridge Drive, Suite 400 North, Fairfax, VA, 22033, (800) 488-7284, http://www.sirweb.org.

Vascular Disease Foundation, 1075 S. Yukon Street, Suite 320, Lakewood, CO, 22033, (888) 833-4463, info@vdf.org, http://www.vdf.org.

Liz Swain

Intermittent explosive disorder

Definition

Intermittent explosive disorder (IED) is a mental disturbance that is characterized by specific and repeated episodes of violent and aggressive behavior that may involve harm to others or destruction of property. Throwing and breaking of objects are often part of the behavior. Often the anger and violence seen in such an individual reaches a point of uncontrollable rage. Such behavior seems out of context to the situation at hand during such outburst. Common signs of IED are temper tantrums, domestic **abuse**, and road rage. IED is sometimes grouped together as an impulse–control disorder with other such behavioral disorders such as kleptomania, pyromania, and pathological gambling.

A person must meet certain specific criteria to be diagnosed with IED:

- There must be several separate episodes of failure to restrain aggressive impulses that result in serious assaults against others or property destruction.
- The degree of aggression expressed must be out of proportion to any provocation or other stressor prior to the incidents.
- The behavior cannot be accounted for by another mental disorder, substance abuse, medication side effects, or such general medical conditions as epilepsy or head injuries.

Many psychiatrists do not place intermittent explosive disorder into a separate clinical category but consider it a symptom of other psychiatric and mental disorders. In many cases individuals diagnosed with IED do in fact have a dual psychiatric diagnosis. IED is frequently associated with mood and **anxiety disorders**, **substance abuse** and **eating disorders**, and narcissistic, paranoid, and antisocial **personality disorders**.

Demographics

With regard to sex and age group, the majority of individuals diagnosed with IED in the United States are adolescent and adult males. Women do experience IED, however, and have reported it as part of **premenstrual syndrome** (PMS). IED may appear in childhood but is usually misdiagnosed as temper tantrums. Later in life, it often goes undiagnosed for years because it is a relatively rare condition.

According to researchers at the National Institutes of Health, in 2006, approximately 2.2 million persons in the United States (about 7.3% of the total population) met the criteria for IED, with a total of 11.5 to 16 million meeting the lifetime criteria for the disorder.

Description

People diagnosed with IED sometimes describe strong impulses to act aggressively prior to the specific incidents reported to the doctor and/or the police. They may experience racing thoughts or a heightened energy level during the aggressive episode, with **fatigue** and depression developing shortly afterward. Some report various physical sensations, including tightness in the chest, **tingling** sensations, increased energy, tremor, hearing echoes, irritability, or a feeling of pressure inside the head.

Many people diagnosed with IED appear to have general problems with anger or other impulsive behaviors between explosive episodes. Some are able to control aggressive impulses without acting on them while others act out in less destructive ways, such as screaming at someone rather than attacking them physically.

Causes and symptoms

Causes

As with other impulse–control disorders, the cause of IED has not been determined. As of 2010, researchers disagree as to whether it is learned behavior (environmental in nature), the result of biochemical or neurological abnormalities (biological in nature), or a combination of factors. Some scientists have reported abnormally low levels of serotonin, a neurotransmitter that affects mood, in the cerebrospinal fluid of some anger–prone persons, but the relationship of this finding to IED is not clear. Generally, IED patients also have higher levels of the hormone testosterone in the systems. Similarly, some individuals diagnosed with IED have a medical history that includes migraine headaches, seizures, attention–deficit hyperactivity disorder, or developmental problems of various types, but it is not clear that these cause IED, as most persons with migraines, learning problems, or other neurological disorders do not develop IED.

Some psychiatrists who take a cognitive approach to mental disorders believe that IED results from rigid beliefs and a tendency to misinterpret other people's behavior in accordance with these beliefs. According to American psychologist Aaron Beck (1921–), a pioneer in the application of cognitive therapy to violence–prone individuals, most people diagnosed with IED believe that other people are basically hostile and untrustworthy, that physical force is the only way to obtain respect from others, and that life in general is a battlefield. Beck also identifies certain characteristic errors in thinking that go along with these beliefs:

- Personalizing. The person interprets others' behavior as directed specifically against him or her.
- Selective perception. The person notices only those features of situations or interactions that fit his or her negative view of the world rather than taking in all available information.
- Misinterpreting the motives of others. The person tends to see neutral or even friendly behavior as either malicious or manipulative.
- Denial. The person blames others for provoking his or her violence while denying or minimizing his or her own role in the fight or other outburst.

Symptoms

The symptoms that can precede episodes of IED, or can accompany the disorder, include:

- Rage.
- Increased energy.
- Tingling.
- Tremors.
- Palpitations.
- Irritability.
- Headache, or feeling of pressure in the head.
- Tightness in the chest.

Risks

People with increased risk of having intermittent explosive disorder may have these other characteristics:

- Substance abuse (more likely to have abused drugs or alcohol).
- Age (younger people are more prone to IED).
- Gender (men are more likely than women to have IED).
- Other mental health problems (people with other mental illnesses, such as anxiety attacks or depression, are more likely to also have IED).
- Previous physical abuse (people previously abused physically as children are at higher risk of IED).

Diagnosis

The diagnosis of IED is basically a diagnosis of exclusion, which means that the doctor will eliminate such other possibilities as neurological disorders, mood or substance abuse disorders, **anxiety** syndromes, and personality disorders before deciding that the patient meets the DSM–IV criteria for IED. In addition to taking a history and performing a **physical examination** to rule out general medical conditions, the doctor may administer one or more psychiatric inventories or screeners to determine whether the person meets the criteria for other mental disorders.

In some cases the doctor may order imaging studies or refer the person to a neurologist to rule out brain tumors, traumatic injuries of the nervous system, **epilepsy**, or similar physical conditions.

Patients diagnosed with IED are also usually diagnosed with at least one other disorder, such as personality disorders, substance abuse, or neurological disorders.

Along with these other evaluations, the doctor will also investigate the personal and professional history of the patient. People with IED often have problems in school, keeping a job, and interpersonal relationships (including divorce), along with numerous automobile accidents and law enforcement crimes.

Treatment

Emergency room treatment

A person brought to a hospital emergency room by family members, police, or other emergency personnel after an explosive episode will be evaluated by a psychiatrist to see whether he or she can safely be released after any necessary medical treatment. If the patient appears to be a danger to him/herself or others,

KEY TERMS

Cognitive therapy—A form of short–term psychotherapy that focuses on changing people's patterns of emotional reaction by correcting distorted patterns of thinking and perception.

Delirium—An acute but temporary disturbance of consciousness marked by confusion, difficulty paying attention, delusions, hallucinations, or restlessness. Delirium may be caused by drug intoxication, high fever related to infection, head trauma, brain tumors, kidney or liver failure, or various metabolic disturbances.

Kleptomania—A mental disorder characterized by impulsive stealing.

Neurotransmitter—Any of a group of chemicals that transmit nerve impulses across the gap (synapse) between two nerve cells.

Pyromania—A mental disorder characterized by setting fires.

Serotonin—A neurotransmitter or brain chemical that is responsible for transporting nerve impulses.

the person may be involuntarily committed for further treatment. In terms of legal issues, a doctor is required by law to notify the specific individuals as well as the police if the patient threatens to harm particular persons. In most states, the doctor is also required by law to report suspected abuse of children, the elderly, or other vulnerable family members.

The doctor will perform a thorough medical examination to determine whether the explosive outburst was related to substance abuse, withdrawal from drugs, head trauma, **delirium**, or other physical conditions. If the patient becomes assaultive inside the hospital, he or she may be placed in restraints or given a tranquilizer (usually either lorazepam [Ativan] or diazepam [Valium]), usually by injection. In addition to the physical examination, the doctor will obtain as detailed a history as possible from the family members or others who accompanied the patient.

Medications

Medications that have been shown to be beneficial in treating IED in nonemergency situations include lithium, carbamazepine (Tegretol), propranolol (Inderal), and such **selective serotonin reuptake inhibitors** as fluoxetine (Prozac) and sertraline (Zoloft). Adolescents diagnosed with IED have been reported to respond well to clozapine (Clozaril), a drug normally used to treat **schizophrenia** and other psychotic disorders.

Psychotherapy

Some persons with IED benefit from cognitive therapy in addition to medications, particularly if they are concerned about the impact of their disorder on their education, employment, or interpersonal relationships. Psychoanalytic approaches are not useful in treating IED.

Prognosis

The prognosis of IED depends on several factors that include the individual's socioeconomic status, the stability of his or her family, the values of the surrounding neighborhood, and his or her motivation to change. As some patients age the disorder tends to decrease in its severity. However, in others the disorder becomes chronic.

Prevention

There is not a clear way to prevent this disorder. It is also difficult to diagnose until symptoms begin to appear. Since the causes of IED are not fully understood as of the early 2010s, preventive strategies should focus on treatment of young children (particularly boys) who may be at risk for IED before they enter adolescence. Teaching self–control skills at a young age is been shown helpful in controlling the disorder.

Resources

BOOKS

Aboujaoude, Elias, and Lorrin M. Koran. *Impulse Control Disorders*. New York: Cambridge University Press, 2010.

Beers, Mark H., ed. *The Merck Manual of Diagnosis and Therapy*, 18th ed., Whitehouse Station, NJ: Merck Research Laboratories, 2006.

Diagnostic and Statistical Manual of Mental Disorders, 4th ed. St. Paul, MN: Thomson/West, 2009.

Grant, Jon E. *Impulse Control Disorders: A Clinician's Guide to Understanding and Treating Behavioral Addictions* . New York: W. W. Norton, 2008.

Hollander, Eris, and Dan J. Stein, eds. *Clinical Manual of Impulse–Control Disorders*. Arlington, VA: American Psychiatric, 2006.

OTHER

"Intermittent Explosive Disorder." Mayo Clinic. (June 10, 2010), http://www.mayoclinic.com/health/intermittent–explosive–disorder/DS00730. (accessed September 5, 2010).

"Intermittent Explosive Disorder Affects up to 16 Million Americans." National Institutes of Health. (June 5, 2006), http://www.nih.gov/n ews/pr/jun2006/nimh–05.htm. (accessed September 5, 2010).

ORGANIZATIONS

American Academy of Child and Adolescent Psychiatry, 3615 Wisconsin Ave., NW, Washington, DC, 20016–3007, (202) 966–7300, (202) 966–2891, http://www.aacap.org.

American Psychiatric Association, 1000 Wilson Blvd, Suite 1825, Arlington, VA, 22209, 888) 357–7924, http://www.psych.org.

National Institute of Mental Health, 6001 Executive Blvd., Room 8184, MSC 9663, Bethesda, MD, 20892–9663, (866) 615–6464, http://www.nimh.nih.gov.

Janie F. Franz
Rebecca Frey, PhD

Internal fetal monitoring *see* **Electronic fetal monitoring**

Internuclear ophthalmoplegia *see* **Ophthalmoplegia**

Interpositional reconstruction *see* **Arthroplasty**

Intersex states

Definition

Intersex states are conditions where a newborn's sex organs (genitals) look unusual, making it impossible to identify the sex of the baby from its outward appearance.

Description

All developing babies start out with external sex organs that look female. If the baby is male, the internal sex organs mature and begin to produce the male hormone testosterone. If the hormones reach the tissues correctly, the external genitals that looked female change into the scrotum and penis. Sometimes, the genetic sex (as indicated by chromosomes) may not match the appearance of the external sex organs. About 1 in every 2,000 births results in a baby whose sex organs look unusual.

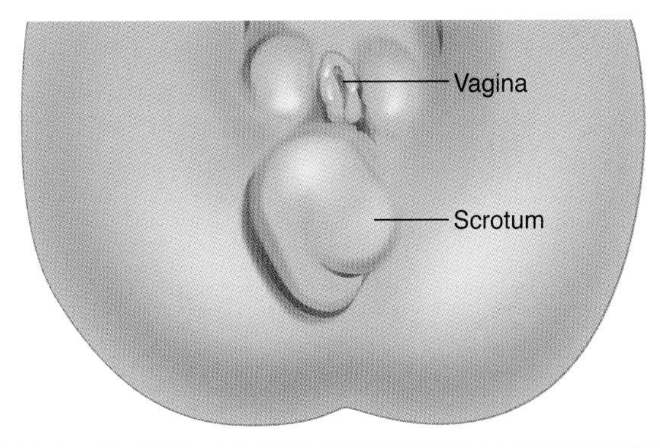

An illustration depicting an infant born with both male and female genitalia. Such a condition can make identification of gender impossible from outward appearance. *(Illustration by Electronic Illustrators Group. Reproduced by permission of Gale, a part of Cengage Learning.)*

Patients with intersex states can be classified as a true hermaphrodite, a female pseudohermaphrodite, or a male pseudohermaphrodite. This is determined by examining the internal and external structures of the child.

A true hermaphrodite is born with both ovaries and testicles. They also have mixed male and female external genitals. This condition is extremely rare.

A female pseudohermaphrodite is a genetic female. However, the external sex organs have been masculinized and look like a penis. This may occur if the mother takes the hormone progesterone to prevent a **miscarriage**, but more often it is caused by an overproduction of certain hormones.

A male pseudohermaphrodite is a genetic male. However, the external sex organs fail to develop normally. Intersex males may have testes and a female-like vulva, or a very small penis.

Causes and symptoms

Any abnormality in chromosomes or sex hormones, or in the unborn baby's response to the hormones, can lead to an intersex state in a newborn.

Intersex states may also be caused by a condition called **congenital adrenal hyperplasia**, which occurs in about 1 out of every 5,000 newborns. This disease blocks the baby's metabolism and can cause a range of symptoms, including abnormal genitals.

KEY TERMS

Chromosomes—Spaghetti-like structures located within the nucleus (or central portion) of each cell. Chromosomes contain the genetic information necessary to direct the development and functioning of all cells and systems in the body. They pass on hereditary traits from parents to child (like eye color) and determine whether the child will be male or female.

Diagnosis

When doctors are uncertain about a newborn's sex, a specialist in infant hormonal problems is consulted as soon as possible. Ultrasound can locate a uterus behind the bladder and can determine if there is a cervix or uterine canal. Blood tests can check the levels of sex hormones in the baby's blood, and chromosome analysis (called karyotyping) can determine sex. Explorative surgery or a biopsy of reproductive tissue may be necessary. Only after thorough testing can a correct diagnosis and determination of sex be made.

Treatment

Treatment of intersex states is controversial. Traditional treatment assigns sex according to test results, the potential for the child to identify with a sex, and the ease of genital surgery to make the organs look more normal. Treatment may then include **reconstructive surgery** followed by hormone therapy. Babies born with congenital adrenal hyperplasia can be treated with cortisone-type drugs and sometimes surgery.

Counseling should be given to the entire family of an intersex newborn. Families should explore all available medical and surgical options. Counseling should also be provided to the child when he or she is old enough.

Prognosis

Since the mid-1950s, doctors have typically assigned a sex to an intersex infant based on how easy reconstructive surgery would be. The American Academy of Pediatrics states that children with these types of genitals can be raised successfully as members of either sex, and recommends surgery within the first 15 months of life.

Some people are critical of this approach, including intersex adults who were operated on as children. The remolded genitals do not function sexually and can be the source of lifelong **pain**. They suggest that surgery be delayed until the patient can make informed choices about surgery and intervention.

ORGANIZATIONS

Ambiguous Genitalia Support Network, P.O. Box 313, Clements, CA, 95227, 209 727-0313.

Intersex Society of North America, 979 Golf Course Drive #282, Rohnert Park , CA, 94928, 801 348-5350, http://www.isna.org/.

Carol A. Turkington

Interstitial microwave thermal therapy

Definition

Interstitial microwave thermal therapy is a type of hyperthermia treatment for **cancer**, in which heat produced by microwaves (which are a non-ionizing form of radiation) is used in conjunction with other cancer treatments, such as radiation or **chemotherapy**, to kill cancer cells associated with tumors located deep with the body.

Purpose

The purpose of interstitial microwave thermal therapy is to damage and kill cancer cells associated with tumors that are deep within the body. Interstitial microwave therapy is a type of hyperthermia cancer treatment procedure (also called thermal therapy or thermotherapy) in which body tissue and the cancerous tumor are exposed to high temperatures (up to 113°F). Hyperthermia kills cancer cells with usually only minimal injury to normal tissues by damaging proteins and structures within the cells. Thermal therapy is usually used with other forms of cancer therapy, such as radiation and chemotherapy. The increased temperatures may make some cancer cells more sensitive to radiation or may harm some cancer cells that radiation cannot damage.

Precautions

If a patient has become insensitive to **pain** due to disease, radiation, surgery, anesthetics, or other conditions, hyperthermia treatment cannot be used to treat tumors. Also the excessive heating of normal surrounding tissue is prevented by normal blood perfusion, so hyperthermia should not be used in patients with known circulatory problems in the heated areas or in patients who are taking vasoconstrictive drugs.

Description

Interstitial microwave thermal therapy is used to treat tumors that are deep within the body, such as brain, cervical, breast, prostate, and neck tumors. This technique allows the tumor to be heated to higher temperatures than external thermal therapy techniques allow. Probes or needles are inserted into the tumor, guided by the use of imaging techniques, such as ultrasound, to make sure that the probe is properly located within the tumor. A new type of microwave generator includes electronic phase control that allows the operator to electronically direct and shape the pattern of hyperthermia treatments based on the positioning the microwave antennae array that is used in treating the tumor. The treatment pattern can be electronically targeted on the tumor position, shape, and size.

Tissues are heated as the electromagnetic energy produced by the microwave treatment results in heating through molecular excitation. This energy is dissipated in normal living tissue by the blood that perfuses through the tissue. However, since large solid malignant tumors have less blood perfusion than the surrounding normal tissue, for a given absorbed thermal dose, the tumor reaches a higher temperature than the normal tissue. Tumors present within normal tissue will therefore be preferentially heated and will reach higher temperatures than the surrounding tissue.

As cancerous tumors grow rapidly, their need for blood quickly begins to exceed the available blood supply, and major portions of the tumors become blood-starved. These blood-starved tumors are resistant to both radiation and chemotherapy. Chemotherapy drugs carried through the blood cannot effectively penetrate tumors that have poor blood flow. Poor blood flow also means that the tumors are oxygen-starved (hypoxic), making it difficult for **radiation therapy** to make the oxygen radicals that are needed to destroy the DNA of cancer cells. Hypoxic cancer cells, which are an especially dangerous type of cancer, for they have a tendency to metastasize and spread the cancer to other parts of the body, are three times more resistant to ionizing radiation than are normal cells.

When the tumor is heated to **fever** levels through the use of microwave thermal therapy, its blood vessels expand so that more blood can flow into the tumor in order to carry away the excess heat. With the increased blood flow, more blood-borne chemotherapy drugs can be carried into the tumor. Blood is also the source of oxygen for tumors, so with increased blood flow due to the thermal therapy, radiation therapy can form the necessary oxygen radicals to kill the cancer cells. The increased temperature also acts as a drug activator, accelerating chemical reactions and pulling increased oxygen molecules into the tumor tissue for chemical reactions with the chemotherapy drug. **Hypothermia** also enhances the effectiveness of chemotherapy drugs encapsulated in liposomes, increasing the penetration of the drug into the tumor.

When tumors are heated to higher temperatures for at least an hour, the tumors in some cases have been shown to decrease in size and to exhibit necrosis (**death** of the tumor cells). Therefore, hyperthermia by itself also tends to shrink tumors, often dramatically, due to the collapse of dead cancer cells, making it easier to remove the tumor by surgical techniques. For tumors of the head and neck, a smaller tumor due to hyperthermia treatment may reduce the disfiguration associated with surgical removal of the tumor.

Hyperthermia is being studied as a means of enhancing **gene therapy** by acting as an activator to turn on new biological therapies, by speeding up gene production by thousands of times. In addition, hyperthermia is used as an essential tool to turn on anti-tumor vaccines that are based on heat shock proteins. Hyperthermia has been shown to prevent a cancererous tumor from growing new blood vessels to expand its blood supply. With regards to quality of life, hyperthermia lessens pain and stimulates the immune system, thus helping patients recover from toxic cancer therapies such as ionizing radiation and chemotherapy. Even in patients with terminal cancer, hyperthermia can provide benefits through the alleviation of bleeding, pain, and infection.

The use of hyperthermia alone and in conjunction with radiation therapy has been approved by the United States Food and Drug Administration for the treatment of advanced, recurrent, and persistent tumors, upon authorization of a licensed practitioner. When used with radiation, the treatment regimen usually consists of 10 hyperthermia treatments delivered twice a week, at 72 hour intervals. The prescribed radiation is administered within 30 minutes of the hyperthermia treatment. During each heat treatment, the temperature within the tumor is usually maintained at 42.5 °C for 60 minutes. The use of hyperthermia in conjunction with chemotherapy is presently investigational in the United States.

The effectiveness of treatment is related to the temperature achieved during the treatment process, the length of the treatment, and cell and tissue characteristics. The temperature within the tumor must be monitored to ensure that the appropriate temperature is achieved, but not exceeded, in the treatment area.

KEY TERMS

Blood perfusion—A physiological term that refers to the process of nutritive delivery of arterial blood to a capillary bed in the biological tissue.

Hyperthermia therapy—A type of treatment in which body tissue is exposed to high temperatures to damage and kill cancer cells or to make cancer cells more sensitive to the effects of radiation and certain anticancer drugs.

Non-ionizing radiation—Rays of energy that move in long, slow wave patterns and do not penetrate cells.

Ionizing radiation—Any electromagnetic or particulate radiation capable of producing ions, directly or indirectly, in its passage through matter.

Monitoring is accomplished by inserting small needles or tubes with small thermometers into the treatment area. Imaging techniques such as computed tomography (CT) are used to make sure that the temperature probes are positioned appropriately.

Preparation

The safety and effectiveness of hyperthermia treatment is dependent on careful placement of the temperature probes and careful monitoring of tissue temperatures during treatment.

Aftercare

During the treatment period, which may last for weeks, the patient must be instructed in proper care of implanted catheters and temperature probe sites to avoid the risk of infection.

Risks

Excessive heating of normal tissues may result in areas of thermal aseptic necrosis that will require medical care. The electromagnetic radiation from the microwave equipment can interfere with electronic devices such as cardiac **pacemakers** or other implanted electronic devices. Thermal treatment of tumors in the neck or head may result in inadvertent heating of thermoregulatory centers in the brain stem, thus resulting in overheating of the body, beyond levels that the patient can tolerate. Metallic implants, such as joint protheses or dental braces may become excessively and preferentially overheated and adversely affect the patient.

Normal results

The effectiveness of interstitial microwave thermal therapy varies among cancer patients. For example, studies have shown in Phase III clinical trials, when hyperthermia was used with ionizing radiation treatment, that the following treatment improvements were seen, as compared to the use of ionizing radiation therapy alone:

- complete response for recurrent breast cancer increased from 38% to 60%
- 2-year survival for globlastoma (brain cancer) increased from 15% to 31%
- complete response for advanced cervical cancer increased from 57% to 83%

Known side effects of hypothermia are associated with direct effects of heat on tissues and indirect effects of tumor necrosis. These side effects, as determined in various medical studies, include:

- surface burns and blistering in the area of application of heat by the microwave applicators; experienced in about 10% of the tumor sites studied.
- localized and temporary pain in the area of and during the delivery of the heat by the microwave applicators; experienced in about 8% of the tumor sites studied.
- ulceration from rapid tumor necrosis following successful hyperthermia treatment, resulting in fever from toxemia and patient discomfort through drainage and bleeding; experienced in about 4% of the tumor sites studied.
- local and systematic (rarely) infections from placement of the temperature probes and from ulceration related to tumor necrosis; experienced in about 2% of the tumor sites studied.

Abnormal results

Hyperthermia has the potential for producing the following adverse reactions as a result of exposure to electromagnetic radiation:

- cataracts
- permanent or temporary male sterility
- exacerbation of existing diseases due to additional systemic stress
- enhanced drug activity
- thermal stress

Resources

BOOKS

Ko, Andrew, Malin Dollinger, and Ernest H. Rosenbaum. *Everyone's Guide to Cancer Therapy*. 5th ed. Kansas City, KS: Andrews McMeel, 2008.

PERIODICALS

Falk, M.H., and Issels, R.D. "Hyperthermia in Oncology." *International Journal of Hyperthermia*. 2001, (17): 1–18.

van der Zee, J. "Heating the Patient: A Promising Approach?" *Annals of Oncology* 2002, (13): 1173–1184.

Wust, P., Hildebrandt, B., Sreenivasa, G. et al. "Hyperthermia in Combined Treatment of Cancer." *The Lancet Oncology* 2002, (3): 487–497.

ORGANIZATIONS

Society for Thermal Medicine, PO Box 1897, Lawrence, KS, 66044-1897, 785 843-1274, 800 627-0326, stm@ allenpress.com, http://www.thermaltherapy.org.

Judith L. Sims

Intestinal culture *see* **Stool culture**

Intestinal lymphangiectasia *see* **Malabsorption syndrome**

Intestinal obstructions

Definition

Intestinal obstructions, sometimes also called bowel obstructions, refers to the partial or complete mechanical or non–mechanical blockages of fluids or foods of the small or large intestine (which includes the colon, cecum, and rectum). When such obstructions occur, they can lead to reduced or blocked passage of digested materials through the intestines. They are often caused by intestinal **adhesions**, hernias, or tumors.

Demographics

The disorder occurs in people of all ages, genders, and ethnic backgrounds.

Description

There are two types of intestinal obstructions, mechanical and non–mechanical. Mechanical obstructions occur because the bowel (intestines) is physically blocked and its contents cannot get past the obstruction. Mechanical obstructions can occur for several reasons. Sometimes the bowel twists on itself (volvulus) or telescopes into itself (**intussusception**). Mechanical obstruction can also result from hernias, impacted feces, abnormal tissue growth, the presence of foreign bodies in the intestines (including **gallstones**), or inflammatory bowel disease (**Crohn's disease**). Non–mechanical obstruction, called **ileus**, occurs because the wavelike muscular contractions of the intestine (peristalsis) that ordinarily move food through the digestive tract stop.

Mechanical obstruction in infants

Infants under one year of age are most likely to have intestinal obstruction caused by meconium ileus, volvulus, and intussusception. Meconium ileus, which is the inability to pass the first fecal excretion after birth (meconium), is a disorder of newborns. It is an early clue that the infant has **cystic fibrosis**, but may also occur in very low birth weight (VLBW) infants. In meconium ileus, the material that is blocking the intestine is thick and stringy, rather than the collection of mucus and bile that is passed by normal infants. The abnormal meconium must be removed with an enema or through surgery.

Volvulus is the medical term for twisting of either the small or large bowel. The twisting may cut off the blood supply to the bowel, leading to tissue **death (gangrene)**. This development is called a strangulating obstruction.

In intussusception, the bowel telescopes into itself like a radio antenna folding up. Intussusception is most common in children between the ages of three and nine months, although it also occurs in older children. Almost twice as many boys suffer intussusception as girls. It is, however, difficult for doctors to predict which infants will suffer from intestinal obstruction.

Mechanical obstruction in adults

Obstructions in adults are usually caused by tumors, trauma, volvulus, the presence of foreign bodies such as gallstones, or hernias, although they have also been reported in adults with cystic fibrosis. Volvulus occurs most often in elderly adults and psychiatrically disturbed patients. Intussusception in adults is usually associated with tumors in the bowel, whether benign or malignant.

More recently, gastroenterologists have described a postsurgical complication known as early postoperative small bowel obstruction, or EPSBO. Although this condition was at one time confused with postoperative ileus, it is now known to be caused by mechanical obstructions resulting from **radiation therapy** for **cancer** or laparoscopic surgery. Most cases can be successfully treated within 10–14 days of surgery.

Causes and symptoms

Causes

Causes of intestinal obstructions can be subdivided into two primary groups: small bowel obstruction and large bowel obstruction. Causes of small bowel obstruction include:

- adhesions (usually from abdominal surgery, but sometimes present at birth)
- hernias (protrusion of intestines through cavity that contains it)
- Crohn's disease (inflammatory disease of the intestines)
- neoplasm (abnormal growth of tissue mass)
- intussusception (layering [telescoping] of sections of intestines within other sections, children only)
- volvulus (abnormal twist in bowel)
- superior mesenteric artery syndrome (compression of part of duodenum by abdominal aorta and superior mesenteric artery)
- intestinal atresia (narrowing or absence of part of intestine)
- carcinoid (neuroendocrine tumor)
- foreign bodies (such as gall stones or swallowed objects)
- ischaemic stricture (abnormal narrowing of intestines usually at outlet from stomach)

Large bowel obstruction can be caused by the following:

- neoplasm
- hernias
- cancer
- inflammatory bowel disease (inflammation of the colon)
- diverticulitis (small pouches in digestive tract become inflamed or infected)
- colonic volvulus (twist in colon)
- fecal impaction (blocked, impacted feces in rectum)
- intestinal atresia
- endometriosis (uterine tissue found outside of uterus, in women only)

Almost all of the causes of intestinal obstructions occur in the small intestines rather than the large intestines.

Symptoms

One of the earliest signs of mechanical intestinal obstruction is abdominal **pain** or cramps that come and go in waves. Infants typically pull up their legs and cry in pain, then stop crying suddenly. They will then behave normally for as long as 15–30 minutes, only to start crying again when the next cramp begins. The cramping results from the inability of the muscular contractions of the bowel to push the digested food past the obstruction.

Vomiting is another symptom of intestinal obstruction. The speed of its onset is a clue to the location of the obstruction. **Vomiting** follows shortly after the pain if the obstruction is in the small intestine but it is delayed if found in the large intestine. The vomited material may be fecal in character. When the patient has a mechanical obstruction, the doctor will first hear active, high–pitched gurgling and splashing bowel sounds while listening with a stethoscope. Later these sounds decrease, and then stop. If the blockage is complete, the patient will not pass any gas or feces. If the blockage is only partial, however, the patient may have **diarrhea**. Initially there is little or no **fever**.

When the material in the bowel cannot move past the obstruction, the body reabsorbs large amounts of fluid and the abdomen becomes sore to the touch and swollen. The balance of certain important chemicals (electrolytes) in the blood is upset. Persistent vomiting can cause the patient to become dehydrated. Without treatment, the patient can suffer **shock** and kidney failure.

Strangulation occurs when a loop of the intestine is cut off from its blood supply. Strangulation occurs in about 25% of cases of small bowel obstruction. It is a serious condition that can progress to gangrene within six hours.

Risks

The following pre–existing conditions can add to the risk of contracting intestinal obstructions:

- Crohn's disease
- abdominal or pelvic surgeries
- long–lasting constipation
- malrotation (congenital condition in which intestines do not develop normally)

If someone has advanced intestinal obstruction of one type or the other, certain symptoms will be apparent due to infection within the lining of the abdominal cavity (a condition known as **peritonitis**). These symptoms include:

- tenderness, pain, and swelling in abdominal area
- thirst, but low urine output
- fluid in abdomen
- vomiting and nausea

KEY TERMS

Electrolytes—Salts and minerals that ionize in body fluids. Electrolytes control the body's fluid balance as well as performing other important functions.

Gangrene—The death of soft tissue in any part of the body when the blood supply is obstructed.

Ileus—Obstruction of the intestines caused by the absence of peristalsis.

Intussusception—The slipping or telescoping of one part of the intestine into the section next to it.

Meconium—A greenish fecal material that constitutes the first bowel movement of an infant.

Peristalsis—The waves of muscular contraction in the intestines that push the food along during the process of digestion.

Strangulated obstruction—An obstruction in which a loop of the intestine has its blood supply cut off.

Volvulus—A twisting of the intestine that causes an obstruction.

- fever and chills
- inability to pass gas or have a bowel movement

When advanced peritonitis occurs, more severe symptoms occur. They include:

- weak, rapid pulse
- either abnormally slow, shallow breathing or rapid breathing
- pale, clammy skin
- inability to pass gas or have a bowel movement
- dilated pupils in the eyes
- eyes that stare off into the distance

If such symptoms occur, the patient has most likely gone into shock, and immediate emergency care should be sought.

Diagnosis

Imaging studies

If the doctor suspects intestinal obstruction based on the **physical examination** and patient history, he or she will order x rays, a computed tomography scan (CT scan), or an ultrasound evaluation of the abdomen. In many cases the patient is given a **barium enema**. A suspension of barium sulfate, which is a white powder, is inserted through the rectum, and the intestinal area is photographed. Barium acts as a contrast material and allows the location of the obstruction to be visualized on film.

Laboratory tests

The first blood test of a patient with an intestinal obstruction usually gives normal results, but later tests indicate electrolyte imbalances. There is no way to determine if an obstruction is simple or strangulated except by performing surgery.

Treatment

Initial assessment

All patients with suspected intestinal obstruction are hospitalized. Treatment must be rapid, because strangulating obstructions can be fatal. The first step in treatment is inserting a nasogastric tube to suction out the contents of the stomach and intestines. The patient is then given intravenous fluids to prevent **dehydration** and correct electrolyte imbalances.

Nonsurgical approaches

Surgery can be avoided for some patients. In some cases of volvulus, guiding a rectal tube into the intestines will straighten the twisted bowels. In infants, a barium enema may reverse intussusception in 50–90% of the cases. An air enema is sometimes used instead of a barium enema. This treatment successfully relieves the obstruction in many infants. The children are usually hospitalized for observation for two to three days after these procedures. In patients with only partial obstruction, a barium enema may dissolve the blockage.

Surgical treatment

If these efforts fail, surgery is necessary. Strangulated obstructions require emergency surgery. The obstructed area is removed and part of the bowel is cut away. If the obstruction is caused by tumors, polyps, or scar tissue, they are removed. Hernias, if present, are repaired. **Antibiotics** are given to reduce the possibility of infection.

Alternative treatment

Alternative practitioners offer few suggestions for treatment. They focus on preventive strategies, particularly the use of high–fiber **diets** to keep the bowels healthy through regular elimination.

Prognosis

The prognosis for intestinal obstructions depends on age, previous illnesses (especially lung, heart, or kidney problems), and the specific cause of the obstruction within the intestines. Generally, healthy people have good prospects. However, when intestinal obstructions are associated with cancer, the prognosis is not as favorable.

Mortality

Untreated intestinal obstructions can be fatal. Delayed diagnosis of volvulus in infants has a mortality rate of 23–33% with prompt diagnosis and treatment the mortality rate is three to nine percent. The bowel either strangulates or perforates, causing massive infection. Tissues within the intestines soon die, which leads to perforation of the intestines and infection. The patient eventually goes into shock. With prompt treatment, however, most patients recover successfully without complications.

Recurrence

As many as 80% of patients whose volvulus is treated without surgery have recurrences. Recurrences in infants with intussusception are most likely to happen during the first 36 hours after the blockage has been cleared. The mortality rate for unsuccessfully treated infants is one to two percent.

Prevention

Most cases of intestinal obstruction are not preventable. Surgery to remove tumors, polyps, or gallstones helps prevent recurrences. Other medical treatments and therapies may help to reduce the risk from many forms of intestinal obstructions.

Resources

BOOKS

Beers, Mark H., et al., eds. *The Merck Manual of Diagnosis and Therapy*, 18th ed. Whitehouse Station, NJ: Merck Research Laboratories, 2006.

Feldman, Mark., et al., eds. *Sleisenger and Fordtran's Gastrointestinal and Liver Disease: Pathophysiology/Diagnosis/Management*. Philadelphia: Saunders/Elsevier, 2006.

Townsend, C. M, et al. eds. *Sabiston Textbook of Surgery: The Biological Basis of Modern Surgical Practice*, 18th ed. Philadelphia: Saunders/Elsevier, 2008.

OTHER

Heller, Jacob L. "Intestinal Obstruction." Medline Plus, U.S. National Library of Medicine and National Institutes of Health. (July 23, 2008), http://www.nlm.nih.gov/medlineplus/ency/article/000260.htm. (accessed September 5, 2010).

"Intestinal Obstruction." Mayo Clinic. (July 8, 2010), http://www.mayoclinic.com/health/intestinal–obstruction/DS00823. (accessed September 5, 2010).

"Intestinal Obstruction—Overview." University of Maryland Medical Center. http://www.umm.edu/ency/article/000260.htm (accessed September 5, 2010).

Tish Davidson, A.M.
Rebecca Frey, PhD

Intestinal polyps

Definition

The word polyp refers to any overgrowth of tissue from the surface of mucous membranes. Intestinal polyps, sometimes also called colorectal polyps (or sometimes just colon polyps), grow out of the lining of the small and large bowels (intestines). Polyps come in a variety of shapes—round, droplet, and irregular being the most common. They also come in many sizes, from those smaller than a pea to others as large as a golf ball. Most are harmless but in a small percentage of cases they can become cancerous (colorectal **cancer**, or

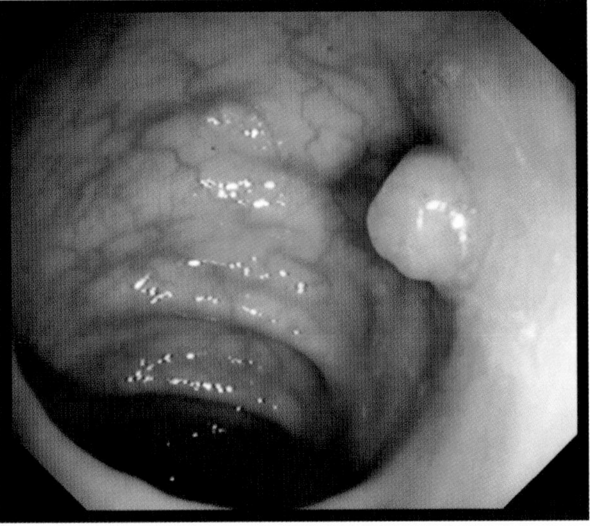

A benign polyp in a patients colon, viewed through an endoscope. *(Custom Medical Stock Photo, Inc. Reproduced by permission.)*

cancers of the colon and rectum) and dangerous to one's health and well–being, especially as one grows older.

Demographics

Intestinal polyps can occur in anyone, regardless of age or other characteristics. However, as one ages the likelihood of developing them increases. In fact, 50 years of age and older is the time when polyps are more likely to develop in humans. The risks from intestinal polyps can be reduced by eating a high–fiber, low–fat diet. A family history of intestinal polyps also increases one's risk of getting them.

The National Cancer Institute (NCI) predicted that about 102,900 new cases of **colon cancer** and approximately 39,670 new cases of **rectal cancer** would occur in the United States in 2010. In addition, NCI predicted that, in the same year, about 51,370 deaths would occur because of colon and rectal cancers (or, colorectal cancer).

Description

Polyps are one of many forms of tissue overproduction that can occur in the body. Cells in many body tissues sometimes keep growing beyond their usual limits. Medical scientists call this process *neoplasia*, which means simply "new growth." An individual overgrowth is called a neoplasm. In most cases these growths are limited, and the result is a benign swelling or mass of cells called a tumor. If the new growth occurs on the surface of the tissue instead of inside an organ it is often called a polyp. Cancer is another type of neoplasm marked by unlimited tissue growth. The essential feature that distinguishes cancer from nonmalignant neoplasms is that it does not stop growing.

Intestinal polyps are a common form of neoplasm. All intestinal polyps arise from the inner lining of the intestinal wall. This layer of mucosal tissue does the work of digestion. About 30% of the general population will develop intestinal polyps at some point in life, with the likelihood increasing with age. Most of these polyps are never noticed during a person's lifetime because they do not cause problems. They are often discovered accidentally at **autopsy**. The primary importance of intestinal polyps is that one percent of them become cancerous. Because the polyps that eventually turn malignant cannot be identified in advance, they are all suspect.

Location of intestinal polyps

The chances of a polyp's becoming cancerous depend to some extent on its location within the digestive tract.

COLON. Ninety–five percent of all intestinal polyps develop inside the large bowel. Several hereditary diseases produce large numbers of intestinal polyps. These disorders include:

- Familial polyposis of the colon.
- Gardner's syndrome.
- Lynch's syndrome.
- Turcot's syndrome.
- Peutz–Jeghers syndrome.
- Juvenile polyposis.

All of these disorders are inherited in an autosomal dominant pattern. This pattern means that the disorders are not sex–linked and that a child can inherit the disorder from either parent. In all of these hereditary disorders, the intestinal polyps appear during or after **puberty**. The first four diseases on the list have such a high rate of cancer of the large bowel (colon)—virtually 100% by the age of 40 years of age—that persons diagnosed with any of them should have the colon removed surgically in early adulthood.

STOMACH. The stomach's lining is host to polyps of a similar appearance, but there is no agreement as to their potential for becoming **stomach cancer**.

SMALL INTESTINE. Polyps in the small bowel do not seem to have malignant potential. Instead, they can produce obstruction in either of two ways. A large polyp can obstruct the bowel by its sheer size. Smaller polyps can be picked up by the rhythmic contractions (peristalsis) of the intestines and pull the part of the bowel to which they are attached into the adjoining section. The result is a telescoping of one section of bowel into another, called **intussusception**.

Causes and symptoms

Population studies of colon cancer suggest that age and diet play an important role in the disease, and, by implication, in the formation of colon polyps. Increased risk of colon cancer begins at the age of 40 years. Most people who have colon cancer are in their 50s or older. The most consistent interpretation of colon cancer data is that animal fats—though not vegetable fats—are the single most important dietary factor the raises the risk of colon polyps. Lack of fiber in the diet may also contribute to polyp formation. Primarily, a person is at elevated risk for colon polyps if their diet consists of high fat, high percentage of red meat, and low fiber.

A family history of colon polyps or cancer also is a factor. The presence of inflammatory intestinal conditions, such as **Crohn's disease** and ulcerative **colitis**, also increases the risk of colon polyps. African Americans and Ashkenazi Jews of Eastern European descent are two groups of people with higher risk for colon cancer.

KEY TERMS

Autosomal dominance—A pattern of heredity in which a trait is inherited without respect to sex and from either parent. The hereditary diseases associated with intestinal polyps are all autosomal dominant.

Colectomy—Surgical removal of the large bowel.

Intussusception—The slipping of one section of the intestine inside an adjoining section. Intussusception can be caused by small intestinal polyps.

Mucosal—Refers to tissues that produce mucus, such as the digestive, genital and urinary tracts.

Neoplasm—A new growth of abnormal tissue.

Peristalsis—The rhythmic contractions of muscular tubes like the intestines that carry the contents along the tube.

Sigmoid—The S–shaped curve of the large intestine where the colon joins the rectum.

Lifestyle and the environment are also factors. Increased risk occurs when a person smokes tobacco products, drinks alcoholic beverages, and is obese (excessively overweight). In fact, smokers are approximately 20% more likely to develop colon polyps than are non–smokers. The more inactive one's lifestyle is, the more likely one will develop colon cancer. Exposure to carcinogenic substances (those known to cause cancer), such as asbestos, increases risks for colon cancer.

Three primary types of colon polyps occur: adenomatous polyps (most polyps are of this kind, but only a few become cancerous); hyperplastic polyps (second most frequent polyps, and they often occur in left colon and rectum); and inflammatory polyps (usually occur after ulcerative colitis or Crohn's disease). Most smaller sized polyps do not cause symptoms. However, larger ones eventually cause intestinal obstruction, which produces cramping abdominal **pain** with **nausea and vomiting**. As colon polyps evolve into cancers, they begin to produce symptoms that include rectal bleeding, blood in the stool, and altered bowel habits (including **constipation**, **diarrhea**, or narrowing of the stool).

Rectal bleeding may occur after a bowel movement. Such bleeding may be due to colon polyps, but may also be the result of **hemorrhoids** or minor tears in the anus. Blood in the stool, which may show up as red streaks within the stool or turn the stool black, can be an indication of colon polyps, but they may also be the result of eating red–colored foods (red streaks in the stool) or iron supplements and various anti–diarrhea medications (black stool). A change in bowel conditions can indicate the presence of colon polyps but can also be the result of other unrelated medical conditions.

Diagnosis

Routine screening for bowel cancer is recommended for everyone over the age of 50 years, and for those with a history of colorectal cancer over the age of 40 years. Medical professionals can test for some diseases that increase the risk for colorectal cancer, such as familial adenomatous polyposis (FAP) which increases one's risk for developing multiple colon polyps. Screening may be as simple as testing the stool for blood (such as through a **fecal occult blood test** [FOBT]) or as elaborate as **colonoscopy**. The FOBT is a noninvasive test that is often performed at the doctor' office or at home. Although it tests only for blood in the stool, the FOBT is a good beginning point for diagnosis.

A stool DNA test detects cancer cells that are present in the stool. Such cancer cells will have altered DNA, which makes this test advantageous for detecting pre–cancerous polyps and colon cancer. As of July 2010, this test has not been approved by the U.S. Food and Drug Administration (FDA).

Most polyps are in the lower segment of the colon, called the sigmoid colon. These polyps can be seen with a shorter scope (tube) called a flexible sigmoidoscope. Flexible **sigmoidoscopy** is a procedure that uses a narrow, lighted tube to examine the rectum and sigmoid (the last third of the colon). A **barium enema** is a diagnostic tool that evaluates the entire large intestine with a barium dye placed inside the colon and an x–ray image. The colon is filled with barium sulfate (a white substance) that shows up as a shadow when imaged by an x–ray film. The colon can also be filled with barium sulfate and air, which is called a double contrast study.

Colonoscopy is a procedure in which the doctor threads an instrument called a colonoscope up through the entire large bowel. The colonoscope is a long, narrow tube attached to a video camera (for imaging inside the colon) and monitor (for viewing outside by the medical team). If one or more polyps are discovered during the examination, they can be removed. Computerized tomographic colonography (CTC) is a colonoscopy that is performed virtually (that is, without actually inserting an instrument inside the colon). It involves a computerized tomography scan of the colon. This three–dimensional look of the colon allows the medical professionals to make a detailed analysis of the colon. However, for this technique, any polyps discovered are not able to be removed.

Because polyps take about ten years to turn into cancers, routine examinations are recommended every three to five years.

Treatment

All polyps should be removed as preventive care. Most of them can be taken out through a colonoscope, in which the larger polyps are snared with a wire loop and the smaller ones are cauterized with an electrical current. Complications like obstruction and intussusception are surgical emergencies. The largest of the polyps can be removed with laparoscopic techniques, in which small incisions are cut into the abdominal wall so tiny instruments can be used to remove such polyps. Endoscopic mucosal resection (EMR) is a specialized procedure for removing large polyps with a colonoscope. The polyp is separated from other tissue with an injected liquid so the procedure can take place.

Chemotherapy, radiation, or a combination of the two is also used to treat colorectal cancer. In serious cases, parts of the colon may have to be removed. In more severe cases, a total proctocolectomy is performed, one in which all of the colon and rectum is removed.

Prognosis

Patients with intestinal polyps have an excellent outlook for the future once the polyps are removed. However, polyps left within the intestines can develop into cancer over time.

Prevention

Patients with hereditary disorders associated with polyps must undergo total colectomy early in adult life. All children of parents with these disorders should be screened early in adulthood, because half of them will have the same disease. For the bulk of the population, increased consumption of dietary fiber and decreased consumption of animal fat are the best preventives known at present. For the occasional intestinal polyp that arises in spite of good dietary habits, routine screening should prevent it from becoming cancerous.

Overall, the following are recommended to reduce the chances of developing colon polyps:

- Consume calcium and vitamin D, such as in no–fat or low–fat milk and other dairy products; some fish, and vitamin supplements.
- Consume fruits and vegetables, especially those high in antioxidants; those with deep green, dark yellow, dark orange colorings, such as squash, sweet potatoes, spinach, and broccoli; and those with lycopene such as tomatoes and red bell peppers and others with red colorings.
- Eat whole grains, such as those found in breads.
- Reduce unhealthy fats such as saturated fats and trans fats to less than 10% per day and total fats to less than 30% daily. When eating fats, select healthy ones such as unsaturated fats (monounsaturated and polyunsaturated fats).
- Limit alcohol consumption to one drink per day for women and two drinks per day for men.
- Stop using tobacco products such as cigarettes.
- Be as physically active as possible.
- Maintain a healthy mass to body index (BMI).

Resources

BOOKS

Bub, David S., Susannah Rose, and W. Douglas Wong. *100 Questions and Answers About Colorectal Cancer*. Sudbury, MA: Jones and Bartlett, 2008.

Fauci, Anthony S., et al, eds. *Harrison's Principles of Internal Medicine*, 17th ed. New York: McGraw-Hill, 2008.

Hayat, M. A., ed. *Colorectal Cancer*. Dordrecht, Netherlands: Springer, 2009.

Kim, Daren E., ed. *Early Detection and Prevention in Colorectal Cancer*. Thorofare, NJ: SLACK, 2009.

OTHER

"Colon Polyps." Mayo Clinic. (July 8, 2010), http://www.mayoclinic.com/health/colon–polyps/DS00511. (accessed September 5, 2010).

"Colon and Rectal Cancer." National Cancer Institute. http://www.cancer.gov/cancertopics/types/colon–and–rectal. (accessed September 5, 2010).

"Colorectal Cancer." National Library of Medicine and National Institutes of Health. (July 9, 2010), http://www .nlm.nih.gov/medlineplus/colorectalcancer.html. (accessed September 5, 2010).

J. Ricker Polsdorfer, MD

Intestinal strangulation *see* **Intestinal obstructions**

Intoxication confusional state *see* **Delirium**

Intracavity therapy *see* **Radioactive implants**

Intracranial abscess *see* **Brain abscess**

Intrapartum monitoring *see* **Electronic fetal monitoring**

Intrauterine device *see* **IUD**

Intrauterine growth retardation

Definition

Intrauterine growth retardation (IUGR) occurs when the unborn baby (fetus) is at or below the 10th weight percentile for his or her gestational age (in weeks). In other words, the unborn baby is developing poorly (more slowly then normal) within the womb. After being born, these babies usually have low weights and are likely to continue having health problems later in life.

Description

There are standards or averages in weight for unborn babies according to their age in weeks. When the baby's weight is at or below the 10th percentile for his or her age, it is called intrauterine growth retardation, or fetal growth restriction. These babies are smaller than they should be for their age. How much a baby weighs at birth depends not only on how many weeks old it is, but the rate at which it has grown. This growth process is complex and delicate. There are three phases associated with the development of the baby. During the first phase, cells multiply in the baby's organs. This occurs from the beginning of development through the early part of the fourth month. During the second phase, cells continue to multiply and the organs grow. In the third phase (after 32 weeks of development), growth occurs quickly and the baby may gain as much as seven ounces (200 grams) per week. If the delicate process of development and weight gain is disturbed or interrupted, the baby can suffer from restricted growth.

IUGR is usually classified as symmetrical or asymmetrical. In symmetrical IUGR, the baby's head and body are proportionately small. In asymmetrical IUGR, the baby's brain is abnormally large when compared to the liver. In a normal infant, the brain weighs about three times as much as the liver. In asymmetrical IUGR, the brain can weigh five or six times as much as the liver.

Causes and symptoms

Doctors think that the two types of IUGR may be linked to the time during development that the problem occurs. Symmetrical IUGR may occur when the unborn baby experiences a problem during early development. Asymmetrical IUGR may occur when the unborn baby experiences a problem during later development. While not true for all asymmetrical cases, doctors think that sometimes the placenta may allow the brain to get more oxygen and **nutrition** while the liver gets less.

There are many IUGR risk factors involving the mother and the unborn baby. A mother is at risk for having a growth restricted infant if she:

- Has had a previous baby who suffered from IUGR
- Has poor weight gain and lack of nutrition (malnutrition) during pregnancy
- Is socially deprived
- Uses substances (like tobacco, narcotics, alcohol, and some prescription drugs, such as anticonvulsants) that can cause abnormal development or birth defects
- Has a vascular disease (like chronic hypertension [high blood pressure], preeclampsia [hypertension during pregnancy], or heart disease)
- Has chronic kidney disease
- Has sickle cell anemia
- Has a coagulation/antibody disorder called antiphospholipid antibody syndrome that causes blood clots
- Has a serious lung disease
- Has a low total blood volume during early pregnancy
- Is pregnant with more than one baby (multiple pregnancies)

A mother that is very small in size (weight) is more likely to have a fetus that is underweight when compared to normally sized unborn babies. Such a situation is not always caused by IUGR. About one out of three babies born smaller than normal have IUGR, while the other two are born smaller usually because the mother is smaller herself.

Additionally, an unborn baby may suffer from IUGR if it has:

- Exposure to an infection, including German measles (rubella), cytomegalovirus, tuberculosis, syphilis, or toxoplasmosis
- A defect in the kidneys, abdominal wall, or in the cardiovascular system
- A chromosome defect, especially trisomy 18 (Edwards' syndrome), Down syndrome, or anencephaly (missing parts of the brain)
- A primary disorder of bone or cartilage
- A chronic lack of oxygen during development (hypoxia), such as from living at high altitudes
- Placenta or umbilical cord defects such as placenta previa (placenta too low in uterus) or placental abruption (placenta detaching from uterus)
- Developed outside of the uterus.

KEY TERMS

Preeclampsia—Hypertension (high blood pressure) during pregnancy.

Diagnosis

IUGR can be difficult to diagnose and in many cases doctors are not able to make an exact diagnosis until the baby is born. A mother who has had a growth-restricted baby is at risk of having another during a later **pregnancy**. Such mothers are monitored closely during pregnancy. The length in weeks of the pregnancy must be carefully determined so that the doctor will know if development and weight gain are appropriate.

Checking the mother's weight and abdomen measurements can help diagnose cases when other risk factors are not present. Measuring the girth of the abdomen is often used as a tool for diagnosing IUGR. During pregnancy, the healthcare provider will use a tape measure to record the height from the pubic bone to the top of the uterus (the uterine fundal height, in centimeters).

As the pregnancy continues and the baby grows, the uterus stretches upward in the direction of the mother's head. Between 18 and 30 weeks of gestation, the uterine fundal height equals the weeks of gestation. For example, if the mother is 26 weeks pregnant, then the fundal height should be about 26 centimeters. If the uterine fundal height is more than two to three centimeters below normal, then IUGR is suspected. Ultrasound is used to evaluate the growth of the baby. Usually, IUGR is diagnosed after week 32 of pregnancy. This is during the phase of rapid growth when the baby should be gaining more weight. IUGR caused by genetic factors or infection may sometimes be detected earlier.

Treatment

Treatment is not available that improves fetal growth, but IUGR babies who are at or near term have the best outcome if delivered promptly. If IUGR is caused by a problem with the placenta and the baby is otherwise healthy, early diagnosis and treatment of the problem may reduce the chance of a serious outcome. Pregnant women suspected of carrying a fetus with IUGR will be monitored closely with several ultrasounds during the course of the pregnancy.

Measurements of movement, blood flow, growth, and fluid surrounding the fetus, will be carefully taken. Fetal monitoring is one test that indicates the health of a fetus. **Amniocentesis**, where a tiny amount of amniotic fluid is withdrawn from the uterus, is a way to test for chromosomal abnormalities.

A fetus that cannot tolerate the **stress** of natural labor may be delivered by **cesarean section** (c-section).

Prognosis

Babies who suffer from IUGR are at an increased risk for intrauterine (inside the womb) **death**, stress during vaginal delivery, abnormally high red blood cell count, low blood sugar (**hypoglycemia**), low body temperature (**hypothermia**), lower resistance to infection, difficulty maintaining body temperature, and abnormal development of the nervous system. These risks increase with the severity of the growth restriction. The growth that occurs after birth cannot be predicted with certainty based on the size of the baby when it is born. Infants with asymmetrical IUGR are more likely to catch up in growth after birth than are infants who suffer from prolonged symmetrical IUGR.

However, doctors cannot reliably predict an infant's future progress. Each case is unique. Some infants who have IUGR will develop normally, while others will have complications of the nervous system or intellectual problems like **learning disorders**. If IUGR is related to a disease or a genetic defect, the future of the infant is related to the severity and the nature of that disorder. Generally, most IUGR babies will attain a normal weight and height within two years of birth.

Prevention

The risk factors that can complicate pregnancies should be strictly controlled. Avoid alcohol, tobacco products, and drugs that are not part of the pregnancy. Make sure that regular prenatal care is obtained from medical professionals.

Movement of the unborn baby inside the mother is a reliable way to indicate its general health. A healthy baby moves and kicks often. Your caregiver may request a fetal kick count in between prenatal appointments to check on the number of kicks. A baby that has moved frequently in the past but has stopped kicking may be a sign of a problem. In such cases, call the pediatrician or other medical profession caring for the mother and baby.

The more nutrients that the mother takes in means the more nutrients for the unborn baby. Eat healthy foods and always go by the amount of calories recommended by the doctor. Plenty of rest is essential. At least eight hours of sleep each night should be taken by the mother, and naps during the day are also helpful.

Resources

BOOKS

Bianchi, Diana W., et al. *Fetology: Diagnosis and Management of the Fetal Patient*. New York: McGraw-Hill Medical, 2010.

Cunningham, F. Gary, et al. *Williams Obstetrics*, 22nd ed. Stamford, CT: Appleton & Lange, 2005.

Kiess, Wieland, et al. *Small for Gestational Age: Causes and Consequences*. Basel, Switzerland: Karger, 2009.

Preedy, Victor R., and Ronald R. Watson, eds. *Handbook of Disease Burdens and Quality of Life Measures*. New York: Springer, 2010.

OTHER

"Intrauterine Growth Restriction." FamilyDoctor.org. (April 2008). http://familydoctor.org/online/famdocen/home/women/pregnancy/fetal/313. html. (accessed September 21, 2010).

"Intrauterine Growth Restriction." Medline Plus, U.S. National Library of Medicine and National Institutes of Health. (February 19, 2009). http://www.nlm.nih.gov/medlineplus/ency/article/001500.htm. (accessed September 21, 2010).

"Intrauterine Growth Restriction (IURG)." BabyCenter L.L.C. (May 2006). http://www.babycenter.com/0_intrauterine-growth-restriction-iugr_142740 6.bc. (accessed September 21, 2010).

Linda Jones

Intravenous nutrition *see* **Nutrition through an intravenous line**

Intravenous pyelography *see* **Intravenous urography**

Intravenous rehydration

Definition

Rehydration is the process of replenishing the human body with water, or water and electrolytes, which have been previously lost through **dehydration**. This process can be performed orally or intravenously. With mild dehydration, oral rehydration is usually used. However, for more severe cases, which can cause serious and permanent injury or even **death**, intravenous rehydration is the method of choice within the medical community. For the method of intravenous (IV) rehydration, a sterile water solution containing small amounts of salt or sugar (and usually essential **minerals** and **vitamins**), are injected into the body through a tube attached to a needle, which is inserted into a vein.

Purpose

Fever, **vomiting**, and **diarrhea** can cause a person to become dehydrated fairly quickly. Infants and children are especially vulnerable to dehydration because of their smaller body weights and of a higher turnover of water and electrolytes, and due to their increased susceptibility to sicknesses such as those involving **vomiting** and diarrhea. Adult patients can become dehydrated due to an illness, surgery, or accident. Athletes, who have overexerted themselves and, thus, become dehydrated, may also require rehydration with IV fluids. An IV for rehydration can be used for several hours to several days, and is generally used if a patient cannot drink fluids.

Precautions

Patients receiving IV therapy need to be monitored to ensure that the IV solutions are providing the correct amounts of fluids and minerals needed. People with kidney and heart disease are at increased risk for **overhydration**, so they must be carefully monitored when receiving IV therapy.

Demographics

Because dehydration is common throughout the human population, intravenous rehydration may be used on any persons in need of such medical treatment. Infants and children, due to their young age, are at greater risk of becoming dehydrated. Adults recovering from surgeries and those that are sick are also vulnerable for dehydration. Athletes that overexert themselves may also become dehydrated. Hot weather, accidents, and medical problems can also cause a person to become dehydrated.

Description

Basic IV solutions are sterile water with small amounts of **sodium** chloride (salt) or dextrose (sugar) supplied in bottles or thick plastic bags that can hang on a stand mounted next to the patient's bed. Additional minerals like potassium, phosphate, magnesium, chloride, **calcium**, vitamins, or drugs can be added to the IV solution by injecting them into the bottle or bag with a needle.

Risks

There is a small risk of infection at the injection site. It is possible that the IV solution will not provide all of the nutrients needed, leading to a deficiency or an imbalance. If the needle becomes dislodged, it is possible that the solution may flow into tissues around the injection site rather than into the vein.

Causes and symptoms

Initial symptoms of dehydration that indicate the possible need for intravenous rehydration include:

- Headache
- Flushing in the face
- Dry, warm skin
- Muscle cramps, especially in the legs and arms
- Lower than normal, and sudden decrease, in blood pressure
- Dizziness or fainting when standings
- Abnormal thirst or the inability to drink
- Decreased urine output and unusually dark yellow-colored urine
- Tiredness, weakness, sleepiness, lethargic
- Irritability, confusion
- Dry mouth, dry tongue with thick saliva

More serious symptoms of dehydration that indicate a more critical need for intravenous rehydration include:

- Low blood pressure
- Delirium
- Unconsciousness/comotose
- Swelling of the tongue
- No urine output
- Lethargy or extreme sleepiness
- Fainting
- Rapid, deep breathing
- Weak, fast pulse
- Severe muscle contractions, especially in the arms, legs, back, and stomach
- Bloated stomach
- Dry eyes, sunken look to eyes
- Wrinkly look to skin, a lost firmness (elasticity) to the skin

Diagnosis

Anyone who exhibits signs and symptoms of moderate to severe dehydration should be taken promptly to an emergency medical professional for appropriate care. At the medical facility, the team will observe for physical characteristics as to indicate low blood pressure, rapid heart rate, appearance of **shock**, poor skin features (lack of elasticity), delayed capillary refill (rate at which blood refills capillaries), and other such signs that indicate dehydration.

Tests that may be performed to indicate moderate to severe dehydration include: **complete blood count** (CBC), creatinine, blood urea nitrogen (BUN), urine specific gravity, and various blood chemistries (such as those indicating sodium, bicarbonate, and potassium).

Treatment

Moderate and (especially) severely dehydrated persons should be initially treated by emergency personnel. Take such people to an emergency room at the hospital or other such facility where immediate emergency care can be given. The person should receive intravenous rehydration with salts and fluids through the vein (intravenously) because such a method provides a fast way to introduce water and essential nutrients into the body. This is especially important in life-threatening situations.

Preparation

A doctor orders the IV solution and any additional nutrients or drugs to be added to it. The doctor also specifies the rate at which the IV will be infused. The IV solutions are prepared under the supervision of a doctor, pharmacist, or nurse, using sanitary techniques that prevent bacterial contamination. Just like a prescription, the IV is labeled clearly to show its contents and the amounts of any additives. The skin around the area where the needle is inserted is cleaned and disinfected. Once the needle is in place, it will be taped to the skin to prevent it from dislodging.

The vein usually used are those in the arm, however, those veins in the back of the hand or the median cubital vein on the inside of the elbow can also be used. Generally, any appropriate vein can be used.

KEY TERMS

Intravenous—Into a vein; a needle is inserted into a vein in the back of the hand, inside the elbow, or some other location on the body. Fluids, nutrients, and drugs can be injected.

Aftercare

Patients need to take fluids by mouth before an IV solution is discontinued. After the IV needle is removed, the site should be inspected for any signs of bleeding or infection.

Prognosis

People with mild to serious dehydration will usually recover when they are given intravenous rehydration promptly and effectively at the first signs of being dehydrated. However, seizures, permanent brain damage and, even, death can result to people who are not given such treatment.

Prevention

To prevent the need for intravenous rehydration, make sure the body is properly hydrated. Consume plenty of fluids on a daily basis, along with foods that are high in water content such as fruits and vegetables. When exercising or performing other strenuous activities, make sure sufficient water is consumed before, during, and after such events. If a person is overly sweating and feels overheated during hot conditions, stop all activity and rest in a shady area to lower the body temperature. Drink fluids to replace any that have been lost. However, do not consume too much water because such a condition can also cause problems.

Fluids can be lost in the body in cold weather, not only in hot weather. **Exercise** or strenuous activity in cold weather, while wearing insulated clothing, can cause sweating and, thus, lost of hydration in the body. Even conditions inside involving very low humidity can contribute to a person's losing moisture within the body. In addition, locations of high altitudes, usually over 8,200 feet, or 2,500 meters, can cause a body to need more fluids.

During illnesses, such as those that include vomiting or diarrhea, make sure water or other fluids that can replenish lost electrolytes are taken promptly and regularly.

Resources

BOOKS

Kliegman, Robert, and Waldo E. Nelson. *Nelson Textbook of Pediatrics*. Philadelphia: Saunders, 2007.

Marx, John A., et al., eds. *Rosen's Emergency Medicine: Concepts and Clinical Practice*. Philadelphia: Mosby/Elsevier, 2010.

Shils, Maurice, et al., eds. *Modern Nutrition in Health and Disease*. Philadelphia: Lippincott Williams and Wilkins, 2006.

OTHER

"Dehydration." Mayo Clinic. (July 25, 2009), www.mayoclinic.com/health/dehydration/DS00561. (accessed July 17, 2010).

"Dehydration." Medline Plus, National Library of Medicine and National Institutes of Health. www.nlm.nih.gov/medlineplus/ency/article/000982.htm. (accessed July 17, 2010).

Altha Roberts Edgren

Intravenous urography

Definition

Intravenous urography is a test which x rays the urinary system using intravenous dye for diagnostic purposes.

Of the many ways to obtain images of the urinary system, the intravenous injection of a contrast agent has been traditionally considered the best. The kidneys excrete the dye into the urine. X rays can then create pictures of every structure through which the urine passes.

The procedure has several variations and many names.

- Intravenous pyelography (IVP).
- Urography.
- Pyelography.
- Antegrade pyelography differentiates this procedure from "retrograde pyelography," which injects dye into the lower end of the system, therefore flowing backward or "retrograde." Retrograde pyelography is better able to define problems in the lower parts of the system and is the only way to get x rays if the kidneys are not working well.
- Nephrotomography is somewhat different in that the x rays are taken by a moving x ray source onto a film moving in the opposite direction. By accurately coordinating the movement, all but a single plane of tissue is blurred, and that plane is seen without overlying shadows.

Every method available gives good pictures of this system, and the question becomes one of choosing among many excellent alternatives. Each condition has special requirements, while each technique has distinctive benefits and drawbacks.

- Nuclear scans rely on the radiation given off by certain atoms. Chemicals containing such atoms are injected into the bloodstream. They reach the kidneys, where images are constructed by measuring the radiation emitted. The radiation is no more dangerous than standard x rays. The images require considerable training to interpret, but unique information is often available using this technology. Different chemicals can concentrate the radiation in different types of tissue. This technique may require several days for the chemical to concentrate at its destination. It also requires a special detector to create the image.

- Ultrasound is a quick, safe, simple, and inexpensive way to obtain views of internal organs. Although less detailed than other methods, it may be sufficient.
- Retrograde pyelography is better able to define problems in the lower parts of the system and is the only way to get x rays if the kidneys are not working well. Dye is usually injected through an instrument (cystoscope) passed into the bladder through the urethra.
- Computed tomography scans (CT or CAT scanning) uses the same kind of radiation used in x rays, but it collects information by computer in such a way that three dimensional images can be constructed, eliminating interference from nearby structures. CT scanning requires a special apparatus.
- Magnetic resonance imaging (MRI) uses magnetic fields and radio frequency signals, instead of ionizing radiation, to create computerized images. This form of energy is entirely safe as long as the patient has no metal in his or her body. The technique is far more versatile than CT scanning. MRI requires special apparatus and, because of the powerful magnets needed, even a special building all by itself. It is quite expensive.

Purpose

Most diseases of the kidneys, ureters, and bladder will yield information to this procedure, which actually has two phases. First, it requires a functioning kidney to filter the dye out of the blood into the urine. The time required for the dye to appear on x rays correlates accurately with kidney function. The second phase gives detailed anatomical images of the urinary tract. Within the first few minutes the dye "lights up" the kidneys, a phase called the nephrogram. Subsequent pictures follow the dye down the ureters and into the bladder. A final film taken after urinating reveals how well the bladder empties.

IVPs are most often done to assess structural abnormalities or obstruction to urine flow. If kidney function is at issue, more films are taken sooner to catch the earliest phase of the process.

- Stones, tumors and congenital malformations account for many of the findings.
- Kidney cysts and cancers can be seen.

KEY TERMS

Contrast agent—Any substance that causes shadows on x rays, also known as contrast dye or medium.

Intravenous—Into a vein.

- Displacement of a kidney or ureter suggests a space-occupying lesion like a cancer pushing it out of the way.
- Bad valves where the ureters enter the bladder will often show up.
- Bladder cancers and other abnormalities are often outlined by the dye in the bladder.
- An enlarged prostate gland will show up as incomplete bladder emptying and a bump at the bottom of the bladder.

Precautions

The only serious complication of an IVP is allergy to the iodine-containing dye that is used. Such an allergy is rare, but it can be dramatic and even lethal. Emergency measures taken immediately are usually effective.

Description

IVPs are usually done in the morning. In the x ray suite, the patient will undress and lie down. There are two methods of injecting the dye. An intravenous line can be established, through which the dye will be consistently fed through the body during the procedure. The other method is to give the dye all at once through a needle that is immediately withdrawn. X rays are taken until the dye has reached the bladder, an interval of half an hour or less. The patient will be asked to empty the bladder before one last x ray.

Preparation

Emptying the bowel with **laxatives** or **enemas** prevents bowel shadows from obscuring the details of the urinary system. An empty stomach prevents the complications of **vomiting**, a rare effect of the contrast agent. Therefore, the night before the IVP the patient will be asked to evacuate the bowels and to drink sparingly.

Risks

Allergy to the contrast agent is the only risk. Anyone with a possible iodine allergy or a previous reaction to x ray dye must be particularly careful to inform the x ray personnel.

Resources

BOOKS

Tanagho, Emil A., Jack W McAninch, and Donald Ridgeway Smith.*Smith's General Urology*. New York: McGraw-Hill Medical, 2008.

J. Ricker Polsdorfer, MD

Intussusception

Definition

Intussusception is the enfolding of one segment of the intestine within another. It is characterized and initially presents with recurring attacks of cramping abdominal **pain** that gradually become more painful.

Description

Intussusception occurs when part of the bowel or intestine is wrapped around itself producing a mass-like object on the right side of the abdomen during palpation (a procedure used during a **physical examination**, when the examiner touches the abdomen with his/her hand, usually feeling for mass, pain, or discomfort). The number of new cases of intussuscetion is approximately 1.5 to four cases per 1,000 live births. The onset of abdominal pain is usually abrupt and severe. Just as fast as the onset of pain appears, it disappears and the child resumes activity normally. This process of sudden severe abdominal pain appearing out of the blue then disappearing is repeated with duration of painful attacks. The pain usually increases after approximately five hours of recurrent cycles of severe abdominal pain followed by relaxation. **Vomiting** and **diarrhea** occur in about 90% of cases within six to 12 hours after initial onset of symptoms.

Physical examination and palpation usually reveal a sausage shaped mass of enfolded bowel in the right upper mid portion of the abdomen. Within a few hours approximately 50% of cases have bloody, mucus filled bowel movements. At about this time the child is visibly very ill with **fever**, tenderness, and distended abdomen. Intussusception is the most frequent cause of intestinal obstruction during the first two years of life and commonly affects children between three to 12 months of age. The disease is three times more common in males than in females. In about 85% of cases the cause is idiopathic (meaning unknown). The remaining 15% of cases can be caused by a variety of other diseases such as tumors of the lymph nodes (lymphoma), fat tumors (lipomas), foreign bodies/objects, or from infections that mobilize immune cells to the area causing an inflammatory reaction and intestinal blockage. Most cases of intussusception do not strangulate the affected bowel within the first 24 hours. If the disease is not treated after this time, the possibility of intestinal **gangrene**, **shock**, and **death** increases.

Causes and symptoms

The major symptom of intussusception is when a healthy child suddenly and without warning experiences severe abdominal pain that subsides and usually results in continuation of normal activities such as playing. The duration of the painful attacks increases as the hours go by. Usually, the child develops **nausea**, **vomiting**, and diarrhea soon afterwards in about 90% of all cases. The child becomes weak, exhausted, and develops a fever. The affected child may also expel bloody, mucus-like bowel movements. These blood filled bowel movements are usually due to impaired blood flow to the obstructed area. During palpation there may be a sausage-shaped mass located on the upper right mid portion of the abdomen. If the disease progresses and is undetected, the child may develop death of cells within the affected area. Additionally, there may be perforation or hole in the intussusception bowel that can cause a life threatening infection in the peritoneum (a layer of tissue that protects the organs and intestines within the abdominal cavity). This infection of the peritoneum is called **peritonitis**. Some patients may exhibit altered states of consciousness or seizures.

Diagnosis

A presumed diagnosis can be made by history alone. If the clinician suspect's intussusception x-ray films should be performed, which may reveal a mass in the right upper mid abdominal region. Two classical clinical signs are mucus-blood filled stools and a "coiled string" appearance in the affected bowel as visualized during an x ray with a **barium enema**. Blood chemistry analysis is not specific for intussusception. Depending on vomiting and blood loss through the stools, blood chemistry may reflect signs of **dehydration** and anemia.

Treatment

Treating intussusception by reduction (alleviating the source of blockage) is an emergency procedure. The barium examination is not only the diagnostic tool of choice, but also frequently curative. Infusion

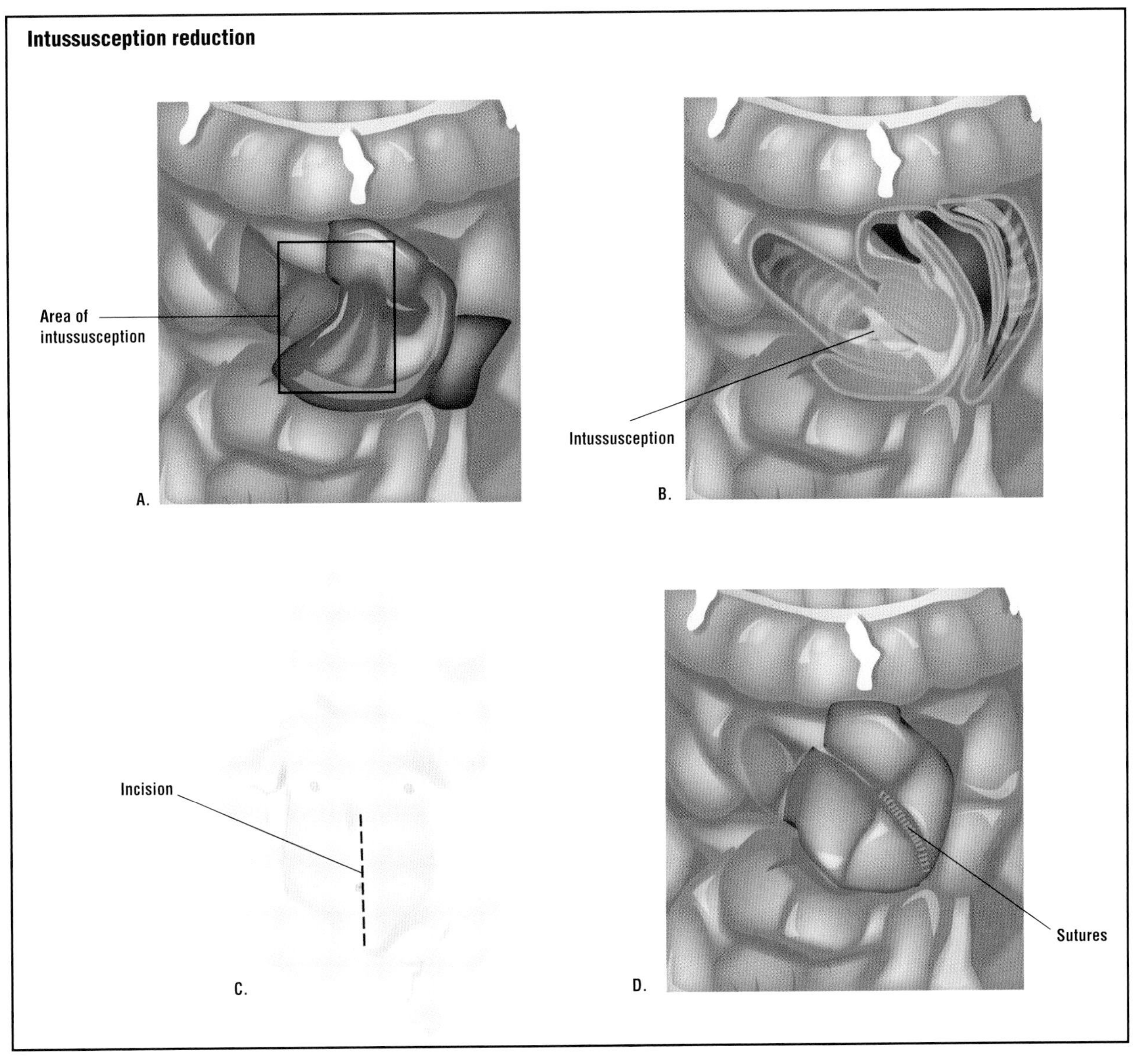

Intussusception of the bowel results in the bowel telescoping onto itself (A and B). To repair it, an incision is made in the baby's abdomen to expose the bowel (C). If the surgeon cannot manipulate the bowel into a normal shape manually, the area of intussusception will be removed and remaining bowel sutured together (D). *(Illustration by PreMediaGlobal. Reproduced by permission of Gale, a part of Cengage Learning.)*

by gravity from a catheter placed in the rectum will tend to relieve pressure buildup. If this does not relieve the area, then air can be pumped into the colon to clear blockage. If these procedures are unsuccessful then surgery is required. Approximately 25% of affected children require surgical intervention. Surgery in the affected bowel is advantageous since the actual cause can be removed, and the procedure decreases the possibility of recurrences. In general without surgical correction of the affected bowel, there is a 5–10% chance of recurrence. Recurrence usually appears within the first 24 to 48 hours after barium procedure.

Prognosis

The outcome of intussusception depends on the duration of symptoms before treatment initiation. Most infants will recover if treatment is initiated within the first 24 hours. Untreated intussusception is almost always fatal. Overall even with treatment, approximately 1–2% of affected children will die.

Prevention

Prevention of death can be accomplished with immediate medical care, within the first 24 hours.

KEY TERMS

Barium—A chemical used in certain radiological studies to enhance visualization of anatomical structures.

Obstruction—A blockage that prevents movement.

Once intussusception is suspected, emergency measures should be initiated. Untreated intussusception is almost always fatal. There is an increased chance for death if the disorder is not treated within 48 hours.

Resources

BOOKS

Kliegman, Robert M., and Waldo Emerson Nelson.*Nelson Textbook of Pediatrics*. 18th ed. Philadelphia: Saunders, Elsevier, 2007.

Sabiston, David C., et al.*Sabiston Textbook of Surgery: The Biological Basis of Modern Surgical Practice*. Philadelphia: Saunders/Elsevier, 2008.

OTHER

"University of Maryland." 2001. http://www.umm.edu.

Laith Farid Gulli, M.D.

Iodine *see* **Antiseptics**

Iodine uptake test *see* **Thyroid nuclear medicine scan**

Ipecac

Definition

Ipecac syrup is a bitter tasting medicine that was formerly given to induce **vomiting** in cases of accidental **poisoning**.

Purpose

Nowadays, **activated charcoal** and gastric lavage (pumping the stomach) are more rapid and effective means of preventing serious illness and **death** from accidental poisoning.

In cases of acute poisoning, contact either the local poison control center, local hospital emergency room, or family doctor for instructions.

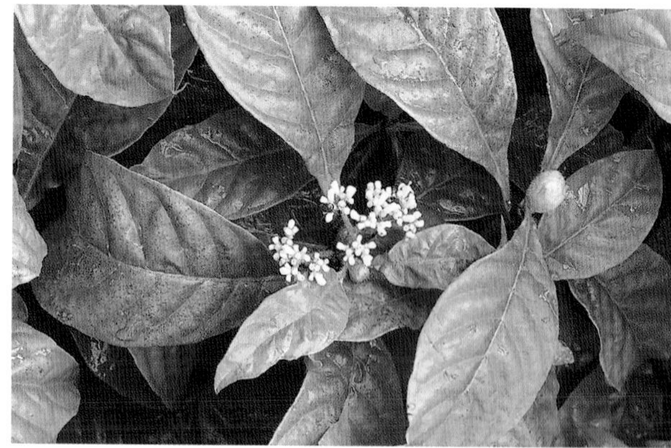

Ipecac plant (*Cephaelis ipecacuanha*). *(© Plantaphile.)*

Ipecac syrup should *never* be used to induce **vomiting** if the poison is

- strong alkali (lye)
- strong acids (bleach)
- strychnine
- crude oil products like kerosene, fuel oil, gasoline, coal oil, paint thinner, or cleaning fluids

Ipecac should never be given to people who are drowsy, unconscious, or having difficulty swallowing.

Ipecac syrup is sometimes used to induce vomiting for weight control. This is dangerous and can cause heart problems and death. Additionally, violent retching and vomiting can cause tears in the esophagus resulting in vomiting blood, seizures, or even death.

Resources

OTHER

Mayo Clinic online. http://www.mayoclinic.com.

James Waun, MD, RPh

Ipratropium *see* **Bronchodilators**

I.Q. tests *see* **Stanford-Binet intelligence scales; Wechsler intelligence test**

Iridocyclitis *see* **Uveitis**

Iritis *see* **Uveitis**

Iron-binding capacity test *see* **Iron tests**

Iron-utilization anemias *see* **Sideroblastic anemia**

Iron deficiency anemia

Definition

Anemia is a condition, which is the result of insufficient numbers of healthy red blood cells, that can be caused by iron deficiency, folate deficiency, vitamin B_{12} deficiency, and other causes. The term iron deficiency anemia means anemia that is due to iron deficiency—that is, the insufficient dietary intake or absorption of iron in the body. Iron deficiency anemia is characterized by the production of smaller than normal red blood cells and less than the normal number of red cells in the blood. When examined under a microscope, the red blood cells also appear pale or light colored due to too little iron in the blood. For this reason, the anemia that occurs with iron deficiency is also called hypochronic microcytic anemia. Because fewer healthy red blood cells are produced (which causes less hemoglobin to be produced and, thus, less oxygen to be carried throughout the body), people with iron deficiency anemia often experience a lack of energy throughout their daily lives.

Demographics

Anyone has the potential for acquiring iron deficiency anemia. In the United States, approximately 20% of all women of child-bearing years, about 50% of pregnant women, and between 2 and 3 % of all men of similar ages have iron deficiency anemia. Women are generally at higher risk for iron deficiency anemia because they lose iron during menstruation.

Description

Iron deficiency anemia is the most common type of anemia throughout the world. In the United States, iron deficiency anemia occurs to a lesser extent than in developing countries because of the higher consumption of red meat and the practice of food fortification (addition of iron to foods by manufacturers). Anemia in the United States is caused by a variety of sources, including excessive losses of iron in menstrual fluids and excessive bleeding in the gastrointestinal tract. The condition can also be produced by **lead poisoning**, often in children ingesting lead-based paints while playing. In developing countries located in tropical climates, the most common cause of iron deficiency anemia is infestation with hookworm.

Risks

The following groups have more chance of getting iron deficiency anemia than other groups: women, infants and children, and people with certain medical conditions. The following are factors that can contribute to increased risk of getting iron deficiency anemia: **pregnancy** (additional iron is needed for support of the fetus), heavy menstrual periods (which depletes iron in the body), low iron diet (such as vegetarian **diets** in which iron in allowed foods, such as vegetables, are not absorbed as well as iron in not-allowed foods, such as meat), and internal bleeding (such as from an ulcer or polyps). Donating blood and eating unhealthy foods on a regular basis are also other ways to increase one' risk of iron deficiency anemia.

Causes and symptoms

Infancy is a period of increased risk for iron deficiency. The human infant is born with a built-in supply of iron, which can be tapped during periods of drinking low-iron milk or formula. Both human milk and cow milk contain rather low levels of iron (0.5–1.0 milligrams of iron per liter [mg iron/L]). However, the iron in human milk is about 50% absorbed by the infant, while the iron of cow milk is only 10% absorbed. During the first six months of life, growth of the infant is made possible by the milk in the diet and by the infant's built-in supply. However, premature infants have a lower supply of iron and, for this reason, it is recommended that pre-term infants (beginning at 2 months of age) be given oral supplements of 7 mg iron/day, as ferrous sulfate. Iron deficiency can be provoked where infants are fed formulas that are based on unfortified cow milk. For example, unfortified cow milk is given free of charge to mothers in Chile. This practice has the fortunate result of preventing general **malnutrition**, but the unfortunate result of allowing the development of mild iron deficiency.

The normal rate of blood loss in the feces is 0.5–1.0 milliliter per day (mL/day). These losses can increase with colorectal **cancer**. About 60% of colorectal cancers result in further blood losses, where the extent of blood loss is 2–10 mL/day. Cancer of the colon and rectum can provoke losses of blood, resulting in iron deficiency anemia. The fecal blood test is widely used to screen for the presence of cancer of the colon or rectum. In the absence of testing, colorectal cancer may be first detected because of the resulting iron deficiency anemia.

Infection with hookworm can provoke iron deficiency and iron deficiency anemia. The hookworm is a parasitic worm. It thrives in warm climates, including in the southern United States. The hookworm enters the body through the skin, as through bare feet. The hookworm then migrates to the small intestines where it attaches itself to the villi (small sausage-shaped structures in the intestines that are used for the absorption of all nutrients). The hookworm provokes damage to the villi, which results in blood loss. They also produce anti-coagulants, which promote continued bleeding. Each worm can provoke the loss of up to 0.25 mL of blood per day.

Bleeding and blood losses through gastrointestinal tract can be provoked by colorectal cancer and hookworms, as mentioned above, but also by **hemorrhoids**, anal fissures, **irritable bowel syndrome**, aspirin-induced bleeding, blood clotting disorders, and **diverticulosis** (a condition caused by an abnormal opening from the intestine or bladder). Several genetic diseases exist which lead to bleeding disorders, and these include **hemophilia** A, hemophilia B, and von Willebrand's disease. Of these, only von Willebrand's disease leads to gastrointestinal bleeding.

The symptoms of iron deficiency anemia include weakness and **fatigue**. These symptoms result because of the lack of function of the red blood cells, and the reduced ability of the red blood cells to carry iron to exercising muscles. Iron deficiency can also affect other tissues, including the tongue and fingernails. Prolonged iron deficiency can result in changes of the tongue; such as, it may become smooth, shiny, and reddened. This condition is called glossitis. The tongue may also become sore and inflamed. The fingernails may grow abnormally, acquiring a spoon-shaped appearance. They may also grow out brittle in texture and appearance.

The whites of the eyes may appear bluish in color. Other symptoms can include irritability, **headache**, cravings of food and other unusual substances while generally having a overall poor appetite, pale skin color, **shortness of breath**, irregular heartbeat, dizziness/lightheadedness, cold feeling of the extremities (hands and feet), and irritability. If iron deficiency anemia is mild, however, symptoms may not appear. Symptoms begin to show up as the condition worsens.

Decreased iron intake is a contributing factor in iron deficiency and iron deficiency anemia. The iron content of cabbage, for example, is about 1.6 milligrams per kilogram (1.6 mg/kg) food, while that of spinach (33 mg/kg), lima beans (15 mg/kg), potatoes (14 mg/kg), tomatoes (3 mg/kg), apples (1.5 mg/kg), raisins (20 mg/kg), whole wheat bread (43 mg/kg), eggs (20 mg/kg), canned tuna (13 mg/kg), chicken (11 mg/kg), beef (28 mg/kg), corn oil (0.6 mg/kg), and peanut butter (6.0 mg/kg), are indicated. One can see that apples, tomatoes, and vegetable oil are relatively low in iron, while whole wheat bread, spinach, and beef are relatively high in iron. The assessment of whether a food is low or high in iron can also be made by comparing the amount of that food eaten per day with the recommended dietary allowance (RDA), which is part of the Dietary Reference Intakes (DRIs), for iron. The RDA for iron for the adult male (19 to 50 years of age) is 8 milligram per day (mg/day), while that for the adult woman (of the same age range) is 18 mg/day. For adult males and females (51 years and older) the RDA for iron is 8 mg/day. The RDA during pregnancy is 27 mg/day. The RDA for infants of 7 to 12 months of age is 11 mg/day, for children 1 to 3 years of age it is 7 mg/day, for children 4 to 8 years it is 10 mg/day, for children 9 to 13 years it is 8 mg/day, and for children 14 to 18 years it is 11 mg/day for males and 15 mg/day for females. The RDA values are based on the assumption that the consumer eats a mixture of plant and animal foods.

The above list of iron values alone may be deceptive, since the availability of iron in fruits, vegetables, and grains is very low, while that the availability from meat is much higher. The availability of iron in plants ranges from only 1–10%, while that in meat, fish, chicken, and liver is 20–30%. The term availability means the percent of dietary iron that is absorbed via the gastrointestinal tract to the bloodstream. Non-absorbed iron is lost in the feces.

Interactions between various foods can influence the absorption of dietary iron. Vitamin C can increase the absorption of dietary iron. Orange juice is a rich source of vitamin C. Thus, if a plant food, such as rice, is consumed with orange juice, then the orange juice can enhance the absorption of the iron of the rice. Vitamin C is also added to infant formulas, and the increased use of formulas fortified with both iron and vitamin C has led to a marked decline in anemia in infants and young children in the United States. In contrast, if rice is consumed with tea, certain chemicals in the tea (tannins) can reduce the absorption of the iron. Phytic acid is a chemical that naturally occurs in legumes, cereals, and nuts. Phytic acid, which can account for 1–5% of the weight of these foods, is a potent inhibitor of iron absorption. The increased availability of the iron in meat products is partly due to the fact that heme-iron is absorbed to a greater extent than free iron salts, and to a greater extent than iron in the phytic acid/iron complex. Nearly all of the iron in plants is nonheme-iron. Much of the iron in meat is nonheme-iron as well. The nonheme-iron in meat, fish, chicken and liver may be about 20% available. The heme-iron of meat may be close to 30% available. The most available source of iron is human milk (50% availability).

KEY TERMS

Hematocrit—The proportion of whole blood in the body, by volume, that is composed of red blood cells.

Hemoglobin—An iron-containing protein that resides within red blood cells. Hemoglobin accounts for about 95% of the protein in the red blood cell.

Protoporphyrin IX—A protein. The measurement of this protein is useful for the assessment of iron status. Hemoglobin consists of a complex of a protein plus heme. Heme consists of iron plus protoporphyrin IX. Normally, during the course of red blood cell formation, protoporphyrin IX acquires iron, to generate heme, and the heme becomes incorporated into hemoglobin. However, in iron deficiency, protophoryrin IX builds up.

Recommended Dietary Allowance (RDA)—The quantities of nutrients of the diet that are required to maintain human health. RDAs are established by the Food and Nutrition Board of the National Academy of Sciences and may be revised every few years.

Diagnosis

Iron deficiency anemia in infants is defined as a hemoglobin level below 109 mg/mL of whole blood, and a **hematocrit** (percentage of blood volume with respect to red blood cells) of under 33%. Anemia in adult males is defined as a hemoglobin under 130 mg/mL and a hematocrit of under 39%. Anemia in adult females is defined as hemoglobin under 120 mg/mL and a hematocrit of under 35%. Anemia in pregnant women is defined as hemoglobin of under 110 mg/mL and hematocrit of under 31%.

When an abnormally high presence of blood is found in the feces during a **fecal occult blood test**, the physician needs to examine the gastrointestinal tract to determine the cause of bleeding. Here, the diagnosis for iron deficiency anemia includes the examination using a sigmoidoscope. The sigmoidoscope is an instrument that consists of a flexible tube that permits examination of the colon to a distance of 60 centimeters (cm). A **barium enema**, with an x ray, may also be used to detect abnormalities that can cause bleeding.

The diagnosis of iron deficiency anemia should include a test for oral iron absorption, where evidence suggests that oral iron supplements fail in treating anemia. The oral iron absorption test is conducted by eating 64 mg iron (325 mg ferrous sulfate) in a single dose. Blood samples are then taken after 2 hours and 4 hours. The iron content of the blood serum is then measured. The concentration of iron should rise by an increment of about 22 micromolar, where iron absorption is normal. Lesser increases in concentration mean that iron absorption is abnormal, and that therapy should involve injections or infusions of iron.

Treatment

Oral iron supplements (pills) may contain various iron salts. These iron salts include ferrous sulfate, ferrous gluconate, or ferrous fumarate. These pills are most effective if they are taken on an empty stomach. Milk and **antacids** should not be taken with such pills. However, vitamin C, such as in orange juice, increases the absorption of iron. Injections and infusions of iron can be carried out with a preparation called iron dextran. In patients with poor iron absorption (by the gut), therapy with injection or infusion is preferable over oral supplements. Intravenous injections are often made into a vein or muscle. Treatment of iron deficiency anemia sometimes requires more than therapy with iron. Where hemorrhoids provoke iron deficiency, surgery may prove essential to prevent recurrent iron deficiency anemia. Where iron deficiency is provoked by bleeding due to **aspirin** treatment, aspirin should be discontinued. Where iron deficiency is provoked by hookworm infections, therapy for this parasite should be used, along with protection of the feet by wearing shoes whenever walking in hookworm-infested soil.

Prognosis

The prognosis for treating and curing iron deficiency anemia is excellent. Perhaps the main problem is failure to take iron supplements. With adequate treatments most cases of iron deficiency anemia goes away in a few weeks. In cases of pregnant women, the health care worker may recommend taking 100–200 mg iron/day. This dose is rather high, and can lead to **nausea**, **diarrhea**, or abdominal **pain** in 10–20% of women taking this dose. The reason for using this high dose is to affect a rapid cure for anemia, where the anemia is detected at a mid-point during the pregnancy. The above problems of side effects and noncompliance can be avoided by taking iron doses (100–200 mg) only once a week, where supplements are initiated some time prior to conception, or continuously throughout the fertile period of life. The problem of compliance is not an issue where infusions are used, however a fraction of patients treated with iron infusions experience side effects, such as flushing, headache, nausea, **anaphylaxis**, or seizures. A number of studies have shown that iron deficiency anemia in infancy can result in reduced intelligence, where intelligence was measured in early childhood. It is not certain if iron supplementation of children with reduced intelligence, due to iron-deficiency anemia in infancy, has any influence in allowing a "catch-up" in intellectual development.

If left untreated, iron deficiency anemia can lead to heart problems such as irregular or rapid heartbeat (as the heart tries to pump more blood that contains less oxygen) or **angina** (chest pains that occur then the heart does not receive sufficient oxygenated blood). It can also cause complications during pregnancy in women and delayed mental and physical growth spurts in children.

Prevention

In the healthy population, all of the mineral deficiencies can be prevented by the consumption of inorganic nutrients at levels defined by the RDA. Iron deficiency anemia in infants and young children can be prevented by the use of fortified foods. Liquid cow milk-based infant formulas are generally supplemented with iron (12 mg/L). The iron in liquid formulas is added as ferrous sulfate or ferrous gluconate. Commercial infant cereals are also fortified with iron, and here small particles of elemental iron are added. The levels used are about 0.5 gram iron/kg dry cereal. This amount of iron is about 10-fold greater than that of the iron naturally present in the cereal. Foods that are rich in iron include, poultry, red meat (such as liver), pork, seafood, egg yolks, whole-grain breads, raisins, legumes (such as beans and peas), dark green leafy vegetables (such as spinach), nuts and seeds and dried fruits (such as apricots and raisins). Many other foods are fortified with iron (such as breakfast foods).

Resources

BOOKS

Null, Gary, and Amy McDonald, eds. *Be a Healthy Woman!* New York: Seven Stories Press, 2009.

Rosenfeld, Gary C. and David S. Loose. *Pharmacology*. Philadelphia: Wolters Kluwer Health/Lippincott Williams and Wilkins, 2010.

Shils, Maurice, et al., eds. *Modern Nutrition in Health and Disease*. Philadelphia: Lippincott Williams and Wilkins, 2006.

OTHER

" Dietary Supplement Fact Sheet: Iron." Office of Dietary Supplements, National Institutes of Health. (August 24, 2007), http://ods.od.nih.gov/factsheets/iron. asp. (accessed July 17, 2010).

"Iron Deficiency Anemia." Mayo Clinic. (March 24, 2009), www.mayoclinic.com/health/iron-deficiency-anemia/DS00323. (accessed July 17, 2010).

"Iron Deficiency Anemia." Medline Plus, National Library of Medicine and National Institutes of Health. (March 21, 2010), www.nlm.nih.gov/medlineplus/ency/article/000584.htm. (accessed July 17, 2010).

Tom Brody, PhD

Iron overload *see* **Hemochromatosis**

Iron tests

Definition

Iron tests are a group of blood tests that are done to evaluate the iron level in blood serum, the body's capacity to absorb iron, and the amount of iron actually stored in the body. Iron is an essential trace element; it is necessary for the formation of red blood cells and certain enzymes. At the other extreme, high levels of iron can be poisonous.

Purpose

There are four different types of tests that measure the body's iron levels and storage. They are called iron level tests, total iron-binding capacity (TIBC) tests, ferritin tests, and transferrin tests. These tests are given for several reasons:

- To help in the differential diagnosis of different types of anemia.
- To assess the severity of anemia and monitor the treatment of patients with chronic anemia.
- To evaluate protein depletion and other forms of malnutrition.
- To check for certain liver disorders.
- To evaluate the possibility of chronic gastrointestinal bleeding. Blood loss from the digestive tract is a common cause of iron deficiency anemia.
- To help diagnose certain unusual disorders, including iron poisoning, thalassemia, hemosiderosis, and hemochromatosis.

A serum iron test can be used without the others to evaluate cases of iron **poisoning**.

Precautions

Patients should not have their blood tested for iron within four days of a blood **transfusion** or tests and treatments that use radioactive materials. Recent high **stress** levels or **sleep deprivation** are additional reasons for postponing iron tests.

Blood samples for iron tests should be taken early in the morning because serum iron levels vary during the day. This precaution is especially important in evaluating the results of iron replacement therapy.

Description

Iron tests are performed on samples of the patient's blood, withdrawn from a vein into a vacuum tube. The amount of blood taken is between 6 mL and 10 mL (1/3 of a fluid ounce). The procedure, which is called a venipuncture, takes about five minutes.

Iron level test

The iron level test measures the amount of iron in the blood serum that is being carried by a protein (transferrin) in the blood plasma.

Medications and substances that can cause *increased* iron levels include chloramphenicol, estrogen preparations, dietary iron supplements, alcoholic beverages, methyldopa, and birth control pills.

Medications that can cause *decreased* iron levels include ACTH, colchicine, deferoxamine, methicillin, and testosterone.

Total iron-binding capacity (TIBC) test

The TIBC test measures the amount of iron that the blood would carry if the transferrin were fully saturated. Since transferrin is produced by the liver, the TIBC can be used to monitor liver function and **nutrition**.

Medications that can cause *increased* TIBC levels include fluorides and birth control pills.

Medications that can cause *decreased* TIBC levels include chloramphenicol and ACTH.

Transferrin test

The transferrin test is a direct measurement of transferrin–which is also called siderophilin–levels in the blood. Some laboratories prefer this measurement to the TIBC. The saturation level of the transferrin can be calculated by dividing the serum iron level by the TIBC.

Ferritin test

The ferritin test measures the level of a protein in the blood that stores iron for later use by the body.

Medications that can cause *increased* ferritin levels include dietary iron supplements. In addition, some diseases that do not directly affect the body's iron storage can cause artificially high ferritin levels. These disorders include infections, late-stage cancers, lymphomas, and severe inflammations. Alcoholics often have high ferritin levels.

Preparation

Patient history

Before patients are tested for iron, they should be checked for any of the following factors:

- Prescription medications that affect iron levels, absorption, or storage
- Blood transfusion or radioactive medications within the last four days
- Recent extreme stress or sleep deprivation
- Recent eating habits. Test results can be affected by eating large amounts of iron-rich foods shortly before the blood test.

Fasting

Patients scheduled for an iron level, TIBC, or transferrin test should fast for 12 hours before the blood is drawn. They are allowed to drink water. Patients scheduled for a ferritin test do not need to fast but they should not have any alcoholic beverages before the test.

Aftercare

Aftercare consists of routine care of the area around the venipuncture.

Risks

The primary risk is the possibility of a bruise or swelling in the area of the venipuncture. The patient can apply moist warm compresses if there is any discomfort.

Normal results

Iron level test

Normal serum iron values are as follows:

- Adult males: 75–175 micrograms/dL
- Adult females: 65–165 micrograms/dL
- Children: 50–120 micrograms/dL
- Newborns: 100–250 micrograms/dL.

KEY TERMS

Anemia—A disorder marked by low hemoglobin levels in red blood cells, which leads to a deficiency of oxygen in the blood.

Ferritin—A protein found in the liver, spleen, and bone marrow that stores iron.

Hemochromatosis—A disorder of iron absorption characterized by bronze-colored skin. It can cause painful joints, diabetes, and liver damage if the iron concentration is not lowered.

Hemosiderosis—An overload of iron in the body resulting from repeated blood transfusions. Hemosiderosis occurs most often in patients with thalassemia.

Iron poisoning—A potentially fatal condition caused by swallowing large amounts of iron dietary supplements. Most cases occur in children who have taken adult- strength iron formulas. The symptoms of iron poisoning include vomiting, bloody diarrhea, convulsions, low blood pressure, and turning blue.

Plasma—The liquid part of blood.

Siderophilin—Another name for transferrin.

Thalassemia—A hereditary form of anemia that occurs most frequently in people of Mediterranean origin.

Transferrin—A protein in blood plasma that carries iron derived from food intake to the liver, spleen, and bone marrow.

TIBC test

Normal TIBC values are as follows:

- Adult males: 300–400 micrograms/dL
- Adult females: 300–450 micrograms/dL.

Transferrin test

Normal transferrin values are as follows:

- Adult males: 200–400 mg/dL
- Adult females: 200–400 mg/dL
- Children: 203–360 mg/dL
- Newborns: 130–275 mg/dL.

Normal transferrin saturation values are between 30–40%.

Ferritin test

Normal ferritin values are as follows:

- Adult males: 20–300 ng/mL
- Adult females: 20–120 ng/mL
- Children (one month): 200–600 ng/mL
- Children (two to five months): 50–200 ng/mL
- Children (six months to 15 years): 7–140 ng/mL
- Newborns: 25–200 ng/mL.

Abnormal results

Iron level test

Serum iron level is *increased* in **thalassemia**, **hemochromatosis**, severe hepatitis, **liver disease**, **lead poisoning**, acute leukemia, and **kidney disease**. It is also increased by multiple blood transfusions and intramuscular iron injections.

Iron levels above 350–500 micrograms/dL are considered toxic; levels over 1000 micrograms/dL indicate severe iron poisoning.

Serum iron level is *decreased* in **iron deficiency anemia**, chronic blood loss, chronic diseases (lupus, **rheumatoid arthritis**), late **pregnancy**, chronically heavy menstrual periods, and thyroid deficiency.

TIBC test

The TIBC is *increased* in iron deficiency anemia, **polycythemia vera**, pregnancy, blood loss, severe hepatitis, and the use of birth control pills.

The TIBC is *decreased* in **malnutrition**, severe **burns**, hemochromatosis, anemia caused by infections and chronic diseases, **cirrhosis** of the liver, and kidney disease.

Transferrin test

Transferrin is *increased* in iron deficiency anemia, pregnancy, **hormone replacement therapy** (HRT), and the use of birth control pills.

Transferrin is *decreased* in protein deficiency, liver damage, malnutrition, severe burns, kidney disease, chronic infections, and certain genetic disorders.

Ferritin test

Ferritin is *increased* in liver disease, iron overload from hemochromatosis, certain types of anemia, acute leukemia, Hodgkin's disease, **breast cancer**, thalassemia, infections, inflammatory diseases, and hemosiderosis.

Ferritin levels may be normal or slightly above normal in patients with kidney disease.

Ferritin is *decreased* in chronic iron deficiency and severe protein depletion.

Resources

BOOKS

Pagana, Kathleen Deska, and Timothy J. Pagana.*Mosby's Manual of Diagnostic and Laboratory Tests.* 4th ed. St. Louis: Mosby, 2009.

Rebecca J. Frey, PhD

Irregular bite *see* **Malocclusion**

Irritable bowel syndrome

Definition

Irritable bowel syndrome (IBS) is a common intestinal condition characterized by abdominal **pain** and cramps; changes in bowel movements (**diarrhea**, **constipation**, or both); gassiness; bloating; **nausea**; and other symptoms. There is no cure for IBS. Much about the condition remains unknown or poorly understood; however, dietary changes, drugs, and psychological treatment are often able to eliminate or substantially reduce its symptoms.

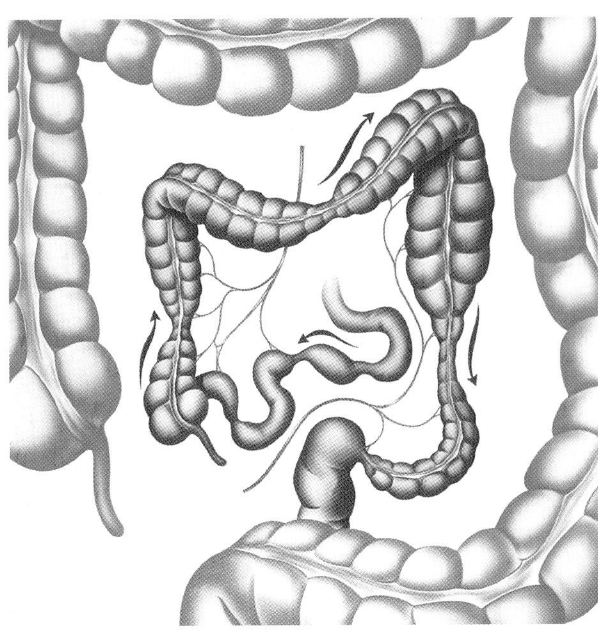

Normal and diseased (center) colons. Areas of constriction in the colon cause constipation, while areas of distention cause diarrhea. *(Custom Medical Stock Photo, Inc. Reproduced by permission.)*

Demographics

No one knows for sure how many Americans suffer from IBS. Surveys indicate a range of 10–20%, with perhaps as many as 30% of Americans experiencing IBS at some point in their lives. IBS normally makes its first appearance during young adulthood, and in half of all cases symptoms begin before age 35. Women with IBS outnumber men by two to one, for reasons that are not yet understood. IBS is responsible for more time lost from work and school than any medical problem other than the **common cold**. It accounts for more than half of all the patients seen by specialists in diseases of the digestive system (gastroenterologists). Yet only half–possibly as few as 15%–of IBS sufferers ever consult a doctor.

Description

IBS is the name people use today for a condition that was once called–among other things–colitis, mucous **colitis**, spastic colon, nervous colon, spastic bowel, and functional bowel disorder. Some of these names reflected the now outdated belief that IBS is a purely psychological disorder, a product of the patient's imagination. Although modern medicine recognizes that **stress** can trigger IBS attacks, medical specialists agree that IBS is a genuine physical disorder–or group of disorders–with specific identifiable characteristics.

Causes and symptoms

Symptoms

The symptoms of IBS tend to rise and fall in intensity rather than growing steadily worse over time. They always include abdominal pain, which may be relieved by defecation; diarrhea or constipation; or diarrhea alternating with constipation. Other symptoms–which vary from person to person–include cramps; gassiness; bloating; nausea; a powerful and uncontrollable urge to defecate (urgency); passage of a sticky fluid (mucus) during bowel movements; or the feeling after finishing a bowel movement that the bowels are still not completely empty. The accepted diagnostic criteria–known as the Rome criteria–require at least three months of continuous or recurrent symptoms before IBS can be confirmed. According to Christine B. Dalton and Douglas A. Drossman in the *American Family Physician,* an estimated 70% of IBS cases can be described as "mild;" 25% as "moderate;" and 5% as "severe." In mild cases the symptoms are slight. As a general rule, they are not present all the time and do not interfere with work and other normal activities. Moderate IBS occasionally disrupts normal activities and may cause some psychological problems. People with severe IBS often find living a normal life impossible and experience crippling psychological problems as a result. For some the physical pain is constant and intense.

Causes

Researchers remain unsure about the cause or causes of IBS. It is called a functional disorder because it is thought to result from changes in the activity of the major part of the large intestine (the colon). After food is digested by the stomach and small intestine, the undigested material passes in liquid form into the colon, which absorbs water and salts. This process may take several days. In a healthy person the colon is quiet during most of that period except after meals, when its muscles contract in a series of wavelike movements called peristalsis. Peristalsis helps absorption by bringing the undigested material into contact with the colon wall. It also pushes undigested material that has been converted into solid or semisolid feces toward the rectum, where it remains until defecation. In IBS, however, the normal rhythm and intensity of peristalsis is disrupted. Sometimes there is too little peristalsis, which can slow the passage of undigested material through the colon and cause constipation. Sometimes there is too much, which has the opposite effect and causes diarrhea. A Johns Hopkins University study found that healthy volunteers experienced 6–8 contractions of the colon each day, compared with up to 25 contractions a day for volunteers suffering from IBS with diarrhea, and an almost complete absence of contractions among constipated IBS volunteers. In addition to differences in the number of contractions, many of the IBS volunteers experienced powerful spasmodic contractions affecting a larger-than-normal area of the colon–"like having a Charlie horse in the gut," according to one of the investigators.

DIET. Some kinds of food and drink appear to play a key role in triggering IBS attacks. Food and drink that healthy people can ingest without any trouble may disrupt peristalsis in IBS patients, which probably explains why IBS attacks often occur shortly after meals. Chocolate, milk products, **caffeine** (in coffee, tea, colas, and other drinks), and large quantities of alcohol are some of the chief culprits. Other kinds of food have also been identified as problems, however, and the pattern of what can and cannot be tolerated is different for each person. Characteristically, IBS symptoms rarely occur at night and disrupt the patient's sleep.

STRESS. Stress is an important factor in IBS because of the close nervous system connections between the brain and the intestines. Although researchers do not yet understand all of the links between changes in the nervous system and IBS, they point out the similarities between mild digestive upsets and IBS. Just as healthy people can feel nauseated or have an upset stomach when under stress, people with IBS react the same way, but to a greater degree. Finally, IBS symptoms sometimes intensify during menstruation, which suggests that female reproductive hormones are another trigger.

Diagnosis

Diagnosing IBS is a fairly complex task because the disorder does not produce changes that can be identified during a **physical examination** or by laboratory tests. When IBS is suspected, the doctor (who can be either a family doctor or a specialist) needs to determine whether the patient's symptoms satisfy the Rome criteria. The doctor must rule out other conditions that resemble IBS, such as **Crohn's disease** and ulcerative colitis. These disorders are ruled out by questioning the patient about his or her physical and mental health (the medical history), performing a physical examination, and ordering laboratory tests. Normally the patient is asked to provide a stool sample that can be tested for blood and intestinal parasites. In some cases x rays or an internal examination of the colon using a flexible instrument inserted through the anus (a sigmoidoscope or colonoscope) is necessary. The doctor also may ask the patient to try a lactose-free diet for two or three weeks to see whether **lactose intolerance** is causing the symptoms.

Treatment

Dietary changes, sometimes supplemented by drugs or **psychotherapy**, are considered the key to successful treatment. The following approach, offered by Dalton and Drossman, is typical of the advice found in the medical literature on IBS. The authors tie their approach to the severity of the patient's symptoms:

Mild symptoms

Dalton and Drossman recommend a low-fat, high-fiber diet. Problem-causing substances such as lactose, caffeine, beans, cabbage, cucumbers, broccoli, fatty foods, alcohol, and medications should be identified and avoided. Bran or 15-25 grams a day of an over-the-counter psyllium laxative (Metamucil or Fiberall) may also help both constipation and

KEY TERMS

Anus—The opening at the lower end of the rectum.

Crohn's disease—A disease characterized by inflammation of the intestines. Its early symptoms may resemble those of IBS.

Defecation—Passage of feces through the anus.

Feces—Undigested food and other waste that is eliminated through the anus. Feces are also called fecal matter or stools.

Lactose—A sugar found in milk and milk products. Some people are lactose intolerant, meaning they have trouble digesting lactose. Lactose intolerance can produce symptoms resembling those of IBS.

Peristalsis—The periodic waves of muscular contractions that move food through the intestines during the process of digestion.

Ulcerative colitis—A disease that inflames and causes breaks (ulcers) in the colon and rectum, which are parts of the large intestine.

diarrhea. The patient can still have milk or milk products if lactose intolerance is not a problem. People with irregular bowel habits–particularly constipated patients–may be helped by establishing set times for meals and bathroom visits.

Moderate symptoms

The advice given by Dalton and Drossman in mild cases applies here as well. They also suggest that patients keep a diary of symptoms for two or three weeks, covering daily activities including meals, and emotional responses to events. The doctor can then review the diary with the patient to identify possible problem areas.

Although a high-fiber diet remains the standard treatment for constipated patients, such **laxatives** as lactulose (Chronulac) or sorbitol may be prescribed. Loperamide (Imodium) and cholestyramine (Questran) are suggested for diarrhea. Abdominal pain after meals can be reduced by taking **antispasmodic drugs** such as hyoscyamine (Anaspaz, Cystospaz, or Levsin) or dicyclomine (Bemote, Bentyl, or Di-Spaz) before eating.

Dalton and Drossman also suggest psychological counseling or behavioral therapy for some patients to reduce **anxiety** and to learn to cope with the pain and other symptoms of IBS. Relaxation therapy, hypnosis, **biofeedback**, and **cognitive-behavioral therapy** are examples of behavioral therapy.

Severe symptoms

When IBS produces constant pain that interferes with everyday life, **antidepressant drugs** can help by blocking pain transmission from the nervous system. Dalton and Drossman also underscore the importance of an ongoing and supportive doctor-patient relationship.

Alternative treatment

Alternative and mainstream approaches to IBS treatment overlap to a certain extent. Like mainstream doctors, alternative practitioners advise a high-fiber diet to reduce digestive system irritation. They also suggest avoiding alcohol, caffeine, and fatty, gassy, or spicy foods. Recommended stress management techniques include **yoga**, **meditation**, hypnosis, biofeedback, and **reflexology**. Reflexology is a technique of foot massage that is thought to relieve diarrhea, constipation, and other IBS symptoms.

Alternative medicine also emphasizes such herbal remedies as ginger (*Zingiber officinale*), buckthorn (*Rhamnus purshiana*), and enteric-coated peppermint oil. Enteric coating prevents digestion until the peppermint oil reaches the small intestine, thus avoiding irritation of the upper part of the digestive tract. Chamomile (*Matricaria recutita*), valerian (*Valeriana officinalis*), rosemary (*Rosemarinus officinalis*), lemon balm (*Melissa officinalis*), and other herbs are recommended for their antispasmodic properties. The list of alternative treatments for IBS is in fact quite long. It includes **aromatherapy**, homeopathy, **hydrotherapy**, juice therapy, **acupuncture**, **chiropractic**, **osteopathy**, **naturopathic medicine**, and Chinese traditional herbal medicine.

Prognosis

IBS is not a life-threatening condition. It does not cause intestinal bleeding or inflammation, nor does it cause other bowel diseases or **cancer**. Although IBS can last a lifetime, in up to 30% of cases the symptoms eventually disappear, and symptoms decrease significantly with treatment in about 60%. Even if the symptoms cannot be eliminated, with appropriate treatment they can usually be brought under control to the point where IBS becomes merely an occasional inconvenience. Treatment requires a long-term commitment, however; six months or more may be needed before the patient notices substantial improvement.

Prevention

Because the cause of IBS is not understood, there are no definitive ways to prevent it. However, some of the following may generally improve digestion:

- Drink sufficient water, about 8 glasses per day
- Follow a high-fiber diet
- Avoid foods that make you feel uncomfortable. For some people, these include highly acidic or spicy foods, caffeinated beverages, and alcohol.
- Physical activity can help improve digestion
- Learn to avoid and cope with stress in your life
- Eating many small meals a day is preferable to eating fewer very larfge meals
- Be aware of medications that you may take that could cause constipation, or irritate your stomach

Resources

BOOKS

Berkowitz, Jonathan M. *A Victim No More: Overcoming Irritable Bowel Syndrome: Safe, Effective Therapies for Relief From Bowel Complaints*. North Bergen, NJ: Basic Health Publications, 2003.

Dean, Carolyn and L. Christine Wheeler. *IBS for Dummies*. Hoboken, NJ: Wiley Pub., 2006.

Feldman, M, et al. *Sleisenger & Fordtran's Gastrointestinal and Liver Disease*. 8th ed. St. Louis: Mosby, 2005.

Nicol, Rosemary. *Irritable Bowel Syndrome: A Natural Approach*. Berkeley, CA: Ulysses Press, 2007

Peikin, Steven R. *Gastrointestinal Health: The Proven Nutritional Program to Prevent, Cure, or Alleviate Irritable Bowel Syndrome (IBS), Ulcers, Gas, Constipation, Heartburn, and Many Other Digestive Disorders*. rev ed. New York, NY: Perennial Currents, 2004.

Talley, Nicholas J. *Conquering Irritable Bowel Syndrome: A Guide to Liberating Those Suffering with Chronic Stomach or Bowel Problems*. Hamilton, Ontario: BC Decker, 2006.

OTHER

El-Baba, Mohammad F. "Irritable Bowel Syndrome." eMedicine.com, April 4, 2007. http://www.emedicine.com/ped/topic1210.htm

International Foundation for Functional Gastrointestinal Disorders "Frequently Asked Questions." April 9, 2007. http://www.aboutibs.org/site/about-ibs/faq

Lichtenstein, Gary R. and Jenifer K. Leher. "Irritable Bowel Syndrome." eMedicineHealth.com, October 26, 2005. http://www.emedicinehealth.com/irritable_bowel_syndrome/article_em.htm

Mayo Clinic Staff. "Irritable Bowel Syndrome." MayoClinic.com, April 10, 2007. http://www.mayoclinic.com/health/irritable-bowel-syndrome/DS00106

Medline Plus. "Irritable Bowel Syndrome." U. S. National Library of Medicine, April 11, 2007. http://www.nlm.nih/gov/medlineplus/irritablebowelsyndrome .html

National Digestive Diseases Information Clearinghouse (NDDIC). "Irritable Bowel Syndrome." February 2006. http://digestive.niddk.nih.gov/ddiseases/pubs/ibs

ORGANIZATIONS

American College of Gastroenterology, P.O. Box 342260, Bethesda, MD, 20827-2260, (301) 263-9000, http://www.acg.gi.org.

American Gastroenterological Association, 4930 Del Ray Avenue, Bethesda, MD, 20814, (301) 654-2055, (301) 654-5920, http://www.gastro.org.

IBS Self Help and Support Group, 1440 Whalley Avenue, New Haven, CT, 06515, http://www.ibsgroup.org.

International Foundation for Functional Gastrointestinal Disorders, P. O. Box 170864, Milwaukee, WI, 53217, (888) 964-2001, (414) 964-7176, http://www.iffgd.org.

National Digestive Diseases Information Clearinghouse (NDDIC), 2 Information Way, Bethesda, MD, 20892-3570, (800) 891-5389, (703) 738-4929, http://digestive.niddk.nih.gov.

Howard Baker

Ischemia

Definition

Ischemia is an insufficient supply of blood to an organ, usually due to a blocked artery.

Description

Myocardial ischemia is an intermediate condition in **coronary artery disease** during which the heart tissue is slowly or suddenly starved of oxygen and other nutrients. Eventually, the affected heart tissue will die. When blood flow is completely blocked to the heart, ischemia can lead to a **heart attack**. Ischemia can be silent or symptomatic. According to the American Heart Association, up to four million Americans may have silent ischemia and be at high risk of having a heart attack with no warning.

Symptomatic ischemia is characterized by chest **pain** called **angina** pectoris. The American Heart

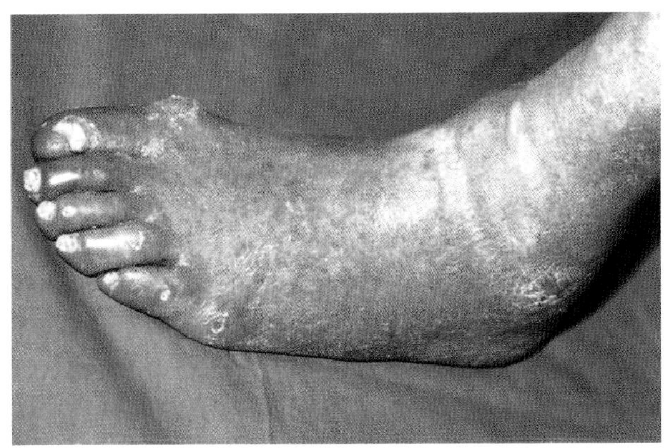

This patient's foot is affected with ischemia. Ischemia occurs when there is an insufficient supply of blood to a specific organ or tissue. *(Dr. P. Marazzi/Photo Researchers, Inc.)*

Association estimates that nearly seven million Americans have angina pectoris, usually called angina. Angina occurs more frequently in women than in men, and in blacks and Hispanics more than in whites. It also occurs more frequently as people age–25% of women over the age of 85 and 27% of men who are 80–84 years old have angina.

People with angina are at risk of having a heart attack. Stable angina occurs during exertion, can be quickly relieved by resting or taking nitroglycerine, and lasts from three to twenty minutes. Unstable angina, which increases the risk of a heart attack, occurs more frequently, lasts longer, is more severe, and may cause discomfort during rest or light exertion.

Ischemia can also occur in the arteries of the brain, where blockages can lead to a **stroke**. About 80–85% of all strokes are ischemic. Most blockages in the cerebral arteries are due to a blood clot, often in an artery narrowed by plaque. Sometimes, a blood clot in the heart or aorta travels to a cerebral artery. A **transient ischemic attack** (TIA) is a "mini-stroke" caused by a temporary deficiency of blood supply to the brain. It occurs suddenly, lasts a few minutes to a few hours, and is a strong warning sign of an impending stroke. Ischemia can also effect intestines, legs, feet and kidneys. Pain, malfunctions, and damage in those areas may result.

Causes and symptoms

Ischemia is almost always caused by blockage of an artery, usually due to atherosclerotic plaque. Myocardial ischemia is also caused by **blood clots** (which tend to form on plaque), artery spasms or contractions, or any of these factors combined. Silent ischemia is usually caused by emotional or mental **stress** or by exertion, but there are no symptoms. Angina is usually caused by increased oxygen demand when the heart is working harder than usual, for example, during **exercise**, or during mental or physical stress. According to researchers at Harvard University, physical stress is harder on the heart than mental stress. A TIA is caused by a blood clot briefly blocking a cerebral artery.

Risk factors

The risk factors for myocardial ischemia are the same as those for coronary artery disease. For TIA, coronary artery disease is also a risk factor.

- Heredity. People whose parents have coronary artery disease are more likely to develop it. African Americans are also at higher risk.
- Sex. Men are more likely to have heart attacks than women, and to have them at a younger age.
- Age. Men who are 45 years of age and older and women who are 55 years of age and older are considered to be at risk.
- Smoking. Smoking increases both the chance of developing coronary artery disease and the chance of dying from it. Second hand smoke may also increase risk.
- High cholesterol. Risk of developing coronary artery disease increases as blood cholesterol levels increase. When combined with other factors, the risk is even greater.
- High blood pressure. High blood pressure makes the heart work harder, and with time, weakens it. When combined with obesity, smoking, high cholesterol, or diabetes, the risk of heart attack or stroke increases several times.
- Lack of physical activity. Lack of exercise increases the risk of coronary artery disease.
- Diabetes mellitus. The risk of developing coronary artery disease is seriously increased for diabetics.
- Obesity. Excess weight increases the strain on the heart and increases the risk of developing coronary artery disease, even if no other risk factors are present. Obesity increases blood pressure and blood cholesterol, and can lead to diabetes.
- Stress and anger. Some scientists believe that stress and anger can contribute to the development of coronary artery disease. Stress increases the heart rate and blood pressure and can injure the lining of the arteries. Angina attacks often occur after anger, as do many heart attacks and strokes.

Angina symptoms include:

- A tight, squeezing, heavy, burning, or choking pain that is usually beneath the breastbone—the pain may spread to the throat, jaw, or one arm

- A feeling of heaviness or tightness that is not painful
- A feeling similar to gas or indigestion
- Attacks brought on by exertion and relieved by rest.

If the pain or discomfort continues or intensifies, immediate medical help should be sought, ideally within 30 minutes.

TIA symptoms include:

- Sudden weakness, tingling, or numbness, usually in one arm or leg or both the arm and leg on the same side of the body, as well as sometimes in the face
- Sudden loss of coordination
- Loss of vision or double vision
- Difficulty speaking
- Vertigo and loss of balance.

Diagnosis

Diagnostic tests for myocardial ischemia include: resting, exercise, or ambulatory electrocardiograms; scintigraphic studies (radioactive heart scans); **echocardiography**; coronary **angiography**; and, rarely, **positron emission tomography**. Diagnostic tests for TIA include physician review of symptoms, **computed tomography scans** (CT scans), carotid artery ultrasound (**Doppler ultrasonography**), and **magnetic resonance imaging**. Angiography is the best test for ischemia of any organ.

An electrocardiogram (ECG) shows the heart's activity and may reveal a lack of oxygen. Electrodes covered with conducting jelly are placed on the patient's chest, arms, and legs. Impulses of the heart's activity are recorded on paper. The test takes about 10 minutes and is performed in a physician's office. About 25% of patients with angina have normal electrocardiograms. Another type of electrocardiogram, the exercise **stress test**, measures response to exertion when the patient is exercising on a treadmill or a stationary bike. It is performed in a physician's office or an exercise laboratory and takes 15 to 30 minutes. This test is more accurate than a resting ECG in diagnosing ischemia. Sometimes an ambulatory ECG is ordered. For this test, the patient wears a portable ECG machine called a Holter monitor for 12, 24, or 48 hours.

Myocardial perfusion scintigraphy and radionuclide angiography are nuclear studies involving the injection of a radioactive material (e.g., thallium) which is absorbed by healthy tissue. A gamma scintillation camera displays and records a series of images of the radioactive material's movement through the heart. Both tests are usually performed in a hospital's nuclear medicine department and take about 30 minutes to an hour. A perfusion scan is sometimes performed at the end of a stress test.

An echocardiogram uses sound waves to create an image of the heart's chambers and valves. The technician applies gel to a handheld transducer then presses it against the patient's chest. The heart's sound waves are converted into an image on a monitor. Performed in a cardiology outpatient diagnostic laboratory, the test takes 30 minutes to an hour. It can reveal abnormalities in the heart wall that indicate ischemia, but it doesn't evaluate the coronary arteries directly.

Coronary angiography is the most accurate diagnostic technique, but it is also the most invasive. It shows the heart's chambers, great vessels, and coronary arteries by using a contrast solution and x-ray technology. A moving picture is recorded of the blood flow through the coronary arteries. The patient is awake, but sedated, and connected to ECG electrodes and an intravenous line. A local anesthetic is injected. The cardiologist then inserts a catheter into a blood vessel and guides it into the heart. Coronary angiography is performed in a **cardiac catheterization** laboratory and takes from half an hour to two hours.

Positron emission tomography (PET) is a noninvasive nuclear test used to evaluate the heart tissue. A **PET** scanner traces high-energy gamma rays released from radioactive particles to provide three-dimensional images of the heart tissue. Performed at a hospital, it usually takes from one hour to one hour and 45 minutes. PET is very expensive and not widely available.

Computed tomography scans (CT scans) and magnetic resonance imaging (MRI) are computerized scanning methods. CT scanning uses a thin x-ray beam to show three-dimensional views of soft tissues. It is performed at a hospital or clinic and takes less than a minute. MRI uses a magnetic field to produce clear, cross-sectional images of soft tissues. The patient lies on a table which slides into a tunnel-like scanner. It is usually performed at a hospital and takes about 30 minutes.

Treatment

Angina is treated with drug therapy and surgery. Drugs such as nitrates, beta-blockers, and **calcium channel blockers** relieve chest pain, but they cannot clear blocked arteries. **Aspirin** helps prevent blood clots. Surgical procedures include percutaneous transluminal coronary **angioplasty** and **coronary artery bypass graft surgery**.

Nitroglycerin is the classic treatment for angina. It quickly relieves pain and discomfort by opening the coronary arteries and allowing more blood to flow to the heart. **Beta blockers** reduce the amount of oxygen required by the heart during stress. **Calcium** channel blockers help keep the arteries open and reduce blood pressure. Aspirin helps prevent blood clots from forming on plaques.

Percutaneous transluminal coronary angioplasty and coronary artery bypass graft surgery are invasive procedures which improve blood flow in the coronary arteries. Percutaneous transluminal coronary angioplasty is a non-surgical procedure in which a catheter tipped with a balloon is threaded from a blood vessel in the thigh into the blocked artery. The balloon is inflated, compressing the plaque to enlarge the blood vessel and open the blocked artery. The balloon is deflated and the catheter is removed. The procedure is performed by a cardiologist in a hospital and generally requires a two-day stay. Sometimes a metal stent is placed in the artery to prevent closing of the artery.

In coronary artery bypass graft, called bypass surgery, a detour is built around the coronary artery blockage with a healthy leg vein or chest wall artery. The healthy vein or artery then supplies oxygen-rich blood to the heart. Bypass surgery is major surgery appropriate for patients with blockages in two or three major coronary arteries or severely narrowed left main coronary arteries, as well as those who have not responded to other treatments. It is performed in a hospital under **general anesthesia** using a heart-lung machine to support the patient while the healthy vein or artery is attached to the coronary artery.

There are several experimental surgical procedures: **atherectomy**, where the surgeon shaves off and removes strips of plaque from the blocked artery; laser angioplasty, where a catheter with a laser tip is inserted to burn or break down the plaque; and insertion of a metal coil, called a stent, that can be implanted permanently to keep a blocked artery open. This stenting procedure is becoming more common. Another experimental procedure uses a laser to drill channels in the heart muscle to increase blood supply.

TIAs are treated by drugs that control high blood pressure and reduce the likelihood of blood clots and surgery. Aspirin is commonly used and anticoagulants are sometimes used to prevent blood clots. In some cases, carotid **endarterectomy** surgery is performed to help prevent further TIAs. The procedure involves removing arterial plaque from inside blood vessels.

The use of **chelation therapy**, a long-term injection by a physician of a cocktail of synthetic amino acid, ethylenediaminetetracetric acid, and **anticoagulant drugs** and nutrients, is controversial.

Alternative treatment

Ischemia can be life-threatening. Although there are alternative treatments for angina, traditional medical care may be necessary. Prevention of the cause of ischemia, primarily **atherosclerosis**, is primary. This becomes even more important for people with a family history of heart disease. Dietary modifications, especially the reduction or elimination of saturated fats (primarily found in meat), are essential. Increased fiber (found in fresh fruits and vegetables, grains, and beans) can help the body eliminate excessive cholesterol through the stools. Exercise, particularly aerobic exercise, is essential for circulation health. Not **smoking** will prevent damage from smoke and the harmful substances it contains.

Abana, a mixture of herbs and **minerals** used in **Ayurvedic medicine**, can reduce the frequency and severity of angina attacks. Western herbal medicine recommends hawthorn (*Crataegus laevigata* or *C. oxyacantha*) to relieve long-term angina, since it strengthens the contractility of the heart muscles. **Nutritional supplements** and botanical medicines that act as **antioxidants**, for example, **vitamins** C and E, selenium, gingko (*Gingko biloba*), bilberry (*Vaccinium myrtillus*), and hawthorn, can help prevent initial arterial injury that can lead to the formation of plaque deposits. Cactus (*Cactus grandiflorus*) is a homeopathic remedy used for pain relief during an attack. Mind/body relaxation techniques such as **yoga** and **biofeedback** can help control strong emotions and stress.

Prognosis

In many cases, ischemia can be successfully treated, but the underlying disease process of atherosclerosis is usually not "cured." New diagnostic techniques enable doctors to identify ischemia earlier. New technologies and surgical procedures can prevent angina from leading to a heart attack or TIA from resulting in a stroke. The outcome for patients with silent ischemia has not been well established.

Prevention

A healthy lifestyle, including eating right, getting regular exercise, maintaining a healthy weight, not smoking, drinking in moderation, not using illegal drugs, controlling **hypertension**, and managing stress are practices that can reduce the risk of ischemia progressing to a heart attack or stroke.

A healthy diet includes a variety of foods that are low in fat, especially saturated fat; low in cholesterol;

KEY TERMS

Atherosclerosis—A process in which the walls of the arteries thicken due to the accumulation of plaque in the blood vessels. Atherosclerosis is the cause of most coronary artery disease.

Coronary artery disease—A narrowing or blockage, due to atherosclerosis, of the arteries that provide oxygen and nutrients to the heart. When blood flow is cutoff, the result is a heart attack.

Plaque—A deposit of fatty and other substances that accumulate in the lining of the artery wall.

Stroke—A sudden decrease or loss of consciousness caused by rupture or blockage of a blood vessel by a blood clot or hemorrhage in the brain. Ischemic strokes are caused by blood clots in a cerebral artery.

and high in fiber. Plenty of fruits and vegetables should be eaten and **sodium** should be limited. Fat should comprise no more than 30% of total daily calories. Cholesterol should be limited to about 300 mg and sodium to about 2,400 mg per day.

Moderate aerobic exercise lasting about 30 minutes four or more times per week is recommended for maximum heart health, according to the Centers for Disease Control and Prevention and the American College of Sports Medicine. Three 10-minute exercise periods are also beneficial. If any risk factors are present, a physician's clearance should be obtained before starting exercise.

Maintaining a desirable body weight is also important. People who are 20% or more over their ideal body weight have an increased risk of developing coronary artery disease or stroke.

Smoking has many adverse effects on the heart and arteries, so should be avoided. Heart damage caused by smoking can be improved by quitting. Several studies have shown that ex-smokers face the same risk of heart disease as non-smokers within five to ten years of quitting.

Excessive drinking can increase risk factors for heart disease. Modest consumption of alcohol, however, can actually protect against coronary artery disease. The American Heart Association defines moderate consumption as one ounce of alcohol per day–roughly one cocktail, one 8-ounce glass of wine, or two 12-ounce glasses of beer.

Commonly used illegal drugs can seriously harm the heart and should never be used. Even stimulants like ephedra and **decongestants** like pseudoephedrine can be harmful to patients with hypertension or heart disease.

Treatment should be sought for hypertension. High blood pressure can be completely controlled through lifestyle changes and medication. Stress, which can increase the risk of a heart attack or stroke, should also be managed. While it cannot always be avoided, it can be controlled.

ORGANIZATIONS

American Heart Association National Center, 7272 Greenville Avenue, Dallas, TX, 75231, 800 242-8721, Review.personal.info@heart.org.

National Heart Lung and Blood Institute Health Information Center, P.O. Box 30105, Bethesda, MD, 20824-0105, 301 592-8573, 240 629-3246, http://www.nhlbi.nih.gov.

Texas Heart Institute. Heart Information Service, MC 3-116, PO Box 20345, Houston, TX, 77225, 832 355-4011, 800 292-2221, http://www.texasheart.org.

Lori De Milto

Isocarboxazid *see* **Monoamine oxidase inhibitors**

Isolation

Definition

Isolation refers to the precautions that are taken in the hospital to prevent the spread of an infectious agent from an infected or colonized patient to susceptible persons.

Purpose

Isolation practices are designed to minimize the transmission of infection in the hospital, using current understanding of the way infections can transmit. Isolation should be done in a user friendly, well-accepted, inexpensive way that interferes as little as possible with patient care, minimizes patient discomfort, and avoids unnecessary use.

Precautions

The type of precautions used should be viewed as a flexible scale that may range from the least to the most demanding methods of prevention. These methods should always take into account that differences exist in the way that diseases are spread. Recognition and understanding of these differences will avoid use of insufficient or unnecessary interventions.

Description

Isolation practices can include placement in a private room or with a select roommate, the use of protective barriers such as masks, gowns and gloves, a special emphasis on handwashing (which is always very important), and special handling of contaminated articles. Because of the differences among infectious diseases, more than one of these precautions may be necessary to prevent spread of some diseases but may not be necessary for others.

The Centers for Disease Control and Prevention (CDC) and the Hospital Infection Control Practice Advisory Committee (HICPAC) have led the way in defining the guidelines for hospital-based infection precautions. The most current system recommended for use in hospitals consists of two levels of precautions. The first level is Standard Precautions which apply to all patients at all times because signs and symptoms of infection are not always obvious and therefore may unknowingly pose a risk for a susceptible person. The second level is known as Transmission-Based Precautions which are intended for individuals who have a known or suspected infection with certain organisms.

Frequently, patients are admitted to the hospital without a definite diagnosis, but with clues to suggest an infection. These patients should be isolated with the appropriate precautions until a definite diagnosis is made.

Standard Precautions

Standard Precautions define all the steps that should be taken to prevent spread of infection from person to person when there is an anticipated contact with:

- Blood
- Body fluids
- Secretions, such as phlegm
- Excretions, such as urine and feces (not including sweat) whether or not they contain visible blood
- Nonintact skin, such as an open wound
- Mucous membranes, such as the mouth cavity.

Standard Precautions includes the use of one or combinations of the following practices. The level of use will always depend on the anticipated contact with the patient:

- Handwashing, the most important infection control method
- Use of latex or other protective gloves
- Masks, eye protection and/or face shield
- Gowns
- Proper handling of soiled patient care equipment
- Proper environmental cleaning
- Minimal handling of soiled linen
- Proper disposal of needles and other sharp equipment such as scalpels
- Placement in a private room for patients who cannot maintain appropriate cleanliness or contain body fluids.

Transmission Based Precautions

Transmission Based Precautions may be needed in addition to Standard Precautions for selected patients who are known or suspected to harbor certain infections. These precautions are divided into three categories that reflect the differences in the way infections are transmitted. Some diseases may require more than one isolation category.

AIRBORNE PRECAUTIONS. Airborne Precautions prevent diseases that are transmitted by minute particles called droplet nuclei or contaminated dust particles. These particles, because of their size, can remain suspended in the air for long periods of time; even after the infected person has left the room. Some examples of diseases requiring these precautions are **tuberculosis**, **measles**, and **chickenpox**.

A patient needing Airborne Precautions should be assigned to a private room with special ventilation requirements. The door to this room must be closed at all possible times. If a patient must move from the isolation room to another area of the hospital, the patient should be wearing a mask during the transport. Anyone entering the isolation room to provide care to the patient must wear a special mask called a respirator.

DROPLET PRECAUTIONS. Droplet Precautions prevent the spread of organisms that travel on particles much larger than the droplet nuclei. These particles do not spend much time suspended in the air, and usually do not travel beyond a several foot range from the patient. These particles are produced when

KEY TERMS

Colonized—This occurs when a microorganism is found on or in a person without causing a disease.

Disinfected—Decreased the number of microorganisms on or in an object.

Latex—A rubber material which gloves and condoms are made from.

Phlegm—Another word for sputum; material coughed up from a person's airways.

Stethoscope—A medical instrument for listening to a patient's heart and lungs.

a patient coughs, talks, or sneezes. Examples of disease requiring droplet precautions are meningococcal **meningitis** (a serious bacterial infection of the lining of the brain), **influenza**, **mumps**, and German measles (**rubella**).

Patients who require Droplet Precautions should be placed in a private room or with a roommate who is infected with the same organism. The door to the room may remain open. Health care workers will need to wear masks within 3 ft of the patient. Patients moving about the hospital away from the isolation room should wear a mask.

CONTACT PRECAUTIONS. Contact Precautions prevent spread of organisms from an infected patient through direct (touching the patient) or indirect (touching surfaces or objects that have been in contact with the patient) contact. Examples of patients who might be placed in Contact Precautions are those infected with:

- Antibiotic-resistant bacteria
- Hepatitis A
- Scabies
- Impetigo
- Lice-

This type of precaution requires the patient to be placed in a private room or with a roommate who has the same infection. Health care workers should wear gloves when entering the room. They should change their gloves if they touch material that contains large volumes of organisms such as soiled **dressings**. Prior to leaving the room, health care workers should remove the gloves and wash their hands with medicated soap. In addition, they may need to wear protective gowns if there is a chance of contact with potentially infective materials such as **diarrhea** or wound drainage that cannot be contained or if there is likely to be extensive contact with the patient or environment.

Patient care items, such as a stethoscope, that are used for a patient in Contact Precautions should not be shared with other patients unless they are properly cleaned and disinfected before reuse. Patients should leave the isolation room infrequently.

Resources

BOOKS

Jarvis, William R.*Bennett and Brachman's Hospital Infections*. Philadelphia: Wolters Kluwer Health/Lippincott Williams & Wilkins, 2007.

Suzanne M. Lutwick, MPH

Isoniazid *see* **Antituberculosis drugs**

Isosorbide dinitrate *see* **Antiangina drugs**

Isotretinoin *see* **Antiacne drugs**

Isradipine *see* **Calcium channel blockers**

Itching

Definition

Itching is an intense, distracting irritation or tickling sensation that may be felt all over the skin's surface, or confined to just one area. The medical term for itching is pruritus.

Description

Itching instinctively leads most people to scratch the affected area. Different people can tolerate different amounts of itching, and anyone's threshold of tolerance can be changed due to **stress**, emotions, and other factors. In general, itching is more severe if the skin is warm, and if there are few distractions. This is why people tend to notice itching more at night.

Causes and symptoms

The biology underlying itching is not fully understood. It is believed that itching results from the interactions of several different chemical messengers. Although itching and **pain** sensations were at one time thought to be sent along the same nerve pathways, researchers reported the discovery in 2003 of itch-specific nerve pathways. Nerve endings that are specifically sensitive to itching have been named pruriceptors.

Research into itching has been helped by the recent invention of a mechanical device called the Matcher, which electrically stimulates the patient's left hand. When the intensity of the stimulation equals the intensity of itching that the patient is experiencing elsewhere in the body, the patient stops the stimulation and the device automatically records the measurement. The Matcher was found to be sensitive to immediate changes in the patient's perception of itching as well as reliable in its measurements.

Stress and emotional upset can make itching worse, no matter what the underlying cause. If emotional problems are the primary reason for the itch, the condition is known as psychogenic itching. Some people become convinced that their itch is caused by a parasite; this conviction is often linked to burning sensations in the tongue, and may be caused by a major psychiatric disorder.

Generalized itching

Itching that occurs all over the body may indicate a medical condition such as **diabetes mellitus**, **liver disease**, kidney failure, **jaundice**, thyroid disorders (and rarely, **cancer**). Blood disorders such as leukemia, and lymphatic conditions such as Hodgkin's disease may sometimes cause itching as well.

Some people may develop an itch without a rash when they take certain drugs (such as **aspirin**, codeine, **cocaine**); others may develop an itchy red "drug rash" or **hives** because of an allergy to a specific drug. Some medications given to cancer patients may also cause itching.

Itching also may be caused when any of the family of hookworm larvae penetrate the skin. This includes swimmer's itch and creeping eruption caused by cat or dog hookworm, and ground itch caused by the "true" hookworm.

Many skin conditions cause an itchy rash. These include:

- Atopic dermatitis
- Chickenpox
- Contact dermatitis
- Dermatitis herpetiformis (occasionally)
- Eczema
- Fungus infections (such as athlete's foot)
- Hives (urticaria)
- Insect bites
- Lice
- Lichen planus
- Neurodermatitis (lichen simplex chronicus)
- Psoriasis (occasionally)
- Scabies.

On the other hand, itching all over the body can be caused by something as simple as bathing too often, which removes the skin's natural oils and may make the skin too dry and scaly.

Localized itching

Specific itchy areas may occur if a person comes in contact with soap, detergents, and wool or other rough-textured, scratchy material. Adults who have **hemorrhoids**, anal fissure, or persistent **diarrhea** may notice itching around the anus (called "pruritus ani"). In children, itching in this area is most likely due to worms.

Intense itching in the external genitalia in women ("pruritus vulvae") may be due to **candidiasis**, hormonal changes, or the use of certain spermicides or vaginal suppositories, ointments, or deodorants.

It is also common for older people to suffer from dry, itchy skin (especially on the back) for no obvious reason. Younger people also may notice dry, itchy skin in cold weather. Itching is also a common complaint during **pregnancy**.

Diagnosis

Itching is a symptom that is quite obvious to its victim. Someone who itches all over should seek medical care. Because itching can be caused by such a wide variety of triggers, a complete physical exam and medical history will help diagnose the underlying problem. A variety of blood and stool tests may help determine the underlying cause.

Treatment

Antihistamines such as diphenhydramine (Benadryl) can help relieve itching caused by hives, but will not affect itching from other causes. Most antihistamines also make people sleepy, which can help patients sleep who would otherwise be awake from the itch.

Specific treatment of itching depends on the underlying condition that causes it. In general, itchy skin should be treated very gently. While scratching may temporarily ease the itch, in the long run scratching just makes it worse. In addition, scratching can lead to an endless cycle of itch–scratch–more itching.

To avoid the urge to scratch, a person can apply a cooling or soothing lotion or cold compress when the urge to scratch occurs. Soaps are often irritating to the skin, and can make an itch

KEY TERMS

Atopic dermatitis—An intensely itchy inflammation often found on the face of people prone to allergies. In infants and early childhood, it is called infantile eczema.

Creeping eruption—Itchy irregular, wandering red lines on the foot made by burrowing larvae of the hookworm family and some roundworms.

Dermatitis herpetiformis—A chronic very itchy skin disease with groups of red lesions that leave spots behind when they heal. It is sometimes associated with cancer of an internal organ.

Eczema—A superficial type of inflammation of the skin that may be very itchy and weeping in the early stages; later, the affected skin becomes crusted, scaly, and thick. There is no known cause.

Hodgkin's disease—A type of cancer characterized by a slowly-enlarging lymph tissue; symptoms include generalized itching.

Lichen planus—A noncancerous, chronic itchy skin disease that causes small, flat purple plaques on wrists, forearm, ankles.

Neurodermatitis—An itchy skin disease (also called lichen simplex chronicus) found in nervous, anxious people.

Pruriceptors—Nerve endings specialized to perceive itching sensations.

Pruritus—The medical term for itching.

Psoriasis—A common, chronic skin disorder that causes red patches anywhere on the body. Occasionally, the lesions may itch.

Scabies—A contagious parasitic skin disease characterized by intense itching.

Swimmer's itch—An allergic skin inflammation caused by a sensitivity to flatworms that die under the skin, causing an itchy rash.

worse; they should be avoided, or used only when necessary.

Creams or ointments containing cortisone may help control the itch from insect **bites**, **contact dermatitis** or **eczema**. Cortisone cream should not be applied to the face unless a doctor prescribes it.

Probably the most common cause of itching is dry skin. There are a number of simple things a person can do to ease the annoying itch:

- Do not wear tight clothes
- Avoid synthetic fabrics
- Do not take long baths
- Wash the area in lukewarm water with a little baking soda
- For generalized itching, take a lukewarm shower
- Try a lukewarm oatmeal (or Aveeno) bath for generalized itching
- Apply bath oil or lotion (without added colors or scents) right after bathing.

Itching may also be treated with whole-body medications. In addition to antihistamines, some of these systemic treatments include:

- tricyclic antidepressants
- sedatives or tranquilizers
- such selective serotonin reputake inhibitors as paroxetine (Paxil) and sertraline (Zoloft)
- binding agents (such as cholestyramine which relieves itching associated with kidney or liver disease).
- aspirin
- cimetidine

People who itch as a result of mental problems or stress should seek help from a mental health expert.

Alternative and complementary therapies

A well-balanced diet that includes carbohydrates, fats, **minerals**, proteins, **vitamins**, and liquids will help to maintain skin health. Capsules that contain eicosapentaenoic acid, which is obtained from herring, mackerel, or salmon, may help to reduce itching. Vitamin A plays an important role in skin health. Vitamin E (capsules or ointment) may reduce itching. Patients should check with their treating physician before using supplements.

Homeopathy has been reported to be effective in treating systemic itching associated with hemodialysis.

Baths containing oil with milk or oatmeal are effective at relieving localized itching. Evening primrose oil may soothe itching and may be as effective as **corticosteroids**. Calendula cream may relieve short-term itching. Other herbal treatments that have been recently reported to relieve itching include sangre de drago, a preparation made with sap from a South American tree; and a mixture of honey, olive oil, and beeswax.

Distraction, **music therapy**, relaxation techniques, and visualization may be useful in relieving itching. Ultraviolet **light therapy** may relieve itching associated with conditions of the skin, kidneys, blood, and gallbladder. There are some reports of the use of **acupuncture** and transcutaneous electrical nerve stimulators (TENS) to relieve itching.

Prognosis

Most cases of itching go away when the underlying cause is treated successfully.

Prevention

There are certain things people can do to avoid itchy skin. Patients who tend toward itchy skin should:

- Avoid a daily bath
- Use only lukewarm water when bathing
- Use only gentle soap
- Pat dry, not rub dry, after bathing, leaving a bit of water on the skin
- Apply a moisture-holding ointment or cream after the bath
- Use a humidifier in the home.

Patients who are allergic to certain substances, medications, and so on can avoid the resulting itch if they avoid contact with the allergen. Avoiding insect bites, bee **stings**, **poison ivy** and so on can prevent the resulting itch. Treating sensitive skin carefully, avoiding overdrying of the skin, and protecting against diseases that cause itchy **rashes** are all good ways to avoid itching.

Resources

BOOKS

Beers, Mark H., Robert S. Porter, and Thomas V. Jones, eds. *The Merck Manual of Diagnosis and Therapy*. 18th ed. Whitehouse Station, NJ: Merck Research Laboratories, 2006.

PERIODICALS

Al-Waili, N. S. "Topical Application of Natural Honey, Beeswax and Olive Oil Mixture for Atopic Dermatitis or Psoriasis: Partially Controlled, Single-Blinded Study." *Complementary Therapies in Medicine* 11 (December 2003): 226–234.

Browning, J., B. Combes, and M. J. Mayo. "Long-Term Efficacy of Sertraline as a Treatment for Cholestatic Pruritus in Patients with Primary Biliary Cirrhosis." *American Journal of Gastroenterology* 98 (December 2003): 2736–2741.

Cavalcanti, A. M., L. M. Rocha, R. Carillo Jr., et al. "Effects of Homeopathic Treatment on Pruritus of Haemodialysis Patients: A Randomised Placebo-Controlled Double-Blind Trial." *Homeopathy* 92 (October 2003): 177–181.

Ikoma, A., R. Rukwied, S. Stander, et al. "Neurophysiology of Pruritus: Interaction of Itch and Pain." *Archives of Dermatology* 139 (November 2003): 1475–1478.

Jones, K. "Review of Sangre de Drago (*Croton lechleri*)—A South American Tree Sap in the Treatment of Diarrhea, Inflammation, Insect Bites, Viral Infections, and Wounds: Traditional Uses to Clinical Research." *Journal of Alternative and Complementary Medicine* 9 (December 2003): 877–896.

Ochoa, J. G. "Pruritus, a Rare but Troublesome Adverse Reaction of Topiramate." *Seizure* 12 (October 2003): 516–518.

Stener-Victorin, E., T. Lundeberg, J. Kowalski, et al. "Perceptual Matching for Assessment of Itch; Reliability and Responsiveness Analyzed by a Rank-Invariant Statistical Method." *Journal of Investigative Dermatology* 121 (December 2003): 1301–1305.

Zylicz, Z., M. Krajnik, A. A. Sorge, and M. Costantini. "Paroxetine in the Treatment of Severe Non-Dermatological Pruritus: A Randomized, Controlled Trial." *Journal of Pain and Symptom Management* 26 (December 2003): 1105–1112.

Carol A. Turkington
Rebecca J. Frey, PhD

IUD

Definition

An IUD is an intrauterine device made of plastic and/or copper that is inserted into the womb (uterus) by way of the vaginal canal. One type releases a hormone (progesterone), and is replaced each year. The second type is made of copper and can be left in place for five years. The most common shape in current use is a plastic "T" which is wrapped with copper wire.

Purpose

IUDs are used to prevent **pregnancy** and are considered to be 95-98% effective. It should be noted that IUDs offer no protection against the acquired immune deficiency syndrome (**AIDS**) virus or other **sexually transmitted diseases** (STDs).

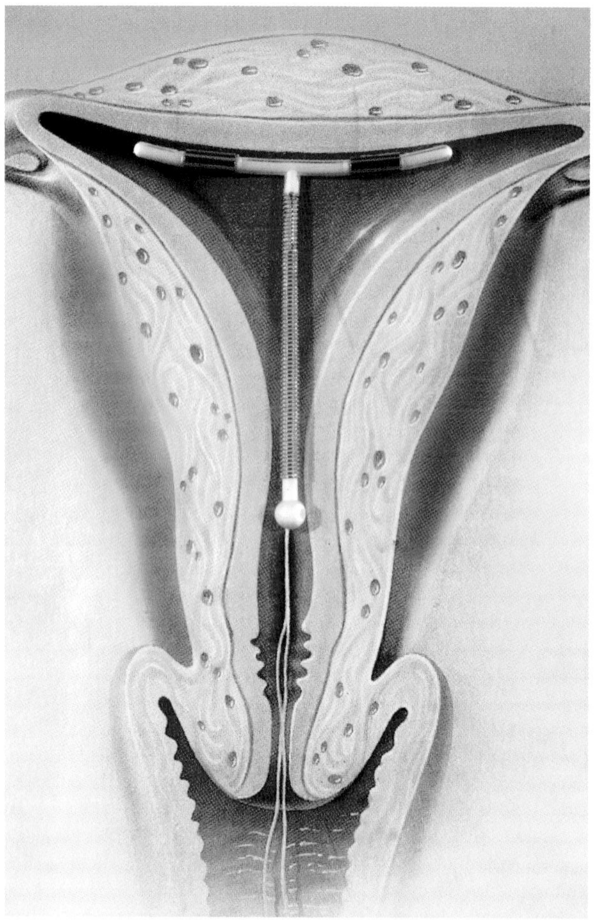

An intrauterine device, inserted and used as a form of birth control. *(© Spencer Grant/Alamy.)*

Precautions

IUDs are placed in the uterus by physicians. Prior to placement the doctor will take a medical history, do a **physical examination**, and take a **Pap test**. Women who have had tubal pregnancies, an abnormal Pap smear, or abnormal vaginal bleeding are generally disqualified from using this form of **contraception**. Also, women who have STDs, an allergy to copper, severe **pain** with periods (menstruation), sex with multiple partners, or who are currently pregnant are not eligible for an IUD. There are no age restrictions.

Description

There is continuing controversy over exactly how IUDs prevent pregnancy. Some researchers think pregnancy is controlled by preventing conception (fertilization), while others believe that the devices prevent embryo attachment to the uterine wall (implantation).

KEY TERMS

Antiseptic—A chemical that prevents the growth of germs.

Hormone—Chemicals that are produced in an organ or gland and then are carried by the blood to another part of the body where they produce a special effect for which they were designed.

Pap test—A procedure by which cells are collected from the cervix and vagina by inserting a swab into the vaginal canal. These cells are then examined under a microscope in order to detect signs of early cancer.

IUDs which release a hormone may prevent pregnancy in several ways. Since one hormonal response is a thickening of the mucous at the entrance to the uterus, it is more difficult for the sperm to gain entry. This prevents the sperm from reaching an ovum. At the same time, the lining of the uterus becomes thinner, making it more difficult for a fertilized egg to implant itself in the uterus. The copper device slowly releases copper which is believed to weaken and perhaps kill sperm. An alternate explanation is that these objects "sweep" the uterus, dislodging any fertilized egg that attempts to implant itself. In addition, both devices tend to cause a mild inflammatory reaction in the lining of the uterus which also has an adverse impact on implantation.

Preparation

After the physician approves the use of an IUD, the woman's genital area is washed thoroughly with soap and water in preparation of IUD insertion. The opening into the uterus (cervix) will also be cleaned with an antiseptic such as an iodine solution. Actual IUD insertion takes about five minutes, during which a **local anesthesia** is used to reduce any discomfort associated with the procedure. A plastic string connected to the IUD will hang out of the uterus into the vagina. The string is used to periodically check the position of the IUD.

Aftercare

The woman will be taught to watch for the signs and symptoms of potential complications and how to check the string, which should be done at least once a week. To check the string, the woman should first wash her hands with soap and water. From a squatting position, or with one foot elevated (such as on a chair), she should gently insert her finger into the vagina until she nears the cervix. If she cannot feel the string, if the string feels longer than it should, or if she can feel part of the IUD, she should notify her physician immediately. Additional information that needs to be reported includes painful intercourse and unusual discharge from the vagina.

Risks

Serious risks are rare, but include heavy bleeding, pain, infection, cramps, **pelvic inflammatory disease**, perforation of the uterus, and **ectopic pregnancy**.

ORGANIZATIONS

Planned Parenthood Federation of America, Inc., 434 West 33rd St., New York, NY, 10001, (212)541-7800, (212) 245-1845, (800) 230-7526, http://search.plannedparenthood.org.

Donald G. Barstow, RN

Ivory bones *see* **Osteopetroses**
Ivy method *see* **Bleeding time**

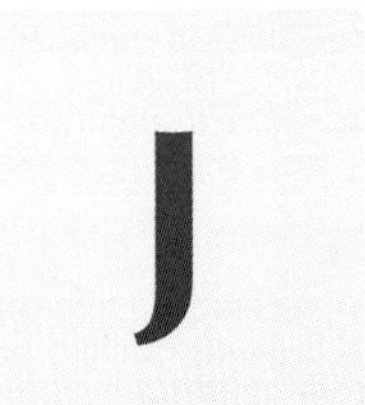

Japanese encephalitis

Definition

Japanese **encephalitis** is an infection of the brain caused by a virus. The virus is transmitted to humans by mosquitoes.

Demographics

Many of these areas are in Asia, including Japan, Korea, China, India, Thailand, Indonesia, Malaysia, Vietnam, Taiwan, and the Philippines. Areas where the disease-causing arbovirus is always present are referred to as being endemic for the disease. In such areas, blood tests will reveal that more than 70% of all adults have been infected at some point with the arbovirus.

Because the virus that causes Japanese encephalitis is carried by mosquitoes, the number of people infected increases during those seasons when mosquitoes are abundant. This tends to be in the warmest, rainiest months. In addition to humans, wild birds and pigs are susceptible to infection with this arbovirus. Because the specific type of mosquito carrying the Japanese encephalitis arbovirus frequently breeds in rice paddies, the disease is considered to be primarily a rural problem.

About 45,000 cases of Japanese encephalitis are reported each year; however, the disease is thought to be seriously underreported. The disease is about 1.5 times more common in men than in women, possibly because men are likely to spend more time outdoors in areas where the disease is endemic. Cases in the United States are exceedingly rare (less than 1 case per year) and usually occur in military personnel or other Americans who have returned home after living in affected areas.

Description

The virus that causes Japanese encephalitis is called an arbovirus, which is an arthropod-borne virus. Mosquitoes are a type of arthropod. Mosquitoes in a number of regions carry this virus. The virus is passed to humans when the mosquitoes bite them. The disease cannot be passed directly from human to human, nor can it be passed directly from animals infected with the virus to human. Not all infections cause severe symptoms; in many cases the only symptoms are a **fever** and **headache**. In areas where the virus is common, most people become infected by the time they are young adults.

Causes and symptoms

The virus is transferred to a human when an infected mosquito sucks that person's blood. Once in the body, the virus travels to various glands where it multiplies. The virus can then enter the bloodstream. Ultimately, the virus settles in the brain, where it causes serious problems.

The time from becoming infected to starting to show symptoms (incubation period) usually is 5–15 days. Serious cases of Japanese encephalitis begin abruptly with fever, severe headache, **nausea**, and **vomiting**. As the tissue covering the brain and spinal cord (the meninges) becomes infected and swollen, the patient will develop a stiff and painful neck. By day two or three, the patient begins to suffer the effects of swelling in the brain. These effects include:

- problems with balance and coordination
- paralysis of some muscle groups
- tremors
- seizures
- lapses in consciousness
- a stiff, mask-like appearance of the face.

The patient becomes dehydrated and loses weight. If the patient survives the illness, the fever will decrease by about day seven and the symptoms will begin to improve by about day 14. Other patients will continue to have extremely high fevers and their symptoms will get worse. In these cases, **coma** and then **death** occur

KEY TERMS

Encephalitis—A swelling of the brain, potentially causing serious brain damage.

Endemic—Naturally and consistently present in a certain geographical region.

in 7–14 days. Many patients who recover have permanent disabilities due to brain damage.

Diagnosis

Most diagnostic techniques for Japanese encephalitis do not yield results very quickly. The diagnosis is made primarily on the basis of the patient's symptoms and the knowledge of the kinds of illnesses endemic to a particular geographic region.

Tests

Immunofluorescence tests, where special viral markers react with human antibodies that have been tagged with a fluorescent chemical, are used to verify the disease. However, these results tend to be unavailable until week two of the infection. Other tests involve comparing the presence and quantity of particular antibodies in the blood or spinal fluid during week one with those present during week two of the illness.

Treatment

There are no treatments available to stop or slow the progression of Japanese encephalitis. Only the symptoms of each patient can be treated. Fluids are given to decrease **dehydration** and medications are given to decrease fever and **pain**. Medications are available to attempt to decrease brain swelling. Patients in a coma may require mechanical assistance with breathing.

Prognosis

While the majority of people infected with arbovirus never become seriously sick, those who develop Japanese encephalitis become very ill. Death ranges can range from 30–60%. A variety of long-term problems may haunt those who recover from the illness. These problems include:

- movement difficulties where the arms, legs, or body jerks or writhes involuntarily
- shaking
- paralysis
- inability to control emotions
- loss of mental abilities
- mental disturbances, including schizophrenia (which may affect as many as 75% of Japanese encephalitis survivors).

Young children are most likely to have serious, long-term problems after an infection.

Prevention

Two different vaccines are available for immunization against Japanese encephalitis. A three-dose vaccine is available for Japanese encephalitis and is commonly given to young children in areas where the disease is endemic. A two-dose vaccine can be give to people age 17 and older. Both vaccines are given over the period of a 28–30 days and should be completed at least 7–10 days before entering an area where the Japanese encephalitis virus is common.

The vaccine is not 100% effective, thus controlling the mosquito population with insecticides is an essential preventive measure. Visitors to regions with high rates of Japanese encephalitis should take precautions (like using mosquito repellents such as DEET and sleeping under a bed net) to avoid contact with mosquitoes.

Resources

OTHER

Jani, Asim A. and Alexander J. Kallin. Japanese Encephalitis. eMedicine.com. May 6, 2009. http://emedicine.medscape. com/article/233802-overview

Japanese Encephalitis vaccine. MedlinePlus. March 22, 2010. http://www.nlm.nih.gov/medlineplus/druginfo/meds/a607019.html

Japanese Encephalitis. United States Centers for Disease Control and Prevention. March 12, 2010. http://www.cdc.gov/ncidod/dvbid/jencephalitis/

The Yellow Book. Chapter 2—The Pre-Travel Consultation: Travel-related Vaccine Preventable Diseases. United States Centers for Disease Control and Prevention. January 25, 2010 (and frequently updated). http://wwwnc.cdc.gov/travel/yellowbook/2010/chapter-2/japanese-encephalitis.aspx

ORGANIZATIONS

United States Centers for Disease Control and Prevention (CDC), 1600 Clifton Road, Atlanta, GA, 30333, (404) 639-3534, 800-CDC-INFO (800-232-4636). TTY: (888) 232-6348, inquiry@cdc.gov, http://www.cdc.gov.

World Health Organization, Avenue Appia 20, 1211 Geneva 27, Switzerland, +22 41 791 21 11, +22 41 791 31 11, info@who.int, http://www.who.int.

Rosalyn Carson-DeWitt, MD
Tish Davidson, A.M.

Jaundice

Definition

Jaundice is a condition in which the skin and whites of the eyes turn yellowish from increased levels of a waste product called bilirubin. Although jaundice is common in newborn infants, at any time after the first few weeks of life it can be a symptom of a serious underlying condition. Jaundice is sometimes called hyperbilirubinemia or icterus from the Greek word for the condition.

Demographics

Newborn jaundice affects more than half of all full-term newborns and 80% of premature newborns within the first few days of life, although only about 10% of newborns require treatment. Jaundice is often more severe in Asian and Native American infants. **Biliary atresia**, a congenital defect in the bile ducts that can cause severe hyperbilirubinemia in otherwise healthy infants, occurs in about one in every 15,000 live births and girls are slightly more at risk than boys.

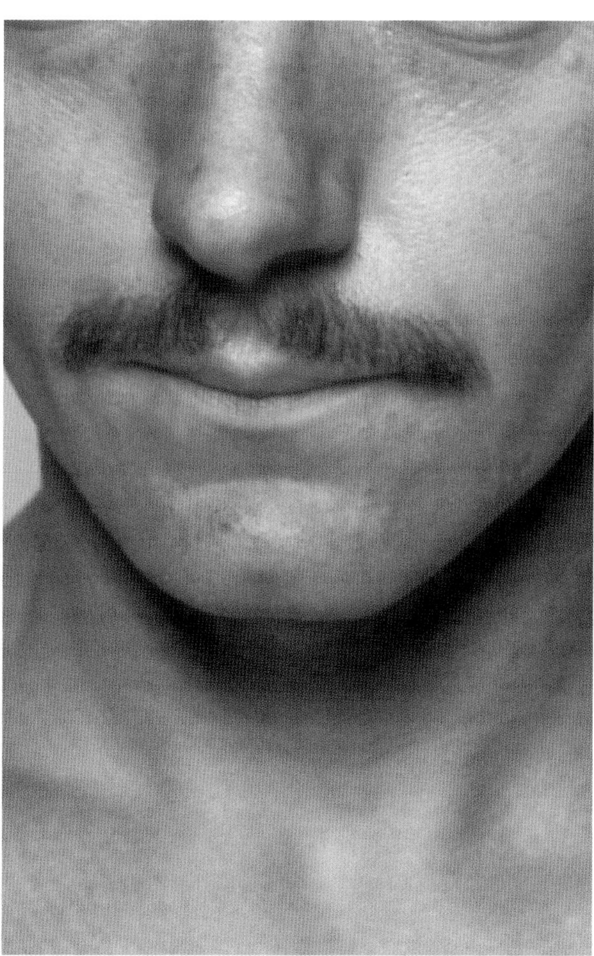

This patient suffers from obstructive jaundice, which is often caused by gallstones. *(Custom Medical Stock Photo, Inc. Reproduced by permission.)*

Description

Bilirubin is a yellow pigment that is formed from the breakdown of hemoglobin—the oxygen-carrying protein in red blood cells (RBCs). RBCs normally are removed from the blood and broken down in the spleen and other parts of the body after about 120 days in circulation. About 1% of RBCs are normally broken down and replaced each day. Bilirubin is carried to the liver where it is attached or conjugated to another molecule and added to bile. Conjugated bilirubin is known as direct or soluble bilirubin and unconjugated bilirubin is known as indirect or insoluble bilirubin.

Bile that is formed in the liver passes into the network of hepatic bile ducts, which join to form a single tube. One branch of this tube carries bile to the gallbladder where it is stored and concentrated. When food enters the stomach, the gallbladder is stimulated to release bile to the intestines through the common bile duct. Before the common bile duct reaches the intestines, it is joined by a duct from the pancreas. Bile and pancreatic juice enter the intestine through a valve called the ampulla of Vater. After entering the intestine, bile and pancreatic secretions assist in digestion and bile is excreted in the stool. However if bilirubin accumulates in the blood rather than being excreted, it discolors tissues, turning the skin and whites of the eyes yellow.

Risk factors

Risk factors for newborn jaundice include:

- Asian or Native American parentage
- a parent or sibling who had high bilirubin levels at birth
- maternal diabetes
- premature birth
- induced labor
- birth at a high altitude
- bruising during birth
- excessive weight loss during the first few days after birth

Causes and symptoms

Although jaundice is always caused by a buildup of bilirubin in the blood and tissues, there are many different causes for this buildup. The causes can be divided into three categories based on where they

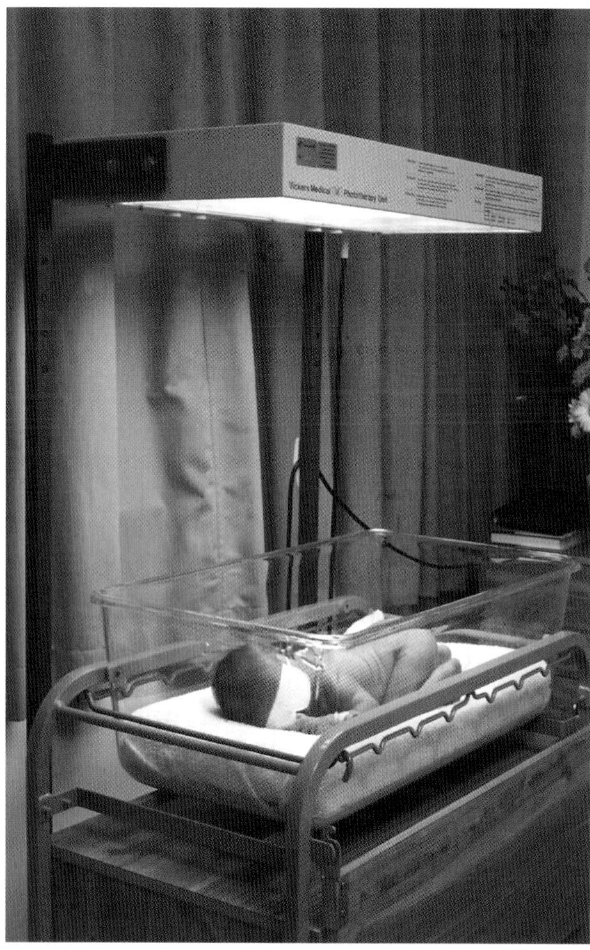

A newborn baby undergoes phototherapy with visible blue light to treat his jaundice. *(Ron Sutherland/SPL/ Photo Researchers, Inc.)*

occur in the bilirubin cycle: before, in, or after the liver—pre-hepatic, hepatic, or post-hepatic.

The pre-hepatic cause of jaundice is hemolysis—the **death** of RBCs at a faster-than-normal rate, which releases hemoglobin and causes bilirubin to accumulate. The many causes of hemolysis include:

- Malaria. The malaria parasite develops inside RBCs and destroys them when it matures. Bilirubin can enter the urine in sufficient quantities to cause "blackwater fever," which is often lethal.
- Certain drugs. Hemolysis is a rare but sudden side effect of some antibiotics, anti-tuberculosis medications, drugs that regulate heartbeat, and levodopa for treating **Parkinson's disease**.
- Certain drugs in combination with an inherited deficiency in the enzyme glucose-6-phosphate dehydrogenase (G6PD). G6PD deficiency affects more than 200 million people worldwide. Some of the drugs listed above, as well as certain others, especially vitamins C and K and anti-malarial medications such as quinine, can cause hemolysis in people with G6PD deficiency.
- Poisons. Snake and spider venoms, certain bacterial toxins, copper, and some organic industrial chemicals cause hemolysis by directly attacking RBC membranes.
- Artificial heart valves. The inflexible moving parts of artificial heart valves damage RBCs.
- Hereditary RBC disorders. Sickle cell disease, which results in abnormal hemoglobin, spherocytosis, which weakens the outer membrane of RBCs, and various other inherited defects that affect the internal chemistry of RBCs can all cause hemolysis.
- Enlargement of the spleen. The spleen filters the blood and destroys old RBCs. If it becomes enlarged, healthy RBCs also are filtered out resulting in hemolysis. A wide variety of conditions can cause enlargement of the spleen.
- Diseases of the small blood vessels. As the RBCs move through diseased capillaries they can be damaged by rough surfaces on the inside of vessel walls.
- Immune reactions. The immune system can produce antibodies that destroy RBCs.
- Blood transfusions. Hemolysis can result from a transfusion with an incompatible blood type.
- Kidney failure and other serious diseases. Several diseases cause defective blood coagulation that destroys RBCs.
- Erythroblastosis fetalis. This results from too many immature RBCs (erythroblasts) in a newborn, usually because of a blood factor incompatibility between the mother and infant that causes maternal antibodies to destroy the newborn's RBCs.

Newborn jaundice results from both pre-hepatic and hepatic sources of excess bilirubin. At birth the newborn immediately begins converting from fetal to adult-type hemoglobin. The removal of the fetal hemoglobin can overload the immature liver for a week or two after birth, resulting in excess bilirubin and jaundice. Bilirubin gives a newborn's stools their yellow color. Jaundice usually appears first on the face, on the third or fourth day after birth, and progresses downward to the chest, abdomen, legs, and feet. If newborn feeding is delayed for any reason, such as illness, a digestive tract problem, or low fluid intake due to inefficient **breastfeeding**, the infant produces fewer stools, which can result in critically high blood levels of bilirubin and severe jaundice.

Jaundice at birth or within the first 24 hours can be a sign of abnormal jaundice, which can be very dangerous, particularly in preterm or unhealthy

KEY TERMS

Ampulla of Vater—The widened portion of the duct through which bile and pancreatic juices enter the intestine. Ampulla is a Latin word for a bottle with a narrow neck that opens into a wide body.

Anemia—A deficiency in hemoglobin, red blood cells, or total blood volume.

Bile—A liquid secreted by the liver and passed through ducts to the small intestine where it aids in the digestion and absorption of fats.

Biliary atresia—The underdevelopment or absence of bile ducts.

Biliary system/bile ducts—The gall bladder and the system of tubes that carries bile from the liver into the intestine.

Bilirubin—A reddish-yellow pigment that is a breakdown product of hemoglobin and is excreted by the liver into the bile.

Cirrhosis—Disruption of liver function due to damage from chronic progressive disease.

Crigler-Najjar syndrome—A moderate to severe form of hereditary jaundice.

Erythroblastosis fetalis—A disorder of newborn infants marked by a high level of immature red blood cells (erythroblasts).

Gilbert's syndrome—A mild hereditary form of jaundice.

Glucose-6-phosphate dehydrogenase (G6PD) deficiency—A hereditary disorder that, in combination with certain medications, can lead to episodes of hemolytic anemia.

Hemoglobin—The red substance in blood cells that carries oxygen.

Hemolysis—The destruction or breakdown of red blood cells.

Hepatic—Referring to the liver.

Hepatitis—Inflammation of the liver or the disease or condition causing liver inflammation.

Hyperbilirubinemia —An excess of bilirubin in the blood.

Icterus—Jaundice.

Microangiopathic—Pertaining to disorders of the small blood vessels.

Pancreas—The organ beneath the stomach that produces digestive juices, insulin, and other hormones.

Sickle cell disease—A hereditary defect in hemoglobin that changes the shape of red blood cells.

Splenectomy—Surgical removal of the spleen.

newborns. **Erythroblastosis fetalis** is the most common cause of abnormal newborn jaundice.

Other causes of hepatic jaundice include a variety of liver diseases in which the damaged organ cannot to keep up with bilirubin processing. These hepatic causes of jaundice include:

- starvation
- circulating (systemic) infections
- certain medications
- hepatitis
- cirrhosis
- hereditary defects in liver chemistry, including Gilbert's syndrome and Crigler-Najjar syndrome

Obstructive jaundices are post-hepatic forms caused by failure of soluble bilirubin to reach the intestines after leaving the liver. The most common cause of obstructive jaundice is **gallstones** in the ducts of the biliary system. Other causes of obstructive jaundice include:

- birth defects such as biliary atresia or infections that damage the bile ducts
- drugs
- cancers
- physical injury
- certain drugs—and rarely, pregnancy—that simply cause the bile in the ducts to stop flowing

Jaundice has no symptoms other than discoloration of the skin and eyes and is usually harmless, although the underlying condition may cause other symptoms and complications. However if unconjugated bilirubin reaches the newborn brain, it can cause permanent damage. Prolonged jaundice can also upset the balance of chemicals in the bile and cause the formation of stones.

Diagnosis

Examination

Jaundice is usually evident from the yellowish tint of the eyes and complexion. All newborns are examined under good light for signs of jaundice. The physician will feel (palpate) the liver and spleen to check for enlargement and evaluate any abdominal **pain**. The location and severity of abdominal pain and the presence or absence of **fever** help distinguish between hepatic and obstructive jaundice.

Tests

Blood tests measure the levels of total and/or conjugated bilirubin in the blood. Total bilirubin in the blood serum is normally between 0.3 milligrams (mg) per deciliter (dL) and 1.9 mg/dL. Conjugated or direct bilirubin is normally 0–0.3 mg/dL. Jaundice occurs when the total bilirubin level rises to 3 mg/dL or higher. It may be necessary to repeatedly measure bilirubin levels in jaundiced newborns because of the danger of insoluble bilirubin reaching the brain. An instrument called a bilirubinometer can be held against the infant's skin to assess the level of jaundice, eliminating the need for blood tests.

Additional tests may include:

- blood cell counts to detect anemia
- tests for blood-clotting function
- tests for excess destruction of RBCs
- blood tests to assess liver function
- urine and stool samples to check for signs of bacterial or viral infection

Procedures

Various procedures may be used to diagnose a disorder underlying jaundice:

- Sometimes a bone marrow biopsy is necessary to diagnose blood-formation disorders.
- Ultrasound or a nuclear scan may be used to evaluate the spleen.
- A liver biopsy may be necessary to diagnose liver disease. A thin needle is used to remove a tiny core of liver tissue, which is sent to the laboratory for microscopic examination.
- Computed tomography (CT) or magnetic resonance imaging (MRI) scans are very useful for imaging certain conditions such as cancers in and around the liver or gallstones in the common bile duct.
- Various imaging techniques can be used to diagnose diseases of the biliary system. X rays for obtaining functional as well as anatomical information are taken one day after swallowing a contrast agent that is secreted into the bile. Alternatively contrast dye can be injected directly into the bile ducts, through a thin needle pushed into the liver or through a scope that is passed through the stomach to inject the dye into the ampulla of Vater.

Treatment

Traditional

Jaundice itself is treated only in newborns with dangerously high bilirubin levels. In the past it was necessary to exchange most of the infant's blood. Now the newborn can be fitted with eye protection and placed under a high-intensity, cool, blue-fluorescent light. The light is absorbed by the bilirubin and converts it into a harmless form than can be excreted in the bile and urine. Other **phototherapy** methods—such as a fiber optic bilirubin blanket—incorporate the light into a blanket so that the child can be breastfed during treatment or treated at home. Frequent feedings lead to more frequent stools, which reduces the reabsorption of bilirubin from the intestines into the blood. The infant also may be given additional fluids, possibly intravenously, to help remove bilirubin.

Obstructive jaundice frequently requires surgery. Surgery for biliary atresia must be performed within the first few weeks of life to prevent fatal liver damage. A common technique is to stitch an open piece of intestine over a bare patch of liver. Tiny bile ducts in that part of the liver will begin to discharge their bile into the intestine and pressure from the obstructed ducts elsewhere will release in that direction. As the bile flow increases, the ducts grow to accommodate it until all of the bile is redirected through the open pathways.

There are a variety of treatments for other conditions underlying jaundice:

- Any medications that are causing hemolysis or arresting the flow of bile are stopped immediately.
- Hemolytic diseases are treated, if at all, with medications and blood transfusions, except in the case of an enlarged spleen. Surgical removal of the spleen (splenectomy) can sometimes cure hemolytic anemia.
- Although there are no specific cures for most liver diseases, the liver can recover from even severe damage and regenerate from only a small remnant of original tissue.

Prognosis

Prognosis depends on the condition underlying the jaundice. Normal newborn jaundice is not harmful and disappears after one–two weeks. In cases of severe newborn jaundice, phototherapy usually returns bilirubin levels to normal within a few days. Infants with a duct obstruction within the liver itself usually require a liver transplant by the age of two.

Prevention

Prevention of jaundice involves preventing the underlying condition:

- Malaria in tropical or subtropical countries can often be prevented by precautions such as bed nets treated with insecticides or mosquito repellants and prophylactic drugs such as mefloquine.
- Hemolytic side effects from medications can be minimized with early detection and immediate cessation of the drug.
- G6PD-deficiency hemolysis can be prevented by testing patients before administering the causative drugs.
- Erythroblastosis fetalis can be prevented by treating an Rh-negative mother with a gamma-globulin solution called RhoGAM if there is a possibility that she is developing antibodies against her baby's blood.

The American Academy of Pediatrics recommendations for identifying and managing **neonatal jaundice** include:

- assessing all newborns for risk of severe jaundice, including measuring bilirubin levels before hospital discharge
- a follow-up visit within three–five days after birth when bilirubin levels are likely to peak
- breastfeeding a newborn at least eight–12 times per day, since effective breastfeeding significantly reduces the risk of hyperbilirubinemia

Resources

BOOKS

Sargent, Suzanne. *Liver Diseases: An Essential Guide for Nurses and Health Care Professionals*. Ames, IA: Wiley-Blackwell, 2009.

Valman, H. B., and Roslyn Thomas. *ABC of the First Year*, 6th ed. Hoboken, NJ: Wiley-Blackwell, 2009.

PERIODICALS

Charles, Katie. "Yellow Alert for Parents" *New York Daily News* (February 18, 2009): 27.

Jacobi, Tillmann. "Jaundice in an Adult." *GP* (March 27, 2009): 35.

Moerschel, Sarah K., Lauren B. Cianciaruso, and Lloyd R. Tracy. "A Practical Approach to Neonatal Jaundice." *American Family Physician* 77, no. 9 (May 1, 2008): 1255–1262.

OTHER

American Association for Clinical Chemistry. "Bilirubin." *Lab Tests Online*. http://www.labtestsonline.org/understanding/analytes/bilirubin/test.html.

American Association for Clinical Chemistry. "Jaundice." *Lab Tests Online*. http://www.labtestsonline.org/understanding/conditions/jaundice.html.

"Jaundice." *freeMD*. http://www.freemd.com/jaundice/visit-virtual-doctor.htm.

"Jaundice." *MedlinePlus*. http://www.nlm.nih.gov/medlineplus/jaundice.html.

Questions and Answers: Jaundice and Your Newborn.American Academy of Pediatrics. http://www.aap.org/family/jaundicefaq.htm.

ORGANIZATIONS

American Academy of Pediatrics, 141 Northwest Point Blvd., Elk Grove Village, IL, 60007-1098, (874) 434-4000, (874) 434-8000, kidsdocs@aap.org, http://www.aap.org.

American Liver Foundation, 75 Maiden Lane, Suite 603, New York, NY, 10038, (212) 668-1000, (212) 483-8179, http://www.liverfoundation.org.

National Institute of Diabetes and Digestive and Kidney Diseases, Building 31, Room 9A06, 31 Center Drive, MSC 2560, Bethesda, MD, 20892-2560, (301) 496-3583, http://www2.niddk.nih.gov.

J. Ricker Polsdorfer, MD
Teresa G. Odle
Margaret Alic, PhD

Jaw wiring

Definition

Jaw wiring, also known as maxillomandibular fixation, is a surgical procedure where metal pins and wires are anchored into the jaw bones and surrounding tissues to keep the jaw from moving.

Purpose

Sports injuries, automobile accidents, falls, or fistfights are a few of the situations where the jaw might be fractured or broken. In these cases, jaw wiring may be necessary to keep the bones aligned and stable while the jaw heals. The presence of **cancer** or other diseased tissues may make removal and reconstruction of the jaw necessary. Wiring the jaws shut has been used in the past as a weight loss aid in cases of extreme **obesity** where other treatments had failed, although this procedure is rarely used for that purpose today.

Precautions

Traumatic injuries to the face can cause damage to facial nerves and salivary glands and ducts. These injuries can also leave **scars** that may require additional surgery to correct.

KEY TERMS

Oral and maxillofacial surgeon—A dentist who is trained to perform surgery to correct injuries, defects, or conditions of the mouth, teeth, jaws, and face.

Otolaryngologist—A doctor who is trained to treat injuries, defects, or conditions of the head and neck.

Description

Jaw wiring surgery can be performed by an oral or maxillofacial surgeon (a specially trained dentist), or by an otolaryngologist (a doctor specializing in surgeries of the head and neck). The procedure may be done in a medical or dental office if the office is staffed and equipped to handle this type of surgery. More often, this surgery is performed in a hospital or medical center surgical area. If jaw wiring is required due to an injury, the surgeon may set the fracture immediately before swelling sets in. It is also possible to wait (up to several weeks) until the swelling goes down and some of the soft tissue injuries have healed, prior to wiring the jaw fracture.

The surgeon realigns the fractured bones. Every effort is made to restore the shape and appearance of the original jaw line. If any teeth were damaged, repair or replacement may be done at the same time. Small incisions may be made through the skin and surrounding tissue so the pins and wires can be set into the jawbone to hold the fracture together. To prevent the lower jaw from moving during healing, pins and wires may be inserted into the top jaw, as well. The upper and lower jaws are then wired together in order to stabilize the fracture.

As with other types of bone **fractures**, the jaw may take several weeks to heal. Another type of jaw immobilization that has been developed more recently, rigid fixation uses small metal plates and screws rather than pins and wires to secure the jaw bones. The main benefit of this technique is that the jaws do not have to be wired shut, allowing the patient to return to a more normal lifestyle sooner.

Preparation

X rays of the fractured area may be taken prior to surgery. Depending on the extent of the facial injury or condition to be corrected, the patient may receive a sedative for relaxation, a local anesthetic drug to numb the area, and/or an anesthetic agent to induce unconsciousness prior to the surgery.

Aftercare

A patient whose jaw has been wired will not be able to eat solid foods for several weeks. In order for the bone and surrounding tissues to heal, it is important to maintain adequate **nutrition**. A liquid diet that can be consumed through a straw, will be required. Soft, precooked foods can be liquefied in a blender, however, it may be difficult for the patient to consume adequate calories, protein, **vitamins**, and **minerals** with this type of diet. Liquid diet formulas may be a good alternative. The patient will also have to be taught how to care for the mouth, teeth, and injured area while the wires are in place.

Risks

It is possible that scarring may occur due to the need to make small incisions in the skin in order to insert the wires. With any surgical procedure, there are risks associated with the anesthetic drugs used and the possibility of infection. If there is a risk that the patient may vomit, the jaw wiring may pose a **choking** hazard. It may be recommended that wire cutters be kept available in case the wires need to be cut in an emergency situation.

Resources

OTHER

"Know the Score on Facial Sports Injuries." *The Virtual Hospital Page*. University of Iowa. http://www.entassociates.com/facial_injuries.htm.

"Topic: Maxillofacial Trauma." *Connecticut Maxillofacial Surgeons Page*. http://www.cmsllc.com/toptrm.html.

ORGANIZATIONS

American Association of Oral & Maxillofacial Surgeons, 9700 West Bryn Mawr Avenue, Rosemont, IL, 60018-5701, (847) 678-6200, (847) 678-6286, (800) 822-6637, http://www.aaoms.org.

American Dental Association, 211 E. Chicago Ave., Chicago, IL, 60611-2678, (312) 440-2500, http://www.ada.org.

Altha Roberts Edgren

JC virus infection *see* **Progressive multifocal leukoencephalopathy**

Jejunostomy *see* **Enterostomy**

Jet lag

Definition

Jet lag, also sometimes called desynchronosis, is a physiological condition marked by **fatigue**, **insomnia**, and irritability that is caused by air travel—usually going from east to west or from west to east—through many changing time zones. It is classified as a circadian rhythm sleep disorder because it alters (disrupts) the natural circadian rhythm ("internal body clock") in humans. The temporary condition is primarily caused by air travel across several time zones, but can also be caused by shift work or other factors. Jet lag comes about from the inability of the internal body clock to adjust quickly enough to drastic changes in the normal sleep and wake cycle. Usually it lasts only for a few days but it can last longer depending on the length of travel and the steps taken to counter it.

Generally, jet lag lasts longer when traveling west to east, than it does when flying east to west. A general relationship is: jet lag lasts two-thirds of a day for each time zone crossed while flying eastward, and lasts one-half of a day for each time zone crossed while heading westward. Thus, flying westward across two time zones would cause jet lag for about one day for the average air traveler.

Demographics

The condition called jet lag can occur in air travelers of all ages and genders when they travel across several time zones. Prior research does not support the contention that it affects those of one age more than another. However, medical studies do show that women are at higher risk than men for getting jet lag, primarily due to the higher levels of estrogen in women's bodies. Exposure to natural light after completing a long trip usually helps to accelerate the adaption process, especially when travel is over three or more time zones.

Description

The natural circadian rhythm in humans is located in the suprachiasmatic nuclei at the base of the hypothalamus, all within the brain. The suprachiasmatic nuclei contain receptors that receive melatonin, which is manufactured in the pineal gland. Melatonin is released based on the amount of darkness or light in one's local environment. More of it is released during the night and less during the day. Consequently, a person's sleep and wake cycle (or "internal body clock") is established by this relationship with the manufacture and release of melatonin based on dark and light cycles.

Over millions of years living organisms have become accustomed to periods of night and day alternating at set intervals. Thus, they (both plants and animals) have a tendency to operate on an approximate 24-hour cycle based on the cycles of sunlight and darkness. Most of the human body's regulating hormones follow this cycle, known as circadian rhythm. The word circadian comes from the Latin, *circa*, meaning about, and *dies*, meaning day. These cycles are not exactly 24 hours long, hence the "circa." Each chemical has its own cycle of highs and lows, interacting with and influencing the other cycles. Characteristics such as body temperature, sleepiness, thyroid function, growth hormone, metabolic processes, adrenal hormones, and the sleep hormone melatonin cycle with daylight. A direct connection exists between the retina (where light hits the back of the eye) and the part of the brain that controls all these hormones. Artificial light has some effect, but sunlight has much more.

When people are without clocks in a compartment that is completely closed to sunlight, most of them fall into a circadian cycle of about 25 hours. Normally, all the regulating chemicals follow one another in order like threads in a weaving pattern. Every morning the sunlight resets the cycle, stimulating the leading chemicals and thus compensating for the difference between the 24-hour day and the 25-hour innate rhythm.

When traveling through a number of time zones, most people reset their rhythms within a few days, demonstrating the adaptability of the human species. Some people, however, have upset rhythms that last much longer. Whatever the period of adjustment, the experience can cause biological and brain wave activity that tries to cope with the new situation. During this coping period, the human undergoing jet lag may feel irritable, fatigue, and disorientiation.

Causes and symptoms

Jet lag is primarily caused by the direction of travel and the number of time zones crossed. However, it can also be affected by a person's ability (or inability) to sleep just before, during, and just after traveling; tolerance (or intolerance) to air travel, and the similarity (or difference) of the natural day-and-night cycle between the departing and arriving locations.

Flying north or south, such as from Chicago, Illinois, to Houston, Texas, does not generally cause jet lag because a time zone has not been changed and periods of night and day have not changed. However, flying east or west, such as from New York City to Los Angeles, does cause jet lag in people. Traveling west to east is generally considered to be more disruptive than travel from east to west. This difference occurs because the circadian cycle is pushed forward (earlier time zone) rather than back (later time zone) when traveling west to east as compared to traveling east to west. Thus, as people travel to places where daylight and darkness are different from what they are used to, then the body's clock becomes disrupted and jet lag occurs. However, flying north or south can cause jet jag when travel changes the normal period of darkness to daytime and the normal period of sunlight to night–time, such as when traveling from Denver, Colorado, in the Northern Hemisphere, to Lima, Peru, in the Southern Hemisphere.

When jet lag occurs, the body's natural pattern is upset. Such things as sleep, body temperature, and hormone regulation are no longer in synchronization to the new environment. Consequently, it takes the human body a period of adjustment to realign itself to its new locality. Traveling through a few time zones at a time is not as disruptive to circadian rhythms as traveling around the world can be. The foremost symptom of jet lag is altered sleep pattern—sleepiness during the day, and insomnia during the night. Jet lag may also include **indigestion** and trouble concentrating. Individuals afflicted by jet lag will alternate in and out of a normal day-night cycle.

It may take one person several days to adjust to a new time zone, while another person may not even experience any problems. Generally, one or two new time zones will not cause problems, but more than that number will usually cause some symptoms identified with jet lag.

Symptoms associated with jet lag include: fatigue, insomnia, irritability, **anxiety** or mild depression, **nausea**, **headache**, disorientation, loss of appetite, **diarrhea** or **constipation** (along with general gastrointestinal disturbances), reduced ability (or inability) to perform common physical and mental tasks, and decreased ability to concentrate. Disorientation and fatigue are the two most common symptoms of jet lag.

Shift work is another cause of what is called jet lag, although it has nothing to do with flying in an airplane. Many people work shifts that are not the customary time during the daylight hour, which is usually called first shift (or day work). They may work a second shift from late in the afternoon to the middle of the night, say, from 5 p.m. to 2 a.m. In another scenario, a person might work a third shift from the middle of the night to early in the morning, for example, from midnight to 8 a.m. In either case, such changes in the normal schedule of being awake during sunlight hours and sleeping during darkness can cause symptoms very similar to jet lag. These symptoms can be worsened when shift work is changed over a week, for instance, five days of working third shift but a two-day weekend where the worker tries to resume a normal life.

Treatment

Current treatments

In cases of short-term insomnia triggered by jet lag, a physician may recommend over-the-counter (OTC) sleeping pills or prescription medication. These medicines may help to counter the biological imbalance caused by jet lag. However, they can cause adverse side effects. Thus, such medication should only be taken under the guidance of a health care professional.

Investigational treatments

A medication that is considered investigational is a melatonin agonist known as LY 156735 (PD–6735). An agonist is a drug that stimulates activity at cell receptors that are normally stimulated by such naturally occurring substances as melatonin. LY 156735 was found to speed up the re–adaptation time of volunteer subjects following a simulated nine–hour time shift. As of 2010, it is still under development as a treatment for jet lag, insomnia, and other such **sleep disorders**. Melatonin is thought to increase the ability to drift off to sleep but it not believed to help in increasing the amount of sleep one gets. It is not regulated by the Food and Drug Administration (FDA) but may be bought at health food stores and other such retail stores. Consult a medical professional before trying such drugs.

Another area of research involves the genes that encode the proteins governing circadian rhythms. It is known that differences among individuals in adaptability to time zone changes are to some extent genetically determined. Targeting the genes that affect this adaptability may yield new treatments for jet lag and other disorders of circadian rhythm. As of 2010, these medical studies are still underway.

Alternative treatment

Exposure to bright morning sunlight cures jet lag after a few days in most people. A few will have prolonged sleep phase difficulties. For these, a curious treatment has achieved success. By forcing one's self into a 27-hour day, complete with the appropriate stimulation from bright light, all the errant chemical cycles will be able to catch up during one week.

When selecting an international flight, individuals should try to arrange an early evening arrival in their destination city. When an individual is traveling to a destination in the east, he or she can try going to bed and waking up a few hours earlier several days before

KEY TERMS

Agonist—A medication that has an affinity for and stimulates the activity of cell receptors that are normally stimulated by naturally occurring substances, including melatonin.

Circadian—Pertaining to biological rhythms occurring at approximately 24-hour intervals. Jet lag is caused by a disruption of the human body's circadian clock.

Hormone—A chemical made in one part of the body that has an effect on another part.

Melatonin—A hormone that helps to regulate circadian rhythms.

their flight. If travel is to the west, going to bed and waking up later than usual can help the body start to adjust to the upcoming time change.

The following precautions taken during an international flight can help to limit or prevent jet lag:

- Stay hydrated. Drink plenty of water and juices to prevent dehydration. Beverages and foods with caffeine should be avoided because of their stimulant properties. Alcohol should also be avoided.
- Stretch and walk. As much movement as possible during a flight helps circulation, which moves nutrients and waste through the body and aids in elimination.
- Stay on time. Set watches and clocks ahead to the time in the destination city to start adjusting to the change.
- Eat a light snack upon arrival at the destination.
- Get as much natural sunlight as possible to help reset one's biological clock. Do not stay inside because avoidance of sunlight makes matters worse.
- Sleep smart. Draw the shade and sleep during the evening hours in the destination city, even if it is still daylight outside of the airplane. Earplugs and sleep masks may be helpful in blocking noise and light. Many airlines provide these items on international flights.
- Dress comfortably. Wear or bring comfortable clothes that will make sleeping during the flight easier.

Once arriving in their destination city, individuals should spend as much time outdoors in the sunlight as possible during the day to reset their internal clock and lessen the symptoms of jet lag. Bedtime should be postponed until at least 10 P.M., with no daytime naps. If a daytime nap is absolutely necessary, it should be limited to no more than two hours.

To promote a restful sleeping environment in a hotel setting, individuals should request that the hotel desk hold all phone calls. Because sleeping in too late can also prolong jet lag, an early wake-up call should be requested if an alarm clock is not available. If the hotel room is noisy, a portable white noise machine can help to block outside traffic and hallway noises. A room air conditioner or fan can serve the same purpose. The temperature in the room should also be adjusted for sleeping comfort.

All **antioxidants** help to decrease the effects of jet lag. Extra doses of **vitamins** A, C, and E, as well as zinc and selenium, two days before and two days after a flight help to alleviate jet lag. Melatonin, a hormone which helps to regulate circadian rhythms, can also help to combat jet lag. Melatonin is available as an over-the-counter supplement in most health food stores and pharmacies, but no more than 3 milligrams (mg) should be used in a 24-hour period.

If weather prevents an individual from spending time in the sunlight, **light therapy** may be beneficial in decreasing jet lag symptoms. Light therapy, or **phototherapy**, uses a device called a light box, which contains a set of fluorescent or incandescent lights in front of a reflector. Typically, the patient sits for 30 minutes next to a 10,000-lux box (which is about 50 times as bright as an ordinary indoor light; lux is a measurement for illuminance). Light therapy is safe for most people, but those with eye diseases should consult a healthcare professional before undergoing the treatment.

Prognosis

Jet lag usually lasts 24–48 hours after travel has taken place. In that short time period, the body adjusts to the time change, and with enough rest and daytime exposure to sunlight, it returns to normal circadian rhythm.

According to the American Sleep Association, almost 93% of travelers will experience jet lag at some point in their travels. Generally, the human body will take one–half to one day to completely adapt to its new surroundings for every one time zone crossed. However, this relationship can vary drastically depending on individuals. For instance, frequent air travelers may have not have any symptoms of jet lag after years of flying, while people on their first flight may be already very nervous and anxious about their trip and may experience debilitating jet lag.

Prevention

One cannot prevent jet lag, but it can be minimized with the following recommendations. Eat a nutritious diet (foods do not have an effect on jet lag but eating healthy can assist the body to counter changes that it experiences while flying), and get plenty of rest and **exercise** before the flight. Exercising and sleeping are also two excellent ways to minimize jet lag. For any medical conditions that may cause problems during and after the flight, visit the doctor beforehand to prepare for such problems. It is always advisable to start preparing for one's new time zone before actually going. Adapt to the new time gradually over the days, or weeks, before the flight.

During the flight, do not drink alcoholic beverages and drinks with **caffeine**. Both beverages can increase the symptoms of jet lag. On the other hand, drink plenty of water to avoid **dehydration** that is present in the cabin of airplanes. For long journeys, move around inside the airplane on a regular basis. While in the seat, exercise the legs. For travelers able to take extra time in their flight, stay overnight in an in-between city.

Melatonin is still under consideration by the U.S. Food and Drug Administration (FDA) as to being effective or not in minimizing or even preventing jet lag. The nutritional supplement has been shown in some medical studies to be effective when 0.5 to 5 milligrams (mg) of melatonin are taken during the first few days of air travel. However, as of July 2010, the FDA does not regulate it, and caution is advised for its use in countering jet lag. The FDA has also found that some melatonin products, especially those found on the Internet, have been found to contain contaminants that may cause unforeseen problems if taken by unsuspecting air travelers.

Resources

BOOKS

Daryal, Mark. *Jet Lag Relief: It's About Time* Amazon.com: CreateSpace, 2010.

Lee-Chiong, Teofilo L, editor. *Sleep Medicine Essentials*. Hoboken, NJ: Wiley-Blackwell, 2009.

Rosenfeld, Gary C. and David S Loose. *Pharmacology*. Philadelphia: Wolters Kluwer Health/Lippincott Williams and Wilkins, 2010.

Scanlon, Lynne Waller, and Charles F. Ehret. *The Cure for Jet Lag*. New York City: Back2Press Books, 2009.

Shils, Maurice, et al., editors. *Modern Nutrition in Health and Disease*. Philadelphia: Lippincott Williams and Wilkins, 2006.

Sutton, Amy L. editor. *Sleep Disorders Sourcebook*. Detroit: Omnigraphics, 2005.

OTHER

"Jet Lag and Sleep." National Sleep Foundation. http://www.sleepfoundation.org/article/sleep-topics/jet-lag-and-sleep (accessed September 5, 2010).

"Sleep and Circadian RhythmDisorders." WebMD. (September 14, 2008), http://www.webmd.com/sleep-disorders/guide/circadian-rhythm-disorders-cause. (accessed September 5, 2010).

Yanni, Emad. "Jet Lag." Centers for Disease Control and Prevention. (July 27, 2009), http://wwwnc.cdc.gov/travel/yellowbook/2010/chapter-2/jet-lag.aspx (accessed September 5, 2010).

ORGANIZATIONS

American Academy of Sleep Medicine, 2510 North Frontage Rd., Darien, IL, 60561, (630) 737-9700, (630) 737-9790, http://www.aasmnet.org.

National Sleep Foundation, 1522 K St., NW, Suite 500, Washington, DC, 20005, (202) 347-3471, (202) 347-3472, nsf@sleepfoundation.org, http://www.sleepfoundation.org.

Paula Anne Ford-Martin
Rebecca J. Frey, PhD

Jock itch

Definition

Also known as *Tinea cruris*, jock itch is a growth of fungus in the warm, moist area of the groin.

Description

Although there are many causes of jock itch, this term has become synonymous with *tinea cruris*, a common fungal infection that affects the groin and inner thighs of men and woman. *Tinea* is the name of the fungus; *cruris* comes from the Latin word for leg. Jock itch can develop when tight garments trap moisture and heat. This creates an environment in which fungi multiply and flourish. Athletes often get jock itch but non-athletic men who sweat a lot can also get it. Jock itch occurs more commonly in men, but can affect women as well. The jock itch fungus may cause a rash on the upper and inner thighs, the armpits, and the area just underneath the breasts. Many people with *tinea cruris* also have **athlete's foot**. Athlete's foot is called *tinea pedis*.

KEY TERMS

Fungus—A single-celled or multi-celled organism without chlorophyll that reproduces by spores and lives by absorbing nutrients from organic matter.

Scrotum—The external pouch of skin and muscle containing the testes (testicles).

Vaginal yeast infection—An overgrowth of fungus in the vaginal area.

Causes and symptoms

The rash of jock itch starts in the groin fold usually on both sides. If the rash advances, it usually advances down the inner thigh. The advancing edge is redder and more raised than areas that have been infected longer. The advancing edge is usually scaly and very easily distinguished or well demarcated. The skin within the border turns a reddish-brown and loses much of its scale. Jock itch can spread to the pubic and genital regions and sometimes to the buttocks.

Jock itch caused by *T. rubrum* does not involve the scrotum or penis. If those areas are involved, the most likely agent is *Candida albicans*, the same type of yeast that causes vaginal yeast infections.

Diagnosis

Often a case of jock itch can be identified based on the characteristic description previously described. If assessed by a conventional doctor, the area of affected skin may be scraped onto a glass slide for definitive diagnosis under the microscope. In order to determine the exact type of fungus present, a small piece of affected skin maybe sent off to the lab for further study.

Treatment

Typical conventional treatment for jock itch involves the use of an anti-fungal cream, spray, or powder twice a day for about two weeks. Three commonly used, over-the-counter anti-fungals are *miconazole* (Micatin), *clotrimazole* (Lotrimin) and *tolnaftate* (Tinactin). While the tendency to discontinue treatment once **itching** disappears is common, it is important to use the anti-fungal for a full two-week course in order to prevent recurrence of the infection.

Alternative treatment

Topical treatments include poultices of peppermint, oregano, or lavender. Tea tree oil, diluted with a carrier oil of almond oil, can be applied to the rash several times per day. Cedarwood and jasmine oils can relieve itching when applied in the same manner. Grapefruit seed extract can be taken as a strong solution of 15 drops in 1 oz of water.

Another alternative remedy for jock itch is to wash the groin area with the diluted juice of a freshly squeezed lemon, which can help dry up the rash. A hair dryer on the cool setting can also be used on the area after showering to dry it thoroughly. A warm bath relieves itching in many patients. The affected area should kept clean and dry, and loose-fitting, cotton underwear is recommended.

Prognosis

Treatment for jock itch is quick and usually effective, but the condition often comes back. With treatment, jock itch improves in two or three days and is completely gone in three or four weeks. The following people should be especially vigilant to prevent the problem from returning:

- Athletes
- People with fungal infections that affect other parts of the body (such as athlete's foot)
- People who wear tight clothing
- People with damaged or altered immune systems, including people with HIV or AIDS

Prevention

The best prevention of jock itch is cleanliness and sanitation. This includes keeping the groin area dry, wearing loose-fitting rather than tight clothing, wear boxer shorts rather than briefs, change sweat-covered clothes as soon as possible, showering immediately after working out or playing a sport and then applying talc, and washing workout clothes or sports uniforms after each use.

Resources

BOOKS

Jameson T. K. *Secrets Of Ringworm Treatment: Everything You Ever Needed to Know about Ringworm, Athletes Foot, Jock Itch, Other Forms of Fungal Infection and How to Treat Them.* Seattle: CreateSpace, 2010.

PERIODICALS

Grin, Caron. "Tinea: Diagnostic Clues, Treatment Keys." *Consultant* (February 2004): 214-216.

"Jock Itch." *Clinical Reference Systems* (January 1, 2004): 1859.

Schmitt, B. D. "Jock Itch for Teenagers." *Clinical Reference Systems* (January 1, 2004): 1858.

OTHER

"Tinea Infections." MedlinePlus. November 23, 2010. http://www.nlm.nih.gov/medlineplus/tineainfections.html (accessed November 24, 2010).

ORGANIZATIONS

American Academy of Dermatology, PO Box 4014, Schaumburg, IL, 60168-4014, (847) 240-1859, (866) 503-SKIN (7546), http://www.aad.org.

Ken R. Wells,

Joint aspiration *see* **Joint fluid analysis**

Joint biopsy

Definition

A joint or synovial membrane biopsy refers to a procedure where a sample of the joint lining or synovial membrane is taken.

Purpose

A joint biopsy is performed to determine why a joint is painful or swollen. It is usually reserved for more difficult cases where the diagnosis is not clear. The test can be used to diagnose bacterial or fungal infections, an abnormal buildup of iron, **cancer**, or other diseases.

Precautions

The procedure must be done under very sterile conditions to reduce the risk of infection.

Description

The test is performed either in the doctor's office, clinic, or hospital by a surgeon. There are many different ways to perform this biopsy: through an incision in the joint; with a scope inserted in the joint; or, more typically, by the insertion of a sharp instrument through the skin. The procedure can be taken from any joint, but the most common joint requiring biopsy is the knee. A sharp instrument (trocar) is pushed into the joint space. A needle with an attached syringe is inserted into the joint to withdraw fluid for laboratory analysis. The surgeon may instill numbing medicine into the joint and along the needle track before the needle is withdrawn. The trocar and then the biopsy needle is inserted and specimens taken. After the specimen is taken, both the trocar and the biopsy needle are removed, a bandage is placed over the joint, and the samples are sent to pathology for analysis.

KEY TERMS

Joint—The point where two bones meet.

Pathology—The branch of medicine that looks at abnormal changes in cells and tissues which signal disease.

Synovial membrane—Membrane lining a joint.

Trocar—A sharp pointed tube through which a needle can be inserted.

Preparation

Blood tests will be done to check that **blood clots** properly. A mild sedative may be given before the procedure. With the patient lying down, the skin over the joint is disinfected and a local anesthetic is injected into the skin and tissue just below the skin.

Aftercare

The joint will need rest for at least one day. Normal activity can resume if there is no increased **pain** or swelling.

Risks

There is a chance of joint swelling or tenderness. Rarely, bleeding and infection can occur in the joint, or the biopsy needle could break off or strike a nerve or blood vessel. The risk of infection is higher if the patient has an immune deficiency.

Resources

BOOKS

Firestein, Gary S., et al. *Kelley's Textbook of Rheumatology*. Philadelphia: Saunders/Elsevier, 2009.

Jeanine Barone

Joint endoscopy *see* **Arthroscopy**

Joint fluid analysis

Definition

Joint fluid analysis, also called synovial fluid analysis, or arthrocentesis, is a procedure used to assess joint-related abnormalities, such as in the knee or elbow.

KEY TERMS

Aspirate—The removal by suction of a fluid from a body cavity using a needle.

Bursae—A closed sac lined with a synovial membrane and filled with fluid, usually found in areas subject to friction, such as where a tendon passes over a bone.

Hematoma—A localized mass of blood that is confined within an organ or tissue.

Synovial fluid—A transparent lubricating fluid secreted in a sac to protect an area where a tendon passes over a bone.

Purpose

The purpose of a joint fluid analysis is to identify the cause of swelling in the joints, to relieve **pain** and distention from fluid accumulation in the joint, and to diagnose certain types of arthritis and inflammatory joint diseases. The test is also a method to determine whether an infection, either bacterial or fungal, exists within the joint.

Precautions

Joint fluid analysis should not be performed on any patient who is uncooperative, especially if the patient cannot or will not keep the joint immobile throughout the procedure. Patients with certain infections should be excluded from the procedure, particularly those who have a local infection along the proposed needle track. The joint space should be accessible. Therefore, a poorly accessible joint space, such as in hip aspiration in an obese patient, should not be subject to this procedure.

Description

The test is also called arthrocentesis, joint tap, and closed joint aspiration. Normal synovial fluid is a clear or pale-yellow fluid found in small amounts in joints, bursae (fluid-filled sac found on points of friction, like joints), and tendon sheaths. The procedure is done by passing a needle into a joint space and sucking out (aspirating) synovial fluid for diagnostic analysis. When the sample is sent to the laboratory, the fluid is analyzed for color, clarity, quantity, and chemical composition. It is also examined microscopically to check for the presence of bacteria and other cells.

The procedure takes about 10 minutes. Prior to the procedure, any risks that are involved should be explained to the patient. No intravenous pain medications or sedatives are required, although the patient will be given a local anesthetic.

The patient is asked to lie on their back and remain relaxed. The local anesthetic, typically an injection of lidocaine, is then administered. The clinician is usually seated next to the patient. Then the clinician marks exactly where the needle is to enter. As the needle enters the joint, a "pop" may be felt or heard. This is normal. Correct placement of the needle in the joint space is normally painless. At this point, the clinician slowly drains some of the fluid into the syringe. The needle is then withdrawn and adhesive tape is placed over the needle site.

Preparation

Glucose, or sugar, in the joint can be a signal of arthritis. If the clinician will be doing a glucose test, the patient will be asked to fast for 6–12 hours preceding the procedure. If not, there is no special preparation required for a joint fluid analysis.

Aftercare

Some post-procedural pain may be experienced. For this reason, the patient should arrange to be driven home by someone else. Aftercare of the joints will depend on the results of the analysis.

Risks

While joint fluid analysis is generally a safe procedure, especially when performed on a large, easily accessible joint, such as the knee, some risks are possible. Some of the complications to the procedure, although rare, include infection at the site of the needle stick, an accumulation of blood (hematoma) formation, local pain, injury to cartilage, tendon rupture, and nerve damage.

Normal results

The results of a normal joint fluid analysis include fluid of a clear or pale-yellow color and the absence of bacteria, fungus, and other cells, such as white blood cells.

Abnormal results

The results of an abnormal joint fluid analysis include fluid that is turbid, or cloudy. Also, white blood cells and other blood cells may be found, from which the clinician can make a diagnosis and arrive at a treatment for the joint problem. An abnormal result can indicate an infection caused by a bacteria, or **tuberculosis**. Or, there might be inflammation that is caused by **gout**, **rheumatoid arthritis**, or **osteoarthritis**.

Resources

BOOKS

Cecil, Russell L., Lee Goldman, and D. A. Audiello. *Cecil Medicine*. 23rd ed, Philadelphia: Saunders Elsevier, 2008.

Ron Gasbarro

Joint infection *see* **Infectious arthritis**
Joint radiography *see* **Arthrography**

Joint replacement

Definition

Joint replacement is the surgical replacement of a joint with an artificial prosthesis.

Great advances have been made in joint replacement since the first hip replacement was performed in the United States in 1969. Improvements have been made in the endurance and compatibility of materials used and the surgical techniques to install artificial joints. Custom joints can be made using a mold of the original joint that duplicate the original with a very high degree of accuracy.

The most common joints to be replaced are hips and knees. There is ongoing work on elbow and other joint replacement, but some joint problems are still treated with joint resection (the surgical removal of the joint in question) or interpositional reconstruction (the reassembly of the joint from constituent parts).

Purpose

Seventy percent of joint replacements are performed because arthritis has caused the joint to stiffen and become painful to the point where normal daily activities are no longer possible. If the joint does not respond to conservative treatment such medication, weight loss, activity restriction, and use of walking aids such as a cane, joint replacement is considered appropriate.

Patients with **rheumatoid arthritis** or other connective tissue diseases may also be candidates for joint replacement, but the results are usually less satisfactory

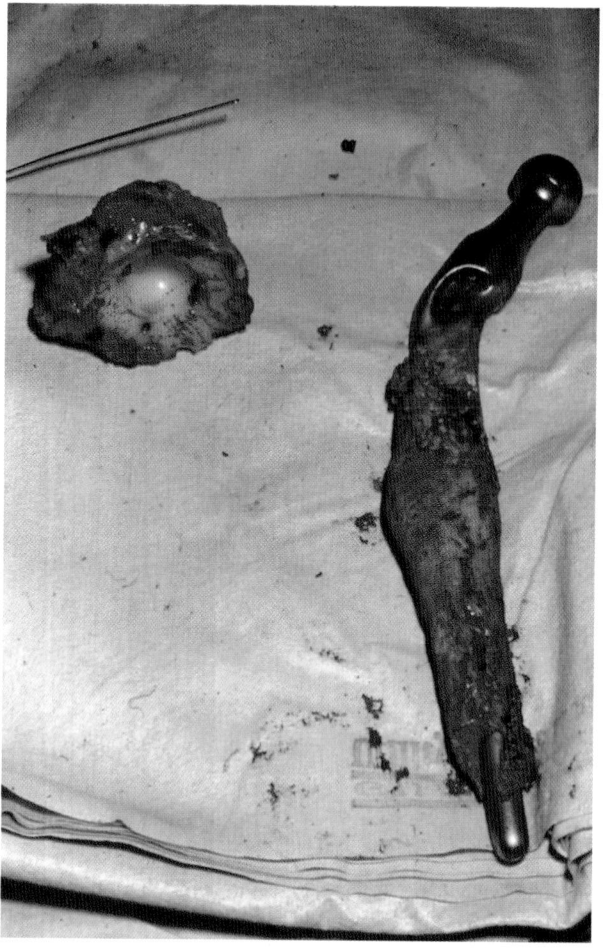

The components of a prosthetic hip joint, removed due to loosening. On the right is the metal shaft encased in the cement which fixed it to the inside of the femur. On the left is the plastic socket. *(Custom Medical Stock Photo, Inc. Reproduced by permission.)*

in those patients. Elderly people who fall and break their hip often undergo hip replacement when the probability of successful bone healing is low.

More than 773,000 hip and knee replacements are performed in the United States each year. Since the lifetime of the artificial joint is limited, the best candidates or joint replacement are over age 60.

Changing demographics will likely place new emphasis on joint replacement procedures in the healthcare system. For example, the demand for joint replacement surgery in younger people is rising dramatically as rising **obesity** rates stress younger joints. According to the American Academy of Orthopedic Surgeons, more than half of patients needing hip or knee replacements will be under 65 by 2016. Also, total joint replacement surgeries, now including shoulder and ankle replacements, are greatly rising at a time

KEY TERMS

Catheterization—Inserting a tube into the bladder so that a patient can urinate without leaving the bed.

Prosthesis—A synthetic replacement for a missing part of the body, such as a knee or a hip.

Rheumatoid arthritis—A joint disease of unknown origins that may begin at an early age causing deformity and loss of function in the joints.

when fewer doctors are choosing **orthopedic surgery** as a career.

Description

Joint replacements are performed under general or regional anesthesia in a hospital by an orthopedic surgeon. Some medical centers specialize in joint replacement, and these centers generally have a higher success rate than less specialized facilities. The specific techniques of joint replacement vary depending on the joint involved.

Hip Replacement

During a hip replacement, the surgeon makes an incision along the top of the thigh bone (femur) and pulls the thigh bone away from the socket of the hip bone (the acetabulum). An artificial socket made of metal coated with polyethylene (plastic) to reduce friction is inserted in the hip. The top of the thigh bone is cut, and a piece of artificial thigh made of metal is fitted into the lower thigh bone on one end and the new socket on the other.

The artificial hip can either be held in place by synthetic cement or by natural bone in-growth. The cement is an acrylic polymer. It assures good locking of the prosthesis to the remaining bone. However, bubbles left in the cement after it cures may act as weak spots, causing the development of cracks. This promotes loosening of the prosthesis later in life. If additional surgery is needed, all the cement must be removed before additional surgery can be performed.

An artificial hip fixed by natural bone in-growth requires more precise surgical techniques to assure maximum contact between the remaining natural bone and the prosthesis. The prosthesis is made so that it contains small pores that encourage the natural bone to grow into it. Growth begins 6 to 12 weeks after surgery. The short-term outcome with non-cemented hips is less satisfactory, with patients reporting more thigh **pain**, but the long-term outlook is better, with fewer cases of hip loosening in non-cemented hips. The current trend is to use the non-cemented technique. Hospital stays last from four to eight days.

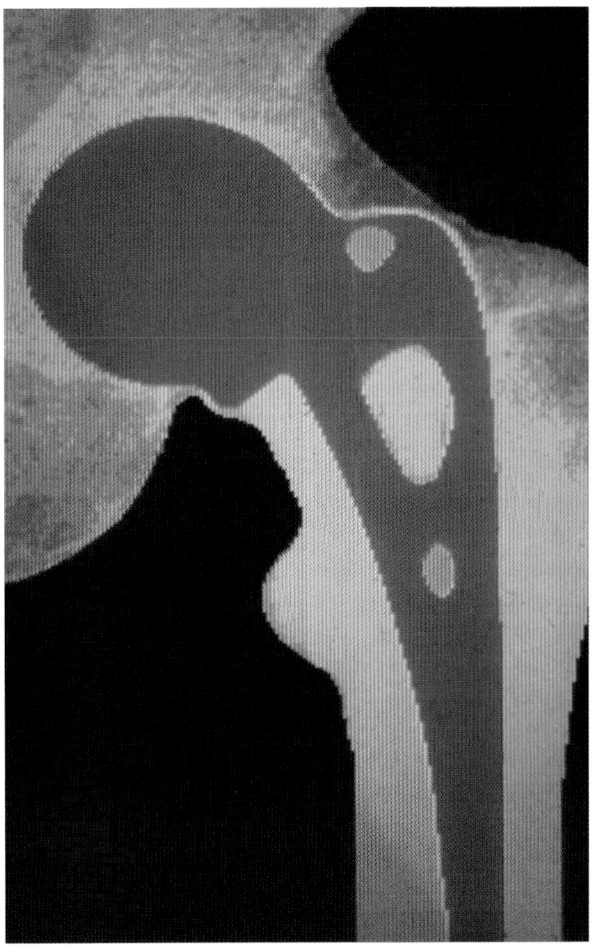

A false color x-ray image of the human pelvis showing a prosthetic hip joint. *(Custom Medical Stock Photo, Inc. Reproduced by permission.)*

Knee Replacement

The doctor puts a tourniquet above the knee, then makes a cut to expose the knee joint. The ligaments surrounding the knee are loosened, then the shin bone and thigh bone are cut and the knee removed. The artificial knee is then cemented into place on the remaining stubs of those bones. The excess cement is removed, and the knee is closed. Hospital stays range from three to six days.

In both types of surgery, preventing infection is very important. **Antibiotics** are given intravenously and continued in pill form after the surgery. Fluid and blood loss can be great, and sometimes blood transfusions are needed.

Preparation

Many patients choose to donate their own blood for **transfusion** during the surgery. This prevents any blood incompatibility problems or the transmission of bloodborne diseases.

Prior to surgery, all the standard preoperative blood and urine tests are performed, and the patient meets with the anesthesiologist to discuss any special conditions that affect the administration of anesthesia. Patients receiving **general anesthesia** should not eat or drink for ten hours prior to the operation.

Aftercare

Immediately after the operation the patient will be catheterized so that he or she will not have to get out of bed to urinate. The patient will be monitored for infection. Antibiotics are continued and pain medication is prescribed. **Physical therapy** begins (first passive exercises, then active ones) as soon as possible using a walker, cane, or crutches for additional support. Long term care of the artificial joint involves refraining from heavy activity and heavy lifting, and learning how to sit, walk, how to get out of beds, chairs, and cars so as not to dislocate the joint.

Risks

The immediate risks during and after surgery include the development of **blood clots** that may come loose and block the arteries, excessive loss of blood, and infection. Blood-thinning medication is usually given to reduce the risk of clots forming. Some elderly people experience short term confusion and disorientation from the anesthesia.

Although joint replacement surgery is highly successful, there is an increased risk of nerve injury. Dislocation or fracture of the hip joint is also a possibility. Infection caused by the operation can occur as long as a year later and can be difficult to treat. Some doctors add antibiotics directly to the cement used to fix the replacement joint in place. Loosening of the joint is the most common cause of failure in hip joints that are not infected. This may require another joint replacement surgery in about 12% of patients within a 15-year period following the first procedure.

Joint replacements are performed successfully on an older-than-average group of patients. People with diseases that interfere with blood clotting are not good candidates for joint replacement. Joint replacement surgery should not be done on patients with infection, or any heart, kidney or lung problems that would make it risky to undergo general anesthesia.

Results

More than 90% of patients receiving hip replacements achieve complete relief from pain and significant improvement in joint function. The success rate is slightly lower in knee replacements, and drops still more for other joint replacement operations.

Resources

BOOKS

Kennon, Robert E., MD. *Hip and Knee Surgery: A Patient's Guide To Hip Replacement, Hip Resurfacing, Knee Replacement, and Knee Arthroscopy*. Lulu.com, 2008.

Shanbhag, Arun S., Rubash, Harry E., and Jacobs, Joshua J. *Joint replacement and Bone Resorption : Pathology, Biomaterials, and Clinical Practice*. New York: Taylor & Francis, 2006.

OTHER

National Institutes of Health. "Knee Replacement." *Medline Plus*. http://www.nlm.nih.gov/medlineplus/kneereplacement.html (accessed February 2, 2010).

ORGANIZATIONS

Arthritis Foundation, P.O. Box 7669, Atlanta, GA, 30357–0669, (404) 872–7100, (800) 283–7800, http://www.arthritis.org.

National Institute of Arthritis and Musculoskeletal and Skin Diseases (NIAMS), 1 AMS Circle, Bethesda, MD, 20892–3675, (877) 22–NIAMS (226–4267), (301) 718–6366, NIAMSinfo@mail.nih.gov, http://www.niams.nih.gov.

Tish Davidson, A.M.
Brenda W. Lerner

Joint resection *see* **Arthroplasty**

Joint x rays *see* **Arthrography**

Juvenile arthritis

Definition

Juvenile arthritis (JA) is not a single disorder but a group of arthritides (plural of arthritis) that affect children and teenagers below the age of 16. JA has been known by various names since 1970, including juvenile **rheumatoid arthritis** (JRA), juvenile idiopathic arthritis (JIA), and juvenile chronic arthritis (JCA). All the conditions included under the general term of JA strike children under age 16, and all have immune-mediated joint inflammation as their major manifestation. The International League of Associations for Rheumatology

(ILAR) has tried to bridge these differences with a unifying set of criteria to define juvenile arthritis.

Demographics

According to the American College of Rheumatology (ACR), as of 2010 about one child in every 1,000 in the United States develops some form of JA. Doctors estimate that around 300,000 children in the United States have been diagnosed with JIA. Native Americans in both Canada and the United States have somewhat higher rates of JA than members of other racial and ethnic groups. Internationally, Norway and Australia have the highest rates of JA, while Africa and individuals of African ancestry appear to have lower than average rates. The reason for these differences is not yet known.

Description

The skeletal system of the body is made up of different types of the strong, fibrous tissue known as connective tissue. Bone, cartilage, ligaments, and tendons are all forms of connective tissue that have different compositions, and thus different characteristics.

The joints are structures that hold two or more bones together. Some joints (synovial joints) allow for movement between the bones being joined (called articulating bones). The simplest model of a synovial joint involves two bones, separated by a slight gap called the joint cavity. The ends of each articular bone are covered by a layer of cartilage. A tough tissue called the articular capsule surrounds both articular bones and the joint cavity. The articular capsule has two components: the fibrous membrane on the outside, and the synovial membrane (or synovium) on the inside. The fibrous membrane may include tough bands of fibrous tissue called ligaments, which are responsible for providing support to the joints. The synovial membrane has special cells and many capillaries (tiny blood vessels). This membrane produces a supply of synovial fluid that fills the joint cavity, lubricates it, and helps the articular bones move smoothly about the joint.

In JA, the synovial membrane becomes intensely inflamed. Usually thin and delicate, the synovium becomes thick and stiff, with numerous infoldings on its surface. The membrane becomes invaded by white blood cells, which produce a variety of destructive chemicals. The cartilage along the articular surfaces of the bones may be attacked and destroyed, and the bone, articular capsule, and ligaments may begin to be worn away. These processes severely interfere with movement in the joint.

JA specifically refers to chronic arthritic conditions that affect a child under the age of 16 years and last for a minimum of three to six months. JA is often characterized by a waxing and waning course, with flares separated by periods during which no symptoms are noted (remission). Some of the medical literature refers to JA as juvenile rheumatoid arthritis, although most types of JA differ significantly from the adult disease called rheumatoid arthritis, in terms of symptoms, progression, and prognosis.

Risk factors

The two major risk factors for JA are sex and race. Most forms of JA are more common in girls than in boys (the major exception being eye disorders), and more common in Caucasian and Native American children than in children of other races.

Causes and symptoms

Causes

A number of different causes have been sought to explain the onset of JA. There seems to be some genetic link, because the tendency to develop JA sometimes runs in a particular family, and because certain genetic markers are more frequently found in patients with JA and other related diseases. Genes that have been linked to increased susceptibility to JA as of 2010 include the *IL2RA/CD25* gene and the *VTCN1* gene.

Many researchers have looked for some infectious cause for JA, but no clear connection to a particular organism has ever been made. JA is considered by some to be an autoimmune disorder. **Autoimmune disorders** occur when the body's immune system mistakenly identifies the body's own tissue as foreign and goes about attacking those tissues as if trying to rid the body of an invader (such as a bacteria, virus, or fungi). While an autoimmune mechanism is strongly suspected, certain markers of such a mechanism (such as rheumatoid factor, often present in adults with such disorders) are rarely present in children with JA.

Symptoms

Joint symptoms of arthritis may include stiffness, **pain**, redness and warmth of the joint, and swelling. Bone in the area of an affected joint may grow too quickly, or too slowly, resulting in limbs that are of different lengths. When the child tries to avoid moving a painful joint, the muscle may begin to shorten from disuse. This is called a contracture.

Symptoms of JA depend on the particular subtype. According to criteria published by the American College of Rheumatology (ACR) in 1973 and modified in 1977,

KEY TERMS

Articular bones—Two or more bones connected with each other via a joint.

Biologics—A class of drugs produced by means of biological processes involving recombinant DNA technology.

Congenital—Present at birth.

Contracture—Shortening of a muscle or joint due to a disease condition or injury.

Flare—A recurrence or worsening of the symptoms of JA.

Idiopathic—Of unknown cause or spontaneous origin. JRA is sometimes called juvenile idiopathic arthritis or JIA because its causes are still not fully known.

Joint—A structure that holds two or more bones together.

Rheumatology—The branch of medicine that specializes in the diagnosis and treatment of disorders affecting the muscles and joints.

Synovial joint—A particular type of joint that allows for movement in the articular bones.

Synovial membrane—The membrane that lines the inside of the articular capsule of a joint and produces a lubricating fluid called synovial fluid.

Uveitis—Inflammation of the pigmented vascular covering of the eye, which includes the choroid, iris, and ciliary body. Uveitis is a common complication of JRA.

JRA is classified by the symptoms that appear within the first six months of the disorder:

- Pauciarticular JA: This is the most common and the least severe type of JA, affecting about 40–60% of all JA patients. This type affects fewer than four joints, usually the knee, ankle, wrist, and/or elbow. Other more general (systemic) symptoms are usually absent, and the child's growth usually remains normal. Very few children (less than 15%) with pauciarticular JA end up with deformed joints. Some children with this form of JA experience painless swelling of the joint. Some children with JA have a serious inflammation of structures within the eye, which if left undiagnosed and untreated could lead to blindness. This condition is known as uveitis, and affects about 20% of children diagnosed with JRA. While many children have cycles of flares and remissions, in some children the disease completely and permanently resolves within a few years of diagnosis.
- Polyarticular JA: About 40% of all cases of JA are of this type. More girls than boys are diagnosed with this form of JA. This type is most common in children up to age three or after the age of 10. Polyarticular JA affects five or more joints simultaneously. It usually affects the small joints of both hands and both feet, although other large joints may be affected as well. Some patients with arthritis in their knees experience a different rate of growth in each leg. Ultimately, one leg will grow longer than the other. About half of all patients with polyarticular JA have arthritis of the spine and/or hip. Some patients with polyarticular JA have other symptoms of a systemic illness, including anemia (low red blood cell count), decreased growth rate, low appetite, low-grade fever, and a slight rash. The disease is most severe in those children who are diagnosed in early adolescence. Some of these children test positive for a marker present in other autoimmune disorders, called rheumatoid factor (RF). RF is found in adults who have rheumatoid arthritis. Children who are positive for RF tend to have a more severe course, with a disabling form of arthritis that destroys and deforms the joints. This type of arthritis is thought to be the adult form of rheumatoid arthritis occurring at a very early age.
- Systemic-onset JA: Sometimes called Still disease (after a physician who originally described it), this is a type of JA that occurs in about 10–20% of all patients with JA. Boys and girls are equally affected, and diagnosis is usually made between the ages of 5–10 years. The initial symptoms are not usually related to the joints. Instead, these children have high fevers; a rash; decreased appetite and weight loss; severe joint and muscle pain; swollen lymph nodes, spleen, and liver; and serious anemia. Some children experience other complications, including inflammation of the sac containing the heart (pericarditis); inflammation of the tissue lining the chest cavity and lungs (pleuritis); and inflammation of the heart muscle (myocarditis). The eye inflammation often seen in pauciarticular JA is uncommon in systemic onset JA. Symptoms of actual arthritis begin later in the course of systemic onset JA, and they often involve the wrists and ankles. Many of these children continue to have periodic flares of fever and systemic symptoms throughout childhood. Some children will go on to develop a polyarticular type of JA.

- Enthesis-related arthritis (sometimes called spondyloarthropathy): This type of JA most commonly affects boys older than eight years of age. The arthritis occurs in the knees and ankles, moving over time to include the hips and lower spine. Inflammation of the eye may occur occasionally, but usually resolves without permanent damage.
- Psoriatic JA: This type of arthritis usually shows up in fewer than four joints, but spreads to include multiple joints (appearing similar to polyarticular JA). Hips, back, fingers, and toes are frequently affected. A skin condition called psoriasis accompanies this type of arthritis. Children often have pits or ridges in their fingernails. The arthritis usually progresses to become a serious, disabling problem.

There is some disagreement among specialists about the classification of JRA. Some prefer the EULAR classification, introduced in 1977, to the ACR system. More recently the International League of Associations for Rheumatology (ILAR) has identified a unifying set of criteria to define juvenile arthritis. As of 2010, inconsistencies in naming the specific types of juvenile arthritis and their criteria for diagnosis continue to exist.

Diagnosis

The diagnosis of JA is not always obvious and may be delayed because some children do not complain of pain, and swelling of the joints may not be obvious.

Diagnosis of JA is usually made on the basis of the child's collection of symptoms together with elimination of other possible causes of the symptoms. Disorders to be ruled out include lupus, **Lyme disease**, certain bone disorders, infections, and childhood **cancer**. The diagnosis will usually involve a referral from the child's pediatrician to a rheumatologist, a physician specializing in disorders of the muscles and joints).

Examination

Symptoms of JA that the doctor can observe or measure during an office physical include:

- limping
- fever
- difficulty in moving or using an arm or leg
- swollen joint(s)
- skin rash on the chest, arms, or legs that comes and goes with fever
- swollen lymph nodes
- enlarged liver and spleen
- red eyes
- pain when a bright light is shone in the eye.

Tests

There is no blood test as of 2010 that can be used to diagnose JA, and other laboratory tests often show normal results. A blood test may be useful in ruling out certain infections as a cause of the child's symptoms. Some nonspecific indicators of inflammation may be elevated, including **white blood cell count**, **erythrocyte sedimentation rate**, and a marker called **C-reactive protein**. As with any chronic disease, anemia may be present. Children with an extraordinarily early onset of the adult type of rheumatoid arthritis will have a positive test for rheumatoid factor.

Imaging studies (most often x rays) may be taken to rule out broken or fractured bones, congenital defects in the joints, tumors, or some types of **infectious disease**. X-ray studies may also be done to monitor the development of the child's bones. **Magnetic resonance imaging** (MRI) and ultrasound are used increasingly as of 2010 to detect damage caused by JA in order to prevent further damage to the child's joints.

Procedures

In some cases the doctor may tap a swollen joint by inserting a small hollow needle into the joint to withdraw some of the fluid. This fluid can be analyzed to help determine the cause of the arthritis. In addition, withdrawing fluid may ease the discomfort in the joint.

Treatment

Traditional

Mainstream treatment of JA involves the use of appropriate medications together with physical and **occupational therapy** as needed. Some children with JA may eventually need surgery, including **joint replacement**, and others may require psychological counseling to cope with depression or anger related to their symptoms. The goal of therapy is to control symptoms, maintain functioning of the child's joints, and prevent damage to the joints.

Drugs

Treating JA involves efforts to decrease the amount of inflammation in order to preserve movement. Medications that can be used for this include such nonsteroidal anti-inflammatory agents (NSAIDs) as ibuprofen (Motrin, Ibuprin), naproxen (Aleve, Naprelan, Naprosyn), diclofenac (Voltaren, Cataflam), and Tolmetin (Tolectin). Oral steroid medications are effective but have many serious side effects with long-term use. Injections of **steroids** into an affected joint can be helpful. Steroid eye drops are used to treat eye inflammation.

Occasionally, splints are used to rest painful joints and to try to prevent or improve deformities.

Children who do not respond to treatment with NSAIDs may be given disease-modifying **antirheumatic drugs** or DMARDs. DMARDs include such medications as hydroxychloroquine (Plaquenil), sulfasalazine (Azulfidine), and methotrexate (Rheumatrex). More recent agents used to treat JA include biologics, which are drugs produced using recombinant DNA technology. Biologics used to treat JA include etanercept (Embrel), infliximab (Remicade), adalimumab (Humira), and abatacept (Orencia). Biologics work by blocking high levels of proteins that cause inflammation in the body.

Alternative

Juice therapy has been suggested as an alternative treatment for arthritis. It works to detoxify the body, helping to reduce JA symptoms. Some recommended fruits and vegetables to include in the juice are carrots, celery, cabbage, potatoes, cherries, lemons, beets, cucumbers, radishes, and garlic. Tomatoes and other vegetables in the nightshade family (potatoes, eggplant, red and green peppers) are discouraged.

As an adjunct therapy, **aromatherapy** preparations use cypress, fennel, and lemon. Massage oils include rosemary, benzoin, chamomile, camphor, juniper, and lavender. Other types of therapy that have been used include **acupuncture**, **acupressure**, and bodywork.

Nutritional supplements that may be beneficial include large amounts of **antioxidants** (**vitamins** C, A, E, zinc, selenium, and flavenoids), as well as B vitamins and a full complement of **minerals** (including boron, copper, manganese). Other nutrients that assist in detoxifying the body, including methionine, cysteine, and other amino acids, may also be helpful. A number of autoimmune disorders, including JA, seem to have a relationship to **food allergies**. Identification and elimination of reactive foods may result in a decrease in JA symptoms. Constitutional homeopathy can work to quiet the symptoms of JA and bring about balance to the whole person. None of these alternative treatments, however, have been proven effective in clinical trials that meet the standards of conventional Western medicine.

Prognosis

The prognosis for pauciarticular JA is quite good, as is the prognosis for spondyloarthropathy. Polyarticular JA carries a somewhat worse prognosis; children who have many joints involved, or who have a positive rheumatoid factor are more likely to have chronic pain, disability, and problems with school attendance. Systemic onset JA has a variable prognosis, depending on the organ systems affected, and the progression to polyarticular JA. JRA is rarely life-threatening; however, about 1–5% of all JA patients die of such complications as infection, inflammation of the heart, or **kidney disease**. In addition, depression and other psychological problems are common in children with JA, particularly when they enter their teen years. Many children benefit from support groups and special summer camp programs for children with JA.

Prevention

Because so little is known about the causes of JA, there are no recommendations as of 2010 for preventing its development.

Resources

BOOKS

Huff, Charlotte. *Raising a Child with Arthritis*. 2nd ed. Atlanta, GA: Arthritis Foundation, 2008.

Rouba, Kelly. *Juvenile Arthritis: The Ultimate Teen Guide*. Lanham, MD: Scarecrow Press, 2009.

Szer, Ilona S., et al., eds. *Arthritis in Children and Adolescents: Juvenile Idiopathic Arthritis*. New York: Oxford University Press, 2006.

PERIODICALS

Angeles-Han, S., and S. Prahalad. "The Genetics of Juvenile Idiopathic Arthritis: What Is New in 2010?" *Current Rheumatology Reports* 12 (April 2010): 87–93.

Damasio, M.B., et al. "Synovial and Inflammatory Diseases in Childhood: Role of New Imaging Modalities in the Assessment of Patients with Juvenile Idiopathic Arthritis." *Pediatric Radiology* 40 (June 2010): 985–98.

Haber, L., et al. "Clinical Manifestations and Treatment of the Pediatric Rheumatoid Patient." *Clinics in Podiatric Medicine and Surgery* 27 (April 2010): 219–33.

Kalinina Ayuso, V., et al. "Male Gender as a Risk Factor for Complications in Uveitis Associated with Juvenile Idiopathic Arthritis." *American Journal of Ophthalmology* 149 (June 2010): 994–99.

Oen, K., et al. "Early Outcomes and Improvement of Patients with Juvenile Idiopathic Arthritis Enrolled in a Canadian Multicenter Inception Cohort." *Arthritis Care and Research* 62 (April 2010): 527–36.

Philpott, J.F., et al. "Physical Activity Recommendations for Children with Specific Chronic Health Conditions: Juvenile Idiopathic Arthritis, Hemophilia, Asthma, and Cystic Fibrosis." *Clinical Journal of Sport Medicine* 20 (May 2010): 167–72.

Shin, S.T., et al. "Nutritional Status and Clinical Characteristics in Children With Juvenile Rheumatoid Arthritis." *Journal of Microbiology, Immunology, and Infection* 43 (April 2010): 93–98.

OTHER

Abramson, Leslie. "Arthritis in Children." American College of Rheumatology (ACR). June 2008. http://

www.rheumatology.org/practice/clinical/patients/diseases_and_conditions/juvenilearthritis.asp (accessed September 25, 2010).

Borigini, Mark James. "Juvenile Rheumatoid Arthritis." *MedlinePlus*. May 31, 2009. http://www.nlm.nih.gov/medlineplus/ency/article/000451.htm (accessed September 25, 2010).

"Juvenile Arthritis Fact Sheet." JA Alliance. http://www.arthritis.org/ja-fact-sheet.php (accessed September 25, 2010).

"Juvenile Rheumatoid Arthritis." *MayoClinic*. October 16, 2009. http://www.mayoclinic.com/health/juvenile-rheumatoid-arthritis/DS00018 (accessed September 25, 2010).

Rabinovich, C. Egla. "Juvenile Rheumatoid Arthritis." *eMedicine*. June 1, 2010. http://emedicine.medscape.com/article/1007276-overview (accessed September 25, 2010).

ORGANIZATIONS

American College of Rheumatology (ACR), 2200 Lake Boulevard NE, Atlanta, GA, 30319, (404) 633-3777, (404) 633-1870, acr@rheumatology.org, http://www.rheumatology.org.

Arthritis Foundation, PO Box 7669, Atlanta, GA, 30357-0669, (800) 283-7800, http://www.arthritis.org.

European League against Rheumatism (EULAR), Seestrasse 240, Zürich, Switzerland, CH 8802 Kächberg, +41 44 716 30 30, +41 44 716 30 39, http://www.eular.org.

International League of Associations for Rheumatology (ILAR), ndavidai@rheumatology.org, http://www.ilar.org.

National Institute of Arthritis and Musculoskeletal and Skin Diseases (NIAMS), 1 AMS Circle, Bethesda, MD, 20892-3675, (301) 495-4484, (877) 22-NIAMS, (301) 718-6366, NIAMSinfo@mail.nih.gov, http://www.niams.nih.gov.

Rosalyn Carson-DeWitt, MD
Rebecca J. Frey, PhD
Tish Davidson, AM

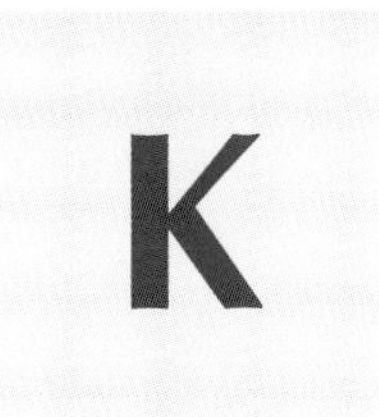

Kala-azar *see* **Leishmaniasis**

Kaposi's sarcoma

Definition

Kaposi's sarcoma (KS) is a form of **cancer** that is manifested by lesions on the skin and can also progress to involve internal organs. It most often is found in patients with acquired **immunodeficiency** syndrome (**AIDS**) and can be fatal.

Demographics

The incidence of KS was very rare in the United States before the AIDS epidemic with only 19 cases reported in men between the ages of 20 and 54 years in the years 1975 to 1980. In 1981, an aggressive form of KS began to appear in homosexual men. At that time, almost half of homosexual men diagnosed with AIDS also developed KS. Incidence of KS peaked in 1989 and has decreased significantly since that time as a result of safer sexual practices and the introduction of highly active antiretroviral therapy (HAART). Among transplant patients, the incidence rate is about one in every 200 patients. At this time about 2500 new cases of KS are diagnosed each year in the United States, although there may be some underreporting of cases in the AIDS population.

Internationally, the incidence of KS remains very high in Africa. The highest rates of classic KS are found in Sicily and in Sardinia. These cases are, in general, unrelated to AIDS.

Description

Kaposi's sarcoma (KS) was once a very rare form of cancer, primarily affecting elderly men of Mediterranean and eastern European background, until the 1980s, when it began to appear among AIDS patients. It manifests in four distinct forms. The first form, called classic or sporadic KS, was described by the Austrian dermatologist Moritz Kaposi more than a century ago. Classic KS usually affects older men of Mediterranean or eastern European ancestry by producing tumors on the lower legs. Though at times painful and disfiguring, the tumors generally are not life–threatening. The second form of the disease, African endemic KS, affects boys and men primarily. It can appear as classic KS, or in a more deadly form that quickly spreads to tissues below the skin, the bones, and lymph system, leading to **death** within a few years of diagnosis. Another form of KS, immunocompromised KS, is observed in kidney and liver transplant patients who take immunosuppressive drugs to prevent rejection of their organ transplant.

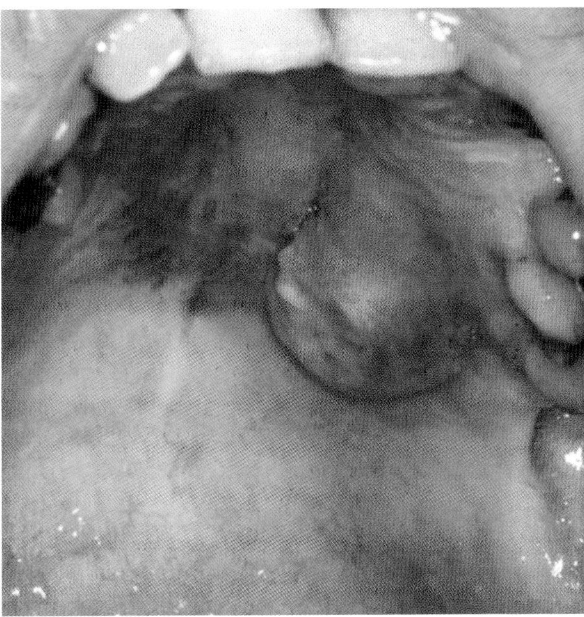

This HIV-positive patient is afflicted with Kaposi's sarcoma inside the mouth. *(Custom Medical Stock Photo, Inc. Reproduced by permission.)*

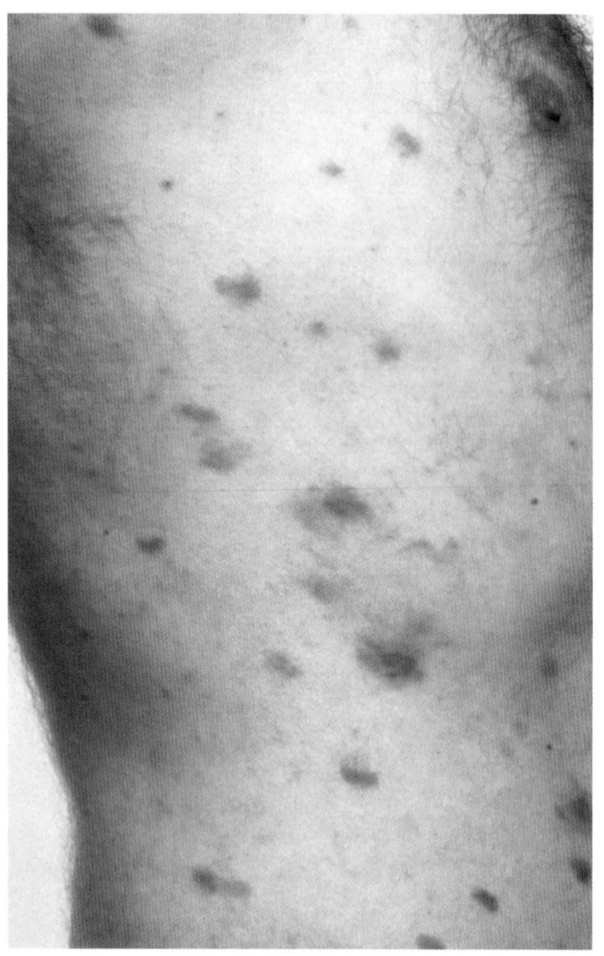

Kaposi's sarcoma usually appears on the lower extremities, as evidenced on this patient's hip. *(Custom Medical Stock Photo, Inc. Reproduced by permission.)*

MORIZ KAPOSI (1837–1902)

Moriz Kohn Kaposi was born in 1837 to very poor Hungarian parents. He studied dermatology under Ferdinand von Hebra at the University of Vienna, earning his medical degree in 1861. Kaposi took a position in Hebra's clinic and ultimately became a lecturer where he was responsible for educating numerous dermatologists. Kaposi and Hebra coauthored *The Handbook of Diseases of the Skin* which had great success. Kaposi married Hebra's daughter and the couple had one son, Hermann (1872). When Hebra died, Kaposi filled the vacant spot as director of the skin clinic and as Vienna's most renowned dermatologist.

Between 1872 and 1887, Kaposi discovered nine skin diseases that had not been previously documented. His discovery of a malignant disease that strikes the lymph nodes and skin (Kaposi's sarcoma 1872) has been documented as the most noteworthy. This disease was seen relatively rarely in the United States until the 1980s when it was tied to AIDS. This sarcoma has been the most common tumor found in AIDS patients. In 1872, Kaposi also studied cases of lupus erythematosus, which had no previous documentation. Kaposi was a prolific writer who published *Pathology and Treatment of Diseases of the Skin* in addition to numerous other publications, which he completed individually and with other authors. Kaposi died in 1902.

Immunocompromised KS usually reverses after the immunosuppressive drug is stopped. The fourth form of KS, epidemic AIDS–related KS, emerged as one of the first illnesses observed among those with AIDS. Unlike classic KS, AIDS–related KS tumors occur in advanced HIV infection and generally appear on the upper body, including the head, neck, and back. Tumors also can appear on the soft palate and gum areas of the mouth. In more advanced cases, they can be found in the stomach and intestines, the lymph nodes, and the lungs.

Causes and symptoms

Classic KS, which typically results in a disease course which is long and generally indolent, is thought to be caused by immune system dysregulation (a combination of factors which lead to immune suppression and immune activation) although the exact cause has not yet been identified. Currently, it is thought that this type of KS may be caused by suppression of the immune system as the individual ages, as a result of the genetic makeup of the patient, as a result of diagnosis with another type of cancer in the same individual and possibly results from concurrent malarial infection in some people.

The cause of immunocompromised KS appears to be directly related to treatment with immunosuppressive drugs following organ transplant or in patients receiving immunosuppressive therapies. These patients' risk for developing KS is increased by 100 times. Most patients develop this type of KS within 15–30 months following transplant. As stated earlier, once the patient stops taking the immunosuppressive drugs, the KS may regress. A newer antirejection drug, sirolimus (Rapamune), has been shown to have a dual effect which is advantageous to transplant patients who have been diagnosed with KS. Sirolimus appears to have an immunosuppressive effect as well as an antitumor (anti–KS) effect. A small group of kidney transplant patients who were diagnosed with KS post–transplant were switched from the immunosuppressive drug cyclosporine to sirolimus. All of the patients in this study experienced regression of their KS; all cutaneous KS lesions in all of the patients

KEY TERMS

African endemic Kaposi's sarcoma—A form of KS that affects men and boys and that can appear like classic KS or in a more lethal form.

AIDS–related Kaposi's sarcoma—A form of KS that emerged as one of the first illnesses associated with AIDS patients. Tumors usually appear on the upper body, the soft palate and gum areas, and, as the disease advances, in the lymph nodes, stomach, intestines, and lungs.

Apoptosis—Cell death.

Classic Kaposi's sarcoma—A form of KS that usually affects older men of Mediterranean or eastern European backgrounds and produces tumors on the lower legs.

Cytokines—Regulatory proteins that are produced by the immune system.

Human herpesvirus 8—Also called Kaposi's sarcoma–associated herpesvirus (KSHV), this virus is thought to be a cause for KS.

Iatrogenic Kaposi's sarcoma—A form of KS that develops in transplant patients who take immunosuppressive drugs to prevent rejection of their organ transplant.

MCH–1—Major histocompatibility complex proteins that protect cells from invasion.

disappeared. In addition, none of these patients experienced rejection.

The cause of African KS is also linked to immune dysregulation. This type of KS occurs primarily in men but also occurs in African women and children, often in individuals who are not HIV positive. The course of this type of KS can be aggressive or indolent. African KS involves the lymph nodes more often than the classic form of KS. In African children who are not HIV positive and who are diagnosed with African KS, lymph node involvement may also be accompanied by visceral KS. This KS disease pattern results in an extremely poor prognosis; virtually 100% of the children with this disease profile are dead within three years.

Epidemic AIDS–related KS is the most aggressive form of KS and is associated with patients with advanced HIV infection who are severely immunocompromised. It appears that infection with human herpes virus 8 (HHV–8) must be present for this type of KS to develop. HHV–8 is transmitted via saliva. It is not yet known whether the virus can be spread via blood–borne transmission. KS may be caused by HHV–8 and activation of other immune system factors including oncostatin M, IL–1, IL–6, fibroblast growth factor, tumor necrosis factor, and the HIV–tat protein, which act as co–stimulants, as well as other abnormal cytokines. A patient infected with HHV–8 who is co–infected with HIV, appears to be much more susceptible to an aggressive KS disease course. Patients who are co–infected with HHV–8 and HIV are 500 to 10,000 times more likely to develop KS.

Therefore, a very complex combination of factors appears to contribute to the development of all four variants of KS. This combination of factors is likely to include environmental factors, immune system factors, infection with human herpesvirus 8 (HHV–8) and in some individuals, co–infection with HIV.

Symptoms of Kaposi's sarcoma vary depending on the extent of the disease. KS produces pink, purple, or brown tumors on the skin, mucous membranes, or internal organs. Other symptoms which may be present, depending on the extent of the disease, include tumor–associated **lymphedema**, **pain** associated with walking if lesions are present on the feet, a variety of gastrointestinal symptoms if the lesions are present in the gastrointestinal tract, as well as **cough**, difficulty breathing, coughing up blood, and chest pain if pulmonary involvement is present.

Diagnosis

Many physicians diagnose KS based on the appearance of the skin tumors and the patient's medical history. Unexplained cough or chest pain, as well as unexplained stomach or intestinal pain or bleeding, can suggest that the disease has moved beyond the skin. The most certain diagnosis can be achieved by taking a biopsy sample of a suspected KS lesion and examining it under high–power magnification. For suspected involvement of internal organs, physicians use a bronchoscope to examine the lungs or an endoscope to view the stomach and intestinal tract. Tests such as the CD4 lymphocyte count and plasma HIV viral–load studies may be conducted on patients diagnosed with HIV.

Treatment

Treatment goals for KS are simple: to reduce the severity of symptoms, shrink tumors, and prevent disease progression. The advent of HAART has resulted in marked advancements in the treatment of KS and is generally the first therapy initiated. Most patients respond very well to HAART although response is dependent on stage of disease. Patients diagnosed with KS that has not affected the visceral organs may receive HAART as the sole treatment modality.

Patients whose disease has spread to the visceral organs and who are considered to be poor risk KS patients may be treated with a variety of modalities including **chemotherapy** which is used with palliative intent. Chemotherapy drugs approved by the FDA to treat AIDS–related KS include liposomal doxorubicin (Doxil), used in patients who have been previously treated; liposomal daunorubicin (DaunoXome), which is approved as a first–line treatment option; and paclitaxel (Taxol), also approved for patients who have been previously treated. These drugs have resulted in high response rates often with less toxicity as compared to other drugs.

In addition, **radiation therapy** may be used and is often very effective in treating lesions that are considered to be advanced and symptomatic. Surgery may be an option to remove small superficial KS lesions. Some KS lesions may be treated with chemotherapy such as vincristine or vinblastine injected directly into the lesion (intralesional therapy) although the lesions are likely to recur in other areas. Systemic infusion of chemotherapy drugs may be more effective. Other treatment options which may be employed include **cryotherapy** with liquid nitrogen applied topically to treat small facial lesions, laser photocoagulation to shrink small lesions, and application of topical retinoids such as alitretinoin (Panretin) gel to lesions.

Interferon–alfa, interferon combined with chemotherapy, interleukin–12, and chemotherapy using a variety of agents have been used as palliative agents to treat KS that is symptomatic or life–threatening. Treatment options being explored in clinical trials include therapy with thalidomide and other antiangiogenesis agents. Other trials are focused on investigating whether antiviral therapy utilizing drugs such as foscarnet and ganciclovir may be effective because of the link between human herpesvirus and KS.

Prognosis

The prognosis for patients with classic KS is good. Tumors can frequently be controlled and patients frequently die of other causes before any serious spread. African endemic KS can progress rapidly and lead to premature death, despite treatment. In AIDS–related KS, milder cases can frequently be controlled; the prognosis for more advanced and rapidly progressing cases is less certain and dependent on the patient's overall medical condition. There are indications that KS can be stabilized or reversed in patients whose level of HIV in the blood is reduced to undetectable levels via combined antiretroviral therapy.

Prevention

Safer sex practices may help to prevent AIDS–related KS by decreasing the risk of transmission of HHV–8 through sexual means. Treatment with antiretrovirals may help to preserve the function of the immune system in HIV patients and delay the appearance and progression of KS lesions. In fact, since the introduction of HAART in those infected with HIV, KS has decreased substantially. However, it still remains the most common cancer among those infected with HIV.

Resources

BOOKS

DeVita, A. "AIDS–related Malignancies." In: DeVita, V., and T. Vincent, Jr. editors. *Cancer Principles and Practice of Clinical Oncology*, vol.8, 5th Ed. Philadelphia,PA: Lippincott, Williams, and Wilkins, 2008.

PERIODICALS

DiLorenzo, G., et al. "Management of AIDS–related Kaposi's Sarcoma." *Lancet Oncology*. 8(2) (February 2008): 167–76.

Grabar, S., et al. "Differential Impact of Combination Antiretroviral Therapy in Preventing Kaposi's Sarcoma With and Without Visceral Involvement." *Journal of Clinical Oncology*. 24(21) (2006): 3408–14.

Little, R.F., et al. "Activity of Subcutaneous Interleukin–12 in AIDS–related Kaposi Sarcoma." *Blood*. 107(12) (2006): 4650–7.

Singh, N.B., R.H. Lakier, and B. Donde. "Hyperfractionated Radiation Therapy in the Treatment of Epidemic Kaposi Sarcoma–A Prospective Randomized Trial." *Radiotherapy & Oncology*. 88(2) (2008): 211–6.

OTHER

"Kaposi Sarcoma Treatment (PDQ)." National Cancer Institute. (April 28, 2008). http://www.cancer.gov/cancertopics/pdq/treatment/Kaposis/patient (accessed September 13, 2010).

Rose, L.J., A.D. Fishman, and J.A. Sparano. "Kaposi Sarcoma." eMedicine (August 19, 2008). http://www.emedicine.medscape.com (accessed September 13, 2010).

Janie F. Franz
Teresa G. Odle
Melinda Granger Oberleitner, RN, DNS, APRN, CNS

Kawasaki syndrome

Definition

Kawasaki syndrome is a potentially fatal inflammatory disease that affects several organ systems in the body, including the heart, circulatory system, mucous membranes, skin, and immune system. It occurs primarily in infants and children but has also been identified in adults as old as 34 years. Its cause is unknown.

Description

Kawasaki syndrome, also called mucocutaneous lymph node syndrome (MLNS), is an inflammatory disorder with potentially fatal complications affecting the heart and its larger arteries. Nearly twice as many males are affected as females. Although persons of Asian descent are affected more frequently than either black or white individuals, there does not appear to be a distinctive geographic pattern of occurrence. Eighty percent of cases involve children under the age of four. Although the disease usually appears in individuals, it sometimes affects several members of the same family and occasionally occurs in small epidemics.

Causes and symptoms

The specific cause of Kawasaki syndrome is unknown, although the disease resembles infectious illnesses in many ways. It has been suggested that Kawasaki syndrome represents an allergic reaction or other unusual response to certain types of infections. Some researchers think that the syndrome may be caused by the interaction of an immune cell, called the T cell, with certain poisons (toxins) secreted by bacteria.

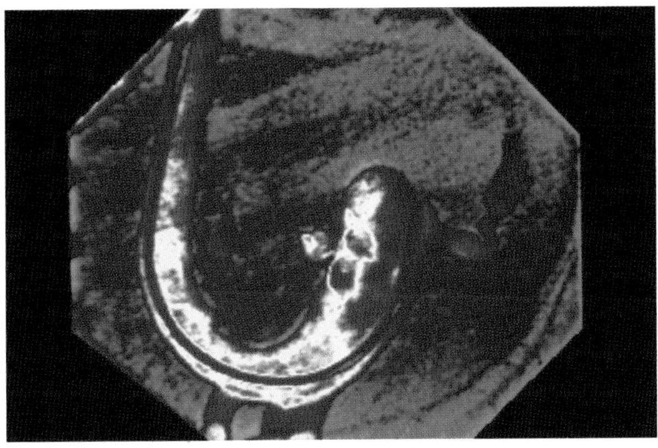

An angiogram showing abnormal coronary arteries in a child suffering from Kawasaki's disease. The coronary arteries are abnormal and weakened in that they bulge into balloon shapes, or aneurysms, along their lengths. This illness afflicts children between the ages of 1–2 years. *(Mehau Kulyk/SPL/Photo Researchers, Inc.)*

Kawasaki syndrome has an abrupt onset, with **fever** as high as 104°F (40°C) and a rash that spreads over the patient's chest and genital area. The fever is followed by a characteristic peeling of the skin beginning at the fingertips and toenails. In addition to the body rash, the patient's lips become very red, with the tongue developing a "strawberry" appearance. The palms, soles, and mucous membranes that line the eyelids and cover the exposed portion of the eyeball (conjuntivae) become purplish-red and swollen. The lymph nodes in the patient's neck may also become swollen. These symptoms may last from two weeks to three months, with relapses in some patients.

In addition to the major symptoms, about 30% of patients develop joint pains or arthritis, usually in the large joints of the body. Others develop **pneumonia**, **diarrhea**, dry or cracked lips, **jaundice**, or an inflammation of the membranes covering the brain and spinal cord (**meningitis**). A few patients develop symptoms of inflammation in the liver (hepatitis), gallbladder, lungs, or tonsils.

About 20% of patients with Kawasaki syndrome develop complications of the cardiovascular system. These complications include inflammation of the heart tissue (**myocarditis**), disturbances in heartbeat rhythm (**arrhythmias**), and areas of blood vessel dilation (aneurysms) in the coronary arteries. Other patients may develop inflammation of an artery (arteritis) in their arms or legs. Complications of the heart or arteries begin to develop around the tenth day after the illness begins, when the fever and rash begin to subside. A few patients may develop **gangrene**, or the **death** of soft tissue, in their hands and feet. The specific causes of these complications are not yet known.

Diagnosis

Because Kawasaki syndrome is primarily a disease of infants and young children, the disease is most likely to be diagnosed by a pediatrician. The physician will first consider the possible involvement of other diseases that cause fever and skin **rashes**, including **scarlet fever**, **measles**, **Rocky Mountain spotted fever**, **toxoplasmosis** (a disease carried by cats), juvenile **rheumatoid arthritis**, and a blistering and inflammation of the skin caused by reactions to certain medications (Stevens-Johnson syndrome).

Once other diseases have been ruled out, the patient's symptoms will be compared with a set of diagnostic criteria. The patient must have a fever lasting

KEY TERMS

Aneurysm—Dilation of an artery caused by thinning and weakening of the vessel wall.

Arrythmia—Abnormal heart rhythm.

Arteritis—Inflammation of an artery.

Cardiomegaly—An enlarged heart.

Conjunctivae—The mucous membranes that cover the exposed area of the eyeball and line the inner surface of the eyelids.

Exanthem—A skin eruption associated with a disease, usually one accompanied by fever as in Kawasaki syndrome.

Gangrene—The death of soft tissue in a part of the body, usually caused by obstructed circulation.

Hepatitis—Inflammation of the liver.

Meningitis—Inflammation of the membranes, called the meninges, covering the brain and spinal cord.

Mucocutaneous lymph node syndrome (MLNS)—Mucocutaneous lymph node syndrome, another name for Kawasaki syndrome. The name comes from the key symptoms of the disease, which involve the mucous membranes of the mouth and throat, the skin, and the lymph nodes.

Myocarditis—Inflammation of the heart muscle.

Stevens-Johnson syndrome—A severe inflammatory skin eruption that occurs as a result of an allergic reaction or respiratory infection.

T cell—A type of white blood cell that develops in the thymus gland and helps to regulate the immune system's response to infections or malignancy.

five days or longer that does not respond to **antibiotics**, together with four of the following five symptoms:

- Inflammation of the conjunctivae of both eyes with no discharge
- At least one of the following changes in the mucous membranes of the mouth and throat: "strawberry" tongue; cracked lips; or swollen throat tissues
- At least one of the following changes in the hands or feet: swelling caused by excess fluid in the tissues; peeling of the skin; or abnormal redness of the skin
- A skin eruption or rash associated with fever (exanthem) on the patient's trunk
- Swelling of the lymph nodes in the neck to a size greater than 1.5 cm.

Since the cause of Kawasaki syndrome is unknown, there are no laboratory tests that can confirm the diagnosis. The following test results, however, are associated with the disease:

- Blood tests show a high white blood cell count, high platelet count, a high level of protein in the blood serum, and mild anemia
- Chest x ray may show enlargement of the heart (cardiomegaly)
- Urine may show the presence of pus or an abnormally high level of protein
- An electrocardiogram may show changes in the heartbeat rhythm

In addition to these tests, it is important to take a series of echocardiograms during the course of the illness because 20% of Kawasaki patients will develop coronary aneurysms or arteritis that will not appear during the first examination.

Treatment

Kawasaki syndrome is usually treated with a combination of **aspirin**, to control the patient's fever and skin inflammation, and high doses of intravenous immune globulin to reduce the possibility of coronary artery complications. Some patients with heart complications may be treated with drugs that reduce blood clotting or may receive corrective surgery.

Follow-up care includes two to three months of monitoring with chest x rays, **electrocardiography**, and **echocardiography**. Treatment with aspirin is often continued for several months.

Prognosis

Most patients with Kawasaki syndrome will recover completely, but about 1–2% will die as a result of **blood clots** forming in the coronary arteries or as a result of a **heart attack**. Deaths are sudden and unpredictable. Almost 95% of fatalities occur within six months of infection, but some have been reported as long as 10 years afterward. Long-term follow-up of patients with aneurysms indicates that about half show some healing of the aneurysm. The remaining half has a high risk of heart complications in later life.

Resources

BOOKS

McPhee, Stephen, and Maxine Papadakis.*Current Medical Diagnosis and Treatment, 2010*, 49th ed. New York: McGraw–Hill Medical, 2009.

Rebecca J. Frey, PhD

Keloids

Definition

Keloids are excessive (overgrowths) of fibrous tissue or **scars** that can occur after an injury to the skin has healed (such as a burn), at the site of intentional alterations of the skin (such as an ear **piercing**), or as the result from medical procedures or illnesses (such as a **vaccination** or the **chickenpox**). Sometimes, they develop without any apparent cause. These heavy, sometimes irregular, and often very noticeable scars are also called cheloid, keloid, or hypertrophic scars. In individuals prone to keloids, even minor traumas to the skin, such as ear piercing, can cause keloids. The word "keloid" itself comes from the Greek word for a crab's claw; it was first used by a French physician to describe the way that keloids grow sideways into normal skin. The term keloidosis is intended to describe the situation when many keloids have occurred in one individual.

Demographics

Keloids are somewhat common in women and young people under the age of 30 years. They are also commonly found in families, with the malady inherited from one generation to the next. They occur most frequently in individuals of African–American descent and in those with darker skin. They are more common in Polynesians and Chinese than in people from India or Malaysia. Caucasians are the least frequently affected by keloids. Other risk factors include a family history of keloids, surgery, **acne**, **burns**, ear piercing, vaccinations, or insect bites. Spontaneous keloids have been reported occasionally in siblings. Keloids are infrequently found among the elderly.

Although the association of keloids with darker skin pigmentation suggests a genetic linkage of some sort, no specific genes have been identified in connection with keloids as of the early 2010s.

Description

Keloids usually start out as a small bump or raised spot on the skin. The size of the bump gradually becomes larger over time, and eventually becomes a mature keloid. Keloids can occur anywhere on the body, but they are most common on the earlobes, upper back, shoulders, and chest. The pattern of distribution of keloids differs according to race, with facial keloids more common in Caucasians and relatively uncommon in Asians. African Americans are more likely to develop keloids on the legs or feet than among either Asians or Caucasians. In general, keloids consist of hard, raised scars that may be slightly pink or whitish. They may itch and be painful, and some keloids can grow to be quite large.

Causes and symptoms

Although the cause of keloids is unknown, it is thought that they are due to the body's failure to turn off the healing process needed to repair skin. When this occurs, extra collagen forms at the site of the scar, and keeps forming because healing does not shut down, resulting in keloid formation. Scientists working on genomics, or the determination of the entire DNA (deoxyribonucleic acid) sequence of organisms, may one day learn the cause(s) of keloids.

Initially, keloids begin as a small lump where the skin has been injured. This lump grows and can eventually become very large and cosmetically unacceptable. Keloids often result from the following conditions:

- Chickenpox
- Acne
- Burns
- Piercings
- Scratches
- Cuts from surgeries
- Wounds
- Vaccinations

The symptoms associated with keloids include lesions that are:

- Flesh–colored, red, or pink
- Nodular or ridged
- At the site of an injury or wound
- Itchy while growing

Diagnosis

A dermatologist can usually make the diagnosis of a keloid based on looking at the scar or the appearance of the skin. In some cases, however, a biopsy may be necessary to rule out other types of **skin lesions**, such as tumors.

Treatment

Most keloids do not need treatment. When they do, several options are available. The treatment of choice for keloids is usually an injection of corticosteroid drugs such as cortisone directly into the lesion. These injections cause the keloid to become atrophic, or thinner, and are repeated every three to four weeks until the keloid has been resolved to the individual's satisfaction. Other therapies include laser treatment or **radiation therapy**, and topical treatments are undergoing study.

Surgery is often used in combination with corticosteroid injections. The injections are given for several weeks, and then the keloid is surgically removed. The injections are then continued for several weeks. Surgical removal of the keloid may also be used in conjunction with radiation therapy, which delivers small amounts of radiation to the affected area.

Another surgical option is cryosurgery, in which liquid nitrogen is used to freeze the tissues in the keloid. The treatment may need to be repeated to remove as much of the keloid as possible; however, cryosurgery prevents keloids from recurring in about 70% of patients.

Newer approaches include silastic gel sheeting, which makes use of pressure to flatten the keloid. The patient is advised to apply a silastic gel each night for several months. The gel is then kept securely in place with tape, cloth, or a bandage. The dressing is changed daily for seven to 10 days for minor cases, and for as long as 12 months in very serious cases.

Finally, researchers are now studying a type of tape that has been soaked with **steroids**, which are released slowly into the keloid, causing it to thin over time.

Newer treatments include injections of interferon directly into the keloid, and local application of five percent imiquimod cream, which induces the skin where it is applied to produce interferon. The imiquimod cream is reported to lower the risk of keloid recurrence significantly.

Prognosis

Although keloids are unsightly, they are not life–threatening nor medically dangerous. Keloids do not have a tendency to develop into malignancies, but they can become cosmetically unacceptable. Keloids can gradually lessen after treatment, but many recur. And just as they can occur spontaneously, they can also resolve spontaneously. Over time, many keloids become smaller and less noticeable. When surgery is performed, a scar usually forms at the sight of the keloid. Sometimes the scar is larger in area than the original keloid. Imiquimod cream is now used to minimize the possibilities of keloids forming after surgery. Often, the area surrounding and at the keloid site can become tender and feel uncomfortable to the person. This sensation is often caused by irritation from the rubbing of clothing or other personal articles that the person is wearing.

People who have keloids can prevent them from discoloring by protecting them from sunlight, or using sunblock when exposing them to sunlight.

KEY TERMS

Atrophy—A wasting away of, becoming thinner, less strong.

Corticosteroids—Any of several steroid medications used to suppress inflammation, allergic, or immune responses of the body.

Cryosurgery—The use of extreme cold to kill or remove tissue.

Prevention

Preventive measures include avoiding any trauma to the skin, and compression pressure dressing for high–risk patients who have suffered burns to their skin. Proper care of the skin on a daily basis is also important, including the prompt treatment of skin abrasions and cuts. Such treatment includes cleaning the site, applying antibiotic medicine on and around the affected skin, placing a protective dressing over the wound, and applying stitches to the cut if deemed medically necessary. Patients with a tendency to form keloids should avoid any sort of elective surgery. Individuals who are prone to develop keloids or who have a history of keloids should immediately care for any cuts or abrasions they may sustain.

To lower the risk of keloids, surgeons are advised to close incisions with as little tension on the sutures as possible, and to use buried sutures whenever possible.

Resources

BOOKS

Beers, Mark H., et al. *The Merck Manual of Diagnosis and Therapy*. Whitehouse Station, NJ: Merck Research Laboratories, 2006.

Frankel, David H., editor. *Field Guide to Clinical Dermatology*. Philadelphia: Lippincott Williams and Wilkins, 2006.

Hom, David B. et al. *Essential Tissue Healing of the Face and Neck*. Shelton, CT: People's Medical Publishing House, 2009.

Schwarzenberger, Kathryn, Andrew E. Werchniak, and Christine J. Ko., editors. *General Dermatology*. Edinburgh, Scotland: Saunders Elsevier, 2009.

OTHER

"Keloids." Black Women's Health. http:/ /www.blackwomenshealth.com/2006/articles.php?id = 75. (accessed September 6, 2010).

"Keloid." Medline Plus, National Library of Medicine and National Institutes of Health. (October 3, 2008), http://www.nlm.nih.gov/medlineplus/ency/article/000849.htm. (accessed September 6, 2010).

"The Skin Site." SkinSite.com. (May 18, 2010), http://www.skinsite.com (accessed September 6, 2010)

ORGANIZATIONS

American Academy of Dermatology, 930 E. Woodfield Rd., PO Box 4014, Schaumburg, IL, 60168–4014, (847) 330–0230, (866) 503–7546, (847) 240–1859, http://www.aad.org.

U.S. Food and Drug Administration, 10903 New Hampshire Ave., Silver Spring, MD, 20993–0002, (888) INFO–FDA (463–6332), http://www.fda.gov.

Liz Meszaros
Rebecca J. Frey, PhD

Keratitis

Definition

Keratitis is an inflammation of the cornea, the transparent dome–shaped membrane that covers the colored part of the eye (iris) and the pupil of the eye. Keratitis can be the result of an infection caused by bacteria, virus, fungi or parasites. Noninfectious Keratitis can be caused by a scratch or abrasion to the eye or by prolonged contact lens usage.

There are differing degrees of Keratitis. If only the upper layers of the cornea are involved, a condition known as superficial keratitis, there is usually no permanent damage. However, when keratitis affects the lower layers of the cornea, a condition called deep keratitis, the damage caused may leave a scar in the cornea permanently impair vision.

Description

There are many types and causes of keratitis. Organisms cannot generally invade an intact, healthy cornea. However, certain conditions can allow an infection to occur. For example, a scratch can leave the cornea open to infection. A very dry eye can also decrease the cornea's protective mechanisms.

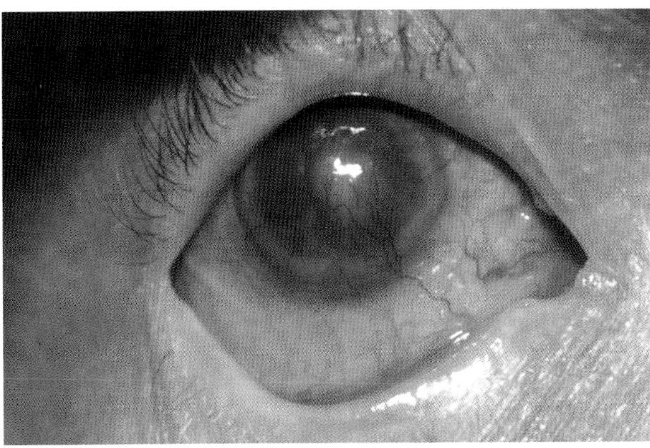

Close-up of a damaged cornea due to complications following cataract surgery. *(Custom Medical Stock Photo, Inc. Reproduced by permission.)*

Risk factors that increase the likelihood of developing this condition include:

- poor contact lens care; overuse of contact lenses
- illnesses or other factors that reduce the body's ability to overcome infection (compromised immune system, such as from diabetes)
- previous injuries
- cold sores, genital herpes, and other viral infections
- crowded, dirty living conditions; poor hygiene
- warm climates, especially if it is humid
- corticosteroids that treat eye problems
- poor nutrition (especially a deficiency of Vitamin A, which is essential for normal vision)

Some common types of keratitis are listed below.

Herpes simplex keratitis

A major cause of adult eye disease, herpes simplex keratitis may lead to:

- chronic inflammation of the cornea
- development of tiny blood vessels in the eye
- scarring
- loss of vision
- glaucoma

This infection generally begins with inflammation of the membrane lining the eyelid (conjunctiva) and the portion of the eyeball that comes into contact with it. Subsequent infections are characterized by a pattern of lesions that resemble the veins of a leaf. These infections are called dendritic keratitis and aid in diagnosis of the condition.

Recurrences may be brought on by **stress**, **fatigue**, or ultraviolet (UV) light exposure. Repeated episodes of dendritic keratitis can cause sores, permanent scarring, and **numbness** of the cornea.

Recurrent dendritic keratitis is often followed by disciform keratitis. This condition is characterized by clouding and deep, disc–shaped swelling of the cornea and by inflammation of the iris.

It is very important not to use topical **corticosteroids** with herpes simplex keratitis as it can make the condition much worse, possibly leading to blindness.

Bacterial keratitis

People who have bacterial keratitis wake up with their eyelids stuck together. There can be pain, sensitivity to light, redness, tearing, and a decrease in vision. This condition, which is usually aggressive, can be caused by wearing soft contact lenses overnight. One study found that overnight wear can increase risk by 10 to 15 times more than daily wear. Improper lens care is also a factor. Contaminated makeup can also contain bacteria.

Bacterial keratitis usually is caused by the bacteria *Staphylococcus aureus* and *Pseudomonas aeruginosa* (especially for wearers of contact lenses). The infection makes the cornea cloudy, and may also cause abscesses to develop in the stroma, which is located beneath the outer layer of the cornea.

Fungal keratitis

Usually a consequence of injuring the cornea in a farm–like setting or in a place where plant material is present, fungal keratitis often develops slowly. This condition:

- usually affects people with weakened immune systems
- often results in infection within the eyeball
- may cause stromal abscesses

This type of keratitis is usually caused by the fungus *Aspergillus fumigatus* or by one of many fungus species within the genus *Fusarium*. It can also be caused by species within the yeast genus of *Candida*. The symptoms of fungal keratisis include red, painful eyed, blurred vision, increased sensitivity to light, and excessive discharge around the eye or increased production of tears. The condition usually does not improve when contact lenses are removed or when an antibiotic treatment is used. Fungal keratisis is a relatively rare disorder.

Peripheral ulcerative keratitis

Peripheral ulcerative keratitis is also called marginal keratolysis or peripheral rheumatoid ulceration. This condition is often associated with active or chronic disorders such as:

- rheumatoid arthritis
- relapsing polychondritis (connective–tissue inflammation)
- Wegener's granulomatosis, a rare condition characterized by kidney disease and development of nodules in the respiratory tract

Superficial punctate keratitis

Often associated with the type of viruses that cause upper respiratory infection (adenoviruses), superficial punctate keratitis is characterized by destruction of pinpoint areas in the outer layer of the cornea (epithelium). One or both eyes may be affected.

Acanthamoeba keratitis

This pus–producing condition, also called amoebic keratitis, is very painful. It is a common source of infection of the cornea. It is especially troublesome in people who wear soft or rigid contact lenses. This type of keratitis is caused by the bacterium *Acanthamoeba*. It can be found in tap water, soil, and swimming pools.

Photokeratitis

Photokeratitis, sometimes also called ultraviolet keratitis or snowblindness, is caused by excess exposure to natural or artificial UV light without proper eye protection. This condition can occur at high altitudes from sunlight reflecting off of snow fields or from, sun–tanning lamps, or welding arcs. It is very painful because it causes a type of "sunburn" to the cornea. The condition may occur several hours after exposure, and may last one to two days. In all cases, symptoms include pain in the eyes and increased production of tears.

Interstitial keratitis

Also called parenchymatous keratitis, interstitial keratitis is a chronic inflammation of tissue deep within the cornea. Interstitial keratitis is rare in the United States. Interstitial keratitis affects both eyes and usually occurs as a complication of congenital or acquired **syphilis**. In congenital syphilis, it can occur between the age of two years and **puberty**. It may also happen in people with **tuberculosis**, **leprosy**, or other diseases.

Causes and symptoms

In summary, keratitis can be caused by:

- contaminated contact lenses
- bacterial, fungal, or parasitic infections

- viral infections, such as from the herpes virus and other viruses that cause chlamydia
- dry eyes resulting from disorders of the eyelid or diminished ability to form tears
- exposure to very bright light
- contaminated water
- foreign object injury
- upper respiratory infection
- sensitivity or allergic reactions
- vitamin A deficiency

Symptoms of keratitis include, but are not limited to:

- excessive tearing or discharge from eyes
- pain in and around eyes
- swelling of eyes
- itchy or burning feeling in eyes
- feeling of foriegn object in eye
- difficulty opening eyelids
- sensitivity to light
- inflammation of the eyelid
- decrease in vision
- redness of the eyes

Diagnosis

A case history will be taken and vision will be tested. Examination with a slit lamp, an instrument that is a microscope and focuses a beam of light on the eye, is important for diagnosis. The cornea can be examined with fluorescein, a yellow dye that highlights defects in the cornea. Deeper layers of the cornea can also be analyzed with the slit lamp. Infiltrates, hazy looking areas in the cornea, can be seen by the doctor and aid in the diagnosis. Samples of infectious matter removed from the eye will be sent for laboratory analysis.

Treatment

Antibiotic, antifungal, or antiviral oral medication are used to treat the appropriate organism. Broad–spectrum **antibiotics** are used immediately, but once the laboratory analysis determines the offending organism, the medication may be changed. Sometimes more than one medication is necessary.

A sterile, cotton–tipped applicator may be used to gently remove infected tissue and allow the eye to heal more rapidly. **Laser surgery** is sometimes performed to destroy unhealthy cells, and some severe infections require corneal transplants.

Antifungal, antibiotic, or antiviral eyedrops or ointments are usually prescribed for keratitis, but they should be used only by patients under a doctor's care. Inappropriate prescriptions or over–the–counter preparations can make symptoms more severe and cause tissue deterioration. Topical corticosteroids can cause great harm to the cornea in patient's with herpes simplex keratitis.

A patient with keratitis may wear a patch to protect the healing eye from bright light, **foreign objects**, the lid rubbing against the cornea, and other irritants. The patient will probably return every day to the eye doctor to check on the progress.

Although early detection and treatment can cure most forms of keratitis, the infection can cause:

- glaucoma
- permanent scarring
- ulceration of the cornea
- blindness

Prognosis

When treated promptly and effectively, keratitis can be treated without loss of vision. However, when minor cases of keratitis are left untreated they can lead to serious complications that may permanently damage or eliminate vision in the eyes. Such complications include chronic or recurrent viral infections of the cornea, corneal swelling or scarring, blindness, open corneal sores, and chronic corneal inflammation.

Prevention

Contact lenses should only be worn as recommended by an eye care professional and cleaned using sterile lens–cleaning and disinfecting solutions. Tap water is not sterile and should not be used to clean contact lenses. Always, wash, rinse, and dry one's hands before handling contact lenses. It is important to go for follow–up checkups because small defects in the

KEY TERMS

Abscess—A collection of pus.

Glaucoma—An eye disease characterized by an increase of pressure in the eye. Left untreated, blindness may result.

Infiltrate—A collection of cells not usually present in that area. In the cornea, infiltrates may be a collection of white blood cells.

Inflammation—A localized response to an injury. May include swelling, redness, and pain.

cornea can occur without the patient' being aware of it. Remove lenses if eyes become red or irritated. Replace contact lenses as scheduled. Proteins and other materials can deposit on the contacts, leading to an increased risk of infection. Clean contact lens cases as directed and replace contact lens cases every three months. Do not wear contact lenses while swimming or in a hot tub.

Eating a well–balanced diet and wearing protective glasses when working or playing in potentially dangerous situations can reduce anyone's risk of developing keratitis. Protective goggles should be worn while mowing the lawn so that if twigs are tossed up they cannot hurt the eyes. Goggles or sunglasses with UV coatings can help protect against damage from UV light.

Avoid touching the eyes if one has an infection, such as a cold sore, to prevent infection within the eyes. Discontinue wearing contact lenses if keratitis occurs frequently. Minimize the use of corticosteroid eye drops, which increase the risks of viral infections.

Resources

BOOKS

Fekrat, Sharon, and Jennifer S. Weizer, editors. *All About Your Eyes*. Durham, NC: Dike University Press, 2006.

Reinhard, Thomas, and Frank Larkin, editors. *Cornea and External Eye Disease*. Berlin, Germany: Springer, 2008.

Williams, David L. *Ophthalmic Immunology and Immune–mediated Disease*. Philadelphia: Saunders, 2008.

OTHER

"Corneal Disorders." Medline Plus, National Library of Medicine and National Institutes of Health. (July 2, 2010), http://www.nlm.nih.gov/medlineplus/corneal disorders.html. (accessed September 6, 2010).

"Facts about the Corneal and Corneal Disease." National Eye Institute. (February 2010), http://www.nei.nih. gov/health/cornealdisease/index.asp. (accessed September 6, 2010).

"Keratitis." Mayo Clinic. (July 15, 2010), http://www.mayoclinic.com/health/keratitis/DS01190/rss = 1. (accessed September 6, 2010).

ORGANIZATIONS

American Academy of Ophthalmology, PO Box 7424, San Francisco, CA, 94120–7424, (415) 561–8500, http://www.aao.org.

American Optometric Association, 243 North Lindbergh Blvd., St. Louis, MO, 63141, (314) 991–4100, (800) 365–2219, http://www.aoanet.org.

National Eye Institute, 2020 Vision Pl., Bethesda, MD, 20892–3655, (301) 496–5248, http://www.nei.nih.gov.

Prevent Blindness America, 211 West Wacker Dr., Suite 1700, Chicago, IL, 60606, (800) 331–2020, http://www.preventblindness.org.

Maureen Haggerty

Keratosis pilaris

Definition

Keratosis pilaris is a common skin condition that looks like small, rough goose bumps (patches), which are actually dead skin cells that build up around the hair follicle. Also called follicular keratosis, or simply KP, it is a commonly found follicular condition that most frequently appears on the back and outer sides of the upper arms, thighs, and buttocks. KP can also be located on the lower arms, hands, legs, and lower back. It never appears on the soles of the feet or the palms of the hands. It is rarely present on the face. When it does appear on the face (especially on the cheeks), KP is commonly mistaken for **acne**. It is also described as 'chicken bumps' and 'chicken skin'. Although the appearance of keratosis pilaris on the body is not desirable, it does not pose a medical risk. It is considered to be completely harmless to the human body.

Demographics

KP can be contracted by anyone all over the world but it is often considered a fairly common condition of children and adolescents. Consequently, more adolescents are at risk for it (about 50% to 80% worldwide) than are adults (about 40%). It is also more commonly found on women than it is on men. It appears equally in all races. Generally, KP improves with age. About 30% to 50% of people who have keratosis pilaris also have a family history for it. People who are obese or have troubling long–term health issues are at increased risk for contracting KP. However, people of normal weight and otherwise good health have also been found to have keratosis pilaris.

Description

Keratosis pilaris is called a hyperkeratinization of the skin because the buildup of keratin on the skin is thought by the medical community to cause the rough bumps and the overall poor skin appearance that characterize the condition. For people with KP, the process called keratinization is defective; that is, the formation of the epidermal skin is not normal, which causes bumps to form. Why this happens is not known to medical professionals, although various assumptions have been made as to why keratosis pilaris occurs on some people but not on others.

KP is a disorder that occurs around the hair follicles of the upper and lower arms, hands, lower back, thighs, legs, and sometimes the buttocks. It presents as small, benign bumps or papules that are actually waxy build–ups of keratin. Normally the skin sloughs (sheds) them off. However, around the hair follicle where the papules form, the keratinized skin cells slough off at a slower rate, clogging the follicles.

The disorder is generally thought to be genetic in nature, although the symptoms of keratosis pilaris are often seen with **ichthyosis** (a disease in which the skin becomes dry, scaly and thick) and allergic **dermatitis** (a form of dermatitis associated with an allergic reaction). It is also observed in people of all ages who have inherited the condition or who have a **vitamin A deficiency** or dry skin. Keratosis pilaris is a self–limiting disorder that usually disappears as the person ages. It can become more severe when conditions are dry such as during the winter months or in dry, arid climates.

A localized area on the skin may show an appearance of between 10 to 100 bumps that may give the area a sandpaper–looking appearance. Some of the bumps may appear slightly red in color, which indicates that they are inflamed. Most bumps are white in color, and are from one to two millimeters in diameter.

Causes and symptoms

The specific causes of this disorder are unknown. However, they are known to exist as keratin builds up. Keratin is a hard protein that helps to protect the skin from infections and harmful substances. When keratin builds up it forms a scaly plug that blocks the opening to the hair follicle. These blockages cause the small, rough bumps associated with keratosis pilaris. Since this disorder sometimes runs in families, it is thought to be a hereditary condition, one in which people have a genetic predisposition for it. If one child has KP then his or her siblings seem to be more likely to acquire it, too, especially among children of multiple births. Keratosis pilaris is not a serious disorder and is not contagious. Dry skin seems to make the condition worsen. Consequently, cold winter months are more troublesome for people with KP than are the warm summer months.

The symptoms of keratosis pilaris are based on the development of small white papules (or acne–like bumps) the size of a grain of sand on the upper arms, thighs, and occasionally the buttocks and face. The papules occur around a hair follicle and are firm and white. They feel a little like coarse sandpaper (that is, like dry, rough patches of skin), but they are not usually painful and **itching** is not usually associated with them. They are sometimes reddish in color, which indicates inflammation. They are easily removed and the material inside the papule usually contains a small, coiled hair.

Diagnosis

The diagnosis for keratosis pilaris is often made by a dermatologist or physician while making a **physical examination** of unrelated skin conditions. Laboratory tests or skin tests have yet to be developed to identify keratosis pilaris. A medical professional can easily diagnose this disorder by examining the skin and reviewing the patient's medical history and family background with respect to skin conditions. During the physical examination, the physician looks for the signs and symptoms associated with KP.

Treatment

There is no cure for keratosis pilaris. It is treatable but usually the treatment is difficult. To treat keratosis pilaris patients can try several strategies to lessen the bumps. First, the patient can supplement the natural removal of dry skin and papules by using a loofah or another type of scrub for showering or bathing. A mild cleanser is recommended. A long–term skin care program that is used regularly seems to produce the best results. Sometimes several skin care plans are used in combination to produce more desirable results.

Most of the treatment options center around (1) topical exfoliants, including medicated creams that include alpha–hydroxy, lactic or salicylic acids, or urea, which moisturize and soften dry skin and remove dead skin cells; (2) topical **corticosteroids**, such as hydrocortisone type substances, which suppress the immune system and decrease the production of skin cells; and (3) topical retinoids, such as tretinoin and tazarotene, which increase the production of skin cells and help to prevent the plugging up of hair follicles.

A variety of different over–the–counter (OTC) lotions, ointments, and creams can also be applied after showering while the skin is still moist and then used several times a day to keep the area moist. Medicated lotions with urea, 15% alpha hydroxy acids, or tretinoin (Retin A) can also be prescribed by the dermatologist and applied one to two times daily. Systemic (oral) medications are not prescribed for keratosis pilaris. However if papules are opened and become infected, **antibiotics** may be necessary to treat the infection.

Lactic acid lotions such as AmLactin and Lac–Hydrin may be prescribed. In addition, salicylic acid (Salex lotion or cream) and topical steroid creams (triamcinolone acetonide 0.1%, or hydrocortisone butyrate [Locoid Lipocream]) may also be prescribed as possible treatments for KP. Sometimes, these lotions are manufactured so they combine more than one of these ingredients in case the prescribing physician or

KEY TERMS

Benign—Not cancerous.

Dermatologist—A physician who specializes in diseases and disorders of the skin.

Ichthyosis—A group of congenital disorders of keratinization characterized by dryness and scaling of the skin.

Keratin—The hard, waxy material that is made by the outer layer of skin cells.

dermatologist uses combination plans. Many other treatment options are also available. Each should be used only under the direction of a physician.

Sometimes minor surgical procedures are used for keratosis pilaris when KP persists even though multiple treatments have been attempted. Gentle acne extraction is one such procedure that can help to correct the problem. Microdermabrasion is another procedure that can be performed, usually in an in–office environment. The procedure exfoliates the skin with a gentle rubbing of abrasive particles (such as aluminum crystals) along with the lifting off the extracted skin with a vacuum. Chemical peels (a chemical solution to remove the top layer of dead skin), **photodynamic therapy** (PDT, consisting of a photosensitizer, light, and tissue oxygen), blue–light lasers (which emits electromagnetic radiation at a wavelength of between 360 and 480 nanometers), and intense pulsed light (IPL) instruments (which produce electromagnetic radiation at high intensities for very short periods) are also used as treatments. Other procedures are also available. It is always important that such procedures are used with the approval and under the direction of a physician.

Prognosis

Unfortunately, the treatment for keratosis pilaris is often disappointing. Although extreme cases of keratosis pilaris can occasionally be unsightly, the disorder is not life threatening and usually begins to disappear as the patient ages. Overall, however, many cases resolve themselves as the person gets older. KP usually disappears by the age of 30 years. In others, the problem persists with chronic reoccurrences and remissions of keratosis pilaris. Although treatment of keratosis pilaris is often frustrating to the patient, prescription medications and skin care measures can improve the appearance of the affected skin areas with consistency and persistence.

Prevention

Since keratosis pilaris is thought to be a genetic disorder and is observed in several members of the same family, there is nothing that can be done to prevent this disorder. Following the treatment advice above can alleviate the outward characteristics of keratosis pilaris. Mild soaps and cleansers help to minimize the problem. Do not aggressively rub the skin because such action will irritate the condition. When washing and bathing or showering, use warm water. Hot water dries the skin more. Keep a bath or shower to less than 15 minutes in duration. Gently dry off with a patting motion, and do not use harsh rubbing motions. The regular application of emollients is also helpful. Preventing dry skin is also recommended. Use a moisturizing lotion or lubricating cream on a regular basis, especially right after drying off from washing. The application of lactic acid, an over–the–counter product, has been shown to help remove excess keratin from the skin. Maintain humidified air within the home to avoid dry air, which will aggravate the problem.

Resources

BOOKS

Beers, Mark H., et al. *The Merck Manual of Diagnosis and Therapy*. Whitehouse Station, NJ: Merck Research Laboratories, 2006.

Frankel, David H., editor. *Field Guide to Clinical Dermatology* Philadelphia: Lippincott Williams and Wilkins, 2006.

Rook, Arthur, and Tony Bums. *Rook' Textbook of Dermatology*. Chichester, UK: Wiley–Blackwell, 2010.

Schwarzenberger, Kathryn, Andrew E. Werchniak, and Christine J. Ko., editors. *General Dermatology* Edinburgh, Scotland: Saunders Elsevier, 2009.

OTHER

"Keratosis Pilaris." eMedicine, WebMD. (May 13, 2010), http://emedicine.medscape.com/article/1070651–overview. (accessed September 6, 2010).

"Keratosis Pilaris." Mayo Clinic (July 10, 2010), http://www.mayoclinic.com/health/keratosis–pilaris/DS00769. (accessed September 6, 2010).

ORGANIZATIONS

American Academy of Dermatology, 930 East Woodfield R.d, PO Box 4014, Schaumburg, IL, 60168–4014, (847) 330–0230, (866) 503–7546, (847) 240–1859, http://www.aad.org.

Sally C. McFarlane–Parrott

Kidney biopsy

Definition

Kidney biopsy is a medical procedure in which a small piece of tissue is removed from the kidney for microscopic examination.

Purpose

The test is usually done to diagnose **kidney disease** and to evaluate the extent of damage to the kidney. A biopsy is also frequently ordered to detect the reason for acute renal failure when normal office procedures and tests fail to establish the cause. In addition, information regarding the progression of the disease and how it is responding to medical treatment can be obtained from a biopsy. Occasionally a biopsy may be done to confirm a diagnosis of **kidney cancer**, to determine its aggressiveness, and decide on the mode of treatment.

Precautions

The biopsy is not recommended for patients who have any uncontrollable bleeding disorders. Platelets are blood cells that play an important role in the blood clotting process. If the bleeding disorder is caused by a low **platelet count** (less than 50,000 per cubic millimeter of blood), then a platelet **transfusion** can be done just before performing the biopsy.

Description

The kidneys, a pair of organsas shaped like kidney beans that are lie on either side of the backbone, just above the waist. The periphery (parenchyma) of the kidney is made up of tiny tubes. These tubes filter and clean the blood by taking out the waste products and making urine. The urine is collected in the central portion of the kidney. Tubes called ureters drain the urine from the kidney into the bladder, where it is held until it is voided from the body.

A kidney specialist (nephrologist) performs the biopsy. It can be done either in the doctor's office or in a local hospital. The patient may be given a calming drug before the procedure to help him relax. The skin and muscles on the back overlying the site that is to be biopsied may be numbed with **local anesthesia**.

The patient will be asked to lie face down and a pad or a rolled towel may be placed under the stomach. Either the left or the right kidney may be biopsied depending on the results of the imaging tests: x rays, **computed tomography scans** (CT scans), **magnetic resonance imaging** (MRI), and ultrasound. The area that will be biopsied is cleaned with an antiseptic solution and sterile drapes are placed on it. The skin is numbed with local anesthesia. A small incision is made on the skin with a scalpel blade. Using a long needle, the physician injects local anesthesia into the incision so that it infiltrates down to the kidney. The biopsy needle is then advanced slowly through the incision. The patient is asked to hold his or her breath each time the needle is pushed forward. Once the wall (capsule) of the kidney has been penetrated, the patient can breathe normally. The tissue is collected for examination and the needle is withdrawn. The needle may be re-inserted into another part of the kidney so that tissue is collected from at least three different areas. The tissue samples are sent to the laboratory for examination. The entire procedure may last about an hour.

Preparation

Before performing the biopsy, the doctor should be made aware of all the medications that the patient is taking. The doctor should also be told whether the patient is allergic to any medications. The procedure and the risks of the procedure are explained to the patient and the necessary consent forms are obtained. The patient should be told that a kidney biopsy requires a 24-hour stay in the hospital after the biopsy.

Some doctors order blood tests to check for clotting problems before performing the biopsy. The patient's blood type may also be determined in case a transfusion becomes necessary.

Aftercare

Immediately after the biopsy, pulse, respiration, and temperature (vital signs) are measured. If they are stable, the patient is instructed to lie flat in bed for at least 12 hours. The pulse and blood pressure are checked at regular intervals by the nursing staff. All urine voided by the patient in the first 12–24 hours is examined in the laboratory for blood cells.

If bleeding is severe, iron levels in the blood drop significantly, or the patient complains of severe **pain** at the biopsy site, the physician should be contacted immediately. After the patient goes home, he should avoid heavy lifting, vigorous **exercise**, and contact sports for at least one or two weeks.

Risks

The risks of a kidney biopsy are very small. Severe bleeding may occur after the procedure. There is also a slight chance that an infection or a lump of blood under the skin that looks black and blue (hematoma)

KEY TERMS

Biopsy—The surgical removal and microscopic examination of living tissue for diagnostic purposes.

Computed tomography (CT) scan—A medical procedure in which a series of x rays are taken and put together by a computer in order to form detailed pictures of areas inside the body.

Magnetic resonance imaging (MRI)—A medical procedure used for diagnostic purposes in which pictures of areas inside the body can be created using a magnet linked to a computer.

Nephrologist—A doctor who specializes in the diseases and disorders of the kidneys.

Renal ultrasound—A painless and non-invasive procedure in which sound waves are bounced off the kidneys. These sound waves produce a pattern of echoes that are then used by the computer to create pictures of areas inside the kidney (sonograms).

may develop. In most cases, the hematoma disappears by itself and does not cause any pain. However, severe pain or a drop in blood pressure and iron levels in the blood indicates that the hematoma is expanding. This condition could lead to complications and should be reported immediately to the doctor.

Very rarely, the patient may develop high blood pressure (**hypertension**), and the bleeding may be severe enough to require a transfusion. In extremely rare circumstances, the kidney may rupture, or the surrounding organs (pancreas, bowel, spleen, and liver) may be punctured. **Death** occurs in about one in 3000 cases.

Normal results

The results are normal if no abnormalities can be seen in the tissue samples with the naked eye, with an electron microscope or through staining with a fluorescent dye (immunofluorescence).

Abnormal results

Any abnormalities in the size, color, and consistency of the sample will be reported as an abnormal result. In addition, any change in the structure of the renal tubules, the presence of red blood cells, or abnormalities in the cells are considered an abnormal result. If cancerous changes are detected in the kidney cells, they are further characterized in order to determine the stage of the tumor and decide on the appropriate mode of treatment.

ORGANIZATIONS

National Kidney Cancer Association, P.O. Box 96503, Washington, DC, 20090, (800) 850-9132, kidney.cancer@hotmail.com, http://www.kidneycancer.org.

National Kidney Foundation, Inc. , 30 East 33rd Street, New York, NY, 10016, (212) 889-2210, (212) 689-9261, (800) 622-9010, http://www.kidney.org.

Lata Cherath, PhD

Kidney cancer

Definition

Kidney **cancer** is a disease in which the cells in certain tissues of the kidney start to grow uncontrollably and form tumors. Renal cell carcinoma, which occurs in the cells lining the kidneys (epithelial cells), is the most common type of kidney cancer. Eighty-five percent of all kidney tumors are renal cell carcinomas. **Wilms' tumor** is a rapidly developing cancer of the kidney most often found in children under four years of age.

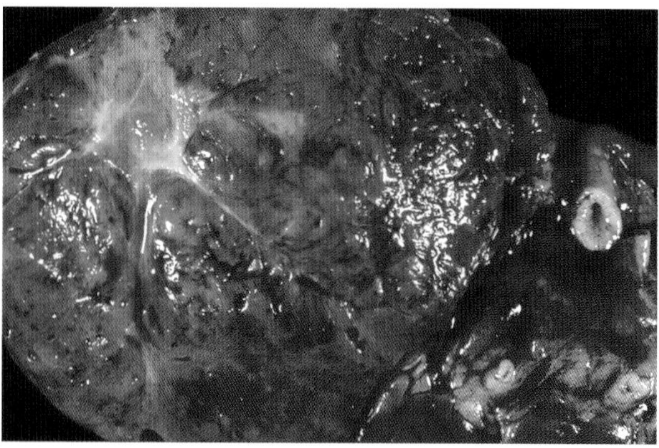

An extracted cancerous kidney. *(Custom Medical Stock Photo, Inc. Reproduced by permission.)*

Description

The kidneys are a pair of organs that lie on either side of the spine just above the waist. Inside each kidney are tiny tubes (tubules) that filter and clean the blood, taking out the waste products and making urine. The urine that is made by the kidney passes through a tube called the ureter into the bladder. Urine is held in the bladder until it is discharged from the body. Renal cell carcinoma generally develops in the lining of the tubules that filter and clean the blood. Cancer that develops in the central portion of the kidney (where the urine is collected and drained into the ureters) is known as transitional cell cancer of the renal pelvis. Transitional cell cancer is similar to **bladder cancer**.

Kidney cancer accounts for approximately 2–3% of all cancers. In the United States, kidney cancer is the tenth most common cancer and the incidence has increased by 43% since 1973; the **death** rate has increased by 16%. According to the American Cancer Society, 35,710 Americans were diagnosed with kidney cancer in 2004, and 12,480 died from the disease. RCC accounts for 90–95% of malignant neoplasms that originate from the kidney.

Causes and symptoms

The causes of kidney cancer are unknown, but men seem to have a greater risk than women of contracting the disease; the male:female ratio in the United States and Canada is 3:2 as of the early 2000s. There is a strong association between cigarette **smoking** and kidney cancer. Cigarette smokers are twice as likely as non-smokers are to develop kidney cancer. Working around coke ovens has been shown to increase people's risk of developing this cancer. Certain types of painkillers that contain the chemical phenacetin are associated with kidney cancer. The United States government discontinued use of **analgesics** containing phenacetin about 20 years ago. **Obesity** may be yet another risk factor for kidney cancer. Some studies show a loose association between kidney cancer and occupational exposure to cadmium, petroleum products, lead, dry-cleaning solvents, trichloroethylene (TCE), and asbestos. Other risk factors for the development of kidney cancer include Hispanic heritage and preexisting von Hippel-Lindau disease.

The most common symptom of kidney cancer is blood in the urine (hematuria). Other symptoms include painful urination, **pain** in the lower back or on the sides, abdominal pain, a lump or hard mass that can be felt in the kidney area, unexplained weight loss, **fever**, weakness, **fatigue**, and high blood pressure.

Other symptoms may occur if the cancer has spread beyond its original location. Spread of kidney cancer most commonly occurs to the lung (55%), liver (33%), bone (33%), adrenal (20%), and opposite kidney (10%). Lymph node spread is also common, occurring in about 25% of patients).

Diagnosis

A diagnostic examination for kidney cancer includes taking a thorough medical history and making a complete **physical examination** in which the doctor will probe (palpate) the abdomen for lumps. Blood tests will be ordered to check for changes in blood chemistry caused by substances released by the tumor. Laboratory tests may show abnormal levels of iron in the blood. Either a low red blood cell count (anemia) or a high red blood cell count (erythrocytosis) may accompany kidney cancer. Occasionally, patients will have high **calcium** levels.

If the doctor suspects kidney cancer, an intravenous pyelogram (IVP) may be ordered. An IVP is an x-ray test in which a dye in injected into a vein in the arm. The dye travels through the body, and when it is concentrated in the urine to be discharged, it outlines the kidneys, ureters, and the urinary bladder. On an x-ray image, the dye will reveal any abnormalities of the urinary tract. The IVP may miss small kidney cancers.

Renal ultrasound is a diagnostic test in which sound waves are used to form an image of the kidneys. Ultrasound is a painless and non-invasive procedure that can be used to detect even very small kidney tumors. Imaging tests such as **computed tomography scans** (CT scans) and **magnetic resonance imaging** (MRI) can be used to evaluate the kidneys and the surrounding organs. These tests are used to check whether the tumor has spread outside the kidney to other organs in the abdomen. If the patient complains of bone pain, a special x ray called a **bone scan** may be ordered to rule out spread to the bones. A **chest x ray** may be taken to rule out spread to the lungs.

A **kidney biopsy** is used to positively confirm the diagnosis of kidney cancer. During this procedure, a small piece of tissue is removed from the tumor and examined under a microscope. The biopsy will give information about the type of tumor, the cells that are involved, and the aggressiveness of the tumor (tumor stage).

Treatment

Each person's treatment is different and depends on several factors. The location, size, and extent of the tumor have to be considered in addition to the patient's

KEY TERMS

Biopsy—The surgical removal and microscopic examination of living tissue for diagnostic purposes.

Bone scan—An x-ray study in which patients are given an intravenous injection of a small amount of a radioactive material that travels in the blood. When it reaches the bones, it can be detected by x ray to make a picture of their internal structure.

Chemotherapy—Treatment with anticancer drugs.

Computed tomography (CT) scan—A medical procedure in which a series of x-ray images are made and put together by a computer to form detailed pictures of areas inside the body.

Cryoablation—A technique for removing tissue by destroying it with extreme cold.

Hematuria—Blood in the urine.

Immunotherapy—Treatment of cancer by stimulating the body's immune defense system.

Intravenous pyelogram (IVP)—A procedure in which a dye is injected into a vein in the arm. The dye travels through the body and concentrates in the urine to be discharged. It outlines the kidneys, ureters, and the urinary bladder. An x-ray image is then made and any abnormalities of the urinary tract are revealed.

Magnetic resonance imaging (MRI)—A medical procedure used for diagnostic purposes in which pictures of areas inside the body can be created using a magnet linked to a computer.

Nephrectomy—A medical procedure in which the kidney is surgically removed.

Radiation therapy—Treatment with high-energy radiation from x-ray machines, cobalt, radium, or other sources.

Renal ultrasound—A painless and non-invasive procedure in which sound waves are bounced off the kidneys. These sound waves produce a pattern of echoes that are then used by the computer to create pictures of areas inside the kidney (sonograms).

age, general health, and medical history. In addition, much has changed in the treatment and management of kidney cancer since the 1980s, including new surgical techniques, new **anticancer drugs**, and the development of effective treatments for advanced disease.

The primary treatment for kidney cancer that has not spread to other parts of the body, which is a Stage I, II, or III tumor, is surgical removal of the diseased kidney (**nephrectomy**). Because most cancers affect only one kidney, the patient can function well with the remaining one. Two types of surgical procedure are used. Radical nephrectomy removes the entire kidney and the surrounding tissue. Sometimes, the lymph nodes surrounding the kidney are also removed. Partial nephrectomy removes only part of the kidney along with the tumor. This procedure is used either when the tumor is very small or when it is not practical to remove the entire kidney. It is not practical to remove a kidney when the patient has only one kidney or when both kidneys have tumors. There is a small (5%) chance of missing some of the cancer. Nephrectomy can also be useful for Stage IV cancers, but alternative surgical procedures such as transarterial angioinfarction may be used.

The rapid development and widespread use of laparoscopic techniques has made it possible for surgeons to remove small tumors while sparing the rest of the kidney. Most tumors removed by **laparoscopy** are 4 cm (1.6 in) in size or smaller. Laparoscopy also allows the surgeon to remove small tumors with cryoablation (destroying the tumor by freezing it) rather than cutting.

Radiation therapy, which consists of exposing the cancer cells to high-energy gamma rays from an external source, generally destroys cancer cells with minimal damage to the normal tissue. Side effects are **nausea**, fatigue, and stomach upsets. These symptoms disappear when the treatment is over. In kidney cancer, radiation therapy has been shown to alleviate pain and bleeding, especially when the cancer is inoperable. However, it has not proven to be of much use in destroying the kidney cancer cells. Therefore radiation therapy is not used very often as a treatment for cancer or as a routine adjuvant to nephrectomy. Radiotherapy, however, is used to manage metastatic kidney cancer.

Treatment of kidney cancer with anticancer drugs (**chemotherapy**) has not produced good results. However, new drugs and new combinations of drugs continue to be tested in clinical trials. One new drug, semaxanib (SU5416), is reported to have good results in treating patients with kidney cancer. However, semaxanib is still undergoing clinical trials in the United States.

Immunologic therapy (or immunotherapy), a form of treatment in which the body's immune system is harnessed to help fight the cancer, is a new mode of therapy that is being tested for kidney cancer. Clinical trials with substances produced by the immune cells (aldesleukin and interferon) have shown some promise in destroying kidney cancer cells. These substances have been approved for use but they can be very toxic and produce severe side effects. The benefits derived from the treatment have to be weighed very carefully against the side effects in each case. Immunotherapy is the most promising systemic therapy for metastatic kidney cancer.

Prognosis

Because kidney cancer is often caught early and sometimes progresses slowly, the chances of a surgical cure are good. Length of survival depends on the size of the original tumor, the aggressiveness of the specific cells making up the tumor, and whether the cancer cells spread from the kidney to surrounding or distant tissues.

Kidney cancer is also one of the few cancers for which there are well-documented cases of spontaneous remission without therapy. Unfortunately, recurrences can occur even as long as ten years after the original diagnosis and treatment, and cancer can also crop up in the other, previously unaffected kidney.

Prevention

The exact cause of kidney cancer is not known, so it is not possible to prevent all cases. However, because a strong association between kidney cancer and tobacco has been shown, avoiding tobacco is the best way to lower one's risk of developing this cancer. Using care when working with cancer-causing agents such as asbestos and cadmium and eating a well-balanced diet may also help prevent kidney cancer.

Resources

BOOKS

Beers, Mark H., Robert S. Porter, and Thomas V. Jones, eds. *The Merck Manual of Diagnosis and Therapy*. 18th ed. Whitehouse Station, NJ: Merck Research Laboratories, 2006.

Rakel, Robert E., Edward T. Bope, and Howard F. Conn.*Conn's Current Therapy 2004: Latest Approved Methods of Treatment for the Practicing Physician*. Philadelphia: Saunders, 2004.

PERIODICALS

Brauch, H., G. Weirich, B. Klein, et al. "VHL Mutations in Renal Cell Cancer: Does Occupational Exposure to Trichloroethylene Make a Difference?" *Toxicology Letters* 151 (June 15, 2004): 301–310.

Griffiths, T. R., and J. K. Mellon. "Evolving Immunotherapeutic Strategies in Bladder and Renal Cancer." *Postgraduate Medical Journal* 80 (June 2004): 320–327.

Jennens, R. R., M. A. Rosenthal, G. J. Lindeman, and M. Michael. "Complete Radiological and Metabolic Response of Metastatic Renal Cell Carcinoma to SU5416 (Semaxanib) in a Patient with Probable von Hippel-Lindau Syndrome." *Urologic Oncology* 22 (May–June 2004): 193–196.

Lam, J. S., O. Svarts, and A. J. Pantuck. "Changing Concepts in the Surgical Management of Renal Cell Carcinoma." *European Urology* 45 (June 2004): 692–705.

Lotan, Y., D. A. Duchene, J. A. Cadeddu, et al. "Changing Management of Organ-Confined Renal Masses." *Journal of Endourology* 18 (April 2004): 263–268.

Moon, T. D., F. T. Lee, Jr., S. P. Hedican, et al. "Laparoscopic Cryoablation under Sonographic Guidance for the Treatment of Small Renal Tumors." *Journal of Endourology* 18 (June 2004): 436–440.

ORGANIZATIONS

American Cancer Society, 1599 Clifton Rd. NE, Atlanta, GA, 30329, (800) 227-2345, http://www.cancer.org.

Cancer Research Institute (National Headquarters), One Exchange Plaza, 55 Broadway, Suite 1802, New York, NY, (212) 688-7515, (212) 832-9376, (800) 992-2623, http://www.cancerresearch.org.

National Cancer Institute (National Institutes of Health), NCI Office of Communications and Education, 6116 Executive Blvd. Suite 300, Bethesda, MD, 20892-8322, (800) 4-CANCER (422-6237), cancergovstaff@mail.nih.gov, http://www.cancer.gov.

National Kidney Cancer Association, P.O. Box 96503, Washington, DC, 20090, (800) 850-9132, kidney.cancer@hotmail.com, http://www.kidneycancer.org.

National Kidney Foundation, Inc. , 30 East 33rd Street, New York, NY, 10016, (212) 889-2210, (212) 689-9261, (800) 622-9010, http://www.kidney.org.

Rosalyn Carson-DeWitt, MD
Rebecca Frey, PhD

Kidney dialysis *see* **Dialysis, kidney**

Kidney disease

Definition

Kidney disease is a general term for any damage that reduces the functioning of the kidney. Kidney disease is also called renal disease.

Description

The kidneys are a pair bean-shaped, fist-sized organs that are located below the rib cage near the middle of the back. In adults they filter about 200 quarts (190 L) of blood every day to remove waste products that result from the normal activities of tissues in the body. These wastes circulate in the blood. and if not removed they would damage the body. The kidneys also play a crucial role in regulating the amount of water and chemicals (electrolytes) in the body such as **sodium**, potassium and phosphorous.

Inside the kidneys are about one million tiny units called nephrons. Inside each nephron is a very thin blood vessel called a capillary that twists around a very thin tube called a tubule. This combination of capillary and tubule inside the nephron is called a glomerulous and it is here that the blood is filtered. Water, electrolytes, and waste products (but not red blood cells) can pass across the capillary wall and into the tubule. The kidney then regulates how much water and which other substances can pass back into the blood in the capillary to keep the body in balance. Waste products, excess water, and excess electrolytes remain in the tubule and eventually leave the body as urine.

The kidneys also release three regulatory chemicals—erythropoietin, renin, and calcitriol—that affect other functions in the body. Erythropoietin stimulates the bone marrow to produce new red blood cells. Renin helps regulate blood pressure, and calcitriol is a form of vitamin D and is important in maintaining bones and the level of **calcium** in the body.

Because the kidney has many functions, there are many types of kidney disease. Congenital kidney diseases are disorders that are present at birth. **Polycystic kidney disease** (PKD) is a rare disorder in which children inherit defective genes from both parents that cause cysts full of fluid to develop in the kidneys and replace the blood filtering units. As a result, the kidneys cannot adequately remove wastes from the body. There are two other types of PDK. One is inherited, but does not appear until adulthood, and the other develops as a result of long-term kidney damage. In total, about half a million people in the United States have some form of PKD. Hereditary disease and **birth defects** are the most common causes of kidney disease in children up to age 14.

Acute kidney diseases are problems that develop suddenly. Many acute kidney diseases can be cured, but some may cause permanent damage. Common acute kidney diseases include kidney infection, hemolytic uremic syndrome, **nephrotic syndrome** in children, and damage caused by injury to the kidney or poisoning. Hemolytic uremic syndrome is a rare disease that usually affects children under age ten and is caused by eating food contaminated with bacteria. The bacteria release a poison that damages the kidney and causes **acute kidney failure**. Most children who develop this disease recover and their kidney function returns to normal.

Chronic kidney disease is disease that is slow to develop and usually does not show any symptoms until kidney damage is permanent. The National Kidney and Urologic Disease Information Clearinghouse, a federal agency, estimates that about 4.5% of people over age 20 have chronic kidney disease as indicated by tests that measure kidney function. The most common cause of chronic kidney disease in the United States is diabetes. It accounts for between 33% and 40% of all new cases of chronic kidney disease in the United States. In diabetes, the body cannot break down glucose (sugar). This extra glucose in the blood damages the nephrons so that they no longer filter blood effectively.

High or uncontrolled blood pressure (**hypertension**) is the second leading cause of chronic kidney disease. It accounts for between 27% and 30% of all new cases of chronic kidney disease. High blood pressure damages the capillaries in the nephron, so that they can no longer work with the tubules to filter the blood. Glomerulonephtitis is a term for several different chronic kidney diseases where damage to the nephrons causes protein or red blood cells pass into the urine. **Kidney cancer** is uncommon, accounting for only 2% of **cancer** cases.

Over-the-counter **analgesics** (pain medications) such as **aspirin**, **acetaminophen** (Tylenol), ibuprofen (Advil), naxopren sodium (Aleve), and similar medications that can be bought without a prescription may make kidney disease worse in individuals who already have kidney damage or cause kidney damage in healthy individuals who take these medications daily for several years. The chance of damage is increased when these pain medications are taken in combination with each other or with **caffeine** or codeine (Some painkilling tablets are a combination of pain medications and caffeine or codeine). Individuals who take these painkillers regularly or who have been told they have kidney damage should discuss the risk of these medications with their physician.

Chronic kidney disease can lead to end-stage renal disease (ESRD), in which there is almost total failure of the kidneys. If renal function is reduced to only 25% of normal, serious illness results. When this drops to 10–15% of normal, **death** occurs unless the individual receives dialysis or a kidney transplant. In 2002, there were over 100,300 new cases of ESRD, 44% of which were caused by diabetes. Treatment of ESRD in the United States cost about $25.2 billion in 2002.

Causes and symptoms

Causes of kidney disease are many and varied. Leading causes are diabetes, high blood pressure, inherited disease, and infection. Acute kidney disease is often marked by a lack of urination and increased fluid build up in the body. Chronic kidney disease is often called a "silent" killer, because no obvious symptoms develop until the kidneys are permanently damaged. The National Kidney Foundation estimated in 2005 that 20 million Americans had undetected moderate chronic kidney disease. Chronic kidney disease most often results from other diseases such as diabetes or hypertension.

Diagnosis

Simple blood and urine tests can indicated kidney disease, but more extensive testing may be needed to determine the exact nature of the disease. A blood test that measures serum creatinine, a waste product, can indicate how well the kidneys are working. Although normal levels of creatinine vary (an average range is 0.6–1.2 mg/dL), a higher than expected level in the blood may indicate kidney damage. A blood urea nitrogen (BUN) blood test measures waste products circulating in the blood. Normal levels range from 7%–20 mg/dL. The less well the kidney is working, the higher the BUN.

A 24-hour urine collection test will accurately measure how much urine the kidneys are producing in a day. A **urinalysis** can determine if protein or red blood cells are leaking into the urine indicating abnormal kidney function. A creatinine clearance test compares the amount of creatinine in a 24-hour urine sample with the amount of creatinine in the blood to determine how much blood the kidneys are filtering each minute.

Based on the results of blood and urine tests, other tests such as a CT scan, MRI, or **kidney biopsy** may be ordered.

Treatment

Most treatment for kidney disease involves treating the underlying cause of the disease, such as controlling high blood pressure or diabetes. Diuretic medication ("water pills") may be given to help relieve fluid accumulation. **Antibiotics** are used to treat kidney infections. Other drugs may be given to treat specific kidney diseases.

KEY TERMS

Congenital—Present at birth.

Diuretic—A substance that stimulates the kidney to excrete water.

Glomerulous—A twisted mass of blood capillaries and urine tubules in the kidney where filtering of waste products occurs.

Hormone—A chemical produced by living cells that travels through the circulatory system and affects tissue at some distance from where it was released.

Hypertension—High blood pressure.

Nephron—The smallest functional unit of the kidney involved in the removal of waste products and excess water from the blood.

Diet and lifestyle changes are an important part of controlling kidney disease. **Obesity** increases blood pressure, so losing weight can help limit kidney damage, as can stopping **smoking**. Reducing sodium (salt) in the diet also helps control blood pressure. In certain kinds of kidney disease, potassium is removed in abnormally large quantities by the kidneys and excreted in urine. Eating more foods such as bananas, dried beans and peas, nuts, and potatoes that are high in potassium or taking a potassium supplement pill help reverse this effect. When protein is found in the urine, some physicians recommend reducing the amount of protein (mainly found in meat) in the diet.

When kidneys fail completely in ESRD, there are only two alternatives: dialysis or kidney transplant. There are two types of dialysis. Peritoneal dialysis uses a membrane in the individual's abdomen to filter waste products. The most common kind of peritoneal dialysis is continuous ambulatory peritoneal dialysis (CAPD), in which the individual is hooked up to a bag of dialysis fluid that he carries with him, allowing continuous dialysis. The fluid is changed four times a day. In another form of peritoneal dialysis, the abdomen is filled with dialysis fluid. Wastes filter into the fluid for several hours often while the individual is asleep, the then the fluid is drained from the body. Peritoneal dialysis can be done at home without the need for a health care professional.

In hemodialysis, the individual must go to a dialysis center about three times a week. His blood is sent through a machine that filters out the waste and then returns the cleansed blood to his body. The process takes three to four hours and is done by a health care professional.

Kidney transplants can come from either a living donor or a deceased donor. Donors are matched with recipients based on blood type and must take drugs to prevent their immune system from rejecting the kidney after transplantation. The United Network for Organ Sharing (UNOS) coordinates matching donor kidneys with appropriate recipients. More than 100 clinical trials are enrolling patients with various types of kidney disease.

Alternative treatment

Alternative treatments tend to focus on removing excess water from the body, but have limited effect on serious disease. Asparagus (*Asparagus officinalis*) birch tea (*Betula* species), goldenrod infusion (*Solidago* species), horsetail (*Equisetum arvense*), and stinging nettle (*Urtica dioica*) all are used to stimulate urine production.

Prognosis

Many individuals recover normal kidney function after developing acute kidney disease, although in some cases, such as poisoning and injury, kidney damage may be permanent. Chronic kidney disease tends to get progressively worse as the individual ages. More than 15,000 kidney transplants are done each year, and there is a often long waiting list for donated kidneys. 80.6% of individuals receiving a transplant from a deceased donor survive for at least 5 years, and 90.4% of individuals receiving a kidney donated from a living donor survive for at least 5 years.

Prevention

Maintaining a healthy body weight, getting regular **exercise**, and not smoking all promote kidney health. Controlling underlying diseases such as diabetes and high blood pressure are important in preventing chronic kidney diseases.

Resources

OTHER

"About Kidney Disease." National Kidney Disease Education Program. June 30, 2010 (accessed October 16, 2010). http://www.nkdep.nih.gov/patients/kidney_disease_information.htm.

ORGANIZATIONS

American Association of Kidney Patients, 3505 E. Frontage Road, Suite 315, Tampa, FL, 33607, (813) 636-8122, (800) 749-2257, info@aakp.org, http://www.aakp.org.

American Urological Association Foundation, 1000 Corporate Blvd., Linthicum, MD, 21090, (410) 689-3700, (410) 689-3800, (866) 746-4282, auafoundation@auafoundation.org, http://www.urologyhealth.org.

National Institute of Diabetes and Digestive and Kidney Diseases, NIDDK, NIH Bldg 31, Rm 9A06 31 Center Drive, MSC 2560, Bethesda, MD, 20892-2560, (301) 496.3583, http://www2.niddk.nih.gov.

National Kidney Foundation, Inc. , 30 East 33rd Street, New York, NY, 10016, (212) 889-2210, (212) 689-9261, (800) 622-9010, http://www.kidney.org.

United Network for Organ Sharing (UNOS), 700 N. 4th Street; PO Box 2484, Richmond, VA, 23218, (804) 782-4800, (804) 782-4817, (888) 894-6361, http://www.unos.org.

Tish Davidson, A.M.

Kidney failure *see* **Acute kidney failure; Chronic kidney failure**

Kidney function tests

Definition

Kidney function tests is a collective term for a variety of individual tests and procedures that can be done to evaluate how well the kidneys are functioning.

Purpose

The kidneys, the body's natural filtration system, perform many vital functions, including removing metabolic waste products from the bloodstream, regulating the body's water balance, and maintaining the pH (acidity/alkalinity) of the body's fluids. Approximately one and a half quarts of blood per minute are circulated through the kidneys, where waste chemicals are filtered out and eliminated from the body (along with excess water) in the form of urine. Kidney function tests help to determine if the kidneys are performing their tasks adequately.

Precautions

A complete history should be taken prior to kidney function tests to assess the patient's food and drug intake. A wide variety of prescription and over-the-counter medications can affect blood and urine kidney function test results, as can some food and beverages.

Description

Many conditions can affect the ability of the kidneys to carry-out their vital functions. Some lead to a rapid (acute) decline in kidney function; others lead to a gradual (chronic) decline in function. Both result in a build-up of toxic waste substances in the blood. A number of clinical laboratory tests that measure the levels of substances normally regulated by the kidneys can help determine the cause and extent of kidney dysfunction. These tests are done on urine samples, as well as on blood samples.

Urine tests

There are a variety of urine tests that assess kidney function. A simple, inexpensive screening test, called a routine **urinalysis**, is often the first test administered if kidney problems are suspected. A small, randomly collected urine sample is examined physically for things like color, odor, appearance, and concentration (specific gravity); chemically for substances such as protein, glucose, and pH (acidity/ alkalinity); and microscopically for the presence of cellular elements (red blood cells, white blood cells, and epithelial cells), bacteria, crystals, and casts (structures formed by the deposit of protein, cells, and other substances in the kidneys' tubules). If results indicate a possibility of disease or impaired kidney function, one or more of the following additional tests is usually performed to more specifically diagnose the cause and the level of decline in kidney function.

- Creatinine clearance test. This test evaluates how efficiently the kidneys clear a substance called creatinine from the blood. Creatinine, a waste product of muscle energy metabolism, is produced at a constant rate that is proportional to the muscle mass of the individual. Because the body does not recycle it, all of the creatinine filtered by the kidneys in a given amount of time is excreted in the urine, making creatinine clearance a very specific measurement of kidney function. The test is performed on a timed urine specimen—a cumulative sample collected over a two to twenty-four hour period. Determination of the blood creatinine level is also required to calculate the urine clearance.
- Urea clearance test. Urea is a waste product that is created by protein metabolism and excreted in the urine. The urea clearance test requires a blood sample to measure the amount of urea in the bloodstream and two urine specimens, collected one hour apart, to determine the amount of urea that is filtered, or cleared, by the kidneys into the urine.
- Urine osmolality test. Urine osmolality is a measurement of the number of dissolved particles in urine. It is a more precise measurement than specific gravity for evaluating the ability of the kidneys to concentrate or dilute the urine. Kidneys that are functioning normally will excrete more water into the urine as fluid intake is increased, diluting the urine. If fluid intake is decreased, the kidneys excrete less water and the urine becomes more concentrated. The test may be done on a urine sample collected first thing in the morning, on multiple timed samples, or on a cumulative sample collected over a twenty-four hour period. The patient will typically be prescribed a high-protein diet for several days before the test and asked to drink no fluids the night before the test.
- Urine protein test. Healthy kidneys filter all proteins from the bloodstream and then reabsorb them, allowing no protein, or only slight amounts of protein, into the urine. The persistent presence of significant amounts of protein in the urine, then, is an important indicator of kidney disease. A positive screening test for protein (included in a routine urinalysis) on a random urine sample is usually followed-up with a test on a 24-hour urine sample that more precisely measures the quantity of protein.

Blood tests

There are also several blood tests that can aid in evaluating kidney function. These include:

- Blood urea nitrogen test (BUN). Urea is a by-product of protein metabolism. This waste product is formed in the liver, then filtered from the blood and excreted in the urine by the kidneys. The BUN test measures the amount of nitrogen contained in the urea. High BUN levels can indicate kidney dysfunction, but because blood urea nitrogen is also affected by protein intake and liver function, the test is usually done in conjunction with a blood creatinine, a more specific indicator of kidney function.
- Creatinine test. This test measures blood levels of creatinine, a by-product of muscle energy metabolism that, like urea, is filtered from the blood by the kidneys and excreted into the urine. Production of creatinine depends on an individual's muscle mass, which usually fluctuates very little. With normal kidney function, then, the amount of creatinine in the blood remains relatively constant and normal. For this reason, and because creatinine is affected very little by liver function, an elevated blood creatinine is a more sensitive indication of impaired kidney function than the BUN.
- Other blood tests. Measurement of the blood levels of other elements regulated in part by the kidneys can also be useful in evaluating kidney function. These include sodium, potassium, chloride, bicarbonate, calcium, magnesium, phosphorus, protein, uric acid, and glucose.

Preparation

Patients will be given specific instructions for collection of urine samples, depending on the test to be performed. Some timed urine tests require an extended

KEY TERMS

Blood urea nitrogen (BUN)—The nitrogen portion of urea in the bloodstream. Urea is a waste product of protein metabolism in the body.

Creatinine—The metabolized by-product of creatine, an organic acid that assists the body in producing muscle contractions. Creatinine is found in the bloodstream and in muscle tissue. It is removed from the blood by the kidneys and excreted in the urine.

Osmolality—A measurement of urine concentration that depends on the number of particles dissolved in it. Values are expressed as milliosmols per kilogram (mOsm/kg) of water.

Urea—A by-product of protein metabolism that is formed in the liver. Because urea contains ammonia, which is toxic to the body, it must be quickly filtered from the blood by the kidneys and excreted in the urine.

collection period of up to 24 hours, during which time the patient collects all urine voided and transfers it to a specimen container. Refrigeration and/or preservatives are typically required to maintain the integrity of such urine specimens. Certain dietary and/or medication restrictions may be imposed for some of the blood and urine tests. The patient may also be instructed to avoid **exercise** for a period of time before a test.

Aftercare

If medication was discontinued prior to a urine kidney function test, it may be resumed once the test is completed.

Risks

Risks for these tests are minimal, but may include slight bleeding from a blood-drawing site, hematoma (accumulation of blood under a puncture site), or **fainting** or feeling light-headed after venipuncture. In addition, suspension of medication or dietary changes imposed in preparation for some blood or urine tests may trigger side-effects in some individuals.

Normal results

Normal values for many tests are determined by the patient's age and sex. Reference values can also vary by laboratory, but are generally within the ranges that follow.

Urine tests

- Creatinine clearance. For a 24-hour urine collection, normal results are 90-139 mL/min for adult males less than 40 years old, and 80-125 mL/min for adult females less than 40 years old. For people over 40, values decrease by 6.5 mL/min for each decade of life.
- Urea clearance. With maximum clearance, normal is 64–99 mL/min.
- Urine osmolality. With restricted fluid intake (concentration testing), osmolality should be greater than 800 mOsm/kg of water. With increased fluid intake (dilution testing), osmolality should be less than 100 mOSm/kg in at least one of the specimens collected.
- Urine protein. A 24-hour urine collection should contain no more than 150 mg of protein.

Blood tests

- Blood urea nitrogen (BUN). 8–20 mg/dL.
- Creatinine. 0.8–1.2 mg/dL for males, and 0.6–0.9 mg/dL for females.

Abnormal results

Low clearance values for creatinine and urea indicate diminished ability of the kidneys to filter these waste products from the blood and excrete them in the urine. As clearance levels decrease, blood levels of creatinine and urea nitrogen increase. Since it can be affected by other factors, an elevated BUN, by itself, is suggestive, but not diagnostic, for kidney dysfunction. An abnormally elevated blood creatinine, a more specific and sensitive indicator of **kidney disease** than the BUN, is diagnostic of impaired kidney function.

Inability of the kidneys to concentrate the urine in response to restricted fluid intake, or to dilute the urine in response to increased fluid intake during osmolality testing may indicate decreased kidney function. Because the kidneys normally excrete almost no protein in the urine, its persistent presence, in amounts that exceed the normal 24-hour urine value, usually indicates some type of kidney disease as well.

ORGANIZATIONS

National Kidney Foundation, Inc., 30 East 33rd Street, New York, NY, 10016, (212) 889-2210, (212) 689-9261, (800) 622-9010, http://www.kidney.org.

Paula Anne Ford-Martin

Kidney nuclear medicine scan

Definition

A kidney nuclear medicine scan, or study, is a simple outpatient test that involves administering small amounts of radioactive substances, called tracers, into the body and then imaging the kidneys and bladder with a special camera. The images obtained can help in the diagnosis and treatment of certain kidney diseases.

Purpose

While many tests, such as x rays, ultrasound exams, or **computed tomography scans** (CT scans), can reveal the structure of the kidneys (its anatomy), the kidney nuclear medicine scan is unique in that it reveals how the kidneys are functioning. This is valuable information in helping a doctor make a diagnosis. Therefore, the kidney nuclear medicine scan is performed primarily to see how well the kidneys are working and, at the same time, they can identify some of the various structures that make up the kidney.

Precautions

If a patient is pregnant, it is generally recommended that she not have a kidney nuclear medicine scan. The unborn baby is more sensitive to radiation than an adult. If a woman thinks she might be pregnant, she should inform her doctor of this too.

Women who are **breastfeeding** should also inform their doctor. The doctor may recommend the woman stop breastfeeding for a day or two after a kidney nuclear medicine scan, depending on the particular tracer that was used since the tracer can accumulate in breast milk.

Description

Nuclear medicine is a branch of radiology that uses radioactive materials to diagnose or treat various diseases. These radioactive materials (tracers) may also be called radiopharmaceuticals, and they accumulate (collect) in specific organs in the body. Radiopharmaceuticals are able to yield valuable information about the particular organ being studied.

Whether outside the body or inside the body, tracers emit radioactive signals, called gamma rays, which can be collected and counted by a special device, called a gamma camera. The images of the kidney that the camera produces are called renal scans.

The kidney nuclear medicine scan can be performed on an outpatient basis, usually by a nuclear medicine technologist. The technologist helps prepare the patient for the exam by positioning him or her on an exam table or cart in the imaging area. The patient's position is usually flat on the back. The patient must lie still during imaging to prevent blurring of the images that will be taken. The technologist positions the camera as close to the kidney (or kidneys) as possible to obtain the best images.

In the next step of the procedure, the technologist injects the radiopharmaceutical into the patient. This may be done with one single injection or through an intravenous (IV) line. Immediately after the tracer is injected, imaging begins. It is important to obtain images right away because the tracer's radioactivity begins to diminish (decay). The time required for one-half of the tracer's activity to decay is called the tracer's half-life (T 1/2). The half-life is unique to each radiopharmaceutical. Also, it is important to see the kidney in its immediate state.

Serial pictures are taken with the gamma camera and may be seen on a computer or TV-like screen. The camera doesn't emit radiation, it only records it. The images then are stored on film.

A kidney nuclear medicine scan ranges from 45 minutes to three hours in length, depending on the goals of the test. But the test typically takes about an hour to an hour-and-a-half.

Once the images and curves are obtained, the nuclear medicine physician or radiologist analyzes, or reads, them. Various information can be provided to the doctor through these, depending on the test that was performed. A variety of kidney nuclear medicine studies are available for a doctor to help in making diagnoses. It is important to understand that kidney nuclear medicine scans are good at identifying when there is an abnormality, but they do not always identify the specific problem. They are very useful in providing information about how the various parts of the kidneys function, which, in turn, can assist in making a diagnosis.

Studies may be performed to determine the rate at which the kidney's are filtering a patient's blood. These studies use a radiopharmaceutical, called Technetium DTPA (Tc 99m DTPA). This radiopharmaceutical also can identify obstruction (blockage) in the collecting system. To study how well the tubules and ducts of the kidney are functioning, the radiopharmaceutical Technetium MAG3 is used. Studying tubular function is a good indicator of overall renal function.

KEY TERMS

Intravenous pyelogram (IVP)—X-ray technique using dye to image the kidneys, ureters, and bladder.

Renal—Having to do with the kidneys.

Renal artery stenosis—Narrowing or constriction of the artery that supplies the kidney with blood.

In many renal diseases, one of the first things that disappears or diminishes is the tubular function.

Candidates for a kidney nuclear medicine scan are patients who have:

- Renal failure or chronic renal failure
- Obstruction in their urine collection systems
- Renal artery stenosis
- A kidney transplant.

Preparation

No preparation is necessary for a kidney nuclear medicine scan. The doctor may ask the patient to refrain from certain medications, however, before the scan if the medications might interfere with the test. For example, if a scan is being performed to study **renal artery stenosis**, the patient may have to refrain from taking medications for **hypertension**.

Aftercare

Patients can resume their normal daily activities immediately after the test. Most tracers are passed naturally from the body, though drinking fluids after a kidney nuclear medicine scan can help flush the tracer into the urine and out of the body more quickly.

Risks

Nuclear medicine procedures are very safe. Unlike some of the dyes that may be used in x-ray studies, radioactive tracers rarely cause side effects. There are no long-lasting effects of the tracers themselves, because they have no functional effects on the body's tissues.

Normal results

The test reveals normal kidney function for age and medical situation.

Abnormal results

The test reveals a change in function that may be attributable to a disease process, such as obstruction or a malfunctioning kidney. If the test is abnormal, the patient may be recalled another day for a repeat study, performed differently, to narrow the list of causes.

ORGANIZATIONS

Society of Nuclear Medicine (SNM), 1850 Samuel Morse Dr., Reston, VA, 20190, (703) 708-9000, (703) 708-9015, http://www.snm.org.

Collette L. Placek

Kidney removal *see* **Nephrectomy**

Kidney stones

Definition

Kidney stones are solid accumulations of material that form in the tubal system of the kidney. Kidney stones cause problems when they block the flow of urine within the kidney or urinary tract. When the stones move through the ureter, they can cause severe **pain**.

Description

Urine is formed by the kidneys. Blood flows into the kidneys, and nephrons (specialized tubes) within the kidneys allow a certain amount of fluid from the blood, along with certain substances dissolved in that fluid, to flow out of the body as urine. Sometimes, a problem causes the dissolved substances to become

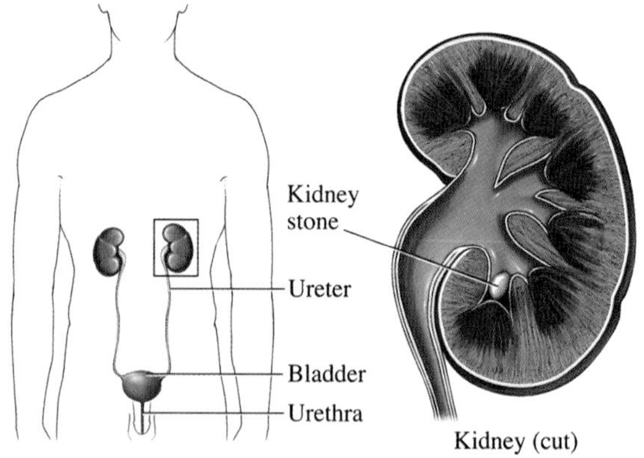

Kidney stones can occur in the ureter near the bladder or kidney. *(© Nucleus Medical Art, Inc./Alamy.)*

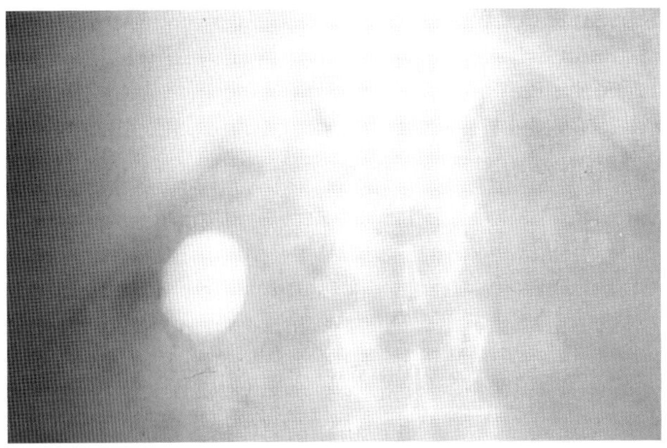

X ray of kidney stone. *(Custom Medical Stock Photo, Inc. Reproduced by permission.)*

solid again. Tiny crystals then form in the urine, meet, and cling together to create a larger solid mass called a kidney stone.

Many kidney stones are small enough that the kidney continues to function normally, and the stones never cause any pain. These are called "silent stones." Kidney stones cause problems when they interfere with the normal flow of urine. They can obstruct (block) the flow through the ureter. The kidney is not accustomed to experiencing any pressure. When pressure builds from backed-up urine, the kidney may swell (**hydronephrosis**). If the kidney is subjected to this pressure for some time, there may be damage to delicate kidney structures. When the kidney stone is lodged further down the ureter, the backed-up urine may also cause the ureter to swell (hydroureter). Because the ureter is a muscular tube, the presence of a stone makes the tube spasm, causing severe pain.

About 10% of all people have a significant kidney stone during their lifetime. Kidney stones are most common among white men over age 30, people who have previously had kidney stones, and people whose family members are prone to developing kidney stones. Eating a lot of animal protein and drinking too few fluids are also thought to contribute to the development of kidney stones.

Causes and symptoms

Kidney stones can be composed of a variety of substances. The most common types of kidney stones are described here.

Calcium stones

About 80% of all kidney stones are **calcium** stones. These stones are composed of either calcium and phosphate, or calcium and oxalate. People with calcium stones may have other diseases that cause them to have increased blood levels of calcium. These diseases include primary parathyroidism, **sarcoidosis**, **hyperthyroidism**, **renal tubular acidosis**, **multiple myeloma**, hyperoxaluria, and some types of **cancer**.

Struvite stones

Struvite stones account for 10% of all kidney stones. Struvite stones are composed of magnesium ammonium phosphate. These stones occur most often in patients who have had repeated urinary tract infections caused by certain types of bacteria. These bacteria produce a substance called urease that increases the urine pH and makes the urine more alkaline. This chemical environment allows struvite to settle out of the urine, forming stones.

Uric acid stones

About 5% of all kidney stones are uric acid stones. These occur when increased amounts of uric acid circulate in the bloodstream. When the uric acid content becomes very high, it can no longer remain dissolved and solid particles of uric acid settle out of the urine. A kidney stone is formed when these particles cling to each other within the kidney, slowly forming a solid mass. About half of all patients with this type of stone also have deposits of uric acid elsewhere in their bodies, commonly in the joint of the big toe. This painful disorder is called **gout**. Other causes of uric acid stones include **chemotherapy** for cancer, bone marrow disorders in which certain types of blood cells are over-produced, and an inherited disorder called **Lesch-Nyhan syndrome**.

Cystine stones

Cystine stones account for 2% of all kidney stones. Cystine is a type of amino acid, and people with this type of kidney stone have an abnormality in the way their bodies process amino acids in the diet.

Patients who have kidney stones usually do not have symptoms until the stone passes into the ureter. Before this, some people may notice blood in their urine. Once the stone is in the ureter, however, most people experience bouts of very severe pain. The pain is crampy, spasmodic, and intense. It usually begins in the flank region, the area between the lower ribs and the hip bone. As the stone moves closer to the bladder, a patient will often feel the pain radiating along the inner thigh. Women may feel the pain in the vulva, while men often feel pain in the testicles. **Nausea**, **vomiting**, frequent and painful urination, and blood in the urine are common. **Fever** and chills usually mean that the ureter has become obstructed, allowing bacteria to become trapped in the kidney and cause a kidney infection (**pyelonephritis**).

Diagnosis

Most often in a healthy adult, diagnosis of kidney stones is based on the patient's pattern of severe, distinctive pain. Diagnosis may include laboratory examination of a urine sample and an x-ray examination. During the passage of a stone, examination of the urine usually reveals blood. A number of imaging tests can, if necessary, be used to diagnose kidney stones. A plain x ray of the kidneys, ureters, and bladder may or may not reveal the stone. An ultrasound can also be used to detect renal blockage. The use of computed tomography (CT) scans has been added to diagnose of some kidney stones.

When a patient is passing a kidney stone, the urine is strained through a special sieve to catch the stone. If the stone can be located (often it cannot), it can then be sent to a laboratory for analysis to determine the chemical composition of the stone. After the kidney stone has been passed, other tests may be done to understand the underlying condition that may have caused the stone to form. Collecting urine for 24 hours, followed by careful analysis of its chemical makeup, can often determine the reason for stone formation.

Treatment

It is believed that stones will pass more quickly if the patient is encouraged to drink large amounts of water (2–3 quarts per day). Cranberry (*Vaccinium macrocarpon*) juice has been a traditional remedy for the treatment and prevention of kidney stones. Although clinical trials have found that cranberry juice has some effect on urinary tract infections, its effectiveness in treating kidney stones is unproven.

Herbal remedies that have anti-lithic (stone-dissolving) action can assist in dissolving small kidney stones. These include gravel root (*Eupatorium purpureum*), hydrangea (*Hydrangea aborescens*), and wild carrot (*Daucus carota*). Starfruit (*Averrhoa carambola*) is recommended to increase the amount of urine a patient passes and to relieve pain.

A Chinese herbal practitioner may use herbs such as *Semen Abutili seu Malvae*, *Semen plantaginis*, and *Herba lygodii japonici* for urinary stones. Dietary changes can be made to reduce the risk of future stone formation and to facilitate the resorption of existing stones. Supplementation with magnesium, a smooth muscle relaxant, can help reduce pain and facilitate stone passing. **Guided imagery** may also be used to help relieve pain. Large stones may require conventional medical intervention.

Allopathic treatment

The pain associated with a kidney stone sends most patients to the emergency room, and a patient with a kidney stone will say that the most important aspect of treatment is adequate pain relief. Because the pain of passing a kidney stone is so severe, narcotic pain medications are usually required. If the patient is **vomiting** or unable to drink fluids because of the pain, it may be necessary to provide intravenous fluids and anti-emetics (drugs that stop vomiting). If symptoms and urine tests indicate the presence of infection, **antibiotics** are required.

Although most kidney stones pass on their own, some do not. The preferred method of treatment is extracorporeal shock wave **lithotripsy** (ESWL). Shock waves are aimed at the stone. The energy of the shock waves causes the stone to vibrate and fragment into small pieces that can be more easily passed. This procedure is generally done under light anesthesia because the shock waves cause pain. If the stone is lodged in the ureter, the urologist may insert a device into the ureter that can direct laser or ultrasound energy at the stone and pulverize it. If the stone is large and ESWL does not work, the stone may be removed by minimally invasive surgery.

Expected results

A patient's prognosis depends on the underlying disorder causing the development of kidney stones. In most cases, patients with uncomplicated calcium stones recover very well. About 60% of these patients, however, will have other kidney stones. Struvite stones are particularly dangerous because they may grow extremely large, filling the tubes within the kidney. These are called staghorn stones and will not pass out in the urine. They require surgical removal. Uric acid stones may also become staghorn stones.

Prevention

Prevention of kidney stones depends on the type of stone and the presence or absence of an underlying disease. In almost all cases, increasing fluid intake so that a person consistently drinks 2 to 3 quarts (liters) of water a day is an important preventative measure. Drinking a glass of lemonade made with real lemons or real lemon concentrate also helps increase the amount of citrate in the urine. Citrate makes it more difficult for kidney stones to form.

KEY TERMS

Diuretic—A substance that removes water from the body by increasing urine production.

pH—A measure of the acidity of a fluid. On a scale of 1 to 14, a pH of 7 is neutral. Higher pH readings are alkaline and lower pH readings are acidic.

Ureter—A tube that carries urine from the kidney to the bladder.

People with calcium oxalate stones do not need to reduce the amount of calcium in their diet but may reduce the amount of foods containing oxalate. These foods include rhubarb, star fruit, beets, beet greens, collards, okra, refried beans, spinach, Swiss chard, sweet potatoes, sesame seeds, almonds, and soy products. A vegan diet or one very low in animal products also is effective in preventing kidney stones, especially when combined with a very low salt diet.

People prone to form kidney stones may also be given medication to help prevent their formation. A thiazide diuretic can help prevent the formation of calcium stones. Allopurinol (Zyloprim, Aloprim) reduces the amount of uric acid blood and urine and helps prevent the formation of uric acid stones. Sturvite stones often form when the kidney becomes infected, so preventing infection also helps to prevent stone formation. Cystine stones are difficult to prevent.

Resources

BOOKS

Chevallier, Andrew. *Herbal Remedies*. New York: DK Publishing, 2007.

Foster, Steven, and Rebecca Johnson. *National Geographic Desk Reference to Nature's Medicine*. Washington, DC: National Geographic Society, 2006.

Mayo Clinic Book of Alternative Medicine: The New Approach to Using the Best of Natural Therapies and Conventional Medicine. New York: Time Inc. Home Entertainment, 2007.

Rodman, John S. *No More Kidney Stones*, rev. ed. Hoboken, NJ: Wiley, 2006.

OTHER

"Kidney Stones." *eMedicine Health* September 7, 2007. http://www.emedicinehealth.com/kidney_stones/page6_em.htm#Medical%20Treatment

"Kidney Stones." *Mayo Clinic* January 31, 2008. http://www.mayoclinic.com/health/kidney-stones/DS00282/DSECTION=7

ORGANIZATIONS

Alternative Medicine Foundation., PO Box 60016, Potomac, MD, 20859, (301) 340-1960, http://www.amfoundation.org.

American Association of Oriental Medicine., PO Box 162340, Sacramento, CA, 95816, (866) 455-7999, (914) 443-4770, http://www.aaaomonline.org.

American Holistic Medical Association., PO Box 2016, Edmonds, WA, 98020, (425) 967-0737, http://www.holisticmedicine.org.

National Kidney Foundation., 30 East Thirty-third Street, New York, NY, 10016, (800) 622-9010, http://www.kidney.org.

Paula Ford-Martin
Laura Jean Cataldo, RN, Ed.D.

Kidney transplantation

Definition

Kidney transplantation is a surgical procedure to remove a healthy, functioning kidney from a living or brain-dead donor and implant it into a patient with non-functioning kidneys.

Purpose

Kidney transplantation is performed on patients with **chronic kidney failure**, or end-stage renal disease (ESRD). ESRD occurs when a disease, disorder, or congenital condition damages the kidneys so that they are no longer capable of adequately removing fluids

National transplant waiting list by organ type (June 2010)

Organ needed	Persons waiting
Kidney	85,296
Liver	16,031
Heart	3,141
Kidney/Pancreas	2,199
Lung	1,802
Pancreas	1,450
Intestine	242
Heart/Lung	79

SOURCE: U.S. Department of Health and Human Services, Organ Procurement and Transplantation Network. Available online at: http://optn.transplant.hrsa.gov/data/default.asp (accessed June 8, 2010).

(Table by PreMediaGlobal. Reproduced by permission of Gale, a part of Cengage Learning.)

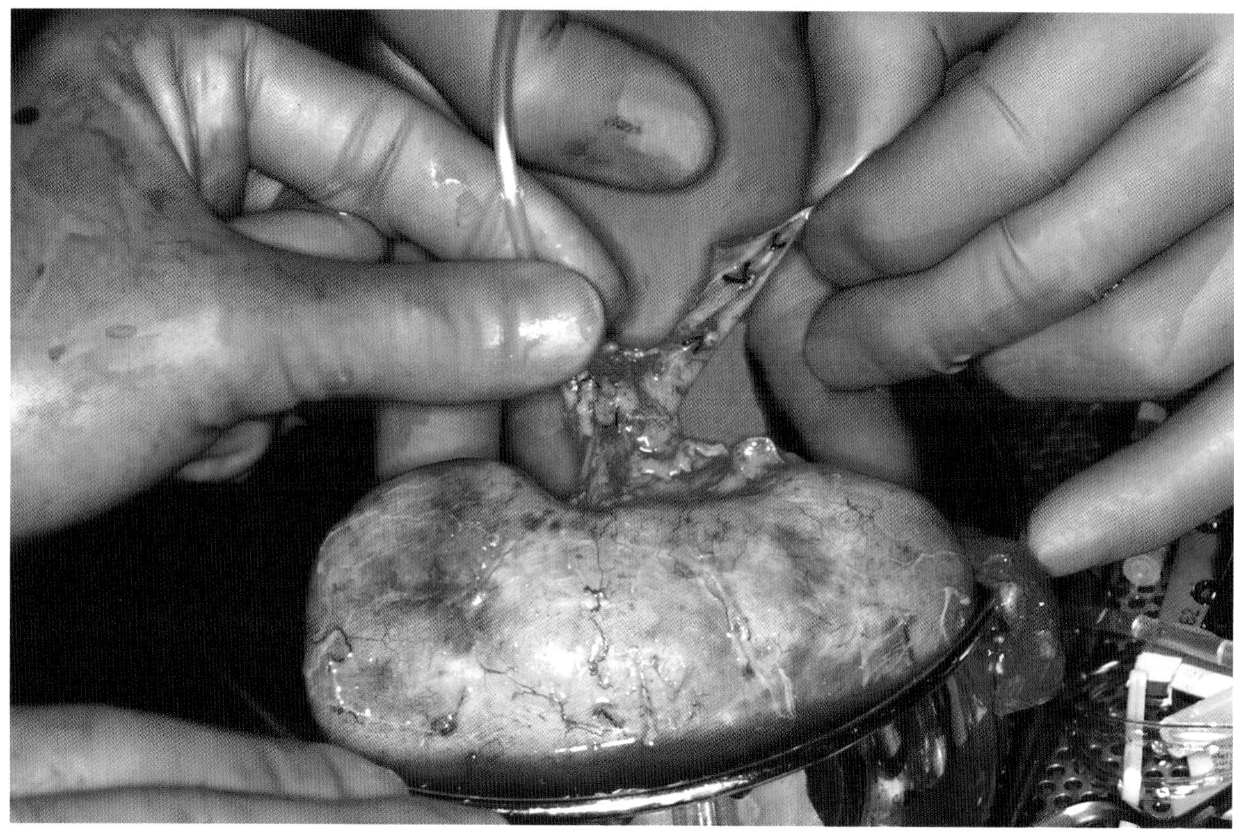

A human kidney is being prepped by medical personnel prior to transplantation. *(Custom Medical Stock Photo, Inc. Reproduced by permission.)*

and wastes from the body or of maintaining the proper level of certain kidney-regulated chemicals in the bloodstream. Without long-term dialysis or a kidney transplant, ESRD is fatal.

Demographics

Diabetes mellitus is the leading single cause of ESRD. **Hypertension** (high blood pressure) is the second leading cause of ESRD in adults, followed by **glomerulonephritis**. African Americans are more likely to develop hypertension-related ESRD than Caucasians and Hispanics. People of Native American and Hispanic descent are at an elevated risk for both **kidney disease** and diabetes.

Among children and young adults under 20 on dialysis, glomerulonephritis is the leading cause of ESRD, followed by hereditary, cystic, and congenital diseases account. According to the United States Renal Data System (USRDS), the average waiting period for a kidney transplant for patients under age 20 is 10 months, compared to the adult wait of approximately two years.

Almost 80,000 people in the U.S. are waiting for a donor kidney on the official transplant list. Less than 25% of that number received a kidney transplant in 2008, while almost 5,000 people died waiting for a transplant. In order to increase the donor pool and reduce the shortage of organs, some scientists advocate an "opt-out" system, where consent for **organ donation** at the time of **death** is presumed unless the person specified otherwise. Currently in the U.S., an "opt in" system requires potential donors to register their consent, which is usually noted on the driver's license. Several countries already have an opt-out system in place, and in Israel, another system is expected to increase donor organs by giving persons who consent to become donors by signing a card priority for a transplant should they need one themselves.

Description

Kidney transplantation involves surgically attaching a functioning kidney, or graft, from a brain-dead organ donor (a cadaver transplant) or from a living donor to a patient with ESRD. Living donors may be

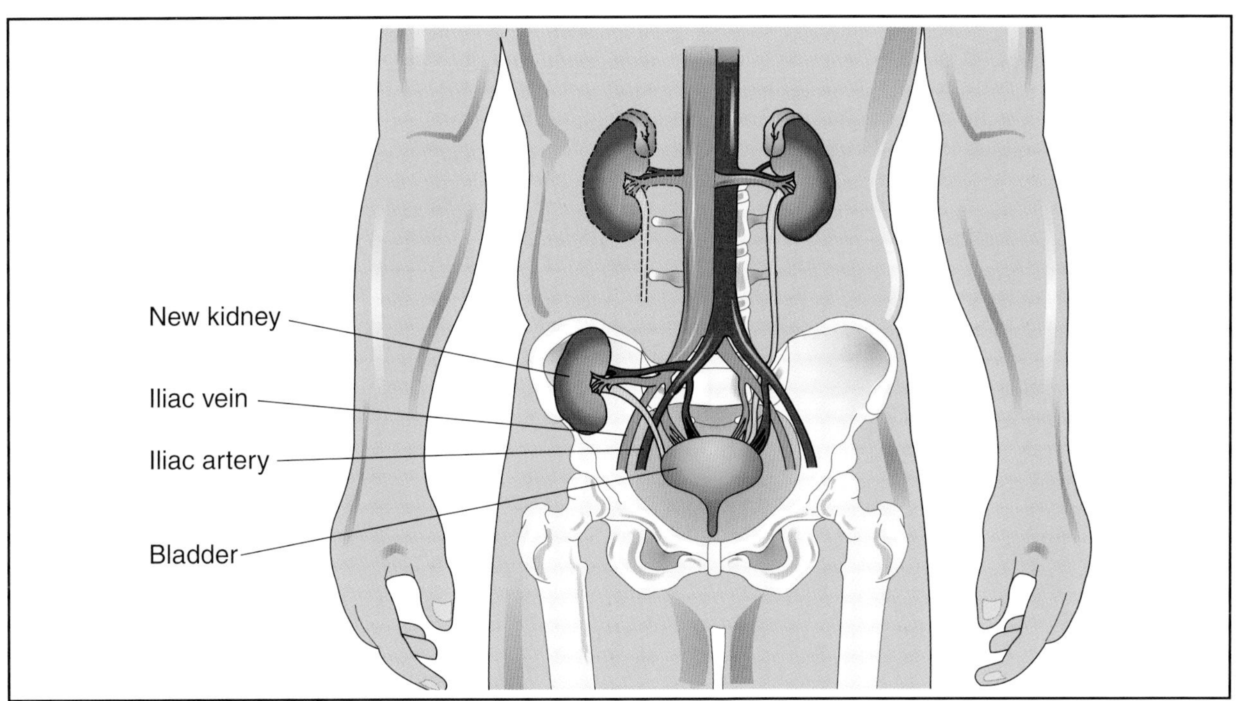

Kidney transplantation involves the surgical attachment of a functioning kidney, or graft, from a donor to a patient with end-stage renal disease (ESRD). During the procedure, the surgeon makes an incision in the patient's flank and implants the new kidney above the pelvic bone and below the non-functioning kidney by suturing the kidney artery and vein to the patient's iliac artery and vein. The ureter of the new kidney is then attached directly to the bladder of the patient.
(Illustration by Electronic Illustrators Group. Reproduced by permission of Gale, a part of Cengage Learning.)

related or unrelated to the patient, but a related donor has a better chance of having a kidney that is a stronger biological match for the patient.

Open nephrectomy

The surgical procedure to remove a kidney from a living donor is called a **nephrectomy**. In a traditional, open nephrectomy, the kidney donor is administered **general anesthesia** and a 6–10 in. (15.2–25.4 cm) incision through several layers of muscle is made on the side or front of the abdomen. The blood vessels connecting the kidney to the donor are cut and clamped, and the ureter is also cut and clamped between the bladder and kidney. The kidney and an attached section of ureter are removed from the donor. The vessels and ureter in the donor are then tied off and the incision is sutured together again. A similar procedure is used to harvest cadaver kidneys, although both kidneys are typically removed at once, and blood and cell samples for **tissue typing** are also taken.

Laparoscopic nephrectomy

Laparoscopic nephrectomy is a form of minimally invasive surgery using instruments on long, narrow rods to view, cut, and remove the donor kidney. The surgeon views the kidney and surrounding tissue with a flexible videoscope. The videoscope and surgical instruments are maneuvered through four small incisions in the abdomen, and carbon dioxide is pumped into the abdominal cavity to inflate it for an improved visualization of the kidney. Once the kidney is freed, it is secured in a bag and pulled through a fifth incision, approximately 3 in. (7.6 cm) wide, in the front of the abdominal wall below the navel. Although this surgical technique takes slightly longer than an open nephrectomy, studies have shown that it promotes a faster recovery time, shorter hospital stays, and less postoperative **pain** for kidney donors.

A modified laparoscopic technique called hand-assisted laparoscopic nephrectomy may also be used to remove the kidney. In the hand-assisted surgery, a small incision of 3–5 in. (7.6–12.7 cm) is made in the patient's abdomen. The incision allows the surgeon to place his hand in the abdominal cavity using a special surgical glove that also maintains a seal for the inflation of the abdominal cavity with carbon dioxide. The technique gives the surgeon the benefit of using his or her hands to feel the kidney and related structures. The kidney is then removed through the incision by hand instead of with a bag.

KEY TERMS

Arteriogram—A diagnostic test that involves viewing the arteries and/or attached organs by injecting a contrast medium or dye, into the artery and taking an x ray.

Congenital—Present at birth.

Dialysis—A blood filtration therapy that replaces the function of the kidneys, filtering fluids, and waste products out of the bloodstream. There are two types of dialysis treatment: hemodialysis, which uses an artificial kidney, or dialyzer, as a blood filter; and peritoneal dialysis, which uses the patient's abdominal cavity (peritoneum) as a blood filter.

Glomerulonephritis—A disease of the kidney that causes inflammation and scarring and impairs the kidney's ability to filter waste products from the blood.

Iliac artery—Large blood vessel in the pelvis that leads into the leg.

Immunosuppressive medication—Drugs given to a transplant recipient to prevent his or her immune system from attacking the transplanted organ.

Rejection—The process in which the immune system attacks foreign tissue such as a transplanted organ.

Videoscope—A surgical camera.

Once removed, kidneys from live donors and cadavers are placed on ice and flushed with a cold preservative solution. The kidney can be preserved in this solution for 24–48 hours until the transplant takes place. The sooner the transplant takes place after harvesting the kidney, the better the chances are for proper functioning.

Kidney transplantation

During the transplant operation, the kidney recipient is typically under general anesthesia and administered **antibiotics** to prevent possible infection. A catheter is placed in the bladder before surgery begins. An incision is made in the flank of the patient, and the surgeon implants the kidney above the pelvic bone and below the existing, non-functioning kidney by suturing the kidney artery and vein to the patient's iliac artery and vein. The ureter of the new kidney is attached directly to the kidney recipient's bladder. Once the new kidney is attached, the patient's existing, diseased kidneys may or may not be removed, depending on the circumstances surrounding the kidney failure. Barring any complications, the transplant operation takes about three to four hours.

Since 1973, Medicare has picked up 80% of ESRD treatment costs, including the costs of transplantation for both the kidney donor and the recipient. Medicare also covers 80% of immunosuppressive medication costs for up to three years. To qualify for Medicare ESRD benefits, a patient must be insured or eligible for benefits under Social Security, or be a spouse or child of an eligible American. Private insurance and state Medicaid programs often cover the remaining 20% of treatment costs.

Patients with a history of heart disease, lung disease, **cancer**, or hepatitis may not be suitable candidates for receiving a kidney transplant.

Precautions

Because the patient's immune system is suppressed with a transplant, he or she is at an increased risk for infection. The incision area should be kept clean, and the transplant recipient should avoid contact with people who have colds, viruses, or similar illnesses. If the patient has pets, he or she should not handle animal waste. The transplant team will provide detailed instructions on what should be avoided post-transplant. After recovery, the patient will still have to be vigilant about exposure to viruses and other environmental dangers.

Transplant recipients may need to adjust their dietary habits. Certain immunosuppressive medications cause increased appetite or **sodium** and protein retention, and the patient may have to adjust his or her intake of calories, salt, and protein to compensate.

Preparation

Patients with chronic renal disease who need a transplant and do not have a living donor registered with United Network for Organ Sharing (UNOS) are placed on a waiting list for a cadaver kidney transplant. UNOS is a non-profit organization that is under contract with the federal government to administer the Organ Procurement and Transplant Network (OPTN) and the national Scientific Registry of Transplant Recipients (SRTR).

Kidney allocation is based on a mathematical formula that awards points for factors that can affect a successful transplant, such as time spent on the transplant list, the patient's health status, and age. The most important part of the equation is that the kidney be compatible with the patient's body. A human kidney has a set of six antigens, substances that stimulate the production of antibodies. (Antibodies then attach to cells they recognize as foreign and attack them.) Donors are tissue matched for 0–6 of the antigens, and compatibility is determined by the number and strength of those matched pairs. Blood type matching is also important. Patients with a living donor who is a close relative have the best chance of a close match.

Before being placed on the transplant list, potential kidney recipients must undergo a comprehensive physical evaluation. In addition to the compatibility testing, radiological tests, urine tests, and a psychological evaluation will be performed. A panel of reactive antibody (PRA) is performed by mixing the patient's serum (white blood cells) with serum from a panel of 60 randomly selected donors. The patient's PRA sensitivity is determined by how many of these random samples his or her serum reacts with; for example, a reaction to the antibodies of six of the samples would mean a PRA of 10%. High reactivity (also called sensitization) means that the recipient would likely reject a transplant from the donor. The more reactions, the higher the PRA and the lower the chances of an overall match from the general population. Patients with a high PRA face a much longer waiting period for a suitable kidney match.

Potential living kidney donors also undergo a complete medical history and **physical examination** to evaluate their suitability for donation. Extensive blood tests are performed on both donor and recipient. The blood samples are used to tissue type for antigen matches, and confirm that blood types are compatible. A PRA is performed to ensure that the recipient antibodies will not have a negative reaction to the donor antigens. If a reaction does occur, there are some treatment protocols that can be attempted to reduce reactivity, including immunosuppresant drugs and **plasmapheresis** (a blood filtration therapy).

The donor's kidney function will be evaluated with a urine test as well. In some cases, a special dye that shows up on x rays is injected into an artery, and x rays are taken to show the blood supply of the donor kidney (a procedure called an arteriogram).

Once compatibility is confirmed and the physical preparations for kidney transplantation are complete, both donor and recipient may undergo a psychological or psychiatric evaluation to ensure that they are emotionally prepared for the transplant procedure and aftercare regimen.

Aftercare

A typical hospital stay for a transplant recipient is about five days. Both kidney donors and recipients will experience some discomfort in the area of the incision after surgery. Pain relievers are administered following the transplant operation. Patients may also experience **numbness**, caused by severed nerves, near or on the incision.

A regimen of immunosuppressive, or anti-rejection, medication is prescribed to prevent the body's immune system from rejecting the new kidney. Common immunosuppressants include cyclosporine, prednisone, tacrolimus, mycophenolate mofetil, sirolimus, baxsiliximab, daclizumab, and azathioprine. The kidney recipient will be required to take a course of **immunosuppressant drugs** for the lifespan of the new kidney. Intravenous antibodies may also be administered after **transplant surgery** and during rejection episodes.

Risks

As with any surgical procedure, the kidney transplantation procedure carries some risk for both a living donor and a graft recipient. Possible complications include infection and bleeding (hemorrhage). A lymphocele, a pool of lymphatic fluid around the kidney that is generated by lymphatic vessels damaged in surgery, occurs in up to 20% of transplant patients and can obstruct urine flow and/or blood flow to the kidney if not diagnosed and drained promptly. Less common is a urine leak outside of the bladder, which occurs in approximately 3% of kidney transplants when the ureter suffers damage during the procedure. This problem is usually correctable with follow-up surgery.

A transplanted kidney may be rejected by the patient. Rejection occurs when the patient's immune system recognizes the new kidney as a foreign body and attacks the kidney. It may occur soon after transplantation, or several months or years after the procedure has taken place. Rejection episodes are not uncommon in the first weeks after transplantation surgery, and are treated with high-dose injections of immunosuppressant drugs. If a rejection episode cannot be reversed and kidney failure continues, the patient will typically go back on dialysis. Another transplant procedure can be attempted at a later date if another kidney becomes available.

The biggest risk to the recovering transplant recipient is not from the operation or the kidney itself, but from the immunosuppressive medication he or she must take. Because these drugs suppress the immune system, the patient is susceptible to infections such as cytomegalovirus (CMV) and varicella (**chickenpox**). Other medications that fight viral and bacterial infections can offset this risk to a degree. The immunosuppressants can also cause a host of possible side effects, from high blood pressure to **osteoporosis**. Prescription and dosage adjustments can lessen side effects for some patients.

Results

Normal results

The new kidney may start functioning immediately, or may take several weeks to begin producing urine. Living donor kidneys are more likely to begin functioning earlier than cadaver kidneys, which frequently suffer some reversible damage during the kidney transplant and storage procedure. Patients may have to undergo dialysis for several weeks while their new kidney establishes an acceptable level of functioning.

Studies have shown that after they recover from surgery, kidney donors typically have no long-term complications from the loss of one kidney, and their remaining kidney will increase its functioning to compensate for the loss of the other.

Morbidity and mortality rates

Survival rates for patients undergoing kidney transplants are 89–98% one year post-transplant, and 67.4–91.4% five years after transplant. About 4,000 patients on the transplant waiting list die annually while awaiting a kidney. The success of a kidney transplant graft depends on the strength of the match between donor and recipient and the source of the kidney. Transplantations using living donor kidneys have a higher rate of success than do cadaver kidney transplantations.

Alternatives

Patients who develop chronic kidney failure must either go on dialysis treatment or receive a kidney transplant to survive.

Resources

BOOKS

Mckay, Dianne, and Steinberg, Steven. *A Guide to the Care of Kidney Transplant Recipients*. Springer Verlag, 2010.

Mancuso, Dominick W. *Progress in Kidney Transplantation*. New York: Nova Science, 2006.

Morris, Peter J., and Stuart J. Knechtle. *Kidney Transplantation: Principles and Practice*. Philadelphia, PA: Saunders/Elsevier, 2008.

Rose, Daniel Asa. *Larry's Kidney: Being the True Story of How I Found Myself in China with My Black Sheep Cousin and His Mail-Order Bride, Skirting the Law to Get Him a Transplant—and Save His Life*. New York: William Morrow, 2009.

PERIODICALS

"Easing the Kidney Transplant Shortage." *New Scientist*. 2649 (2008): 12–13.

Castro M.C.C. "Kidney Transplant." *Nursing*. 39 (2009): 3.

Leichtman AB. "Balancing Efficacy and Toxicity in Kidney-Transplant Immunosuppression." *The New England Journal of Medicine*. 357 (2007): 25, 2625–2627.

Mitka, Mike. "Efforts Under Way to Increase Number of Potential Kidney Transplant Donors." *JAMA : the Journal of the American Medical Association*. 295 (2006): 22, 2588.

Olarte, Ivan G, and Abdelkader Hawasli. "Kidney Transplant Complications and Obesity." *The American Journal of Surgery*. 197 (2009): 3, 424.

Seppa, Nathan. "Two Ways to Boost Kidney-Transplant Viability." *Science News*. 169 (2006): 4, 53.

Waring, R. "After Kidney Transplant." *Chest-Chicago*. 135 (2009): 1, 244.

OTHER

American Kidney Fund. "Kidney Transplant." http://www.kidneyfund.org/kidney-health/kidney-failure/transplant.html (accessed February 6, 2010).

ORGANIZATIONS

American Association of Kidney Patients, 3505 E. Frontage Rd., Suite 315, Tampa, FL, 33607, (800) 749–2257, info@aakp.org, http://www.aakp.org.

American Kidney Fund, 6110 Executive Boulevard, Suite 1010, Rockville, MD, 20852, (800) 638–8299, helpline@akfinc.org.

United Network for Organ Sharing, 700 North 4th St., Richmond, VA, 23219, (888) 894–6361, http://www.transplantliving.org.

Paula Anne Ford-Martin
Brenda W. Lerner

Kidney ultrasound *see* **Abdominal ultrasound**

Kidney, ureter, and bladder x-ray study

Definition

A kidney, ureter, and bladder (KUB) x-ray study is an abdominal x ray. Despite its name, KUB does not show the ureters and only sometimes shows the kidneys and bladder and, even then, with uncertainty.

Purpose

The KUB study is a diagnostic test used to detect **kidney stones** and to diagnose some gastrointestinal disorders. The KUB is also used as a follow-up procedure after the placement of devices such as ureteral stents and nasogastric or nasointestinal tubes (feeding tubes) to verify proper positioning.

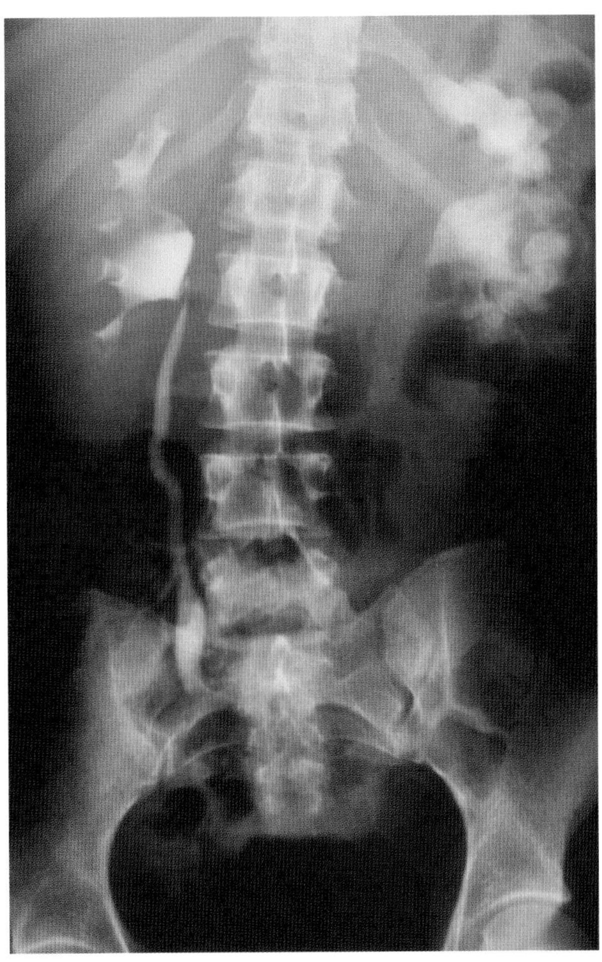

An x-ray image of a human torso and abdomen showing a blocked ureter. *(Custom Medical Stock Photo, Inc. Reproduced by permission.)*

Precautions

Because of the risks of radiation exposure to the fetus, pregnant women are advised to avoid this x-ray procedure.

A KUB study is a preliminary screening test for kidney stones, and should be followed by a more sophisticated series of diagnostic tests [such as an **abdominal ultrasound**, **intravenous urography**, or computed tomography scan (CT scan)] if kidney stones are suspected.

Description

A KUB is typically a single x-ray procedure. The patient lies flat on his back on an x-ray table. An x-ray plate is placed underneath him near the small of the back, and the x-ray camera is aimed at his abdomen.

KEY TERMS

Ureteral stent—A surgical device implanted in patients with damaged ureters that holds the ureter open so that urine can flow freely from the kidneys to the bladder.

The patient is asked to hold his breath and lie still while the x ray is taken. Sometimes a second KUB will be ordered, with the patient standing, or if unable to do so, lying on his side.

Preparation

A KUB study requires no special diet, fluid restrictions, medications, or other preparation. The patient is typically required to wear a hospital gown or similar attire and to remove all jewelry so the x-ray camera has an unobstructed view of the abdomen. A lead apron may be placed over the abdominal areas of the body not being x-rayed to shield the patient from unnecessary radiation.

Aftercare

No special aftercare treatment or regimen is required for a KUB study.

Risks

Because the KUB study is an x-ray procedure, it does involve minor exposure to radiation.

Normal results

Normal KUB x-ray films show two kidneys of a similar size and shape. A normal amount of intestinal gas is seen.

Abnormal results

Abnormal KUB films may show calculi (kidney stones). If both kidneys are visible, it may be possible to diagnose renal size discrepancies. The films may also show too much bowel gas indicating possible obstruction or soft tissue masses.

Resources

BOOKS

Pagana, Kathleen Deska, and Timothy J. Pagana.*Mosby's Manual of Diagnostic and Laboratory Tests*. 4th ed. St. Louis: Mosby, 2009.

Paula Anne Ford-Martin

Kinesiology, applied

Definition

Kinesiology is a series of tests that locate weaknesses in specific muscles reflecting imbalances throughout the body. Then specific massages or **acupressure** techniques are used in an attempt to rebalance what has been revealed by the kinesiology tests. Thus, kinesiology is used as both an assessment tool and as a limited therapeutic modality.

Purpose

Kinesiology claims to be a healing system that detects and corrects imbalances in the body before they develop into a disease, and which restores overall system balance and harmony. It is used to alleviate muscle, bone, and joint problems, treat all manner of aches and pains, and correct many areas of imbalance and discomfort.

KEY TERMS

Acupressure—A form of acupuncture in which certain points of the body are pressed with the fingers and hands to release energy blocks.

Alleviate—To make something easier to be endured.

Complementary—Something that serves to fill out or complete something else.

Deficiency—A shortage of something necessary for health.

Diagnostic—The art or act of identifying a disease from its signs and symptoms.

Flaccid—Flabby, limp, weak.

Meridian—In traditional Chinese medicine, the channels which run beneath the skin through which the body's energy flows.

Spasm—An involuntary, sudden, violent contraction of a muscle or a group of muscles.

Precautions

Since interpretation of the muscle tests is both complex and subjective, it should only be performed by a licensed health professional trained to look for "subclinical" symptoms (those which have not yet become a major problem). Kinesiology, itself, is more of a diagnostic technique and should not be thought of as a cure for any particular problem.

Description

Traditionally, the word "kinesiology" refers simply to the study of muscles and body movement. In 1964, however, American chiropractor George J. Goodheart founded what has become known as applied kinesiology when he linked oriental ideas about energy flow in the body with western techniques of muscle testing. First, Goodheart noted that all muscles are related to other muscles. He observed that for each movement a muscle makes, there is another muscle or group of muscles involved with that movement; one muscle contracts while another one relaxes. So when he was presented with a painful, overly-tight muscle, he would observe and treat the opposite, and necessarily weak, muscle to restore balance. This was then a very new technique.

Further, Goodheart argued that there is a definite and real connection between muscles, glands, and organs, and that by testing the strength of certain muscles he could learn about the health or condition of the gland or organ to which it was related.

Applied kinesiology is based on the idea that the body is an interacting unit made of different parts that interconnect and affect each other. Everything we do affects the body as a whole; therefore, a problem in one area can cause trouble in another area. According to kinesiology, the muscles eventually register and reflect anything that is wrong with any part of the body, whether physical or mental. Thus, a particular digestive problem might show up in the related and corresponding muscles of the legs. By testing the strength of certain muscles, the kinesiologist claims to be able to gain access to the body's communication system, and, thus, to read the health status of each of the body's major components.

The manual testing of muscles or muscle strength is not new, and was used in the late 1940s to evaluate muscle function and strength and to assess the extent of an injury. Applied kinesiology measures whether a muscle is stuck in the "on" position, acting like a tense muscle spasm, or is stuck "off," appearing weak or flaccid. It is called manual testing because it is done without instruments, using only the kinesiologist's fingertip pressure. During the first and longest appointment, which lasts about an hour, the kinesiologist conducts a complete consultation, asking about the patient's history and background. During the **physical examination**, patients sit or lie down, then the kinesiologist holds the patient's leg or arm to isolate a particular muscle. The practitioner then touches a point on the body which he believes is related to that muscle, and, with quick, gentle, and painless pressure, pushes down on the limb. Patients are asked to resist this pressure, and, if they cannot, an imbalance is suspected in the related organ, gland, or body part. This diagnostic technique uses muscles to find the cause of a problem, and is based on **traditional Chinese medicine** and its idea that the body has common energy meridians, or channels, for both organs and muscles. Kinesiologists also claim that they are able to locate muscle weaknesses that stem from a variety of causes such as **allergies**, mineral and vitamin deficiencies, as well as from problems with the lymph system. Once the exact cause is determined, the kinesiologist uses his fingertips to work the appropriate corresponding acupressure points in order to rebalance the flow of energy and restore health. Often he will recommend a complementary program of **nutrition** therapy.

Risks

There are no major risks associated with this gentle, noninvasive therapy. It is generally safe for people of all ages and has no side effects.

Normal results

If applied kinesiology does what it claims, patients should expect muscle testing to discover the cause of their physical complaint and to be told how to correct it.

ORGANIZATIONS

International College of Applied Kinesiology, 17A Lenox Pointe NE, Atlanta, GA, 30324, (404) 634-0201, http://www.icak.com.

Leonard C. Bruno, PhD

Kleine-Levin syndrome *see* **Sleep disorders**

Klinefelter syndrome

Definition

Klinefelter syndrome is a chromosomal disorder that affects only males. People with this condition are born with at least one extra X chromosome. The syndrome was first identified and described in 1942 by Harry Fitch Klinefelter, Jr., an American physician.

Description

Klinefelter syndrome is a condition in which one or more extra X chromosomes are present in a male. Boys with this condition appear normal at birth. They enter **puberty** normally, but by mid puberty have low levels of testosterone causing small testicles and the inability to make sperm. Affected males may also have learning disabilities and behavior problems such as **shyness** and immaturity, and an increased risk for certain other health problems.

Klinefelter syndrome is one of the most common chromosomal abnormalities. About 1 in every 500 to 800 males is born with this disorder; approximately 3000 affected boys are born each year in the United States. About 3% of the infertile male population have Klinefelter syndrome. The condition appears to affect all racial and ethnic groups equally.

Causes and symptoms

Chromosomes are found in the cells in the body. Chromosomes contain genes, structures that tell the body how to grow and develop. Chromosomes are responsible for passing on hereditary traits from parents to child. Chromosomes also determine whether the child will be male or female. Normally, a person has a total of 46 chromosomes in each cell, two of which are responsible for determining that individual's sex. These two sex chromosomes are called X and Y. The combination of these two types of chromosomes determines the sex of a child. Females have two X chromosomes (the XX combination); males have one X and one Y chromosome (the XY combination).

In Klinefelter syndrome, a problem very early in development results in an abnormal number of chromosomes. About 60% of embryos with Klinefelter syndrome do not survive the fetal period. Most commonly, a male with Klinefelter syndrome will be born with 47 chromosomes in each cell, rather than the normal number of 46. The extra chromosome is an X chromosome. This means that rather than having the normal XY combination, the male has an XXY combination. Because people with Klinefelter syndrome have a Y chromosome, they are all male.

Approximately 1/3 of all males with Klinefelter syndrome have other chromosomal abnormalities involving an extra X chromosome. Mosaic Klinefelter syndrome occurs when some of the cells in the body have an extra X chromosome and the others have normal male chromosomes. These males can have the same or milder symptoms than non-mosaic Klinefelter syndrome. Males with more than one additional extra X chromosome, such as 48,XXXY, are usually more severely affected than males with 47,XXY.

Klinefelter syndrome is not considered an inherited condition. The risk of Klinefelter syndrome reoccurring

KEY TERMS

Chromosome—A microscopic thread-like structure found within each cell of the body and consists of a complex of proteins and DNA. Humans have 46 chromosomes arranged into 23 pairs. Changes in either the total number of chromosomes or their shape and size (structure) may lead to physical or mental abnormalities.

Gonadotrophin—Hormones that stimulate the ovary and testicles.

Gynecomastia—Excessive growth of breast tissue in males.

Leydig cells—Cells that make up the endocrine tissue of the testis and produce testosterone. They are named for Franz von Leydig (1821–1908), the German professor of anatomy who first identified them.

Testosterone—Hormone produced in the testicles that is involved in male secondary sex characteristics.

in another **pregnancy** is not increased above the general population risk.

The symptoms of Klinefelter syndrome are variable and not every affected person will have all of the features of the condition. Males with Klinefelter syndrome appear normal at birth and have normal male genitalia. From childhood, males with Klinefelter syndrome are taller than average with long limbs. Approximately 20–50% have a mild intention tremor, an uncontrolled shaking. Many males with Klinefelter syndrome have poor upper body strength and can be clumsy. Klinefelter syndrome does not cause homosexuality. Approximately 1/3 of males with Klinefelter syndrome have **gynecomastia** or breast growth, some requiring **breast reduction** surgery.

Most boys enter puberty normally, though some can be delayed. The Leydig cells in the testicles usually produce testosterone. With Klinefelter syndrome, the Leydig cells fail to work properly causing the testosterone production to slow. By mid-puberty, testosterone production is decreased to approximately half of normal. This can lead to decreased facial and pubic hair growth. The decreased testosterone also causes an increase in two other hormones, follicle stimulating hormone (FSH) and luteinizing hormone (LH). Normally, FSH and LH help the immature sperm cells grow and develop. In Klinefelter syndrome, there are few or no sperm cells. The increased amount of FSH and LH causes hyalinization and fibrosis, the growth of excess fibrous tissue, in the seminiferous tubules, where the sperm are normally located. As a result, the testicles appear smaller and firmer than normal. With rare exception, men with Klinefelter syndrome are infertile because they can not make sperm.

While it was once believed that all boys with Klinefelter syndrome are mentally retarded, doctors now know that the disorder can exist without retardation. However, children with Klinefelter syndrome frequently have difficulty with language, including learning to speak, read, and write. Approximately 50% of males with Klinefelter syndrome are dyslexic.

Some people with Klinefelter syndrome have difficulty with social skills and tend to be more shy, anxious, or immature than their peers. They can also have poor judgment and do not handle stressful situations well. As a result, they often do not feel comfortable in large social gatherings. Some people with Klinefelter syndrome can also have **anxiety**, nervousness and/or depression.

The greater the number of X chromosomes present, the greater the disability; each extra X chromosome lowers the child's IQ by about 15 points. Boys with several extra X-chromosomes have distinctive facial features, more severe retardation, deformities of bony structures, and even more disordered development of male features.

Diagnosis

Diagnosis of Klinefelter syndrome is made by examining chromosomes for evidence of more than one X chromosome present in a male. This can be done in pregnancy with prenatal testing such as a **chorionic villus sampling** or **amniocentesis**. Chorionic villus sampling is a procedure done early in pregnancy (approximately 10–12 weeks) to obtain a small sample of the placenta for testing. An amniocentesis is done further along in pregnancy (from approximately 16–18 weeks) to obtain a sample of fluid surrounding the baby for testing. Both procedures have a risk of **miscarriage**. Usually these procedures are done for a reason other than diagnosing Klinefelter syndrome. For example, a prenatal diagnostic procedure may be done on an older woman to determine if her baby has **Down syndrome**. If the diagnosis of Klinefelter syndrome is suspected in a young boy or adult male, chromosome testing can also be on a small blood or skin sample after birth.

Many men with Klinefelter syndrome go through life without being diagnosed. The two most common complaints leading to diagnosis of the condition are gynecomastia and **infertility**.

Treatment

There is no treatment available to change a person's chromosomal makeup. Children with Klinefelter syndrome may benefit from **speech therapy** for speech problems or other educational interventions for learning disabilities. Testosterone injections started around the time of puberty may help to produce more normal development including more muscle mass, hair growth and increased sex drive. Testosterone supplementation will not increase testicular size, decrease breast growth or correct infertility. Psychiatric consultation may be helpful when the boy reaches adolescence.

Some doctors recommend **mastectomy** as a surgical treatment for gynecomastia, on the grounds that the enlarged breasts are often socially stressful for affected males and significantly increase their risk of **breast cancer**.

Prognosis

While many men with Klinefelter syndrome go on to live normal lives, nearly 100% of these men will be sterile (unable to produce a child). However, a few men with Klinefelter syndrome have been reported who have fathered a child through the use of assisted fertility services.

Males with Klinefelter syndrome have an increased risk of several systemic conditions, including **epilepsy**, **osteoporosis**, such **autoimmune disorders** as lupus and arthritis, diabetes, and breast and **germ cell tumors**. One Danish study reported in 2004 that men with Klinefelter's syndrome have a slightly shortened life span, dying about 2.1 years earlier than men without the syndrome.

Resources

BOOKS

Beers, Mark H., Robert S. Porter, and Thomas V. Jones, eds. *The Merck Manual of Diagnosis and Therapy*. 18th ed. Whitehouse Station, NJ: Merck Research Laboratories, 2006.

Bolch, Andreas. *Klinefelter–Syndrome: Questions. Answers.* 3rd ed. Falkenstein, Germany: Klinefelter–Syndrom–Vereinigung, 2010.

PERIODICALS

Bojesen, A., S. Juul, N. Birkebaek, and C. H. Gravholt. "Increased Mortality in Klinefelter Syndrome." *Journal of Clinical Endocrinology and Metabolism* 89 (August 2004): 3830–3834.

Diamond, M., and L. A. Watson. "Androgen Insensitivity Syndrome and Klinefelter's Syndrome: Sex and Gender Considerations." *Child and Adolescent Psychiatric Clinics of North America* 13 (July 2004): 623–640.

Grosso, S., M. A. Farnetani, R. M. Di Bartolo, et al. "Electroencephalographic and Epileptic Patterns in X Chromosome Anomalies." *Journal of Clinical Neurophysiology* 21 (July-August 2004): 249–253.

Lanfranco, F., A. Kamischke, M. Zitzmann, and E. Nieschlag. "Klinefelter's Syndrome." *Lancet* 364 (July 17, 2004): 273–283.

Tyler, C., and J. C. Edman. "Down Syndrome, Turner Syndrome, and Klinefelter Syndrome: Primary Care throughout the Life Span." *Primary Care* 31 (September 2004): 627–648.

OTHER

Klinefelter Syndrome Support Group Home Page. http://klinefeltersyndrome.org.

ORGANIZATIONS

KS&A, Klinefelter Syndrome, P.O. Box 461047, Aurora, CO, 80046-1047, (303) 400-9040, (888)999-9428, info@genetic.org, http://www.genetic.org.

National Organization for Rare Disorders, P.O. Box 8923, New Fairfield, CT, 06812-8923, (800) 999-6673, http://www.rarediseases.org.

The American Association for Klinefelter Syndrome Information and Support, 2945 W. Farwell Ave, Chicago, IL, 60645-2925, (888) 466-5747, http://www.aaksis.org.

Carin Lea Beltz, MS
Rebecca J. Frey, PhD

Knee injuries

Definition

The knee joint consists of bone, ligaments, cartilage, and fluid. It moves with the help of surrounding muscles and tendons. When any of these structures is degraded, the knee can become injured. According to the Mayo Clinic, nearly one out of three Americans older than 45 years of age have some type of knee **pain**. Whether it is a minor or major problem, it usually involves a certain amount of pain and a degree of difficulty in walking.

The five most common knee problems are arthritis, tendonitis, **bruises**, cartilage tears, and damaged ligaments, with arthritis being the most common problem of the bones of the knee. The ligaments and tendons of the knee can also become injured. Damage to the anterior cruciate ligament (ACL) is a common problem of knee ligaments and tendons. Knee injuries can be caused by accidents, impacts and other such traumas, sudden or awkward movements (misalignments), and gradual wear and tear of the knee joint (degeneration).

Most injuries of the knee are minor and are usually treated at home with rest and ice packs. Serious injuries necessitate treatments by physicians and **rehabilitation** experts. Often, various types of surgeries are needed to correct the worst knee injuries such as a ruptured ligament or tendon.

Demographics

Because the knee joint is both vulnerable and used extensively in many activities, it is prone to injuries in all peoples young and old. The American Academy of Orthopaedic Surgeons (AAOS) estimates that approximately nine million American adults are diagnosed with knee **osteoarthritis** each year. Osteoarthritis of the knee is deterioration (degradation) of the knee joint. Over half of all people with knee osteoarthritis were over the age of 65 years. The AAOS states that knee osteoarthritis is a leading cause of disability in the United States. In some sports including football, skiing, gymnastics, and racket sports, injury rates to avid practitioners can be nearly 50%, and knee injuries are the most common reason patients visit orthopedic doctors. An estimated one in five runners gets a knee injury at some point in their lives. The majority of knee injuries, however, are minor and do not require intensive treatment.

Description

The knee, the largest joint in the body, connects the thighbone (femur) to the lower leg (tibia). It is a complex and efficient joint consisting of ligaments, cartilage, and the bone of the kneecap (patella). All of these parts can be injured. Inside the knee joint is synovial fluid that protects and lubricates the parts, which may increase as the result of an injury, causing swelling. The bursa are sacs in the knee that contain synovial fluid and provide cushioning and lubrication.

Four ligaments comprise the knee joint. The medial collateral ligament (MCL) runs along the inside of the knee, while the lateral collateral ligament (LCL) is on the outside of the knee. The cruciate ligaments cross inside the knee. The anterior cruciate ligament (ACL) is deep inside the knee and limits rotation of the joint. The posterior cruciate ligament (PCL) is also inside the knee and limits the backward movement of the joint. Ligaments in the knee can be partially or completely torn, depending on the extent of the injury.

The minisci cartilage are two thin, oval–shaped tissues that act as cushions between the ends of the leg bones. The medial miniscus is the cartilage closest to the other leg while the lateral miniscus is nearer the outside of the knee. Injuries to the minisci include tears from injuries and impact and degenerative wearing away of the structure. The minisci can be partially or completely torn during injury.

The bones around the knee, including the kneecap, can be broken, fractured, or chipped. The patellar tendon connects the kneecap to the shinbone, while the quadriceps tendon connects the quadriceps muscle to the patella. The patellar tendon can be torn or can develop injury and pain from degeneration. It can also be fully dislocated or partially dislocated (called subluxation). The tendons in the knee may develop pain and inflammation known as tendonitis.

The bones of the knee joint are covered with tissue known as articular cartilage. This cartilage can be injured or fractured, and can also develop a degenerative condition called chondromalacia. Osteoarthritis is the condition associated with the wearing down of this cartilage.

There are many risks that increase one's chance of having a knee injury. These risks include:

- Excessive weight, being obese, because of the additional weight being carried in part by the knees.
- Sports and activities that are considered high risk for knee injuries, such as basketball, racquetball, downhill skiing, and tennis.
- Overuse, repeated activities can lead to fatigue in the muscles around the joints and contribute to tissue damage.
- Neuromuscular abnormalities, such as different lengths for legs and misaligned knees, can increase the likelihood of knee injuries.
- Muscle inflexibility and weakness provides less support for the knee and adds to more stress placed upon the knees.
- Previous injuries to the knee make is more likely that future knee injuries will occur.
- Gender increases the likelihood of certain types of knee problems; that is, males are more likely to have some knee problems (such as a dislocated kneecap), while females are more likely to have others (such as Osgood–Schlatter disease).
- Age increases the likelihood of more knee problems.

Causes and symptoms

Knee injuries are commonly caused by the following: impact (such as from an accident, landing after a fall, and a blow from an object), repeated stress/overuse, sudden motion (excessive turning, pivoting, or stopping), rapidly growing bones, and age–related degeneration.

There are many specific causes of knee injuries. Arthritis may develop from an auto–immune disorder, known as **rheumatoid arthritis**, or may be caused by the gradual wear and tear of the joint, known as osteoarthritis. Symptoms of arthritis in the knee include pain ranging from dull aches to severe pain, and may be accompanied by swelling and range of movement loss. Arthritic symptoms may tend to be worst in the morning and decrease throughout the day as the knee is used. Arthritis can be caused by lupus, **Lyme disease**, and other infections.

Hyperextended knee can occur when the knee is extended beyond its normal range. When this happens the knee bends back on itself, which usually causes minor damage, along with pain and swelling. However, hyperextended knee can also cause a partial or complete tear in a ligament, which produces more problems. Then the patella, the bone that covers the front of the knee, is dislodged from its normal position, so a dislocated kneecap can occur. The kneecap will look obviously out of place, and it can even be moved from side to side with ease. Symptoms of a hyperextended knee include swelling, intense pain, problems straightening the knee, and difficulty walking.

Cartilage injuries may include chondromalacia, with symptoms including dull pain at any time and more intense pain while climbing stairs. Damage to the minisci cartilage often occurs from sudden twists, forceful plants, and awkward movements. (The meniscus is a C–shaped piece of cartilage that curves inside of the knee joint.) A torn cartilage may make a popping sound, and may be accompanied by mild to severe pain, particularly while straightening the leg. Swelling, stiffening, and loss of movement are also symptoms of cartilage tears, as are clicking sounds and friction in the knee during movement. A knee suffering from a cartilage injury may become completely immobile.

Ligament injuries, which produces immediate pain when it occurs, may cause dull or severe pain, swelling, loss of the range of movement of the joint, and loss of the stability and strength of the knee. Ligament injuries typically occur from strong blows and forces applied to the knee. Injuries to the MCL are the most common, often caused by impact to the side of the knee joint. Of the cruciate ligaments, the PCL is less commonly injured than the ACL. Typically, forceful blows to the knee, such as during car accidents, injure the PCL, while the ACL can be injured by impacts and by sudden twists. Torn ligaments may be accompanied by a popping sound indicating the rupture, and may not always cause pain, so that some of them go unnoticed. Torn ligaments may weaken the knee and cause buckling or folding under weight.

Tendon injuries range from tendonitis to torn tendons. Symptoms of tendonitis include pain (which worsens when movement occurs such as running or climbing), irritation, inflammation, inability to completely extend or straighten the knee, and swelling (especially in the front of the knee or just below the kneecap), while ruptured tendons can cause more intense pain, swelling, and loss of movement.

Osgood–Shlatter disease is a condition common in young boys and girls who play running and jumping sports. Symptoms include swelling, tenderness of the tibial tuberosity located below the kneecap, and inflammation of the patellar tendon and pain in the front of the knee during and after strenuous activity.

Iliotibial band syndrome is common in running and other repetitive sports, characterized by a sharp, burning pain at the outer side of the knee caused by **stress** on the band of tendons there. Sometimes this condition causes a snapping sensation when the knee is straightened. Long–distance runners are especially susceptible to illiotibial band syndrome. The pain usually goes away when at rest after running but returns when climbing occurs. Swelling usually does not occur with this problem and normal range of motion within the knee is usually present.

Bursitis is a problem caused by inflammation in the bursa, or the small fluid sacs that cushion the outside of the knee joint. Symptoms of bursitis include redness, swelling, constant pain, stiffness or aching while walking, and added pain when climbing. Infection may also occur within the bursae, which can cause **fever**, and additional pain and swelling.

Diagnosis

Depending on the severity of the condition, family physicians or orthopedic physicians who specialize in the knee joint may be consulted. A complete **physical examination** will be performed, along with a comprehensive review of past medical records. If arthritis is suspected, a rheumatologist may be consulted. The diagnostic process includes taking a complete patient history with details of the pain and the circumstances of the injury. During a physical exam, the doctor will specifically include several manual techniques of moving the knee joint and legs in various positions to help determine the type of injury. An experienced practitioner can often make an accurate diagnosis of injuries by performing a sequence of manual diagnostic tests.

Laboratory tests may be ordered to further or clarify the diagnosis. X rays can show damage to the bones as well as the narrowing of the knee space that may imply cartilage problems. For more in–depth diagnosis, a computerized axial tomographic (CAT) scan is an x–ray technique that can provide three–dimensional views of the bones in the knee. A **magnetic resonance imaging** (MRI) scan gives a computerized portrait of the interior of the knee, and may show damage to the ligaments and cartilage. **Arthroscopy** is a form of minor surgery in which a tiny camera is inserted into the knee, giving a very accurate view of the joint. Radionuclide scanning (bone scans) use radioactive material injected into the bloodstream to monitor the blood flow in particular areas. If infection or rheumatoid arthritis is suspected, a physician may order blood tests for diagnosis. Biopsies, in which pieces of tissue are laboratory tested, may also be used for diagnosis.

Treatment

When a person suspects a knee injury, the first treatment recommended by the Mayo Clinic is a process called P.R.I.C.E., which stands for protection, rest, ice, compression, and elevation. First, the person should "protect" the knee from further motion by using a wrap that immobilizes the knee and/or crutches or braces if necessary. Then, cease the activity that caused the injury and immediately "rest" and immobilize the joint. "Ice" may be applied to reduce pain and swelling, and "compression", such as wraps and braces, may be used to immobilize the knee. "Elevating" the leg is also helpful in reducing swelling and aiding circulation. Immediate care will prevent the worsening of the injury.

Generally, pain relievers such as nonsteroidal anti–inflammatory drugs (NSAIDs) can be used. They include **aspirin**, ibuprofen (such as Advil), and naproxen (such as Aleve). **Physical therapy** may also be necessary so that the knee regains is normal movement.

Treatment options for knee injuries can range from rest and light activity, to physical therapy, to surgery. Most knee injuries are treated with proper rest, **exercise**, and strengthening programs recommended by physicians. For injuries that require surgery or deeper diagnosis, arthroscopy is the least invasive technique and involves a short recovery time. Arthroscopy is commonly used to repair cartilage and partially torn ligaments. For severe knee injuries, **reconstructive surgery** or open knee surgery may be required. Full knee replacements may also be performed for severely damaged knees. After surgery, physical therapy programs for rehabilitation are recommended. Treatment for osteoarthritis includes over–the–counter painkillers, exercise, and weight reduction. For rheumatoid arthritis, more powerful prescription medications, such as **steroids** and stronger painkillers, and intensive physical therapy may be ordered. Knee injuries associated with infection may require **antibiotics**.

KEY TERMS

Lupus—Chronic inflammatory disease caused by immune system disorder.

Lyme disease—Bacterial infection spread by ticks.

Orthopedist—Physician specializing in the diagnosis and treatment of problems involving the skeletal system.

Rheumatologist—Physician specializing in the diagnosis and treatment of arthritis and related conditions.

Alternative treatment

Alternative therapies for knee injuries focus on supporting the body's ability to heal itself. Various therapies may include bodywork and postural adjustments such as **chiropractic** and **Rolfing** work, in addition to physical therapy and gentle exercise routines. Herbal remedies and **nutritional supplements** may be used to aid the healing process and reduce symptoms. **Acupuncture** may be used for pain relief, and **yoga** is a low–impact exercise routine that increases flexibility, good alignment, and strength.

Prevention

The best prevention for knee injuries is being aware of activities that carry high risks for knee injuries and acting carefully. The knees can be strengthened by evenly building the muscles in the quadriceps and hamstrings. Increasing flexibility in the body through stretching can also help reduce injuries. Properly fitting shoes and other sports equipment are essential for preventing injury as well. Finally, before engaging in activities that stress the knee, a thorough and gradual warm–up routine, including aerobic activity and stretching, will lessen the chances of knee injury.

General life–style habits are also recommended to reduce the risk for knee injuries. These include maintaining a health height–to–weight ratio (commonly called the body mass index); exercising on a regular basis (to keep the knees and the surrounding materials strong and flexible); warming up before exercising and cooling down after exercising; not over exercising the knees if they are hurting; and using protective devices when involved in high–risk sports (such as knee pads in basketball). It is also important to wear a seat belt and harness while driving because kneecap injuries are common when automobiles crash into other cars and objects along the road.

Resources

BOOKS

Miller, Mark D., Jennifer A. Hart, and John M. MacKnight, editors. *Essential Orthopaedics*. Philadelphia: Saunders/Elsevier, 2010.

Noyes, Frank R., and Sue D. Barber–Westin, editors. *Noyes' Knee Disorders: Surgery, Rehabilitation, Clinical Outcomes*. Philadelphia: Saunders/Elsevier, 2010.

Starkey, Chad, Sara D. Brown, and Jeffrey L. Ryan. *Examination of Orthopedic and Athletic Injuries*. Philadelphia: F. A. Davis, 2010.

OTHER

"Knee Injuries and Disorders." Medline Plus, National Library of Medicine and National Institutes of Health. (March 1, 2010), http://www.nlm.nih.gov/medlineplus/kneeinjuriesanddisorders.html (accessed September 6, 2010).

"Knee and Leg." American Academy of Orthopaedic Surgeons. http://orthoinfo.aaos.org/menus/leg.cfm (accessed September 6, 2010).

"Knee Osteoarthritis Statistics." American Academy of Orthopaedic Surgeons. (October 2009), http://orthoinfo.aaos.org/topic.cfm?topic = A00399 (accessed September 6, 2010).

"Knee Pain." Mayo Clinic. (September 9, 2008) http://www.mayoclinic.com/health/knee-pain/DS00555 (accessed September 6, 2010).

"Save Your Knees." American Academy of Orthopaedic Surgeons. http://www.saveyourknees.org (accessed September 6, 2010).

ORGANIZATIONS

American Academy of Orthopaedic Surgeons, 6300 North River Rd., Rosemont, IL, 60018–4262, (847) 823–7186, (800) 824–BONE (–2663), (847) 823–8125, http://www.aaos.org.

National Athletic Trainers' Association, 2952 Stemmons Fwy., Suite 200, Dallas, TX, 75247, (214) 637–6282, (214) 637–2206, http://www.nata.org.

American Physical Therapy Association, 1111 North Fairfax St., Alexandria, VA, 22314–1488, (703) 684–APTA (–2782), (800) 999–2782, (703) 684–7343, http://www.apta.org.

Douglas Dupler

Knee replacement *see* **Joint replacement**

Kneecap removal

Definition

Kneecap removal, or patellectomy, is the surgical removal of the patella, commonly called the kneecap.

Purpose

Kneecap removal is done under three circumstances:

- When the kneecap is fractured or shattered
- When the kneecap dislocates easily and repeatedly
- When degenerative arthritis of the kneecap causes extreme pain

A person of any age can break a kneecap in an accident. When the bone is shattered beyond repair, the kneecap is removed. No prosthesis or artificial replacement part is put in its place.

Dislocation of the kneecap is most common in young girls between the ages of 10-14. Initially, the kneecap will pop back into place of its own accord, but **pain** may continue. If dislocation occurs too often, or the kneecap doesn't go back into place correctly, the patella may rub the other bones in the knee, causing an arthritis-like condition. Some people are born with **birth defects** that cause the kneecap to dislocate frequently.

Degenerative arthritis of the kneecap, also called patellar arthritis or *chondromalacia patellae*, can cause enough pain that it is necessary to remove the kneecap. As techniques of **joint replacement** have improved, arthritis in the knee is more frequently treated with total knee replacement.

Precautions

People who have had their kneecap removed for degenerative arthritis and then later have to have a total knee replacement are more likely to have problems with the stability of their artificial knee than those who only have total knee replacement. This is because the realigned muscles and tendons provide less support once the kneecap is removed.

Description

Kneecap removal is performed under either general or **local anesthesia** at a hospital or freestanding surgical center, by an orthopedic surgeon. The surgeon makes an incision around the kneecap. Then, the muscles and tendons attached to the kneecap are cut and the kneecap is removed. Next, the muscles are sewed back together, and the skin is closed with sutures or clips that stay in place about one week. Any hospital stay is generally brief.

KEY TERMS

Degenerative arthritis, or osteoarthritis—A non-inflammatory type of arthritis, usually occurring in older people, characterized by degeneration of cartilage, enlargement of the margins of the bones, and changes in the membranes in the joints.

Preparation

Prior to surgery, x rays and other diagnostic tests are done on the knee to determine if removing the kneecap is the appropriate treatment. Pre-operative blood and urine tests are also done.

Aftercare

Pain relievers may be prescribed for a few days. The patient will initially need to use a cane, or crutches, to walk. **Physical therapy** exercises to strengthen the knee should be begun immediately. Driving should be avoided for several weeks. Full recovery can take months.

Risks

Risks involved with kneecap removal are similar to those that occur in any surgical procedure, mainly allergic reaction to anesthesia, excessive bleeding, and infection.

Normal results

People who have kneecap removal because of a broken bone or repeated **dislocations** have the best chance for complete recovery. Those who have this operation because of arthritis may have less successful results, and later need a total knee replacement.

Resources

BOOKS

Griffith, H. Winter. *The Complete Guide to Symptoms, Illness and Surgery*. 5th ed. New York: Perigee, 2006.

Tish Davidson, A.M.

KOH test

Definition

The KOH test takes its name from the chemical formula for potassium hydroxide (KOH), which is the substance used in the test. The test, which is also called a potassium hydroxide preparation, is done to rapidly diagnose fungal infections of the hair, skin, or nails. A sample of the infected area is analyzed under a microscope following the addition of a few drops of potassium hydroxide.

Purpose

The primary purpose of the KOH test is the differential diagnosis of infections produced by dermatophytes and *Candida albicans* from other skin disorders. Dermatophytes are a type of fungus that invade the top layer of the skin, hair, or nails, and produce an infection commonly known as **ringworm**, technically known as tinea. It can appear as "jock itch" in the groin or inner thighs (tinea cruris); on the feet (tinea pedis); on the scalp and hair (tinea capitis); and on the nails (tinea unguium). Tinea versicolor appears anywhere on the skin and produces characteristic unpigmented patches. Tinea unguium affects the nails.

Similar symptoms of redness, scaling, and **itching** can be caused by other conditions, such as **eczema** and **psoriasis**. The KOH test is a quick, inexpensive test—often done in a physician's office—to see if these symptoms are caused by a dermatophyte. If a dermatophyte is found, treatment is started immediately; further tests are seldom necessary.

A yeast (candidal) infection of the skin or a mucous membrane, such as the mouth, often produces a white cheesy material at the infection site. This type of infection, known as thrush, is also identified with the KOH test.

Description

The KOH test involves the preparation of a slide for viewing under the laboratory microscope. KOH mixed with a blue-black dye is added to a sample from the infected tissues. This mixture makes it easier to see the dermatophytes or yeast under the microscope. The KOH dissolves skin cells, hair, and debris; the dye adds color. The slide is gently heated to speed up the action of the KOH. Finally the slide is examined under a microscope.

Dermatophytes are easily recognized under the microscope by their long branch-like structures. Yeast cells look round or oval. The dermatophyte that causes tinea versicolor has a characteristic spaghetti-and-meatballs appearance.

If the KOH test is done in the doctor's office, the results are usually available while the person waits. If the test is sent to a laboratory, the results will be ready the same or following day. The KOH test is covered by insurance when medically necessary.

KEY TERMS

Dermatophyte—A type of fungus that causes diseases of the skin, including tinea or ringworm.

KOH—The chemical formula for potassium hydroxide, which is used to perform the KOH test. The test is also called a potassium hydroxide preparation.

Thrush—A disease of the mouth, caused by *Candida albicans* and characterized by a whitish growth and ulcers. It can be diagnosed with the KOH test.

Tinea—A superficial infection of the skin, hair, or nails, caused by a fungus and commonly known as ringworm.

Preparation

The physician selects an infected area from which to collect the sample. Scales and cells from the area are scraped using a scalpel. If the test is to be analyzed immediately, the scrapings are placed directly onto a microscope slide. If the test will be sent to a laboratory, the scrapings are placed in a sterile covered container.

Normal results

A normal, or negative, KOH test shows no fungi (no dermatophytes or yeast).

Abnormal results

Dermatophytes or yeast seen on a KOH test indicate the person has a fungal infection. Follow-up tests are usually unnecessary.

Resources

PERIODICALS

Crissey, John Thorne. "Common Dermatophyte Infections. A Simple Diagnostic Test and Current Management." *Postgraduate Medicine* February 1998: 191–192, 197–198, 200, 205.

Nancy J. Nordenson

Korsakoff's psychosis *see* **Korsakoff's syndrome**

Korsakoff's syndrome

Definition

Korsakoff's syndrome is a memory disorder which is caused by a deficiency of vitamin B_1, also called thiamine.

Description

In the United States, the most common cause of thiamine deficiency is **alcoholism**. Other conditions which cause thiamine deficiency occur quite rarely, but can be seen in patients undergoing dialysis (a procedure used primarily for patients suffering from kidney failure, during which the patient's blood circulates outside of the body, is mechanically cleansed, and then is circulated back into the body), pregnant women with a condition called **hyperemesis gravidarum** (a condition of extreme morning sickness, during which the woman vomits up nearly all fluid and food intake), and patients after surgery who are given vitamin-free fluids for a prolonged period of time. Thiamine deficiency is an important cause of disability in developing countries where the main source of food is polished rice (rice with the more nutritious outer husk removed).

An associated disorder, Wernicke's syndrome, often precedes Korsakoff's syndrome. In fact, they so often occur together that the spectrum of symptoms produced during the course of the two diseases is frequently referred to as Wernicke-Korsakoff syndrome. The main symptoms of Wernicke's syndrome include ataxia (difficulty in walking and maintaining balance), **paralysis** of some of the muscles responsible for movement of the eyes, and confusion. Untreated Wernicke's will lead to **coma** and then **death**.

Causes and symptoms

One of the main reasons that alcoholism leads to thiamine deficiency has to do with the high-calorie nature of alcohol. A person with a large alcohol intake often, in essence, substitutes alcohol for other, more nutritive calorie sources. Food intake drops off considerably, and multiple vitamin deficiencies develop. Furthermore, it is believed that alcohol increases the body's requirements for B vitamins, at the same time interfering with the absorption of thiamine from the intestine and impairing the body's ability to store and use thiamine. Direct neurotoxic (poisonous damage to the nerves) effects of alcohol may also play some role.

Thiamine is involved in a variety of reactions which provide energy to the neurons (nerve cells) of the brain. When thiamine is unavailable, these reactions cannot be carried out, and the important end-products of the reactions are not produced. Furthermore, certain other substances begin to accumulate, and are thought to cause damage to the vulnerable neurons. The area of the brain believed to be responsible for the symptoms of Korsakoff's syndrome is called the diencephalon, specifically the structures called the mamillary bodies and the thalamus.

An individual with Korsakoff's syndrome displays much difficulty with memory. The main area of memory affected is the ability to learn new information. Usually, intelligence and memory for past events is relatively unaffected, so that an individual may remember what occurred 20 years previously, but is unable to remember what occurred 20 minutes ago. This memory defect is referred to as anterograde **amnesia**, and leads to a peculiar symptom called "confabulation," in which a person suffering from Korsakoff's fills in the gaps in his or her memory with fabricated or imagined information. For instance, a person may insist that a doctor to whom he or she has just been introduced is actually an old high school classmate, and may have a lengthy story to back this up. When asked, as part of a memory test, to remember the name of three objects which the examiner listed ten minutes earlier, a person with Korsakoff's may list three entirely different objects and be completely convincing in his or her certainty. In fact, one of the hallmarks of Korsakoff's is the person's complete unawareness of the memory defect, and complete lack of worry or concern when it is pointed out.

Diagnosis

Whenever someone has a possible diagnosis of alcoholism, and then has the sudden onset of memory difficulties, it is important to seriously consider the diagnosis of Korsakoff's syndrome. While there is no specific laboratory test to diagnose Korsakoff's syndrome in a patient, a careful exam of the individual's mental state should be rather revealing. Although the patient's ability to confabulate answers may be convincing, checking the patient's retention of factual information (asking, for example, for the name of the current president of the United States), along with the patient's ability to learn new information (repeating a series of numbers, or recalling the names of three objects ten minutes after having been asked to memorize them) should point to the diagnosis. Certainly a patient known to have just begun recovery from Wernicke's syndrome, who then begins displaying memory difficulties, would be very likely to have developed Korsakoff's syndrome. A **physical examination** may also show signs of Wernicke's syndrome, such as **peripheral neuropathy**.

KEY TERMS

Amnesia—Inability to remember events or experiences. Memory loss. Includes: 1) Anterograde amnesia: inability to retain the memory of events occurring after the time of the injury or disease which brought about the amnesic state. 2) Retrograde amnesia: inability to recall the memory of events which occurred prior to the time of the injury or disease which brought about the amnesic state.

Confabulation—An attempt to fill in memory gaps by fabricating information or details.

Diencephalon—A part of the brain that binds the mesencephalon to the cerebral hemispheres. Considered by some as part of the brain stem.

Treatment

Treatment of both Korsakoff's and Wernicke's syndromes involves the immediate administration of thiamine. In fact, any individual who is hospitalized for any reason and who is suspected of being an alcoholic, should receive thiamine. The combined Wernicke-Korsakoff syndrome has actually been precipitated in alcoholic patients hospitalized for other medical illnesses, due to the administration of thiamine-free intravenous fluids (intravenous fluids are those fluids containing vital sugars and salts which are given to the patient through a needle inserted in a vein). Also, the vitamin therapy may be impaired by the feeding of carbohydrates prior to the giving of thiamine; since carbohydrates cannot be metabolized with thiamine.

Prognosis

Fifteen to twenty percent of all patients hospitalized for Wernicke's syndrome will die of the disorder. Although the degree of ataxia nearly always improves with treatment, half of those who survive will continue to have some permanent difficulty walking. The paralysis of the eye muscles almost always resolves completely with thiamine treatment. Recovery from Wernicke's begins to occur rapidly after thiamine is given. Improvement in the symptoms of Korsakoff's syndrome, however, can take months and months of thiamine replacement. Furthermore, patients who develop Korsakoff's syndrome are almost universally memory-impaired for the rest of their lives. Even with thiamine treatment, the memory deficits tend to be irreversible, with less than 20% of patients even approaching recovery. The development of Korsakoff's syndrome often results in an individual requiring a supervised living situation.

Prevention

Prevention depends on either maintaining a diet with a sufficient intake of thiamine, or supplementing an inadequate diet with vitamin preparations. Certainly, one of the most important forms of prevention involves treating the underlying alcohol **addiction**.

ORGANIZATIONS

National Institute on Alcohol Abuse and Alcoholism (NIAAA), 5635 Fishers Lane, MSC 9304, Bethesda, MD, 20892-9304, (301) 443-3860, http://www.niaaa.nih.gov.

Rosalyn Carson-DeWitt, MD

KUB *see* **Kidney, ureter, and bladder x-ray study**

Kuru *see* **Creutzfeldt-Jakob disease**

Kwashiorkor *see* **Protein-energy malnutrition**

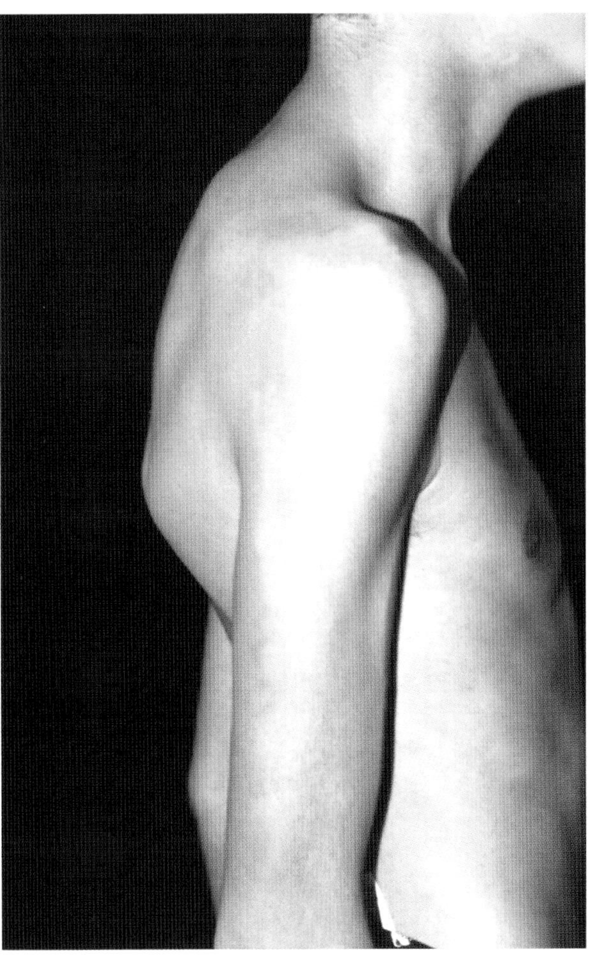

This patient's spine shows excessive backward curvature at the level of the upper chest. *(Custom Medical Stock Photo, Inc. Reproduced by permission.)*

Kyphosis

Definition

Kyphosis is the extreme curvature of the upper back also known as a hunchback.

Description

The upper back bone (thoracic region), is normally curved forward. If the curve exceeds 50° it is considered abnormal (kyphotic).

Causes and symptoms

Kyphosis can be divided into three ages of acquisition—birth, old age, and the time in between.

- Spinal birth defects can result in a fixed, exaggerated curve. Vertebrae can be fused together, shaped wrong, extraneous, or partially missing. Congenital and hereditary defects in bone growth weaken bone and result in exaggerated curves wherever gravity or muscles pull on them. Dwarfism is such a defect.
- During life, several events can distort the spine. Because the natural tendency of the thoracic spine is to curve forward, any weakness of the supporting structures will tend in that direction. A diseased thoracic vertebra (a spine bone) will ordinarily crumble its forward edge first, increasing the kyphotic curve. Conditions that can do this include cancer, tuberculosis, Scheuermann's disease, and certain kinds of arthritis. Healthy vertebra will fracture forward with rapid deceleration injuries, such as in car crashes when the victim is not wearing a seat belt.
- Later in life, kyphosis is caused from osteoporosis, bone weakness, and crumbling forward.

The **stress** caused by kyphosis produces such symptoms as an increase in musculoskeletal pains, tension headaches, back aches, and joint pains.

KEY TERMS

Congenital—Present at birth.

Dwarfism—A congenital disease of bone growth that results in short stature and weak bones.

Orthopedic—Refers to surgery on the supporting structures of the body: bones, joints, ligaments, muscles.

Osteoporosis—A weakening of bones due to calcium loss that affects post-menopausal women.

Scheuermann's disease—Juvenile kyphosis due to damaged bone in the spinal vertebrae.

Diagnosis

A quick look at the back will usually identify kyphosis. X rays of the spine will confirm the diagnosis and identify its cause.

Treatment

Congenital defects have to be repaired surgically. The procedures are delicate, complicated, and lengthy. Often orthopedic hardware must be placed to stabilize the back bone. At other times, a device called a Milwaukee brace can hold the back in place from the outside. Fitting Milwaukee braces comfortably is difficult because they tend to rub and cause sores.

Kyphosis acquired during the younger years requires treatment directed at the cause, such as medications for **tuberculosis**. Surgical reconstruction or bracing may also be necessary.

Kyphosis induced by **osteoporosis** is generally not treated except to prevent further bone softening.

Prognosis

Congenital kyphosis may be alleviated to some extent by surgery and bracing. Kyphosis occurring later in life may worsen over time.

Prevention

Preventing osteoporosis is within the grasp of modern medicine. Menopausal women must start early with estrogen replacement, **calcium** supplementation, and appropriate **exercise**. The treatment must continue through the remainder of life. Evidence suggests that a high calcium intake even during younger years delays the onset of symptomatic osteoporosis. Dairy products are the major dietary sources of calcium.

ORGANIZATIONS

Arthritis Foundation, P.O. Box 7669, Atlanta, GA, 30357-0669, (404) 872-7100, http://www.arthritis.org.

National Osteoporosis Foundation (NOF), 1150 17th Street NW, Suite 850, Washington, DC, 20036-4603, (202) 223-2226, (202) 223-2237, (800) 231-4222, http://www.nof.org.

Osteoporosis and Related Bone Diseases—National Resource Center, 2 AMS Circle, Bethesda, MD, 20892-3676, (202) 223-0344, (202) 293-2356, NIAMSBoneInfo@mail.nih.gov, http://www.niams.nih.gov/Health_Info/bone/default.asp.

J. Ricker Polsdorfer, MD